An Evidence-Based
Clinical Textbook in
Obstetrics & Gynaecology
for
MRCOG-2

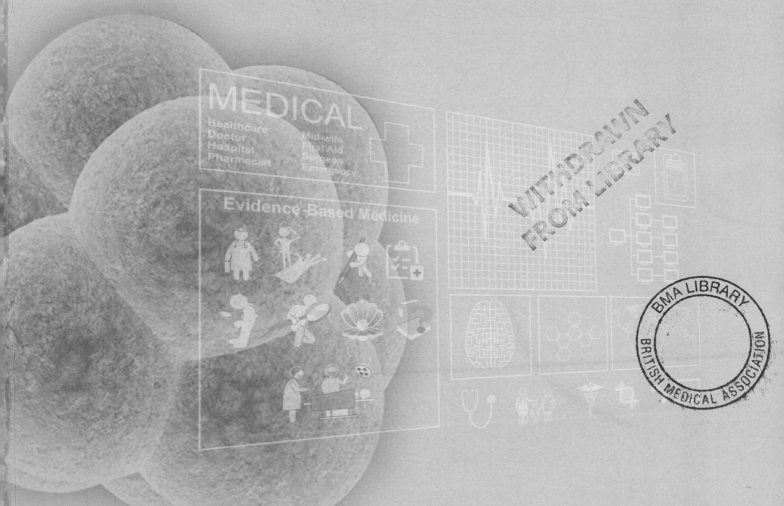

WITHDRAWN FROM LIBRARY

BMA LIBRARY
BRITISH MEDICAL ASSOCIATION

ACQUISITION

D1146836

BDA LIBRARY
BRITISH DENTAL ASSOCIATION

An Evidence-Based
Clinical Textbook in
Obstetrics & Gynaecology
for
MRCOG-2

Richa Saxena
MBBS MD (Obstetrics and Gynaecology)
PG Diploma in Clinical Research
Obstetrician and Gynaecologist
New Delhi, India

The Health Sciences Publisher
New Delhi | London | Panama

Jaypee Brothers Medical Publishers (P) Ltd

Headquarters

Jaypee Brothers Medical Publishers (P) Ltd
4838/24, Ansari Road, Daryaganj
New Delhi 110 002, India
Phone: +91-11-43574357
Fax: +91-11-43574314
Email: jaypee@jaypeebrothers.com

Overseas Offices

J.P. Medical Ltd
83 Victoria Street, London
SW1H 0HW (UK)
Phone: +44 20 3170 8910
Fax: +44 (0)20 3008 6180
Email: info@jpmedpub.com

Jaypee-Highlights Medical Publishers Inc
City of Knowledge, Bld. 235, 2nd Floor, Clayton
Panama City, Panama
Phone: +1 507-301-0496
Fax: +1 507-301-0499
Email: cservice@jphmedical.com

Jaypee Brothers Medical Publishers (P) Ltd
17/1-B Babar Road, Block-B, Shaymali
Mohammadpur, Dhaka-1207
Bangladesh
Mobile: +08801912003485
Email: jaypeedhaka@gmail.com

Jaypee Brothers Medical Publishers (P) Ltd
Bhotahity, Kathmandu, Nepal
Phone: +977-9741283608
Email: kathmandu@jaypeebrothers.com

Website: www.jaypeebrothers.com
Website: www.jaypeedigital.com

© 2017, Jaypee Brothers Medical Publishers

The views and opinions expressed in this book are solely those of the original contributor(s)/author(s) and do not necessarily represent those of editor(s) of the book.

All rights reserved. No part of this publication may be reproduced, stored or transmitted in any form or by any means, electronic, mechanical, photocopying, recording or otherwise, without the prior permission in writing of the publishers.

All brand names and product names used in this book are trade names, service marks, trademarks or registered trademarks of their respective owners. The publisher is not associated with any product or vendor mentioned in this book.

Medical knowledge and practice change constantly. This book is designed to provide accurate, authoritative information about the subject matter in question. However, readers are advised to check the most current information available on procedures included and check information from the manufacturer of each product to be administered, to verify the recommended dose, formula, method and duration of administration, adverse effects and contraindications. It is the responsibility of the practitioner to take all appropriate safety precautions. Neither the publisher nor the author(s)/editor(s) assume any liability for any injury and/or damage to persons or property arising from or related to use of material in this book.

This book is sold on the understanding that the publisher is not engaged in providing professional medical services. If such advice or services are required, the services of a competent medical professional should be sought.

Every effort has been made where necessary to contact holders of copyright to obtain permission to reproduce copyright material. If any have been inadvertently overlooked, the publisher will be pleased to make the necessary arrangements at the first opportunity.

Inquiries for bulk sales may be solicited at: jaypee@jaypeebrothers.com

An Evidence-Based Clinical Textbook in Obstetrics & Gynaecology for MRCOG-2

First Edition: **2017**

ISBN: 978-93-86322-87-6

Printed at Sanat Printers

Dedicated to...

My mother Mrs Bharati Saxena
for always being there.....

"My mother was the most beautiful woman I ever saw. All I am I owe to my mother.
I attribute all my success in life to the moral, intellectual and physical education
I received from her."

—George Washington

Preface

"I wanted a perfect ending. Now I have learnt, the hard way, that some poems don't rhyme and some stories don't have a clear beginning, middle, and end. Life is about not knowing, having to change, taking the moment and making the best of it, without knowing what is going to happen next. It is a delicious ambiguity."

—**Gilda Radner**

Years ago, after acquiring the MD (Obstetrics and Gynaecology) degree, similar to many young Indian doctors, I too wanted to add a foreign qualification in my credentials. Though I had completed part of the process, I could not complete it in entirety because of some health-related issues which prevented me in pursuing my career as a surgeon. However, life has its own ways and here I am writing a book for the doctors wishing to obtain the degree "Membership of Royal College of Obstetricians and Gynaecologists", (MRCOG, UK). For more details related to the MRCOG examination, kindly refer to the Royal College of Obstetricians and Gynaecologists (RCOG) website, https://www.rcog.org.uk. According to the latest RCOG curriculum, the MRCOG is a three-part examination. While parts 1 and 2 are written examinations, part 3 is an objective structured clinical examination, which aims at assessing the candidate's ability to apply core clinical skills in the practice of obstetrics and gynaecology. Part 2 MRCOG is a written examination comprising of SBAs (single best answers) and EMQs (extended matching questions) which help in the evaluation of clinical skills and knowledge pertaining to the subject of obstetrics and gynaecology. Though part 1 MRCOG examination mainly focusses on basic medical sciences, some questions pertaining to the speciality of obstetrics and gynaecology are also asked.

Recently, there has been a growing consensus regarding the use of evidence-based approach for healthcare management. Evidence-based practice has been defined as follows:

"The conscientious, explicit and judicious use of current best evidence in making decisions about the care of the individual patient. It means integrating individual clinical expertise with the best available external clinical evidence from systematic research."

—**Sackett D, 1996**

This book, *An Evidence-Based Clinical Textbook in Obstetrics & Gynaecology for MRCOG-2*, an evidence-based approach, typically focusses on the current standards in healthcare. It helps in the amalgamation of clinical expertise, patient values, and the best research evidence so that it can be used in the decision-making process for patient care. It is intended for the doctors who are planning to appear in MRCOG examination and wish to pursue their specialisation in obstetrics and gynaecology in the UK. This comprehensive textbook comprises of 93 chapters, distributed into 17 sections and is based as per the current MRCOG-2 curriculum (available from https://www.rcog.org.uk/en/careers-training/mrcog-exams/part-2-mrcog/syllabus). Designed into three parts, the textbook covers all the relevant topics related to general principles of medical practice, obstetrics, and gynaecology which are further segregated into sections like general principles, antenatal period, medical disorders during pregnancy, complications specific to pregnancy and those during early pregnancy, foetal complications (diagnosis and management), intrapartum period, delivery and its complications, postpartum period, the newborn infant, general gynaecology, abnormalities of menstruation, reproductive medicine, urogynaecological and pelvic floor abnormalities, gynaecological oncology, gynaecological infections as well as pregnancy prevention. To facilitate easy learning, the text is organised in accordance with a predefined template, including introduction, aetiology/indications, diagnosis, differential diagnosis, management, complications, clinical pearls and evidence-based medicine. An effort has been made to incorporate all the recent most evidence-based guidelines (Green-top Guidelines, NICE Guidelines, etc.) in the text. Numerous flowcharts and diagrams have been incorporated in the text to make it more understandable for the students. The book also includes the latest statistics related to the causes of maternal and neonatal mortality in the UK as published by the MBRRACE UK in December 2016. It also includes details pertaining to the Green-top Guidelines (No. 52) for prevention and management of postpartum haemorrhage (published in December 2016).

The text aptly offers all the required information a specialist registrar or senior house officer requires during his/her training and while preparing for the MRCOG examination. In fact, this book would also assist all the applicants, especially overseas, preparing for MRCOG examination (part 1 as well as parts 2 and 3). It would equip them with the knowledge to answer the SBAs and EMQs asked during MRCOG-2 examination. It would also enhance their clinical knowledge to be able to attempt the OSCES in MRCOG-3 examination. Also, any healthcare professional in the UK interested in learning more about the healthcare of women is likely to benefit from this book. In a nutshell, this book would serve as an invaluable companion not only for the doctors aiming towards higher training in obstetrics and gynaecology, but would also serve as a useful source of ready reference for those in established practice.

Writing a book is a colossal task. It can never be completed without divine intervention and approval. Therefore, I have decided to end this preface with a small prayer of thanks to the Almighty, which I was taught in my childhood.

"Father, lead me day by day, ever in thy own sweet way. Teach me to be pure and good and tell me what I ought to do."

—**Amen**

Simultaneously, I would like to extend my thanks and appreciation to all the related authors and publishers whose references have been used in this book. Book creation is teamwork and I acknowledge the way the entire staff of M/s Jaypee Brothers Medical Publishers (P) Ltd., New Delhi, India, worked hard on this manuscript to give it a final shape. I would especially like to thank Mr Jitendar P Vij (Group Chairman), Mr Ankit Vij (Group President), Ms Tania Banerjee (medical editor), Ms Uma Adhikari (typesetter), Mr Rajesh Ghurkundi (artist), and Ms Seema Dogra (cover designer) for publishing the book. I believe that writing a book involves a continuous learning process. Though extreme care has been taken to maintain the accuracy while writing this book, constructive criticism would be greatly appreciated.

Please e-mail me your comments at the e-mail address: richa@drrichasaxena.com. Also, please feel free to visit my website www.drrichasaxena.com for obtaining information related to various other books written by me and to make use of the free online resources available for the doctors attempting the MRCOG examination.

Richa Saxena
(richa@drrichasaxena.com)
www.drrichasaxena.com

Contents

PART III: GYNAECOLOGY

MRCOG Standards

This comprehensive textbook is based as per the current MRCOG-2 curriculum (available from https://www.rcog.org.uk/en/careers-training/mrcog-exams/part-2-mrcog/syllabus). Described below are various RCOG modules (1 to 18, except for modules 4 and 19 which are not assessed by MRCOG-2 examination), on which different chapters of this textbook are based.

Chapter 1: Principles of Clinical Practice

Module 1: Clinical Skills
- Comprehend the different elements of history taking.
- Developing effective communication skills.
- Understanding the importance and conventions of accurate clinical note keeping.
- Accepting the patterns of symptoms and understanding the importance of risk factors.
- Appreciating the pathological basis for physical signs and clinical investigations.
- Interpreting results of clinical investigations.

Module 2: Teaching, Appraisal and Assessment
- Identifying teaching strategies appropriate to adult learning like principles, needs and styles relevant to medical education.
- Understanding the difference between appraisal, assessment and performance review.
- Demonstrating appropriate skills in education, training and continuing professional development.

Module 3: Information Technology, Clinical Governance and Research

Use of IT, Audit and Standards
- Demonstrating an understanding of common usage of computing systems, including the principles of data collection, storage, retrieval, analysis and presentation.
- Acquiring adequate knowledge for performing, interpreting and using clinical audit cycles.
- Understanding the production and application of clinical standards, guidelines and care pathways and protocols.

Risk Management
- Demonstrating the working knowledge of the principles of risk management and to have an understanding of the context, meaning and implementation of clinical standards and governance.

Research
- Understanding the difference between audit and research.
- Learning how to plan and analyse a research project.
- Demonstrating the skills required to critically appraise scientific trials and literature.
- Gaining knowledge of principles of screening, clinical trial design (multicentre, randomised controlled trials, etc.) and the statistical methods used in clinical research.
- Comprehending levels of evidence, quantification of risk, power of study, level of significance, informed consent and ethical and regulatory approvals in research.
- Understanding principles of safe prescribing, quality control in medicine and the accuracy of tests.

Ethical and Legal Issues
- Awareness about principles and legal issues surrounding informed consent, implications for the unborn child, postmortem examinations, consent to surgical procedures, medical certification, research and teaching.

Confidentiality
- Establishing awareness of the applicable strategies to ensure confidentiality.
- Understanding the role of interpreters and patient advocates.

Chapter 2:   General Principles of Surgery

Module 5: Core Surgical Skills

- Understanding and demonstrating appropriate knowledge, skills and attitudes in relation to basic surgical skills.
- Comprehending issues surrounding informed consent, knowledge of complication rates and risks.
- Learning diagnostic methods and treatment of complications to increase success rates of different gynaecological surgeries.
- Awareness regarding the appropriate use of blood and blood products together with postoperative fluid and electrolyte balance, and the diagnosis of these different postoperative problems.
- Showing familiarity with surgery by discussing the common surgeries together with common surgical instruments and sutures.

Module 6: Postoperative Care

- Understanding and demonstrating appropriate knowledge, skills and attitudes in relation to postoperative care.
- Knowing how to reach a diagnosis and assess a postoperative patient and deal with all aspects of postoperative care, including immediate, short-term and long-term.
- Learning skills for prevention of common postoperative problems.
- Ability to discuss all aspects of surgery, complications and follow-up with patients, their caretakers and relatives and providing psychological support to them.

Module 7: Surgical Procedures

- Demonstrating appropriate knowledge, skills and attitudes in relation to surgical procedures in obstetrics and gynaecology, such as vaginal hysterectomy, diagnostic laparoscopy, hysteroscopy, gynaecological laparotomy for ovarian cysts, ectopic pregnancy, vaginal surgery for prolapse and urinary incontinence.
- Understanding the principles and procedures involved in more intricate gynaecological surgery for endometriosis and cancer.
- Gaining knowledge related to the principles of safe surgery, surgical instruments and sutures as well as the management of common complications of surgery.
- Be informed about the principles of risk management, surgical team working and risk reduction.

Chapter 3:   Routine Antenatal Care
Chapter 4:   Biochemical and Ultrasound Screening for Foetal Anomalies
Chapter 5:   Invasive Prenatal Diagnosis
Chapter 6:   Tests for Foetal Well-being

Module 8: Antenatal Care

- Having a better understanding of normal antenatal processes and progress.
- Recognising and managing complications from preconceptual care through to delivery.
- Dealing with the variety of maternal choices in antenatal and intrapartum care.
- Developing skills in attending and in passing on complex information (e.g. concerning risk).
- Demonstrating skills to communicate with midwives and other health professionals to optimise care of the woman thereby exhibiting empathic teamwork.
- To be well acquainted with the principles of prenatal diagnosis and screening.
- Understanding the ways in which problems may affect the foetus, and be able to interpret and act upon any appropriate investigations.
- Learning how to be well trained in the use of ultrasound in the investigation and treatment of foetal disorders.

Chapter 7:	Hypertensive Disorders during Pregnancy
Chapter 8:	Cardiac Disease in Pregnancy
Chapter 9:	Thyroid Disorders during Pregnancy
Chapter 10:	Connective Tissue Disorders (Autoimmune Disorders)
Chapter 11:	Respiratory Diseases in Pregnancy
Chapter 12:	Epilepsy and Other Neurological Disorders
Chapter 13:	Hepatic and Gastrointestinal Diseases
Chapter 14:	Anaemia and Other Haematological Abnormalities
Chapter 15:	Diabetes Mellitus and Gestational Diabetes
Chapter 16:	Abdominal Pain during Pregnancy
Chapter 17:	Malignancy during Pregnancy
Chapter 18:	Dermatological Disorders during Pregnancy
Chapter 19:	Renal Disease during Pregnancy
Chapter 20:	Infection during Pregnancy
Chapter 21:	Smoking during Pregnancy
Chapter 22:	Alcohol and Drug Usage during Pregnancy

Module 9: Maternal Medicine
- Understanding the epidemiology, aetiology, pathophysiology, clinical characteristics, prognostic features and management of common medical disorders and the effect that pregnancy may have on them, as well as the effect of such disorders on pregnancy (including both medical and obstetric problems). Some such disorders include hypertension, thyroid, epilepsy, neurological, dermatological, connective tissue as well as cardiac, respiratory and renal diseases.
- Developing the skills to liaise effectively with colleagues in other disciplines both clinical and non-clinical to assess and treat these conditions and know when more expert help is required.

Chapter 23:	Multifoetal Gestation
Chapter 24:	Preterm Labour and Premature Rupture of Membranes
Chapter 25:	Antepartum Haemorrhage
Chapter 26:	Rhesus Isoimmunisation
Chapter 27:	Abnormal Presentation
Chapter 28:	Intrauterine Death
Chapter 29:	Recurrent Miscarriage
Chapter 30:	Pregnancy after Previous Caesarean Delivery
Chapter 31:	Post-term Pregnancy (Prolonged Pregnancy)
Chapter 32:	Liquor Abnormalities
Chapter 33:	Maternal Mortality
Chapter 34:	Medications during Pregnancy

Module 10: Management of Labour
- Understanding and demonstrating appropriate knowledge, skills and attitudes in relation to the normal progress of labour.
- Attaining knowledge to demonstrate the appropriate use of protocols and guidelines.
- Skilled initial management of intrapartum problems without direct supervision, including knowledge and understanding of mechanism of normal and abnormal labour and delivery.
- Acquiring expertise in handling multifoetal gestation, preterm labour or premature rupture of membranes, antepartum and intrapartum haemorrhage, prolonged labour, intrauterine death, maternal mortality, etc.
- Being aware of the causes and management of maternal collapse including massive haemorrhage, cardiac problems, pulmonary and amniotic embolism, drug reactions, trauma, etc.
- Learning practical skills relating to normal and abnormal delivery.
- Learning causes, management and complications related to intrauterine death.

Chapter 35: Ectopic Pregnancy
Chapter 36: Spontaneous Miscarriage
Chapter 37: Gestational Trophoblastic Neoplasia

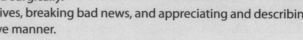

Module 16: Early Pregnancy Care

- Understanding epidemiology, aetiology, pathogenesis and clinical features related to miscarriage and other early pregnancy complications, including diagnosis, investigations, management and psychological support in cases of miscarriage and ectopic pregnancy.
- Ability to assess and manage these conditions both medically and surgically.
- Learning skills to communicate effectively with patients and relatives, breaking bad news, and appreciating and describing the possible long-term consequences for the woman in a sensitive manner.
- Attaining knowledge related to the use of ultrasound for diagnosis and management of complications in the early pregnancy, e.g. trophoblastic disease, ectopic pregnancy , etc.

Chapter 38: Foetal Growth Restriction
Chapter 39: Foetal Infection
Chapter 40: Non-immune Foetal Hydrops
Chapter 41: Foetal Anomalies and Their Management

Module 10: Management of Labour

- Acquiring expertise in assessment of foetal well-being using foetal heart rate monitoring, acid/base balance, and foetal scalp blood sampling.
- Learning causes, mechanisms of action and complications of foetal pulmonary maturity, infection risks and foetal compromise including cord prolapse.

Chapter 42: Normal and Abnormal Progress of Labour
Chapter 43: Induction of Labour
Chapter 44: Anaesthesia and Analgesia in Labour

Module 10: Management of Labour

- Understanding the mechanisms of normal and abnormal labour.
- Attaining expertise in the methods of induction of labour, and understanding its indications, contraindications and complications.
- Getting acquainted with the types and methods of action of regional anaesthesia including epidural and spinal.
- Learning types and methods of action of analgesia and sedation including narcotics, hypnotics, psychotropics, non-steroidal anti-inflammatory drugs, its indications and contraindications.
- Being aware of complications of anaesthesia and analgesia.

Chapter 45: Caesarean Delivery
Chapter 46: Instrumental Vaginal Delivery
Chapter 47: Shoulder Dystocia
Chapter 48: Perineal Injuries
Chapter 49: Antepartum and Intrapartum Foetal Asphyxia

Module 11: Management of Delivery

- Understanding the mechanism and making appropriate decisions in the choice of delivery in partnership with the mother at the same time respecting the views of other healthcare workers especially the midwives.

- Attaining expertise in indications, contraindications and complications related to labour and delivery.
- Learning types and methods of different types of deliveries like caesarean, instrumental vaginal as well as management of complications such as shoulder dystocia.
- Understanding perineal trauma and its repair as well as management of complications such as antepartum and intrapartum foetal asphyxia.

Chapter 50: Postpartum Haemorrhage and Postpartum Collapse
Chapter 51: Puerperal Pyrexia
Chapter 52: Psychiatric Disorders in the Puerperium (Mood Disturbances)
Chapter 53: Problems with Breastfeeding

Module 12: Postpartum Problems (The Puerperium)

- Understanding and demonstrating proper knowledge, skills and attitudes in management of postpartum problems, including resuscitation of both mother and baby and the ability to manage birth trauma and other birth complications.
- Learning techniques for the control of postpartum haemorrhage.
- Showing empathy and developing good counselling skills and an understanding about the role of other professionals.
- Awareness of the breast feeding initiative.

Chapter 54: Asphyxia Neonatorum
Chapter 55: Care of a Newborn Child and Perinatal Mortality

Module 12: Postpartum Problems (The Puerperium)

- Understanding and demonstrating appropriate knowledge, skills and attitudes in relation to the neonatal problems.
- Ability to manage neonatal problems at birth like resuscitation of newborn and other neonatal complications.
- Developing counselling skills regarding the patients who have faced perinatal loss or intrauterine death.

Chapter 56: Normal and Abnormal Embryological Development
Chapter 57: Karyotypic Abnormalities
Chapter 58: Menstrual Cycle
Chapter 59: Adolescent and Paediatric Gynaecology
Chapter 60: Menopause and Hormone Replacement Therapy
Chapter 61: Injuries of the Female Genital Tract and Female Genital Mutilation
Chapter 62: Child Abuse, Sexual Assault and Rape
Chapter 63: Dyspareunia and Other Psychosexual Problems

Module 13: Gynaecological Problems

- Understanding and demonstrating appropriate knowledge, skills and attitudes in relation to common gynaecological disorders such as menstrual disorders, menopause and hormone replacement therapy.
- Demonstrating knowledge of the aetiology, signs, symptoms, investigation and treatment of common gynaecological problems like congenital abnormalities of the genital tract, paediatric gynaecology and puberty-related abnormalities.
- Appreciating the influence of psychosocial factors on the presentation and management of gynaecological problems using a patient-centred approach.
- Being familiar with the laws related to child protection.

Module 13: Gynaecological Problems

Understanding the epidemiology, aetiology, biological behaviour, pathophysiology, clinical characteristics, prognostic features and management of menstrual and endocrine disorders, pelvic pain, dysmenorrhoea as well as premenstrual syndrome and problems of the climacteric like abnormal and postmenopausal bleeding.

Module 14: Subfertility

- Understanding the issues and demonstrating appropriate knowledge, skills and attitudes in relation to subfertility, including comprehending of the epidemiology, aetiology, pathogenesis, clinical treatment and prognosis of all aspects of male and female fertility problems like PCOD, primary and secondary amenorrhoea.
- Gaining knowledge of indications, limitations and interpretation of relative investigations and treatments in relation to both males and females, including disorders of fertility development and endometriosis.
- Learning broad-based and up-to-date knowledge of assisted reproductive technologies, including ovulation induction, in vitro fertilisation, intracytoplasmic sperm injection, gamete donation and surrogacy, and the legal and ethical implications of these procedures.

Module 18: Urogynaecology and Pelvic Floor Problems

- Understanding and demonstrating appropriate knowledge, skills and attitudes in the management of urogynaecology and pelvic floor problems like urinary and faecal incontinence, benign bladder conditions and urogenital prolapse.
- Demonstrating an understanding of the anatomy, pathophysiology, epidemiology, aetiology and investigation of these conditions.
- Develop awareness regarding taking consultation from the experts while managing their patients.
- Ability to discuss clearly all aspects of management of urinary incontinence with patients, carers and other continence care providers.

Chapter 83:   Endometrial Cancer
Chapter 84:   Ovarian Neoplasia (Benign and Malignant)
Chapter 85:   Cervical Intraepithelial Neoplasia
Chapter 86:   Invasive Cervical Cancer
Chapter 87:   Rare Cancers of the Female Genital Organs
Chapter 88:   Vulvar Cancer and Vulval Pain Syndromes

Module 17: Gynaecological Oncology

- Developing detailed understanding related to the aetiology and screening involved in gynaecological oncology, including the international perspective.
- Understanding presenting symptoms of various gynaecological malignancies and their management and have the appropriate competencies for each stage of the diagnostic process, including comprehension of the different roles and skills required at the district lead and gynae oncologist.
- Know the prognosis and treatment options for various gynaecological cancers like vulvar, cervical, endometrial, ovarian, etc.
- Ability to show empathy and to provide counselling for patients with gynaecological cancer.

Chapter 89:   Sexually Transmitted Infections
Chapter 90:   Vaginal Discharge
Chapter 91:   Pelvic Inflammatory Disease

Module 15: Sexual and Reproductive Health

- Understanding and demonstrating appropriate knowledge, skills and attitudes in relation to the diagnosis and management of sexually transmitted infections.
- Demonstrating broad-based recognition of management techniques relating to the sexual health of vulnerable groups, such as young people, asylum seekers, commercial sex workers, drug users and prisoners.
- Learning the basis of national screening programmes and their implementation through local care pathways.

Chapter 92:   Contraception (Temporary and Permanent)
Chapter 93:   Medical Termination of Pregnancy

Module 15: Sexual and Reproductive Health

- Attaining knowledge regarding, reversible, irreversible and emergency contraception and abortion, mode of action, efficacy, indications, contraindications and complications of various contraceptive methods.
- Being familiar with the laws relating to abortion, sexually transmitted infections and consent.

Introduction to the Symbols Used in the Textbook

Promoting evidence-based medicine is the basic purpose of this book. Assembled into three parts, General, Obstetrics and Gynaecology, the comprehensive textbook is divided into 17 sections and 93 chapters that are written as per the current MRCOG-2 curriculum. All the chapters have been organised into various subparts with the help of the symbols as described below.

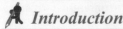 **Introduction**

Abdominal pain during pregnancy may present additional challenges for the obstetrician because he/she needs to consider physiologic or anatomic alterations related to pregnancy, gestational age and foetal well-being. Moreover, the causes of acute abdomen that may be more commonly related to the pregnant state or to the obstetrical complications.

Introduction

A brief description of the disease, its incidence and the probable effects which act as an opening section of the chapter.

Aetiology/Indications

The probable set of causes, risk factors or manner of causation of a disease or condition. The term 'indication' rather than aetiology is used in cases of a surgical condition.

Aetiology/Indications

Heart disease in pregnancy can be due to various causes. According to the Confidential Enquiries into Maternal Deaths (CEMD), UK, the overall rate of mortality due to cardiac disease has risen from 7.3 per million births in the 1982–84 triennium to 22.7 per million births in the 2003–05 triennium.

 Diagnosis

There are two clinical forms of MG: ocular and generalised. In ocular type, weakness is limited to the eyelids and extraocular facial muscles. In generalised type, the weakness involves a variable combination of bulbar, limb, ocular and respiratory muscles. The cardinal clinical feature of the disease is fluctuating muscle weakness often accompanied with true muscle fatigue.

Diagnosis

The process of detecting the disease, based on the clinical findings on general physical and systemic examination as well as on the result of various investigations.

 Differential Diagnosis

Anembryonic gestation:

• Threatened abortion: Both the conditions are associated with vaginal bleeding and similar sonographic findings.

• Presence of fibroid or an ovarian tumour with pregnancy: They may cause the uterine size to be larger in relation to the period of gestation.

Differential Diagnosis

The process of differentiating between two or more medical conditions having similar signs and symptoms.

Management

Women with suspected genital herpes, who are being managed by the midwife, should be referred for review by a genitourinary medicine physician as well as the obstetrician.

Genitourinary medicine physician would help in confirming or disproving the diagnosis by viral PCR.

Management

Plan of prevention, treatment and control of the relevant disease.

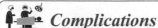 *Complications*

Unlike placenta praevia, vasa praevia carries no major maternal risk but is associated with significant risk to the foetus. When the foetal membranes are ruptured, either spontaneously or artificially, the unprotected foetal vessels are at risk of disruption with consequent foetal haemorrhage and high foetal mortality rates.

Complications

The problems which are likely to occur if the disease remains untreated.

 Clinical Pearls

It is considered good practice to avoid vaginal and rectal examinations in women with placenta praevia because this can sometimes provoke an episode of torrential bleeding. These women must also be advised to avoid penetrative sexual intercourse for similar reasons.

Women having placenta praevia with a previous history of uterine scar are at an increased risk of developing a MAP.

Clinical Pearls

Important bits of clinically relevant information based on experience or observation, or the vast domain of evidence-based medicine, which would be helpful in dealing with clinical problems and making management decisions.

Evidence-Based Medicine

The present evidence supports the safety of conventional antiemetic drugs during pregnancy including the first trimester. There is sufficient evidence in the literature to support the safety of antiemetics, antacids, sucralfate, histamine-2 (H_2) receptor blockers and proton pump inhibitors in pregnancy.

Evidence-Based Medicine

Thorough, clear, sensible and realistic use of modern, best evidence while taking decisions related to the care and management of individual patients.

 References

1. Clausson B, Francis A, Cnattingius S. Perinatal outcome in SGA births defined by customised versus population-based birthweight standards. BJOG. 2001;108(8):830-4.
2. Chang TC, Robson SC, Boys RJ, Spencer JA. Prediction of the small for gestational age infant: which ultrasonic measurement is best? Obstet Gynecol. 1992;80(6):1030-8.

References

This includes the list of sources which have been cited while writing the chapter and help the readers gain deeper insight about the subject

Abbreviations

ACE	Angiotensin-converting Enzyme	ESR	Erythrocyte Sedimentation Rate
ACOG	American College of Obstetricians and Gynecologists	FDA	Food and Drug Administration
AED	Antiepileptic Drug	FDP	Fibrin Degradation Products
AFI	Amniotic Fluid Index	FEV1	Forced Expiratory Volume in 1 Second
AFV	Amniotic Fluid Volume	ffDNA	Free-foetal Deoxyribonucleic Acid
AIDS	Acquired Immune Deficiency Syndrome	fFM	Foetal Fibronectin
ALT	Alanine Aminotransferase	FHR	Foetal Heart Rate
ANA	Antinuclear Antibodies	FHS	Foetal Heart Sound
ANC	Antenatal Care	FIGO	International Federation of Gynecology and Obstetrics
Anti-Sm	Anti-Smith Antibodies	FMH	Foetomaternal Haemorrhage
AP	Anteroposterior	FNAC	Fine-needle Aspiration Cytology
APGAR	Appearance, Pulse, Grimace, Activity and Respiration	FSH	Follicle-stimulating Hormone
APS	Antiphospholipid Antibody Syndrome	GBS	Group B Streptococcus
aPTT/APTT	Activated Partial Thromboplastin Time	GDG	Guideline Development Group
ARB	Angiotensin II Receptor Blockers	GFR	Glomerular Filtration Rate
ARM	Artificial Rupture of Membranes	GI	Gastrointestinal
AST	Aspartate Aminotransferase	GnRH	Gonadotropin-releasing Hormone
BMI	Body Mass Index	GP	General Practitioners
BP	Blood Pressure	GUM	Genitourinary Medicine
bpm	Beats Per Minute	hCG	Human Chorionic Gonadotropin
BPP	Biophysical Profile	HELLP	Haemolysis, Elevated Liver Enzymes and Low Platelet Count
CA-MRSA	Community-acquired methicillin-resistant *Staphylococcus aureus*	HG	Hyperemesis Gravidarum
CBC	Complete Blood Count	HIV	Human Immunodeficiency Virus
CDC	Centre of Disease Control	HLA	Human Leucocyte Antigen
CEMACH	Confidential Enquiries into Maternal and Child Health	HPV	Human Papillomavirus
		HR	Heart Rate
CEMD	Confidential Enquiries into Maternal Deaths	HRT	Hormone Replacement Therapy
CESDI	Confidential Enquiries into Stillbirths and Deaths in Infancy	HSV	Herpes Simplex Virus
		Ig	Immunoglobulin
CI	Confidence Interval	IM	Intramuscular
CMACE	Centre for Maternal and Child Enquiries	INR	International Normalised Ratio
CNS	Central Nervous System	ISSHP	International Society for the Study of Hypertension in Pregnancy
CO	Carbon Monoxide	IUCD	Intrauterine Contraceptive Device
CRP	C-reactive protein	IUGR	Intrauterine Growth Restriction/Retardation
CS	Caesarean Section	IVF	In Vitro Fertilisation
CST	Contraction Stress Test	IV	Intravenous
CT	Computed Tomography	L:S ratio	Lecithin:Sphingomyelin Ratio
CTG	Cardiotocography	LDA	Low-dose Aspirin
DFMC	Daily Foetal Movement Count	LFT	Liver Function Test
DIC	Disseminated Intravascular Coagulation	LH	Luteinising Hormone
DLC	Differential Leucocyte Count	LMWH	Low-molecular-weight Heparin
DVT	Deep Vein Thrombosis	MAP	Morbidly Adherent Placenta
ECG	Electrocardiogram	MCHC	Mean Corpuscular Haemoglobin Concentration
ELISA	Enzyme-linked Immunosorbent Assay		
ERCS	Elective Repeat Caesarean Section	MCH	Mean Corpuscular Haemoglobin
ESHRE	European Society of Human Reproduction and Embryology	MC	Monochorionic
		MCV	Mean Corpuscular Volume

MRI	Magnetic Resonance Imaging	RCT	Randomised Controlled Trial
MS	Multiple Sclerosis	RIA	Radioimmunoassay
NCEPOD	National Confidential Enquiry into Patient Outcome and Death	ROM	Rupture of Membranes
		ROS	Reactive Oxygen Species
NHS	National Health Service	RPF	Renal Plasma Flow
NICE	National Institute for Health and Care Excellence/ National Institute for Clinical Excellence	SC	Subcutaneous
		SLE	Systemic Lupus Erythematosus
		SOGC	Society of Obstetricians and Gynaecologists of Canada
NICU	Neonatal Intensive Care Unit		
NSAIDs	Non-steroidal Anti-inflammatory Drugs	STD	Sexually Transmitted Disease
NST	Non-stress Test	T_3	Tri-iodothyronine
OC	Obstetric Cholestasis	T_4	Thyroxine
OCPs	Oral Contraceptive Pills	TAS	Transabdominal Scan or Sonography
OPD	Outpatient Department	TENS	Transcutaneous Electrical Nerve Stimulation
OR	Odds Ratio	TLC	Total Leucocyte Count
PCOS/PCOD	Polycystic Ovarian Syndrome/Polycystic Ovarian Disease	TORCH	Toxoplasmosis, Other Infections, Rubella, Cytomegalovirus, Herpes Simplex Virus
PCR	Polymerase Chain Reaction	TSH	Thyroid-stimulating Hormone
PEFR	Peak Expiratory Flow Rate	TT	Thrombin Time
PET	Positron Emission Tomography	TTTS	Twin-to-twin Transfusion Syndrome
PFT	Pulmonary Function Test	TVCL	Transvaginal Cervical Length
PGI_2	Prostacyclin/Prostaglandin I_2	TVS	Transvaginal Scan or Sonography
PID	Pelvic Inflammatory Disease	TVT	Tension-free Vaginal Tape
PIH	Pregnancy-induced Hypertension	TXA_2	Thromboxane A_2
POF	Premature Ovarian Failure	UDCA	Ursodeoxycholic Acid
POG	Period of Gestation	UFH	Unfractionated Heparin
PO	Per orally or per os	UNICEF	United Nations Children's Fund
PPH	Postpartum Haemorrhage	US	Ultrasonography
PROM	Premature Rupture of Membranes	UTI	Urinary Tract Infection
PT	Prothrombin Time	UV	Ultraviolet
PV	Per Vaginally	VBAC	Vaginal Birth after Caesarean
RBC	Red Blood Cell	VDRL	Venereal Disease Research Laboratory
RCOG	Royal College of Obstetricians and Gynaecologists	WBC	White Blood Cell
		WHO	World Health Organization
		WY	Women Years

PLATE 1

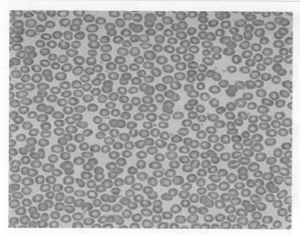

Fig. 14.1: Peripheral smear in case of iron deficiency anaemia

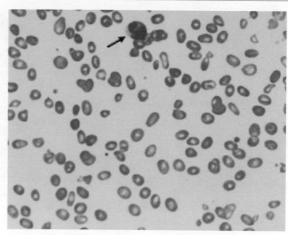

Fig. 14.2: Peripheral smear in case of megaloblastic anaemia
(the arrow points towards hypersegmented neutrophil)

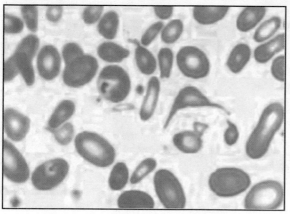

Fig. 14.3: Peripheral smear in case of thalassaemia
(Target cell is indicated by the arrow)

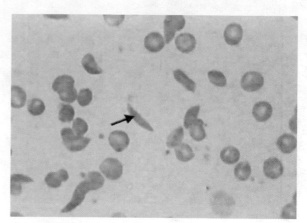

Fig. 14.4: Peripheral smear in case of sickle cell anaemia
(Arrow indicates sickle-shaped cell)

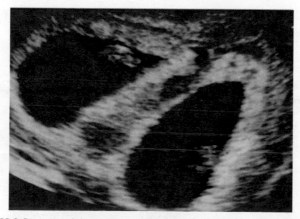

Fig. 23.8: Diamniotic dichorionic twins at 7 weeks of gestation. There are two separate chorionic sacs surrounding each of the two amniotic sacs, with each sac containing an embryo. The intervening membrane between the twins is composed of four layers: two layers of chorion in the middle surrounded by a layer of amnion on either side

PLATE 2

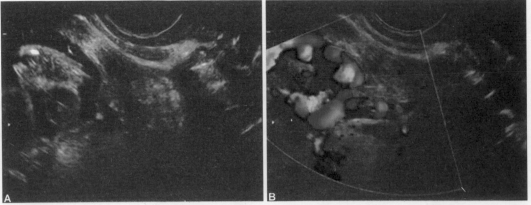

Figs 25.11A and B: Diagnosis of vasa praevia. (A) Transvaginal ultrasound; (B) Doppler ultrasound showing presence of foetal blood vessels in front of the foetal presenting part

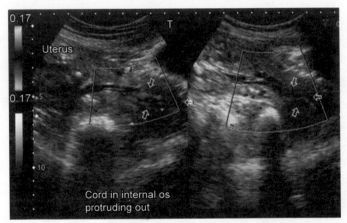

Fig 27.27: Internal os appears dilated with umbilical cord within the cervix; this finding is diagnostic of cord prolapse

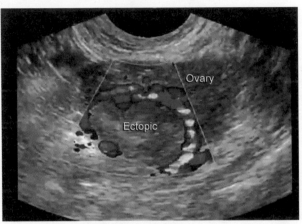

Fig. 35.5B: Doppler ultrasound in the same case showing a 'ring of fire' appearance due to increased vascularity of the surrounding fallopian tube

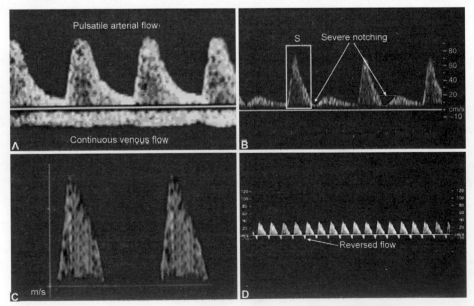

Figs 38.7A to D: Umbilical artery blood flow patterns. (A) Normal umbilical artery Doppler ultrasound waveforms; (B) Early diastolic notching; (C) Absent end diastolic flow; (D) Reversed end diastolic flow

PLATE 3

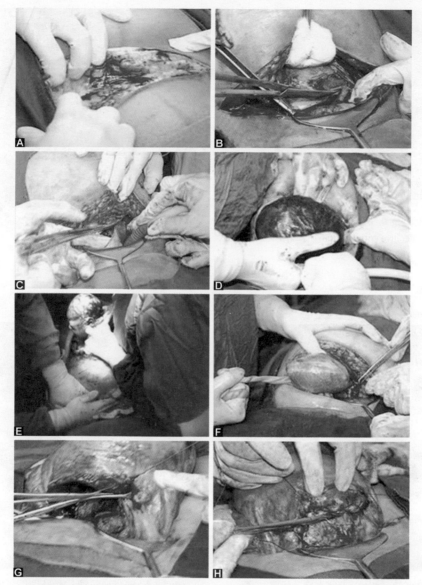

Figs 45.1A to H: Steps of caesarean delivery: (A) Giving an incision over the abdomen and dissecting out different layers of skin; (B) Application of Doyen's retractor after dissection of parietal peritoneum followed by incision of visceral peritoneum; (C) Giving a uterine incision; (D) Delivery of foetal head; (E) Delivery of the entire baby out of the uterine cavity; (F) Delivery of the placenta; (G) Clamping the uterine angles with Green Armytage clamps; (H) Stitching the uterine cavity

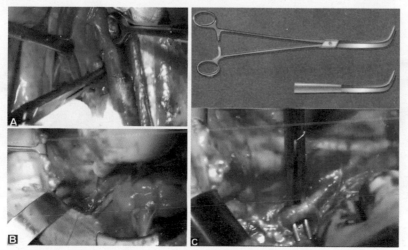

Figs 50.5A to C: Process of internal iliac artery ligation: (A) Dissection of the retriperitoneal tissues to identify the internal iliac artery; (B) Mixter's forceps and placement of Mixter's forceps around the internal iliac artery; (C) The ligation of internal iliac artery

PLATE 4

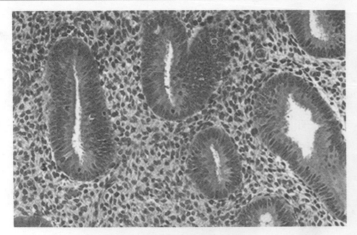

Fig. 58.5: Proliferative endometrium

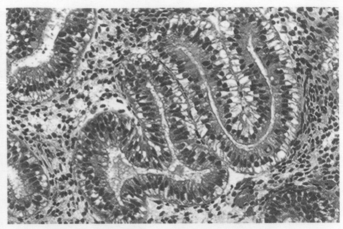

Fig. 58.6: The secretory phase endometrium

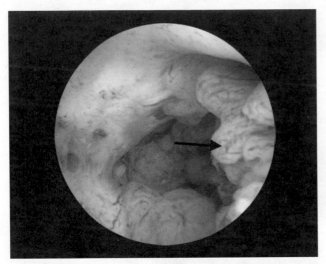

Fig. 64.1: Hysteroscopic appearance of an exophytic endometrial cancer growth (indicated by arrow)

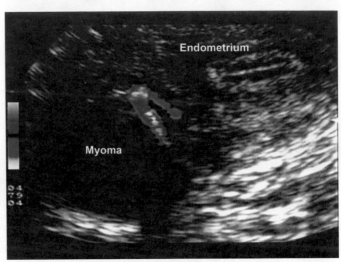

Fig. 65.3: Colour Doppler shows presence of subserosal fibroids with peripheral vascularisation

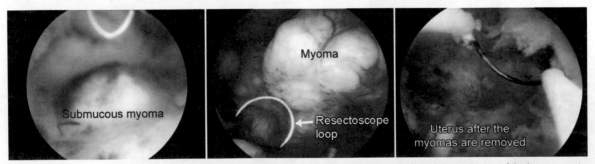

Figs 65.5A to C: Hysteroscopic myomectomy: (A) Hysteroscopic view showing presence of a submucous fibroid; (B) Beginning of the hysteroscopic resection of submucous fibroid; (C) Completion of the hysteroscopic resection of submucous fibroid

PLATE 5

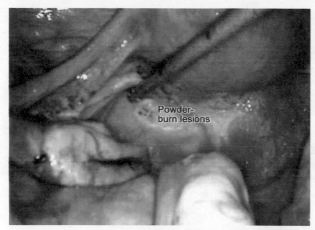

Fig. 68.2: Powder-burn lesions over endometrial surface

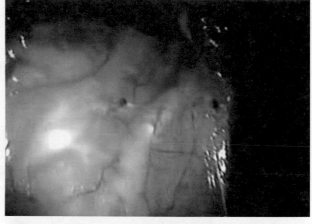

Fig. 68.3: Nodular endometrial lesions

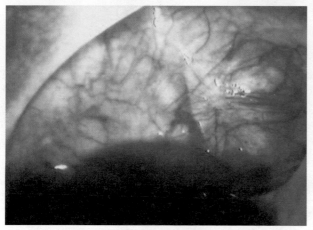

Fig. 68.4: Presence of blood in cul-de-sac

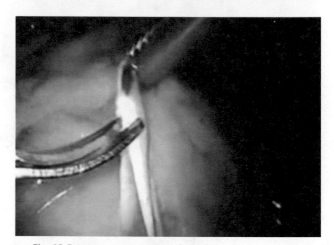

Fig. 68.5: Laparoscopic excision of nodular endometrial lesions overlying the round ligament

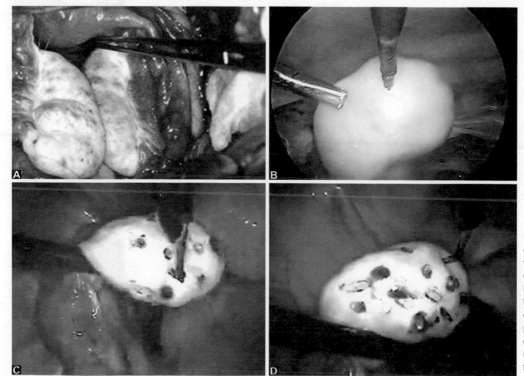

Figs 74.2A to D: Laparoscopic ovarian drilling. (A) Laparoscopic visualisation of the pelvis in an effort to locate the ovaries; (B) Lifting the ovaries out of the ovarian fossa and placing them over the cervicouterine junction; (C) The procedure of laparoscopic ovarian drilling using electrocauterisation; (D) Appearance of the ovary following the procedure

PLATE 6

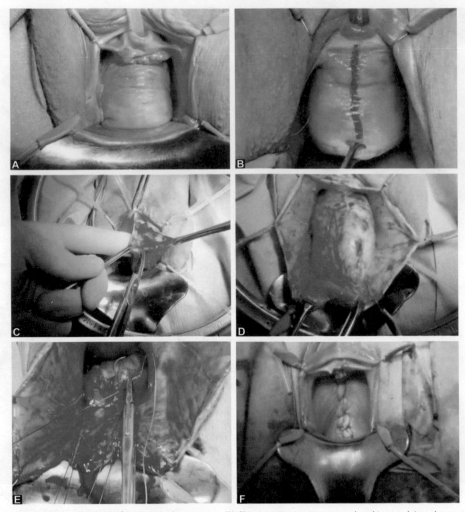

Figs 80.2A to F: (A) Appearance of cystocele just before giving the incision; (B) Skin incision is given over the skin overlying the cystocele; (C) Dissection of the underlying fascia; (D) Dissection of the underlying fascia is continued until the midline defect in pubocervical fascia is visualized; (E) The tissue under the bladder is plicated and pulled together in the midline, thus reducing the bulge. Following the reduction, excess vaginal skin is then cut off, which can create a shortened or constricted vagina; (F) Closure of the vaginal epithelium

PLATE 7

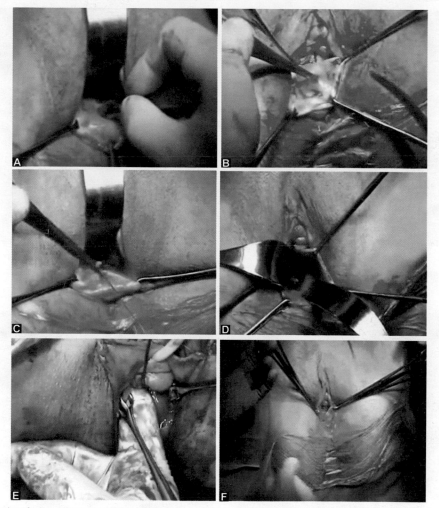

Figs 80.3A to F: (A) Rectocele identified and skin incised: a bulge is apparent on the bottom (posterior) floor of the vagina. The dotted line represents the skin incision, about to be performed in this posterior repair procedure; (B) Identification of the fascia break: the rectocele exists because of a break in the supportive layer known as the rectovaginal fascia. The defect is readily identified and the rectal wall is found protruding through this break in the rectovaginal fascia; (C) The rectovaginal fascia is reattached to the perineal body, where the distal defect was located; (D) The rectovaginal fascial defect has been repaired; (E) The rectovaginal fascia is reattached to the iliococcygeal muscles bilaterally with permanent sutures; (F) Closure of the vaginal epithelium (skin) completes the operation

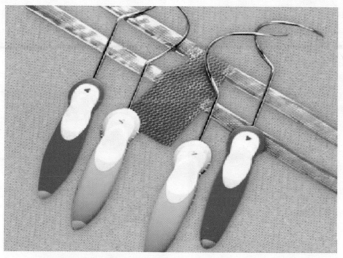

Fig. 80.11: Perigee system for transobturator cystocele repair

PLATE 8

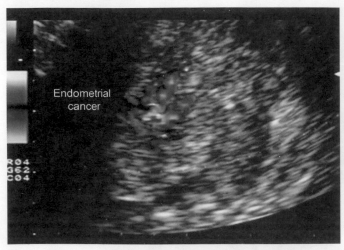

Fig. 83.2: Thick heterogeneous endometrium with proliferation of blood vessels on colour Doppler. This was found to be advanced stage of endometrial cancer

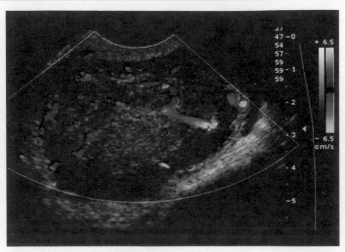

Fig. 86.3: Colour Doppler of the same patient showing randomly distributed irregular vessels in the mass arising from the posterior aspect of the cervix

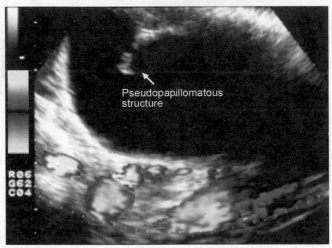

Fig. 91.1: Chronic hydrosalpinx: dilated fallopian tube with thin-walled incomplete septations

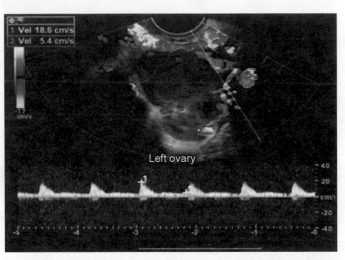

Fig. 91.2: Tubo-ovarian mass: complex cystic solid structure showing prominent vascular perfusion with low-moderate vascular impedence on colour flow Doppler

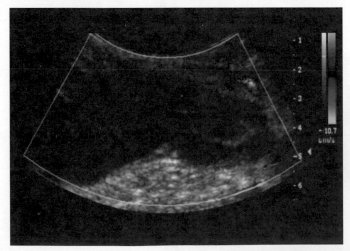

Fig. 91.3: Retort-shaped tubal mass suggestive of hydrosalpinx

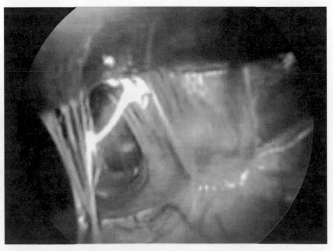

Fig. 91.4: Fitz-Hugh-Curtis syndrome

SECTION 1

General Principles

GENERAL

Principles of Clinical Practice

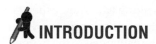 **INTRODUCTION**

Effort must be made towards improving the maternity care and gynaecological practice as much as possible. Adverse outcomes occurring in maternity care are often avoidable and may be due to reasons such as poor recognition of obstetric emergencies, failure to recognize problems at the correct time, failure to seek input from the seniors, poor communication, etc. Obstetricians are also likely to confront numerous ethical challenges in clinical practice. It is also important for all doctors to be well acquainted with the practice of evidence-based medicine, which combines clinical expertise and external scientific evidence. All these important principles of clinical practice have been discussed in this chapter.

ETHICAL PRACTICE OF MEDICINE

'I will use treatments for the benefit of the ill in accordance with my ability and my judgment, but from what is to their harm and injustice I will keep them.'

—**Hippocratic Oath**

Oaths, codes and guidelines for the ethical practice of medicine date back to the Hippocratic Oath of the 4th century BC. Though this oath was largely forgotten at the time of its composition, it achieved a place of prominence in the 18th and 19th centuries as a result of renewed interest in the field of medical ethics. The 'Hippocratic Oath' is the most durable medical oath of Western civilization, which graduating medical students swear to at most of the medical schools in the world. Other oaths commonly sworn to by new physicians include the 'Declaration of Geneva' (an updated form of the Hippocratic oath formulated by the World Medical Association, Ferney-Voltaire, France).[1] The origins of the Hippocratic Oath presently remain unclear, although most historians agree that the oath's name, 'Hippocrates' was not based on the name of its author. Most historians think that the oath originated from a cult of Greek physicians, who were followers of Pythagoras.[2] Alternatively, many researchers also believe that 'the Hippocratic Oath' was created by physician-priests of the cult of Asclepius in ancient Greece. The main ethical principles set forth by the Hippocratic Oath include beneficence (action that is done for the benefit of others), non-maleficence (doing no harm), confidentiality, and prohibition of abortion, euthanasia and sexual relations with patients.[3]

In the early 19th century, some work in the area of medical ethics was done by Sir Thomas Percival.[4] The American Medical Association (AMA) was formed in 1847, which led to the resurgence of interest in the area of medical ethics.[5] However, the surgeons were excluded from this code of ethics. The American College of Surgeons (ACS), Chicago, Illinois, by Dr Miles F Porter, formed in 1913 had set some of the earliest ethics guidelines for the surgeons.[6,7]

The World Medical Association (WMA) made efforts towards the modernisation of the Hippocratic Oath, following the conclusion of World War II.[8] This issue was raised during the trial of Nazi doctors, who had experimented with Jewish prisoners in concentration camps at the time of World War II. After the conviction of the Nazi physicians, the War Crimes Tribunal had put forth 10 principles relevant to human experimentation, known as the 'Nuremberg Code.'[9] The Nuremberg code included the concepts of informed consent, societal good and volunteerism as the foundation for biomedical research. The Nuremberg code emphasizes the following principles:[10] the voluntary consent of the human subject is absolutely essential before involving a person in biomedical research; the person involved should have legal capacity to give consent and should be given free power of making appropriate choice. There should not be any element of force, fraud, deceit, duress or other concealed form of constraint or coercion involved in taking consent.[11] In order to enable the patient to make an enlightened decision, the patient or research subject must be explained in details about the nature, duration and purpose of the procedure or research; the method and means by which it is to be conducted and the inconveniences, complications and the hazards of the procedure and the likely effects upon the health.

During the coming years, approximately eight more declarations of ethics were published by various international organizations. The first ones were the Declaration of Geneva by the WMA and the International Code of Medical Ethics, which were published in 1948.[12] The Declaration of Helsinki, published in 1964 reemphasized the principle of informed consent for volunteers in biomedical research.

Ethical Principles for Medical Research and Practice

The ethical principles for medical research and practice as highlighted by the Belmont report for the protection of human subjects in the biomedical and behavioural research are as follows:[13]

Respect for the Patients

The doctors must show respect for their patients and research subjects by treating them as autonomous individuals and obtaining informed consent before undertaking surgical procedures or any medical or surgical procedure related to research. In the practice of obstetrics and gynaecology, the doctor needs to develop respect for the patient as an individual as well as a woman.

Beneficence

Beneficence refers to the action which is done for the benefit of others. This is based on the principle of 'avoiding any harm'. The doctors need to favour those procedures and treatments, which are likely to benefit the patients and avoid unnecessary harm.

Justice

The doctor should be fair in the process of selecting subjects or the patients. They should be treated fairly in the distribution of benefits and burden.

The Ethical Confidentiality

Trust is the foundation of physician-patient relationship. This is based on the fact that the patient has the right to privacy, which must be always respected. Patients may disclose their private information to the doctor. This is especially the case in the gynaecological practice, where the patients share sensitive information related to intimacy and sexuality with their doctors. Confidentiality, therefore, forms an important aspect of successful therapeutic relationship. According to the code of ethics of American Medical Association (1957), 'A physician may not reveal the confidences entrusted to him in the course of medical attendance or the deficiencies he may observe in the character of patients, unless he is required to do so by the law or unless it becomes absolutely necessary to protect the welfare of the individual or the community.'[14] The parameters within which the breach of confidentiality would be justified are still controversial. Reporting of STDs, which may pose to be serious risk to the public health, may be permitted in some US states. In gynaecological practice,

a variety of complex and difficult situations may arise, where the doctor is faced with the dilemma of whether or not to maintain patient confidentiality. For example, when a woman seeks a medical termination of pregnancy (MTP) or sterilization and requests confidentiality from her partner, the doctor may be faced with a dilemma. In most cases, obligation to patient confidentiality predominates.

Informed Consent

Before undertaking any gynaecological surgery or obstetric procedure, it is important for the obstetrician gynaecologist to take informed consent from the patient. Nowadays, the informed consent is required for all operative procedures. The process involves counselling the patient about the various available surgical options so that the patient can select the best surgical procedure out of the various available options. In practice, the informed consent involves informing the patient about the diagnosis, degree of certainty regarding the diagnosis, the surgery that would be recommended in that case and possible alternatives along with their expected outcomes, risks and benefits. The patient outcome, if no therapy is administered, must also be explained to the patient. The consent should be taken well in advance of surgery in a comfortable setting. The patient must be given adequate time to absorb the information, ask any questions if she feels so and then to make an informed decision. Effective communication between the patient and the surgeon is of utmost importance, while counselling the patient regarding various available treatment options. The surgeon may make use of written material (self-explanatory patient leaflets), visual aids (models), websites, etc. to explain the procedure to the patients. The patients must also be informed about the advantages, disadvantages, success and failure rates and complications of the various procedures. The patient must be counselled even regarding the rare complications that are serious and may affect the individual's life. The patient should be given adequate time to interpret and absorb the information presented to her before making the final decision. At no point must it be taken for granted that the patient would be herself able to understand the general risks of surgery, e.g. anaesthetic complications.

Elements of Informed Consent

The informed consent requires the following pieces of information: nature of the procedure, rationale of doing the procedure, advantages and disadvantages of doing the procedure and availability of alternatives. If the surgeon encounters an additional pathology at the time of surgery in addition to one for which the informed consent was taken, then the surgeon must first finish the planned surgery and discuss the condition later with the patient. The exception to this rule is the discovery of a life-threatening pathology in which case the surgeon can legally perform surgery in the patient for that condition. The elements of informed consent are as follows:[14]

❖ *Disclosure of information*: The patients must be explained about their diagnosis and also briefed about the various available treatment options, including no treatment and various medical, surgical and alternative therapies. Risks and benefits of each modality need to be explained in sufficient details so that a reasonable adult patient can understand the situation and make an informed choice.

❖ *Comprehension by the patient*: The language and the descriptive material, which is used to explain the situation to the patient, must be appropriate to the patient's level of comprehension. The patients must be asked questions in between, to ensure that they understand what they have been told.

❖ *Voluntariness*: While making a decision, the patient must be free of coercion or constraints and must be able to choose freely. The patient should be mentally competent to be able to make a choice and there must be no evidence of limitation in her ability to understand the information. She must be in a condition to act independently on the basis of information that has been disclosed.

❖ *Validation*: A written consent form must be given to the patient, which must be duly signed by her. Consent must be taken for each procedure, which is going to be performed even if they are being performed in a single setting. If an additional pathology is discovered at the time of surgery, the surgeon can legally operate on it, only if the condition is life-threatening. On the other hand, if the condition is not life-threatening then the surgeon must finish the planned surgery and discuss the condition later with the patient. There are four exceptions to the informed consent:[15]

1. *Emergency situations*: If the relatives are unavailable, the patient is unconscious and is suffering from an emergency life-threatening condition.

2. *Intentional relinquishing by the patient*: Waiver may be given by the patient in case of research projects or exploratory laparotomy.

3. *The patient is mentally incompetent,* i.e. the patient has been declared mentally unsound to be able to understand and take decisions appropriately. In this case, the court takes the responsibility for the patient.

4. *Therapeutic privilege*: In case the patient is unconscious or is in the state of confusion and there are no relatives, the physician can act in the patient's benefit without taking her consent.

Surgical Competence as a Moral Commitment

Competence of the surgeon is a moral commitment towards the patient, especially if the surgeon wants to undertake a new procedure. It is essential that the surgeon has been appropriately trained in the clinical sciences and surgical techniques, especially before any new procedure is introduced into clinical medicine.

PATIENT COMMUNICATION AND COUNSELLING

In order to communicate effectively, the surgeon needs to develop the art and skill of listening. The surgeon must tell the patient regarding what will be done to her body at the time of surgery and what are the consequences, surgery can have on her life postoperatively.[16] When the patient expresses her feelings, this results in the revelation of her knowledge, fears and biases. The surgeon can help her cope up with them by supplementing her knowledge with the appropriate explanations regarding the anatomy and physiology of her body parts. The usual preoperative, operative and postoperative routines must also be described in detail. The surgeon must also explain the patient about various physical sensations (pain, discomfort, inability to walk, etc.), bandages, incisions, catheters, tubing and medications. Patients own role in her convalescence and recovery must also be defined. The most common complications, which are likely to occur as a result of surgery must be explained to the patient. Before undergoing surgery, the woman may feel lonely, frightened and sick. It is the duty of the surgeon to make her feel more relaxed, calm and peaceful, by allaying all her fears and anxieties. The therapeutic laying on of the surgeon's hands over the patient's shoulders or head may work wonders at time. A healing touch can often comfort the distressed patient when the words may not prove to be adequate.

In the multicultural society, it is important for the clinician to comprehend if there is any cultural issue which is influencing her decision. For example, some women may have regional or cultural concerns regarding being examined by a male gynaecologist.

The patient's family is an important part of her support system. If the patient so desires, the surgeon must involve the patient's family in decision-making process. They should be provided with an adequate amount of information, reassurance, support and attention. If the patient requests the presence of family members, they should be allowed wherever feasible. The surgeon's contact details must be available to the patient, in case she wants to contact him or her for further clarification or information.

Verbal Communication

Verbal communication with the patient must be based on the following parameters:

❖ The doctor must use the vocabulary which the patient understands.

❖ The doctor must provide appropriate amount of information to the patient, neither too less nor too much that results in information overload. One of the most difficult questions for the clinicians to answer is, 'how much is too much?' The problem is further aggravated due to perceptions regarding litigations.

❖ The clinicians should make sure that they properly greet the patient before they start taking the history.

❖ The doctor must ensure that the patient is at ease, by using an appropriate body posture and facial expression. Besides the patient-doctor communication, the surgeon also needs to pay attention towards the doctor-doctor and doctor-nurse communication, all of which are equally important.

Non-verbal Communication

Besides the verbal communication, there are certain non-verbal components of communication that may be perceived by the patients and may reflect the doctor's attitude towards them. This may include the way the doctor greets the patient, their facial expression, their posture, etc.

Written Communication

These include maintaining the patient's records and sending letters to other healthcare professionals.

Clinical Records

Well-maintained clinical records help in maintaining communication with other professionals and in the protection of the patients. They may serve to protect against the future medicolegal litigations. Poor quality records are likely to confuse other healthcare professionals, thereby endangering the patient's life. Records must be either typed or written in legible handwriting. Preferably, these records must be dated, timed and signed. Concise information must be presented in these records. The physician must not try to present any information, which is not based on evidence. Multidisciplinary team approach must also be practiced and other clinicians may be involved, if the gynaecologist feels the requirement.

Communication with an Angry or Complaining Patient

Observation of good communication principles as described previously may help in addressing an angry or a complaining patient. At all times, the doctor must try to remain as calm and patient as possible.

Patient Counselling

The surgeon can help prepare the patient psychologically, by providing counselling in form of reassurance, information and any other form of support to help her deal with the emotional distress related to gynaecological surgery. The patient is likely to react to surgery in the same way she had reacted to the stressful events in her life. Once the surgeon has come to know about this, while counselling the patient, he or she can start the psychological preparation of the patient. Psychological preparation for surgery is supposed to be effective by reducing negative impact of surgery on the quality of life, pain, medication use, behavioural recovery and physiological function. The surgeon should be with the patient at the time of administering anaesthesia. Simply holding the patient's hand at the time of administering anaesthesia would help her feel safe. Psychosexual rehabilitation may be important after gynaecological surgery to help restore her sexual function, sexual identity, body image and self-esteem. Common emotional responses to surgery or medical treatment are described next.

Insecurity

Feelings of insecurity and vulnerability are common among women undergoing surgery. The surgeon can diminish these feelings by ensuring the patient that the surgery is likely to improve the quality of life by providing improvement in the various parameters, such as relief of pain, removal of cancer, improvement in the quality of life, restoration of fertility, etc. If the patient is convinced that she would be better than she is before surgery, she is likely to trust and believe her surgeon and feel less insecure.

Anxiety or Fear

The patient faces fear of unknown at the time of hospitalisation. Proper information about the surgery and recovery process would help allay this fear and anxiety. Surgeon is also responsible to ensure that the rest of the hospital staff involved in the surgery also behaves positively with the patient. There is also fear regarding the loss of economic competence for an uncertain length of time. This may be especially important if the patient is the only earning member of the family.

Regression and Dependency

People who are ill or who undergo surgery tend to regress into a more dependent state. It may be difficult for the family to deal with a woman, who is no longer self-sufficient or is emotionally unstable. This can lead to anger and frustration on part of the relatives and friends. The prospects of surgery as well as feelings of non-health are likely to contribute to emotional fragility, including the feelings of sadness, depression, tearfulness and irritability. These women are vulnerable to attack on all personal and professional fronts.

Grief and Depression

Grief is a normal, natural reaction to illness or loss of any kind. Grief is essential for emotional healing. By recognising the various stages of grief, the surgeon is able to help the patient understand, regarding what is happening to her.

Postsurgical depression is also a common finding in patients who have undergone surgery. She may experience the feelings of helplessness, hopelessness and worthlessness. Other symptoms of depression may include midnight depression, insomnia, nightmares, loss of appetite or excessive eating, lethargy, difficulty in making decisions, psychosomatic symptoms and fatigue.

CLINICAL GOVERNANCE

Clinical governance can be described as a systematic approach for sustaining and improving the quality of patient care within the National Health System (NHS).[17] The six elements of clinical governance are described in Figure 1.1 and are as follows:

1. Practice of evidence-based medicine and effectiveness
2. Research and development
3. Risk management

Important elements of clinical governance

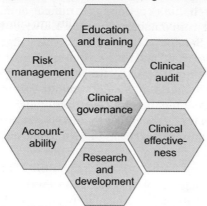

Fig. 1.1: Elements of clinical governance

4. Clinical audit
5. Education, training and continuing professional development
6. Openness or accountability.

Each of these elements has been described in details next in the text.

Practice of Evidence-based Medicine

This is an approach to medical practice, which aims at integrating individual clinical expertise with the best available external clinical evidence from systematic research in form of well-designed and conducted research trials. The term 'evidence-based medicine' was coined by Guyatt in 1991. The coined term subsequently appeared in 1991 in the editorial of American College of Physicians (ACP) Journal Club.[18] However, its roots go much further back. Evidence-based medicine incorporates a broad range of topics, from clinical epidemiology to biomedical informatics to evidence-based guidelines.

Evidence-based medicine involves the conscientious, explicit and judicious use of current best evidence in making decisions about the care of individual patients. On the other hand, clinical expertise implies the proficiency and judgement that the individual clinicians acquire through clinical experience and clinical practice. Evidence-based medicine is a guide only and we should not assume that all patients should be treated similarly according to the results of clinical trials. It is used to make decisions about the care of individual patients. Each patient is an individual, and the clinician must remember this while initiating treatment. All types of clinical trials are included in the practice of evidence-based medicine. However, the methods must be critically appraised in order to assess the validity of the evidence. Objective measurements of disease outcome eliminate bias, are more scientific relative to subjective measures, and are therefore applicable to the practice of evidence-based medicine. Strongest degree of evidence coming from meta-analysis, systemic reviews and randomised controlled trials (RCTs) can yield the strongest recommendations, whereas evidence in form of case-control trials can yield only weak recommendations. Often an RCT will be conducted to assess the benefits or risks associated with a new, expensive treatment. Though RCTs reveal a strong degree of evidence, they are not the only trials that contribute to evidence-based medicine. Prospective trials, observational and cross-sectional studies, all provide vital information that guides the process of daily decision-making.[19] Grading criteria for various levels of evidence are described in Table 1.1 and Figure 1.2.

Traditionally, surgical practice had been experiential and based on the contemporary understanding of basic mechanisms of disease. Surgery was considered as an art and was largely based on experience. There was a change in this trend with the emergence of 'evidence-based medicine' in the 1980s. There is no doubt that the use of evidence-based medicine has been beneficial, but over-reliance on RCTs and the scientific evidence may not prove to be useful for providing individualised medical care to the patients. There has been a continuing debate between the practice of 'experience' or 'evidence-based medicine', while providing care to the patients. The situation is improving, but inevitable tensions remain between the clinician committed towards providing individualised patient care and the clinical researcher, whose focus is on the results of RCTs.

The ethical principles, which must be kept in surgeon's mind before administering treatment to any patient, include the following: the interests of their patients must always

Table 1.1: Grading criteria for levels of evidence

Levels of evidence	Grading criteria	Grading of recommendations
1a	Systematic review of RCTs including meta-analysis	A
1b	Individual RCT with narrow confidence interval	A
1c	All or none studies	B
2a	Systematic review of cohort studies	B
2b	Individual cohort studies and low quality RCT	B
2c	Outcome research studies	C
3a	Systematic review of case-control studies	C
3b	Individual case-control studies	C
4	Case series, poor quality cohort and case-control studies	C
5	Expert opinion	D

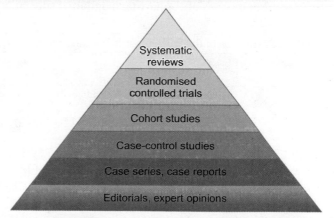

Fig. 1.2: Pyramid showing various levels of evidence

CHAPTER 1

be paramount; any recommendation to a patient must be supported by the best available evidence; before implementing any new intervention or procedure, it must have been properly compared with the currently accepted method(s).

Steps of Evidence-based Medicine

The practice of evidence-based medicine comprises of the following steps:

1. Asking the right question
2. Searching for best evidence
3. Appraising the evidence for its validity
4. Acting on the basis of findings associated with evidence
5. Evaluating the clinical practice and efficacy of the above steps through the process of audit.

Asking the right question: In order to define the clinical problem, correct question must be asked from the patient. The question should be as clear and focussed as possible, in terms of the four elements described by the abbreviation PICO (patient, intervention, comparison and outcome) and summarised in Table 1.2.

For comparison regarding a specific intervention or a treatment strategy, the best quality evidence is available from the RCTs. On the other hand, for comparison related to the exposure to a particular risk factor, cohort studies, which are followed up for a specified period of time, provide the best evidence. Therefore, in case of cohort studies, the abbreviation can be modified as PECOT (Patient, Exposure, Comparison, Outcome and Time).

Searching for evidence: Finding the evidence to the focussed question may require an extensive search. As previously mentioned, the best quality evidence comes from the RCTs. Evidence can be searched from many databases, where the published research studies are indexed. There are several large databases that include citations of published studies. One of the larger ones is PubMed[20] or Medline, produced by the US Library of Medicine, which contains over 23 million articles. These may comprise different types of studies including case reports, observational studies, RCTs, systematic reviews, etc. Several other online databases are also available for search. Excerpta Medica dataBASE (EMBASE) is a biomedical and pharmacological database of published literature, indexing primarily European studies. This has been designed to support information managers and pharmacovigilance specialists

in conforming to the regulatory requirements of a licensed drug. Research studies pertaining to nursing or midwifery can be obtained from databases such as Midwives Information & Resource Service [(MIDIRS), (midwifery digest)], British Nursing Index (BNI) and Current Index to Nursing and Allied Health Literature (CINAHL). Research studies pertaining to psychological literature may be obtained from psycLIT (a CD-ROM version of psychological abstracts) or psycINFO. PsycLIT was merged into the PsycINFO online database in 2000. It contains research studies from not only the field of psychology, but also sociology, linguistics, medicine, law, psychiatry and anthropology. PROSPERO (International Prospective Register of Systematic Reviews) is another open access international database of prospectively registered systemic reviews in health and social care. The best resource for the high-quality systemic reviews is the Cochrane library (ISSN 1465–1858), which has a collection of six databases containing different types of high-quality independent evidence. This information is likely to enable healthcare professionals in evidence-based decision-making process. It also has a seventh database which provides information about Cochrane groups. These seven databases are as follows:

1. *Cochrane Database of Systemic Reviews (CDSR)*: This is the leading resource for systematic reviews in health care. The CDSR includes Cochrane Reviews (the systematic reviews) and protocols for Cochrane Reviews as well as editorials.
2. *Cochrane Central Register of Controlled Trials (CENTRAL)*: This is a source of randomised and quasi-randomised controlled trials.
3. *Cochrane Methodology Register (CMR)*: This register comprises a bibliography of publications which report on methods used while conducting controlled trials.
4. *Database of Abstracts of Reviews of Effects (DARE)*: This is a database containing abstracts of systematic reviews which have been quality-assessed. DARE complements the CDSR by assessing the quality and summarising reviews, which have not yet been carried out by Cochrane.
5. *Health Technology Assessment (HTA) Database*: This includes UK and international health technology assessments (studies of the medical, social, ethical and economic implications of healthcare interventions). The aim of the HTA database is the development of the quality and cost-effectiveness of healthcare services.

Table 1.2: Description of the four elements of asking a focussed question

Letter of abbreviation	Full form	Explanation	Example question: Does aspirin reduce the risk of death after a heart attack in adults?
P	The *patient* or problem being addressed	Description of the appropriate patient characteristics (e.g. age, parity, gender, etc.)	Adults who have suffered a heart attack in the past month
I	The *intervention* being considered	This is the main action being implemented (e.g. diagnostic test or a treatment strategy or modification of a risk factor)	Administration of aspirin
C	The *comparison* intervention or exposure when relevant	The comparison group could be a placebo or an alternate treatment	No treatment/placebo
O	The clinical *outcomes* of interest	Change in health expected as a result of an intervention	Prevention of death

6. *NHS Economic Evaluation Database (EED)*: This database assists decision-makers by systematically identifying economic evaluations from around the world. It not only appraises their quality, but also highlights their relative strengths and weaknesses.
7. *About The Cochrane Collaboration Database*: This database contains information related to various Cochrane groups within Cochrane.

The DARE and HTA database are available on the websites, www.tripdatabase.com and www.cr.york.ac.uk. There are two online databases pertaining to the international guidelines: (1) AHRQ (Agency for Healthcare Research and Quality) National Guidelines Clearinghouse and; (2) the Guidelines International Network Library. In the UK, national guidelines pertaining to obstetrics and gynaecology are produced by the following societies:

❖ Scottish Intercollegiate Guidelines Network (SIGN)
❖ National Institute for Health and Care Excellence (NICE)
❖ Royal College of Obstetricians and Gynaecologists (RCOG).

Appraising the evidence for its validity: It is important to critically appraise the available evidence for its validity because different types of studies reported in the literature are likely to have different strengths and weaknesses. The clinician needs to decide if a particular research study would be clinically significant for their patients. A particular research study can be critically appraised by asking the following questions:

❖ Is the study valid [i.e. are the results of the study reliable and what kind of research study (study methodology) was carried out]?
❖ What are the results of the study?
❖ Would the results of the study help the clinicians in looking after their patients?

Generally, larger studies are preferred over the smaller ones because the results of larger studies are less likely to be due to chance. A systematic review of the RCTs is the most important component in the practice of evidence-based medicine.[21] Clinical guidelines are usually based on systematic reviews. A systematic review is a type of literature review, which collects and critically analyses multiple research studies. These mainly include RCTs. However, at times, there also may be observational studies. The method of systematic review must be clear, specific and well-structured. It must include the clearly-defined PICO questions. An extensive search of literature must be carried out followed by the critical appraisal of the studies located after searching with a specific criterion. Finally, these research studies must be analysed using appropriate methods. Data from each of these individual studies may be pooled and statistically analysed using a technique known as the meta-analysis.

While systematic reviews and meta-analyses are essential for summarising the evidence related to efficacy and safety of healthcare interventions, the clarity and transparency of these studies at times may be suboptimal. In order to improve the system for reporting and conduct of the systematic reviews and meta-analysis, the quality of reporting of meta-analysis (QUOROM) statement was published in 1999. Since then, there has been publication of several statements for improving the standards for primary and secondary research, such as preferred reporting items for systematic reviews and meta-analyses (PRISMA); Consolidated Standards of Reporting Trials (CONSORT); The Standards for Reporting of Diagnostic Accuracy (STARD) and Strengthening the Reporting of Observational Studies in Epidemiology (STROBE).[22-25]

Acting on the basis of findings associated with evidence: Decisions related to treatment must be based on the results of the appraised evidence after considering both the benefits and harms of treatment and helping the patient make a choice, i.e. the shared decision-making process.

Audit: *Evaluation of the clinical practice and efficacy of the previous steps*: Audit has been described in details later in the text.

Research and Development

Due to occurrence of technological advancements in the field of medicine over time, clinicians need to keep themselves abreast with the latest advancements and research in the field of medicine. Techniques for using and implementing the results of these research studies in clinical practice include critical appraisal of literature, development of guidelines, protocols, application of strategies, etc.

Different Types of Trials or Research Studies in Clinical Practice

Double-blind trials: Double-blind study refers to a type of research study in which neither the study participants nor the person giving the treatment knows which treatment a particular subject is receiving. This helps in alleviating potential bias through randomisation of patients to the drug or placebo without either the doctor or the patient knowing which agent is being used. In this way, both the researchers and the study participants are 'blind' to which subject is receiving what type of treatment during the study. This method helps the researchers to get more accurate results from their research. Double blinding allows researchers to 'control' a study for the psychological effects that sometimes help people feel better, simply because they expect to feel better when they receive a medication. In other words, double blinding helps the researchers to separate the 'power of suggestion' from the real effects of a medication or therapy. Placebo-controlled studies are most appropriately undertaken in a double-blind fashion with both the observer and the patient blinded to treatment. Although one might think that placebo has no effect, in fact, there may well be a huge placebo (psychological) effect. Placebo studies are undertaken in patients with cancer, particularly to establish the palliative value of drugs or the effectiveness of a new treatment where none exists. As a variation of this theme, patients can be randomised to receive either the new drug or an established therapy. Example of a double-blinded trial is a study conducted amongst a group of 500 patients for assessing the effectiveness of a new antirheumatic agent. The drug company randomises the patients to receive either placebo or the active drug although neither the patients nor investigators know which treatment they are receiving.

Single-blind trial: This is a single-blind study where the patient does not know which arm of therapy they are receiving. However, the investigator does have this information. For example, a study is undertaken assessing the effects of a cholesterol-lowering agent on cardiovascular disease. Patients are randomised by the investigators to receive either the drug or the placebo. However, the patients are unaware regarding the kind of treatment they would receive.

Randomised controlled trials: Randomised control trials form the heart of evidence-based medicine because these trials help in evaluating the effectiveness of a particular therapeutic method and are likely to be associated with least bias. A typical RCT involves the following steps (Fig. 1.3):

1. Enrolment of the subjects who meet the eligibility criteria into the study
2. Random allocation of the subjects into the treatment and control groups
3. Administration of the treatment to the 'treatment group', while no treatment or placebo is administered to the 'control group'.
4. Follow-up of both the groups
5. Analysis of the results.

Subjects with a particular condition, who meet the inclusion criteria for entry into the trial, are randomly allo-cated to either receive treatment or some form of control (either no treatment or the current, 'gold standard' treatment). A computer programme is used for randomising the data in different participating centres. Various participating centres are also linked with telephone services to request the randomisation procedure. Wherever possible, double blinding should be performed, i.e. both the subjects and investigators must be blinded to the randomised allocation and the control group should be provided with some form of placebo. The outcome of interest is measured to evaluate if one group experiences any benefit over the others. The main advantage of the RCT is the concealment of the treatment allocation and thus minimisation of the selection bias and low chances of confounding. These studies are, however, time-consuming and expensive. Also, there can be an appreciable loss to follow-up if the infrastructure is not in place to ensure good data collection.

Parameters which decide the validity of these studies include the following: Random allocation of the subjects into the treatment and control groups; group selection in a way that the characteristics (age, parity, sample size, etc.) of both the groups should be similar; equal treatment of both the groups and inclusion of all the patients while analysis of results and formulation of conclusion.

Case-control study: This is a study comparing the character-istics of subjects selected on the basis of their disease status. A case-control study compares two groups of people: those with the disease or condition under study (cases) and a very similar group of people who do not have the disease or condition (controls). While the cohort study can be visualised as a prospective study, following subjects forward through time, case-control study is a retrospective study. This study involves the recruitment of cases (subjects with the disease) and a group of control (subjects without the disease), both of which are looked back through time to compare their exposures to evaluate if any of the exposure appears to relate to the disease development. Case-control studies are relatively cheap in comparison with the cohort studies and can be used to investigate a number of different exposures simultaneously. The main difficulty associated with this type of study is the selection of the control group. Also, these studies can be often associated with considerable problems related to the selection bias and observer or recall bias. These studies differ from the cohort studies regarding the fact that cohort studies are not good at investigating rare exposures as a large number of subjects need to be recruited to obtain enough evidence of the exposure. Moreover, case-control studies cannot be used for making estimates of disease incidence and are not very helpful in investigating the series of events resulting in the disease diagnosis. Presence of confounding factors can also pose further problems.

Cross-sectional studies: In these studies, the data are collected from a sample of subjects at a given point of time and comparisons are made between the variables to investigate the extent of disease of interest or to assess which exposures may be linked with the disease. These studies represent a snapshot in time and therefore the prevalence is generally the main outcome measure. Moreover, no information is obtained on the disease incidence over time.

Open study: Open study is a type of study in which both the researchers and the participants know which treatment is being administered. For example, a study compares the effect of low-molecular-weight heparin versus aspirin in the prevention of deep vein thrombosis (DVT) amongst postoperative gynaecological patients. Patients are randomised by the study coordinator to receive treatment as either a tablet or injection. This study assessing DVT postoperatively is an open study as patients and investigators will know which treatment they are receiving as it is either an injection or a tablet. If, however, they wished to create a double-blind study then patients could be

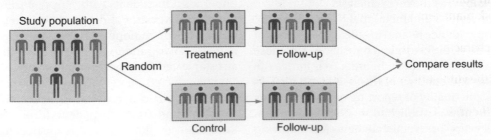

Fig. 1.3: Steps involved in a randomised controlled trial

randomised to receive injection plus placebo tablet or aspirin plus placebo injection.

Cohort studies: Cohort studies or longitudinal studies involve the follow-up of individuals. Subjects are recruited into cohort studies and followed up over time to assess the incidence of a particular disease. In case of a disease that has already been diagnosed, disease progression can be assessed. A cohort study is prospective in the sense that the individuals who are exposed and non-exposed to a putative risk factor are followed up over a defined period of time and the disease experience of the exposed group at the end of follow-up is compared with that of the non-exposed group. Cohort studies are more important than the cross-sectional studies because they provide far more information on the incidence of events. These studies also allow temporal assessments to be made regarding whether the exposure preceded the outcomes of interest or not. A cohort study may also be historical (retrospective or non-concurrent). Cohort studies are, however, not useful at investigating rare studies. They are frequently used when the disease is common and the effects of various exposures are not well understood.

Meta-analysis: Analysis of data from published literature is termed as meta-analysis. Meta-analysis is a common way of assessing the effect of treatment or the potential risks of treatment by reviewing and assessing all the data published in the medical literature. Many of the guidelines are published through meta-analysis.

Risk Management

Over recent years, there has been a growing appreciation that a small but significant proportion of patients may experience adverse events, as a result of an error on the part of the healthcare workers, e.g. errors in the route of administration or dosage of medicines by the nurses. Sometimes, these events may prove to be serious or even life-threatening. Over the past few decades, there has been an increasing trend towards application of principles of risk management in healthcare organisations. Since small errors can result in particularly disastrous and costly adverse outcomes in both obstetrics and gynaecology, it is appropriate to review clinical risk management issues. Risk management involves the ways in which these errors can be identified, analysed and subsequently reduced. It involves examining the various procedures, right from the beginning until their end. The various incidents and accidents are analysed to prevent their occurrence. This is based on the principle that simple system errors can result in some of the most devastating mistakes. The concept of risk management is based on the following strategies:[26]

❖ Identification, characterisation and assessment of potential threats

❖ Assessment of the vulnerability of critical assets to specific threats

❖ *Determining the risk*: This involves assessment of the expected consequences of specific types of attacks on various assets

❖ Identifying ways to reduce those risks

❖ Prioritising risk reduction measures.

An educational and supportive environment, rather than a blame culture, helps in encouraging the reporting of adverse incidents. This encourages the staff to learn from the adverse outcomes. Reduction in the adverse events, which occur in healthcare institutions helps in improving the overall quality of patient care. Within the NHS, risk is managed best within a framework, called RADICAL framework, which incorporates all elements of clinical governance. The RADICAL (Raise Awareness, Design for safety, Involvement of users, Collection and Analysis of safety data, and Learning from patient safety incidents) framework for risk management in the healthcare system is described in Flow chart 1.1.[27]

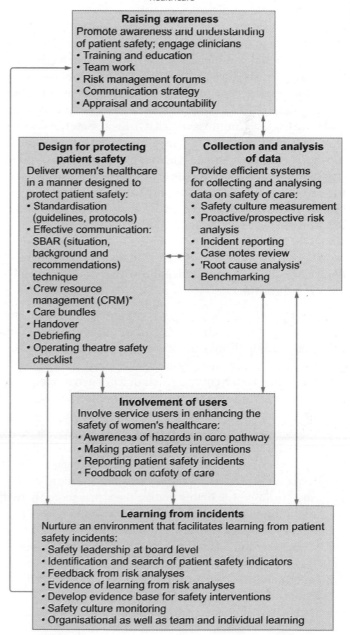

Flow chart 1.1: The RADICAL framework for the management of risk in healthcare[27]

Raising awareness
Promote awareness and understanding of patient safety; engage clinicians
• Training and education
• Team work
• Risk management forums
• Communication strategy
• Appraisal and accountability

Design for protecting patient safety
Deliver women's healthcare in a manner designed to protect patient safety:
• Standardisation (guidelines, protocols)
• Effective communication: SBAR (situation, background and recommendations) technique
• Crew resource management (CRM)*
• Care bundles
• Handover
• Debriefing
• Operating theatre safety checklist

Collection and analysis of data
Provide efficient systems for collecting and analysing data on safety of care:
• Safety culture measurement
• Proactive/prospective risk analysis
• Incident reporting
• Case notes review
• 'Root cause analysis'
• Benchmarking

Involvement of users
Involve service users in enhancing the safety of women's healthcare:
• Awareness of hazards in care pathway
• Making patient safety interventions
• Reporting patient safety incidents
• Feedback on safety of care

Learning from incidents
Nurture an environment that facilitates learning from patient safety incidents:
• Safety leadership at board level
• Identification and search of patient safety indicators
• Feedback from risk analyses
• Evidence of learning from risk analyses
• Develop evidence base for safety interventions
• Safety culture monitoring
• Organisational as well as team and individual learning

*Set of training procedures for use in environments where human error can have overwhelming effects

Process of Risk Management

The process of risk management involves the following steps: risk identification; compilation of a risk register; risk analysis and risk control.

Risk identification: There must be formal processes for identifying anything that might interfere with the delivery of safe, good-quality maternity services. If something goes wrong, the clinicians can identify the risk by looking back at the series of events to identify the things that went wrong. Risks could also be identified through internal or external sources. Internal sources for identifying risk refer to risk assessment conducted in all clinical (wards, clinics, theatre, delivery suite, day assessment unit, etc.) as well as non-clinical areas (secretarial office, canteen, etc.). Risk assessment can also be obtained through reporting of incidents; record of complaints and claims; consultation with the staff in form of workshops, surveys, interviews and clinical audit, etc. External sources identify the risk at national level and include national confidential enquiries, Clinical Negligence Scheme for Trusts (CNST) standards, RCOG guidelines, NICE guidelines, protocols and visitation, National Patient Safety Agency Alerts (NPSA), postgraduate dean's specialty site visits and Care Quality Commission (CQC). Each maternity as well as gynaecology unit should have a trigger list for reporting of incidents (Tables 1.3 and 1.4). Staff must be encouraged to complete incident forms for these various triggers. To optimise the reporting of incidents, an organisation should have a culture wherein staff should be aware and motivated about reporting of adverse events. They should be aware that they would be listened to and not blamed for the adverse event. In fact, they should be provided with an accurate feedback because feedback drives motivation, which would eventually help in improvement.

Compilation of a risk register: Risks identified through the processes described above should be entered in the risk registers, which should be preferably maintained in the clinical area of each maternity and gynaecology unit. Example of various risks, which could be included in a gynaecology risk register, may include the risks identified in the care pathways for management of gynaecological emergencies, etc. However, risk registers are not merely limited to clinical issues. Non-clinical issues such as those related to breakdown of building, heating system, etc. can also be noted in the risk register. Once the risk is identified, it is graded within a standard matrix described in Table 1.5. In this matrix, the risk is scored in two ways. First one is the seriousness or consequences of risk (from being a negligible event to a catastrophic event, which can result in multiple fatalities). Levels of severity are locally defined, taking into account the extent of harm caused to the patient and the organisation. The second score reflects the probability of the occurrence of an event (from being impossible to occur to occurring certainly). Both these scores are multiplied to reach a risk score, which helps to quantify the level of risk. Within this matrix, a risk with a score of 20

Table 1.3: Suggested trigger list for incident reporting in maternity[27]

Maternal incident	Foetal/neonatal incident	Organisational incidents
• Death of the mother	• Death of the neonate	• Unavailability of health record
• Undiagnosed breech presentation	• Stillbirth >500 g	• Delay in responding to call for assistance
• Shoulder dystocia	• Apgar score <7 at 5 minutes	
• Blood loss >1,500 mL	• Birth trauma	• Unplanned home birth
• Return to theatre	• Foetal laceration at the time of operative delivery	• Faulty equipment
• Eclampsia		• Conflict over case management
• Hysterectomy/ laparotomy	• Cord pH <7.05 arterial or <7.1 venous	• Potential service/ user complaint
• Anaesthetic complications	• Neonatal seizures	• Medication error
• Intensive care admission	• Term baby admitted to neonatal unit	• Retained swab or instrument
• Venous thromboembolism	• Undiagnosed foetal anomaly	• Hospital-acquired infection
• Pulmonary embolism		• Violation of local protocol
• Third-/fourth-degree perineal tears		
• Unsuccessful attempt at forceps or ventouse assisted delivery		
• Uterine rupture		
• Re-admission of mother		

Table 1.4: Suggested trigger list for incident reporting in gynaecology[27]

Clinical incident	Organisational incidents
• Damage to structures (e.g. ureter, bowel, vessel)	• Delay following call for assistance
• Delayed or missed diagnosis (e.g. ectopic pregnancy)	• Faulty equipment
• Anaesthetic complications	• Conflict over case management
• Venous thromboembolism	• Potential service user complaint
• Failed procedures (e.g. termination of pregnancy, sterilisation)	• Medication error
• Unplanned intensive care admission	• Retained swab or instrument
• Omission of planned procedures (failure to insert planned intra-uterine contraceptive device after a hysteroscopy)	• Violation of local protocol
• Unexpected operative blood loss >500 mL	
• Moderate/severe ovarian hyperstimulation (assisted conception)	
• Procedure performed without consent (e.g. removal of ovaries at hysterectomy)	
• Unplanned return to theatre	
• Unplanned return to hospital within 30 days	

or higher is usually considered to represent an unacceptable risk. Residual risks exceeding a preset threshold are entered into a departmental or a directorate register. Significant risks from that register are then in turn mentioned in a hospital or trust-wide risk register. Ideally, a risk register should be in electronic format. A risk register is not a static document; it must be continually reviewed. It is modified as older risks are treated or new ones appear. Steps must be taken for reduction of risk either by reducing the frequency of its occurrence or by reducing its severity.

Risk analysis: Once the risks have been identified, they are noted in the risk register, following which they are assigned a risk score as previously described (Table 1.5). This helps in identifying the risks or incidents that require in-depth investigation or those that require immediate action for correction.

The incident must be investigated using the Reason's organisational 'Swiss cheese' model of accident causation (Fig. 1.4). This model illustrates that there are many layers of defence between the hazards to accidents. Alignment of flaws in each of the layers allows the accident to occur. This model has been adopted by the NPSA and used as the 'fishbone tool' for root cause analysis. Fishbone diagrams (Fig. 1.5) are often used by the NPSA for identifying the contributory factors.[28] It helps to categorise the potential sources of defects or the root causes. Various components of a fishbone are as follows:

❖ *Head of the fish*: Effect or the outcome
❖ *Horizontal branches*: Causes (various causes can be divided into non-service processes such as methods,

Table 1.5: Standard matrix for grading risk[27]

Consequences	Probability				
Severity of risk	Rare (1)	Unlikely (2)	Moderate (3)	Likely (4)	Certain (5)
Multiple fatalities (5)	5	10	15	20	25
Fatality (4)	4	8	12	16	20
Major (3)	3	6	9	12	15
Serious (2)	2	4	6	8	10
Minor (1)	1	2	3	4	5

Note: Scores obtained from the matrix can be graded as follows:
■ 1–3: Low risk; ■ 4–6: Moderate risk; ■ 8–12: High risk; ■ 15–25: Extreme risk

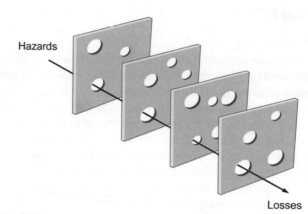

Hazards

Losses

Fig. 1.4: Reason's organisational Swiss cheese model of accident causation

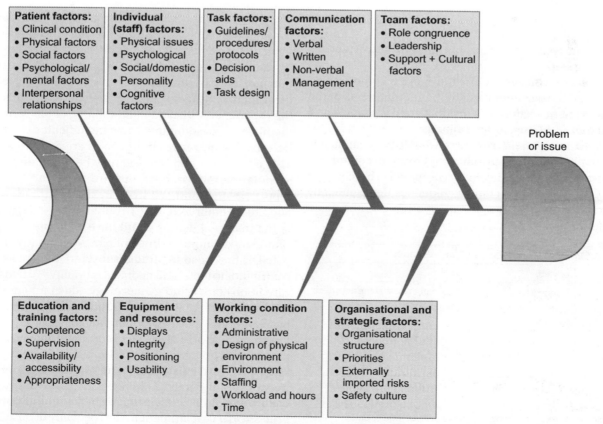

Patient factors:
• Clinical condition
• Physical factors
• Social factors
• Psychological/ mental factors
• Interpersonal relationships

Individual (staff) factors:
• Physical issues
• Psychological
• Social/domestic
• Personality
• Cognitive factors

Task factors:
• Guidelines/ procedures/ protocols
• Decision aids
• Task design

Communication factors:
• Verbal
• Written
• Non-verbal
• Management

Team factors:
• Role congruence
• Leadership
• Support + Cultural factors

Problem or issue

Education and training factors:
• Competence
• Supervision
• Availability/ accessibility
• Appropriateness

Equipment and resources:
• Displays
• Integrity
• Positioning
• Usability

Working condition factors:
• Administrative
• Design of physical environment
• Environment
• Staffing
• Workload and hours
• Time

Organisational and strategic factors:
• Organisational structure
• Priorities
• Externally imported risks
• Safety culture

Fig. 1.5: Fishbone diagram for root cause analysis[28]

PART I

materials, people, equipment, technique, environment and service processes such as policy, procedures, plan and people)
❖ *Sub-branches*: Reasons.

Risk control: Following the appropriate analysis of risk, measures must be put in place for controlling these risks. Selection of the appropriate treatment plan is dependent on the risk rating. Lessons learned from the identification and treatment of risk should be shared with the healthcare professionals in other parts of the hospital or trust through several routes such as multidisciplinary team meetings, ward meetings, safety alerts, newsletters, intranet and educational meetings. Both the NPSA and the RCOG have communication channels which can be used for this purpose.

Clinical Audit

Definition

Audit is the process of quality improvement of the healthcare services, thereby improving the overall quality of life. It aims at improving the patient care and outcome by assessing, evaluating and improving the care of the patients. This is achieved through the systematic review of care against set criteria. Based on the findings of the review, the changes are identified and implemented. Where indicated, the identified changes are implemented at an individual, team or service level. Further monitoring is implemented to confirm if these changes result in an improvement towards the delivery of healthcare services. Difference between audit and research has been described in Table 1.6.

Steps of Audit Cycle

A typical audit cycle is described in Figure 1.6 and comprises the following steps:

1. *Initial needs assessment*: The audit cycle comprises an initial needs assessment where the requirements of the department or section or individual are determined and the actual audit itself is determined.
2. *Identification of standards*: Then what is to be audited is decided upon; it is important to identify the standards against which the audit will be compared. These can be national standards or clinical guidelines determined by the national bodies or comparisons can even be made within the department.

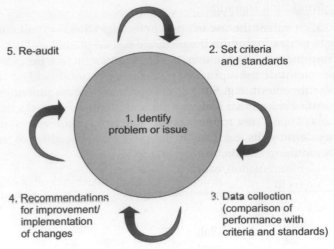

Fig. 1.6: The audit cycle

3. *Data collection*: Once the standards are set, data collection is undertaken, with selection of retrospective or prospective data followed by data analysis.
4. *Recommendations*: The results can then be presented, compared to the standards and from this, recommendations for improvements or implementation of changes are made.
5. *Re-audit*: Finally, to assess how effectively these recommendations have been implemented, a re-audit is suggested in the future.

Education, Training and Continuing Professional Development

Obstetric emergencies are not a common occurrence. However, they often may be unpredictable. Successful management of these emergencies requires coordinated functioning by the experienced staff. Management of the patient must function as a part of an efficient multidisciplinary team. The most important factor behind the success of this team is the experience, education and training of the various team members. This sometimes may be difficult to be acquired because the obstetric emergencies are a rare occurrence. This experience and training may be best gained through stimulation and practice. According to the most recent report, 'saving mothers' lives' by the Centre for Maternal and Child Enquiries (CMACE) published in 2011, nearly 50% of the maternal deaths could have been prevented.[29] The Confidential Enquiries into Stillbirths and Deaths in Infancy (CESDI) have also identified substandard care as a major contributor to foetal and neonatal mortality.[30, 31] Substandard care in obstetrics and gynaecology adds immensely to the NHS expenditure because maternity claims are responsible for the highest-value litigation complains reported to the NHS Litigation Authority (NHSLA). Most important causes of the maternity claims have been mistakes in the interpretation of foetal heart, mistakes in the management of labour, prevention of cerebral palsy etc. This further highlights the importance of training, education and continuing professional development in the speciality of obstetrics and gynaecology.

Table 1.6: Difference between audit and research

Characteristic	Research	Audit
Definition	Discovers and defines the right thing to do	Determines whether the right thing is being done
Aims	Aims for the generalisation of the findings	It is never possible to generalise the findings because each report deals with an individual situation
Special feature	Each project stands alone	Involves a cyclical series of reviews
Methodology	Collection of complex and unique data	Collection of routine data

Stimulation Training

This involves the use of stimulation models for training in obstetrics including bony pelvis and advanced full body birthing simulators having accurate anatomy and functionality to facilitate multiprofessional obstetric training of birth management, e.g. SimMom, Noelle, PRactical Obstetric Multi-Professional Training (PROMPT) birth stimulator, etc. Simple part-task trainers can be used for teaching specific obstetric skills, e.g. instrumental delivery, manoeuvres for shoulder dystocia, manoeuvres for breech delivery, etc. Hybrid stimulation, which involves the use of simple part-task trainers in combination with full body birthing simulators, is also used. Computer-based virtual reality simulation models, which provide both kinaesthetic and visual feedback to the trainers, are also available.

Simple and advanced simulation models can be used for teaching advanced obstetric skills within the structured simulation-based training courses. One such structured simulation-based training course, the Advanced Life Support in Obstetrics (ALSO) course was introduced in the US in 1991.[32] This was followed by the Managing Obstetric Emergencies and Trauma (MOET) course in 1998.[33] This course aimed at teaching advanced skills to the obstetricians and anaesthetists. Both these courses resulted in a significant improvement in obstetric emergency management. PROMP course has been developed in the UK to provide practical training to the obstetricians, midwives and the anaesthetists.[34] Other obstetric emergency courses, which have been described, include Multidisciplinary Obstetric Simulated Emergency Scenarios (MOSES), and Training in Obstetric Emergency Scenarios (TOES).[35,36] Training programmes should be specifically focussed towards the development of specific clinical skills (e.g. management of eclampsia, shoulder dystocia, cord prolapse, postpartum haemorrhage, conducting instrumental deliveries, etc.), communication skills, team working and awareness of an individual's role within the team. Some of the important features of Stimulation-Based Medical Education (SBME) include the following:[37]

❖ *Active participation of all team members*: These training programmes must aim at the training of all staff within the maternity and gynaecological unit including the doctors, midwives, healthcare assistants, porters, etc. Training should be provided in a non-threatening environment and as per the individual's specific role in the team. Constructive feedback must be provided to the various team members for the purpose of improvement.

❖ *Provision of local (in-house) training*: The training should be preferably provided to the staff locally within their unit. This is not only likely to be less expensive, but also helps in recognition of the safety issues within the environment, and helps the staff to become familiar with their working environments.

❖ *Use of realistic simulation models*: As far as possible, real-appearing simulation models (e.g. trousers with bleeding red material, demonstrating PPH; perineum with prolapsed cord; etc.) must be used for these training programmes.

❖ *Provision of incentives for training*: Institutions should help in implementing and subsequently running a training program by funding its cost. The NHS has schemes in which maternity hospitals having a high standard of training, guidelines and audit are rewarded with reduced insurance premiums.

❖ *Interprofessional clinical training with an integrated team approach*: Training should be provided to the various members of the team in accordance to their specific roles in the team so that they function as a part of the multidisciplinary team. People are likely to make fewer errors when they work as part of an integrated team.

❖ *Multiprofessional 'fire-drill' training*: According to the recommendations by the RCOG and the Royal College of Midwives in their report, 'Safer Childbirth: Minimum Standards for the Organisation and Delivery of Care in Labour', there is a requirement for regular multiprofessional 'fire-drill' training in the management of labour ward emergencies such as cord prolapse, vaginal breech delivery, shoulder dystocia, antepartum haemorrhage, severe postpartum haemorrhage, etc.[38]

❖ *Provision of evidence-based training*: Training should be based on the practice of evidence-based medicine.

❖ *Evaluation of the training programme*: The training programme must be formally evaluated to assess its effectiveness.

Levels of Training

Kirkpatrick has described four levels for evaluating the efficacy of training programmes (Table 1.7).[39]

Openness or Accountability

It is often believed that poor performance and practice often flourishes behind closed doors. Accountability is based on five core principles: responsibility, explainability, accuracy, auditability and fairness.

LEGAL RIGHTS OF WOMAN, UNBORN AND NEWBORN CHILDREN

Unborn babies have little by way of legal rights. Although the human foetus is worthy of respect, according to law it does not have any right prior to birth.[40] With the increasing use of foetal imaging in clinical practice, the foetus is commonly being regarded as a separate patient with unique rights. According to law, if the woman is legally competent, her wishes must be respected. She should not be treated any different from other competent adults. A pregnant woman cannot be made to have treatment unless she gives her consent for it, e.g. caesarean

Table 1.7: Kirkpatrick levels for evaluation of the efficacy of training programmes

Level	Description
Level 1: Reaction	Satisfaction of learners
Level 2: Learning	Factual and applied knowledge, attitudes
Level 3: Behaviour	Patient care and satisfaction
Level 4: Results	Patient outcomes and infrastructural/organisational changes

section, even if this means that her baby will die or come to serious harm. However, this may sound harsh and may not always be accepted by the clinicians taking caring for that particular patient. As a result, problems may sometimes arise with the doctors taking legal help. This has led to a grey zone and there have been cases where the decision of a competent woman regarding the management of her pregnancy and labour may not always be respected.

Sometimes, a woman's decision or behaviour may threaten the survival of an otherwise healthy foetus. According to law, the clinician needs to respect the decision of a competent woman, even if it results in her death or death of an otherwise viable foetus. Similarly, a competent refusal by the pregnant patient of the treatment designed to save the life of her foetus (and or herself) must be respected. In particular, a mother cannot be made to put herself at risk or through unpleasant or unwanted procedures just for the benefit of the child.

On the other hand, the interests of the foetus and the embryo are not completely ignored by the law. The embryo or foetus can be offered benefit without breaching the rights of others, particularly the mother. Once a child is born, it acquires the same rights as others. Children are entitled to sue for the damage they had sustained during the prenatal period. However, this does not imply that the foetus has rights before birth.

Refusal of the parents to give consent for treatment of their newborn child is dealt with in the 'Department of Health' document. The key feature is that clinicians and parents may not always agree on what is best for a child. Usually, if parents refuse treatment for their child, then treatment will not go ahead. However, if the clinicians and their colleagues believe that it is crucial for the child to have the treatment in question, for example, if they think that the child would die or suffer serious permanent injury without the treatment, then the courts can be asked to decide what would be best in the child's interests. Applications to court can be made at short notice if necessary. If the emergency is such that there is no time to apply to court, any doubts should be resolved in favour of the preservation of life.

The Mental Capacity Act 2005

The main aim of this act is to provide a legal framework for making decisions on behalf of those adults who lack the capacity for making a particular decision by themselves.[41] Every possible step to confirm capacity must be taken before deciding that someone lacks capacity. If there is doubt about whether the patients have capacity or not, the health professional must get an expert-opinion from consultant psychiatrist or psychologist having a background in dealing with patients having learning difficulties. If following assessment, there remains a serious doubt about the patient's competence, legal advice must be sought.

The legalities in such cases are wrapped up in the Mental Capacity Act 2005. A court order will be usually required to provide treatment in these cases. The court would normally expect to make a 'one-off' decision relating to a particular treatment for an individual lacking capacity. If the court foresees that further decisions may be needed, it can

appoint a 'Deputy' to act on behalf of an individual who lacks capacity. The Deputy will have lasting power to make decisions on the patient's behalf over all matters, including medical care. In an emergency situation, treatment can be provided without a court order. However, in these cases, it is sensible to get a second opinion to confirm that it is an emergency and that urgent treatment is necessary. In these cases, relatives and carers are not able to give consent. However, the health professional in charge can use 'consent form 4' from the Department of Health to authorise the investigation or treatment. The health professional must be acting only in the best interest of the patient by consulting the relatives, carers, etc. and the Trust's legal department. A second opinion should also be obtained from a colleague. There are a number of serious situations that must be referred to the Court for their judgement. For example, if it was felt that a young woman (who lacks capacity) would be incapable of rearing a child, the parents might wish her to be sterilised. The courts view removal of fertility as extremely serious. Any decision of this kind would have to come from the Court and it would be illegal for the health professional to use the consent form 4. However, in case of an adult woman who lacks capacity to give consent or withholds consent to treatment, it is alright for the health professional to carry out hysterectomy for dealing with menorrhagia by using the consent form 4 if he or she is able to demonstrate that they are acting in the patient's best interest even though the procedure would render the woman infertile. The Mental Capacity Act (2005) also extends 'powers of attorney' to cover medical matters. 'Power of attorney' implies that individuals give someone else the legal power to make decisions on their behalf. For example, old persons may realise that their brain is beginning to fail. The 'power of attorney' may be given to their children, but it could also be given to a trusted friend or lawyer. An individual can arrange for someone to have 'lasting power of attorney' in the event of his or her losing capacity.

 CLINICAL PEARLS

❖ Over the centuries, with the changing medical practice and increased emphasis placed on patient autonomy, managed care and rapidly developing technologies, the long-practiced ethical concepts from the Hippocratic Oath and AMA Code of Medical Ethics have been largely altered. These new forces have caused surgeons to seek greater responsibility in discussing and deciding various bioethical issues.

❖ Taking informed consent from the patients prior to an obstetric or gynaecological procedure ensures that the patient's autonomy is respected.

❖ Clinicians are responsible for maintaining their medical and surgical competence.

❖ The patient's confidentiality must be protected at each stage. It can be overridden only under exceptional circumstances.

❖ Attempts by the law to enforce clinical decisions upon a pregnant woman are a departure from the basic legal principles and must be best resisted.

❖ Simulation-based training of maternity staff in obstetric emergencies appears to be the most effective strategy to help reduce the rate of complications in obstetrics and gynaecology practice.

EVIDENCE-BASED MEDICINE

Training in obstetrics: Several studies evaluating the effectiveness of skills training for dealing with obstetric emergencies have presented with conflicting results.[42,43] Though various training methods in obstetrics and gynaecology have been developed, described and evaluated, further well-designed RCTs for evaluation of training in obstetrics are urgently required.

A systematic review of obstetric emergency training in the UK (2003) evaluated six obstetric emergency courses.[44] There was little evidence demonstrating the direct benefit of obstetric emergency training. The Simulation and Fire-drill Evaluation (SaFE) study, a large RCT commissioned by the Department of Health comprised 140 individuals (95 midwives and 45 doctors) who were randomly recruited from six hospitals across the southwest of England. The study evaluated the methods of multiprofessional obstetric emergency training. The results of the study showed that practical, multiprofessional, obstetric emergency training is likely to increase the knowledge of midwives and doctors regarding the management of obstetric emergencies.[45] However, neither of the factors such as the location of training (in a simulation centre or in local hospitals), nor the use of teamwork training is likely to cause any significant difference in the level of knowledge regarding the management of obstetric training acquired by the healthcare professionals.

REFERENCES

1. Marketos SG, Diamandopoulos AA, Bartsocas CS, Poulakou-Rebelakou E, Koutras DA. The Hippocratic Oath. Lancet. 1996;347(8994):101-2.
2. Robin ED, McCauley RF. Cultural lag and the Hippocratic Oath. Lancet. 1995;345(8962):1422-4.
3. Blume E. Hippocratic oath versus managed care: physicians caught in ethical squeeze. J Natl Cancer Inst. 1997;89(8):543-5.
4. Thomas Percival (1740-1804) codifier of medical ethics. JAMA. 1965;194(12):1319-20.
5. Baker R, Caplan A, Emanuel LL, Latham SR. Crisis, ethics, and the American Medical Association 1847 and 1997. JAMA.1997;278(2):163-4.
6. Hanlon CR. Ethics in surgery. J Am Coll Surg. 1998;186(1):41-9.
7. Fearnside MR. A code of ethics for the college. Aust N Z J Surg. 1994;64(4):226.
8. Kassirer JP. Managing care—should we adopt a new ethic? N Engl J Med. 1998;339(6):397-8.
9. Shuster E. The Nuremberg Code: Hippocratic ethics and human rights. Lancet. 1998;351(9107):974-7.
10. Pellegrino ED. The metamorphosis of medical ethics: A 30-year retrospective. JAMA. 1993;269(9):1158-62.
11. Pellegrino ED. Ethics. JAMA. 1996;275(23):1807-9.
12. Royal Australasian College of Surgeons. Code of Ethics: September 1993. Arch Surg. 1996;131(8):900-1.
13. Health and human rights: a call to action on the 50th anniversary of the Universal Declaration of Human Rights. The Writing Group for the Consortium for Health and Human Rights. JAMA. 1998;280(5):462-4, 469-70.
14. Beecher HK. Ethics and clinical research. N Engl J Med. 1966;274(24):1354-60.
15. Royal College of Obstetricians and Gynaecologists. Obtaining valid consent. Clinical Governance Advice No. 6. London: RCOG; 2015.
16. General Medical Council. Good Medical Practice. Manchester: RCOG; 2013.
17. Scally G, Donaldson LJ. Clinical governance and the drive for quality improvement in the new NHS in England. BMJ. 1998;317(7150):61-5.
18. Guyatt GH. Evidence-based medicine. ACP J Club. 1991;114: A–16.
19. Smith R, Rennie D. Evidence based medicine––an oral history. BMJ. 2014;348:g371.
20. Anonymous. US National Library of Medicine, National Institutes of Health. [online] Available from www.ncbi.nlm.nih.gov/pubmed [Accessed October, 2016].
21. Evans I, Thornton H, Chalmers I, Glasziou P. Testing Treatments: Better Research for Better Healthcare, 2nd edition. London: Printer and Martin; 2011.
22. Liberati A, Altman DG, Tetzlaff J, Mulrow C, Gøtzsche PC, Ioannidis JP, et al. The PRISMA statement for reporting systematic reviews and meta-analyses of studies that evaluate healthcare interventions: explanation and elaboration. BMJ. 2009;339:b2700.
23. Schulz KF, Altman DG, Moher D. CONSORT 2010 statement: updated guidelines for reporting parallel group randomised trials. BMJ. 2010;340:c332.
24. Bossuyt PM, Reitsma JB, Bruns DE, Gatsonis CA, Glasziou PP, Irwig LM, et al. The STARD initiative: standards for reporting of diagnostic accuracy. Toward complete and accurate reporting of studies of diagnostic accuracy. Clin Chem. 2003;49(1):1-6.
25. von Elm E, Altman DG, Egger M, Pocock SJ, Gøtzsche PC, Vandenbroucke JP. STROBE initiative. The strengthening the reporting of observational studies in epidemiology (STROBE) statement: guidelines for reporting observational studies. BMJ. 2007;335(7624):806-8.
26. NHS litigation Authority. Ten years of maternity claims: An analysis of NHS litigation authority data. London: NHSLA; 2012.
27. Royal College of Obstetricians and Gynaecologists. Improving patient safety: risk management for maternity and gynaecology. Clinical Governance Advice No. 2. London: RCOG; 2009.
28. National Patient Safety Agency. (2010). Root cause analysis: fishbone template. [online] Available from http://www.nrls.npsa.nhs.uk/resources/?entryid45=75605 [Accessed November, 2016].
29. Office of the Public Guardian. Mental Capacity Act Code of Practice. London: TSO; 2016.
30. Maternal and Child Health Research Consortium. CESDI 5th Annual Report—Focus Group Shoulder Dystocia 1996. London: MCHRC.
31. Maternal and Child Health Research Consortium. CESDI 6th Annual Report—The '4kg and over' Enquiries 1997. London: MCHRC.

PART I

32. Beasley JW, Damos JR, Roberts RG, Nesbitt TS. The advanced life support in obstetrics course: a national programme to enhance obstetric emergency skills and to support maternity care practice. Arch Fam Med. 1994;3(12):1037-41.

33. Johanson RB, Menon V, Burns E, Kargramanya E, Osipov V, Israelyan M, et al. Managing obstetric emergencies and trauma (MOET): structured skills training using models and reality-based scenarios. BMC Medical Education. 2002;2:5.

34. Sibanda T, Crofts JF, Barnfield S, Siassakos D, Epee MJ, Winter C, et al. PROMPT education and development: saving mothers' and babies lives in resource-poor settings. BJOG. 2009;116(6):868-9.

35. Johannsson H, Ayida G, Sadler C. Faking it? Simulation in the training of obstetricians and gynaecologists. Curr Opin Obstet Gynecol. 2005;17557-61.

36. Royal College of Obstetricians and Gynaecologists, Royal College of Midwives. The Clinical Learning Environment and Recruitment. Report of a Joint Working Party. London: RCOG Press; 2008.

37. Siassakos D, Crofts JF, Winter C, Weiner CP, Draycott TJ. The active components of effective training in obstetric emergencies. BJOG. 2009;116(8):1028-32.

38. Royal College of Obstetricians and Gynaecologists, Royal College of Anaesthetists, Royal College of Midwives, Royal College of Paediatrics and Child Health. Safer Childbirth: Minimum Standards for the Organisation and Delivery of Care in Labour. London: RCOG Press; 2007.

39. Kirkpatrick D. Technique for evaluating training program. J AM Soc Training Dev. 1959;13:11-2.

40. Centre for Maternal and Child Enquiries (CMACE). Executive summary, eighth report of the confidential enquiries into maternal deaths in the UK. BJOG. 2011;118 (Suppl 1):e12-21.

41. Harrison MR. Unborn: historical perspective of the foetus as patient. Pharos Alpha Omega Alpha Honor Med Soc. 1982;45(1):19-24.

42. Markova V, Sørensen JL, Holm C, Nørgaard A, Langhoff-Roos J. Evaluation of multiprofessional obstetric skills training for postpartum hemorrhage. Acta Obstet Gynecol Scand. 2012;91(3):346-52.

43. Nielsen PE, Goldman MB, Mann S, Shapiro DE, Marcus RG, Pratt SD, et al. Effects of team work training on adverse outcomes and process of care in labour and delivery. Obstet Gynecol. 2007;109(1):48-55.

44. Black RS, Brocklehurst P. A systematic review of training in acute obstetric emergencies. BJOG. 2003;110:837-41.

45. Siassakos D, Crofts J, Winter C, Draycott T. Multiprofessional 'fire-drill' training in the labour ward. Obstet Gynaecol. 2009;11:55-60.

General Principles of Surgery

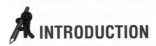 INTRODUCTION

For the success of any surgical process, besides the surgical procedure per se, the preoperative preparation of the patient, administration of anaesthesia, techniques of surgery and postoperative care of the patient play an equally important role in contributing towards the overall success of surgery. All these parameters shall be discussed in details in this chapter. Surgeons also need to understand the principles related to the working of equipment they use during surgery to minimise the occurrence of complications. This especially applies to the use of diathermy at the time of surgery. Therefore, surgical equipment such as diathermy, hysteroscopy and laparoscopy are also discussed briefly in this chapter.

PREOPERATIVE PRINCIPLES IN SURGERY

The main aim of preoperative assessment before anaesthesia and surgery is to help improve the final outcome. This is achieved by identifying potential anaesthetic difficulties; identifying existing medical conditions; improving safety by assessing and quantifying risk; planning of perioperative care; providing the opportunity for explanation and discussion and by allaying the patient's fear and anxiety. Proper preoperative preparation helps in ensuring the optimal outcome of the operative gynaecological procedures. Good preoperative preparation comprises adequate patient assessment through appropriate clinical history and examination, and preanaesthetic evaluation. The clinical examination must include a complete gynaecological examination as well as complete evaluation of the pulmonary, cardiovascular, gastrointestinal, urinary, musculoskeletal and neurological systems. Sometimes, the symptoms of gastrointestinal disease can resemble the symptoms related to the diseases of the reproductive tract. In these cases, a proper gastrointestinal tract history and investigations usually help in arriving at the correct diagnosis. At the time of preoperative counselling, the surgeon must ensure that the patients have access to easily understood information. Such information may be conferred to the patient in the form of information booklets or sheets in an appropriate language. Adequate preoperative patient preparation comprises of the following components:

Confidentiality and Informed Consent

The principles of confidentiality and informed consent have already been discussed in Chapter 1 (Principles of Clinical Practice). Guidelines for obtaining consent are available on the GMC website.[1] The patient must be counselled regarding the various available treatment options, with the help of written information (booklets, leaflets, etc.) or visual aids. Prior to taking consent, the patient must be informed about the advantages, disadvantages, success and failure rates, and the complications and risks associated with various procedures. The adequacy of consent must be assessed by the concept of material risk.[2] The doctor is obliged to discuss all material risks with the patient implying that the clinician needs to address even the rare complications, which are serious or may have a significant impact over the patient's quality of life. The patients should be given appropriate time before taking an appropriate decision. While dealing with the foreign patients, interpretators can be used. According to the GMC's guidelines, the responsibility of taking informed consent from the patient lies in the hands of the person performing the procedure.

History

A concise, but accurate history must be taken from the patient. Besides the history of presenting complaints, an accurate menstrual history must be taken from the patient. In case of discrepancy between the menstrual dates and findings of pelvic examination, pregnancy must be ruled out. Additionally, a proper obstetric history, sexual history and a complete urological history must also be taken. This must be followed by complete general physical, gynaecological and abdominal examination. The history must be taken in a non-judgemental, sensitive and thorough manner.[3] Detailed history and clinical vaginal examination forms an important aspect of a normal gynaecological check-up.

Importance must be given towards maintenance of patient-physician relationship. It is important for the gynaecologist to maintain good communication with the patient in order to elicit proper history and to accurately be able to recognise her problems. The manner of speaking, the words used, the tone of speaking and the body language are important aspects of the patient-physician interaction.[4] Kindness and courtesy must be maintained at all times. These aspects are especially important in case of male gynaecologists because the gynaecological history entails asking some private and confidential questions from the female patients. Also, the women may be reluctant while telling the history regarding her menstrual cycles to a male gynaecologist. It is important for a male gynaecologist to take the history and perform the vaginal examination in presence of a third party or a chaperone (a female nurse or the patient's female relative or friend).[5] The clinician must adopt both an empathetic and analytical attitude towards the patient. The patient's privacy must be respected at all costs. The gynaecologist must refrain from asking personal questions until appropriate patient confidence has been established.[6] The gynaecologist needs to listen more and talk less while taking the patient's history.

If any serious condition (e.g. malignancy) is suspected, the diagnosis must not be disclosed to the patient until it has been confirmed by performing investigations. Bad news must be preferably told to the patient when she is being accompanied by someone (relative, friend or spouse). The seriousness and urgency of the situation must be explained without causing undue alarm and fright to the patient. The clinician must never give false reassurance to the patient. Honest advice and opinion must always be provided.[7] It is important to elicit the following history at the time of examination:

❖ *Past medical history*: History of medical illnesses such as hypertension, hepatitis, diabetes mellitus, cancer, heart disease, pulmonary disease and thyroid disease needs to be taken. Patient's previous medical and surgical problems may have a bearing on her present complaints. For example, a history of longstanding diabetes could be responsible for development of genital candidiasis and associated pruritus. A patient with previous medical history of severe anaemia or cardiovascular heart disease may require special anaesthetic preparation (e.g. correction of anaemia, or treatment of cardiovascular pathology) before undergoing a major gynaecological surgery (e.g. hysterectomy). If the woman gives history of a recent myocardial infraction, the surgery should be delayed for at least 6 months after the episode of myocardial infarction (MI) due to high risk of reinfarction during the first 6 months.[8]

Triad of diabetes, hypertension and obesity is associated with an increased risk of endometrial carcinoma. A history of sexually transmitted disease (especially infection with Chlamydia) may have a direct bearing on future infertility. Previous history of PID or puerperal sepsis could be responsible for producing gynaecological complaints such as menstrual disturbances, lower abdominal pain, congestive dysmenorrhoea and infertility. Presence of endocrinological disorders (e.g. thyroid dysfunction) could be responsible for menstrual irregularities. Patients with diabetes, thyroid dysfunction and increased body mass index (BMI) are also at an increased risk during the administration of anaesthesia. Therefore, such conditions are discussed below in details.

- *History of diabetes*: History of diabetes can be associated with significant metabolic derangements in the patient. A proper management of diabetes in the preoperative period helps in preventing complications such as metabolic aberrations, impaired wound healing and increased risk of postoperative infections. Stress of surgery is likely to release counter-regulatory hormones such as glucagon, growth hormone, epinephrine, cortical hormones, etc. which are further likely to exacerbate hyperglycaemia. On the other hand, diabetic patients are particularly prone to hypoglycaemia because they may be fasting and may not receive certain medications in the perioperative period. Therefore, it becomes important for the surgeon to monitor the patient's blood glucose levels during the perioperative period in order to strike a balance between prevention of both hyperglycaemia and hypoglycaemia in the postoperative period. In the perioperative period, various medical agents such as insulin with or without oral hypoglycaemic agents may be used in order to achieve control of blood glucose levels. The aim of this treatment is to maintain blood glucose levels in the range of 120–200 mg/dL.

- *Obesity*: Patients with an increased BMI are prone to develop complications such as hypertension, diabetes, atherosclerotic disease, obstructive sleep apnoea syndrome, etc. In these cases, apart from a routine preoperative chest X-ray and electrocardiography (ECG), pulmonary function tests and a baseline arterial blood gas analysis may also be essential. Use of narcotics and sedatives must be avoided in these cases and regional anaesthesia be used wherever possible.

- *Thyroid dysfunction*: Since disorders of thyroid function, particularly hyperthyroidism, are likely to affect the cardiovascular system (CVS), the thyroid levels must be controlled by the use of medicines in the preoperative period.

- *Haematopoietic dysfunction*: In the presence of complications such as easy bruising and episodes of prolonged or excessive bleeding (epistaxis, menorrhagia, bleeding from the gums, etc.), the coagulation profile must be determined. This must comprise the following tests: bleeding time, clotting time, prothrombin time, activated partial prothrombin time and a platelet count.

❖ *Past treatment history*: The patient should also be asked about the various medicines she has been consuming. The details of various medicines including their dosage, route of administration, frequency and duration of use need to be asked. The patient must be specifically asked about the various medicines she has been taking, including prescription drugs, over-the-counter drugs, herbal drugs and any therapy related to alternative medicine. History of allergy to any medication also needs to be asked. If the woman has been using combined oral contraceptive pills, she must be advised to stop using them at least 1 month prior to the major surgery.

❖ *History of surgery*: History of undergoing previous abdominal surgery like caesarean section, removal of appendix, excision of ovarian cyst, myomectomy, etc. may result in the development of pelvic adhesions. These may not only make any subsequent surgery difficult, but also may be the cause of common gynaecological problems like pelvic and abdominal pain, infertility, menstrual disturbances and dyspareunia.

❖ *Family history*: Certain gynaecological cancers (e.g. cancer of ovary, uterus and breast) have a genetic predisposition. A woman may be at a high risk of development of such cancers in the future if there is a positive family history of such cancers in her first-degree relatives (especially mother and sister).

❖ *Marital and sexual history*: Details of the woman's marital life including her age at the time of marriage, how long she has been married and sexual history need to be asked. Details of the woman's sexual history are particularly important. Some such details include her age at the time of first sexual intercourse; her current sexual activities (vaginal, oral, anal and manual); frequency of her sexual intercourses; is she currently seeking a pregnancy; is she presently using any method of contraception, if yes, the type of contraception used; is she or her partner experiencing any sexual dysfunction (frigidity in the woman or impotence or premature ejaculation in the male or problems with libido, arousal, lubrication or orgasm in both males and females); current frequency of her sexual activities; past sexual activities; number of sexual partners (currently and in the past); sexual preferences (heterosexual, homosexual or both); pain at the time of sexual intercourse (dyspareunia), etc.

❖ *Obstetric history*: Details of every pregnancy conceived irrespective of its ultimate outcome, need to be recorded. Number of previous live births, stillbirths, deaths, miscarriages (both spontaneous and induced), history of recurrent miscarriages if any, medical termination of pregnancies and number of children living at present need to be noted.

Clinical Examination

General Physical Examination

General physical examination involves the observation of the patient's general appearance, orientation in time, place and person, nutritional status and patient's demeanour (calm, anxious or aggressive). The following features need to be observed at the time of general physical examination.[9,10]

Vital signs: Patient's vital signs such as temperature, blood pressure, pulse, respiratory rate, height and weight need to be measured.

Height and weight: Height of the patient (in meters) and her weight (in kilograms) can be used for calculation of BMI.

Table 2.1: Classification of weight according to body mass index

Weight for height status	Body mass index (kg/m²)
Very low	<16.5
Low	16.5–19.8
Normal	19.8–25.9
High	26.0–29.9
Very high	>30.0

The classification of the woman as underweight, normal weight and obese has been described in Table 2.1. Calculation of BMI is especially important in women who appear underweight or overweight. Underweight women may commonly suffer from amenorrhoea and other menstrual irregularities, whereas overweight women are at an increased risk for endometrial cancer.

Anaemia and dehydration: Excessive blood loss may result in the development of anaemia. Excessive loss of body fluids may result in the development of dehydration, which causes dryness of mucous membranes and loss of skin turgor.

Signs suggestive of hyperandrogenaemia: Signs suggestive of hyperandrogenaemia such as hirsutism (presence of facial hair), deepening of voice, etc. may be related to the presence of androgen-secreting tumours or chronic anovulatory states (polycystic ovarian disease).

Blood pressure: Blood pressure that is persistently greater than or equal to 140 mmHg (systolic), or greater than or equal to 90 mmHg (diastolic) is considered as elevated.

Neck examination: Local examination of the neck may reveal enlargement of thyroid gland or lymph nodes of the neck. Neck examination should also involve palpation of cervical and supraclavicular lymph nodes.

Lymphadenopathy: Lymphadenopathy could be a sign of advanced metastatic disease associated with malignancy. The neck, axilla and groins must also be palpated for the presence of enlarged lymph nodes.

Thyroid examination: It is important to examine the thyroid gland because menstrual abnormalities may be commonly associated with thyroid dysfunction. While hypothyroidism is commonly associated with oligomenorrhoea, hyperthyroidism may be responsible for menorrhagia.

Breast examination: Examination of the breast should be carried out in three positions: (1) with patient's hands on her hips (to accentuate the pectoral muscles); (2) with her arms raised and then (3) in supine position. Both the breasts must be inspected for symmetry, skin or nipple retraction, presence of any obvious growth or mass and skin changes such as dimpling, retraction, crusting or Peau d'orange appearance. Both the breasts must be then palpated bilaterally for the presence of lumps, masses and tenderness. The nipples are assessed for the presence of discharge.

Axillary and supraclavicular regions are palpated for the presence of any lymphadenopathy. The points which need to be particularly observed on examination of breast are described next.

❖ Breast examination may reveal changes indicative of early pregnancy. This is especially important in cases where pregnancy is not suspected, e.g. in young unmarried girls.

❖ *Staging of breast development*: This could be important in women who have yet not attained sexual maturity.

❖ In all women and especially those above the age of 30 years, breast must be routinely palpated to exclude tumour formation.

❖ Bilateral milk discharge from the nipples may indicate galactorrhoea due to hyperprolactinaemia. Ruling out the presence of galactorrhoea is especially important in cases that are infertile and suffer from oligomenorrhoea or amenorrhoea.

❖ Unilateral bloody nipple discharge could be associated with an intraductal papilloma.

Systemic Examination

Cardiovascular system examination: Routine examination of CVS involves palpation of cardiac impulse and auscultation of the heart at the apex for presence of any sounds, murmurs, clicks, etc. Detailed examination of the CVS is required in cases of history of cardiovascular disease or complaints suggestive of a possible cardiovascular pathology. Cardiovascular examination may be important in some patients, where they may be at a risk of myocardial hypoxia at the time of gynaecological surgery, especially in cases of previous history of cardiovascular diseases. The occurrence of cardiac risk increases in the presence of previous history of MI. In order to evaluate the patient's risk of developing cardiac complications during surgery, Goldman's cardiac risk index has been devised (Table 2.2).[11] This is a point system, which classifies the patient's risk for perioperative cardiac morbidity and mortality in terms of points. If the total score is less than or equal to 5, the risk of cardiac complications is only 1%. If the total adds up to 12, the risk increases to 5%; with the counts up to 25, the risk increases to 11%.

Hypertension: The patients with mild-to-moderate hypertension (systolic BP = 140–150 mmHg and diastolic BP = 90–110 mmHg) can proceed to surgery without undergoing any treatment. However, in patients with severe hypertension (systolic BP > 150 mmHg and diastolic BP > 110 mmHg), the blood pressure should be first controlled over a period of 6 months before proceeding for the surgery. The antihypertensive medication must be continued until the morning of surgery and started as soon as possible in the postoperative period.

Pulmonary system: Examination of the pulmonary system may be required to detect the presence of wheezes, rales, rhonchi and bronchial breath sounds. Presence of a pulmonary pathology such as chronic obstructive pulmonary disease (COPD) in a patient predisposes her to develop pulmonary complications in the postoperative period.[12] Pulmonary function tests must be performed in the preoperative period to help decide the ventilatory settings in the postoperative period. Use of sedatives and general anaesthesia (GA) may result in the development of hypoxia in these patients. Therefore, it is preferable to perform surgery under local or epidural anaesthesia in these patients. Application of strategies such as cessation of smoking, use of chest physiotherapy or bronchodilators may help in improving pulmonary function in these patients. This can be attributed to the fact that postoperative complications are more common in patients with history of chronic smoking and COPD.[13] Two most important pulmonary complications such as atelectasis and bronchitis can be prevented by instructing the patient to make use of deep breathing exercises postoperatively.

Pelvic examination: Pelvic examination forms an important aspect of the gynaecological check-up of a woman. If the patient is virginal, the opening of the hymen may be wide enough to allow only one finger or narrow speculum examination. As far as possible, a per vaginal examination must be avoided in virginal women.[14] The prerequisites before performing a pelvic examination are described below:

❖ The patient must be asked to empty her bladder before lying down on the table for the examination. In case of complaints of urinary incontinence, examination must be performed with a full bladder in the lithotomy and erect positions to demonstrate stress incontinence.

❖ Gloves and instruments, if not disposable, should be sterilised by autoclaving before reuse.

❖ Since this is an intimate examination, it requires patient's full cooperation. The patient must be described the procedure of pelvic examination and her informed consent be taken before proceeding with the examination.

❖ Both male and female examiners should be chaperoned by a female assistant.

Laboratory Investigations

Medical and anaesthetic problems are identified more efficiently by taking a detailed history and by the physical examination of patients. No special investigations are required prior to minor surgery in an otherwise healthy patient.[15] Routine investigations, which need to be performed even in otherwise healthy patients are described next. An ECG should be performed on every patient with a cardiac disease or related history but is not indicated for asymptomatic males under the age of 40 years or asymptomatic females under the

Table 2.2: Goldman's index of cardiac risk

Cardiovascular risk factor	No. of points
Jugular venous distension (evidence of congestive cardiac failure)	11 points
Recent myocardial infarction in 6 months	10 points
Premature ventricular contractions (5 or more per minute)	7 points
Rhythm other than sinus	7 points
Age above 70 years	5 points
Emergency surgery, aortic valvular stenosis	4 points
Poor medical condition or surgery within the chest or abdomen	3 points

age of 50 years. All patients undergoing elective surgery must be screened for methicillin-resistant *Staphylococcus aureus* (MRSA).

Routine Investigations

The investigations, which are routinely performed include haemoglobin level, haematocrit, total leukocyte count (TLC), differential leukocyte count (DLC) and complete urine analysis. In the presence of underlying or suspected renal or hepatic diseases, kidney function test (KFT) or liver function test (LFT) must be ordered respectively. Baseline electrolyte levels must be done for all patients who would be undergoing extensive pelvic surgery in order to decide postoperative fluid and electrolyte replacement therapy.[16] In case of women undergoing any pelvic procedure, screening for STI and bacterial vaginosis should be performed prior to the surgery.

Other Investigations

Depending on the particular pathology, other preoperative investigations can be ordered. For example, in case of patients with a gynaecological malignancy, a CT scan or MRI may be ordered to evaluate the spread of malignancy. If the renal system or the gastrointestinal system appears to be involved, investigations such as intravenous pyelography or barium enema respectively may help to evaluate the spread of malignancy.

Preoperative Management Prior to Surgery[17]

One Day Prior to Surgery

Fasting: For safety reasons, patients should not eat or drink immediately prior to anaesthesia. The Association of Anaesthetists of Great Britain and Ireland (AAGBI) recommends the minimum fasting periods based on the American Society of Anesthesiologists (ASA) guidelines:

❖ Six hours for solid food, infant formula, or other milk
❖ Four hours for breast milk
❖ *Two hours for clear non-particulate and non-carbonated fluids*: For all practical purposes, the patient may be allowed to have a light and easily digestible diet, the night before the morning of surgery. After midnight, the patient must be nil per orally (NPO) and must not eat or drink anything. It is important that the elderly women, who have undergone bowel preparation, children and breastfeeding mothers, should not be left for long periods without hydration. They may require intravenous fluids prior to surgery.

Sedation: Mild sedative drugs may be administered on the night before the surgery to help allay the patient's anxiety.

Bowel preparation: In women undergoing abdominal surgery in which entry into the bowel is anticipated, complete bowel preparation must be performed by use of laxatives or preoperative enema, either the evening before or on the morning of surgery. Before undertaking an elective major surgery, which is likely to involve the bowel, mechanical cleansing of the large intestines is required. In these cases, cleansing enemas may be given in the early morning to ensure emptying of bowel before the morning of surgery.

Advice related to smoking: The patient should be advised to stop smoking at least 24 hours prior to the surgery in order to reduce the levels of carboxyhaemoglobin in their bodies and to minimise the cardiovascular effects of nicotine in the body.[18]

Screening for MRSA: All patients undergoing elective surgery must be screened for MRSA.

Preoperative antibiotics: Preoperative prophylactic broad-spectrum antibiotics are frequently used prior to undertaking gynaecological surgery for preventing infection. A single dose of antibiotics immediately prior to the surgery is sufficient for most of the cases. A repeat dose may be required if the surgery is likely to last for longer than 8 hours.[19] The most optimal method of antibiotic administration appears to be IV administration of antibiotics. The antibiotics most commonly used include the new generation cephalosporins (ceftazidime or cefotaxime 2 grams IM/IV), semisynthetic penicillin or β-lactamase antibiotics, which are usually prescribed 2 hours prior to the surgery.[20] Besides the use of antibiotics, principles such as maintenance of adequate haemostasis and gentle handling of the tissues must be followed. Previously, the patients were administered parenteral antibiotics 48–72 hours preoperatively, followed by oral antibiotics for at least 5 days postoperatively. Nowadays, more emphasis is given towards maintenance of asepsis rather than antisepsis. Prophylactic antibiotics are now administered in 1–4 doses at 12-hourly intervals, starting 20 minutes prior to surgery.[21]

Thromboprophylaxis: Adequate prophylactic action must be taken for the prevention of thromboembolism because gynaecological surgery may be associated with a high incidence of deep vein thrombosis and pulmonary embolism (PE). Venous thromboembolism (VTE) can be considered as one of the most serious complications of surgery. All units in various hospitals in the UK must have clear protocols for thromboprophylaxis. According to the recommendations by NICE (2008), all patients at the time of admission must be assessed to identify those who are at an increased risk of VTE.[22]

Medical patients are considered to be at an increased risk of VTE if they have had or are expected to have significantly reduced mobility for 3 days or more or are expected to have ongoing reduced mobility relative to their normal state and have one or more of the risk factors shown in Box 2.1.[22] Surgical patients and patients with trauma are at an increased risk of VTE if they have undergone a surgical procedure with a total anaesthetic and surgical time of more than 90 minutes, or 60 minutes if the surgery involves the pelvis or lower limb or have one or more of the risk factors shown in Box 2.1. Measures for reducing the risk of VTE include the following:

❖ Adequate hydration must be maintained.
❖ The patient must be encouraged to mobilise as soon as possible.
❖ Temporary inferior vena caval filters may be offered to the patients who are at very high risk of VTE and for whom mechanical and pharmacological VTE prophylaxes are contraindicated.

Box 2.1: Risk factors for venous thrombosis

Age
- ❑ <40 years (major surgery)
- ❑ 60 years (non-major surgery)

Obesity
- ❑ *Moderate obesity*: 75–90 kg or >20% above the ideal weight
- ❑ *Morbid obesity*: 115 kg or >30% above the ideal weight with reduced fibrinolysins and immobility

Immobility
- ❑ *Preoperative immobility*: Prolonged hospitalisation, dehydration, venous stasis
- ❑ *Intraoperative immobility*: Prolonged operative time, loss of pump action of the calf muscles, compression of vena cava
- ❑ *Postoperative immobility*: Prolonged periods of confinement to the bed, venous stasis, admission to the critical care unit

Trauma
- ❑ Damage to the walls of the pelvic veins
- ❑ *Radical pelvic surgery/malignancy*: Release of tissue thromboplastins

Activation of factor X
- ❑ Prior radiation therapy, diabetes mellitus
- ❑ *Reduced fibrinolysin*: Radiation, medical disease, cardiac disease, heart failure, severe varicose veins, previous venous thrombosis

Comorbid conditions
- ❑ Known thrombophilias
- ❑ One or more significant medical comorbidities (for example: heart disease; metabolic, endocrine or respiratory pathologies; acute infectious diseases; inflammatory conditions)
- ❑ Varicose veins with phlebitis

Family history
- ❑ Personal history or first-degree relative with a history of VTE

Treatment history
- ❑ Use of hormone replacement therapy
- ❑ Use of oestrogen-containing contraceptive therapy

❖ Mechanical prophylaxis for VTE comprises one of the following: antiembolism stockings (thigh or knee length); foot impulse devices, or intermittent pneumatic compression devices (thigh or knee length). Mechanical VTE prophylaxis must be continued until the patient no longer has significantly reduced mobility.

❖ Pharmacological VTE prophylaxis can be considered for patients who are at a low risk of major bleeding, taking into account the patient's clinical condition. Patients at risk of bleeding must be offered pharmacological VTE prophylaxis in situations where the risk of VTE outweighs the risk of bleeding. Clinicians can use either low-molecular-weight heparin (LMWH) or unfractionated heparin (UFH) for VTE prophylaxis. Pharmacological VTE prophylaxis must be continued until the patient no longer has significantly reduced mobility (generally 5–7 days). This can be extended to 28 days postoperatively for patients who have had major cancer surgery in the abdomen or pelvis.

Preoperative showering or washing: Patient should be advised to have a shower or a bath using standard soap either the day before or on the day of surgery.

ROLE OF THE ANAESTHETIST

Ruling out the presence of pre-existing medical disease: This is important because the morbidity and mortality related to surgery and anaesthesia is increased in women with coexisting diseases, such as ischaemic heart disease, hypertension, chronic respiratory diseases, cardiac arrhythmias, etc. In case there is a presence of concurrent illness, the surgeon must liaise with the anaesthetist and other specialists, in order to evaluate the complexity of the patient's situation.

Before selecting a particular anaesthetic technique or before performing surgery, the patients must be classified based on their physical state or the degree of sickness based on the classification system devised by the ASA (Table 2.3).[23]

During the preanaesthetic check-up performed prior to the surgery, the anaesthetist gets the opportunity to discuss with the patient, the choice of anaesthetic method in the light of the patient's preferences, his or her clinical state, the surgery itself and the anaesthetist's own preferences and special skills. This discussion also helps in highlighting various risks and benefits of different types of anaesthesia that can be used. The advantages and complications of each type of anaesthetic procedure must be explained to the patient. This is also the time during which the patient can clear all her doubts and even raise questions about any aspect of anaesthetic care. During this time, the anaesthetist must also gain the patient's consent for the anaesthetic procedure. The anaesthetists can make use of questionnaires for obtaining basic background information from the patients. These questionnaires may be given to the patient at the surgical outpatient clinic to be completed immediately or taken home for completion and returned by post. During the preanaesthetic check-up, the patient should preferably get an opportunity to talk to the anaesthetist, who would be administering the anaesthesia. The patient should also have an opportunity to meet other healthcare professionals who may be involved in her care.

The preanaesthetic check-up is the perfect time for building the patient's trust and confidence. This trust is likely to play an important role in making the patient feel safe, reassured and relaxed when she sees the doctor again in the operation

Table 2.3: American Society of Anesthesiologists (ASA) Physical Status Classification System[23]

ASA PS classification	Definition
ASA PS 1	Normal healthy patient
ASA PS 2	Patients with mild controlled systemic disease, which does not affect normal activity
ASA PS 3	Patients with severe systemic disease, which limits activity
ASA PS 4	Patients with severe systemic disease that is a constant threat to life
ASA PS 5	Moribund patients who are not expected to survive with or without the operation
ASA PS 6	A declared brain-dead patient whose organs are being removed for donor purposes

theatre. The discussion between the anaesthetist and the patient must involve the following details: how the patient will get to theatre (if inpatient) or when and where she should report on reaching the hospital (if outpatient); what are the things she is likely to experience in the anaesthetic room; what time the operation is scheduled; what will be experienced in the recovery room and how the postoperative and postdischarge pain be managed. The patient should be explained about the epidural or patient-controlled analgesia (PCA), intravenous lines, oxygen mask, urinary catheters, etc. if these things are likely to be used.

Types of Anaesthesia

There are a number of options available to women for pain relief during obstetric or gynaecologic surgery.[24] Various methods used for obtaining pain relief during labour are enumerated in Table 2.4. Pain medications given intravenously or intramuscularly help to decrease the amount of pain during childbirth or other obstetric procedures. The types of anaesthesia used most commonly for the obstetric and gynaecological surgeries include GA and regional anaesthesia (spinal, epidural or combined spinal and epidural).[25] Various types of anaesthetic agents and analgesia techniques used during labour have been described in details in Chapter 44 (Anaesthesia and Analgesia in Labour) and are summarised in Table 2.4. Local anaesthesia blocks (pudendal nerve block and paracervical blocks) are also commonly used for minor surgeries. Types of nerve blocks used in various obstetric and gynaecological procedures are illustrated in Figure 2.1.

Regional anaesthesia has currently become the most effective means of providing analgesia during labour.[26] In some instances, use of GA may be indicated.

General Anaesthesia

General anaesthesia can be more rapidly administered in the case of an emergency (e.g. severe foetal distress, cord prolapse, etc.). If the mother has a coagulation disorder or hypotension, GA would be the better alternative to use

Table 2.4: Methods for labour analgesia

Non-pharmacological therapy	Pharmacological therapy	
	Systemic	**Regional**

• Transcutaneous electrical nerve stimulation (TENS)
• Relaxation/ breathing techniques
• Biofeedback and physical therapies
• Hypnosis
• Massage
• Acupuncture
• Hydrotherapy (use of hot or cold packs)
• Use of birthing ball (Swiss ball/Bobath ball)
• Music therapy
	Inhalational anaesthetic agents
	• Nitrous oxide
	• Enflurane
	• Isoflurane
	• Desflurane
	• Sevoflurane
	Systemic analgesics
	• Opioid analgesics
	  – Pethidine
	  – Morphine
	  – Fentanyl
	  – Sufentanil
	  – Alfentanil
	  – Remifentanil
	• Tranquilizers/ sedatives
	  – Barbiturates
	  – Phenothiazines
	  – Benzodiazepines
	• Dissociative/ amnesic drugs
	  – Ketamine
	  – Scopolamine
		• Lumbar epidural
		• Combined spinal epidural analgesia (CSEA)
		• Continuous spinal analgesia (CSA)
		• Alternative regional technique
		  – Lumbar sympathetic block
		  – Pudendal block
		  – Paracervical block

rather than regional anaesthesia. GA with endotracheal intubation and controlled ventilation helps in providing adequate relaxation of muscles and analgesia, thereby resulting in optimal operative outcomes. The advantage of using GA is that the patient's airways are secured and adequate oxygenation is ensured. The disadvantages include cardiovascular depression, reduced protective reflexes, prolonged psychomotor impairment, and nausea, vomiting and grogginess in the patient.[27] Patients given GA have a higher risk of hypoxia and pulmonary aspiration (in the event of a difficult/failed intubation) especially during an emergency caesarean section, when the patient is likely to be full stomach.

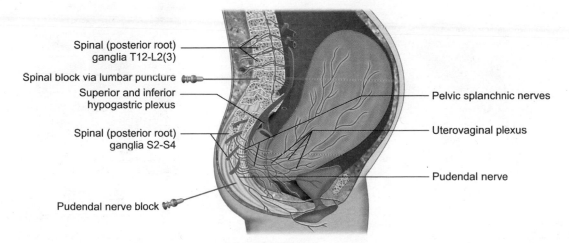

Fig. 2.1: Various types of nerve blocks

Due to the risk of aspiration when administered in 'full stomach', GA for caesarean section usually involves a crash induction. In these cases, an inducing agent along with a rapidly acting muscle relaxant is administered whilst the application of cricoid pressure. Following this, the endotracheal tube is inserted and its cuff inflated. Anaesthesia is continued with oxygen, nitrous oxide and a low concentration of volatile agent like isoflurane together with a longer-acting muscle relaxant. Narcotics are not administered until after the delivery of the baby because of their potential for causing foetal distress. Various medications given to the patient while administering GA include the following:

❖ *Preanaesthetic medications*: The drugs used for preanaesthetic medication commonly include an anxiolytic (to allay anxiety the night before surgery); antiemetic (to reduce nausea and vomiting); H2 blockers (to reduce the pH and volume of gastric secretions) and glycopyrrolate/atropine to reduce the amount of gastric secretions. Analgesic drugs such as non-steroidal anti-inflammatory drugs (NSAIDs) and opioids, etc. can also be used.

❖ *Inducing agent*: The most commonly used intravenous inducing agent for GA is thiopentone sodium. Lately, propofol has also gained popularity as an inducing agent. It is associated with reduced grogginess and has an inherent antiemetic property, which results in reduced amount of nausea and vomiting. Ketamine is another agent, which can be used, but must be avoided in those with hypertension and cardiovascular disease.[28]

❖ *Muscle relaxants*: Succinylcholine is used as a muscle relaxant during endotracheal intubation. The main drawbacks associated with its use include myalgia and muscle fasciculations, which can cause a rise in serum potassium levels. The main advantage with its use is a quick onset of intubating conditions. Non-depolarising group of muscle relaxants such as pancuronium, vecuronium and atracurium can also be used for intubating the patients. They are free from the drawbacks of succinylcholine and also help in providing relaxation during the entire course of surgery.

Local Anaesthesia

Some common minor obstetrical and gynaecological procedures can be performed under local anaesthesia.[29] Local anaesthesia can be administered either in the form of a pudendal or a paracervical block. The two main complications associated with the use of local anaesthetics are systemic toxicity and delayed haemorrhage (especially if combined with adrenaline). The patient must be observed for at least 2 hours prior to discharge.

❖ *Pudendal block*: The pudendal nerve, which is derived from the 2nd, 3rd and 4th sacral nerve is blocked with local anaesthetic administered using a special needle introduced via a needle guide (Fig. 2.2). Though the anaesthesia may prove excellent for minor surgical procedures, the failure rate of the procedure is high, approaching almost 50%.

❖ *Paracervical block*: Nowadays, paracervical block anaesthesia is being more often used in the practice of obstetrics and gynaecology. It has been accepted as a simple, safe and effective method for anaesthetic administration. This block helps in preventing transmission through the paracervical plexus bilaterally (Fig. 2.3).[30] Though this block helps in providing complete relief against the pain of the first stage of labour, additional anaesthesia is required at the time of delivery. This is an ideal method of anaesthetic administration for dilatation and curettage. Paracervical block can also be used in other minor procedures such as cervical repair, conisation and Shirodkar or Wurm operations. However, the main disadvantage associated with its use is the high incidence of foetal bradycardia along with the several reports of foetal deaths. With the gaining popularity of epidural and spinal anaesthesia, the use of paracervical blocks has greatly declined.

Conscious Sedation

The aim of conscious sedation is to produce a level of sedation at which the patient is calm and relaxed. She is not able to experience pain because she has also been administered

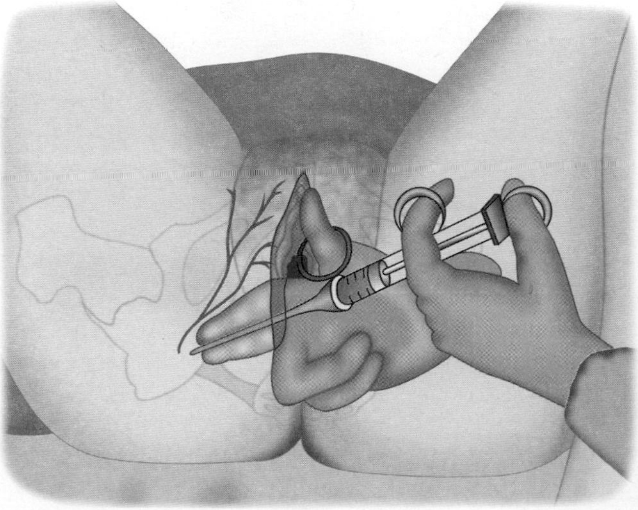

Fig. 2.2: Pudendal nerve block

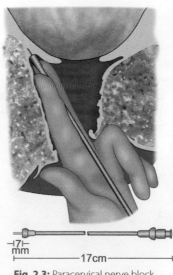

Fig. 2.3: Paracervical nerve block

an anaesthetic. The patient does not become unconscious, and verbal communication is possible. The patient must be monitored using a pulse oximeter while undergoing surgery under the effect of conscious sedation. The patient should be preferably observed for 2 hours prior to discharge.

Preparation Just Prior to Surgery

Before undertaking any gynaecological surgery, the surgeon must be well versed with the abdominal and pelvic anatomy. In case of distorted anatomy, all attempts must be made to restore the normal anatomy as far as possible. The preoperative preparation just prior to the surgery comprises the following steps:

1. The bladder is catheterised.
2. The patient is anaesthetised.
3. A careful bimanual examination is performed under anaesthesia so that the surgeon can obtain valuable information, which may otherwise not be possible.
4. The vulva, vagina and perineum must then be cleaned and scrubbed with a sterile sponge soaked in non-alcohol-based antiseptic solution. The abdominal area to be surgically prepared extends superiorly from the inferior limit of the rib cage and inferiorly up to the mid thighs (Figs 2.4A and B). The lateral margins of the skin preparation extend to the anterior iliac crest, inferiorly, and the anterior axillary line, superiorly. Umbilicus is prepared first using a sterile cotton-tipped applicator dipped in antiseptic solution. This should be discarded after use. A separate applicator should be used for applying antiseptic solution over rest of the abdomen.
5. The most commonly used antiseptic solutions include povidone iodine or chlorhexidine solution. The antiseptic solution (alcohol-based or aqueous) should be applied using a painting technique from the proposed site of incision to the periphery using light pressure. It should not be blotted or wiped out, but allowed to air-dry completely.

INTRAOPERATIVE CARE PRINCIPLES

Some of the important things, which must be kept in the mind at the time of surgery, include the following:
- Surgery must be done along the lines of tissue planes.
- Tissues must be handled gently.
- Adequate access to the operation field and good source of light are important prerequisites before undertaking any surgery. A senior surgeon may be called for a difficult

surgery in order to obtain adequate access at the time of surgery.
- Use of appropriate retractors and bowel packing helps in obtaining adequate access.
- Maintenance of asepsis is an important principle, which must be kept in mind at the time of surgery.

Principles of Asepsis

Asepsis may be defined as prevention of the exposure of the incision site with microorganisms, thereby preventing the risk of development of infection. Three important principles, which are required for achieving asepsis, are reduction of time, trauma and trash.[26]

Time: The time duration during which the surgical procedure is performed, is an important factor. The longer the procedure, greater would be the possibility of infection and contamination.

Trauma: Trauma to the tissues as a result of rough handling, drying and desiccation of tissues upon exposure to room temperature, creation of excessive dead space, use of implants or foreign bodies or non-optimal temperature is likely to contribute to infection.

Trash: Trash refers to the contamination of tissues by bacteria or foreign bodies.

Handwashing for 3–5 minutes prior to any surgical procedure is important for the maintenance of asepsis. Precautions to be taken at the time of surgery to minimise the tissue harm are as follows.[31]

Gentle handling of the tissues: Prolonged surgical time results in drying of the tissues and compromises blood flow through them. Tissues damaged by crushing, drying, excessive use of sutures or other surgical implants serve as a nidus of infection.

Surgeon must carry out meticulous dissection: Proper haemostasis must be obtained. If electrocautery is being used, it must be switched off immediately, when not in use. Use of toothed or crushing instruments must be avoided as far as possible.

Appropriate suturing techniques: The surgeon must make use of appropriate suturing techniques. Sutures must be placed as close to the tissue edge as possible. In order to prevent the obstruction of blood flow, the sutures must be placed no more than 1 cm from the edge. Sutures should be tightened enough to oppose the tissue edges. If the sutures are tighter, they are likely to further obstruct the blood supply, resulting in dehiscence. All the dead space between the tissues must be removed at the time of closure.

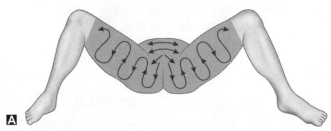 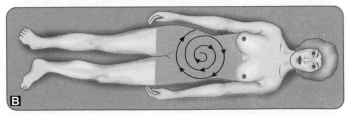

Figs 2.4A and B: Extent of abdominal and perineal site pre-operative preparation with antiseptic solution: (A) Perineum; (B) Abdomen

PART I

Among the various steps taken to maintain asepsis, use of preoperative shaving has not been observed to alter the rate of wound infection.

Use of a single dose of antibiotics preoperatively helps in preventing wound infection or septicaemia. Prolonged course of antibiotics or unnecessary use of antibiotics must be avoided to prevent the development of antibiotic resistance and an increased risk of infection with *Clostridium difficile.* According to the recommendations by NICE (2016), antimicrobial prophylaxis against infective endocarditis (IE) is not recommended in patients undergoing urological, gynaecological and obstetric procedures where infection is not already present.[32] If infection is present, patients at high risk of IE should receive antibiotics against the organisms responsible for causing IE. Patients at an increased risk of IE include the patients with acquired valvular heart disease, those who have undergone valve replacement in the past, those with structural congenital heart disease, patients with hypertrophic cardiomyopathy and those with a previous history of IE.

SURGICAL EQUIPMENT

Diathermy

Diathermy/electrosurgery implies the use of electricity to generate heat in the tissues. It is used at the time of surgery to vaporise the tissues for cutting purposes or for coagulating the tissues to achieve haemostasis or for destroying the tissues. Diathermy (or Bovie) is a device used to pass an electric current through tissues, which causes coagulation, cutting and tissue destruction by heating effect. It uses alternating current with a frequency of 500 KHz–10 MHz. This frequency is much higher than that of mains electricity, which in the UK is low-frequency AC current of approximately 50 Hz. Low-frequency currents cause depolarisation and neuromuscular stimulation. On the other hand, the high-frequency current is too fast to stimulate nerve fibres. Therefore, it does not cause depolarisation. This prevents spasm or paralysis of muscles. However, the high-frequency current does cause excitation of ions, resulting in heat production.

Cutting with the help of diathermy is achieved using constantly flowing current having low voltage, but high frequency. On the other hand, coagulation is achieved using intermittently flowing current having both high voltage and frequency. Cutting current is associated with a lower risk of inadvertent current discharge as a result of lower voltage. Cutting current is therefore safer than the coagulation current.

Two types of diathermy are commonly used in gynae-cological surgery: unipolar and bipolar (Figs 2.5A and B). The current density is higher in bipolar (e.g. bipolar diathermy forceps) in comparison to unipolar or monopolar diathermy.

Bipolar diathermy: Bipolar diathermy is a very safe form of diathermy. It is usually employed at the time of using forceps. The current only flows between the tips of the forceps, from the active electrode to the neutral electrode. So, there is less

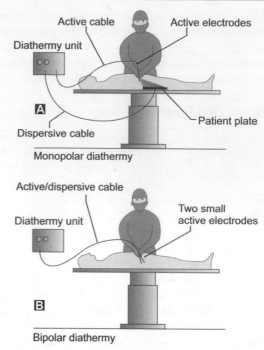

Figs 2.5A and B: Diathermy: (A) Monopolar diathermy; (B) Bipolar diathermy

risk of stray currents damaging tissues other than those, which are being aimed at. Diathermy employs use of continuous current at low voltage: 500–1,000 volts. The water in the cells is turned to steam, so the cells vaporise giving a cutting effect. The best effect will occur when the current flows through the smallest tissue volume. This can be produced by using a clean needlepoint. The low voltage (500–1,000 volts) current flows continuously. Since the effect is relatively superficial and the tissues are vaporised, not coagulated, there is no great haemostasis. This is used in laparoscopic surgery for dividing adhesions, myomectomy, etc. The total tissue damage is less, so smoke production is less.

Unipolar diathermy: This is the type of diathermy that is most often used in surgery, including open, minimally invasive, colposcopic and hysteroscopic. In these cases, electrons are driven via a circuit, from the surgeon's handheld 'active electrode' (connected to the diathermy machine) through the patient and leave the patient via the return electrode attached to the patient. Once the device is applied to the patient, the current will flow from the point of contact and spreads out as it passes through the patient, heading for the 'return' pad, which is usually attached to the patient's thigh. From there, it runs back to the diathermy machine, so completing the circuit. Tissues will be heated according to the amount of electric current running through them. The greatest current per cubic centimetre of tissue will be at the point of contact of the active electrode. The tissue in this area will usually be coagulated or vaporised. Away from the immediate point of contact of the active electrode, the current spreads out. So, the amount of current passing through any cubic centimetre will be small and the temperature rise will be insufficient to cause tissue damage.

Precautions

Precautions to be taken while using diathermy include the following:

❖ The colon contains hydrogen and methane. Therefore, use of diathermy on the colon may be associated with an explosive risk.

❖ Only the surgeon wielding the active electrode should activate the machine. The dial setting should be checked by the surgeon operating before the operation starts.

❖ Placing the active electrode in an insulating quiver prevents inadvertent burns.

❖ If diathermy performance is poor, the plate and lead should be checked and replaced if necessary.

Complications of Diathermy

❖ *Risks of the surgical procedures per se*: Laparoscopy, hysteroscopy and open surgery have their own risks, to which are added the risks of diathermy. The same problems with the use of diathermy can occur during laparoscopic and hysteroscopic surgery as with open surgery. The risks are greater with the latter. The medium used to distend the abdomen at laparoscopy must be non-combustible. At hysteroscopy, the medium used should be non-conductive if diathermy is to be used, so the electric current is not dissipated. Normal saline is conductive. Therefore, it is best avoided.

❖ *Operator error*: The main problem associated with the use of diathermy is operator error. This could either involve treating the wrong tissue or allowing super-heated tissue after treatment to come into contact with other tissue, such as bowel, which may inflict thermal damage to the surrounding tissues. Precautions such as proper training/servicing and checking equipment can help prevent these errors. The following precautions may be required:

  • All staff requires proper training.
  • The equipment used must be modern and up-to-date (e.g. employing diathermy systems based on solid-state isolated generators greatly help in preventing thermal injury).
  • The equipment must be regularly serviced and thoroughly checked before each use.

❖ *Thermal injury*: With bipolar diathermy, the risks of thermal injury are minimal. The current only flows between the tips of the instrument, so heat is generated only at the tips. There is no risk of stray currents. There is a small risk of damage from heated tissue coming into contact with other tissues. Unipolar diathermy, on the other hand, is associated with considerable risk of inadvertent damage. Direct coupling is one of the major complications associated with unipolar diathermy and refers to the tissue damage caused by the electrode touching another nearby conducting instrument. This may be sometimes secondary to the insulation failure, which can occur due to damaged equipment or the use of excessive voltage with coagulation current. In order to minimise the occurrence of side effects, strict adherence to the safety protocols must be followed. The whole of the probe is not in the field of view, so faulty insulation out of the field of view might cause unseen damage. Therefore, most damage is not seen or appreciated at the time. There is a requirement for careful assessment if recovery from surgery does not occur as per the norm. Other causes of diathermy burns include careless technique, use of spirit-based skin antiseptic lotions, not checking the dial setting before use or someone other than the surgeon activating the current flow. Also, the thigh pad has to be applied over an area large enough to prevent burns.

❖ *Capacitance coupling*: Capacitance coupling is an important cause of thermal burns due to diathermy. A capacitor can be formed by two conductors separated by an insulator; for example, an insulated laparoscopic instrument passing through a metallic port, forms a capacitor. The current stored in the capacitor can discharge to the tissues, resulting in thermal burns. Greater the amount of current passing through the instrument, higher would be the capacitance current. Use of plastic laparoscopic ports also does not completely remove this risk because the patient's bowel or omentum may sometimes act as the second conductor. Capacitance coupling can be avoided by using active electrode monitoring systems.

Laparoscopy

This minimally invasive procedure has become a preferred method of choice for diagnosis and treatment of several gynaecological surgical conditions. Laparoscopic surgery is likely to be associated with several advantages over laparotomy such as reduced duration of hospital stay and earlier discharge from the hospital, reduced postoperative pain and reduced blood loss. Furthermore, the advent of robotic laparoscopic surgery appears to be changing the approach to many gynaecological surgery cases. The robotic system allows surgeons to perform procedures that previously would have been performed via laparotomy using modified laparoscopic procedures. However, presently there is no robust evidence in form of randomised trials supporting these previously-mentioned advantages of laparotomy. Various complications likely to occur with laparoscopy include, gas embolism, abdominal wall vessel injury, retroperitoneal vessel injury, intestinal injury, urologic injuries, incisional hernia, nerve injuries, anaesthetic complications, etc. Steps to be taken to reduce the complications related to laparoscopic surgery are as follows:[33]

❖ The patient should be lying flat at the time of surgery.

❖ The bladder must be empty.

❖ The abdomen must be palpated to rule out presence of any abdominal mass.

❖ The primary incision should be either subumbilical or at the base of the umbilicus.

❖ Two distinct pops must be felt at the time of insertion of the Veress needle, if it enters the peritoneal cavity. The entry of the needle into the peritoneal cavity and its proper placement can be ascertained with help of the signs described next.

- *Sound of air*: As the needle enters the peritoneal cavity, there would be a hissing sound of air being sucked inside.
- *Palmer's test*: A 20-mL syringe is half-filled with saline and is attached to the hub of Veress needle. The plunger is first drawn back. Aspiration of blood or bowel contents implies that the needle is in a major splanchnic structure such as bowel or blood vessel. If no blood or bowel contents are aspirated back, 10 mL of saline contained inside the syringe can be flushed back inside the peritoneal cavity. This can occur easily without resistance if the needle is positioned properly inside the peritoneal cavity. As the saline enters the peritoneal cavity, it cannot be aspirated back. The last phase of this test comprises of withdrawing the plunger again. When the needle is positioned properly, no fluid would be sucked back into the syringe. However, if the needle tip is lying within the adhesions or in the abdominal wall, the saline is likely to have collected in form of a pool and can be drawn back.
- *Hanging drop test*: This test is done by placing a drop of saline at the open end of the Veress needle. The abdominal wall is then elevated, while observing if the saline drop disappears into the shaft or not. The drop of saline instilled into the needle will be sucked in if the needle is inside the peritoneal cavity. However, if the needle is extraperitoneal, the saline drop would remain there.

Hysteroscopy

Hysteroscopy-guided surgery has now become an important tool for the gynaecological surgeon. Hysteroscope can be used both for diagnostic and therapeutic purposes. It is a form of minimally invasive surgery that helps in avoiding giving a scar on the patient's abdomen and sometimes also helps in preventing hysterectomy. With the help of hysteroscope, the surgeon gains entry into the endometrial cavity via the cervix. Since the procedure does not require opening up of the patient's abdomen or peritoneal cavity, it is associated with minimal postoperative morbidity and mortality in comparison to that associated with laparotomy. The surgeon should be well versed in the technique of hysteroscopy before performing the procedure to reduce the rate of potential complications associated with it. Complications due to hysteroscopy are tabulated in Box 2.2.

POSTOPERATIVE CARE

Introduction

Postoperative care begins immediately after the surgery when the patient is shifted from the operation theatre into the recovery room. Postoperative care continues throughout the recovery period, even after the patient is discharged home. Critical concerns during the postoperative period include airway clearance, pain control, mental status examination and wound healing. Other important concerns

---

Box 2.2: Complications due to hysteroscopy

Instrument-related complications
- ❏ Cervical trauma
- ❏ Uterine perforation
- ❏ Bleeding
- ❏ Infection

Complications related to the use of distension media
- ❏ CO_2: Hypercarbia resulting in arrhythmias and shoulder pain
- ❏ Glycine (1.5%): Dilutional hyponatraemia and pulmonary oedema
- ❏ Dextran: Anaphylactic shock, ascites
- ❏ Dextrose (5%): Dilutional hyponatraemia and pulmonary oedema
- ❏ Sorbitol: Cerebral oedema

---

in this period include prevention of various surgery-related complications such as blood pressure variability (hypotension or hypertension), urinary retention, constipation and deep venous thrombosis.[34] Various postoperative considerations are dependent on the presence of underlying medical conditions. For example, in patients with diabetes, blood glucose levels need to be monitored every 1–4 hourly until patients become conscious and responsive. The patients, in whom the surgery is performed under GA, must be extubated before leaving the operating room. Patients should not be shifted from the operation theatre to the recovery room until they can clear and protect their airways.[35] The intubated patients with normal lungs and trachea may have a mild cough for 24 hours after extubation. In patients with a previous history of bronchitis or smoking, postextubation coughing is likely to last longer. Hypoxic dyspnoea is treated with oxygen. Non-hypoxic dyspnoea may be treated with anxiolytics or analgesics. Controlling the pain is an important aspect of postoperative management. Opioids are typically the first-line choice and can be given orally or parenterally. The patients may be briefly confused when they come out of anaesthesia. The first 72 hours after the surgery is the most critical period for the patient. During this period, precise monitoring of the patient's cardiovascular, renal and respiratory system provides valuable information regarding the patient's postoperative status. Due to the extreme importance of postoperative care, this chapter would be briefly discussing the major concerns in the postoperative care of patients who have undergone gynaecological or obstetric surgery.

No standard postoperative orders can be followed for each patient. They need to be customised according to the individual patient's needs and requirements. It is important that each patient must be evaluated before being transferred to the recovery room. The frequency of checking patient's vitals must be based on the severity of the patient's condition. All patients must be evaluated on the evening of surgery and appropriate documentation recorded in their chart. This should include thorough evaluation of the vital signs, catheter drainage (nasogastric, peritoneal and Foley's), evaluation of the pulmonary status and performance of an abdominal examination. Postoperative care can be divided into three phases, discussed here.

Table 2.5: Modified Early Warning Score[36]

Score	3	2	1	0	1	2	3
Respiratory rate (per minute)		≤8		9–14	15–20	21–29	>30
Heart rate (per minute)		≤40	41–50	51–100	101–110	111–129	>129
Systolic BP (mmHg)	≤70	71–80	81–100	101–199		≥200	
Urine output (mL/kg/h)	Nil	<0.5					
Temperature (°C)		≤35	35.1–36	36.1–38	38.1–38.5	≥38.6	
Neurological				Alert	Reacting to voice	Reacting to pain	Unresponsive

1. Immediate Postoperative Care (Theatre Recovery)

This involves the period immediately following surgery when the patient is still in the operation theatre. The parameters such as airway, breathing and circulation (ABC) must be monitored soon after the surgery. All the healthcare professionals involved in the patient care at this stage must be well versed in life-support skills. The patient must be eventually shifted to the recovery area. The patients' vitals should have stabilised and adequate pain relief been provided when the patient is shifted to the recovery area. It is important that each patient must be evaluated before being transferred from the recovery room. If the patient does not appear ready for transfer, efforts must be made to stabilise the patient or to transfer her to the ICU.

2. Early Postoperative Care

This involves the period after the patient is shifted from the recovery area to the ward, until the time of discharge from the hospital. The care in the ward can be summarised by acronym SOAP, which can be described as follows:

S: *Subjective*: How does the patient feel?
O: *Objective*: Assessment of objective parameters such as BP, temperature and fluid balance
A: *Assessment*: Physical examination
P: *Plan*: Plan of care for the next 24 hours.

Initially, the patient's pulse and BP must be recorded after every 15 minutes and thereafter every 30 minutes. Features such as tachycardia (>100/min), falling BP, pallor, gasping for breath, etc. may indicate internal or external blood loss. Patient's temperature must be recorded at least twice daily. The rise of temperature by 37–38°C in the first 36 hours after surgery could be related to pyrogen release, caused due to massive intraperitoneal haemorrhage or trauma. In cases of suspected infection, the following investigations need to be performed: urine culture and sensitivity; culture and sensitivity of pus from wound; and vaginal swab culture and sensitivity. Chest X-ray may indicate atelectasis or patchy lung consolidation or pleural effusion. Presence of calf tenderness could be indicative of phlebothrombosis. In lactating mothers, there could be breast engorgement, mastitis or breast abscess formation. In cases of urinary tract infection (UTI), fever is associated with rigor, increased frequency of micturition and dysuria. The presence of pelvic hematoma, abscess or infection must be ruled out on clinical examination.

Modified early warning scores: The Modified Early Warning Score (MEWS) is a simple, physiological score which aims at preventing the delay in intervention and facilitating the transfer of critically ill surgical ward patients (Table 2.5).[36] The scores for each parameter are recorded at the time of taking observations. The ward doctor is informed if the total is 4 or more. The use of this scoring system helps in improving the quality of care and ensuring the safety of management provided to surgical ward patients. A MEWS score of 5 or more is associated with a statistically significant increased risk of admission to the intensive therapy unit (ITU) or high dependency unit (HDU).

Various patients' requirements, which must be looked after during this period, include analgesic medications for pain relief, maintenance of fluid electrolyte balance and nutrition and dietary requirements.

Medications: The use of analgesic medications is particularly important during this period. Adequate analgesia must be prescribed. These may include oral medicines such as paracetamol and NSAIDs, PCA, opioids, epidural analgesia, etc. In case, the patient complains about nausea, she should be administered antiemetic medications. The type of medicine, the route of administration, and the dosage need to be specified. The other medications, which must be prescribed, include antibiotics and prophylactic therapy for DVT.

Fluid and electrolyte balance: Maintenance of fluid balance is important during this phase. The nursing care professionals must be instructed to inform the surgeon in case the urinary output becomes less than 30 cc per hour. Average fluid intake for a healthy person is about 750 mL in the form of food and 1,500 mL in the form of fluid. Insensible loss of about 1–1.5 litres occurs every day in the form of breathing and sweating. Urinary excretion is about 1,500 mL per day and loss through stools is about 150–200 mL per day. The fluid loss through vomitus and drainage via drains also needs to be taken into account. Proper fluid balance, therefore, needs to be maintained in order to avoid fluid and electrolyte imbalance. Most gynaecological patients can tolerate up to 2,500 mL of fluid intake per day. Daily requirements for sodium and potassium are 1 mmol/kg. If the patient is on IV fluids, serum electrolyte levels must be checked every 24–48 hours. Central venous pressure (CVP) monitoring may be required if maintenance of fluid balance appears to be difficult. Colloids or whole blood should be used for volume

CHAPTER 2

expansion in surgical patients. As a result of surgical trauma, increased amount of potassium may be excreted in the urine. In case of poor muscle tone and lethargy, K⁺ deficiency must be replaced. Protein catabolism is accelerated due to surgical trauma resulting in an increased urea excretion. If 100 g of glucose can be administered by oral or IV route, protein loss can be spared. NICE provides useful algorithms for the management of IV fluid therapy postoperatively.[37]

Nutrition and dietary requirements: Patient who had uncomplicated surgery may be given a regular diet on the first postoperative day if the bowel sounds are present; abdominal examination reveals no distension and the patient is no longer nauseated from anaesthesia. In case the bowel sounds are absent or abdominal distension is present, the patient can be started on IV fluids or kept NPO depending upon the other clinical findings.

3. Late Postoperative Care

This involves the period after which the patient is discharged home and comprises of the following components, as given below.

Wound Care

The surgeon must individualise care of each wound, but the sterile dressing placed in the operating room is generally left intact for 24 hours unless signs of infection (e.g. increasing pain, erythema and drainage) develop. After 24 hours, the site should be checked twice a day, if possible, for signs of infection. If they occur, wound exploration and drainage of abscesses, systemic antibiotics, or both may be required. Topical antibiotics are usually not helpful. A drain tube, if present, must be monitored for quantity and quality of the fluid collected. Sutures, skin staples, and other closures are usually left in place for 7 days or longer depending on the site and the type of surgery.

Requirement for Hormone Replacement Therapy

Oestrogen deficiency may occur in patients who have undergone bilateral oophorectomy at the time of surgery. In those cases, hormone replacement therapy may be administered.

Prophylactic oophorectomy is sometimes performed in women approaching menopause due to the likely risk of developing ovarian malignancy in the future. Some of the complications as a result of bilateral ovary removal include vasomotor symptoms, osteoporosis, genitourinary atrophy, etc. Ideally, the patients should have been counselled about these adverse effects prior to the surgery. Moreover, the benefits and risks of using HRT post-hysterectomy should also have been explained.

Physical Activity

The patient should be encouraged to ambulate as early as possible in the postoperative period in order to reduce the risk of development of VTE.

Discharge from the Hospital

At the time of discharge, the patient should be given a discharge sheet which adequately summarises all the postoperative instructions which the patient must observe. The patient should be given instructions regarding various activities, such as when to return to work; when to resume social activities, driving and sexual intercourse, and when to appear for follow-up visits for detection of potential complications and providing ongoing treatment. The GP should be informed about the patient's treatment. This can be done by giving a brief discharge letter to the patient, which she can give to her GP. This must preferably be followed by a formal letter to the GP. The social services, Macmillan nurses or district nurses may be occasionally involved in the discharge process.

Follow-up Visits

The requirement for follow-up visits depends on the type of surgery performed. Not all surgical procedures may require a follow-up visit. Common conditions requiring follow-up visit include the following: uncontrolled hypertension (BP > 140/100 mmHg); cardiac failure; history of MI, transient ischaemic attack, cerebrovascular accident, in the past 6 months; severe asthma/respiratory disease; type 1 diabetes mellitus or poorly controlled type 2 diabetes; renal or hepatic disease, etc. Follow-up visits help in proactive detection of complications, provision of ongoing treatment and for completing the treatment cycles. These visits are also useful for the audit purposes. However, these visits may result in considerable costs to the healthcare services as well as the patient (cost of travelling and time off work). They may also result in unnecessary patient anxiety.

 ## POSTOPERATIVE COMPLICATIONS

The events occurring at the time of surgery and anaesthesia can result in postoperative complications, which can alter the outcome of surgery and result in significant operative morbidity and mortality. Some complications are described next.

Haemorrhage

The minimum haemoglobin level at the time of surgery must be about 10 g/dL. In patients with severe anaemia prior to the surgery, blood must be transfused. In the patients with mild anaemia, blood must be kept arranged, even though the actual transfusion may not be required. Elective surgery is usually not performed until the patient's haemoglobin levels have been built up.[38] Therefore, blood transfusions are rarely required as a result of anaemia in the patient. Nevertheless, intraoperative blood transfusion may be required in the circumstances where there is excessive blood loss at the time of surgery. This may result in haemodynamic instability, poor intravascular volume and a state of collapse. Blood transfusion is usually lifesaving in the cases of shock. It helps in increasing the oxygen carrying capacity of blood by the addition of red blood cells, restoration of blood volume and the raising of plasma proteins in the blood. It also helps in the provision of the coagulation factors. While awaiting blood transfusion, fluids such as Ringer's lactate or plasma expanders such as haemaccel or hetastarch can be used.

Additionally, some precautions may be observed at the time of surgery. The surgery must be performed carefully, quickly and gently in order to minimise blood loss and tissue damage. The ligatures on the pedicles should be properly secured. The evaluation of blood loss at the time of surgery can be made by calculating the number of soaked sponges, weights of wet swabs and variation in the pulse and BP. In case of extensive surgery such as Wertheim's, blood transfusion may be required in the theatre.

Primary Haemorrhage

Primary haemorrhage due to arterial blood loss may occur at the time of surgery due to slipping of ligatures and retraction of vessels in it. Double ligatures must therefore be tied and an unduly thick pedicle in single suture be avoided. Transfixation of sutures may also be helpful. The loss of venous blood is usually in the form of ooze from an ill-defined area of dissection around a mass or adhesion. This is usually encountered in case of pelvic floor surgery. To prevent this, the dissection should be blunt and preferably in the line of cleavage. If required, tight compression or vaginal packing may be done. In case of retractable internal haemorrhage, internal iliac artery ligation may be required.

Reactionary haemorrhage: Reactionary haemorrhage is a type of prolonged primary haemorrhage, which does not occur immediately as it is originally masked by the hypotensive effect of drug or anaesthesia. However, when the blood pressure reverts to normal, vasodilatation occurs and oozing begins.

Secondary Haemorrhage

It usually occurs on 7th–10th postoperative day. The usual cause is the sepsis, which erodes the blood vessels and bleeding starts from the infected granulation tissues. The haemorrhage may begin as dirty discharge and dark clots, which proceed to fresh red profuse bleeding. This may eventually result in haemodynamic instability and shock. Broad-spectrum intravenous antibiotics must be started in these cases. Since the use of sutures would be ineffective due to the presence of infected tissues, tight compression helps in achieving haemostasis in these cases. This helps in tiding over the emergency until the sepsis settles.

Postoperative Febrile Morbidity

The common cause of fever is a high metabolic rate that occurs due to the stress of a surgical procedure. Other causes of fever may include pneumonia, UTIs and wound infections. Precautionary steps such as incentive spirometry, deep breathing exercises and periodic coughing can help to reduce the risk of pneumonia.

Pulmonary Complications

Upper respiratory tract infections such as acute bronchitis or pneumonitis must be treated prior to elective surgery, especially if planned under GA. Most important pulmonary complications after pelvic or abdominal surgery include atelectasis, pneumonia and pulmonary thromboembolic diseases. Some of the risk factors for the development of postoperative pulmonary complications in gynaecological surgery patients include, those with age greater than 60 years, cancer, congestive cardiac failure, smoking within 8 weeks of surgery, upper abdominal incision, vertical incision and length of incision greater than 20 cm.[39] Some of the pulmonary complications are described next. Complications such as lung abscesses, pleurisy and empyema are rare as a result of improved anaesthesia techniques and prophylactic antibiotic cover.

Atelectasis: The diagnosis of atelectasis is based on the following parameters: impaired oxygenation, unexplained temperature of more than 38°C and chest radiography showing the evidence of volume loss or new airspace opacity.[40] Risk factors for development of atelectasis include advanced age, obesity, intraperitoneal sepsis, prolonged anaesthesia time, nasogastric tube placement and smoking. Steps, which can be taken to prevent the occurrence of atelectasis, include cessation of smoking, 8 weeks prior to the elective surgery; deep breathing exercises; mobilization; adequate analgesia (epidural or PCA) and selective gastric compression. Chest physiotherapy is usually not recommended, as it is associated with numerous disadvantages such as exhaustion, pain in the chest, bronchospasm and transient hypoxaemia.[41] Moreover, it has not been shown to be superior over deep breathing exercises in the prevention of atelectasis.[42]

Postoperative pneumonia: Hospital-acquired pneumonia develops 48 hours or more after hospital admission and is caused by an organism that was not incubating at the time of hospitalisation. Common pathogens, which are responsible for causing hospital-acquired pneumonias, can include *Streptococcus pneumoniae, methicillin-sensitive Staphylococcus aureus, Haemophilus influenzae, Escherichia coli, Klebsiella pneumoniae, Enterobacter* species, etc. Some interventions to reduce the risk for the hospital-acquired pneumonia include strict adherence to infection control procedures, early removal of invasive devices (e.g. catheters), semi-recumbent positioning of the patient, restriction of acid suppression therapy, restrictive red blood cell transfusion strategy and the strict control of hyperglycaemia. Procedures for control of infection include use of alcohol-based hand disinfection and appropriate barrier precautions.

Postoperative bronchitis: Postoperative bronchitis may present with dyspnoea and persistent cough with expectoration.

Mendelson syndrome: This may result from the inhalation of regurgitated gastric contents during the time of anaesthesia. It may present in the form of acute respiratory distress with cyanosis due to bronchospasm and pulmonary oedema. This may lead to hypotension and cardiovascular collapse, which may even prove to be fatal.

Lung collapse: This may occur due to the blockage of the alveoli with tenacious mucous plugs. It may present with dyspnoea, chest constriction, cyanosis of varying degrees and fever with resultant tachycardia. The chest on the affected side has restricted movements with reduced air entry. The trachea and the mediastinum may be displaced ipsilaterally and the diagnosis may be confirmed on chest X-ray. Though chest physiotherapy does not prove to be effective, deep breathing exercises may prove to be effective.

Urinary Tract Complications

Urinary Infection

It may commonly occur after vaginal surgery, prolonged or intermittent repeated catheterisation, bladder surgery or elective gynaecological cancer surgery. Aseptic precautions must be observed while performing urethral catheterisation to prevent the occurrence of infections. Poor voiding after surgery or extensive bladder dissection may result in an increased residual volume in the bladder causing cystitis. This may present as hypogastric pain, increased frequency of micturition, dysuria, etc. In these cases, urine routine and microscopy, and urine culture and sensitivity must be performed. Rarely, the infection may ascend high up in the urinary tract to cause acute pyelonephritis. The patient may be acutely ill having high fever with rigors, vomiting and anorexia. The pain is localised to the loin and the renal angle may be tender to palpation.

Urinary Retention

Urinary retention may commonly occur after surgery. Causes include use of anticholinergics or opioids, immobility and decreased oral intake. Patients must be monitored for urinary retention. Direct catheterisation is typically necessary for patients who have a distended bladder and are uncomfortable or who have not urinated for 6–8 hours after surgery.

Gastrointestinal Complications

Slight postoperative nausea and vomiting due to the use of anaesthetic agents is common problem amongst post-operative patients. Two other common gastrointestinal complications include postoperative ileus and postoperative intestinal obstruction. Excessive vomiting may result from paralytic ileus. This could be as a result of pelvic haematoma, peritonitis, bladder/rectal injury or hypokalaemia. It initially may contain only gastric content; later on, it becomes bilious and lastly may become offensive and dark coloured and may contain faecal matter. Vomiting is usually effortless and is associated with a fall in BP and electrolyte imbalance. The causative factor must be treated vigorously. Use of bowel stimulants such as enema is strictly prohibited until the condition has reversed and bowel sounds have reappeared.

Postoperative Ileus

Postoperative ileus can be considered as an inevitable consequence of abdominal surgery. Paralytic ileus is a form of non-mechanical intestinal obstruction, which occurs due to reduced peristaltic activity of the intestines. It is important to differentiate between postoperative ileus and postoperative obstruction. In case of postoperative ileus, there is discomfort from distension, but crampy pains are not present. In case of postoperative obstruction, cramping progressively increases in severity. Postoperative ileus occurs 48–72 hours after the surgery; while in case of intestinal obstruction, the onset may be delayed for up to 5–7 days after surgery. There may be nausea, vomiting and distension in both the cases. While bowel sound may be absent or hypoactive in case of postoperative ileus, high-pitched bowel sounds and borborygmi with peristaltic rushes may be present in case of postoperative obstruction. In paralytic ileus, abdominal radiography shows presence of distended loops of small and large bowel. Gas is usually present in the colon. On the other hand, in postoperative obstruction, abdominal radiographs may show single or multiple loops of distended bowel (usually small bowel) with air-fluid levels. In case of postoperative paralytic ileus, treatment is mainly conservative with the use of nasogastric suction, enemas and cholinergic stimulations. However, in case of postoperative obstruction, the mainstay of treatment is surgical. In the initial stages, conservative management with nasogastric decompression may be done. Serial monitoring of the white blood cell count and differential count is an important method for differentiating between bowel obstruction and paralytic ileus.

Intestinal Obstruction

Mechanical intestinal obstruction is suspected when the patient has severe colicky abdominal pain and visible peristalsis with loud and exaggerated bowel sounds in the area of gut proximal to the site of obstruction. There may be some abdominal distension and vomiting of gastric or bilious contents. This condition requires immediate surgical intervention.

Venous Thrombotic Events

One of the most common postoperative complications is the venous thrombotic events such as DVT and PE. PE can be considered as one of the most important causes of postoperative mortality.[43] DVT is also associated with considerable morbidity and mortality. PE may be characterised by rapid onset of respiratory distress, hypotension, chest pain and cardiac arrhythmias. The major sites of thrombus formation are soleal venous sinuses of the calf and venous arcade, which join the posterior tibial and peroneal veins draining the soleal muscle.[44] Due to confluence of large veins in this area, the local stasis is marked. This results in formation of large friable thrombus, which grows rapidly and has minimal intimal anchorage. Once the thrombus is dislodged, it may rapidly embolise via the inferior vena cava to reach the cardiopulmonary sites. Presence of thrombus along with accompanying inflammation of the blood vessels may result in the development of DVT. This may be associated with a small, but persistent rise in the temperature and pulse rate on the third postoperative day, aches or pain in the lower limbs and calf tenderness. The flexion and extension of the ankle joints may elicit pain (i.e. Homan's sign positive). Duplex ultrasonography of the calf muscle blood flow helps in establishing the diagnosis.[45,46] In cases where the clot embolises, if the clot is small, it can produce symptoms such as slight chest pain, moderate cyanosis, dyspnoea or pleural effusion with bloodstained sputum. If the clot is large, it may result in symptoms such as intense pain in the chest, acute dyspnoea, cyanosis, tachycardia and shock. Massive clots can prove to be fatal, resulting in profuse haemoptysis, gasping and collapse.

Various factors, which are thought to lead to postoperative thrombosis, are venous stasis, changes in the blood constituents, and impaired function of the vessel wall. Venous stasis can be considered as the most important factor in the genesis of postoperative thrombosis. Venous stasis in the pelvis and lower extremity promotes the adhesion of the platelets to the endothelial cells lining the vessels, which encourage the development of the thrombus. Another factor which could be responsible for producing venous stasis during the prolonged surgery, is the use of tight packing of the intestines in the upper abdomen resulting in the obstruction of the underlying vena cava.[47]

Doppler ultrasound has become the most widely used investigation for the diagnosis of DVT. It helps in measuring blood flow velocity through the major blood vessels. In the presence of thrombosis, reduced signal is produced. Colour enhancement can be used for identifying arteries (red) and veins (blue). This technique helps in identification of DVT in the iliac, femoral or popliteal veins.

Prevention

Prevention is the most important tool in the treatment of VTE. Some of the preventive measures, which can be taken to reduce the risk of embolism, include preoperative and postoperative prophylaxis with UFH or LMWH and concomitant use of embolic stockings or intermittent pneumatic compression stockings.[48,49] Early mobilisation in the postoperative period encourages the muscle pumping function of the legs, thereby reducing venous stasis.

Unfractionated heparin: The mainstay of prophylactic treatment had been low-dose UFH. Since it does not affect activated partial thromboplastin time (APTT), it does not cause any increase in postoperative bleeding. The main effect of low-dose heparin is exerted via antithrombin through factor Xa, as well as directly on thrombin. The commonly used dosage is 5,000 IU, 2 hours before surgery and then 5,000 IU every 12 hourly for the next 5 days. For the high-risk patients, the dosage must be used at every 8-hourly interval. There is a risk of heparin-induced thrombocytopenia and requires monitoring of APTT when used for treatment. The various anticoagulant therapies, which can be used for treatment of VTE, are as follows:

Warfarin: Warfarin can be used for the long-term treatment and prevention of VTE. Due to its teratogenic action, it is contraindicated in pregnancy. It requires anticoagulation monitoring and is associated with a high risk of bleeding.[50]

Low-molecular-weight heparin: They have now become the mainstay of prophylactic treatment and have replaced all other forms of the drug therapy. These drugs have a longer half-life than UFH and are therefore much more biopredictable.[51,52] They have a much more reliable pharmacokinetic profile. LMWH mainly act by inhibiting factor Xa and have very little activity against thrombin. They have a much longer half-life than UFH and measurement of APTT does not reflect its anticoagulation state. The main advantage of LMWH is that they are associated with a lower incidence of heparin-induced thrombocytopenia and postoperative bleeding.

Inferior vena caval filters: Inferior vena caval filters help in trapping large emboli. These can be used for the prevention of PE when anticoagulation therapy fails or is contraindicated. It can be used prior to pulmonary embolectomy or pulmonary endarterectomy.

External pneumatic leg compression: They are used as a prophylactic agent for DVT. They help in preventing venous stasis and stimulate the fibrinolytic system.[52-55]

Postoperative Infection

In the majority of cases, the cause of pelvic and abdominal wound infection is the bacteria found amongst the endogenous microflora of the lower genital tract. Other risk factors include the patient's age, socioeconomic status, type of surgery, site of incision, duration of surgery, use of implants, obesity, presence of concurrent comorbid conditions such as diabetes mellitus, history of surgery, radiotherapy, chemotherapy, prolonged hospitalisation or use of inappropriate antibiotic prophylaxis. Common postoperative infections include the following:

❖ Pelvic infections such as pelvic cellulitis, vaginal cuff haematoma and/or abscess, pelvic vein thrombosis, postoperative adnexal abscess, cellulitis, osteomyelitis pubis, incisional wound infection and cystitis. In case of pelvic cellulitis, the patients present with fever on 2nd–5th postoperative days after hysterectomy. Other findings may include abdominal tenderness, peritoneal signs or postoperative ileus. Induration may be present on pelvic examination. Also, no fluctuant mass is present in the majority of cases. However, in case of vaginal cuff haematoma and/or abscess, there may be purulent discharge and/or a fluctuant mass may be palpated at the vaginal cuff.

Presence of postoperative febrile morbidity, not responding to antimicrobial therapy is suggestive of septic pelvic thrombophlebitis. In these cases, usually there is no evidence of abscess on pelvic examination or investigations such as CT or ultrasonography. Full heparin anticoagulation must be administered to the patient for about a week. Response may be observed within 24–48 hours of the start of therapy.

In case of adnexal abscesses, the patient presents with fever and abdominal pain. There may be a tender palpable adnexal mass on pelvic examination.

- Non-pelvic infections may include infections such as pneumonia, bacteraemia, pyelonephritis, etc.
- The most commonly used antibiotics for the treatment of postoperative infections include semisynthetic penicillins, cephalosporins (third generation) or aminoglycosides in combination with clindamycin or one of new large spectrum penicillin (third generation, e.g. carbenicillin and ticarcillin and fourth generation, e.g. piperacillin).

Prevention

Steps, which can be taken to reduce the incidence of post-operative infection, are as follows:

- Prophylactic antibiotics 30 minutes prior to the incision or at the time of induction of anaesthesia.[56]
- Use of meticulous surgical techniques at the time of surgery.
- Ensuring adequate haemostasis at the time of surgery. Drains must not be used as an alternative against good haemostasis.
- Judicious use of cautery at the time of surgery.
- Gentle handling of the tissues.
- Sterilisation of the operation theatre and high-level disinfection of the instruments.

Wound Infection at the Incision Site

The wound infections could be of two types: (1) early onset wound infections or (2) late onset wound infections. Early onset wound infections are caused by group β-haemolytic streptococci and respond to high doses of parenteral penicillin. Late onset wound infections, on the other hand, become apparent by 5th–7th postoperative day. There may be a single high spike of the fever in the afternoon or early morning. Treatment consists of drainage, irrigation, dressing and systemic antibiotics. Continuing wound sepsis may result in development of burst abdomen by second postoperative week. This may be associated with the peeping out of the gut and omentum through the incision line. The treatment for burst abdomen includes emergency single-layered closure along with resuturing. The various factors, which may influence wound healing, include malnourishment, anaemia, chronic diseases, diabetes, malignancy, sepsis and massive corticosteroid therapy. Incisional hernia may occur due to the herniation of abdominal contents, usually gut and omentum through a gap in the rectus sheath as a result of partial or complete wound dehiscence. The treatment comprises repairing the hernia and strengthening with inlay or sublay of prosthetic mesh as an elective procedure at a later date.

Cystitis

This may occur if appropriate precautions are not taken at the time of urethral catheterisation or in cases where the urinary output is less than 2,500 mL in 24 hours. The presentation is in the form of fever with chills and rigors, and pain and tenderness over the hypogastrium. Urine culture and sensitivity must be done and antibiotics started appropriately.

POSTOPERATIVE ANALGESIA

Satisfactory postoperative pain management is an important component of patient care. Pain is a subjective experience, which may be defined as 'an unpleasant sensory and emotional experience associated with actual or potential tissue damage.' Since the sensation of pain can be influenced by many physiological and psychological factors, management of pain is a complex process and would be discussed in details in this section.

Effects of Postoperative Pain

Besides being the major cause of discomfort, pain in the postoperative period can affect the different organ systems resulting in the development of postoperative complications such as atelectasis, sputum retention and hypoxaemia; myocardial ischaemia, tachycardia and dysrhythmia; decreased gastric emptying, reduced gut motility and constipation; urinary retention; hyperglycaemia and metabolic acidosis; increased protein catabolism; complications related to reduced mobility such as difficulty in getting out of bed, physiotherapy, and changing of dressing, etc. resulting in impaired wound healing, development of pressure sores and increased risk of DVT; and psychological complications such as anxiety and fatigue. Both pharmacological and non-pharmacological treatment modalities are now available for postoperative pain control. The pain medications can be administered by various routes including intramuscular, subcutaneous, intravenous, oral, rectal or transdermal.[57] For control of postoperative pain, analgesic medications can be either administered in the form of continuous infusions of opioids and/or NSAIDs; patient-controlled administration of opioids and/or NSAIDs; and intermittent boluses and/or continuous infusion of epidural or intra-thecal opioids.

Non-pharmacological Methods

Non-pharmacological methods of pain relief comprise of the methods such as relaxation therapy, hypnosis, cold or heat massage, splinting of wounds, transcutaneous electrical nerve stimulation (TENS), etc. Preoperative explanation and patient education plays an important role in preparing the patient prior to surgery and helps in reducing the pain perception.

Pharmacological Management

Oral NSAIDs form the first line of management for mild-to-moderate pain. For patients who cannot tolerate NSAIDs or who require stronger dosage of analgesic, combinations of paracetamol and opioids are the next best choice. For more severe pain, injectable opioids may be required. For high-risk surgery, spinals and epidurals using combinations of local anaesthetic and opioid analgesics may help in reducing the morbidity related to the pain of surgery.[58]

Non-steroidal Anti-inflammatory Agents

These form the first line of pharmacological management for mild-to-moderate postoperative pain. Some commonly used NSAIDs include aspirin, ibuprofen, ketoprofen, naproxen, mefenamic acid, piroxicam, ketorolac, paracetamol, etc. NSAIDs act by inhibiting the enzyme cyclooxygenase, which helps in reducing the production of inflammatory mediators such as prostaglandin, prostacyclin and thromboxane at the site of tissue injury. Their use can produce certain side effects such as gastric irritation and peptic ulceration; impairment of renal function; platelet dysfunction; exacerbation of aspirin-induced asthma, poor bone or wound healing, etc. Furthermore, NSAIDs may not appear as an adequate analgesic agent for severe pain. They appear to best work in conjunction with other agents. For example, administration of ketorolac helps in reducing the requirements of morphine by nearly 50% in patients recovering from abdominal surgery. NSAIDs can be administered either via oral or parenteral route. At times, NSAIDs can also be administered via alternative routes such as per rectal route.

Paracetamol: Paracetamol (acetaminophen) is the most commonly used NSAID, which also has a weak anti-inflammatory activity. It can be administered both by oral or rectal routes. It is usually prescribed on an 'as and when required' basis. In comparison to other NSAIDs (especially aspirin), paracetamol does not stimulate respiration or affect the acid-base balance or has an effect on cellular metabolism. In normal dosage, paracetamol is usually safe and well tolerated. However, it has the potential to cause paracetamol poisoning in large doses (>150 mg/kg body weight in an adult). Dosage greater than 250 mg/kg body weight can even prove to be fatal. Overdose of paracetamol may result in hepatic necrosis. Paracetamol is often prescribed in combination with other weak opiates.

Opiates

The most commonly used opiate drugs are diamorphine, morphine and pethidine. Pethidine has only about 10% the analgesic potency of morphine. They act on μ receptors in brain and spinal cord. The main side effect of opiates is their potential to cause respiratory depression. The action of opiate drugs on μ1 receptors is responsible for analgesic action, whereas their action on μ2 receptors is responsible for respiratory depression. Use of opiates can produce side effects such as sedation, nausea and vomiting, vasodilatation and myocardial depression, pruritus, delayed gastric emptying, constipation, urinary retention, etc.

Opiates can be administered by oral, subcutaneous, intramuscular or intravenous, and epidural or spinal routes. Opiates can also be used for PCA, where the patient determines her own analgesic requirement all by herself. Opioids, which can be administered by oral route, include dihydrocodeine, oxycodone, codeine, tramadol and morphine. Opioids such as morphine sulphate and meperidine hydrochloride (pethidine) can be administered by the intramuscular, subcutaneous or IV routes.[59] However, the main disadvantage of administering intramuscular injections is that it can be extremely painful. On the other hand, use of subcutaneous injections may help in providing effective pain relief. Moreover, the injection is less painful and the effect lasts longer.

Patient-Controlled Analgesia

Patient-controlled analgesia is a mechanism of drug delivery in which the analgesic medicine (e.g. pethidine) is delivered intravenously. The drug is released in the blood only when the patient feels the need of a painkiller medicine and pushes the button of the pump. The physician, however, can determine the dosage of this intermittent injection. Moreover, the physician can also determine the minimal length of time that must elapse between two consecutive doses as well as the amount of drug that can be injected in a specified period of time (1–4 hours).

Opioid drugs can also be administered by epidural or intrathecal route. This can help reduce the dosage of opioids required for adequate pain relief, especially if administered in association with local anaesthetics. While using the epidural route, a catheter can be used to maintain analgesia in the postoperative period.

CLINICAL PEARLS

❖ All units in hospitals across the UK should have clear protocols for thromboprophylaxis.
❖ All healthcare workers must be immunised against hepatitis B.
❖ Facilities must be available to manage an anaesthetised patient postoperatively.
❖ Even if the surgery has been performed under local anaesthesia and sedation, the patient must be observed for at least 2 hours prior to discharge.
❖ Two laser systems are commonly used in the gynaecological practice: CO_2 laser and Nd:YAG (neodymium:yttrium-aluminium-garnet) laser.
❖ There is requirement for accurate fluid deficit during the hysteroscopic procedures because fluid and electrolyte imbalance may result in the development of serious complications.

EVIDENCE-BASED MEDICINE

❖ *Enhanced recovery programmes*: Enhanced recovery programmes (ERPs) have been established over the past 10 years in the UK to help improve patient outcomes and to hasten recovery following surgery. This programme, which was initially started in colorectal surgery, is now being increasingly used in gynaecological surgery. Enhanced recovery after surgery (ERAS) protocols are multimodal perioperative care pathways for attaining early recovery after surgical procedures by maintaining preoperative organ function and reducing the intense stress response following surgery. The main elements of ERAS protocols include adequate preoperative patient assessment, planning, counselling and preparation prior to admission, optimization of nutrition, standardised analgesic and anaesthetic regimens, and early mobilisation. A meta-analysis comprising a total of 5,099 participants, showed that ERPs are likely to reduce the primary length of hospital stay as well as the risk of all postoperative complications within 30 days. There was no evidence of a reduction in mortality rates or patient outcomes. Despite the significant body of evidence indicating improved outcomes with ERAS protocols, their implementation in clinical practice is slow.[60]

❖ *Use of drains at the time of surgery:* Presently, there is lack of availability of good-quality evidence to support the routine use of drains at the time of surgery. Drains can be used depending upon the clinical indication. However, their use does not serve as an alternative to adequate haemostasis. Drains can be used in cases where there is repair of urinary tract injury to prevent urinary leakage.[61]

REFERENCES

1. General Medical Council. (2008). Consent: patients and doctors making decisions together. [online] Available from http://www.gmc-uk.org/GMC_Consent_0513_Revised.pdf_52115235.pdf. [Accessed October, 2016].
2. Lim V. Changing trends in informed consent. IeJSME. 2014;8(1):3-7.
3. Hammond, Charles B. Gynecology: The female reproductive organs. In: Sabiston Textbook of Surgery. Philadelphia: WB Saunders Company; 2001.
4. Department of Health. Best practice guidance for doctors and other health professionals on the provision of advice and treatment to young people under 16 on contraception, sexual and reproductive health. London: DH; 2004.
5. General Medical Council. (2001). Good Medical Practice, London. [online] Available from www.gmc-uk.org/gmp_2001.pdf_25416526.pdf [Accessed August, 2014].
6. Bates B. A Guide to Physical Examination and History Taking, 6th edition. Philadelphia: JB Lippincott Company; 1995.
7. Department of Health. Confidentiality: NHS code of practice. London: DH; 2003.
8. Portal RW. Elective surgery after myocardial infraction. Br Med J (Clin Res Ed). 1982;284(6319):843-4.
9. Nestel D, Kneebone R. Please don't touch me there: the ethics of intimate examinations: integrated approach to teaching and learning clinical skills. BMJ. 2003;326(7402):1327.
10. Oakeshott P, Hay P. Best practice in primary care. BMJ. 2006;333(7560):173-4.
11. Bonnar J. Venous thromboembolism and gynecologic surgery. Clin Obstet Gynecol. 1985;28(2):432-46.
12. Wightman JA. A prospective survey of the incidence of postoperative pulmonary complications. Br J Surg. 1968;55(2):85-91.
13. Anderson DO, Ferris BG. Role of tobacco smoking in the causation of chronic respiratory disease. N Engl J Med. 1962;267:787-94.
14. Selby M. Please don't touch me there: The ethics of intimate examinations: informed consent failed to protect me. BMJ. 2003;326(7402):1326.
15. Roizen MF. Pre-operative Testing. In: Sweitzer BJ (Ed). Handbook of Preoperative Assessment and Management. Philadelphia: Lippincott Williams & Wilkins; 2000.
16. McKee RF, Scott EM. The value of routine preoperative investigations. Ann R Coll Surg Engl. 1987;69(4):160-2.
17. Perez A, Planell J, Bacardaz C, et al. Value of routine preoperative tests: a multicentre study in four general hospitals. Br J Anaesth. 1995;74(3):250-6.
18. Perioperative smoking. Conference of experts. Short text. 2005. Ann Fr Anesth Reanim. 2006;25(4):479-81.
19. Ledger WJ. Prevention, diagnosis and treatment of post-operative infections. Obstet Gynecol. 1980;55(5 Suppl):203S-206S.
20. Hoeprich PD. Current principles of antimicrobic therapy. Obstet Gynecol. 1980;55(5 Suppl):121S-127S.
21. Berger SA, Nagar H, Gordon M. Antimicrobial prophylaxis in obstetric and gynecologic surgery: a critical review. J Reprod Med. 1980;24(5):185-90.
22. National Institute of Clinical Excellence. Venous thrombo-embolism: reducing the risk for patients in hospital. Clinical guideline CG92. London: NICE; 2010.
23. American Society of Anesthesiologists. (1941). ASA Physical Status Classification System. [online] Available from https://www.asahq.org/resources/clinical-information/asa-physical-status-classification-system. [Accessed October, 2016].
24. Chamberlain G, Wraight A, Steer P. Pain and its relief in childbirth. Report of the 1990 NBT Survey. Edinburgh (UK): Churchill Livingstone; 1993.
25. Reynolds F. Pain relief in labour. Br J Obstet Gynaecol. 1993;100(11):979-83.
26. Gamlin FM, Lyons G. Spinal analgesia in labour. Int J Obstet Anesth. 1997;6(3):161-72.
27. Hawkins JL, Chestnut DH, Gibbs CP. Obstetric Anesthesia. In: Chestnut DH, Gibbs CP (Eds). Obstetrics: Normal & Problem Pregnancies. Philadelphia: Churchill Livingstone; 2002.
28. Chan YK, Ng KP. A survey of the current practice of obstetric anaesthesia and analgesia in Malaysia. J Obstet Gynaecol Res. 2000;26(2):137-40.
29. Chan YK, Ng KP. Regional Analgesia in Obstetrics in the Far East. In: Reynolds F (Ed). Regional Analgesia in Obstetrics—a millennium update. London: Springer-Verlag; 2000. pp. 73-8.
30. Shibli KU, Russell IF. A survey of anaesthetic techniques used for caesarean section in the UK in 1997. Int J Obstet Anesth. 2000;9(3):160-7.
31. Paul J. Epidural analgesia for labor. In: David J Birbach, Stephen Gatt, Sanjay Datta (Eds). Textbook of Obstetric Anesthesia. Philadelphia: Churchill Livingstone; 2000. pp. 145-56.
32. NICE. Prophylaxis against infective endocarditis. Clinical Guidelines 634. London: NICE; 2016.
33. Royal College of Obstetricians and Gynaecologists. Preventing entry related gynecological laparoscopic injuries. Green-Top guidelines No 49. London: RCOG; 2008.
34. Djokovic JL, Hedley-Whyte J. Prediction of outcome of surgery and anesthesia in patients over 80. JAMA. 1979;242(21):2301-6.
35. Korttila K. Recovery from outpatient anaesthesia. Factors affecting outcome. Anaesthesia. 1995;50 Suppl:22-8.
36. Gardner-Thorpe J, Love N, Wrightson J, Walsh S, Keeling N. The Value of Modified Early Warning Score (MEWS) in Surgical In-Patients: A Prospective Observational Study. Ann R Coll Surg Engl. 2006;88(6):571-5.
37. NICE. Intravenous fluid therapy in adults in hospital, NICE clinical guideline 174. London: NICE; 2016.

38. Twombly GH. Hemorrhage in gynecologic surgery. Clin Obstet Gynecol. 1973;16(2):135-61.

39. Schlueter DP. High-risk gynecology: pulmonary risks. Clin Obstet Gynecol. 1973;16(2):91-110.

40. Ashbaugh DG, Bigelow DB, Petty TL, Levine BE. Acute respiratory distress in adults. Lancet. 1967;2(7511):319-23.

41. Kirilloff LH, Owens GR, Rogers RM, Mazzocco MC. Does chest physical therapy work? Chest. 1985;88(3):436-44.

42. Stiller KR, Munday RM. Chest physiotherapy for the surgical patient. Br J Surg. 1992;79(8):745-9.

43. Adar R, Papa MZ, Amsterdam E, Bass A, Schneiderman J. Antithrombosis routines and hemorrhagic complications: a seven year survey comparing vascular and general surgical operations. J Cardiovasc Surg. 1985;26(3):275-9.

44. Becker DM. Venous thromboembolism: epidemiology, diagnosis, prevention. J Gen Intern Med. 1986;1(6):402-11.

45. Aitken AG, Godden DJ. Real-time ultrasound diagnosis of deep vein thrombosis: a comparison with venography. Clin Radiol. 1987;38(3):309-13.

46. Cranley JJ, Canos AJ, Sull WJ. The diagnosis of deep venous thrombosis. Fallibility of clinical symptoms and signs. Arch Surg. 1976;111(1):34-6.

47. Gallus AS, Hirsh J, Hull R, Aken WG. Diagnosis of venous thromboembolism. Semin Thromb Hemost. 1976;2(4):203-31.

48. Adolf J, Buttermann G, Weidenbach A, et al. Optimization of postoperative prophylaxis of thrombosis in gynecology. Geburtshilfe Frauenheilkd. 1978;38(2):98-104.

49. Allan A, Williams JT, Bolton JP, Le Quesne LP. The use of graduated compression stockings in the prevention of post-operative deep vein thrombosis. Br J Surg. 1983;70(3):172-4.

50. Peterson CE, Kwann HC. Current concepts of warfarin therapy. Arch Intern Med. 1986;146(3):581-4.

51. Baertschi U, Schaer A, Bader P, Huber L, Morf P. A comparison of low dose heparin and oral anticoagulants in the prevention of thrombo-phlebitis following gynaecological operations. Geburtshilfe Frauenheilkd. 1975;35(10):754-60.

52. Bergqvist D, Burmark US, Frisell J, Hallböök T, Lindblad B, Risberg B, et al. Low molecular weight heparin once daily compared with conventional low-dose heparin twice daily: a prospective double-blind multicentre trial on prevention of postoperative thrombosis . Br J Surg. 1986;73(3):204-8.

53. Allenby F, Boardman L, Pflug JJ, Calnan JS. Effects of external pneumatic intermittent compression on fibrinolysis in man. Lancet. 1973;2(7843):1412-4.

54. Baker WH, Mahler DK, Foldes MS, Michelini MA, Hayes AC, Littooy FN, et al. Pneumatic compression devices for prophylaxis of deep venous thrombosis (DVT). Am Surg. 1986;52(7):371-3.

55. Mittelman JS, Edwards WS, McDonald JB. Effectiveness of leg compression in preventing venous stasis. Am J Surg. 1982;144(6):611-3.

56. Pollock AV. Surgical prophylaxis: the emerging picture. Lancet. 1988;1(8579):225-30.

57. Crews JC. Multimodal pain management strategies for office-based and ambulatory procedures. JAMA. 2002;288(5):629-32.

58. Schecter WP, Bongard FS, Gainor BJ, Weltz DL, Horn JK. Pain control in outpatient surgery. J Am Coll Surg. 2002;195(1):95-104.

59. Taylor MS. Managing postoperative pain. Hosp Med. 2001;62(9):560-3.

60. Nicholson A, Lowe MC, Parker J, Lewis SR, Alderson P, Smith AF. Systematic review and meta-analysis of enhanced recovery programmes in surgical patients. Br J Surg. 2014;101(3):172-88.

61. Patsner B. Closed-suction drainage versus no drainage following radical abdominal hysterectomy with pelvic lymphadenectomy for stage IB cervical cancer. Gynecol Oncol. 1995;57(2):232-4.

CHAPTER 2

Antenatal Period

OBSTETRICS

Routine Antenatal Care

INTRODUCTION

Antenatal care is a type of preventive healthcare strategy, which provides regular health check-ups to the pregnant women with the aim of detecting and treating any potential healthcare problem throughout the course of pregnancy and simultaneously, also promoting a healthy lifestyle for both the mother and the baby.[1] A woman centred approach, with an emphasis on providing choice, easy access and continuity of care, must be implemented for provision of antenatal services to the women during their pregnancies.[2,3] The aim of ANC is to identify risk factors related to the development of various complications during pregnancy, so as to ensure early recognition and treatment of complications which arise during the period.

As per the statistics by WHO, in the year 2015, nearly 830 women died world-wide due to pregnancy-related complications. However, of these only five belonged to the developed countries.[4] Remaining belonged to the high-risk countries. Provision of routine ANC helps in reducing the maternal death rate and miscarriage, as well as neonatal complications such as birth defects, low birth weight, neonatal infections, etc. Management of ANC in the UK must be in guidance with the NICE clinical guidelines and WHO recommendations.[5]

Kindness, respect and dignity must always be maintained on part of the healthcare professionals while dealing with the women, their partners and their families. Efforts must be made to search for their views, beliefs and values in relation to the care of the mother as well as that of her baby. Their views must be respected at all times. The women and her family must be provided with information to enable an improved experience of pregnancy, delivery and neonatal period. During the antenatal period, following the provision of appropriate information, women should be given the opportunity to make informed decisions about their own care and treatment as well as that of their baby. This should be done in partnership with their healthcare professionals. This requires suitable communication between healthcare professionals and women and should be reinforced by evidence-based, written information (patient information leaflets) designed in accordance to the woman's requirements and culture. This information could be related to physiological or biological changes of pregnancy, prenatal nutrition, especially prenatal vitamins, common pregnancy ailments, pregnancy-related complications, etc.[5] Women with additional needs such as physical, sensory or learning disabilities must be provided with information in a manner easily accessible to them. Women with an uncomplicated low-risk pregnancy must be offered midwife-led and GP-led models of care.[6] Midwife-led care can be described as the model of care where a midwife is the leading professional starting from the initial booking appointment till the baby is delivered including the early neonatal period. Routine involvement of obstetricians in the care of women with an uncomplicated low-risk pregnancy at scheduled times is not likely to improve perinatal outcomes. Therefore, obstetricians are involved only when the complications arise. Midwife-led model is likely to be associated with a reduced rate of intervention and higher rates of patient satisfaction in comparison with other models of care.

ANTENATAL APPOINTMENTS

Antenatal care should be promptly and effortlessly made available to all pregnant women, taking into account the requirements of individual women and the local community. The antenatal appointments should take place in an environment comfortable to the woman so as to facilitate her to discuss sensitive issues such as domestic violence, sexual abuse, psychiatric illness, recreational drug use, etc. Structured maternity records should be used for provision of ANC. Maternity services should have a system in place whereby women carry their own case notes.[7] This is likely to be associated with several benefits such as increased maternal control and increased availability of antenatal records during hospital attendance.

A standardised, national maternity record with an agreed minimum data set should be developed and used. This would enable the healthcare professionals to provide evidence-based care to the pregnant women.

Frequency of Antenatal Appointments

The present pattern of ANC in the UK comprises of the following:

❖ Monthly visits during the first two trimesters (from week 1–32)

❖ Fortnightly visits from 32nd week to 36th week of pregnancy

❖ Weekly visits after 36th week until the baby's birth which usually occurs between weeks 38 and 42.

A nulliparous woman with an uncomplicated pregnancy should at the minimum have at least 10 appointments. For a parous woman with an uncomplicated pregnancy, a schedule of seven appointments is likely to be sufficient.[8] Early in the antenatal period, all women should be provided with appropriate written information regarding the likely number, timing, duration and content of the antenatal appointments. Each antenatal appointment should be structured and have focused content.[9] Longer appointments may be required early in pregnancy to enable the midwife to undertake comprehensive assessment and discussion. Wherever possible, routine tests and investigations must be performed at the time of these appointments.[10]

PRINCIPLES OF MATERNAL RISK ASSESSMENT

Principles of risk assessment are enlisted in Table 3.1. Maternal risk assessment aims at the identification of various medical, obstetric or local risk factors in previous or current pregnancies, which are likely to affect the outcomes of present pregnancy. Specific risks which need to be assessed during pregnancy, include presence of significant medical conditions such as hypertension or diabetes, obstetric risk factors, such as previous history of IUGR, antepartum haemorrhage (APH), etc., and important social issues such as the history of domestic violence. This is likely to influence the frequency and level of ANC which should be provided.[11] The identification of risks may result in incorporation of certain changes in pregnancy management plan. The risk assessment should begin at the booking visit and must be then repeated during

Table 3.1: Principles of maternal risk assessment

Principle	Explanation
Step 1	Identification of hazards, i.e. anything that may cause harm
Step 2	Identifying who may be at a risk and how
Step 3	Assessment of the risks and taking action
Step 4	Making a record of the main findings
Step 5	Reviewing the risk assessment

the second and third trimesters to ensure that the woman is receiving appropriate care.

AIMS

Aims of ANC are as follows:

❖ Provision of high quality information in accordance to the woman's requirements and culture in a format which is easily understood by the woman

❖ Identification and screening for specific maternal and foetal pathologies

❖ Provision of informed choice regarding the pathways of ANC

❖ Diagnosis and treatment of maternal and foetal complications

❖ Assessment of maternal and foetal well-being throughout pregnancy

❖ Provision of advice and education related to the normal symptoms of pregnancy.

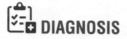 DIAGNOSIS

Clinical Examination

Clinical examination of pregnant women during the antenatal visit should involve the following:

❖ Elicitation of woman's complete medical and obstetric history

❖ Measurement of maternal weight and height at the time of booking appointment

❖ Calculation of the woman's BMI. BMI should be calculated using the given formula [weight (kg)/height(m)^2]

❖ Measurement of mother's blood pressure

❖ Measurement of symphyseal fundal height (SFH) from 24 weeks of gestation onwards[12]

❖ Doppler FHR monitoring

❖ Blood and urine tests of the mother.

Breast Examination

Routine breast examination during ANC for the promotion of postnatal breastfeeding is not recommended.

Abdominal Examination

❖ Symphysis fundal height should be measured and recorded at each antenatal appointment from 24 weeks onwards.[12] The SFH is measured from the woman's pubic bone to the top of the uterus. Plotting the SFH on growth chart can help in the detection of small for gestational age (SGA) babies.

❖ Foetal presentation should be assessed by abdominal palpation at 36 weeks or later, when presentation is likely to influence the mode of delivery. Routine assessment of presentation by abdominal palpation should preferably not be performed before 36 weeks because it is not always accurate and may be uncomfortable to the mother. Ultrasound examination must be used for confirming cases of suspected foetal malpresentations.

Pelvic Examination

Routine pelvic examination during the antenatal period is not recommended because it does not accurately assess gestational age or cephalopelvic disproportion. It also does not accurately predict preterm birth.

Investigations

❖ *Haemoglobin levels*: Pregnant women should be offered screening for anaemia early in pregnancy (at the time of booking appointment) and then at 28 weeks when other blood screening tests are being performed. This allows enough time for treatment if anaemia is detected. The normal UK range for haemoglobin levels during early pregnancy is 11 g per 100 mL and 10.5 g per 100 mL at 28 weeks. Haemoglobin levels outside this range should be investigated and iron supplementation may be prescribed if deemed appropriate.

❖ *Blood grouping and red-cell alloantibodies*: Women should be offered testing for blood group and rhesus D status in early pregnancy. It is recommended that routine antenatal anti-D prophylaxis be offered to all non-sensitised pregnant women who are rhesus D-negative.

❖ *Ultrasound examination*: Ultrasound examination should be used for the accurate assessment of gestational age early during pregnancy between 10^{+0} weeks and 13^{+6} weeks. During this period of gestation, crown-rump length measurement should be used for determining the gestational age. If the crown-rump length is above 84 mm, head circumference should be used for estimating the gestational age. Ultrasound examination is also used for screening of foetal abnormalities during 18^{+0} to 20^{+6} weeks of gestation.[13]

❖ *Urine test*: At the time of booking appointment, urine tests for determination of proteinuria and asymptomatic bacteriuria must be performed.

Screening Tests

At the time of booking appointment (preferably before 10 weeks), arrangements must be made for screening of the following: haemoglobinopathies, foetal anomalies, infection [HIV, hepatitis B virus (HBV), rubella susceptibility and syphilis], pre-eclampsia and gestational diabetes.

Screening for haemoglobinopathies: Screening for various haemoglobinopathies should be offered to all women as early as possible, preferably by 10 weeks during pregnancy. Screening for haemoglobinopathies such as thalassaemias and sickle cell anaemia has been described in Chapter 14 (Anaemia and Other Haematological Abnormalities).

Screening for foetal anomalies: Biochemical screening for Down's syndrome has been described in details in Chapter 4 (Biochemical and Ultrasound Screening for Foetal Anomalies). Screening for Down's syndrome should be offered during the first trimester between 11^{+0} weeks and 13^{+6} weeks using the 'combined test' (measurement of nuchal translucency,

β-human chorionic gonadotropin and pregnancy-associated plasma protein-A).[13] For women who book later in pregnancy, the most clinically and cost-effective serum screening test (triple or quadruple test) should be offered between 15^{+0} weeks and 20^{+0} weeks.

Screening for gestational diabetes: Testing for gestational diabetes in form of a 2-hour 75 g oral glucose tolerance test (OGTT) at 24–28 weeks must be offered to women having risk factors described in Chapter 15 (Diabetes Mellitus and Gestational Diabetes).[14]

Screening for pre-eclampsia: Measurement of blood pressure and urinalysis for protein should be performed during each antenatal visit to screen for pre-eclampsia. Various risk factors for pre-eclampsia are described in Chapter 7 (Hypertensive Disorders during Pregnancy). At the time of booking appointment, the patient should be evaluated for presence of risk factors for pre-eclampsia. Blood pressure should be measured more frequently in pregnant women who have any of the risk factors.[15] Increased surveillance is required in presence of significant hypertension and/or proteinuria.

Screening for preterm birth: Routine screening for preterm labour is usually not offered.

Screening for placenta praevia: Woman whose placenta extends over the internal cervical os at the time of routine anomaly scan should be offered another TAS at 32 weeks. If the TAS is unclear, a TVS should be offered.

Screening for infection: Routine antenatal serological screening is done for various infections such as hepatitis B, HIV, syphilis and rubella [refer to Chapter 20 (Infection during Pregnancy) for details].

❖ *Screening for hepatitis B*: Screening for hepatitis B during pregnancy has been a part of the routine screening programme in the UK since 2000. If the woman is identified as having an active carrier state, she should be referred to the secondary obstetric care. Here, effective postnatal interventions can be undertaken to reduce the risk of mother-to-child (MTC) transmission. Administration of HBV and immunoglobulins to the baby at birth is likely to reduce the risk of MTC by nearly 95%.

❖ *Screening for HIV infection*: Screening for HIV infection is performed early in pregnancy. This helps in identifying women with asymptomatic infection, initiation of treatment with antiretroviral therapy, arranging referral to appropriate specialist services, planning for labour and delivery, and initiation of treatment for the baby. Use of these strategies has helped in reducing the risk of MTC from over 25% in 1993 to less than 1% presently. In addition to the reduction in the risk of transmission, the number of vaginal deliveries of HIV infected women has increased from 15% to 40%.

❖ *Screening for syphilis:* This should also be offered to all the women at the time of booking appointment. This is especially important because MTC of syphilis during pregnancy is associated with neonatal deaths, severe growth restriction and foetal hydrops. Moreover, congenital syphilis may be also associated with long-term disability, preterm births and stillbirths. Effective treatment in the form of parenteral administration of penicillin is available for treatment of pregnant women and successfully helps in preventing MTC.

❖ *Screening for susceptibility to rubella infection*: Pregnant women must be screened for testing their susceptibility to rubella infection early in pregnancy. This would help in the identification of women who are at the risk of contracting rubella infection. Such women must be vaccinated in the postnatal period so that the future pregnancies may be protected from congenital rubella infection.

 MANAGEMENT

Nutritional Advice

❖ *Diet*: It is important to take a healthy, well-balanced diet during pregnancy.[16] Women should be advised that they are likely to gain between 10 kg to 12.5 kg (22–28 lb) of weight during their pregnancy.[17] However, this is likely to vary from woman to woman and it is dependent on the pre-pregnancy weight.

❖ *Nutritional supplements*: Pregnant women and those planning pregnancy should be advised that dietary supplementation with folic acid in the dosage of 400 µg per day, before conception and throughout during the first 12 weeks of gestation helps in reducing the risk of neural tube defects in the baby.

❖ *Iron supplements*: Iron supplementation is not routinely offered to all pregnant women unless the woman is anaemic. Iron supplementation does not prove beneficial either to the mother or the baby. Rather, it may produce unpleasant side effects in the mother.

❖ *Vitamin D supplementation*: All pregnant women at the time of their booking appointment must be informed about the importance of maintaining adequate stores of vitamin D during pregnancy and breastfeeding for their own as well as their baby's health. Women should be advised to take 10 µg of vitamin D per day, as found in the 'Healthy Start multivitamin supplements'.[16] These vitamins contain appropriate amount of recommended dosage of vitamins A, C and D for children aged from 6 months to 4 years. It also contains the appropriate amount of folic acid and vitamins C and D for pregnant and breastfeeding women. Pregnant women, women with a child under 12 months and children aged from 6 months to 4 years who are eligible for 'Healthy Start benefit' are entitled to free 'Healthy Start vitamins'. Women who are not eligible for the 'Healthy Start benefit' should be advised from where they can buy vitamin D supplements. Care must also be taken to identify the risk factors in a woman, which may be associated with an increased risk of developing vitamin D deficiency. Some of these include:
  - Women with darker skin (such as those of African, African-Caribbean or South Asian ethnic origin)

  - Women who have limited exposure to sunlight, such as women who are confined indoors inside their houses for long periods, or those who cover their skin for cultural reasons.

❖ *Prescribed medicines*: Prescription medicines should be used as less as possible during pregnancy. Their use should be limited to the circumstances where the benefits outweigh the risk. Pregnant women should be informed that only a few over-the-counter medicines or complementary therapies have been established as being safe for use during pregnancy. Therefore, over-the-counter medicines and complementary therapies should be used as little as possible during pregnancy.

❖ *Exercise in pregnancy*: Pregnant women should be educated that beginning or continuing a moderate course of exercise during pregnancy is not associated with adverse outcomes. They should be, however, informed about the potential dangers of certain high-impact sports activities during pregnancy, e.g. contact sports, high-impact sports, vigorous racquet sports, scuba diving, etc. These activities may be associated with risks such as abdominal trauma, falls, excessive joint stress, etc. Sports activities such as scuba diving may result in foetal birth defects and foetal decompression disease.

❖ *Sexual intercourse in pregnancy*: Pregnant woman should also be informed that sexual intercourse in pregnancy is not known to be associated with any adverse outcomes. Sexual intercourse should be avoided in presence of conditions such as placenta praevia, premature rupture of membranes, etc.

❖ *Alcohol consumption in pregnancy*: Pregnant women and women planning a pregnancy should be advised to avoid alcohol consumption during the first 3 months of pregnancy due to an increased risk of miscarriage. However, if woman does choose to drink alcohol during pregnancy, she should be advised to consume no more than 1–2 UK units once or twice a week [1 unit equals half a pint of ordinary strength lager or beer, or one shot (25 mL) of spirits. One small (125 mL) glass of wine is equal to 1.5 UK units]. Women should be informed that getting drunk or binge drinking during pregnancy (defined as more than 5 standard drinks or 7.5 UK units on a single occasion) may be harmful to the unborn baby. Adverse effects of alcohol on the baby are described in details in Chapter 22 (Alcohol and Drug Usage during Pregnancy).

❖ *Smoking in pregnancy*: The adverse effects of smoking to the unborn child and the hazards of exposure to second-hand smoke must be explained to the mother during her booking appointment [refer to Chapter 21 (Smoking during Pregnancy) for details]. The benefits of quitting at any stage should be emphasised to the woman and she should be offered personalised information, advice and support regarding quitting smoking, including the risks and benefits of nicotine replacement therapy (NRT) and nicotine patches. The pregnant woman should be advised to use local NHS 'Stop Smoking Services' and the NHS 'pregnancy smoking helpline', by providing details about accessing these services.[18] The midwife should consider

PART II

visiting the pregnant women at home if it is difficult for them to attend specialist services.

Cannabis use is associated with smoking, which is known to be harmful during pregnancy. Therefore, pregnant women should be discouraged from using cannabis during pregnancy. The direct effects of cannabis on the foetus are not known for certain, but are likely to be harmful.

Travelling during Pregnancy

❖ *Air travel during pregnancy*: Pregnant women should be informed to avoid long-haul air travel during pregnancy because it may be associated with an increased risk of venous thrombosis.[19] Use of correctly fitted compression stockings may be helpful in reducing this risk. Pregnant women should also be informed that if they are planning to travel abroad, they should discuss details such as flying, vaccinations and travel insurance with their midwife or doctor.

❖ *Car travel during pregnancy*: Pregnant women should be informed about the correct use of seatbelts, i.e. three-point seatbelts 'above and below the bump, and not over it'.

Management of Common Symptoms of Pregnancy

❖ *Nausea and vomiting in early pregnancy*: Women should be informed that most women might experience nausea and vomiting during the first trimester. However, in most cases this usually resolves spontaneously within 16–20 weeks. Moreover, nausea and vomiting is not generally associated with a poor pregnancy outcome. If a woman requests treatment, the following interventions appear to be effective in reducing symptoms:
  • *Non-pharmacological*: Ginger and P6 (wrist) acupressure
  • *Pharmacological*: Antihistaminic drugs.

❖ *Heartburn*: Women presenting with symptoms of heartburn during pregnancy should be offered information regarding modification of their lifestyle and diet. If the heartburn remains bothersome despite the modifications in lifestyle and diet, she should be offered antacids.

❖ *Constipation*: Women who present with constipation in pregnancy should be offered information regarding dietary modifications, such as supplementation with bran or wheat fibre.

❖ *Haemorrhoids*: In case of pregnant woman presenting with haemorrhoids, she should be offered information concerning dietary modification because presently, there does not appear to be any effective treatment available for management of haemorrhoids during pregnancy. If clinical symptoms remain problematic, standard haemorrhoid creams may be prescribed.

❖ *Varicose veins*: Women should be informed that varicose veins are a common symptom of pregnancy, which is unlikely to cause any harm. Use of compression stockings is likely to cause an improvement in the symptoms. However, it will not prevent new varicose veins from emerging.

❖ *Vaginal discharge*: Women should be informed that an increase in vaginal discharge is a common physiological change that occurs during pregnancy. Investigations may be required if there are signs of infection such as itch, soreness, offensive smelling discharge, painful micturition, etc. A weekly course of a topical imidazole may be prescribed in cases of vaginal candidiasis during pregnancy. The effectiveness and safety of oral treatments for vaginal candidiasis in pregnancy are uncertain and these treatments should not be offered.

❖ *Backache*: Women should be informed that mild to moderate level exercises, swimming, massage therapy, and group or individual back care classes might help in providing relief from backache during pregnancy.

❖ *Female genital mutilation*: Pregnant women who have had female genital mutilation in the past should be identified early in the course of ANC by sensitively tackling this issue. Intrapartum care should be planned based on the findings of antenatal examination.

❖ *Domestic violence*: Healthcare professionals need to be alert regarding the symptoms or signs of domestic violence and women should be given the opportunity to reveal about domestic violence in an environment in which they feel secure.[20]

❖ *Working during pregnancy*: Pregnant women should be informed about their maternity rights and benefits. The majority of women can be reassured that it is safe to continue working during pregnancy. Further information about possible occupational hazards during pregnancy is available from the Health and Safety Executive. A woman's occupation during pregnancy should be ascertained to identify those who are at an increased risk through occupational exposure.

Antenatal Foetal Monitoring

❖ There is no requirement for the routine formal counting of foetal movements.

❖ Routine auscultation of the foetal heart is not recommended because it is unlikely to have any predictive value. However, it can be done if requested by the mother. In these cases auscultation of the foetal heart is likely to provide reassurance to the mother.

❖ The current evidence also does not support the routine use of antenatal electronic FHR monitoring (cardiotocography) for foetal assessment in women with an uncomplicated pregnancy. This is therefore not offered in uncomplicated cases.

❖ The available evidence also does not support the routine use of ultrasound scanning after 24 weeks of gestation in uncomplicated cases and therefore should not be offered.

Provision of Antenatal Information

Information during pregnancy should be given in a form that is easy to understand and accessible to normal pregnant women as well to those with additional needs, such as physical, sensory or learning disabilities, and to pregnant women who cannot speak or read English. Information during the antenatal period should be provided to pregnant women according to the schedule described in Table 3.2.[1]

CHAPTER 3

Table 3.2: Schedule for providing information to women during the antenatal period[1]

At the time of first contact with the healthcare professional	At the time of booking appointment (preferably by 10 weeks)	Before or at 36 weeks	At 38 weeks
• Folic acid supplementation • Food hygiene, including the methods for reducing the risk of a food-acquired infection (e.g. listeriosis, salmonella infection, etc.) • Lifestyle advice, including cessation of smoking, alcohol and recreational drug use • All antenatal screening, including screening for haemoglobinopathies, the foetal anomaly scan, screening for Down's syndrome, screening for infection as well as informing the patient about risks and benefits of the screening tests	• Development of the baby during pregnancy • Advice related to nutrition and diet, including supplementation with vitamin D and details of the 'Healthy Start programme' • Exercise, including pelvic floor exercises • Place of birth • Pregnancy care pathway • Breastfeeding, including workshops • Participant-led antenatal classes • Further discussion of all antenatal screening • Discussion related to the mental health issues	• Information related to breastfeeding, including the technique and good management practices which would help a woman to be able to successfully breastfeed • Preparation for labour and birth, including information about coping with pain in labour and the birth plan • Recognition of signs of active labour • Care of the newborn baby • Prophylaxis with vitamin K • Newborn screening tests • Postnatal self-care • Awareness of mental health issues such as 'baby blues' and postnatal depression	• Options for management of prolonged pregnancy • Supplementation of the information provided at 36 weeks

The information provided to the patient can be further supported by providing information booklets such as 'The pregnancy book' (Department of Health, 2007). Other relevant source of information includes the publications by the UK National Screening Committee and the Midwives Information and Resource Service (MIDIRS).

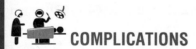

COMPLICATIONS

Pregnancy is a unique physiological condition, which may be associated with complications due to pre-existing medical conditions or those which are specific to gestation itself. Such various complications have been described in Sections 3 (Medical Disorders during Pregnancy) and 4 (Complications Specific to Pregnancy) of this book.

CLINICAL PEARLS

❖ A system of clear referral paths should be established during the antenatal period so that pregnant women who require additional care are managed and treated by the appropriate specialist teams when problems are identified.

❖ Recognition of various risk factors early in pregnancy is important for the success of antenatal, intrapartum and postnatal care planning.

❖ The risk of listeriosis during pregnancy can be reduced by advising the pregnant woman to drink only pasteurised milk and avoiding the consumption of ripened soft cheese such as Camembert, Brie and blue-veined cheese, pâté and uncooked or undercooked ready-prepared meals. There is no risk with hard cheeses, such as Cheddar, or cottage cheese and processed cheese.

❖ The risk of salmonella infection can be reduced by avoiding the consumption of raw or partially cooked eggs, partly cooked meat (especially poultry) or foodstuffs likely to contain this bacteria (e.g. mayonnaise).

EVIDENCE-BASED MEDICINE

❖ Ultrasound estimation of foetal size for suspected large-for-gestational-age unborn babies should not be undertaken during the antenatal period in a low-risk population.[14]

❖ Routine Doppler ultrasound should not be used in low-risk pregnancies.[1,2]

REFERENCES

1. National Institute of Clinical Excellence (NICE). (2016). Antenatal care for uncomplicated pregnancies. NICE clinical guideline CG68. [online] NICE Website. Available from https://www.nice.org.uk/guidance/cg62 [Accessed August, 2016].
2. Department of Health. Changing Childbirth. Report of expert maternity group. London: HMSO; 1993.
3. Department of Health. Maternity Matters, Choice, Access and Continuity of Care in a Safe Service. London: Department of Health; 2006.
4. WHO, UNICEF, UNFPA, World Bank Group and the United Nations Population Division. Trends in Maternal Mortality: 1990 to 2015. Geneva: WHO; 2015.
5. National Collaborating Centre for Woman's and Children's Health. Antenatal care: Routine care for healthy pregnant women. NICE clinical guidelines No. 62, CG062. London: NICE; 2016.

6. Sandall J, Soltani H, Gates S, Shennan A, Devane D. Midwife-led continuity models versus other models of care for childbearing women. Cochrane Database Syst Rev. 2016;(4): CD004667.

7. Brown HC, Smith HJ, Mori R, Noma H. Giving women their own case notes to carry during pregnancy. Cochrane Database Syst Rev. 2015;(10):CD002856.

8. Villar J, Carroli G, Khan-Neelofur D, Piaggio G, Gülmezoglu M. Patterns of routine antenatal care for low-risk pregnancy. Cochrane Database Syst Rev. 2001;(4):CD000934.

9. Dowswell T, Carroli G, Duley L, Gates S, Gülmezoglu AM, Khan-Neelofur D, Piaggio GG. Alternative versus standard package of antenatal care for low risk pregnancy. Cochrane Database Syst Rev. 2010 Oct 6;(10):CD000934.

10. Carroli G, Villar J, Piaggio G, Khan-Neelofur D, Gülmezoglu M, Mugford M, et al. WHO systematic review of randomised controlled trials of routine antenatal care. Lancet. 2001; 357(9268):1565-70.

11. Mbuagbaw L, Medley N, Darzi AJ, Richardson M, Habiba Garga K, Ongolo-Zogo P. Health system and community level interventions for improving antenatal care coverage and health outcomes. Cochrane Database Syst Rev. 2015;(12):1-157.

12. Robert Peter J, Ho JJ, Valliapan J, Sivasangari S. Symphysial fundal height (SFH) measurement in pregnancy for detecting abnormal fetal growth. Cochrane Database Syst Rev. 2015; (9):CD008136.

13. UK National Screening Committee. Fetal Anomaly Screening Programme Standards 2015-16. London: Public Health England; 2016.

14. National Institute of Clinical Excellence (NICE). Diabetes in pregnancy: management from preconception to the postnatal period. NICE guideline NG3. London: NICE; 2015.

15. National Institute of Clinical Excellence (NICE). Hypertension in pregnancy: diagnosis and management. NICE clinical guideline CG107. London: NICE; 2010.

16. National Institute of Clinical Excellence (NICE). Maternal and child nutrition. NICE guideline PH11. London: NICE; 2008.

17. National Institute of Clinical Excellence (NICE). Weight management before, during and after pregnancy. NICE guideline PH27. London: NICE; 2010.

18. National Institute of Clinical Excellence (NICE). Smoking: stopping in pregnancy and after childbirth. NICE guideline PH 26. London: NICE; 2010.

19. Royal College of Obstetricians and Gynecologists (RCOG). Thrombosis and Embolism during Pregnancy and the Puerperium, Reducing the Risk (Green-top Guideline No. 37a). London: RCOG; 2009.

20. National Institute of Clinical Excellence (NICE). Pregnancy and complex social factors: a model for service provision for pregnant women with complex social factors. Clinical guideline CG110. London: NICE; 2010.

CHAPTER 3

Biochemical and Ultrasound Screening for Foetal Anomalies

BIOCHEMICAL SCREENING

BIOCHEMICAL SCREENING FOR NEURAL TUBE DEFECTS

Neural tube defects (NTDs) are a group of defects characterised by the presence of an opening in the spinal cord or brain starting from an early period of human development, e.g. spina bifida, anencephaly, encephalocoele, etc. These lesions may occur anywhere along the spine but are more common in the lumbar and sacral regions. Spina bifida is a congenital defect of the spine resulting from the failure of closure of the neural tube at 3–4 gestational weeks. In cases where the meninges protrude through this defect, it is called a meningocele, and if neural tissue is involved, it is known as a myelomeningocele. The ultrasound diagnosis of spina bifida is based on the evaluation of the foetal spine, which is usually visualised clearly by 16 weeks of gestation in the majority.

In the present time with the widespread use of ultrasound, α-foetoprotein (AFP) screening has a minor role in the detection of foetal NTDs. Though raised level of maternal serum α-foetoprotein (MSAFP) has a good sensitivity, but poor specificity for detection of open neural defects, it is commonly used in areas with a high prevalence of NTDs.[1] In presence of NTDs, ultrasound examination may show the 'lemon sign', in which the foetal frontal bones are distorted. It may also show the 'banana sign' in which shape of the cerebellum is altered. Polyhydramnios may also be associated with NTDs. Children with spina bifida are at risk of having a neuropathic bladder and hence urinary incontinence.

Folic acid taken periconceptually is likely to reduce the incidence of NTDs by approximately 70%. There is evidence that it also reduces the risk of other congenital abnormalities. The recommended dose of folic acid for low-risk women is 400 µg daily. It should be started preconception and continued until at least 12 weeks postconception. High-risk individuals should be prescribed 5 mg of folic acid daily. Folic acid is thought to at least reduce the risk by 50%, but does not eliminate it completely. Fortification of flour with folic acid has been introduced to have good effect in a number of countries. Folic acid fortification of flour has been advocated by many authorities including the RCOG in 1997 and the Committee on Medical Aspects for Food and Nutrition Policy (COMA) in the UK in 2000. COMA recommended fortification of flour in the dosage of 240 µg per 100 g.

Levels of Alpha-foetoprotein

Alpha-foetoprotein, a biochemical marker for NTDs, is a protein produced by the yolk sac and the foetal liver. It crosses into the maternal serum via the placenta. Normal adult level is achieved by 8–12 months. Therefore, accurate determination of gestational age is important before interpreting the measured value of MSAFP. MSAFP levels rise throughout pregnancy, specifically between 12 weeks to 32 weeks of gestation. The optimal time for screening of neural tube disorders is 16–18 weeks. Increased levels of AFP may be associated with other foetal conditions such as multiple pregnancy, spontaneous foetal loss, pre-eclampsia, foetal congenital anomalies such as gastroschisis, exomphalos, bladder exstrophy, congenital nephrosis, and malignancies such as ovarian and testicular malignancies, hepatoma, pregnancy and choriocarcinoma. Occasionally, AFP may be raised in association with breast, pancreatic and secondary hepatic deposits, but levels are usually only slightly elevated. On the other hand, AFP levels may be lowered in conditions such as Down's syndrome (DS), Edwards' syndrome, type 1 diabetes, high maternal weight, etc.

As previously mentioned, increased levels of AFP could be associated with an increased risk of NTDs. An affected parent or an affected sibling is associated with approximately 5% risk, whereas the risk in presence of two affected siblings increases to about 10%. Recurrence risk is also higher for women who have previously given birth to a child with a NTD (2–3%). If there are two previously affected children, the risk is approximately 6%. The prevalence of NTD is estimated to be around 1 in 1,000 births, but there is much racial and geographic variation. For example, prevalence is higher in Wales in comparison to the rest of England. Background levels of MSAFP are higher in Afro-Caribbean women. However, on the contrary, they have a lower incidence of NTDs than Caucasians. Laboratory reports must take this into account. Therefore, once the levels are corrected for ethnicity, Afro-Caribbean women have a reduced risk of NTD. The converse is true of women with insulin-dependent diabetes mellitus (IDDM) and obesity. They have a significantly increased risk of NTD, but lower overall AFP levels.

BIOCHEMICAL SCREENING FOR DOWN'S SYNDROME

Down's syndrome is the most common cause for severe learning disability. Groups at an increased risk of DS include older mothers (>35 years), women who previously gave birth to a baby with DS, parents with a balanced translocation t (14; 21), etc. All pregnant women must be offered screening for DS. DS screening should be discussed at their first encounter with a health professional. Women should be aware that screening is voluntary and should have access to good information about the subject. Informed consent is mandatory before undertaking screening for DS. Screening can be done either in the first trimester or the second trimester.[2] In the early 1980s, increased maternal age (>35 years) was used for antenatal screening. Age-related risk for DS is elaborated in Table 4.1.

Soon after a few years, AFP was the first marker used to improve the age-related risk. The risk of DS is increased by the degree to which the AFP levels lies below the norm. MSAFP levels now form part of the commonly performed triple test. Biochemical screening can be performed both in the first and the second trimesters. However, for the precise utility of these markers, the accurate assessment of the gestational age is important.[3] Also, biochemical screening is applicable only in cases of singleton pregnancies. Due to both these reasons, ultrasound assessment of gestational age becomes mandatory prior to the performance of biochemical tests.

First Trimester Biochemical Screening

First trimester biochemical screening programmes involve the following:
- Assay of pregnancy-associated plasma protein A (PAPP-A) and hCG levels between 8 weeks and 14 weeks of gestation
- Ultrasound for measuring nuchal translucency (NT) is another test for screening in the first trimester (Fig 4.1), which is not good enough to be used on its own.

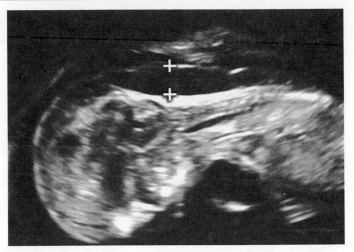

Fig. 4.1: Ultrasound image showing increased nuchal translucency (6.4 mm in this photograph)

In DS the levels of PAPP-A are reduced, whereas the NT is increased. First trimester screening of DS can also be done using increased maternal age and additional ultrasound markers, (e.g. absent nasal bone, reversed a-wave in the ductus venosus and tricuspid regurgitation). A large US-based study of first-trimester DS screening till date, involving 8,514 pregnancies, has shown the detection rate of 79%, with a false positive rate of 5%.[4] Using a combination of both the markers, ultrasound markers as well as the serum markers in the first trimester screening for DS, is likely to be more effective than using either alone. At 11 weeks of gestation, adding the serum markers such as PAPP-A and β-hCG levels to measurement of NT is likely to increase the detection rate of DS from 70% to 87%, at a false positive rate of 5%.[5]

Second Trimester Biochemical Screening

Second trimester biochemical screening programmes involve the following:
- Determination of two components: (1) MSAFP levels and (2) total hCG or free β-hCG
- Determination of three components (triple test): (1) MSAFP, (2) hCG and (3) unconjugated oestriol (UE3) levels
- Determination of four components (quadruple test): (1) MSAFP, (2) hCG, (3) UE3 and (4) inhibin levels.[6]

Second trimester biochemical screening (triple test or quadruple test) is performed in women who were unable to have first trimester combined screening (e.g. late booking) or in cases where the clinician is unable to determine the NT because of high BMI or awkward foetal position. However, since the raised levels of MSAFP are associated with an increased risk for NTDs, triple test also helps in diagnosing the NTDs. One must remember that the pregnancy with raised MSAFP but a normal scan is also a high-risk pregnancy because such pregnancies are associated with an increased risk of IUGR and pregnancy loss. Measurement of different markers in case of various defects is described in Table 4.2. Biochemical screening also gives a risk for Edward's syndrome, (trisomy 18). In this condition, all three main markers AFP, free β-hCG and oestriol levels are low.

CHAPTER 4

Table 4.1: Age-related risk for Down's syndrome

Maternal age (in years)	Risk of Down's syndrome
20	1 in 1,500
35	1 in 350
40	1 in 100
45	1 in 40

Table 4.2: Measurement of different markers in case of various defects

	Alpha-foetoprotein	Unconjugated oestriol	Human chorionic gonadotropin	Inhibin	PAPP-A
Neural tube defects	Increased	—	—	—	—
Down's syndrome	Reduced	Reduced	Increased	Increased	Reduced
Edward's syndrome (Trisomy 18)	Reduced	Reduced	Reduced	—	—
Triploidy	Very high or very low	Low	Very high or very low	—	—

Abbreviation: PAPP, pregnancy-associated plasma protein A

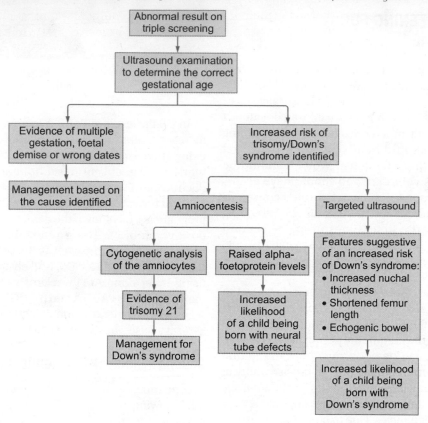

Flow chart 4.1: Management algorithm in case of abnormal results on triple screening tests

As previously mentioned, values of all markers vary with period of gestation. Therefore, multiple of the median (MOM) is used for determining abnormal values of these markers. Second trimester quadruple screening is likely to be associated with a higher false positive rate than first trimester combined screening performed at 11 or 12 weeks.[2]

Management algorithm in case of abnormal results on triple screening tests is described in Flow chart 4.1.

Integrated Screening

More complex options for screening of DS have become available in the present times. These mainly include sequential testing and integrated or hybrid testing. In the sequential testing, screening tests are performed at different times during pregnancy and the results are provided to the patient after each test.[7] On the other hand, integrated screening involves performance of screening tests at different times during pregnancy and a single result is provided to the patient only after all tests have been completed.[7,8]

The results of the FASTER trial (First- and Second-Trimester Evaluation of Risk) have shown high efficacy rates for the first trimester screening for DS. However, the combination of measurements of markers from both the first and the second trimesters is likely to be associated with a higher detection rates and lower false positive rates. Fully integrated screening tests (involving the measurement of NT along with the measurement of serum markers in both the trimesters) were associated with a significantly better performance than either first trimester combined screening or second trimester quadruple screening alone.[2] On the other hand, integrated screening (using the serum markers alone) showed an efficacy similar to that of the first trimester combined screening. This may serve as a useful alternative in cases where the accurate assessment of NT is not possible. The differences in the detection rates between screening tests were not apparent if the false positive rate was set at 5% rather than 1%. According to the SURUSS trial (Serum, Urine and Ultrasound Screening Study), the combined integrated test appears to be most effective and safe method for screening for women who attend in the first trimester.[9] The next best test is the serum integrated test. The quadruple test appears to the best test for women who first attend in the second trimester. There appears to be no good reason for retaining the double or triple tests, or NT alone (with or without maternal age) in antenatal screening for DS.[9]

A major disadvantage associated with an integrated screening is that it prevents the performance of chorionic villus sampling for early definitive diagnosis because the combined results are available only following the measurement of serum markers in the second trimester. On the other hand, with independent sequential screening, first trimester combined screening results are provided immediately. Therefore, women with positive results may decide if they want to undergo chorionic villus sampling.

National Recommendations for Down's Syndrome Screening

According to the current recommendations, a screening test is offered to all women in the UK during early pregnancy to evaluate risk of the baby being born with DS. If the woman's screening test shows that she has a high risk of the baby being born with DS, she may be offered a prenatal diagnostic test. The two main prenatal diagnostic tests, which are available, include amniocentesis and chorionic villus sampling [for details, refer to Chapter 5 (Invasive Prenatal Diagnosis)]. All pregnant women must be preferably offered first trimester screening by 13[+6] weeks). However, if first trimester screening could not be performed, provision should be there to perform screening as late as 20[+0] weeks. Ideally the combined first trimester screening (NT along with serum markers PAPP-A and hCG) should be offered between 11[+0] weeks and 13[+6] weeks of gestation. For women who present for screening in the second trimester, the clinically most effective test (triple test or quadruple test) can be performed between 15[+0] weeks and 20[+0] weeks.

Preimplantation Genetic Diagnosis

Preimplantation genetic screening is increasingly used in embryos produced by IVF prior to implantation. It is particularly used for the detection of X-linked disorders, single gene defects or chromosomal abnormalities. The conditions screened for include cystic fibrosis, Tay–Sachs disease, haemophilia, fragile X syndrome, etc. It is primarily used in women above 35 years of age, when semen has been obtained using intracytoplasmic sperm injection (ICSI) and when there are particular genetic disorders. Preimplantation genetic diagnosis (PIGD) is used to diagnose abnormalities in a fertilised egg before it is implanted in the mother's uterus. One or two cells are removed from the surface of the blastocyst and the removed cells are subjected to a molecular analysis—PCR, fluorescent in situ hybridisation, etc. Therefore, this technique cannot be performed in natural conceptions. This process can prevent the transmission of sex-linked diseases by eliminating all male embryos. This technique is currently available to couples whose offspring are at a high risk (25–50%)

for a specific genetic condition due to one or both parents being carriers or affected by the disease. The limiting factor, however, is that few cells (usually only one to two) are available for diagnosis unlike that following amniocentesis or chorionic villus sampling.

CLINICAL PEARLS

❖ A dating scan is essential prior to the screening for DS.
❖ Measurement of a combination of markers in both the first and the second trimesters is likely to provide the best screening performance for DS.
❖ All pregnant women in the UK must be offered a combined first trimester screening (NT along with serum markers, PAPP-A and hCG)
❖ Mid-trimester screening for DS is also widely available in the UK. Detection rate for DS may vary depending on the markers used.
❖ Patient counselling both after and before the screening tests is extremely important.

EVIDENCE-BASED MEDICINE

❖ The available evidence supports the use of combined first trimester screening for evaluating the risk for DS. Stepwise sequential screening and fully integrated screening are both associated with high detection rates and acceptable false positive rates. The sequential screening is associated with an advantage of earlier diagnosis. This needs to be weighed against the lower false positive rate obtained with integrated screening.[2,9,10]
❖ Present evidence indicates that high-resolution ultrasound is associated with a better detection rate than MSAFP for open NTDs.[1]

ULTRASOUND SCREENING

EARLY PREGNANCY SCAN

The first scan in early pregnancy, referred to as a booking scan, must preferably be undertaken before 15 weeks of gestation. This scan helps in the accurate estimation of the gestational age, foetal viability, number of foetuses and gross foetal anomalies. In case of multiple pregnancies, it also helps in determining the chorionicity or amnionicity.

Routine Ultrasound Scan at 18 to 20[+6] Weeks

A routine ultrasound examination for assessment of congenital anomalies in the UK is recommended between 18 to 20[+6] weeks of gestation. The '20 week' scan offered by a particular antenatal unit should have a minimum standard, which has been summarised in Box 4.1.[11] This information should also be provided to the woman in the form of a leaflet.

Box 4.1: Minimum standard for a '20 week' anomaly scan[11]

❏ *Transverse section through foetal head*: Evaluation of the head shape and internal structures [cavum pellucidum, cerebellum ventricular size at atrium (<10 mm)]
❏ *Spine*: Longitudinal, transverse and coronal views
❏ *Foetal abdomen*: Longitudinal and transverse views (abdominal shape and content at level of stomach)
❏ *Foetal abdomen*: Longitudinal and transverse views (abdominal shape and content at level of kidneys and umbilicus)
❏ Renal pelvis (<5 mm anteroposterior measurement)
❏ *Longitudinal axis*: Abdominal-thoracic appearance (diaphragm/bladder)
❏ *Thorax (transverse view)*: To examine the four-chamber cardiac view and outflow tracts
❏ *Arms*: Three bones and hand (not counting fingers)
❏ *Legs*: Three bones and foot (not counting toes)
❏ Face and lips

Table 4.3: Presence of soft markers on ultrasound examination[12]

Normal variants whose presence does not require further assessment	Soft markers whose presence requires further assessment
• Choroid plexus cyst(s) • Dilated cisterna magna • Echogenic foci in the heart • Two vessel cord	• Nuchal fold (>6 mm) • Ventriculomegaly (atrium >10 mm) • Echogenic bowel (with density equivalent to bone) • Renal pelvic dilatation (antero-posterior measurement >7 mm) • Small measurements compared to dating scan (significantly <5th centile on national charts)

If not previously determined, gestational age can be determined at the time of this scan by measurement of biparietal diameter, head circumference and femur length. The inclusion of abdominal circumference during this scan is optional.

Some minor abnormalities can be identified on ultrasound examination. They were previously known as the soft markers. The term 'soft markers' is no longer used for some of these abnormalities. Instead Foetal Anomaly Screening Programme, UK (FASP) recommends the use of term 'normal variant' (Table 4.3). Women who had been found to be 'lower risk' through testing in either first or second trimesters, or who have declined screening for DS need not be referred for further assessment of chromosomal abnormality even if some normal variants are identified on ultrasound examination. However, there are some ultrasound abnormalities whose presence requires referral for further assessment and treatment (Table 4.3).[12]

Cardiac Anomalies

A transverse section through the foetal chest is likely to demonstrate a four-chamber view. Various cardiac malformations which can be identified on ultrasound scan are listed in Table 4.4. The detection rate for cardiac anomalies varies between 6% to 77%.[13] Addition of the ventricular outlet views to the four-chamber assessment of the heart during the routine foetal anomaly scans between 18 weeks to 22

Table 4.4: Cardiac malformations identified on a four-chamber view

Abnormal four-chamber view	Normal four-chamber view
• Hypoplastic left heart • Hypoplastic right heart • Atrioventricular canal defects • Large ventricular septal defects • Single ventricle • Valve stenosis or atresia • Ebstein's anomaly • Cardiac tumours • Cardiac situs abnormalities	• Interpositioning of the great vessels • Small atrial and ventricular septal defects • Mild stenosis of pulmonary or aortic valves • Mild coarctation of the aorta

weeks is likely to increase the efficacy for prenatal detection of congenital heart disease (CHD).[14]

Thoracic Malformations

These include space occupying solid or cystic lesions of the foetal lungs. Pleural effusion within the pleural cavity may be identified as a result of certain foetal conditions. Cystic lesions of lungs which can be commonly identified include bronchogenic cysts and congenital cystic adenomatous malformations of the lungs (there is overgrowth of terminal bronchioles). Other thoracic malformations which can be identified on ultrasound examination include diaphragmatic hernia, Potter's syndrome, chylothorax, exstrophy of the cloaca, prune-belly syndrome, cystic hygroma, short rib polydactyly syndrome, etc.[15] In foetuses with congenital diaphragmatic hernia, cystic structures may be demonstrated within the chest due to herniation of stomach or other abdominal organs above the level of diaphragm.

Gastrointestinal and Abdominal Wall Malformations

Ultrasound examination may show ventral wall defects such as gastroschisis (paraumbilical defect) and exomphalos (central defect). Both these defects may be associated with elevated levels of MSAFP. Presence of multiple gastrointestinal and abdominal wall malformations is more likely to be associated with abnormal karyotypes in comparison to isolated defects. The prognosis for both these malformations is good with surgical repair when this defect occurs in isolation.[16] On the other hand, prognosis for defects such as large bowel obstruction or absent stomach is relatively poor.

Other intra-abdominal pathologies which may be identified on ultrasound examination include foetal ascites, small and large bowel obstruction, meconium peritonitis, cysts of mesentery, omentum and retroperitoneum, etc.

Urogenital Malformations

The foetal urinary tract can be visualised ultrasonically from 11 weeks onwards. Many foetal renal anomalies are associated with disturbances in amniotic fluid volume. Majority of amniotic fluid is produced by the foetal kidneys by 16 weeks of gestation. Presence of oligohydramnios in the mid-trimester in the absence of the history of rupture of membranes is indicative of renal malformations.

Table 4.5: Structural anomalies of the skeleton which can be identified on the ultrasound examination

Generalised skeletal dysplasias (osteochondrodysplasias)	Localised skeletal anomalies
• Achondrogenesis	• Radial anomalies
• Thanatophoric dysplasia	• Talipes equinovarus
• Fibrochondrogenesis	• Femoral hypoplasia
• Achondroplasia	• Facial clefts
• Osteogenesis imperfecta	• Digital anomalies

Bilateral renal agenesis can be identified on ultrasound examination and shows features such as empty renal fossae, absent filling of the bladder, along with severe oligohydramnios or anhydramnios. A commonly encountered autosomal recessive disease in foetuses is infantile polycystic kidneys. On ultrasound examination, there is presence of bilateral enlarged hyperechogenic kidneys, absent foetal bladder, associated oligohydramnios, etc. This condition is associated with poor prognosis.

Obstructive uropathy may occur due to the obstruction at the urethra or in the ureters. Urethral obstruction can occur due to urethral atresia, posterior urethral valves, etc. In these cases, the foetal bladder may be distended.[17] Hydroureter and hydronephrosis may also be present. In cases of posterior urethral valves, there may be thick bladder walls and a dilated posterior urethra (keyhole sign). Ureter obstruction, on the other hand, can be unilateral or bilateral. There may be presence of hydronephrosis in these cases.

Skeletal Malformations

Complete foetal examination along with skeletal survey is required for the diagnosis of skeletal abnormalities. This involves complete examination of the skull, vertebrae, ribs, long bones and digits of the hand and feet. Malformations of foetal skeleton can be classified into two major categories: generalised skeletal dysplasias which are characterised by abnormalities in multiple bones throughout the foetus; and focal skeletal abnormalities which have a localised pattern of distribution and affect an individual or a small group of bones (Table 4.5).[18,19] Some generalised skeletal dysplasias may even prove lethal especially if there is involvement of thoracic cage, resulting in pulmonary insufficiency or there may be concomitant visceral abnormalities. The localised skeletal abnormalities may often be part of another syndrome, including chromosomal anomalies.

CLINICAL PEARLS

❖ Ultrasound screening of all pregnancies is preferred because nearly 95% of abnormalities may occur in foetuses born to the mothers with no risk.
❖ Anomalies of renal tract may be isolated but can also occur in association with other congenital anomalies. Therefore, if an anomaly of urinary tract is identified, a thorough examination of the other systems is mandatory to exclude other possible genetic disorders.

❖ Prior to the performance of any screening test (biochemical or ultrasound), the parents must be counselled regarding the possible objectives of the screening tests, their limitations and the likely rates of detection with the help of information leaflets.

EVIDENCE-BASED MEDICINE

❖ The present evidence indicates that the ideal time for identification of major structural anomalies in the foetus through ultrasound examination varies between 18 weeks to 21 weeks of gestation.[20,21]
❖ There is no good quality evidence to establish a strong link between ultrasound examination and the possible biological adverse effects of diagnostic ultrasound such as childhood cancer, delayed speech development, reduced birth weight, etc.[22]

REFERENCES

1. Christensen RL, Rea MR, Kessler G, Crane JP, Valdes R. Implementation of a screening program for diagnosing open neural tube defects: selection, evaluation, and utilization of alpha-fetoprotein methodology. Clin Chem. 1986;32(10):1812-7.
2. Malone FD, Canick JA, Ball RH, Nyberg DA, Comstock CH, Bukowski R, et al. First-trimester or second-trimester screening, or both, for Down's syndrome. N Engl J Med. 2005;353(19):2001-11.
3. Wald NJ, Cuckle HS, Densem JW, Kennard A, Smith D. Maternal serum screening for Down's syndrome: the effect of routine ultrasound scan determination of gestational age and adjustment for maternal weight. Br J Obstet Gynaecol. 1992;99(2):144-9.
4. Wapner R, Thom E, Simpson JL, Pergament E, Silver R, Filkins K, et al. First-trimester screening for trisomies 21 and 18. N Engl J Med. 2003;349(15):1405-13.
5. ACOG Practice Bulletin No. 77: screening for fetal chromosomal abnormalities. Obstet Gynecol. 2007;109(1):217-27.
6. Wald NJ, Densem JW, Smith D, Klee GG. Four marker serum screening for Down's syndrome. Prenat Diagn. 1994;14(8):707-16.
7. Wald NJ, Watt HC, Hackshaw AK. Integrated screening for Down's syndrome on the basis of tests performed during the first and second trimesters. N Engl J Med. 1999;341(7):461-7.
8. Wright D, Bradbury I, Benn P, Cuckle H, Ritchie K. Contingent screening for Down syndrome is an efficient alternative to non-disclosure sequential screening. Prenat Diagn. 2004;24(10):762-6.
9. Wald NJ, Rodeck C, Hackshaw AK, Rudnicka A. SURUSS in perspective. BJOG. 2004;111(6):521-31.
10. Benn PA. Advances in prenatal screening for Down syndrome: I. General principles and second trimester testing. Clin Chim Acta. 2002;323(1-2):1-16.
11. Boyd PA, Chamberlain P, Hicks NR. 6-year experience of prenatal diagnosis in an unselected population in Oxford, UK. Lancet. 1998;352(9140):1577-81.
12. UK National Screening Committee. (2015). Fetal Anomaly Screening Programme: programme handbook June 2015. [online] GOV.UK website. Available from www.gov

uk/government/publications/fetal-anomaly-screening programme-handbook [Accessed August, 2016].

13. Kirk JS, Comstock CH, Lee W, Smith RS, Riggs TW, Weinhouse E. Sonographic screening to detect fetal cardiac anomalies: a 5-year experience with 111 abnormal cases. Obstet Gynecol. 1997;89(2):227-32.

14. Carvalho JS, Mavrides E, Shinebourne EA, Campbell S, Thilaganathan B. Improving the effectiveness of routine prenatal screening for major congenital heart defects. Heart. 2002;88(4):387-91.

15. Meizner I, Bar-Ziv J, Insler V. Prenatal ultrasonic diagnosis of fetal thoracic and intrathoracic abnormalities. Isr J Med Sci. 1986;22(5):350-4.

16. Nicolaides KH, Snijders RJ, Cheng HH, Gosden C. Fetal gastro-intestinal and abdominal wall defects: associated malformations and chromosomal abnormalities. Fetal Diagn Ther. 1992;7(2):102-15.

17. Dias T, Sairam S, Kumarasiri S. Ultrasound diagnosis of fetal renal abnormalities. Best Pract Res Clin Obstet Gynaecol. 2014;28(3):403-15.

18. Bowerman RA. Anomalies of the fetal skeleton: sonographic findings. AJR Am J Roentgenol. 1995;164(4):973-9.

19. Krakow D, Lachman RS, Rimoin DL. Guidelines for the prenatal diagnosis of fetal skeletal dysplasias. Genet Med. 2009;11(2):127-33.

20. Whittle MJ. Routine fetal anomaly screening. In: Drife JO, Donnai D (Eds). Antenatal Diagnosis of Foetal Abnormalities. London: Springer-Verlag London; 1991. pp. 35-43.

21. National Institute of Clinical Research. Routine care for healthy pregnant women. Clinical care guidelines No 62. UK: NICE; 2008.

22. Whittle M. Ultrasound screening for foetal anomalies. Report of the RCOG working party. London: RCOG press; 1997.

Invasive Prenatal Diagnosis

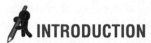

INTRODUCTION

Prenatal testing aims at detecting various anomalies such as structural, chromosomal and genetic disorders in the foetus or the embryo before its birth, while it is still in utero.

Some of these anomalies include neural tube defects, chromosomal anomalies, genetic disorders (cystic fibrosis, Tay-Sachs disease, thalassaemia, sickle cell anaemia, etc.) and other anomalies such as spina bifida, cleft lip, etc. Prenatal diagnostic procedures can be divided into two categories: (1) invasive and (2) non-invasive procedures. Common non-invasive procedures include ultrasound examination and maternal serum screens (e.g. alpha-foetoprotein levels in the serum). The invasive tests include procedures such as amniocentesis, chorionic villus biopsy and cordocentesis. All the three procedures help in providing foetal cells which can be used for determining foetal karyotype. All these three procedures would be discussed in this chapter.

Prenatal diagnostic testing done for foetal karyotyping to identify babies with Down's syndrome most commonly involves amniocentesis at 16–20 weeks of gestation, or chorionic villus sampling (CVS) at 10–12 weeks of gestation.[1,2] The prenatal diagnosis of Down's syndrome by amniocentesis was first reported in 1968[3] and the procedure of CVS was first described later, in the same year.[4] The advantage of the invasive tests over the non-invasive ones is that these tests help in obtaining foetal tissue which would assist in the diagnosis of various chromosomal and genetic disorders of the foetus with the help of various cytogenetics, molecular or biochemical tests. Foetal blood sample obtained through cordocentesis helps in detection of various haematological abnormalities and infections. The choice regarding the exact procedure to be performed is usually based on the period of gestation. CVS is performed at 10–12 weeks, amniocentesis at 16–20 weeks and cordocentesis at 18–24 weeks of gestation. Karyotype evaluation of foetal cells can be done with the help of tests such as fluorescence in situ hybridisation, chromosomal banding, comparative genomic hybridisation (CGH) or array CGH. It is important to inform the patient at the time of counselling, before undertaking any of these prenatal diagnostic cytogenetics tests that even if the results of amniocentesis or CVS report gives finding of normal foetal karyotype and amniotic fluid α-foetoprotein levels are within normal limits, it does not guarantee the birth of a normal newborn. This is so as there are many types of birth defects and mental retardation cases, which might be associated with a normal karyotype. Thus, these defects would be missed on amniocentesis or CVS.

OVERVIEW OF SURGERY

Amniocentesis

Amniocentesis is a prenatal diagnostic procedure, which involves the use of ultrasound-guided, needle-insertion technique for aspiration and sampling of amniotic fluid and is the most common invasive prenatal diagnostic procedure undertaken in the UK.[3]

The procedure of amniocentesis, when performed initially in 1968 was a 'blind' one, involving the palpation of the outline of the uterus and insertion of a needle into the selected spot, with the aim that it would reach the amniotic fluid surrounding the foetus. Amniocytes, obtained from the amniotic fluid are used for cytogenetic and molecular genetics studies. Also, α-foetoprotein levels of amniotic fluid can be determined. Biochemical analysis of amniotic fluid helps in assessment of pulmonary maturity, diagnosis of open neural tube defects and for the assessment of various viral and bacterial infections. Nowadays, this procedure is performed under 'ultrasound guidance', in which the uterine contents and the position of the placenta are visualised prior to the procedure.[3] Amniocentesis has proven to be a safe and effective technique for prenatal diagnosis and can be performed after approximately 11 weeks of gestation. However, it is usually performed between

PART II

15 (15^{+0}) weeks and 17 (17^{+6}) weeks of gestation when the ratio of viable to non-viable cells in the amniotic fluid is the greatest and sufficient amount of amniotic fluid (up to 200–250 mL) is present. Approximately, 15–20 mL of amniotic fluid is aspirated out. Amniocentesis performed before 15 completed weeks of gestation is referred to as 'early amniocentesis'. This helps in providing prenatal diagnosis at an early period of gestation so that if the woman elects to undergo medical termination of pregnancy (MTP) after abnormal results, it can be done easily. However, early amniocentesis may be technically difficult because of reduced amniotic fluid volume. Since the number of amniocytes is fewer at this stage, a longer time may be required to grow an adequate number of cells. Moreover, early amniocentesis performed in the early second trimester has not been shown to be a safe procedure by many research trials.[4] The RCOG has recommended that an early amniocentesis should be undertaken only in exceptional circumstances after the mother has been made fully aware of the potential complications.[5]

Amniocentesis in the third trimester can be carried out for a number of indications, including late karyotyping, amniotic fluid optical density assessments for rhesus disease, amniotic fluid insulin measurements, lung maturity studies (measurement of components of pulmonary surfactant) and detection of indices of suspected preterm labour or ROMs (amniotic fluid fibronectin levels).[6] Amniocentesis in the third trimester is performed under continuous ultrasound guidance. Third-trimester amniocentesis does not appear to be associated with significant risk of emergency delivery. Women should be informed that the third-trimester procedure is associated with a higher rate of complications including multiple attempts and blood-stained fluid in comparison to the mid-trimester procedures.[7-11]

Chorionic Villus Biopsy

Chorionic villus sampling is a prenatal diagnostic technique in which a sample of foetal chorionic tissue is obtained from the chorion frondosum (future placenta) between 11 (11^{+0}) weeks and 13 (13^{+6}) weeks of gestation. CVS should preferably not be performed before 10 (10^{+0}) completed weeks of gestation.

A larger amount of foetal DNA is obtained through CVS in comparison to amniocentesis. With the introduction of first-trimester screening programs, there has been a decline in the rate of CVS, especially amongst women more than 35 years of age. CVS is performed either with the help of a catheter inserted transcervically (transcervical CVS) or a needle inserted transabdominally (transabdominal CVS) under ultrasound guidance. The third type of CVS procedure (transvaginal CVS) is rarely done nowadays. The decision regarding whether CVS is to be performed transabdominally or transcervically is usually made by the obstetrician based on the placental localisation. Majority of CVS procedures are performed by transabdominal route. Since this procedure can be performed during the first trimester, it helps in providing better options for safely terminating a pregnancy. While CVS is commonly performed between 10 weeks to 12 weeks, it can also be performed as early as 6–9 weeks of gestation. However, in order to minimise the teratogenic effects of CVS, it is usually performed from 10 weeks onwards.

Cordocentesis

Cordocentesis, also sometimes called percutaneous umbilical cord blood sampling (PUBS), was performed for the first time in 1974 for diagnosis of haemoglobinopathies. It is a diagnostic test, which aims at detection of foetal anomalies (e.g. blood disorders like haemolytic anaemia, etc.) through direct examination of foetal blood. This test is used for the chromosomal analysis when the period of gestation is so advanced that the tests such as amniocentesis and chorion villus biopsy cannot be carried out. Cordocentesis is usually performed during 18–24 weeks of pregnancy. In cases of foetal anaemia, such as Rh-negative immunised women, and cases of non-immune hydrops, the procedure of cordocentesis helps in estimating the foetal haemoglobin and haematocrit levels. It can be used for the diagnosis of haematological disorders such as thrombocytopenia; diagnosis of congenital infections such as rubella, cytomegalovirus (CMV), toxoplasmosis, etc. and for foetal blood gas analysis. This procedure can also be used for therapeutic purposes such as intrauterine transfusion, drug therapy (in cases of foetal arrhythmias) and for stem cell transplantation.

🐦 INDICATIONS

The indications for various prenatal diagnostic tests are as follows:
- ❖ Advanced maternal age of more than 35 years
- ❖ Family history of genetic disorders/chromosomal anomalies (thalassaemia/haemophilia/Duchenne muscular dystrophy, etc.)
- ❖ History of recurrent miscarriages or stillbirths
- ❖ Ultrasound examination showing presence of congenital anomalies
- ❖ Abnormal results of maternal biochemical screening
- ❖ Early onset intrauterine growth restriction (IUGR) or oligohydramnios of severe degree
- ❖ Maternal congenital infections
- ❖ Exposure to teratogens
- ❖ Amniocentesis in late pregnancy (after 32 weeks) is done for the assessment of foetal lung maturity.

📋 DIAGNOSIS

Investigations

The following investigations must be performed before undertaking any of the prenatal invasive procedure:
- ❖ *Determination of maternal blood group*: Maternal blood group including Rh factor needs to be determined before performing the procedure. If the mother is Rh-negative, she should be administered Rh-immune globulins in order to prevent foetal isoimmunisation.

❖ *Preprocedure ultrasound evaluation*: A comprehensive preprocedure ultrasound examination needs to be performed in order to determine the gestational age, number of gestational sacs, placental localisation, and to rule out multifoetal pregnancy or presence of foetal congenital anomalies. Nowadays, various prenatal diagnostic procedures are usually performed under the 'ultrasound guidance', in which the uterine contents and the position of the placenta are visualised prior to the insertion of needle or catheter and a suitable point on the mother's abdomen for the needle insertion is marked before performing the particular procedure.

❖ *Cervicovaginal cultures*: Cervicovaginal cultures must be obtained prior to transcervical CVS in order to rule out infection with pathogens such as gonorrhoea, chlamydia, group B streptococcus, etc. In case of infection, appropriate antibiotics must be administered.

SURGICAL MANAGEMENT

Preoperative Preparation

Preoperative preparation for all the three procedures is more or less the same and is described here:

❖ *Informed consent*: The procedure should be performed only after the woman has given formal written consent. Use of the Department of Health Consent Form 3 is recommended. Before performing the procedure, the obstetrician must counsel the patient regarding the procedure, indications, advantages, disadvantages, the risks involved to the patient and her baby, and the type of cytogenetic results that would become available.

❖ *Aseptic technique*: Strict asepsis should be maintained at the time of the procedure. After cleaning and draping, the patient is placed in the lithotomy position.

❖ *Local anaesthesia*: Though local anaesthesia is commonly used, there is little evidence regarding the benefit of the use of local anaesthesia or analgesic drugs prior to the procedure.[12]

❖ *Screening tests for blood-borne viruses*: Invasive prenatal procedures should not be carried out without reviewing the reports related to the screening tests of various blood-borne viruses. In cases where women refuse screening for blood-borne viruses, they must be counselled regarding the potential risk of vertical transmission of infection to the foetus. In women who are HIV positive, viral load and treatment regimens must be reviewed prior to performing the invasive prenatal testing.[13-15] If the woman is already on treatment, the clinician must consider delaying the procedure until there is no detectable viral load. Anti-retroviral therapy must be considered prior to prenatal invasive procedures in women not yet on treatment for HIV.

Invasive prenatal testing in the first or second trimester can be carried out in women who are positive for hepatitis B or C.

❖ *Extra preoperative steps in case of cordocentesis*: The following preoperative steps are those, which may be required in cases undergoing cordocentesis:

• *Antenatal glucocorticoids*: Glucocorticoids may be administered at least 24 hours prior to cordocentesis in foetuses between 24 weeks to 34 weeks of gestation in order to enhance foetal lung maturity, in case this has not been previously documented.

• *Intravenous access*: An IV line must be secured in the patient so that she can be administered analgesics, antibiotics and fluids, as required. This may also be required to prepare the patient in the anticipation of procedure-related complications requiring an emergent caesarean delivery.

• *Antibiotic prophylaxis*: Broad-spectrum antibiotic prophylaxis can be administered 30–60 minutes prior to the procedure in order to minimise the risk of intra-amniotic infection, which may sometimes occur after the procedure in case strict asepsis was not maintained during the procedure.

• *Maternal local anaesthesia and sedation*: Local anaesthesia can be optionally used in case of diagnostic procedures. However, it is usually required in cases of therapeutic procedures (e.g. transfusions) to reduce the patient discomfort associated with an increased duration of needle insertion. Maternal sedation is generally not required either for diagnostic or therapeutic procedures.

• *Foetal paralytic drugs*: Restriction of foetal movement is usually not required in cases of diagnostic procedures. However, it may be required in cases of prolonged procedures (e.g. foetal transfusion) where foetal movement is likely to dislodge the needle. In these cases, atracurium (0.4 mg/kg) may be administered intramuscularly in order to produce foetal paralysis for up to an hour, at the same time producing minimal foetal cardiovascular effects.

Surgical Steps

Amniocentesis

❖ The procedure of amniocentesis is described in Figures 5.1A and B. Following the preoperative preparation, the amniocentesis needle is inserted under 'continuous ultrasound control' by using the real-time ultrasound equipment. The current RCOG recommendations are that amniocentesis must be performed under 'continuous ultrasound control' in order to avoid 'bloody taps', because the presence of blood interferes with amniocyte culture.[16-18]

❖ Once the ultrasound examination is complete, sterile preparation of maternal abdomen is done. Since nowadays, the amniocentesis is performed under ultrasonic guidance, the best practice to maintain asepsis during the procedure of amniocentesis is to enclose the ultrasound probe in a sterile bag and to use separate sterile gel for the probe.

❖ The ultrasound scanning during the procedure is usually performed by the same person inserting the needle.

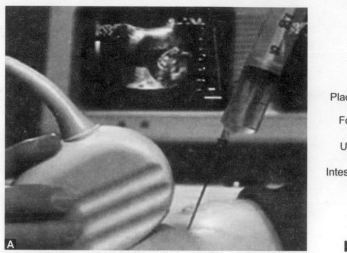
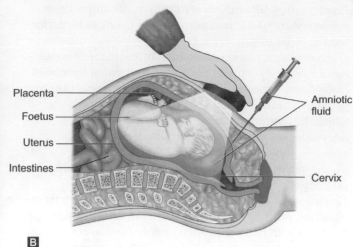

Figs 5.1A and B: (A) Procedure of amniocentesis; (B) Diagrammatic representation of the procedure of amniocentesis

While inserting the needle, the obstetrician must try as much as possible to avoid passing through the placenta. Transplacental passage of the amniocentesis needle should be avoided unless it provides an easy safe access to a pool of liquor.[19-21] Care must be taken to avoid cord insertion. All research studies have emphasised the need to place the needle through the thinnest available part of the placenta. The RCOG has recommended that the outer diameter of the amniocentesis needle used should not be wider than 20 gauge (0.9 mm) and it must be inserted in two rapid, successive steps.[5] A spinal needle having a standard length of 8.9 cm (excluding the hub) is commonly used. Longer needles having a length of 15 cm are also sometimes used. Before the insertion of amniocentesis needle, the area selected for needle insertion should be visualised with colour Doppler to exclude the presence of placental or uterine blood vessels. The point of needle insertion is usually chosen as an area, which shows the presence of a large pocket of amniotic fluid, away from the foetus. Insertion through the placenta must be avoided and the needle tip must be kept away from the foetal face and cord.

❖ On entering the amniotic fluid pocket, the stylet is withdrawn. This causes the amniotic fluid to come out freely through the needle hub. Sometimes, instead of connecting the syringe directly to the needle, a plastic connecting tube is then attached to the needle hub at one end and to a 10 cc plastic syringe at the other end. Presence of the connecting tube helps in preventing abrupt, jerky motion of the needle, thereby preventing foetal needle-related injuries.[22]

❖ A 2-mL syringe is connected to the needle hub. Initial 1–2 mL of fluid, which is withdrawn, is usually discarded due to the possibility of contamination with blood.

❖ Approximately, 15–20 mL of amniotic fluid is then obtained and transferred to the transportation tubes.

❖ The two samples of 10 mL each are taken in two separate aliquots and sent to the laboratory for cytogenetic analysis and α-foetoprotein determination, respectively.

❖ Since the amount of amniotic fluid increases with the increasing period of gestation, a rule of thumb commonly employed for removing an appropriate amount of amniotic fluid is to take a volume (in mL) which is equivalent to the gestational age in weeks (e.g. 17 mL at 17 weeks of gestation).

Chorionic Villus Sampling

There is consensus that CVS, both transabdominal and transcervical, have to be performed under continuous ultrasound control.[5] The two procedures differ from each other in terms of the method of villous aspiration.

Transcervical chorionic villus sampling: The procedure of transcervical CVS is shown in Figure 5.2 and comprises of the following steps:

❖ After the cervix and vagina have been cleaned with an antiseptic solution, a sterile polythene catheter 26 cm long, with an outer diameter of 1.5 mm and a soft stainless steel obturator is inserted inside the endocervical canal so that it lies parallel to the chorion frondosum.

❖ Once the tip of the catheter is in the desirable position, the obturator of the catheter is removed.

❖ Then a 20 mL syringe containing small amount of culture medium is connected to the catheter. The catheter is moved back and forth couple of times, while negative suction pressure is applied to suck in the placental tissue.

❖ The sample of tissue obtained, is sent to the laboratory for cytogenetic analysis.

Transabdominal chorionic villus sampling: This procedure is illustrated in Figure 5.3 and comprises of the following steps:

❖ Under ultrasound guidance, the surgeon visualises the area from where the needle will be punctured. An 18–20 gauge needle, which is 9–12 cm long, with a stylet is used.

❖ The clinician administers local anaesthetic agent around the point of insertion.

❖ Ideally, the area of placenta where needle would be inserted is chosen in such a way that the needle would be

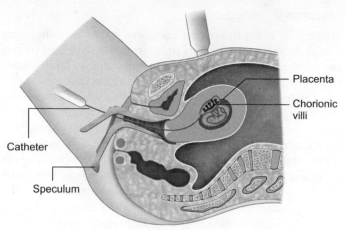

Fig. 5.2: Procedure for transcervical chorionic villus sampling

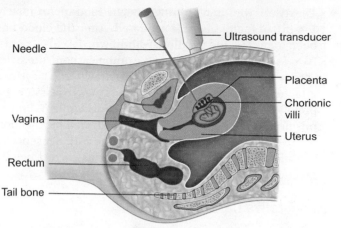

Fig. 5.3: Diagrammatic representation of the procedure of transabdominal chorionic villus sampling

parallel to the long-axis of the placenta. The sampling site is located over the thickest part of the placenta.

❖ The needle is carefully introduced into the placental tissues, taking care not to pierce the amniotic sac. The needle is inserted using a free-hand technique and is slowly moved back and forth a number of times along the chorion frondosum.

❖ A 20-mL syringe containing 1–2 mL of the culture media is attached to the needle, through which the placental tissue is aspirated after application of negative suction pressure. The syringe should fit snugly over the needle in order to create an adequate amount of vacuum.

❖ The needle is rotated several times in order to loosen the villi. Up and down movements are made along the length of placenta about 3–4 times. Villi are slowly aspirated out. Villi with culture medium in the syringe are flushed into a Petri dish and examined.

❖ The aspirated tissue is then sent to the laboratory for analysis. The tissue that gets contaminated with blood, decidua or mucus should be discarded. Irrespective of the route of CVS, the sample must be taken in a strictly sterile container.

Cordocentesis

The procedure of cordocentesis involves the following steps (Fig. 5.4):

❖ A thin needle (20–22 gauge) must be inserted through the abdomen and uterine walls into the umbilical cord under ultrasound guidance. Placental origin of the cord is the best site for cordocentesis. If this site is not accessible, then a full loop of cord can be selected for the puncture. Foetal side of cord should preferably be avoided. Length of the needle is decided on the basis of distance from the skin to the site of puncture.

❖ *Sampling site*: The first step in sampling the umbilical cord is to identify a fixed segment of the cord, preferably where the cord inserts into the placenta. Doppler colour flow ultrasound can be used for confirming the placental cord insertion site. The abdominal insertion site of cord

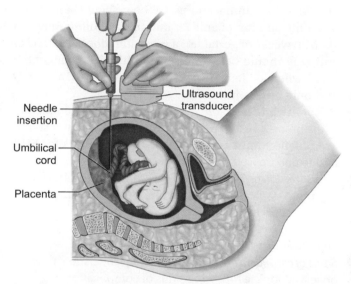

Fig. 5.4: The procedure of cordocentesis

is not chosen because it is likely to become unstable, in case the foetus moves. The main drawback of using the placental insertion site is the possibility of contamination with maternal blood. It is easier and safer to sample the umbilical vein in comparison to the umbilical artery. Moreover, sampling of the umbilical artery is associated with an increased risk of bradycardia and prolonged postprocedural bleeding. The procedure of cordocentesis is easiest when the placenta is anterior; however, this may be associated with an increased risk of foetomaternal haemorrhage (FMH) and foetal loss in case the placenta is penetrated. These complications are less likely to occur in case the placenta is posterior. However, in these cases, the foetus may obstruct access to the target portion of the cord. In these cases, manipulation of the maternal abdomen to move the foetus may help in providing better access to the sampling site.

❖ When the needle tip reaches the cord, a sharp and quick puncture is made over the wall to achieve penetration into the vessel. Tip of the needle can be visualised inside the vessel lumen.

❖ The stylet is withdrawn; syringe attached and approximately 2–4 mL of foetal blood is aspirated. After the blood has been obtained, the needle is withdrawn.

❖ *Blood sample*: Upon entering the umbilical cord, the stylet is removed and foetal blood is withdrawn into a syringe attached to the hub of the needle. The syringe may be preloaded with a small amount of anticoagulant. Proper positioning of the needle can be confirmed by injection of physiological saline solution into the cord. Presence of turbulent flow along the vessel confirms correct needle positioning.

Postoperative Care

The postoperative steps for all the three procedures are more or less the same and involve the following:

❖ *Administration of anti-Rh immunoglobulins*: Any invasive procedure like amniocentesis, CVS, etc. should be followed by administration of anti-Rh immunoglobulins. Between 12 to 20 weeks of gestation, a minimum dose of 250 IU of anti-D Ig should be administered within 72 hours of the event, whereas after 20 weeks of gestation, 500 IU of anti-D Ig should be administered.

❖ *Postprocedural ultrasound examination*: At the completion of the procedure and removal of the needle, an ultrasound examination must be performed again to check for FHR and to ensure well-being of the baby.

❖ *Confirmation of foetal well-being*: Electronic foetal monitoring must be performed after the procedure in order to ensure the foetal well-being. Presence of foetal bradycardia or late decelerations on electronic foetal monitoring may be an indication for emergency caesarean section.

❖ *Signs of complications*: Postoperatively, the patient must be observed for the following signs of complications:
- *Excessive bleeding or discharge per vaginum*: Bleeding is more common following transcervical CVS in comparison to the transabdominal one.
- *Fever*: Fever is more common following transabdominal CVS in comparison to the transcervical one.
- *Bleeding from the puncture site*: In case of cordocentesis, transient bleeding can occur from the puncture site in approximately 10–20% cases. This bleeding is usually self-limiting in nature.

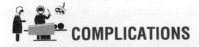

COMPLICATIONS

Amniocentesis

Amniocentesis is a commonly performed invasive procedure. Though it is associated with a low complication rate when performed under ultrasonic guidance, the patients need to be counselled regarding the possibility of a few likely complications. Some of these include, foetal miscarriage, risk of infection, leaking per vaginum, etc. These would be described here in detail.

Miscarriage

One of the most important concerns to both mother and the clinician is the risk of pregnancy loss related to the invasiveness of the procedure. Different studies have shown different rates for spontaneous abortions, with the rates varying from 0.5% to 1% in most cases.[23-27] According to the RCOG guidelines, the rate of miscarriage associated with amniocentesis is approximately 0.5–1% above the normal risk for spontaneous miscarriage among the general population.[5] Some of the factors tend to increase the risk of spontaneous abortion following amniocentesis. These include, increased levels of maternal serum alpha-foetoprotein (MSAFP) before amniocentesis, perforation of the placenta during amniocentesis, withdrawal of discoloured amniotic fluid, avoiding concurrent use of ultrasonic guidance,[22] past histories of one or more previous spontaneous abortions,[29] etc. No statistically significant effect of maternal age or gravidity on the risk of miscarriage following amniocentesis has been detected. The incidence of spontaneous abortion after amniocentesis has been found to be greatest in the first 3 weeks following the procedure.

Chorioamniotic Separation

Chorioamniotic separation can occur as a result of amniocentesis. This however, does not usually affect the pregnancy outcome unless it extends for the entire chorioamniotic surface.

Infection

The risk of infection when amniocentesis is performed under strict aseptic conditions is very low, probably less than 1 in 1,000. However, a few cases of severe sepsis resulting in maternal death have been reported following amniocentesis. Infection can be caused by inadvertent puncture of the bowel, skin contaminants or organisms present on the ultrasound probe or gel.[29] The infection due to presence of skin contaminants or due to organisms present on the ultrasound probe can be avoided by following standard practices for maintaining asepsis. As mentioned previously, the best practice recommended by RCOG for maintaining asepsis during the procedure of amniocentesis is to enclose the ultrasound probe in a sterile bag and to use separate sterile gel for the probe.[5]

Rare Injuries

Rarely, severe injury can result from the amniocentesis procedure, including haemorrhage, gangrenous limbs, pneumothorax, ocular trauma, cardiac tamponade, peripheral nerve damage, fistula formation, intracranial abnormalities, bowel abnormalities, foetal cutaneous scarring, laceration of various internal organs, foetal demise, etc.[25]

Foetal cutaneous scarring: The incidence of foetal cutaneous scarring secondary to amniocentesis is estimated to be approximately 1–3%.[30] However, the actual rate is probably higher, since these marks are often inconspicuous at birth and infants are seldom examined thoroughly for needle puncture scars at that time. The frequency of foetal cutaneous scarring

PART II

significantly increases when women undergo multiple attempts at amniocentesis during a given pregnancy.[31] The areas of cutaneous trauma may be overlying the areas of serious internal injury. Needle injury can result in multiple scars at several locations, particularly the extremities, abdomen, back, buttocks and neck. Some scars are linear, possibly resulting from a tangential path taken by the needle, and some are circular. Though inexperienced surgeons while performing amniocentesis are more likely to result in foetal puncture, sometimes needle punctures may be unavoidable due to abrupt movements of the foetus. Over the past few decades, the use of real-time ultrasonic monitoring during amniocentesis has helped clinicians determine the exact position of the foetus while performing the amniocentesis. This has greatly helped in reducing the chances of injury due to needle puncture.

Preterm Premature Rupture of Membranes and Preterm Labour

The risk for development of preterm premature rupture of membranes is 3% and that for preterm delivery is about 8%. The procedure, however, is not associated with an increased risk of abruption.

Amniotic Fluid Leakage

Minor degree of tears in foetal membranes caused by the amniocentesis needle is likely to result in an increased risk of leaking per vaginum related to amniotic fluid leakage. This is most likely to occur in the first 6 weeks following amniocentesis. However, this does not result in any significant increase in the rate of vaginal bleeding. Rupture of the foetal membranes is common but can be a potentially serious complication of amniocentesis. Quintero has described a technique to seal the defect present in foetal membranes in which intra-amniotic injection of platelets and cryoprecipitate (amniopatch or blood patch) is used for the treatment of amniocentesis induced PROM.[32] The technique is simple and does not require knowledge about the exact location of the defect.[33] However, the appropriate dose of platelets and cryoprecipitate yet needs to be established.

Vertical Transmission

There have been reports of mother-to-infant transmission of viral infections such as hepatitis, CMV, toxoplasmosis, HIV, etc. related to the procedure of amniocentesis.[34,35] The highest risk of transmission is related to HIV infection. The risk appears lowest amongst women receiving highly active antiretroviral therapy (HAART).

Chorionic Villus Sampling

Some of the complications associated with the procedure of CVS are listed below:

❖ *Foetal loss or miscarriage*: The most serious complication, occurring as a result of CVS is foetal damage or loss. CVS may be associated with a pregnancy loss rate of 0.7–2%, which is slightly higher than that associated with amniocentesis. CVS can be considered to be less safe than second-trimester amniocentesis, and the additional risk seems to be limited to transcervical CVS.

❖ Mild transient cramps
❖ Bleeding per vaginum
❖ Infection
❖ Rupture of membranes
❖ *Vertical transmission of maternal infection*: There is also a risk of vertical transmission of maternal infection such as hepatitis, HIV, etc.
❖ *Failure to obtain an adequate sample*: The failure rate of CVS is dependent upon the operator experience. At the first attempt, the success rate is estimated to be about 80% and at the time of second attempt, it is 90%. More than two attempts for a particular procedure at the time of same sitting are usually not recommended.
❖ *Foetal defects*: Chorionic villus sampling, performed before 10 completed weeks of pregnancy, has been found to be associated with foetal defects like oromandibular facial defects, limb hypoplasia, isolated limb disruption defects, etc.[36] In order to reduce the incidence of these defects, the RCOG has recommended that CVS should not be performed before 10 completed weeks of gestation.[5] This risk appears to be very low (1 in 3,000) when CVS is performed after 10 weeks' gestational age.
❖ *Foetomaternal haemorrhage*: Foetomaternal haemorrhage has been recognised and may occur due to an increase in MSAFP levels following CVS. FMH has been suggested as one cause of foetal loss after CVS. This is particularly so in cases where the level of MSAFP is very high or continues to rise after CVS.

Cordocentesis

Cordocentesis is mainly associated with foetal complications, some of which can be even fatal.[37] These may include life-threatening complications such as bleeding, bradycardia and infection. Maternal complications unrelated to the pregnancy are unlikely to occur.

❖ *Haemorrhage*: Bleeding from the puncture site is the most common complication of cordocentesis, occurring in about 20–30% of cases. Puncture of the umbilical artery is associated with a significantly longer duration of bleeding in comparison to venipuncture. Foetuses with defects in platelet number or function are particularly at a significant risk for developing potentially fatal bleeding from the puncture site. A transfusion of 15–20 mL of platelet concentrate helps in increasing the foetal platelet count by 70,000–90,000/µL which is adequate for preventing bleeding from the cord puncture site. If continued bleeding is noted from the puncture site, management comprises of immediate delivery, if considered safe based on gestational age, or attempts must be made for the restoration of foetal volume.
❖ *Cord haematoma*: Cord haematoma is usually asymptomatic, but can be associated with a transient or prolonged sudden foetal bradycardia. Expectant management is recommended in the presence of reassuring FHR monitoring

and a non-expanding haematoma. However, delivery is indicated if signs of non-reassuring foetal status persist.

❖ *Foetomaternal haemorrhage*: A significant foetomaternal transfusion occurs in approximately 40% of cases. These foetomaternal bleeds may be defined by either greater than 50% increase in MSAFP concentration in blood following the procedure or presence of greater than 1 mL of FMH as calculated by Kleihauer-Betke staining of the maternal blood. FMH is more common with an anterior than a posterior placenta, with procedures lasting longer than 3 minutes, and with those requiring two or more needle insertions. The main consequence of a small FMH is an increase in maternal antibody titres when the procedure is performed in cases of red blood cell isoimmunisation.

❖ *Bradycardia*: Transient foetal bradycardia has been reported in 5–10% of foetuses. Most cases resolve without intervention within 5 minutes. This complication occurs due to a vasovagal response caused by local vasospasm.

❖ *Infection*: The procedure may be associated with the maternal risk for the development of chorioamnionitis.

❖ *Failure rate*: Cordocentesis may be associated with a failure rate of 9%.

❖ *Foetal loss*: The procedure has been found to be associated with an overall risk of foetal loss of 1.4% before 28 weeks of gestation, and an additional 1.4% risk of perinatal death after 28 weeks. This loss rate is significantly greater than that related to amniocentesis.

❖ *Vertical transmission of infection*: There is a risk for vertical transmission of infection in women with chronic hepatitis or infection with the HIV undergoing cordocentesis.

CLINICAL PEARLS

❖ It is important for the obstetrician to know the differences between amniocentesis and CVS so that they can use this information to counsel their patients. If the patient chooses to undergo first-trimester CVS over second-trimester amniocentesis, it helps in facilitating the earlier prenatal diagnosis of various genetic and cytogenetic disorders in the foetus, thereby enabling earlier termination of affected pregnancies.

❖ In comparison to amniocentesis, CVS is associated with higher rate of foetal loss. Also, CVS is associated with a greater risk of sampling and technical failures in comparison to amniocentesis.

❖ Operators carrying out amniocentesis and CVS should be trained to the competency level expected by sub-specialty training in maternal and foetal medicine in accordance with the RCOG Foetal Medicine Advanced Training Skills Module (ATSM) or other international equivalent. Operators can maintain their competency level by performing at least 30 ultrasound-guided invasive procedures per annum.

❖ Both the routes of CVS (transabdominal versus transcervical) are associated with comparable results and are performed between 10 weeks and 12 weeks. Transcervical CVS is associated with a higher risk of ascending infection,

risk of threatened abortion and vaginal bleeding. The transcervical CVS has also been found to be associated with poor sampling efficacy in comparison to transabdominal route. Transcervical approach is usually opted in cases where the placenta is posterior and approach through the anterior route may not seem to be feasible.

❖ In case of multifoetal gestation, CVS can be performed by a transabdominal, transcervical or a combined transabdominal, transcervical approach.[38]

EVIDENCE-BASED MEDICINE

❖ Insertion of needle under 'continuous ultrasound control' using real-time ultrasound is the technique of choice for these prenatal diagnostic procedures.[16-18]

❖ Though CVS in general is thought to be more invasive and associated with higher rate of foetal loss in comparison to amniocentesis, the available evidence till date have presented with conflicting results. While a few studies have shown almost identical rate of miscarriage after CVS compared with amniocentesis, most RCTs indicate that the rate of miscarriage following CVS is higher in comparison to the second-trimester amniocentesis.[39-42]

❖ In case of multifoetal gestation, multineedle technique is most commonly adopted for performing invasive diagnostic procedures. In these cases, a separate procedure is performed on each sac identified using prior injection of the dye indigo carmine. Following sac identification, procedure is performed using separate and sequential insertion of a new needle for each amniotic cavity. The available evidence has not shown multineedle technique to be associated with an increased risk of adverse outcomes in comparison to the single needle technique.[43]

REFERENCES

1. Caughey AB, Hopkins LM, Norton ME. Chorionic villus sampling compared with amniocentesis and the difference in the rate of pregnancy loss. Obstet Gynecol. 2006;108(3 Pt 1):612-6.

2. Valenti C, Schutta EJ, Kehaty T. Prenatal diagnosis of Down's syndrome. Lancet. 1968;2(7561):220.

3. Hahnemann N, Mohr J. Genetic diagnosis in the embryo by means of biopsy from extra-embryonic membrane. Bull Eur Soc Hum Genet. 1968;2:23-9.

4. Randomised trial to assess safety and fetal outcome of early and midtrimester amniocentesis. The Canadian Early and Mid-trimester Amniocentesis Trial (CEMAT) Group. Lancet. 1998;351(9098):242-7.

5. Royal College of Obstetricians and Gynecologists. (2010). Amniocentesis and chorionic villus sampling. Green-top Guideline No. 8. [online] RCOG website. Available from www.rcog.org.uk/globalassets/documents/guidelines/gt8amniocentesis0111.pdf [Accessed September, 2016].

6. Crandon AJ, Peel KR. Amniocentesis with and without ultrasound guidance. Br J Obstet Gynaecol. 1979;86(1):1-3.

7. Stark CM, Smith RS, Lagrandeur RM, Batton DG, Lorenz RP. Need for urgent delivery after third-trimester amniocentesis. Obstet Gynecol. 2000;95(1):48-50.

8. Blackwell SC, Berry SM. Role of amniocentesis for the diagnosis of subclinical intra-amniotic infection in preterm premature rupture of the membranes. Curr Opin Obstet Gynaecol. 1999;11(6):541-7.

9. Hausler MC, Konstantinuik P, Dorfer M, Weiss PA. Amniotic fluid insulin testing in gestational diabetes: safety and acceptance of amniocentesis. Am J Obstet Gynecol. 1998; 179(4):917-20.

10. Hodor JG, Poggi SH, Spong CY, Goodwin KM, Vink JS, Pezzulio JC, et al. Risk of third trimester amniocentesis: a case-control study. Am J Perinatol. 2006;23(3):177-80.

11. O'Donoghue K, Giorgi L, Pontello V, Pasquini L, Kumar S. Amniocentesis in the third trimester of pregnancy. Prenat Diagn. 2007;27(11):1000-4.

12. Mujezinovic F, Alfirevic Z. Analgesia for amniocentesis or chorionic villus sampling. Cochrane Database Syst Rev. 2011;(11):CD008580.

13. Mandelbrot L, Mayaux MJ, Bongain A, Berrebi A, Moudoub-Jeanpetit Y, Bénifla JL, et al. Obstetric factors and mother-to-child transmission of human immunodeficiency virus type 1: the French perinatal cohorts. SEROGEST French Pediatric HIN Infection Study Group. Am J Obstet Gynecol. 1996;175:661-7.

14. Tess BH, Ridrigues LC, Newell ML, Dunn DT, Lago TD. Breastfeeding, genetic, obstetric and other risk factors associated with mother-to-child transmission of HIV-1 in Sao Paulo State, Brazil. Sao Paulo Collaborative Study for Vertical Transmission of HIV-1. AIDS. 1998;12:513-20.

15. Maiques V, Garcia-Tejedor A, Perales A, Cordoba J, Esteban RJ. HIV detection in amniotic fluid samples. Amniocentesis can be performed in HIV pregnant women? Eur J Obstet Gynecol Reprod Biol. 2003;108(2):137-41.

16. Crandon AJ, Peel KR. Amniocentesis with and without ultrasound guidance. Br J Obstet Gynaecol. 1979;86(1):1-3.

17. de Crespigny LC, Robinson HP. Amniocentesis: a comparison of monitored versus blind needle insertion. Aust N Z J Obstet Gynaecol. 1986;26(2):124-8.

18. Romero R, Jeanty P, Reece EA, Grannum P, Bracken M, Berkowitz R, et al. Sonographically monitored amniocentesis to decrease intra-operative complications. Obstet Gynecol. 1985;65(3):426-30.

19. Giorlandino C, Mobili L, Bilancioni E, D'Alessio P, Carcioppolo O, Gentili P, et al. Transplacental amniocentesis: is it really a high-risk procedure? Prenat Diagn. 1994;14(9):803-6.

20. Marthin T, Liedgren S, Hammar M. Transplacental needle passage and other risk-factors associated with second trimester amniocentesis. Acta Obstet Gynecol Scand. 1997;76(8):728-32.

21. Alfirevic Z, Sundberg K, Brigham S. Amniocentesis and chorionic villus sampling for prenatal diagnosis. Cochrane Database Syst Rev. 2003;(3):CD003252.

22. Gordon MC, Narula K, O'Shaughnessy R, Barth WH Jr. Complications of third-trimester amniocentesis using continuous ultrasound guidance. Obstet Gynecol. 2002;99(2): 255-9.

23. Esrig SM, Leonardi DE. Spontaneous abortion after amniocentesis in women with a history of spontaneous abortion. Prenat Diagn. 1985;5(5):321-8.

24. Seeds JW. Diagnostic mid-trimester amniocentesis: how safe? Am J Obstet Gynecol. 2004;191(2):607-15.

25. Kong CW, Leung TN, Leung TY, Chan LW, Sahota DS, Fung TY, et al. Risk factors for procedure-related fetal losses after mid-trimester genetic amniocentesis. Prenat Diagn. 2006;26(10):925-30.

26. Odibo AO, Gray DL, Dicke JM, Stamilio DM, Macones GA, Crane JP. Revisiting the fetal loss rate after second-trimester genetic amniocentesis: a single center's 16-year experience. Obstet Gynecol. 2008;111(3):589-95.

27. Horger EO, Finch H, Vincent VA. A single physician's experience with four thousand six hundred genetic amniocenteses. Am J Obstet Gynecol. 2001;185(2):279-88.

28. Jeanty P, Rodesch F, Romero R, Venus I, Hobbins JC. How to improve your amniocentesis technique? Am J Obstet Gynecol. 1983;146(6):593-6.

29. Bruce S, Duffy JO, Wolf JE. Skin dimpling associated with midtrimester amniocentesis. Pediatr Dermatol. 1984;2(2): 140-2.

30. Ahluwalia J, Lowenstein E. Skin dimpling as a delayed manifestation of traumatic amniocentesis. Skinmed. 2005; 4(5):323-4.

31. Erez Y, Ben-Shushan A, Elchalal U, Ben-Meir A, Rojansky N. Maternal morbidity following routine second trimester genetic amniocentesis. Fetal Diagn Ther. 2007;22(3):226-8.

32. Quintero RA, Morales WJ, Allen M, Bornick PW, Arroyo J, LeParc G. Treatment of iatrogenic previable premature rupture of membranes with intra-amniotic injection of platelets and cryoprecipitate (amniopatch): preliminary experience. Am J Obstet Gynecol. 1999;181(3):744-9.

33. Lewi L, Van Schoubroeck D, Van Ranst M, Bries G, Emonds MP, Arabin B, et al. Successful patching of iatrogenic rupture of the fetal membranes. Placenta. 2004;25(4):352-6.

34. Mandelbrot L, Mayaux MJ, Bongain A, Berrebi A, Moudoub-Jeanpetit Y, Bénifla JL, et al. Obstetric factors and mother-to-child transmission of human immunodeficiency virus type 1: the French perinatal cohorts. SEROGEST French Pediatric HIV Infection Study Group. Am J Obstet Gynecol. 1996;175(3 Pt 1): 661-7.

35. Cohen J, Dussaix E, Bernard O. Transmission du virus de l'hepatite C de la mere a l'enfant: une etude de 44 enfants. Gastroenterol Clin Biol. 1998;22:179.

36. Firth HV, Boyd PA, Chamberlain P, MacKenzie IZ, Lindenbaum RH, Huson SM. Severe limb abnormalities after chorionic villus sampling at 56–66 days' gestation. Lancet. 1991;337(8744): 762-3.

37. Ghidini A, Sepulveda W, Lockwood CJ, Romero R. Complications of fetal blood sampling. Am J Obstet Gynecol. 1993;168(5): 1339-44.

38. Pergament E, Schulman JD, Copeland K, Fine B, Black SH, Ginsberg NA, et al. The risk and efficacy of chorionic villus sampling in multiple gestations. Prenat Diagn. 1992;12(5): 377-84.

39. Smidt-Jensen S, Philip J. Comparison of transabdominal and transcervical CVS and amniocentesis: sampling success and risk. Prenat Diagn. 1991;11(8):529-37.

40. Brambati B, Terzian E, Tognoni G. Randomized clinical trial of transabdominal versus transcervical chorionic villus sampling methods. Prenat Diagn. 1991;11(5):285-93.

41. Nicolaides K, Brizot Mde L, Patel F, Snijders R. Comparison of chorionic villus sampling and amniocentesis for fetal karyotyping at 10-13 weeks' gestation. Lancet. 1994;344(8920): 435-9.

42. Nicolaides KH, Brizot ML, Patel F, Snjders R. Comparison of chorion villus sampling and early amniocentesis for karyotyping in 1,492 singleton pregnancies. Fetal Diagn Ther. 1996;11(1):9-15.

43. Weisz B, Rodeck CH. Invasive diagnostic procedures in twin pregnancies. Prenat Diagn. 2005;25(9):751-8.

CHAPTER 5

Tests for Foetal Well-Being

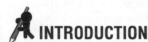 **INTRODUCTION**

Many methods have been developed to assess the antenatal well-being. The primary aim of these methods is to identify foetuses at risk of intrauterine injury and death. This would enable timely delivery to prevent progression to stillbirths. Use of antenatal tests helps in reducing the number of foetal deaths without putting a large number of foetuses at risk of premature delivery and the associated mortality and morbidity.

There is a widespread use of many such methods in clinical practice. With the exception of Doppler ultrasound for monitoring high-risk pregnancies (at risk of placental insufficiency), there is limited evidence regarding the effectiveness of various methods in improving the perinatal outcome.

INDICATIONS

High-risk pregnancies where the antepartum testing is commonly performed are listed in Box 6.1.[1] However, performing the tests for antenatal well-being only in high-risk pregnancies may be inappropriate because nearly 30–50% of perinatal deaths may actually occur in low-risk patients. Therefore, all women are likely to benefit from some form of antepartum foetal testing.

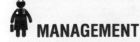 **MANAGEMENT**

❖ Various tests for antepartum foetal assessment late in pregnancy include: biochemical tests for the evaluation of placental function, ultrasound assessment, Doppler ultrasound evaluation, daily foetal movement count (DFMC), evaluation of foetal heart traces with tests such as cardiotocography (CTG), NST and contraction stress test (CST), BPP, modified BPP, etc. Various tests for antepartum

Box 6.1: Indications for antenatal testing in pregnant women[1]

Medical causes
❑ Hypertensive disorders
❑ Hyperthyroidism
❑ Haemoglobinopathies
❑ Cyanotic heart disease
❑ Systemic lupus erythematosus
❑ Chronic renal disease
❑ Diabetes mellitus
❑ Antiphospholipid syndrome

Indications specific to pregnancy
❑ Pre-eclampsia
❑ Oligohydramnios
❑ Polyhydramnios
❑ Post-term pregnancy
❑ Isoimmunisation
❑ Multiple pregnancy
❑ Gestational diabetes
❑ Preterm premature rupture of membranes
❑ Chronic abruption

Foetal causes
❑ Reduced foetal movement
❑ Intrauterine growth restriction
❑ Previous foetal demise/loss

foetal assessment in various high-risk situations during late pregnancy are tabulated in Table 6.1.
❖ Before performing any of these methods, informed consent must be obtained from the mother.
❖ In case of an abnormal test, clinicians must proceed to the second antenatal test. If the second antenatal test is also abnormal, foetal jeopardy is likely to be present. In such cases, decision needs to be taken to deliver the baby.
❖ In cases of suspected foetal prematurity, amniocentesis must be performed for evaluation of L:S ratio for assessment of foetal lung maturity. If the period of gestation is less than 37 completed weeks, she must be administered betamethasone to accelerate the lung maturity.

Table 6.1: Antepartum foetal surveillance in high-risk pregnancy

High-risk pregnancy	Antepartum test to be performed
Gestational diabetes (controlled on insulin)	*NST/AFI*: Weekly starting at 28–32 weeks. *Obstetric ultrasound*: Monthly starting at 32–36 weeks for estimated foetal weight
Pre-eclampsia	*NST/AFI*: Biweekly starting at time of diagnosis
Intrauterine growth retardation	*NST/AFI*: Biweekly *Obstetric ultrasound*: Bimonthly from time of diagnosis (>28 weeks)
Rh isoimmunisation	*NST/AFI*: Weekly *Obstetric ultrasound*: Monthly starting at 28 weeks
Multiple pregnancy	*NST/AFI*: Weekly *Obstetric ultrasound* : Monthly starting at 28–32 weeks
Oligohydramnios (AFI <5)	*NST/AFI*: Biweekly starting at 28 weeks
Chronic placental abruption	*NST/AFI*: Weekly *Obstetric ultrasound*: Monthly starting at time of diagnosis
Placenta praevia	*NST/AFI*: Weekly starting at 34 weeks
Maternal anaemia, sickle cell disease	*NST/AFI*: Weekly starting at 34 weeks
Maternal heart disease	*NST/AFI*: Weekly starting at 34 weeks *Obstetric ultrasound*: Monthly starting at 28 weeks
Maternal renal or collagen vascular disease	*NST/AFI*: Weekly starting at 28–30 weeks *Obstetric ultrasound*: Monthly starting at 28 weeks
Previous foetal demise or stillbirth	*NST/AFI*: Weekly starting at time of IUD or 32 weeks
Post-term pregnancy (>41 weeks)	*NST/AFI*: Biweekly starting at 41 weeks

Abbreviations: NST, non-stress test; AFI, amniotic fluid index; IUD, intrauterine death

❖ Foetal umbilical artery Doppler evaluation for foetal monitoring should be performed in high-risk pregnancies with underlying placental insufficiency.
❖ In the case of acute maternal illness, priority must be given towards stabilising the maternal condition. Foetal retesting may be performed if deemed appropriate.

Biochemical Tests of Placental Function

Prior to the advent of ultrasound for evaluation of foetal well-being, various biochemical tests were employed for assessment of placental and foetal well-being, including measurement of oestrogen, human placental lactogen and hCG in the maternal plasma, serum and urine. Biochemical tests are rarely used nowadays for evaluation of placental and foetal well-being. Cochrane review by Heazell et al.[2] has revealed the presence of inadequate evidence supporting the use of biochemical tests of placental function for reducing perinatal mortality or increasing the identification of small-for-gestational-age infants. Nevertheless, recently there has been a resurgence of interest and ongoing research for the evaluation of several new biochemical markers of placental function, e.g. placental growth factor, plasma protein A, placental protein 13,

pregnancy-specific glycoproteins, progesterone metabolites, etc. While in the past, the clinicians mainly relied on clinical abdominal examination and intermittent auscultation using a foetoscope, stethoscope or hand foetal Doppler's device, good antenatal surveillance today involves a combination of patient education, clinical examination, sonographic assessment, Doppler ultrasound and electronic foetal monitoring (EFM).

Ultrasound Examination

Ultrasound examination in the first trimester is crucial for establishing intrauterine pregnancy, gestational age, early pregnancy failure and to exclude other causes of bleeding, such as ectopic pregnancy, molar pregnancy, missed abortion and incomplete abortion.[3] The role of ultrasound examination in the second trimester is detailed in Table 6.2, and the role of ultrasound monitoring in the third trimester is summarised in Table 6.3. Obstetric ultrasound in the third trimester is the most important modality for assessment and monitoring of the foetal health and for detecting foetal compromise, hypoxaemia and metabolic acidosis, which can result in CNS damage and even prenatal death.

Ultrasound Grading of Placenta

Based on a review of multiple ultrasound evaluations of placental texture over past 4 years, Grannum et al. (1979) has described a classification system of placental maturity in an attempt to sonographically identify placental dysfunction.[4] This classification system classified placentas from grade 0 to 3 in accordance with specific ultrasonic findings at the basal

Table 6.2: Role of ultrasound examination in the second trimester

Role of ultrasound examination	Parameters of foetal well-being
Antenatal monitoring	Biophysical profile (evaluation of foetal movements, tone and breathing) and IUGR
Foetal characteristics	Foetal presentation, foetal viability, foetal biometry, foetal survey, evaluation of amniotic fluid volume, number of foetuses, chorionicity, foetal presentation, etc.
Foetal survey for congenital anomalies	Level I ultrasound (standard examination); level II ultrasound (for those at high risk)
Adjunct to obstetrical procedures	Amniocentesis, chorionic villus sampling, etc.
Amount of liquor	Hydramnios and oligohydramnios
Placental localisation	Placental grading and localisation

Table 6.3: Role of ultrasound monitoring in the third trimester

Role of ultrasound examination	Parameters of foetal well-being
Antenatal monitoring	Biophysical profile (evaluation of foetal movements, tone and breathing), IUGR, macrosomia, etc.
Foetal characteristics	Foetal presentation, foetal viability, foetal biometry, evaluation of amniotic fluid volume
Adjunct to obstetric procedures	External cephalic version procedures

CHAPTER 6

and chorionic plates as well as within the placental substance. This approach is, however, complicated by high intraobserver and interobserver variability. Moreover, there is no clear-cut understanding about the significance of various placental echogenic changes.[5,6] Recent studies have shown that placental characteristics, such as jelly-like placenta and foetal echogenic cystic lesions (ECLs), are related to intervillous thrombosis and fibrin deposition.[7,8] A combination of various placental characteristics, such as placental thickness and morphology, and other investigations, such as uterine Doppler analysis and evaluation of maternal serum alpha-foetoprotein level, may help in efficient screening of high-risk pregnancies for evaluation of foetal well-being. Presence of ECL is associated with poor prognosis in foetuses with severe growth restriction. Presently there is little evidence to indicate if the placental ultrasound grading is likely to reduce perinatal mortality or morbidity.[9] Future studies are required to define the clinical utility of placental ultrasound findings.

Doppler Sonography

Doppler ultrasound is a non-invasive technique which helps in assessing foetoplacental unit by detecting the movement of blood flow through the maternal and foetal vessels. The Doppler examination begins by the second trimester. Both the uterine and foetal circulations have been studied with the help of Doppler sonography. Abnormal Doppler waveform patterns may be associated with conditions that impair blood supply to the placenta and are associated with impaired foetal growth, e.g. pre-eclampsia and maternal hypertension in which adequate trophoblastic invasion of spiral vessels does not take place. This would result in abnormal uterine artery or umbilical artery waveforms on Doppler ultrasound examination.[10,11] Doppler sonography is used to evaluate the blood flow in various foetal vessels in order to identify foetal hypoxia and asphyxia, often seen in combination with IUGR or certain maternal complications such as pre-eclampsia and gestational diabetes. Foetal conditions, such as IUGR and foetal hypoxaemia, can cause alteration in the foetoplacental circulation and produce haemodynamic modifications which can affect specific foetal vessels like umbilical vessels. The Doppler detectable modifications in the foetal circulation associated with IUGR and foetal hypoxaemia include increased resistance to flow in the umbilical artery and foetal peripheral vessels, in association with decreased resistance in the foetal cerebral vessels. This is known as the 'brain-sparing' phenomenon, in which there is preferential perfusion of the brain, heart and adrenals at the expense of the integument and viscera, gut and kidneys in the hypoxic foetuses.

Foetal Movement Count

Cardiff count-to-10 foetal movement screening programme is a simple and effective method for reducing the foetal mortality rate. However, educating the women to monitor foetal movements may be associated with possibly increased maternal anxiety.

Technique: The technique for DFMC is as follows:

❖ The patient is instructed to self-monitor the kick counts daily at home.
❖ She is instructed to perform the count at same time every day. She is free to choose a time when she feels that her foetus is most active. Usually, foetal activity is increased while she is involved in stimulating activities like walking or exercises.
❖ While performing the kick count, she must lie on her left side in a comfortable location.
❖ She is asked to report the time it takes for her to feel 10 movements, no matter how small and is instructed to record them in the form of a chart.
❖ Whenever she feels a foetal movement, she is instructed to mark each movement on the chart until she has marked 10 movements in all. Then, she must note the time. If the woman can feel about 10 movements in 2 hours' time period, it is considered as normal. If she is not able to feel adequate movements, she should have something to eat or drink and lie in the left lateral position. She must also concentrate a little more to feel the foetal movements. In most low-risk normal pregnancies, a woman's general impression that the foetus is moving normally, along with the normal clinical obstetric examination is enough to imply that the foetus is in good condition. If at any time she feels uncertain regarding the perception of foetal movements, she should consult her obstetrician or midwife.

Cardiotocography

Cardiotocography is used for assessing the heart rate both in the antepartum period as well as during labour. CTG has been described in details in Chapter 49 (Antepartum and Intrapartum Foetal Asphyxia). During the antenatal period, CTG can be used in isolation, referred to as NST, or with the stimulation of uterine contractions to see the response of foetal heart in face of uterine contractions. The latter case is known as CST.

Non-stress Test

Indications for Doing a Non-stress Test

Non-stress test is a non-invasive test which indicates whether the foetus is receiving enough oxygen or not. Reduced oxygen supply to the foetus could be related to placental or umbilical cord problems. NST is usually performed after 28 weeks of gestation. The NST is based on the principle that the heart rate of a well-oxygenated, healthy, non-acidotic and neurologically intact foetus should normally accelerate with foetal movements.[12] Continuous carditographic record of FHR obtained by an ultrasound transducer placed on the mother's abdomen and the second transducer placed over the uterine fundus is used to measure the uterine activity. The results of NST can be classified as either reactive or non-reactive (Table 6.4). Now, it is believed that other parameters of electronic foetal heart assessment including baseline rate, variability and the presence or absence of decelerations should also be assessed.

PART II

On the basis of various parameters of foetal heart trace, the Royal Australian and New Zealand College of Obstetricians and Gynaecologists (RANZCOG) and the Royal College of Obstetricians and Gynaecologists (RCOG) has classified NST as normal, atypical or abnormal (Table 6.5).[13,14]

The NST is used widely in current obstetrics practice. The NST is associated with a low false-negative rate ranging from 0.19% to 1%.[15] On the other hand, it may be associated with a false-positive rate as high as 55%.[16] This implies that even with an abnormal test result, the foetus is more likely to be healthy than compromised. Despite a relationship between the features of an abnormal NST-CTG and foetal compromise, the efficiency of NST to predict perinatal mortality and morbidity is less than 40%. A Cochrane review by Grivell et al. has revealed no reduction in the perinatal mortality, but instead an increase in the obstetric interventions with the use of antenatal CTG.[17] Therefore, the results of NST must be cautiously interpreted by the clinicians, particularly at early gestational age when delivery could result in significant neonatal morbidity or mortality.

Since there are large intraobserver and interobserver variations in the manual interpretation of NST-CTG, computerised algorithms have been developed to increase the accuracy of NST-CTG assessment and detect simple changes missed by clinicians on manual interpretation. The most widely adopted system for computerised CTG is the Dawes Redmen's criteria developed in Oxford, UK. This approach emphasises the importance of short-term variability (STV) of 3.75 seconds epoch. STV is a better predictor of foetal compromise in comparison to accelerations or decelerations.[18]

Non-stress test-cardiotocography can be augmented by the vibroacoustic stimulus by holding an acoustic probe over the maternal abdomen and transmitting a sound to the foetus via maternal abdomen. This may result in increased foetal movements, thereby increasing the efficacy of antepartum CTG tracing. Nevertheless, it is safe for the baby.[19]

Contraction Stress Test

The CST or oxytocin challenge test is a test of foetal well-being, first described by Ray et al. in 1972.[20] The CST is usually performed in the presence of an atypical NST in order to test the adequacy of uteroplacental function.[21] The results of this test greatly aid the obstetrician in taking decision regarding the timing and mode of delivery. The CST should not be performed when vaginal delivery is contraindicated. The CST should be performed in a setting where facilities for emergency caesarean section are available.

Principle: The principle of the CST is that if foetal oxygenation is marginal at rest, it will transiently worsen with uterine contractions as the resultant hypoxaemia will lead to late decelerations. This test measures the ability of the placenta to provide enough oxygen to the foetus while under stress (contractions). The CST is based on the effect produced by the uterine contractions on the FHR. It is based on the fact that uterine contractions would produce transient compression of uterine blood vessels resulting in transient reduction of foetal oxygenation. A well-oxygenated foetus would effectively be able to deal with this transient decline in oxygenation. However, in the suboptimally oxygenated foetus, the resultant intermittent worsening in oxygenation may lead to the FHR pattern of late decelerations. The purpose of the test is to see whether the baby would be better off outside the mother's body than inside. Oxytocin is administered through IV route until three uterine contractions are observed, lasting 40–60

Table 6.4: Classification of non-stress test as reactive and non-reactive

Test result	Interpretation
Reactive non-stress result	If there are accelerations of the foetal heart rate of at least 15 bpm over the baseline, lasting at least 15s, occurring within a 20 mins time block
Non-reactive non-stress result	• If these accelerations do not occur, the test is said to be non-reactive. • Additional testing may be required to determine whether the result is truly due to poor oxygenation

Table 6.5: Classification of non-stress test as normal, abnormal and atypical[13,14]

Parameters	Normal NST (previously reactive)	Atypical NST (previously non-reactive)	Abnormal NST (previously non-reactive)
Baseline	110–160 bpm	• 100–110 bpm • >160 bpm • Rising baseline	• Bradycardia <100 bpm • Tachycardia >160 bpm for >30 mins
Variability	6–25 bpm (moderate) ≤5 (absent or minimal) for <40 mins	≤5 (absent or minimal) for 40–60 mins	≤5 for >80 mins; >25 bpm >10 mins; sinusoidal
Decelerations	None or occasional variable <30 s	Variable decelerations 30–60 s duration	Variable decelerations >60 s in duration
Accelerations (term foetus)	• >2 accelerations with acme of ≥15 bpm lasting 15 s <40 mins of testing • ≥2 accelerations with acme of ≥ 10 bpm lasting 10 s <40 mins of testing	• ≤2 accelerations with acme of ≥15 bpm lasting 15 s in 40–80 mins of testing • ≤2 accelerations with acme of ≥ 10 bpm lasting 10 s in 40–80 mins of testing	• ≤2 accelerations with acme of ≥15 bpm lasting 15 s in >80 mins of testing • ≤2 accelerations with acme of ≥10 bpm lasting 10 s in >80 mins of testing
Action	Further assessment is optional and is based on the total clinical picture	Further assessment required	• Urgent action required. An overall assessment of the situation and further investigation with U/S or BPP • Urgent delivery may be required

CHAPTER 6

Table 6.6: Biophysical profile criteria

Components	Score of 2	Score of 0
Amniotic fluid volume	Single vertical pocket of amniotic fluid is greater than 2 cm in two perpendicular planes	Largest vertical pocket of amniotic fluid is 2 cm or less
Foetal breathing movements	One or more episodes of rhythmic foetal breathing movements of 30 s or more within 30 mins	Abnormal, absent or insufficient breathing movements
Foetal movements	Three or more discrete body or limb movements within 30 mins	Abnormal, absent or insufficient movements
Foetal tone	At least one episode of flexion-extension of a foetal extremity with return to flexion, or opening or closing of a hand within 30 mins	Abnormal, absent, or insufficient foetal tone
Non-stress test	Reactive (normal)	Non-reactive (abnormal)

seconds, over a 10 minute period. An IV infusion of dilute oxytocin may be initiated at a rate of 0.5 mU/min and doubled every 20 minutes until an adequate contraction pattern is achieved. The CST is interpreted according to the presence or absence of late FHR decelerations.

Biophysical Profile

The BPP was first described by Manning in 1980.[22] It utilises multiple ultrasound parameters of foetal well-being and the NST. It is more accurate than a single test as it correlates five measurements to give a score. As a result, it is associated with much lower rates of false positives and false negatives.[23] The ultrasound parameters of the test are foetal tone, foetal movement, foetal breathing and amniotic fluid volume. An NST, which is not an ultrasonic measurement, is also performed. Table 6.6 shows the parameters of each observation. Two points are given if the observation is present and zero points are given if it is absent. A BPP test score of at least 8 out of 10 is considered reassuring. A score of 6 or 7 out of 10 is equivocal and must be repeated within 24 hours. A score of 4 or less out of 10 is a positive test and strongly suggests preparing the patient for delivery. The first sign of acidosis (cord arterial pH <7.2) was thought to be an abnormal NST and absent foetal breathing. Advanced or chronic acidosis is thought to compromise foetal tone and movement. Assessment of amniotic fluid volume helps as its reduction in the late second and all through the third trimester is indicative of foetal distress. Amniotic fluid is essentially foetal urine. With uteroplacental dysfunction, redistribution of blood flow takes place. This leads to decreased renal perfusion and thus to oligohydramnios.[24, 25] BPP is recommended for evaluation of foetal well-being in the pregnancies at increased risk for adverse perinatal outcome. If an abnormal result on BPP is obtained, the further management is usually determined by the overall clinical situation. Wherever possible, efforts should be made to deliver the baby as soon as possible.

Modified Biophysical Profile

Manning described the modified BPP in 1990.[26] The modified BPP combines NST (with the option of acoustic stimulation in case of nonreactive NST after 20 minutes) with the amniotic

Table 6.7: Interpretation of modified biophysical profile

	Non-stress test	Amniotic fluid index
Normal result	Reactive	>5 cm
Abnormal result	Non-reactive	<5 cm

fluid index (AFI).[27] While NST or vibroacoustic stimulation test (VAST) is a short-term indicator of foetal acid-base status, the AFI serves as an indicator of long-term placental function. An AFI greater than 5 cm is generally considered to represent an adequate volume of amniotic fluid.[25] Thus, the modified BPP is considered normal, if the NST is reactive and the AFI is more than 5 cm, and abnormal, if either the NST is non-reactive or the AFI is 5 cm or less (Table 6.7). If the result of a modified BPP indicates a possible abnormality, then the full BPP is performed. A Cochrane review has shown that presently, there is insufficient evidence from randomised trials to support the BPP as a test of foetal well-being in high-risk pregnancies.[28]

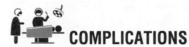

COMPLICATIONS

Foetal compromise during the antenatal period is likely to result in foetal hypoxaemia and metabolic acidosis, which can cause CNS damage (hypoxic ischaemic encephalopathy) and an increased rate of perinatal mortality.

❖ *Perinatal mortality*: Appropriate tests for antenatal well-being are likely to bring about a reduction in perinatal mortality by reducing the number of stillbirths. Perinatal mortality rate (PMR) is defined as the number of stillbirths and deaths in the first week of life per 1,000 total deliveries. It is calculated using the following formula:

$$PMR = \frac{\text{Total mortalities}}{(\text{Total mortalities} + \text{Live births})} \times 1,000$$

In UK, stillbirth can be defined as a baby born after 24 weeks of life, showing no signs of life.

❖ *Hypoxic ischaemic encephalopathy*: For details related to hypoxic ischaemic encephalopathy, kindly refer to Chapter 49 (Antepartum and Intrapartum Foetal Asphyxia).

PART II

CLINICAL PEARLS

❖ Biochemical assessment of placental function is not likely to improve pregnancy outcomes. Presently, there is insufficient evidence to show that the assessment of placental echogenicity by ultrasound is likely to cause a reduction in perinatal mortality.

❖ In case the mother perceives reduced foetal movements, NST-CTG can be used for assessing foetal well-being. Consideration can also be given towards the use of ultrasound examination for the assessment of foetal growth.

❖ Use of BPP in the antepartum period is not likely to improve pregnancy outcomes in comparison to NST-CTG.

EVIDENCE-BASED MEDICINE

❖ There is reliable evidence regarding the use of umbilical artery Doppler in high-risk pregnancy and computerised CTG for confirming foetal well-being or suspected foetal compromise.[29-31] Evidence also suggests that routine measurement of foetal size by ultrasound after 24 weeks and umbilical artery Doppler in low-risk pregnancies is not associated with a reduction in perinatal mortality.

❖ Presently there is no clear evidence regarding the use of antenatal CTG for improving perinatal outcomes.[13-15] Computerised CTG assessment is likely to be more effective than the conventional NST-CTG. There is requirement for future studies focusing on the use of computerised CTG in specific populations of women with an increased risk of complications.

REFERENCES

1. O'neill E, Thorp J. Antepartum evaluation of the fetus and fetal well being. Clin Obstet Gynecol. 2012;55(3):722-30.
2. Heazell AEP, Whitworth M, Duley L, Thornton JG. Use of biochemical tests of placental function for improving pregnancy outcome. Cochrane Database Syst Rev. 2015;(11):CD011202.
3. Paspulati RM, Bhatt S, Nour S. Sonographic evaluation of first-trimester bleeding. Radiol Clin North Am. 2004;42(2):297-314.
4. Grannum PA, Berkowitz RL, Hobbins JC. The ultrasound changes in the maturing placenta and their relation to the fetal pulmonic maturity. Am J Obstet Gynecol. 1979;133(8):915-22.
5. Moran M, Ryan J, Higgins M, Brennan PC, McAuliffe FM. Poor agreement between operators on grading of placenta. J Obstet Gynaecol. 2011;31(1):24-8.
6. Cooley SM, Donnelly JC, Walsh T, McMahon C, Gillan J, Geary MP. The impact of ultrasonographic placental architecture on the antenatal course, labour and delivery in a low-risk primigravid population. J Matern Fetal Neonatal Med. 2011;24(3):493-7.
7. Jauniaux E, Ramsay B, Campbell S. Ultrasonographic investigation of placental morphological characteristics and size during the second trimester of pregnancy. Am J Obstet Gynecol. 1994;170(1 Pt 1):130-7.
8. Proctor LK, Whittle WL, Keating S, Viero S, Kingdom JC. Pathologic basis of echogenic cystic lesions in the human placenta: role of ultrasound-guided wire localization. Placenta. 2010;31(12):1111-5.
9. Viero S, Chaddha V, Alkazaleh F, Simchen MJ, Malik A, Kelly E, et al. Prognostic value of placental ultrasound in pregnancies complicated by absent-end diastolic flow velocity in the umbilical arteries. Placenta. 2004;25(8-9):735-41.
10. Kofinas AD, Penry M, Nelson LH, Meis PJ, Swain M. Uterine and umbilical artery flow velocity waveform analysis in pregnancies complicated by chronic hypertension or pre-eclampsia. South Med J. 1990;83(2):150-5.
11. Zhou R, Li W, Liu S, Tang L. [Pulsed-wave Doppler ultrasound evaluation of flow velocity waveforms of foetal umbilical artery and uterine artery as predictors of neonatal outcome]. Hua Xi Yi Ke Da Xue Xue Bao. 1991;22(4):424-7.
12. Bishop EH. Fetal acceleration test. Am J Obstet Gynecol. 1981;141:905-9.
13. Royal Australian and New Zealand College of Obstetricians and Gynaecologists (RANZCOG). Intrapartum fetal surveillance: Clinical guidelines, 3rd edition. Melbourne: RANZCOG; 2014.
14. Royal College of Obstetricians and Gynaecologist (RCOG). The use of electronic fetal monitoring: The use and interpretation of cardiotocography in intrapartum fetal surveillance. (Evidence-based clinical guideline No 8). London: RCOG; 2001.
15. Blix E, Sviggum O, Koss KS, Øian P. Inter-observer variation in assessment of 845 labour admission tests: comparison between midwives and obstetricians in the clinical setting and two experts. BJOG. 2003;110:1-5.
16. Freeman RK, Anderson G, Dorchester W. A prospective multi-institutional study of antepartum fetal heart rate monitoring. I. Risk of peri-natal mortality and morbidity according to antepartum fetal heart rate test results. Am J Obstet Gynecol. 1982;143(7):771-7.
17. Grivell RM, Alfirevic Z, Gyte GM, Devane D. Antenatal cardiotocography for fetal assessment. Cochrane Database Syst Rev. 2015;(9):CD007863.
18. Dawes GS, Moulden M, Redman CW. System 8000: computerized antenatal FHR analysis. J Perinat Med. 1991; 19(1-2):47-51.
19. Tan KH, Smyth RM, Wei X. Fetal vibroacoustic stimulation for facilitation of tests of fetal well-being. Cochrane Database Syst Rev. 2013;(12):CD002963.
20. Ray M, Freeman R, Pine S, Hesselgesser R. Clinical experience with the oxytocin challenge test. Am J Obstet Gynecol. 1972;114(1):1-9.
21. Lagrew DC. The contraction stress test. Clin Obstet Gynecol. 1995;38(1):11-25.
22. Manning FA, Morrison I, Lange IR, Harman CR, Chamberlain PF. Foetal biophysical profile scoring: Selective use of the nonstress test. Am J Obstet Gynecol. 1987;156:709-12.
23. Rutherford SE, Phelan JP, Smith CV, Jacobs N. The four quadrant assessment of amniotic fluid volume: An adjunct to antepartum foetal heart-rate testing. Obstet Gynecol. 1987;70 (3 Pt 1):353-6.
24. Seeds AE. Current concepts of amniotic fluid dynamics. Am J Obstet Gynecol. 1980;138(5):575-86.
25. Chamberlain PF, Manning FA, Morrison I, Harman CR, Lange IR. Ultrasound evaluation of amniotic fluid volume I. The relationship of marginal and decreased amniotic fluid volumes to perinatal outcome. Am J Obstet Gynecol. 1984; 150(3):245-9.

CHAPTER 6

26. Manning FA, Harman CR, Morrison I, Menticoglou SM, Lange IR, Johnson JM. Fetal assessment based on foetal biophysical profile scoring. IV. An analysis of perinatal morbidity and mortality. Am J Obstet Gynecol. 1990;162:703-9.

27. Miller DA, Rabello YA, Paul RH. The modified biophysical profile: antepartum testing in the 1990s. Am J Obstet Gynecol. 1996;174(3):812-7.

28. Lalor JG, Fawole B, Alfirevic Z, Devane D. Biophysical profile for fetal assessment in high risk pregnancies. Cochrane Database Syst Rev. 2008;(1): CD000038.

29. Karsdorp VH, van Vugt JM, van Geijn HP, Kostense PJ, Arduini D, Montenegro N, et al. Clinical significance of absent or reversed end diastolic velocity waveforms in umbilical artery. Lancet. 1994;344(8938):1664-8.

30. Tyrrell S, Obaid AH, Lilford RJ. Umbilical artery Doppler velocimetry as a predictor of fetal hypoxia and acidosis at birth. Obstet Gynecol. 1989;74(3 Pt 1):332-7.

31. Alfirevic Z, Stampalija T, Gyte GM. Fetal and umbilical Doppler ultrasound in high-risk pregnancies. Cochrane Database Syst Rev. 2010;(1):CD007529.

SECTION 3

Medical Disorders during Pregnancy

OBSTETRICS

Hypertensive Disorders during Pregnancy

The International Society for the Study of Hypertension in Pregnancy (ISSHP), National High Blood Pressure Education Program (NHBPEP, 2000)[1] and the ACOG Task Force for Hypertension in Pregnancy (2013)[2] have classified the hypertensive disorders of pregnancy into the following four groups (Table 7.1 and Flow chart 7.1).

1. Gestational hypertension
2. Pre-eclampsia or eclampsia
3. Chronic hypertension
   - Essential
   - Secondary
4. Pre-eclampsia superimposed on chronic hypertension.

Hypertension can be classified as mild, moderate and severe as described in Table 7.2.

PRE-ECLAMPSIA

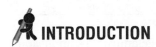 **INTRODUCTION**

Pre-eclampsia can be described as a pregnancy-specific syndrome, which can affect almost every organ system in the body. According to the NHBPEP (2000) working group report on high blood pressure in pregnancy and ACOG, pre-eclampsia can be considered as a potentially serious disorder, which is characterised by high blood pressure ($\geq$140/90 mmHg) and proteinuria (>300 mg/dL or >1+ on the dipstick).[1,2] It has now been recognised that overt proteinuria may not be a feature in some women with pre-eclampsia syndrome.[3] Due to this, the ACOG Task Force (2013) has suggested the use of other diagnostic criteria such as thrombocytopenia, renal dysfunction, hepatic dysfunction, perturbations of the CNS or pulmonary oedema (Box 7.1). A sudden rise in blood pressure later in pregnancy, known as delta hypertension, may also signify pre-eclampsia even if the blood pressure is less than 140/90 mmHg (or in the normotensive range).[4] Such women are at an increased risk of eclamptic seizures or haemolysis, elevated liver enzymes and low platelet count (HELLP) syndrome (even though they may be normotensive).

The diastolic blood pressure corresponds to Korotkoff's V sounds, i.e. disappearance of sound.[5] The measurements must be made on at least two occasions 6 hours apart, but within the span of about a week. Pre-eclampsia usually develops after the 20th week of pregnancy and goes away after the delivery (usually within the 12th postpartum week).

Table 7.1: Characteristic features of various types of hypertensive disorders during pregnancy

	Onset	Subsidence	Blood pressure	Proteinuria
Pre-eclampsia	Develops after 20th week of pregnancy	Goes away after delivery (usually within 12th postpartum weeks)	>140/90 mmHg	Present (Proteinuria is greater than 0.3 g/L in a 24-hour collection)
Gestational hypertension	Develops after 20th week of pregnancy	Goes away after delivery (usually within 12th postpartum weeks)	>140/90 mmHg	Absent
Chronic hypertension	Onset is before pregnancy or before 20th week of pregnancy in absence of gestational trophoblastic disease	The condition does not return to normal within 12th postpartum week	>140/90 mmHg	Absent
Pre-eclampsia superimposed upon chronic hypertension	Onset is before pregnancy or before the 20th week of pregnancy in absence of gestational trophoblastic disease	The condition does not return to normal within 12 weeks of postpartum period	>140/90 mmHg	Onset of proteinuria after 20 weeks of pregnancy

Flow chart 7.1: Classification of hypertensive disorders in pregnancy

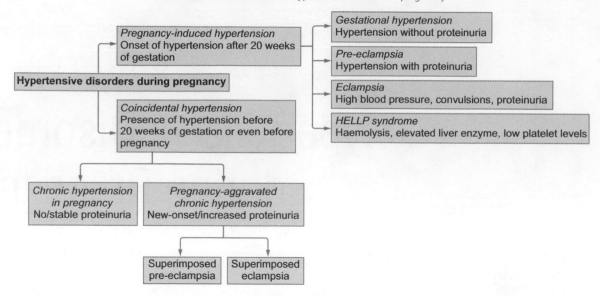

Table 7.2: Classification of hypertension based on its severity

	Mild	Moderate	Severe
Systolic BP	140–149 mmHg	150–159 mmHg	≥160 mmHg
Diastolic BP	90–99 mmHg	100–109 mmHg	≥110 mmHg

Box 7.1: Diagnostic criteria for pre-eclampsia

Hypertension plus proteinuria
❑ Proteinuria ≥300 mg/24 hours
        Or
❑ Protein: creatinine ratio ≥0.3
        Or
❑ Dipstick >1+ persistent proteinuria
        Or
Clinical/biochemical abnormalities
❑ Thrombocytopenia: Platelet <100,000/μL
        Or
❑ Renal insufficiency: Creatinine >1.1 mg/dL or doubling of the baseline
        Or
❑ Liver involvement: Serum transaminases level is twice the normal
        Or
❑ Cerebral symptoms: Headache, visual disturbances, convulsions, etc.
        Or
❑ Pulmonary oedema

Table 7.3: Difference between non-severe and severe pre-eclampsia

Abnormalities	Non-severe	Severe
Diastolic BP	<110 mmHg	≥110 mmHg
Systolic BP	<160 mmHg	≥160 mmHg
Proteinuria	None to positive	None to positive
Headache	Absent	Present
Visual disturbances	Absent	Present
Upper abdominal pain	Absent	Present
Oliguria	Absent	Present
Convulsions (eclampsia)	Absent	Present
Serum creatinine	Normal	Increased
Thrombocytopenia (<100,000 cells/μL)	Absent	Present
Serum transaminases	Minimum elevation	Marked elevation
Foetal growth restriction	Absent	Present
Pulmonary oedema	Absent	Present

Severe pre-eclampsia is pre-eclampsia with severe hypertension and/or with symptoms (headache, visual problems, epigastric or right upper quadrant abdominal pain, eclampsia, etc.) and/or biochemical and/or haematological impairment. Unlike the previous classification comprising of mild, moderate and severe (Table 7.2), the ACOG Task Force discourages the use of term, mild pre-eclampsia. It instead classifies pre-eclampsia as severe versus non-severe. Differentiation between severe and non-severe pre-eclampsia is described in Table 7.3. Non-severe pre-eclampsia probably includes moderate and mild types. Eclampsia, a complication of pre-eclampsia can be defined as convulsions occurring in women with pre-eclampsia, which cannot be attributed to another cause.

Though even in developed countries, deaths due to pre-eclampsia and eclampsia may sometimes occur, mortality due to these conditions is relatively rare in the UK. Nevertheless, cases of severe hypertension and cerebral vascular accident may occasionally occur.

AETIOLOGY

The exact pathophysiology of pre-eclampsia is not yet understood.

The most likely causes for pre-eclampsia and their underlying mechanisms are described in Flow chart 7.2 and Table 7.4 and are enumerated below:[6]

❖ Inadequate trophoblastic invasion

Flow chart 7.2: Pathophysiology of pre-eclampsia

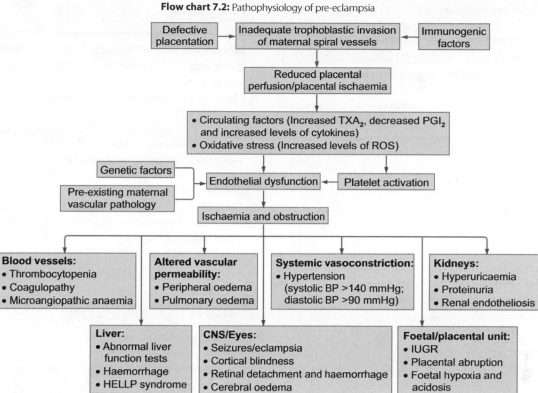

Table 7.4: Pathophysiology of pre-eclampsia	
Likely cause for pre-eclampsia	**Underlying mechanism**
Inadequate trophoblastic invasion	Insufficient blood flow to the uterus
Prostacyclin or thromboxane imbalance	Disruption of the balance of the hormones that maintain diameter of the blood vessels
Endothelial activation and dysfunction	Damage to the endothelial lining of the blood vessels that regulates the diameter of the blood vessels keeping fluid inside and preventing leakage of proteins
Calcium deficiency or insufficient magnesium oxide	Calcium helps maintain vasodilation, so a deficiency would impair the function of vasodilation; magnesium oxide also helps in the regulation of vascular tone because magnesium stabilises vascular smooth muscles
Haemodynamic vascular injury	Injury to the blood vessels due to too much blood flow
Immunological activation	The immune system believes that damage has occurred to the endothelial cells and while trying to rectify the problem, it may result in the formation of scar tissues, thereby worsening the problem
Nutritional problems or poor diet	Insufficient proteins and not enough fresh fruits and vegetables (antioxidants) in the diet may have a role
Genetic factors	Exact gene has yet not been identified

❖ Maternal inflammatory response resulting in vascular endothelial dysfunction

❖ *Hereditary factors*: The exact genetic defect or pre-eclampsia gene has yet not been identified.

Box 7.2: Risk factors for pre-eclampsia
Moderate
❑ First pregnancy
❑ Age 40 years or older
❑ Pregnancy interval more than 10 years
❑ Obesity (BMI 35 kg/m² or more at first visit)
❑ Family history of pre-eclampsia
❑ Multi-foetal gestation
❑ Hyperhomocysteinaemia
❑ Metabolic syndrome
High
❑ Hypertensive disease during previous pregnancy
❑ Chronic kidney disease
❑ Autoimmune disease such as systemic lupus erythematosus or antiphospholipid syndrome
❑ Type 1 or type 2 diabetes
❑ Chronic hypertension

❖ *Immunological factors*: Production of blocking antibodies to various placental antigenic sites is associated with reduced risk.

❖ Endothelial dysfunction and vasospasm due to increased sensitivity to the action of angiotensin II (vasopressor) and due to the imbalance in production of various prostaglandins.

Risk Factors for Pre-eclampsia

Moderate risk factors for pre-eclampsia are enumerated in Box 7.2. Risk of developing pre-eclampsia is high amongst young and nulliparous women. Older women, on the other hand, are at an increased risk of developing chronic hypertension with superimposed pre-eclampsia. Ironically, smoking is associated with a reduced risk of pre-eclampsia. The period of gestation at which the woman presents with hypertension is an important factor in establishing the risk. A woman with late-onset hypertension after 37 weeks of gestation is rarely associated with any serious maternal or foetal morbidity. However, early-onset hypertension, typically that presenting prior to 28 weeks of gestation is likely to result in the development of pre-eclampsia in approximately 50% of the patients.

DIAGNOSIS

Clinical Presentation

❖ *Increased blood pressure*: Presence of an increased blood pressure(>140/90 mmHg) for the first time during pregnancy, after 20 weeks of gestation.[5]

❖ *Proteinuria*: Proteinuria is defined as significant if the excretion of proteins exceeds 300 mg per 24 hours or there is persistent presence of the protein (30 mg/dL or 1+ dipstick) in a random urine sample in the absence of any evidence of urinary tract infection.

❖ *Oedema*: Oedema of hands and face can commonly occur amongst women with pre-eclampsia. Since oedema is a universal finding in pregnancy, it is not considered as a criterion for diagnosing pre-eclampsia.

❖ *Symptoms of severe pre-eclampsia*: Indicators of severe pre-eclampsia during pregnancy are severe headache, visual problems such as blurring or flashing before the eyes, epigastric or right upper quadrant abdominal pain, vomiting, oliguria (urine volume <500 mL/24 hours), convulsions, sudden swelling of the face, hands or feet, papilloedema, signs of clonus (≥3 beats), liver tenderness, HELLP syndrome, platelet count falling to below 100×10^9 per litre, abnormal liver enzymes [alanine aminotransferase (ALT) or aspartate aminotransferase (AST) rising to above 70 IU/L, etc.]. In accordance with the NICE guidelines (2010), pregnant women should be made aware of the requirement to seek immediate advice from a healthcare professional if they experience any of the previously mentioned symptoms of severe pre-eclampsia.

❖ *Shortness of breath or dyspnoea*: This could be reflective of pulmonary oedema or acute respiratory distress syndrome.

❖ *Reduced foetal movements*: This is especially observed in association with intrauterine growth restriction (IUGR) and oligohydramnios.

❖ *Weight gain*: Weight gain of more than 2 pounds per week or 6 pounds in a month can be considered as significant.

Abdominal Examination

There may be evidence of placental insufficiency in the form of oligohydramnios and/or IUGR.

Investigations

❖ *Haematocrit and complete blood count*: The decrease in blood volume in pre-eclampsia can lead to a rise in maternal haemoglobin concentration resulting in an increased haematocrit.

❖ *Platelet count*: Platelet count of less than $150–400 \times 10^9$/litre could be indicative of the HELLP syndrome.

❖ *Kidney function tests*: In severe pre-eclampsia, raised serum creatinine and uric acid levels are associated with a worsening outcome both for the mother and baby.

❖ *Liver function test*: An AST level of above 75 IU/L can be considered as significant.

❖ *Ophthalmoscopic examination*: The abnormalities include presence of retinal oedema, constrictions of the retinal arterioles and alteration of normal ratio of vein: arteriolar diameter.

OBSTETRIC MANAGEMENT

Prevention

There is no evidence regarding the use of any of the following for the prevention of pre-eclampsia:

❖ *Nutritional supplements*: There is no evidence regarding the benefit of nutritional supplements such as magnesium, folic acid, antioxidants (vitamins C and E), fish oils or algal oils, garlic, calcium, etc.[7]

❖ *Dietary changes*: Salt restriction during pregnancy, solely for the prevention of gestational hypertension or pre-eclampsia during pregnancy is not recommended.

❖ *Lifestyle interventions*: The woman must be offered advice related to rest and exercise during the antenatal period.

❖ *Pharmacological interventions*: None of the following must be used to prevent hypertensive disorders in pregnancy: nitric oxide donors, progesterone, diuretics, low-molecular-weight heparin, etc.

❖ *Aspirin*: Women with at least 2 moderate-risk factors or at least 1 high-risk factor for pre-eclampsia must be advised to take aspirin, 75 mg per day from 12 weeks onwards until birth.[8] Aspirin is a cyclooxygenase enzyme inhibitor, which works by reversing the balance between the vasoconstrictor thromboxane A2, and the vasodilator prostacyclin.

Antenatal Care

❖ Women with pre-eclampsia must be assessed during each consultation preferably by a healthcare professional trained in the management of hypertensive disorders of pregnancy.

❖ They must be offered integrated care including admission to hospital, treatment, measurement of blood pressure, testing for proteinuria and performance of investigations (Table 7.5).[9] Management of cases of mild and severe pre-eclampsia has been described in Flow charts 7.3 and 7.4 respectively.

Table 7.5: Management of patients with pre-eclampsia

	Antenatal period		
Parameter	**Mild hypertension (140/90 to 149/99 mmHg)**	**Moderate hypertension (150/100 to 159/109 mmHg)**	**Severe hypertension (160/110 mmHg or higher)**
Hospital admission	Yes	Yes	Yes
Medical treatment required	No	Oral labetalol must be administered as first-line treatment for keeping diastolic blood pressure between 80–100 mmHg and systolic blood pressure <150 mmHg	Oral labetalol must be administered as first-line treatment for keeping diastolic blood pressure between 80–100 mmHg and systolic blood pressure <150 mmHg
Blood pressure measurement	Blood pressure must be measured at least four times a day	Blood pressure must be measured at least four times a day	Blood pressure must be measured more than four times a day, depending on the clinical circumstances
Test for proteinuria	Test for quantification of proteinuria does not require to be repeated	Test for quantification of proteinuria does not require to be repeated	Test for quantification of proteinuria may require to be repeated during the day
Blood tests	The following tests must be performed twice a week: kidney function, electrolytes, full blood count, transaminases, and serum bilirubin levels	The following tests must be performed thrice a week: kidney function, electrolytes, full blood count, transaminases, and serum bilirubin levels	The following tests must be performed thrice a week: kidney function, electrolytes, full blood count, transaminases, and serum bilirubin levels
	Postnatal period		
Blood pressure measurement	Blood pressure must be measured at least four times a day while the woman is an inpatient; at least once between day 3 and day 5 after birth and thereafter every alternate day until normal, if blood pressure was abnormal on days 3–5	Blood pressure must be measured at least four times a day while the woman is an inpatient and thereafter every 1–2 days for up to 2 weeks after transfer to community care until the woman is off treatment and has no hypertension	Blood pressure must be measured at least four times a day while the woman is an inpatient and thereafter every 1–2 days for up to 2 weeks after transfer to community care until the woman is off treatment and has no hypertension

Flow chart 7.3: Management of cases of mild pre-eclampsia

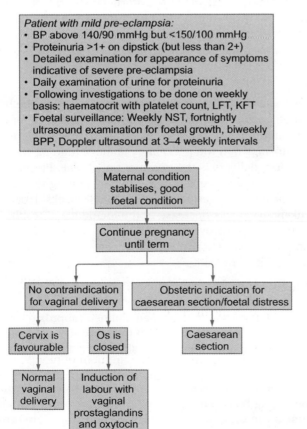

❖ Principles of management in cases of pre-eclampsia include timely delivery of the baby and adequate foetal surveillance. Before taking any decision related to the management of pre-eclampsia, the first task of the clinician is to confirm the diagnosis of pre-eclampsia so as to prevent iatrogenic morbidity related to premature births.

❖ In case of patients admitted in the hospital, bed rest is not required.[10]

❖ In women receiving outpatient care after severe hypertension has been effectively controlled in hospital, blood pressure measurement and test for proteinuria must be done at least two times a week. Blood tests must be carried out on a weekly basis.

Antihypertensive Medications

The aim of treatment must be to maintain diastolic blood pressure between 95 mmHg to 105 mmHg. The most commonly used first-line drugs include labetalol.[11] Antihypertensive treatment with alternative drugs (e.g. methyldopa or nifedipine) other than labetalol must only be offered after considering side-effect profiles for the woman, foetus and newborn baby. Hydralazine may be used for severe hypertension. Though less commonly used in Europe, hydralazine is still used in some National Health Service (NHS) trusts (RCOG, 2006).[12] Use of diuretics, angiotensin-converting enzyme (ACE) inhibitors and angiotensin II receptor blockers (ARBs), should be preferably avoided during pregnancy. Atenolol is licensed for the treatment of hypertension in the postpartum period and is

Flow chart 7.4: Management of cases of severe pre-eclampsia

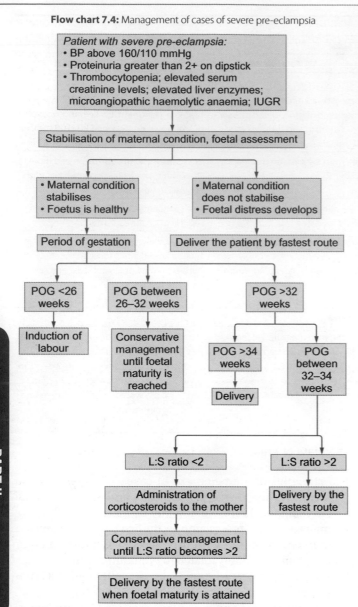

PART II

already used widely in UK postnatal obstetric practice. Loop diuretics can compromise placental perfusion. Therefore, antenatal use of furosemide is limited to the treatment of pulmonary oedema.

Fluid Therapy

Lactated ringer solution is administered at the rate of 60 mL to no more than 125 mL per hour unless there are other ongoing fluid losses (for example, due to haemorrhage). Volume expansion must not be done in women with severe pre-eclampsia unless she had been prescribed hydralazine.

Mode of Birth

Severe pre-eclampsia per se is not an indication for caesarean section. If the cervix is ripe, labour can be induced by using intravenous oxytocin and artificial rupture of the membranes (ARM). In case of presence of unfavourable cervix or other complications (e.g. breech presentation, foetal distress, etc.),

a caesarean section needs to be done. Decision regarding caesarean section versus induction of labour for the women with pre-eclampsia must be based on the clinical circumstances and the woman's preference.[13]

Foetal Monitoring

Due to risk of foetal growth restriction in women with pre-eclampsia, foetal well-being must be carefully considered in all the cases. Symphyseal-fundal height must be carefully measured in women with pre-eclampsia.

Cardiotocography must be performed at the time of diagnosis of severe gestational hypertension or pre-eclampsia. Enquiry about foetal movements must be made every day. If at any time a woman perceives abnormal foetal movements, cardiotocography must be performed. Cardiotocography may also be required if there is vaginal bleeding, abdominal pain or deterioration in maternal condition. Cardiotocography must not be performed more than weekly if the results of all other foetal monitoring tests are normal.

In cases of pre-eclampsia and gestational hypertension, ultrasound-assisted foetal growth and amniotic fluid volume assessment and umbilical artery Doppler velocimetry must be performed starting at 28–30 weeks (or at least 2 weeks before previous gestational age of onset if pre-eclampsia appears prior to 28 weeks). It must be repeated 4 weeks later in women with previous history of severe pre-eclampsia, pre-eclampsia that required birth before 34 weeks, pre-eclampsia with a baby whose birthweight was less than the 10th centile, previous history of intrauterine death or placental abruption. If the results of any of the foetal monitoring tests are abnormal, a consultant obstetrician must be informed. In women with severe gestational hypertension or pre-eclampsia, these tests must be routinely repeated at intervals every 2 weeks or less.

Timing of Birth

The only way to cure pre-eclampsia is to deliver the baby. The pregnancy should not be allowed to continue beyond estimated date of delivery (EDD). In cases of severe pre-eclampsia, when the pregnancy is more than 32 weeks of gestation, delivery is the treatment of choice. Prophylactic steroids should be given to induce foetal lung maturity in case the period of gestation is less than 32 weeks. Treatment is likely to cause a decrease in the incidence of respiratory distress and improved foetal survival. At the same time, administration of corticosteroids does not seem to worsen maternal hypertension.

Period of gestation 32 weeks or more: In women with established diagnosis of pre-eclampsia, delivery should be considered once foetal maturation has been attained (approximately 32 weeks of gestation), especially if there are signs of maternal multiorgan involvement or the signs of foetal compromise becomes apparent.

Period of gestation between 26 weeks and 32 weeks: Women presenting between 26 weeks and 32 weeks of gestation must be managed conservatively without substantial risk to the mother as long as close maternal and foetal supervision is maintained.[14] As far as possible, the clinician must try to manage pregnancy in women with pre-eclampsia conservatively until 34 weeks of gestation. If birth is considered likely within 7 days in women with pre-eclampsia having period of gestation between 24 weeks to 34 weeks, two doses of betamethasone 12 mg intramuscularly must be administered 24 hours apart.[15] Before 34 weeks of gestation, women with pre-eclampsia must be delivered, following discussion with neonatal and anaesthetic teams, if severe hypertension, which is refractory to treatment, develops or there are maternal or foetal indications for delivery.

Women with pre-eclampsia, who have severe hypertension, must be delivered after 34 weeks when their blood pressure has been controlled and a course of corticosteroids has been completed (if appropriate).

Women with pre-eclampsia, who have mild or moderate hypertension at 34[+0] to 36[+6] weeks must be delivered depending on maternal and foetal condition, risk factors and availability of neonatal intensive care. Women with pre-eclampsia, having mild or moderate hypertension must be delivered within 24–48 hours after 37[+0] weeks.

Indications for delivery in women at less than 32 weeks of gestation undergoing conservative management are enlisted in Box 7.3.

Before 26 weeks of gestation: In women with severe pre-eclampsia before 26 weeks of gestation, prolonging the pregnancy at this gestational age may result in grave complications for the mother. Therefore, labour must be induced for pregnancies less than 26 weeks, although the foetus may not survive at this time.

Anticonvulsants

Magnesium sulphate: Magnesium sulphate should be considered for women with pre-eclampsia, especially in whom there is concern about the risk of development of eclampsia.[16] In case of an eclamptic fit, magnesium sulphate is the drug of choice for prophylaxis. Magnesium sulphate must be discontinued 24 hours after delivery. Magpie trial (MAGnesium sulphate for Prevention of Eclampsia) has shown that the use of magnesium sulphate halves the risk of eclampsia and probably also reduces the risk of maternal death. The use of magnesium sulphate is not associated with any substantial short-term adverse effects either on the mother or the baby.[16-18]

Use of magnesium sulphate not only helps in reducing the incidence of further fits, it also proves useful over both diazepam and phenytoin by reducing the requirement of maternal ventilation, pneumonia and fewer admissions to the intensive care unit. When magnesium sulphate is administered, the following parameters must be regularly assessed:
- Urine output (urine output in the previous 4 hours must exceed 100 mL)
- Maternal deep-tendon reflexes (presence of patellar reflex)
- Respiratory rate and oxygen saturation (respirations must not be depressed).

In case of oliguria, care must be taken prior to the administration of magnesium sulphate because it undergoes renal excretion. Toxicity is demonstrated by the absence of patellar reflexes. Ultimately, this may lead to the development of respiratory arrest and muscle paralysis or cardiac arrest. In case of magnesium sulphate toxicity, 10 mL of 10% calcium gluconate or chloride, which serves as an antidote must be slowly administered intravenously.

Simultaneously, the administration of magnesium sulphate must be withheld. In case of severe respiratory depression or arrest, prompt tracheal intubation and mechanical ventilation are lifesaving.

If a woman in a critical care setting has severe hypertension or severe pre-eclampsia or previously had an eclamptic fit, intravenous magnesium sulphate must be administered.

Administration of intravenous magnesium sulphate must also be considered in women with severe pre-eclampsia in a critical care setting where the birth is planned within 24 hours.

The Collaborative Eclampsia Trial regimen must be used for administration of magnesium sulphate. This comprises of a loading dose of 4 g, given intravenously over 5 minutes, followed by an infusion of 1 g/h maintained for 24 hours (Zuspan's regimen).[19] Recurrent seizures should be treated with a further dose of 2–4 g given over 5 minutes. According to the NICE guidelines (2013), diazepam, phenytoin or lytic cocktail must not be used as an alternative to magnesium sulphate in women with eclampsia.

Anaesthesia

Use of general anaesthesia is dangerous in cases of pre-eclampsia because endotracheal intubation can cause hypertension. Regional anaesthesia is the preferred method of analgesia for labour and anaesthesia in case of operative deliveries.[20] However, the clinician needs to rule out coagulopathy prior to its administration. Care must also be taken to avoid arterial hypotension.

Box 7.3: Indications for delivery in women with pre-eclampsia undergoing conservative management

Delivery following maternal stabilisation (Only initial dose of corticosteroid needs to be administered)
- Uncontrollable severe hypertension
- Eclampsia
- Pulmonary oedema
- Placental abruption
- Disseminated intravascular coagulation
- Non-reassuring foetal status
- Foetal demise
- Maternal neurological complications

Delay delivery by 48 hours (Delivery following the administration of two doses of corticosteroids)
- Preterm rupture of membranes or labour
- Thrombocytopenia (<100,000 cells/μL)
- Level of hepatic transaminases twice the upper limit of normal
- Foetal growth restriction
- Oligohydramnios
- Reversed end-diastolic flow in umbilical artery Doppler
- Worsening renal dysfunction

Intrapartum Care

For women with pre-eclampsia, the following need to be done in the intrapartum period:

❖ Blood pressure must be measured every hourly in cases of mild or moderate hypertension. Blood pressure must be continually measured in cases of severe hypertension.

❖ Antenatal hypertensive treatment must be continued during labour.

❖ Haematological and biochemical monitoring must be done according to criteria as described in the antenatal period.

❖ The duration of the second stage of labour must not be limited if blood pressure remains stable.[21]

❖ Second stage of labour must be cut short in women in whom the blood pressure remains high. Vaginal operative birth must be offered in the second stage of labour to women with severe hypertension whose hypertension has not responded to initial treatment.

❖ Before establishing low-dose epidural analgesia and combined spinal epidural analgesia, women who have severe pre-eclampsia must not be overloaded with intravenous fluids.

Postnatal Period

Breastfeeding

❖ The women who still require antihypertensive treatment during the postnatal period must be advised that the following antihypertensive drugs have no known adverse effects on babies receiving breast milk, e.g. labetalol, nifedipine, enalapril, captopril, atenolol and metoprolol.

❖ She should also be informed that presently there is insufficient evidence regarding the adverse effects on babies receiving the following antihypertensive drugs, e.g. ARBs, amlodipine, and ACE inhibitors other than enalapril and captopril.

❖ If the woman is breastfeeding, diuretic treatment for hypertension must be avoided.

❖ If a woman had been prescribed methyldopa to treat pre-eclampsia during the antenatal period, it must be stopped within 2 days of birth.

❖ Clinical well-being of the baby, especially adequacy of feeding, must be assessed at least for the first 2 days after birth.

Weight Management

Women who have had pre-eclampsia must be advised to keep their BMI between 18.5 kg/m² to 24.9 kg/m² before planning their next pregnancy.

Medical Care

❖ Each time blood pressure is measured, the women must be asked about symptoms of severe pre-eclampsia, such as severe headache, epigastric pain, etc.

❖ Women with pre-eclampsia who did not take anti-hypertensive treatment during the antenatal period must be offered antihypertensive treatment if blood pressure

becomes 150/100 mmHg or higher during the postnatal period.

❖ For women with pre-eclampsia who have taken anti-hypertensive treatment in the antenatal period, their antihypertensive treatment must be continued during the postnatal period. The clinician must consider reducing antihypertensive treatment if the blood pressure falls below 140/90 mmHg.

❖ Such women must be transferred to community if there are no symptoms of pre-eclampsia; blood pressure is 149/99 mmHg or lower and blood test results are stable or improving, with or without treatment.

❖ All women who have had pre-eclampsia, must be offered a postnatal medical review 6–8 weeks after birth. Women who still require antihypertensive treatment at the postnatal review must be offered a specialist assessment of their hypertension.

❖ Women who have had gestational hypertension or pre-eclampsia must be counselled at the time of discharge that these conditions are associated with an increased risk of developing high blood pressure and its complications in later life. Such women are also at an increased long-term risk of cardiovascular diseases and end-stage renal disease.[22] Such women are also at an increased risk of recurrence of hypertensive disorders of pregnancy. Women who had gestational hypertension, have an approximately 40% risk of developing gestational hypertension in a future pregnancy. On the other hand, women who had pre-eclampsia, have an approximately 16% risk of developing pre-eclampsia in a future pregnancy.

 COMPLICATIONS

Some of the maternal and foetal complications related to pre-eclampsia are enumerated in Table 7.6. Perinatal mortality is increased in cases of pre-eclampsia. Incidence of IUGR typically increases in association with early onset pre-eclampsia. There also may be an increased incidence of placental abruption due to placental involvement. Since delivery of the baby is the only cure, pre-eclampsia has become the commonest cause of iatrogenic prematurity.

Table 7.6: Complications related to pre-eclampsia

Maternal	Foetal
• HELLP syndrome	• Oligohydramnios
• Abruptio placentae	• Intrauterine death
• Cerebral haemorrhage	• Premature delivery (before 37 weeks of gestation)
• Eclampsia	• Intrauterine growth restriction
• Sepsis/shock	• Risk of recurrence of intrauterine asphyxia and acidosis
• Risk of recurrence of gestational hypertension or pre-eclampsia in future pregnancies	• Infant death
• Pulmonary oedema	
• Maternal death	

HELLP Syndrome

About 20% of women with severe pre-eclampsia may develop a complication called HELLP syndrome (an abbreviation which stands for haemolysis, elevated liver enzymes and low platelet count).[23] Management of HELLP syndrome has been described in Flow chart 7.5. Use of corticosteroids can help treat the laboratory anomalies associated with HELLP syndrome. Presently, the ACOG Taskforce does not recommend the use of corticosteroids for treatment of thrombocytopenia associated with HELLP syndrome.

 CLINICAL PEARLS

❖ Management of cases with pre-eclampsia is important because there is a danger of progression to eclampsia, if the blood pressure remains uncontrollably high.

❖ Umbilical artery Doppler analysis showing absent or reversed end diastolic flow is associated with poor neonatal outcomes and mandates immediate delivery.

ECLAMPSIA

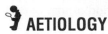 **INTRODUCTION**

Eclampsia can be defined as onset of tonic-clonic convulsions in a pregnant patient with pre-eclampsia, usually occurring in the third trimester of pregnancy, intrapartum period or more than 48 hours postpartum.

AETIOLOGY

Eclampsia is thought to be related to cerebral vasospasm, which can cause ischaemia, disruption of the blood-brain barrier and cerebral oedema.

CHAPTER 7

Flow chart 7.5: Management of cases with HELLP syndrome

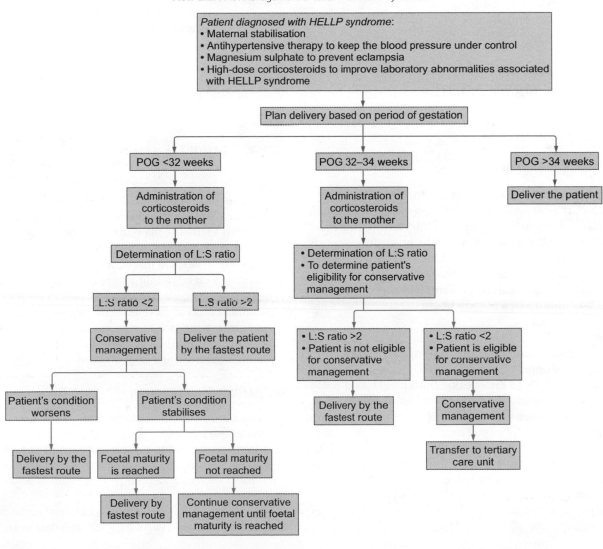

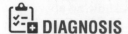 **DIAGNOSIS**

Symptoms

Premonitory stage: In this stage, there is unconsciousness; twitching of the muscles of face, tongue and limbs; and rolling and fixation of eyeballs.

Tonic stage: There is tonic spasm of the body muscles.

Clonic stage: There is alternate contraction and relaxation of the skeletal muscles. Twitching starts from the face onto the extremities and soon involves the whole body.

Coma: This may be present for a brief period or may persist for a longer time.

Investigations

These are same as that described with pre-eclampsia.

 DIFFERENTIAL DIAGNOSIS

❖ Epilepsy, hysteria or poisoning
❖ Meningitis or encephalitis
❖ Cerebral malaria or thrombosis.

 OBSTETRIC MANAGEMENT

Cases with eclampsia are managed as follows and have been summarised in Flow chart 7.6.[5]

Immediate Management

❖ Immediate care involves maintenance of airway, oxygenation, maintenance of circulation and prevention of trauma or injury to the patient. An intravenous line must be secured and the patient must be given intravenous Ringer's lactate or 0.9% normal saline solution. The patient should be shifted to the eclampsia room.
❖ Injury to the patient can be prevented by placing her on a railed bed and using a tongue blade to prevent her from biting her tongue.
❖ Monitoring of vitals including pulse, blood pressure, respiratory rate and oxygen saturation needs to be done at every 15 minutes.
❖ Parameters, such as knee jerks, fluid intake and urine output need to be monitored at every half-hourly interval.
❖ Treatment of choice for convulsions is the administration of magnesium sulphate. The dosage of magnesium sulphate has been previously described. Convulsions must be controlled using an IV administered bolus dose of magnesium sulphate followed by the maintenance dose.
❖ Antihypertensive medicine must be intermittently administered to lower the blood pressure whenever it becomes dangerously high.

Flow chart 7.6: Management of cases of eclampsia

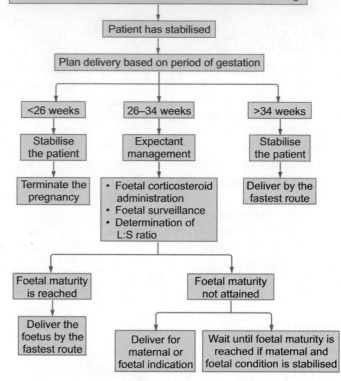

❖ Once the patient has stabilised, an obstetric examination must be performed and foetal status must be evaluated and plan to deliver the patient as soon as possible must be made. Delivery of the foetus is essential to achieve remission in cases of pre-eclampsia.
❖ Continued foetal monitoring is required until the baby is delivered.
❖ Administration of diuretics must be avoided unless there is an obvious pulmonary oedema. Intravenous fluids must be limited unless there is an excessive fluid loss. Hyperosmotic agents are also best avoided.

Intrapartum Management

❖ Strict blood pressure monitoring must be continued throughout labour.
❖ Eclampsia per se is not an indication for caesarean delivery. In case the cervix is not favourable, labour can be induced using vaginal prostaglandins and oxytocin infusion.
❖ Second stage of labour should be cut short through vaginal operative delivery (vacuum or forceps delivery).

PART II

Postnatal Period

- ❖ Following delivery, close monitoring should be continued for a minimum of 24 hours.[24]
- ❖ Since labour and delivery is the likely time for the convulsions to develop, women with pre-eclampsia-eclampsia complex are usually given magnesium sulphate during labour and for 24 hours postpartum.

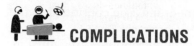
COMPLICATIONS

Maternal

- ❖ Injuries due to fall from bed, tongue bite, etc.
- ❖ *Pulmonary complications*: These include pulmonary oedema, pneumonia, adult respiratory distress, embolism, etc.
- ❖ Hyperpyrexia
- ❖ *Cardiac*: Acute left ventricular failure
- ❖ Renal failure
- ❖ Hepatic necrosis
- ❖ *Cerebral complications*: Cerebral anoxia, cerebral oedema, cerebral dysrhythmia, cerebral haemorrhage, neurological deficits, etc.
- ❖ *Visual complications*: These could be due to retinal detachment or occipital lobe ischaemia.
- ❖ *Haematological complications*: These include thrombocytopenia, DIC, etc.
- ❖ *Postpartum complications*: These include shock, sepsis and psychosis.

Foetal

These are same as those described in the section of pre-eclampsia.

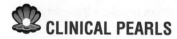
CLINICAL PEARLS

- ❖ In order to prevent the occurrence of eclampsia, women with severe pre-eclampsia (blood pressure >160/110 mmHg along with proteinuria) should be given magnesium sulphate as a prophylactic measure.
- ❖ Occurrence of fits in a quick succession, one after the other is known as status eclampticus.

EVIDENCE-BASED MEDICINE

- ❖ Intravenous magnesium sulphate must be administered if a woman has severe hypertension (blood pressure 160/110 mmHg or higher), severe pre-eclampsia or those who had an eclamptic fit.[16-18]
- ❖ Intravenous administration of magnesium sulphate must also be considered if birth is planned within 24 hours in a woman with severe pre-eclampsia.[16-18]

GESTATIONAL HYPERTENSION

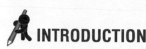
INTRODUCTION

Gestational hypertension can be defined as hypertension (blood pressure at least 140 mmHg systolic or 90 mmHg diastolic) developing for the first time in pregnancy after 20 weeks of gestation, during labour or in the first 24 hours postpartum. It is not accompanied by proteinuria or any other systemic feature of pre-eclampsia in previously normotensive, non-proteinuric women. The blood pressure usually comes back to normal within 3 months postpartum. It can be classified as mild, moderate and severe. In severe gestational hypertension, the systolic blood pressure can be elevated to 160 mmHg or higher and diastolic blood pressure to 110 mmHg or higher on two occasions at least 4–6 hours apart. Diagnosis of this condition is important because women with gestational hypertension need to be monitored for ensuring that they do not develop proteinuria over a period of time, eventually resulting in pre-eclampsia.

AETIOLOGY

The causative features of severe gestational hypertension include:
- ❖ Poor placentation
- ❖ Placental ischaemia and insufficiency
- ❖ Haemodynamic changes characterised by vasoconstriction and reduced cardiac output.

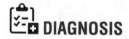
DIAGNOSIS

Clinical Presentation

Increased blood pressure: There is presence of an increased blood pressure (>140/90 mmHg) for the first time during pregnancy, after 20 weeks of gestation. Blood pressure usually returns to normal within 3 months postpartum. There is no accompanying proteinuria.

Abdominal Examination

There may be evidence of placental insufficiency in the form of oligohydramnios and/or IUGR.

Investigations

In mild to moderate cases, there may be no changes in the various blood investigations. However, in severe cases of gestational hypertension, the aberration in various blood parameters may be similar to that described in the section of pre-eclampsia.

CHAPTER 7

OBSTETRIC MANAGEMENT

Antenatal Care

Women with gestational hypertension must be offered an integrated package of care comprising of admission to hospital, treatment, measurement of blood pressure, testing for proteinuria and blood tests as indicated in Table 7.7.

❖ Drugs used for controlling severe gestational hypertension include methyldopa, labetalol and nifedipine.

❖ Women with gestational hypertension must be offered antihypertensive treatment other than labetalol, e.g. methyldopa and labetalol only after considering their side-effect profiles for the woman, foetus and newborn baby.

❖ In women receiving outpatient care for severe gestational hypertension, once the blood pressure has been effectively controlled in hospital and the patient has been discharged home, blood pressure measurement and testing the urine for proteinuria must be done twice weekly. Other blood tests must be carried out on a weekly basis.

❖ Bed rest must not be offered in the hospital as a treatment for gestational hypertension.

Foetal Monitoring

This is same as described in the section of pre-eclampsia.

Timing of Birth

❖ Women with gestational hypertension whose blood pressure is lower than 160/110 mmHg, with or without antihypertensive treatment should preferably not be delivered before 37 weeks of gestation.[25]

❖ For women with gestational hypertension whose blood pressure is lower than 160/110 mmHg after 37 weeks, with or without antihypertensive treatment, timing of birth, and maternal and foetal indications for birth should be agreed upon following discussion between the woman and the senior obstetrician.

❖ Women with refractory severe gestational hypertension must be delivered after a course of corticosteroids has been completed, especially if the period of gestation is less than 32 weeks.

Intrapartum Care

For Women with Mild or Moderate Hypertension

❖ Blood pressure must be measured on an hourly basis.

❖ Antihypertensive treatment must be continued in the intrapartum period.

❖ Haematological and biochemical monitoring must be carried out according to criteria from the antenatal period (Table 7.6).

❖ The duration of the second stage of labour must not be limited if blood pressure is stable.

For Women with Severe Hypertension

❖ Blood pressure must be measured continually.

❖ Antihypertensive treatment must be continued in the intrapartum period.

❖ Haematological and biochemical monitoring must be carried out according to criteria from the antenatal period (Table 7.6).

❖ The duration of the second stage of labour must not be limited if blood pressure is controlled within the normal range. If blood pressure does not respond to initial treatment, operative vaginal birth must be advised.

Postnatal Care

❖ Antenatal antihypertensive treatment must be continued during the postnatal period.

❖ If the patient had not been receiving any antihypertensive treatment in the antenatal period, antihypertensive treatment must be started during the postnatal period if blood pressure becomes 150/100 mmHg or higher.

❖ Blood pressure must be measured daily for the first 2 days after the birth; at least once every 3–5 days thereafter and then as per clinical indications.

Table 7.7: Management in cases with gestational hypertension during the antenatal period

Degree of hypertension	Mild gestational hypertension (140/90 to 149/99 mmHg)	Moderate gestational hypertension (150/100 to 159/109 mmHg)	Severe gestational hypertension (160/110 mmHg or higher)
Admission to the hospital	No	No	Yes (until blood pressure is 159/109 mmHg or lower)
Treatment	No	Oral labetalol must be administered as first line treatment for keeping diastolic blood pressure between 80–100 mmHg and systolic blood pressure less than 150 mmHg	Oral labetalol must be administered as first-line treatment for keeping diastolic blood pressure between 80–100 mmHg and systolic blood pressure less than 150 mmHg
Blood pressure measurement	Not more than once a week	At least twice a week	At least four times a day
Test for proteinuria	Test for proteinuria must be done at each visit using automated reagent-strip reading device or urinary protein: creatinine ratio	Test for proteinuria must be done at each visit using automated reagent-strip reading device or urinary protein: creatinine ratio	Test for proteinuria must be done on daily basis using automated reagent-strip reading device or urinary protein: creatinine ratio
Blood tests	Only those blood tests required for routine antenatal care are done	Blood tests, which need to be performed, include kidney function tests, electrolytes, full blood count, transaminases, and serum bilirubin levels. Further blood tests are not required if there is no proteinuria during subsequent visits	Test at presentation and then monitor weekly: kidney function, electrolytes, full blood count, transaminases, and serum bilirubin levels

PART II

- If methyldopa was used during pregnancy, it should be stopped within 2 days of birth.
- If blood pressure falls to below 130/80 mmHg, the antihypertensive treatment must be reduced.
- If the woman is breastfeeding, the use of diuretics for treatment of hypertension is best avoided.
- A medical review must be offered to women who have had gestational hypertension and remains on antihypertensive treatment 2 weeks after transfer to community care.

 ## COMPLICATIONS

Gestational hypertension is not a benign condition and pregnancy outcomes in severe gestational hypertension may be worse than that in mild pre-eclampsia. This condition may be associated with the following complications:
- Increased maternal and perinatal morbidity due to placental insufficiency
- Increased incidence of obstetric interventions such as induction of labour and caesarean section
- Increased incidence of preterm or small for gestational age (SGA) babies
- Progression to pre-eclampsia which is heralded by the development of proteinuria.

 ## CLINICAL PEARLS

- Diagnosis and management of gestational hypertension is important because nearly 15–25% of women with gestational hypertension may subsequently progress to the development of clinical syndrome of pre-eclampsia.

 ## EVIDENCE-BASED MEDICINE

- The early the period of gestation at which the gestational hypertension is recognised and more severe the hypertension, higher is the risk of developing pre-eclampsia and related morbidity.[26] It is associated with a substantial increase in poor maternal and perinatal outcome.
- On the other hand, onset of gestational hypertension after 35 weeks of gestation is associated with a low risk (approximately 10%) for development of pre-eclampsia. It is also associated with a little increase in the risk of adverse pregnancy outcomes.

CHRONIC HYPERTENSION

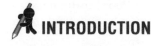 ## INTRODUCTION

Chronic hypertension can be defined as the presence of persistent hypertension, whatever be the cause, before 20th week of gestation (in the absence of hydatidiform mole) or persistent hypertension beyond 6 weeks postpartum. Chronic hypertension can be of two types:

1. Essential or primary hypertension (there is no underlying abnormality)
2. Secondary hypertension (there is an underlying abnormality such as renal parenchymal disease, endocrinological disease, etc.)

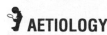 ## AETIOLOGY

Overall, approximately 95% cases of hypertension come in the category of primary hypertension. On the other hand, nearly 5% cases are secondary and could be related to an underlying renal or adrenal disease. Renal causes include glomerulonephritis, tubointerstitial disease such as reflex pyelonephritis, renal stone or renal artery stenosis. Endocrine diseases include Cushing's syndrome, Conn's syndrome, phaeochromocytoma, thyroid disease, etc.[27]

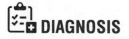 ## DIAGNOSIS

Clinical Presentation

Physical Examination

A physical examination comprising of the following must be performed in cases of chronic hypertension:
- Calculation of the BMI
- Presence of bruits or systolic murmur in association with delayed femoral pulses could be indicative of renal artery stenosis or coarctation of the aorta respectively.
- Polycystic kidneys may be palpable on abdominal examination.
- Fundoscopy to look for the evidence of an arterial disease may reveal retinal changes such as vessel tortuosity, silver wiring, arteriovenous nipping, etc.
- In severe cases, there may be retinal haemorrhages in association with hard exudates, cotton wool spots and papilloedema.

Investigations

The investigations, which need to be performed, include measurement of the urea levels, serum electrolytes, urine analysis, 24-hour urine collection for proteins and creatinine clearance. In severe cases, the following tests need to be done: chest X-ray, electrocardiogram (ECG), testing of antinuclear antibodies, etc. Echocardiography may be required in cases where there is a long-standing history of severe hypertension. In case of history of thromboembolic events or recurrent pregnancy loss, investigation of lupus anticoagulant and anticardiolipin antibodies must be performed.

 ## OBSTETRIC MANAGEMENT

Prevention

- Women with chronic hypertension, similar to those at risk of pre-eclampsia must be advised to take 75 mg of aspirin daily from 12 weeks onwards until the baby's birth.

CHAPTER 7

❖ Women with chronic hypertension must be encouraged to lower their dietary sodium intake or use sodium substitute in their diet.

Antenatal Care

❖ In women with chronic hypertension, additional antenatal consultations may be required based on the individual needs of the woman and her baby.

❖ In pregnant women with uncomplicated chronic hypertension, the main aim during the antenatal period is to keep blood pressure lower than 150/100 mmHg. In case of a pregnant woman having chronic hypertension associated with underlying target-organ damage, the main aim must be to keep the blood pressure lower than 140/90 mmHg.

❖ Patients with chronic hypertension are at an increased risk of developing pre-eclampsia. Since these patients are at an increased risk for development of pre-eclampsia, they must be regularly assessed for proteinuria. The second most important complication in patients with chronic hypertension is placental abruption.

❖ Even women who do not develop overt signs of pre-eclampsia are at an increased risk of pre-eclampsia. Such women must be strictly monitored by checking their blood pressure and urine analysis which must be performed at least after every 2 weeks. Uterine artery Doppler analysis helps in estimating the risk in these individuals. Measurement of platelet count and uric acid levels also help in identification of those individuals who are likely to develop the clinical manifestations of pre-eclampsia as these biochemical abnormalities may precede the development of proteinuria by few weeks.

❖ Pregnant women with chronic hypertension must be offered referral to a medicine specialist dealing with hypertensive disorders.

Timing of Birth

❖ Women with chronic hypertension whose blood pressure is lower than 160/110 mmHg, with or without antihypertensive treatment, should not be preferably delivered before 37 weeks.

❖ Following 37 completed weeks of gestation, the timing of delivery can be agreed upon based on the consultation between the woman and the senior obstetrician.

❖ If the woman has refractory severe chronic hypertension, she should preferably be delivered after a course of corticosteroids (if required) has been completed.

Foetal Monitoring

❖ In women with chronic hypertension, ultrasound-assisted foetal growth and amniotic fluid volume assessment, and umbilical artery Doppler velocimetry should be done between 28 to 30 weeks and between 32 to 34 weeks of gestation respectively. If results are normal, there is no need to repeat these investigations at more than 34 weeks, unless otherwise clinically indicated.

❖ In women with chronic hypertension, cardiotocography must be done only if foetal activity is abnormal.

Antihypertensive Treatment

❖ Various drugs used for the treatment of chronic hypertension in pregnancy are enumerated in Table 7.8.[28] On the other hand, drugs used for urgent control of severe hypertension in pregnancy are described in Table 7.9.[28]

❖ Hypertensive women who had been taking ACE inhibitors, ARBs, and/or chlorothiazide during the antenatal period must be advised about alternative antihypertensive treatment options because these drugs may be associated with an increased risk of congenital abnormalities and neonatal complications if taken during pregnancy.

❖ Women taking ACE inhibitors and ARBs prior to conception must be advised to stop these drugs within 2 days of notification of pregnancy and be prescribed alternative drugs.

❖ Beta-blockers must also be avoided during pregnancy due to the risk of IUGR.

❖ Antihypertensive drugs such as calcium channel blockers (e.g. nifidepine), centrally acting drugs such as methyldopa and labetalol have been commonly used during pregnancy. There appears to be no significant advantage of using one drug over the other. Methyldopa is probably the drug, which is associated with longest most established safety profile. It has not been found to be associated with any adverse effect on the neonatal or long-term outcome. However, methyldopa can be associated with side effects such as depression, tiredness and occasionally liver dysfunction. Therefore, newer antihypertensive drugs like labetalol are increasingly being used.

Intrapartum Care

Mild or Moderate Hypertension

❖ Antenatal antihypertensive treatment must be continued for women with mild or moderate hypertension.

❖ Blood pressure should be measured on an hourly basis.

❖ Haematological and biochemical monitoring must be carried out according to criteria to be followed in the antenatal period.

❖ If blood pressure is stable, the duration of the second stage of labour must not be limited.

Severe Hypertension

❖ Antenatal antihypertensive treatment must be continued for women with severe hypertension.

❖ Blood pressure should be measured continuously.

❖ Haematological and biochemical monitoring must be carried out according to criteria to be followed in the antenatal period.

❖ If blood pressure is stable, the duration of the second stage of labour must not be limited. If blood pressure does not respond to initial treatment, operative vaginal birth must be advised.

Table 7.8: Drugs for chronic hypertension in pregnancy[28]

Drug	Dose	Comments
Methyldopa	0.5–3.0 g/day in 2 divided doses	Drug of choice according to NHBPEP working group. The safety of this drug after the first trimester has been well documented
Labetalol	200–1,200 mg/day in 2–3 divided doses	The use of this drug during pregnancy is gaining popularity because no real adverse effects have been demon-strated
Nifedipine	30–120 mg/day of a slow release preparation	Nifedipine may inhibit labour and has synergistic interaction with magnesium sulphate causing the possible risk of neuromuscular blockade and myocardial depression. There has been little experience with other calcium-channel blockers
Hydralazine	It is used for urgent control of severe hypertension or as a third-line agent for multidrug control of refractory hypertension in the dosage of 50–300 mg/day in 2–4 divided doses	Though there are a few controlled trials, long-term experience with a low risk for adverse events has been documented. It is useful only in combination with sympatholytic agent. Its use may be associated with neonatal thrombocytopenia
β-receptor blockers	• Dosage varies with different agents. Propranolol is initiated at a dosage of 40–60 mg daily. The maximum dosage is 480–640 mg/day • Dosage of labetalol has been previously mentioned	• Use of β-blockers in general may cause foetal bradycardia and reduced uteroplacental blood flow. None of them has been found to be associated with tetratogenicity. However, there is a risk for foetal growth restriction with the use of atenolol in the first or second trimesters. Use of atenolol must be avoided during pregnancy • Presently, labetalol is being considered safer than other β-blockers during pregnancy and it is rapidly becoming the first-line therapy for the treatment of chronic hypertension during pregnancy. Propranolol can also be considered as an effective drug for treatment of chronic hypertension during pregnancy
ACE inhibitors	To be avoided in all trimesters of pregnancy	Exposure during the first trimester has been found to be associated with the congenital malformations of the cardiovascular and central nervous systems. Exposure during the second and third trimesters can result in complications such as oligohydramnios, foetal growth restriction, bony malformations, hypocalvaria, limb contractures, persistent patent ductus arteriosus, pulmonary hypoplasia, etc.
AT1- receptor antagonists	This is classified as category X drug during second and third trimesters of pregnancy. Its use should be avoided in all trimesters of pregnancy	Its use may be associated with various foetal anomalies

Abbreviations: NHBPEP, National High Blood Pressure Education Program; ACE, angiotensin-converting enzyme; AT 1, angiotensin 1

CHAPTER 7

Postnatal Care

❖ The aim of antihypertensive treatment in the postnatal period must be to keep the blood pressure lower than 140/90 mmHg.

❖ Blood pressure must be measured daily for first 2 days after birth; at least once 3–5 days after birth and thereafter as per clinical indications.

❖ If methyldopa was prescribed during pregnancy, it should be stopped within 2 days of birth.

❖ Treatment with diuretics must be avoided in women who are breastfeeding.

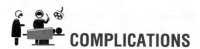

COMPLICATIONS

Complications due to chronic hypertension are as follows: [29]

Complications due to hypertension per se: Some of these Complications include:

❖ Stroke or heart attack

❖ Aneurysm

❖ Heart failure

❖ Renal dysfunction

❖ Metabolic syndrome.

Table 7.9: Drugs used for urgent control of severe hypertension in pregnancy[28]

Drug	Dose and Rate	Comments
Labetalol	20 mg IV, then 20–80 mg every 20–30 minutes, up to a maximum of 300 mg; or constant infusion of 1–2 mg/ minute	Less risk for tachycardia and arrhythmia in comparison to other vasodilators
Hydralazine	5 mg, IV or IM, then 5–10 mg every 20–40 minutes; or constant infusion of 0.5–10 mg/ hour	Drug of choice according to NHBPEP working group; long-term experience of safety and efficacy
Nifedipine	Tablets recommended only; 10–30 mg orally, repeat in 45 minutes if needed	Possible interference with labour

Abbreviation: NHBPEP, National High Blood Pressure Education Program

Complications specific to pregnancy: These include:

❖ Placental abruption
❖ Superimposed pre-eclampsia or pregnancy aggravated hypertension
❖ Complications associated with pre-eclampsia, e.g. eclampsia, oligohydramnios, IUGR, etc.

CLINICAL PEARLS

❖ Treatment of moderate hypertension during pregnancy is associated with a significant reduction in the cases of severe hypertension.
❖ Antihypertensive treatment during pregnancy does not influence the perinatal mortality rate or the subsequent development of pre-eclampsia.

EVIDENCE-BASED MEDICINE

❖ Presently, the limited amount of available evidence has not shown an increased risk of congenital malformations with antihypertensive treatments other than ACE inhibitors, ARBs or chlorothiazide.[27]
❖ Available evidence has indicated an increased risk of congenital malformations and neonatal complications with antihypertensive treatment such as ACE inhibitors, ARBs or diuretics (e.g. chlorothiazide) during pregnancy. Therefore, during pregnancy, it is recommended that these drugs be changed to alternative antihypertensive agents.[27]

REFERENCES

1. NHBPEP (National High Blood Pressure Education Program) working group. Report of the National High Blood Pressure Education Program working group in high blood pressure in pregnancy. Am J Obstet Gynecol. 2000;183: S1-22.

2. American College of Obstetricians and Gynecologists. Hypertension in pregnancy. Report of the American College of Obstetricians and gynecologists taskforce on hypertension in pregnancy. Obstet Gynecol. 2013;122: 1122.

3. Sibai BM. Imitators of severe pre-eclampsia. Obstet Gynecol. 2007;109: 956.

4. Vollard E, Zeeman G, Alexander JA, McIntire DD, Cunningham FG. "Delta eclampsia"—a hypertensive encephalopathy of pregnancy in "normotensive" women. Am J Obstet Gynecol. 2007;197 (6 Suppl): S140.

5. ACOG Committee on Obstetric Practice. ACOG practice bulletin. Diagnosis and management of preeclampsia and eclampsia. Number 33, January 2002. American College of Obstetricians and Gynecologists. Int J Gynaecol Obstet. 2002;77(1): 67-75.

6. Lindheimer MD, Taler SJ, Cunningham FG. Hypertension in pregnancy. J Am Soc Hypertens. 2008;2(6): 484-94.

7. Levine RJ, Hauth JC, Curet LB, Sibai BM, Catalano PM, Morris CD, et al. Trial of calcium to prevent pre-eclampsia. N Engl J Med. 1997;337(2): 69-76.

8. Caritis S, Sibai B, Hauth J, Lindheimer C, Klebanoff M, Thom E, et al. Low dose aspirin to prevent to prevent pre-eclampsia in women at high risk. National institute of child health and human development network of maternal-fetal medicine units. N Engl J Med. 1998;338(11): 701-5.

9. National Institute for Health and Care Excellence. Hypertension in pregnancy: Management of hypertensive disorders during pregnancy. Clinical guideline No. 107. London: RCOG Press; 2010.

10. Abenhaim HA, Bujold E, Benjamin A, Kinch RA. Evaluating the role of bedrest on the prevention of hypertensive disease of pregnancy and growth restriction. Hypertens Pregnancy. 2008;27(2): 197-205.

11. Abalos E, Duley L, Steyn DW, Henderson-Smart DJ. Antihypertensive drug therapy for mild to moderate hypertension during pregnancy. Cochrane Database Syst Rev. 2007;(1): CD002252.

12. Royal College of Obstetricians and Gynaecologists. (2006). The management of severe pre-eclampsia. [online] RCOG website. Available from http: //ncagip.ru/for-experts/snk/RCOG.pdf. [Accessed May 2016].

13. Alanis MC, Robinson CJ, Hulsey TC, Ebeling M, Johnson DD. Early onset severe pre-eclampsia: induction of labour versus elective cesarean delivery and neonatal outcomes. Am J Obstet Gynecol. 2008;199(3): 262.e1-6.

14. Barber D, Xing G, Towner D. Expectant management of severe pre-eclampsia between 24–32 weeks of gestation: a ten-year review. (Abstract No 742). California : 29th Annual Meeting Of The Society For Maternal–Fetal Medicine; 2009.

15. Amorim MM, Santos LC, Faundes A. Corticosteroid therapy for prevention of respiratory distress syndrome in severe pre-eclampsia. Am J Obstet Gynecol. 1999;180(5): 1283-8.

16. Altman D, Carroli G, Duley L, Farrell B, Moodley J, Neilson J, et al. Do women with pre-eclampsia and their babies benefit from magnesium sulphate? The Magpie trial: a randomized placebo controlled trial. Lancet. 2002;359(9321): 1877-90.

17. Magpie trial Follow-up Collaborative Group. The Magpie trial: a randomised trial comparing magnesium sulphate with placebo for pre-eclampsia. Outcome for women at 2 years. BJOG. 2007;114(3): 300-9.

18. Smyth RM, Spark P, Armstrong N, Duley L. Magpie trial in the UK: methods and additional data for women and children at 2 years following pregnancy complicated by pre-eclampsia. BMC Pregnancy Childbirth. 2009;9: 15.

19. The Eclampsia Trial Collaborative Group. Which anti-convulsant for women with eclampsia? Evidence from the Collaborative Eclampsia Trial. Lancet. 1995;345: 1455-63.

20. American College of Obstetrics and Gynecology. ACOG practice bulletin. Obstetric analgesia and anesthesia. Number 36, July 2002. American College of Obstetrics and Gynecology. Int J Gynaecol Obstet. 2002;78(3): 321-35.

21. Duley L, Meher S, Abalos E. Management of pre-eclampsia. BMJ. 2006;332(7539): 463-8.

22. Bellamy L, Casas JP, Hingorani AD, Williams DJ. Pre-eclampsia and risk of cardiovascular disease and cancer later in life: systematic review and metaanalysis. BMJ. 2007;335(7627): 974.

23. Hupuczi P, Nagy B, Sziller I, Rigó B, Hruby E, Papp Z. Characteristic laboratory changes in pregnancies complicated by HELLP syndrome. Hypertens Pregnancy. 2007;26(4): 389-401.

24. Brown CE, Cunningham FG, Pritchard JA. Convulsions in hypertensive, proteinuric primiparas more than 24 hours after delivery: eclampsia or some other cause? J Reprod Med. 1987;32(7): 499-503.

25. Koopmans CM, Bijlenga D, Groen H, Vijgen SM, Aarnoudse JG, Bekedam DJ, et al. Induction of labour versus expectant monitoring for gestational hypertension or mild pre-eclampsia after 36 weeks of gestation (HYPITAT): a multicentric, open label randomised control trial. Lancet. 2009;374(9694): 979-88.

26. Saudan P, Brown MA, Buddle ML, Jones M. Does gestational hypertension become pre-eclampsia? Br J Obstet Gynaecol. 1998;105(11): 1177-84.

27. August P, Jayabalan A, Roberts JM. Chronic hypertension. In: Taylor RN, Roberts JM, Cunningham FG (Eds). Chesley's Hypertensive Disorders in Pregnancy, 4th edition. Amsterdam: Academic Press; 2014.

28. Alpern RJ, Hebert SC. Seldin and Giebisch's The Kidney: Physiology and Pathophysiology, 4th edition. San Diego, California: Academic Press, Elsevier; 2008. p. 2387.

29. Seely EW, Maxwell C. Cardiology patient page. Chronic hypertension in pregnancy. Circulation. 2007;115: e188-90.

CHAPTER 7

Cardiac Disease in Pregnancy

INTRODUCTION

Pregnancy is associated with significant haemodynamic changes (Fig. 8.1 and Table 8.1) that can pose a substantial demand on cardiac function in patients with valvular heart disease and may require the initiation or titration of cardiovascular medications to manage volume overload, hypertension or arrhythmias. Furthermore, pregnancy is a state of relative hypercoagulability, which clearly increases the risk of thromboembolic events.

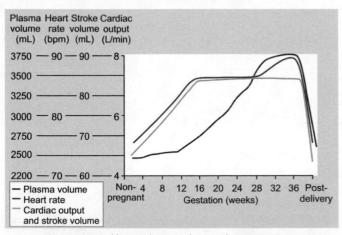

Fig. 8.1: Normal haemodynamic changes during pregnancy

The most common valvular heart disease encountered during pregnancy is mitral stenosis. Chronic mitral regurgitation, most commonly encountered as a result of rheumatic heart disease is usually well-tolerated during pregnancy.

AETIOLOGY

Heart disease in pregnancy can be due to the various causes listed in Table 8.2. According to the Confidential Enquiries into Maternal Deaths (CEMD), UK, the overall rate of mortality due to cardiac disease has risen from 7.3 per million births in the 1982–84 triennium to 22.7 per million births in the 2003–05 triennium.[1,2] Majority of the cases related to heart disease in pregnancy can be attributed to the acquired causes. Rheumatic heart disease is less common in the UK but is increasingly encountered in the immigrant population, especially that belonging to the developing countries. Mitral stenosis is the most common rheumatic heart disease encountered in pregnancy.

DIAGNOSIS

Clinical Presentation

❖ Fatigue, dizziness
❖ Dyspnoea, orthopnoea

Table 8.1: Haemodynamic changes during normal pregnancy

Haemodynamic parameter	Change during antepartum period	Change during labour and delivery	Change during postpartum period
Blood volume	Increases by 40–50%	Increases	Decreases (auto-diuresis)
Heart rate	Increases by 10–15 beats/min	Increases	Decreases
Cardiac output	Increases by 30–50% above the baseline	Additional increase by 50%	Decreases
Blood pressure	Decreases by 10 mmHg	Increases	Decreases
Stroke volume	Increases during the first and second trimesters; decreases during the third trimester	Additional increase of 300–500 mL with each uterine contraction	Decreases
Systemic vascular resistance	Decreases	Increases	Decreases

Table 8.2: Various causes for heart disease in pregnancy

Congenital causes	Acquired causes
• Atrial septal defects • Ventricular septal defects • Patent ductus arteriosus	• Ischaemic heart disease • Rheumatic heart disease • Cardiomyopathies • Aneurysms • Dissection of aorta or its branches: Bicuspid aortic valve, aortic coarctation, Turner's syndrome, Marfan's syndrome, Ehler's Danlos syndrome • Pulmonary hypertension: Idiopathic pulmonary arterial hypertension, Eisenmenger's syndrome

❖ Non-specific chest pain
❖ Peripheral oedema
❖ *Palpitations*: May be due to ectopic beats, atrial fibrillations, supraventricular tachycardia, thyrotoxicosis, anxiety, etc.
❖ Abdominal discomfort and distension
❖ Light-headedness or fainting.

General Physical Examination

❖ *Pulse*: Abnormalities in pulse pattern may be suggestive of underlying cardiac disease. Presence of radiofemoral delay could be suggestive of coarctation of aorta.
❖ *Respiratory rate*: The patient's dyspnoea may be revealed.
❖ *Finger clubbing*: Clubbing of fingers may be associated with the diseases of heart or lungs.
❖ *Cyanosis*: Presence of cyanosis suggests that arterial oxygen saturation is less than 85%. Peripheral cyanosis is detected in the fingertips including underneath the nail beds, whereas central cyanosis may be present in the lips and tongue.
❖ *Features indicative of infective endocarditis*: These may include features, such as splinter haemorrhages, Janeway lesions, Osler's nodes, etc.
❖ *Peripheral oedema*: Presence of oedema in the feet or sacral region could occur as a result of congestive cardiac failure.

Abdominal Examination

Hepatomegaly: Presence of hepatomegaly or ascites on abdominal examination could be due to congestive heart failure.

Examination of Cardiovascular System

❖ *Palpation*: The cardiac apex (normally palpated in the left fifth intercostal space, 1 centimetre medial to the mid-clavicular line) may be shifted downward and outward in cases of left ventricular enlargement.
❖ *Auscultation*: Upon auscultation of the precordial area, normal heart sounds (S1 and S2) can be heard. It is important to note whether or not an additional sound (e.g. murmur, opening snap, click, third or fourth heard sounds, etc.) is present during auscultation.

Investigations

❖ A 12-lead electrocardiogram and a chest radiograph
❖ A transthoracic echocardiogram
❖ An arterial oxygen saturation measurement by percutaneous oximetry.

 MANAGEMENT

Antenatal Care

❖ *Management of mitral stenosis*: Drugs, like digoxin and β-blockers, can be used to reduce heart rate and diuretics can be used to reduce the blood volume and left atrial pressure. With development of atrial fibrillations and haemodynamic deterioration, electrocardioversion can be performed safely.[3] Anticoagulation must be initiated with the onset of atrial fibrillations in order to reduce the risk of stroke. Heart surgery may be necessary when medical treatment fails to control heart failure or symptoms remain intolerable to the patients despite medical therapy. While open heart surgery may be associated with risks to the foetus, closed mitral valvuloplasty (CMV) is a relatively safe procedure. It may be performed in case of severe pulmonary congestion, which is unresponsive to drugs, profuse haemoptysis and any episode of pulmonary oedema before pregnancy. Most patients with mitral stenosis can undergo vaginal delivery.

Women with severe mitral stenosis or those, in whom medical therapy has failed, must be advised to delay pregnancy until after balloon, open or closed mitral valvotomy or mitral valve replacement. Management of women with mitral stenosis during and prior to pregnancy is summarised in Flow chart 8.1.

Flow chart 8.1: Management of women with mitral stenosis during and prior to pregnancy

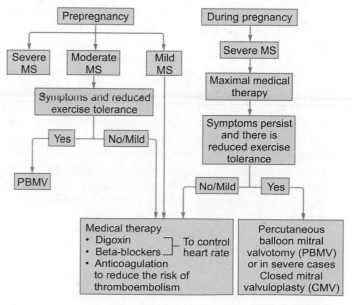

Abbreviation: MS, mitral stenosis

Flow chart 8.2: Management of pregnancy in a patient with prosthetic heart valves

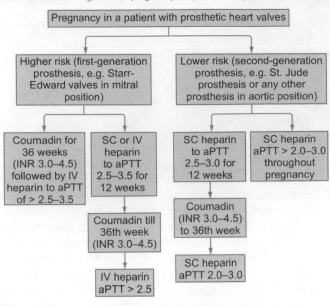

Flow chart 8.3: Regimens for administration of anticoagulation therapy during pregnancy

PART II

❖ *Mechanical heart valves*: Women with heart valve replacement require life-long anticoagulation, which must also be continued during pregnancy due to an increased risk of thrombosis. Management of pregnancy in a patient with prosthetic heart valves is described in Flow chart 8.2. Use of warfarin can result in warfarin embryopathy and increased risk of complications such as miscarriage, stillbirths, foetal intracerebral haemorrhages, etc. Use of heparin, on the other hand, may be associated with an increased risk of thrombosis and thromboembolic events.[4,5] The available evidence advocates the use of warfarin therapy throughout pregnancy.[4,5] Anticoagulation with warfarin is the safest option for the mother because it is most effective in preventing valve thrombosis and thromboembolism. However, use of warfarin may be associated with an increased risk of foetal anomalies. Other management strategies for the administration of anticoagulation therapy during pregnancy are described in Flow chart 8.3. These strategies involve replacement of warfarin with either unfractionated heparin (UFH) or low-molecular-weight heparin (LMWH) during 6–12 weeks of gestation (to avoid warfarin embryopathy) or continuous use of either UFH or LMWH throughout the pregnancy. Heparin does not cross the placenta and therefore does not have any harmful effect over the foetus. However, the risk of thromboembolic complications is high with the continuous use of UFH or LMWH throughout the pregnancy.

No matter what therapy is used, warfarin should be discontinued and replaced with heparin 10 days prior to delivery so that warfarin can get cleared off from the foetal circulation. Just prior to delivery, heparin must also be discontinued. Warfarin must be started again, 2–3 days after the delivery during the postpartum period. In the

event of bleeding in a fully coagulated patient, effects of warfarin can be reversed with fresh frozen plasma and vitamin K and that of heparin with protamine sulphate.

❖ *Aortic dissection*: Aortic dissection is an important cause of cardiac death in pregnancy. Progressive dilatation of the aortic root and its dimensions greater than 4 cm are associated with an increased risk. Systolic hypertension in association with severe chest or interscapular pain is indicative of acute aortic dissection. Systolic hypertension is also an important cause of death in cases of aortic dissection. This emphasises the importance of regular blood pressure monitoring and prompt administration of antihypertensive therapy in pregnancy in case of blood pressure elevation.

❖ *Pulmonary hypertension*: Women with pulmonary hypertension must be advised to avoid pregnancy. In the event of an unplanned pregnancy, a therapeutic termination must be advised. If the woman refuses to get her pregnancy terminated, she should be advised bed rest, oxygen and thromboprophylaxis. Drugs such as endothelin antagonists and sildenafil should be continued in pregnancy despite of the foetal risks associated with endothelin antagonists. Some centres prefer to use nebulised or IV prostacyclin.

❖ *Congenital heart disease*: Women with congenital heart disease should be offered a foetal echocardiogram during the second trimester, preferably carried out by an accredited paediatric or foetal cardiologist.

❖ *Acute myocardial infarction*: Management of acute myocardial infarction during pregnancy is similar to that in non-pregnant women. Coronary angiography must not be withheld in pregnant patients. Percutaneous coronary intervention may prove to be a better alternative to thrombolysis. Aspirin and β-blockers are safe options in pregnancy. However, statins should be discontinued prior to and during pregnancy.

Table 8.3: New York Heart Association functional classification of heart failure

Class I	Patients with cardiac disease, but without resulting limitations of physical activity. Ordinary physical activity does not cause fatigue, palpitations, dyspnoea or anginal pain
Class II	Patients with cardiac disease resulting in slight limitation of physical activity. They are comfortable at rest. Ordinary physical activity results in fatigue, palpitations, dyspnoea or anginal pain
Class III	Patients with cardiac disease resulting in marked limitation of physical activity. They are comfortable at rest. Less than ordinary physical activity results in fatigue, palpitations, dyspnoea or anginal pain
Class IV	Patients with cardiac disease result in an inability to carry out any physical activity without discomfort. Symptoms of cardiac insufficiency may even be present at rest. If any physical activity is undertaken, discomfort is increased

- ❖ *NYHA classification*: Patients can be classified into various New York Heart Association (NYHA) classes based on their underlying functional cardiac status (Table 8.3). Patients with NYHA class III and IV are at a higher risk. In women who have only milder forms of heart disease with no underlying haemodynamic problems, nothing special needs to be done. However, in patients belonging to high risk and having potential or real haemodynamic problems (signs of heart failure or low cardiac output), important decisions including the need for medical termination of pregnancy may be required.
- ❖ *Use of antiarrhythmic medicines during pregnancy*: Pharmacologic treatment is usually reserved for patients with severe symptoms.
- ❖ *Foetal surveillance*: Careful foetal monitoring, mainly in the form of clinical and ultrasound examinations may be required when signs of haemodynamic compromise are present.
- ❖ *Increased frequency of antenatal visits*: In general, prenatal visits should be scheduled every month in women with mild disease and every 2 weeks in women with moderate or severe disease, until 28–30 weeks and weekly thereafter until delivery.
- ❖ *Multidisciplinary team*: Management of a woman with underlying cardiac disease must be carried out by a multidisciplinary team comprising of a cardiologist, obstetrician, physician, haematologist, specialist nurse, etc.
- ❖ *Bed rest*: Bed rest is advised to the women with underlying cardiac disease. However, supine and lithotomy positions must preferably be avoided. Left lateral position is preferred.

Intrapartum Care

- ❖ The main objective of management should be to minimise any additional load on the cardiovascular system from delivery and puerperium by aiming for spontaneous onset of labour and providing effective pain relief with low-dose regional analgesia.
- ❖ Vaginal delivery or assisted vaginal delivery over caesarean section is the preferred mode of delivery for most women with heart disease—whether congenital or acquired. Caesarean section is considered only in the presence of specific obstetric or cardiac considerations which may place the woman at an additional risk during labour.
- ❖ Positioning the patient on the left lateral side helps in reducing associated haemodynamic fluctuations.
- ❖ *Intrapartum endocarditis prophylaxis*: According to the current National Institute for Health and Care Excellence (NICE, 2008) guidelines, antibiotic prophylaxis against infective endocarditis is not required for childbirth.[6] However, previous recommendations by the American Heart Association and British Society for Antimicrobial Chemotherapy (2006) suggested that antibiotic prophylaxis may be required during delivery for women at high risk for developing infective endocarditis (e.g. women with prosthetic heart valves or those with previous history of endocarditis).[7,8] If antibiotics are administered, the subsequent regimen is followed: 1 g amoxicillin (IV) plus 120 mg gentamicin (IV) is administered at the onset of labour or ruptured membranes or prior to caesarean delivery. This is followed by the administration of amoxicillin 500 mg orally (or via IM or IV routes depending on the clinical condition) 6 hours later. For patients allergic to penicillin, 1 g vancomycin (IV) or teicoplanin 400 mg (IV) may be administered.

Postpartum Period

- ❖ *Peripartum cardiomyopathy*: This condition usually presents late in pregnancy or early in puerperium and can occur up to 6 months after delivery. It should be suspected if the pregnant or puerperal woman complains of increasing shortness of breath on lying flat or at night.
- ❖ *Management of the third stage of labour*: During the third stage of labour in women with heart disease, bolus doses of oxytocin can cause severe hypotension and should therefore be avoided. Low-dose oxytocin infusions are safer and may be equally effective. Ergometrine is best avoided in most cases as it can cause acute hypertension. Misoprostol may be safer but it can cause problems such as hyperthermia. At the time of caesarean section, prophylactic compression sutures can be considered instead of oxytocics.

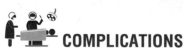

COMPLICATIONS

Maternal: These include the following:
- ❖ Pulmonary oedema and arrhythmias
- ❖ Increased maternal morbidity
- ❖ An increased risk for cardiac complications, such as heart failure, arrhythmias and stroke.

Foetal: These include the following:

❖ Intrauterine growth restriction (mild in cases of patients with rheumatic heart valve disease and severe in cases of lesions associated with cyanosis in the mothers).
❖ Neonatal asphyxia
❖ Respiratory distress
❖ Foetal or neonatal death.

CLINICAL PEARLS

❖ Some cardiac diseases such as pulmonary artery hypertension (due to any cause), severe mitral stenosis, Marfan's syndrome with dilatation of aortic root and severe cardiomyopathy are contraindications for pregnancy.
❖ Angiotensin converting enzyme inhibitors are safe to use in breastfeeding mothers.
❖ There is a small increased risk of IUGR with the use of β-blockers during pregnancy.

EVIDENCE-BASED MEDICINE

❖ The current evidence favours the use of warfarin throughout the pregnancy in order to lower the risk of thromboembolic events.[4,5]
❖ Antibiotic prophylaxis against infective endocarditis is not required for childbirth.[6]

REFERENCES

1. Department of Health and Social Security. Report on Confidential Enquiries into Maternal Deaths in England and Wales, 1982–84. Reports on Health and Social Subjects No. 34. London: HMSO; 1989.
2. Lewis G (Ed). The Confidential Enquiry into Maternal and Child Health (CEMACH). Saving Mothers' Lives: Reviewing Maternal Deaths to Make Motherhood Safer 2003–2005. The Seventh Report on Confidential Enquiries into Maternal Deaths in the United Kingdom. London: CEMACH; 2007.
3. Steer PJ, Gatzoulis MA, Baker P (Eds). Heart Disease and Pregnancy. London: RCOG Press; 2006.
4. Chan WS, Anand S, Ginsberg JS. Anticoagulation of pregnant women with mechanical heart valves. Arch Intern Med. 2000; 160(2):191-6.
5. Sadler L, McCowan L, White H, Stewart A, Bracken M, North R. Pregnancy outcomes and cardiac complications in women with mechanical, biprosthetic and homograft valves. BJOG. 2000;107(2):245-53.
6. NICE. (2008). Prophylaxis against infective endocarditis. [online] NICE website. Available from https://www.nice.org.uk/Guidance/cg64. [Accessed March, 2016].
7. Gould FK, Elliott TSJ, Foweraker J, Fulford M, Perry JD, Roberts GJ, et al. Guidelines for the prevention of endocarditis: report of the Working Party of the British Society for Antimicrobial Chemotherapy. J Antimicrob Chemother. 2006;57:1035-42.
8. American Heart Association Guideline. Prevention of Infective Endocarditis. Circulation. 2007;116:1736-54.

Thyroid Disorders during Pregnancy

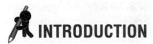 **INTRODUCTION**

Thyroid disease is the most common pre-existing endocrine disease in pregnant women and affects nearly 1% of the population. Thyroid dysfunction can manifest both in the form of hypothyroidism and hyperthyroidism. Thyrotoxicosis occurs in about 1 pregnancy in 500. On the other hand, hypothyroidism occurs in about 1 pregnancy in 100. Both carry risks for the foetus and neonate. Thyrotoxicosis carries bigger risk to the mother.

Functioning of the Thyroid Gland

The thyroid gland is composed of follicular cells (lining the follicles) and the parafollicular or the C cells (which produce the hormone calcitonin). Production of thyroid hormones by the thyroid gland is stimulated by the anterior pituitary hormone, thyroid-stimulating hormone (TSH) and secretion begins from approximately the 12th week of gestation. TSH acts on the thyroid gland to produce the thyroid hormones, thyroxine (T_4) and tri-iodothyronine (T_3) through iodination of tyrosine. Therefore, iodine is essential for the synthesis of thyroid hormones. The thyroid follicles synthesise T_3 and T_4, which is then stored within the colloid at the centre of the thyroid follicles. They are stored attached to thyroglobulin (a glycoprotein in the colloid) and released through proteolysis into the blood wherein, they are mainly transported bound to thyroid-binding globulin (TBG), albumin and transthyretin. The affinity of TBG for binding with the thyroid hormones is quite high, with TBG binding with nearly 75% of the thyroid hormone. The unbound thyroid hormones have the highest biological activity, with 0.04% of T_4 and 0.05% of T_3 being free.[1]

As previously mentioned, thyroid hormones include T_4 and T_3, which are glycoprotein in nature. T_4 is produced within the thyroid gland from the oxidation of four iodide molecules with two tyrosine residues under the influence of peroxidase and iodinase (Fig. 9.1). Out of the two hormones, T_4 and thyronine,

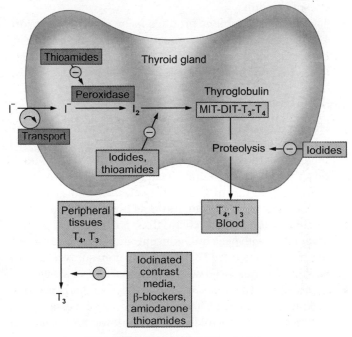

Fig. 9.1: Synthesis of thyroid hormones
Abbreviations: MIT, mono-iodo-tyrosine; DIT, di-iodo-tyrosine; T_3, tri-iodothyronine; T_4, thyroxine; I⁻, iodide, I_2, iodine

thyronine is the most active hormone and is mainly produced by deiodination of thyroxine. In the body, more T_4 than T_3 is produced.

Changes in the Thyroid Gland during Pregnancy

The major changes related to thyroid function during normal pregnancy include the following:

❖ Increase in serum TBG concentrations
❖ Stimulation of the thyrotropin receptor by chorionic gonadotropin
❖ Thyroid-binding globulin excess results in an increase in the concentration of both serum total T_4 and T_3, whereas

free (unbound) serum T_4 and T_3 concentrations remain within normal range. However, these values must be interpreted with pregnancy-specific reference ranges.

❖ Iodine deficiency occurs due to increased loss through glomerular filtration. In absence of adequate iodide content in the diet, this can cause increased iodine uptake by the thyroid gland resulting in thyroid enlargement and goitre.

❖ Maternal iodide pool can also get depleted due to increased foetal thyroid activity wherein iodide moves via diffusion along the concentration gradient.

❖ During the first trimester, foetus requires maternal T_4 for normal brain development. Therefore, small amounts of T_4 may cross the placenta before 12 weeks of gestation. However, otherwise T_3, T_4 and TSH do not cross the placenta. Both T_3 and T_4 are produced by the foetal thyroid gland from 10 weeks onwards. From here onwards, the foetal thyroid axis becomes independent and there is little relationship between maternal and the foetal levels. By 36 weeks of gestation, foetal levels of thyroid hormone reach that of an adult.

❖ The foetus is unable to produce its own thyroxine before 12 weeks. So, there are concerns about embryonic brain development in presence of inadequate maternal thyroxine levels (hypothyroidism).

Thyroid Function Tests during Pregnancy

❖ Human chorionic gonadotropin (hCG) and TSH share a common α subunit and have similar β subunits. TSH receptors are prone to stimulation by the hCG. Due to this, thyroid activity is increased in conditions associated with high serum hCG levels, such as molar gestation, hyperemesis gravidarum, multiple pregnancy, etc.

❖ To balance the thyroid activity, there is a fall in TSH levels in association with peak hCG concentrations even in a normal pregnancy. Since the TSH levels are often supressed, they can only be measured with new ultrasensitive assays.

❖ In pregnancy, there is also an increased placental conversion of T_4 to T_3. Therefore, low levels of T_4 are necessarily not indicative of hypothyroidism. Also, the lower limit of normal for free T_4 is below that on non-pregnant women.

❖ Deiodination also occurs in the trophoblastic and placental tissues, preventing the excessive exposure of thyroid hormone to the baby.

❖ It is important to measure the free levels of T_3 and T_4 and to base the management decisions on these levels.

AETIOLOGY

Hyperthyroidism

The most common cause is Grave's disease, which accounts for about 95% cases of thyrotoxicosis. Less than 5% of cases can occur as a result of toxic thyroid nodule, thyroiditis or a carcinoma. All such patients should be stabilised before pregnancy. Grave's disease is an autoimmune condition, in which antibodies are produced to the TSH receptors in the thyroid cells. These antibodies stimulate the receptors resulting in an increased thyroid activity. The condition is characterised by exophthalmos, evidence of thyroid overactivity and *peau d'orange* appearance of the skin in which the skin is thickened and the pores become prominent. The condition often improves as the pregnancy proceeds because pregnancy is a state of relative immunosuppression. However, the condition reverts back in the puerperium. Diagnosis is based on assay of TSH and T_4. T_4 is raised due to stimulation of the thyroid by autoantibodies. As a consequence of thyroid stimulation, there occurs a fall in TSH levels.

Hyperemesis Gravidarum and Hyperthyroidism

Women with hyperemesis gravidarum have elevated levels of T_4 and suppressed TSH levels. However, there are no clinical signs of thyrotoxicosis and these women do not require treatment with the antithyroid drugs.[2] The condition is related to high hCG levels which stimulate the TSH receptors. The condition is self-limiting and resolves by 20 weeks of gestation with a fall in the levels of β-hCG. A similar picture may be present in cases of gestational trophoblastic disease which is also associated with increased hCG levels.

Hypothyroidism

Hypothyroidism affects about 1% of pregnancies. Hashimoto's disease is the most common cause of hypothyroidism followed by treated Grave's disease. Hashimoto's disease is an auto-immune condition, featuring the presence of microsomal autoantibodies. An important clinical feature is goitre. Hypothyroidism can also result from surgery, radioactive iodine, drugs, etc. Drugs, which can result in hypothyroidism, include carbimazole and thiouracil, radioactive iodine, amiodarone, lithium, etc. De Quervain's thyroiditis is an inflammatory thyroiditis, which can also result in hypothyroidism. Worldwide, the biggest problem related to hypothyroidism is congenital cretinism due to iodine deficiency. In cases of iodine deficiency, the maternal thyroid gland has a greater affinity for iodine in comparison to the placenta. Therefore, the baby may be born with hypothyroidism, cretinism and goitre. The parts of foetal brain, which are particularly sensitive to iodine deficiency, include the cerebral neocortex and the basal ganglia. Iodine deficiency is presently the leading, preventable cause of mental retardation worldwide.[3] In the UK, all newborn babies must be screened for hypothyroidism as part of the Guthrie test. This is a heel-prick bloodspot test. Administration of iodine prior to conception and up to the second trimester is likely to improve the neurological outcome by protecting the foetal brain. This can be achieved through iodination of water, salt or flour. Administration of annual iodide injection to the women of reproductive age groups also appears to be a feasible option.

Though iodine supplementation during pregnancy can help in decreasing the rates of miscarriage and stillbirths, administration of high levels of iodine can also result in foetal hyperthyroidism. Therefore, medicines like cough syrups, eye drops containing iodine, drugs like amiodarone (which is rich in iodine), radiological procedures utilizing iodinated contrast dyes, etc. must be avoided during pregnancy unless absolutely necessary. Amiodarone can lead to both hypothyroidism (amiodarone-induced hypothyroidism) and less commonly hyperthyroidism (amiodarone-induced thyrotoxicosis). Radioactive iodine is capable of destroying foetal thyroid gland and is therefore absolutely contraindicated during pregnancy even in early pregnancy.

Postpartum Thyroiditis

Postpartum thyroiditis is a condition that may develop in approximately 10% of the individuals during the postpartum period. The condition is thought to be autoimmune and usually presents in the postpartum period following a return to normal immunity after delivery. It usually presents with hyperthyroidism. Hyperthyroidism is due to the release of pre-formed hormones as a result of destruction of thyroid follicles. This is followed by hypothyroidism due to the destruction of thyroid gland itself. Hypothyroid phase may last for some months and may present with symptoms such as tiredness, cold intolerance and even goitre. Goitre may be present in approximately 50% cases. These women are predisposed to hypothyroidism in later life. Affected women may present with postnatal depression.[4] All women with postnatal depression should be screened for thyroid function. The condition can be distinguished from Grave's disease with the help of radioactive iodine or technetium uptake tests. While Grave's disease is associated with high uptake of radioactive iodine, postpartum thyroiditis is associated with a reduced uptake. Lactation should be discontinued while the test is being done. Histological testing of the thyroid tissue helps in distinguishing this condition from Hashimoto's thyroiditis, because biopsy reveals a chronic thyroiditis with lymphocytic infiltration in postpartum thyroiditis, while Hashimoto thyroiditis is typically associated with fibrosis.

Treatment should be with β-blockers in symptomatic women with hyperthyroidism. There is no need to prescribe antithyroid drugs in these patients because T_4 production is not increased. In cases of hypothyroidism, a short course of T_4 may be sufficient.

Thyroid Cancer in Pregnancy

Thyroid cancer is encountered 2–3 times more commonly amongst women than in men. Approximately, 50% cases occur in the women of reproductive age group. Pregnancy itself does not appear to affect the survival rate in women diagnosed with thyroid cancer. It is recommended that pregnancy should be delayed after treatment with radioactive iodine probably for a period of 1 year in view of high incidence of congenital anomalies following treatment.[5]

Thyroid function tests and ultrasound are indicated if a pregnant woman presents with a thyroid nodule. Thyro-toxicosis occurring with cystic nodules is unlikely to be malignant. However, any other thyroid nodule must be investigated with help of fine needle aspiration cytology (FNAC). Removal of a thyroid nodule, which is increasing in size, must be considered. Thyroidectomy should be preferably performed in the second trimester.

DIAGNOSIS

Clinical Presentation

Hypothyroidism

The various symptoms include dry skin with yellowing, especially around eyes, hair loss, weakness, tiredness, fatigue, hoarseness, constipation, sleep disturbance, depression, cold intolerance, muscle cramps, weight gain, oedema, dry skin, prolonged relaxation phase of deep tendon reflexes and/or a pathologically enlarged thyroid gland or goitre (in cases of endemic iodine deficiency or Hashimoto's thyroiditis).[6]

Hyperthyroidism

The various symptoms include palpitations, nervousness, irritability, breathlessness, tachycardia, tremors in hands, heat intolerance, insomnia, increased bowel movements, light or absent menstrual periods, weight loss, muscle weakness, warm moist skin, hair loss, nervousness, etc. Typical signs of hyperthyroidism are difficult to elicit in pregnancy. However, signs such as poor weight gain in presence of good appetite or maternal tachycardia that is unresponsive to Valsalva manoeuvre may indicate the disease. There is an association of thyrotoxicosis with hyperemesis gravidarum. Patients with excessive vomiting in early pregnancy should have their thyroid function checked. It is essential to maintain the euthyroid status during pregnancy because uncontrollable maternal disease may be associated with various maternal and foetal complications such as thyroid storm, heart failure, maternal hypertension, premature labour, growth restriction, stillbirths, etc.

Investigations

Hyperthyroidism

The diagnosis of hyperthyroidism in pregnant women should be based primarily on serum TSH value less than 0.01 mU/L and a high serum free T_4 value.[7]

Hypothyroidism

Hypothyroidism is characterised by low T_4 levels and raised TSH levels.

MANAGEMENT

Management of thyroid disorders during pregnancy are well-illustrated in Flow chart 9.1.

CHAPTER 9

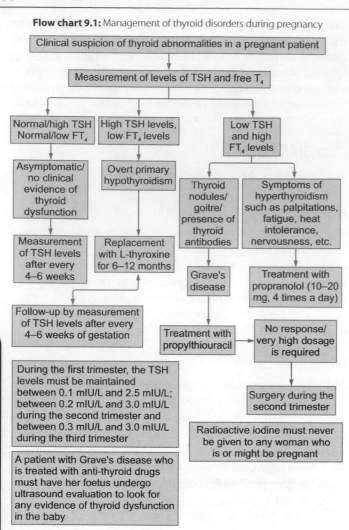

Flow chart 9.1: Management of thyroid disorders during pregnancy

Abbreviations: T$_4$, thyroxine; FT$_4$, free thyroxine; TSH, thyroid-stimulating hormone

Hyperthyroidism

Medical treatment involves blocking the synthesis of thyroid hormones. Thioamides [propylthiouracil (PTU), methimazole and carbimazole] are recommended for the treatment of moderate to severe hyperthyroidism complicating pregnancy. β-blockers may be given to ameliorate the symptoms of moderate to severe hyperthyroidism in pregnant women.

Carbimazole and PTU are the drugs commonly used; carbimazole in the dosage of 15–40 mg daily and thiouracil in the dosage of 150–400 mg daily.

The initial dose is usually gradually reduced after a month to 6 weeks to maintenance levels of carbimazole, 5–15 mg daily, and thiouracil, 50–150 mg daily. If treatment is being started in pregnancy, thiouracil was previously the preferred therapy because it not only inhibited T$_4$ synthesis by blocking the incorporation of iodine into tyrosine, but also by inhibiting the conversion of T$_4$ to T$_3$.[8,9] However, PTU has also been linked with hepatotoxicity.[10] Moreover, both the drugs can cross the placenta in same proportion. According to the present recommendations by the American Thyroid Association and American Association of Clinical Endocrinologists (2011),

use of propylthiouracil therapy during the first trimester must be followed by methimazole beginning in the second trimester.[11,12] However, this may lead to poor controlled thyroid function and therefore, in most National Health Service (NHS) Trusts, the treatment with PTU or carbimazole is continued as such during pregnancy. Both the drugs are non-teratogenic and appear to be equally beneficial and therefore can be continued during pregnancy. Though the evidence is limited, carbimazole is linked to a small risk of teratogenicity. Rare cases of embryopathy, including aplasia cutis, have been reported with use of methimazole (carbimazole) during pregnancy.[13] No such cases have been reported with PTU use during pregnancy. On the other hand, thiouracil has been linked with a small risk of liver diseases. It is advised that the patient be closely monitored for signs of liver problems, especially in the first 6 months of treatment. Carbimazole is also linked to agranulocytosis or bone marrow suppression. Therefore, clinician needs to remain vigilant in patients on carbimazole who develop signs of infection and should stop treatment if there is neutropenia. Both drugs can cause skin rashes in up to 5% individuals. Moreover, both of these drugs can cross the placenta and reach the baby, thereby causing hypothyroidism. Therefore, the baby needs to be closely observed for the signs of hypothyroidism. Treatment with antithyroid drugs must be preferably reduced in the third trimester to prevent foetal hypothyroidism. The dosage can be restored back in the postnatal period.

Breastfeeding: Carbimazole and thiouracil are excreted in small amounts in the breast milk. Usually, there are no consequences and breastfeeding is not contraindicated. However, the baby needs to be observed, particularly if the mother requires high drug doses or breastfeeding is prolonged.

Ablation with radioiodine is absolutely contraindicated during pregnancy due to the possibility of the ablation of foetal thyroid tissue as well, which is usually present by 10–12 weeks of gestation.

In case of failure of medical treatment or clinical suspicion of cancer or compressive symptoms due to goitre, surgery must be considered.

Hypothyroidism

Replacement therapy with levothyroxine is administered in the dosage of 1–2 µg/kg/day (approximately, 100 µg/day) in cases of hypothyroidism. The management is based on the titration of levothyroxine levels against the biochemical parameters. Replacement therapy with levothyroxine is safe during pregnancy and lactation. As long as the patient is clinically euthyroid, thyroid function tests should be performed at intervals of every 2–3 months.[14] More frequent measurements may be required in case of derangement of clinical or biochemical parameters. An increase in therapy is not required during pregnancy in most women. Low level of free T$_4$ rather than free TSH level is more indicative of a requirement for an increase in therapy.

COMPLICATIONS

Hyperthyroidism

This includes complications such as spontaneous abortion or miscarriage, premature labour, low birthweight, stillbirth, pre-eclampsia, heart failure, thyroid storm (rarely), foetal or neonatal hyperthyroidism or hypothyroidism, with or without a goitre, non-immune hydrops and foetal demise. The biggest risk to the mother is the rare 'thyroid storm'. This can cause heart failure and death in up to 30% cases.

Hypothyroidism

This includes complications such as pre-eclampsia, gestational hypertension, placental abruption, non-reassuring foetal heart rate tracing, preterm delivery, low birthweight, increased rate of caesarean section, neuropsychological and cognitive impairment, postpartum haemorrhage (PPH), and overall increased rate of perinatal morbidity and mortality.[15]

CLINICAL PEARLS

- ❖ Grave's disease is the most common cause of hyperthyroidism in pregnancy.
- ❖ Hyperthyroidism during pregnancy can present as hyperemesis gravidarum or rarely as thyroid storm. Therefore, thyroid function tests must be definitely checked in such patients.
- ❖ Serum TSH is the most reliable indicator of genuine hypothyroidism.
- ❖ Overt hypothyroidism complicating pregnancy is unusual because hypothyroidism may be associated with anovulation, as well as a high rate of first trimester spontaneous abortion.

EVIDENCE-BASED MEDICINE

- ❖ Management decisions during pregnancy must be based on the free levels of T_3 and T_4 in the body and not that of the total hormonal levels (bound and free).[1]
- ❖ Women with hypothyroidism should be in the hypothyroid state prior to pregnancy to avoid intellectual impairment in the baby.[3]

REFERENCES

1. Kotarba DD, Garner P, Perkins SL. Changes in serum free thyroxine, free tri-iodothyronine and thyroid stimulating hormone reference intervals in normal term pregnant women. J Obs Gynaecol. 1995;15(1):5-8.
2. Kimura M, Amino N, Tamaki H, Ito E, Mitsuda N, Miyai K, et al. Gestational thyrotoxicosis and hyperemesis gravidarum: possible role of hCG with higher stimulating activity. Clin Endocrinol (Oxf). 1993;38(4):345-50.
3. Cao XY, Jiang XM, Dou ZH, Rakeman MA, Zhang ML, O'Donnell K, et al. Timing of vulnerability of the brain to iodine deficiency in endemic cretinism. N Engl J Med. 1994;331(26):1739-44.
4. Muller AF, Drexhage HA, Berghout A. Postpartum thyroiditis and autoimmune thyroiditis in women of childbearing age: recent insights and consequences for antenatal and postnatal care. Endocr Rev. 2001;22(5):605-30.
5. Shim MH, Mok CW, Chang KH, Sung JH, Choi SJ, Oh SY, et al. Clinical characteristics and outcome of cancer diagnosed during pregnancy. Obstet Gynecol Sci. 2016;59(1):1-8.
6. Hypothyroidism in pregnant women. Drug Bulletin. 2006; 44:53-6.
7. Brent GA. Clinical practice. Grave's disease. N Engl J Med. 2008;358(24):2594-605.
8. Weetman AP. Graves' disease. N Engl J Med. 2000;343(17): 1236-48.
9. Masiukiewicz US, Burrow GN. Hyperthyroidism in pregnancy: Diagnosis and treatment. Thyroid. 1999;9(7):647-52.
10. Wing DA, Millar LK, Koonings PP, Montoro MN, Mestman JH. A comparison of propylthiouracil versus methimazole in the treatment of hyperthyroidism in pregnancy. Am J Obstet Gynecol. 1994;170(1 Pt 1):90-5.
11. Bahn Chair RS, Burch HB, Cooper DS, Garber JR, Greenlee MC, Klein I, et al. Hyperthyroidism and other causes of thyrotoxicosis: management guidelines of American thyroid Association and the American Association of Clinical Endocrinologists. Endocr Pract. 2011;17(3):456-520.
12. Bahn Chair RS, Burch HB, Cooper DS, Garber JR, Greenlee MC, Klein I, et al. Hyperthyroidism and other causes of thyrotoxicosis: management guidelines of the American Thyroid Association and American Association of Clinical Endocrinologists. Thyroid. 2011;21(6):593-646.
13. Karg E, Bereg E, Gaspar L, Katona M, Turi S. Aplasia cutis congenita after methimazole exposure in utero. Pediatr Dermatol. 2004;21(4):491-4.
14. Glinoer D, Abalovich M. Unresolved questions in managing hypothyroidism during pregnancy. BMJ. 2007;335(7614):300-2.
15. Pop VJ, Kuijpens JL, van Baar AL, Verkerk G, van Son MM, de Vijlder JJ, et al. Low maternal free thyroxine concentration during early pregnancy are associated with impaired psychomotor development in infancy. Clin Endocrinol (Oxf). 1999;50(2):149-55.

CHAPTER **10**

Connective Tissue Disorders (Autoimmune Disorders)

Two autoimmune connective tissue disorders are mainly covered in this chapter: systemic lupus erythematosus (SLE) and antiphospholipid antibody syndrome (APS). During pregnancy, there are changes in the immune system. This is associated with suppressed cell-mediated immunity and increased humoral immunity. There also occurs a sudden reduction in the levels of hormones such as oestrogens, progesterone and other hormones in the postpartum period. As a result of these changes, the autoimmune conditions are likely to improve during pregnancy and flare-up during the postpartum period.

SYSTEMIC LUPUS ERYTHEMATOSUS

INTRODUCTION

Connective tissue disorders are characterised by production of antibodies to components of cell nucleus, resulting in autoantibody-mediated connective tissue abnormalities. There is a deposition of immune complexes at specific organ or tissue sites, thereby affecting them. SLE, a heterogeneous autoimmune disorder is one of the commonest connective tissue disorders, characterised by the presence of antinuclear antibodies (ANA) directed against components of cell nucleus.

AETIOLOGY

* Unknown
* Genetic factors (high concordance rate among twins)
* Environmental factors such as sunlight (UV rays), stress, etc.
* Viral or other type of infection
* Drugs (e.g. hydralazine, procainamide and isoniazid).

DIAGNOSIS

Clinical Presentation

Systemic lupus erythematosus can be associated with the following clinical signs and symptoms:[1]
* *Arthritis and arthralgia*: Systemic lupus erythematosus typically affects the joints and is characterised by symmetrical non-erosive peripheral arthritis and arthralgia.
* *Photosensitive malar rash*: Malar rash due to SLE needs to be distinguished from chloasma (dark skin discolouration due to normal pregnancy).
* Fever and fatigue
* Serositis, discoid lupus
* Raynaud phenomenon
* Glomerulonephritis
* Alopecia, vasculitis
* *Haematologic abnormalities*: There may be anaemia, lymphopenia, thrombocytopenia, hypocomplementaemia and a raised erythrocyte sedimentation rate (ESR). Levels of C-reactive protein (CRP) may not be raised.
* Diagnosis of SLE is clinical and may be made using the revised criteria of the American Rheumatism Association (1997) (Box 10.1).[2]

The diagnosis is made if four or more classification criteria are present.

Investigations

* *Detection of autoimmune antibodies*: Identification of ANAs is the best screening test. However, this test is not specific for lupus. Other antibodies, which can be present, include anti-double-stranded (ds)-DNA, anti-Sm (Smith antigen), anti-Sjögren's-syndrome-related antigen A [(anti-SSA), (anti-Ro)], anti-SSB (anti-La), antihistone, antiphospholipid antibodies, etc. Of these, antibodies,

Box 10.1: The revised criteria of the American Rheumatism Association for Systemic Lupus Erythematosus[2]

1. *Malar (butterfly) rash*: Fixed erythema, flat or raised, over malar eminences, with a tendency to spare nasolabial folds
2. *Discoid lupus*: Erythematous raised patches with scaling and follicular plugging
3. *Photosensitivity*: Skin rash resulting from hypersensitivity reaction to sunlight
4. *Oral or nasopharyngeal ulcers*: These are usually painless
5. *Non-erosive arthritis*: Involving two or more peripheral joints, often accompanied with tenderness, and swelling
6. *Serositis*: This could be manifested in the form of pleuritis or pericarditis
7. *Renal involvement*: Persistent proteinuria (>0.5 g/day or 3+ on dipstick) or cellular casts (red cell, haemoglobin, granular, tubular or mixed)
8. *Neurological disorders*: Seizures or psychosis without any underlying organic cause
9. *Haematological disorder*: This may be characterised by haemolytic anaemia with reticulocytosis, or leukopenia (leukocyte count <4,000/mm³ on two occasions) or lymphopenia (absolute lymphocyte count <1,500/mm³ on at least two occasions) or thrombocytopenia (platelet count <100,000/mm³ without any history of using thrombocytopenic drugs)
10. *Immunologic disorder*: This may be characterised by the presence of anti-DNA antibodies (anti-dsDNA) in abnormal titre, anti-Sm antibodies, false-positive VDRL test or positive finding of antiphospholipid antibodies, such as IgG or IgM anticardiolipin antibodies, or positive test for lupus anticoagulant using standard method
11. *Antinuclear antibodies*: Abnormal titres of ANAs in the absence of drugs

such as anti-Sm and dsDNA, are quite specific. There also may be antibodies to extractable nuclear antigens (ENA). Studies must also be done for the estimation of lupus anticoagulant (LA) and anticardiolipin (aCL) antibodies.

❖ *Blood investigations*: There may be a positive Coomb's test due to haemolysis. Blood abnormalities like anaemia, thrombocytopenia, leukopenia, etc. may also be present. Therefore, a complete blood count must be performed.

❖ *D-dimer levels*: Elevated serum D-dimer levels may commonly follow a flare or infection.

❖ *Liver function tests*: Hepatic involvement is suggested by increased serum levels of bilirubin or serum transaminase activity.

❖ Rheumatoid factor

❖ *Renal function tests*: This should include determination of the glomerular filtration rate (GFR), urinalysis, and tests of the urinary protein-to-creatinine (P/C) ratio. Urine must also be tested for proteins because new-onset or worsening of pre-existing proteinuria could be suggestive of the disease.

❖ *Complement studies*: This involves estimation of CH50 or C3 and C4.

❖ *Imaging studies*: Since the foetuses are at an increased risk of growth restriction, ultrasound examination must be done at the time of first prenatal visit to accurately determine the gestational age. Serial foetal echocardiography must be done to detect foetal heart block at an early stage.[3]

 OBSTETRIC MANAGEMENT

❖ *Preconceptional counselling*: Women must be counselled regarding the effect of the disease on the pregnancy outcome. The women should be preferably asked to conceive during the periods of disease remission. Pregnancy may be associated with flaring up of SLE. This may occur anytime during the antenatal or the postpartum period of pregnancy. It may become difficult to recognise the flareups during pregnancy due to the overlap of symptoms between the two. Also, active disease during pregnancy may be associated with an increased risk of complications such as miscarriage, pre-eclampsia, foetal growth restriction, preterm delivery and stillbirths.

❖ *Prenatal visits*: Frequent follow-up with prenatal visits (weekly visits after 28 weeks) are required.

❖ *Foetal surveillance*: In pregnant women, close monitoring of foetal growth needs to be done [e.g. weekly non-stress test (NST) after 28 weeks].

❖ *Patient monitoring*: The patient needs to be regularly monitored for thrombocytopenia and proteinuria.

❖ *Mode of delivery*: There is no need for a routine caesarean delivery in these cases. Caesarean section may be required in cases of obstetric complications or foetuses with congenital heart block.

❖ *Medication*: There is no cure for the disease and complete remission is rare. The drugs, which can be used include non-steroidal anti-inflammatory drugs (NSAIDs) (for relief from mild aches and pains), corticosteroids (for severe flare-ups), immunosuppressive agents (azathioprine), cyclophosphamide, methotrexate (for arthritis), antimalarials (e.g. hydroxychloroquine to control skin disease), etc.

❖ *Breastfeeding*: Breastfeeding is recommended for women with SLE. However, the patients must avoid breastfeeding if they are taking drugs such as azathioprine, methotrexate, cyclophosphamide, or mycophenolate. Hydroxychloroquine is also secreted in breast milk; therefore, it should be used with caution. Hydroxychloroquine may displace bilirubin, resulting in kernicterus. On the other hand, low-dose prednisone (<15–20 mg/d) can be used safely during breastfeeding.

 COMPLICATIONS

Systemic lupus erythematosus during pregnancy can be associated with the following complications: [4,5]

Maternal: These include the following:

❖ Pre-eclampsia
❖ Foetal loss, low-birth-weight infants
❖ Deep vein thrombosis (DVT) or pulmonary embolism
❖ Renal impairment, chronic hypertension
❖ *Recurrence*: Risk of neonatal lupus in subsequent pregnancies is 17%.

Foetal: These include the following:
- Preterm delivery
- Foetal growth restriction
- Stillbirths
- *Neonatal lupus*: This is characterised by lupus dermatitis (red, raised rash on the scalp and around the eyes), a number of haematological and systematic derangements, congenital heart block, etc.
- *Systemic lupus erythematosus complications in babies*: Complete heart block and learning disabilities.

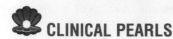 **CLINICAL PEARLS**

- Outcome is best for mother and baby when SLE has been controlled for at least 6 months prior to pregnancy.
- Approximately one-third of the women with SLE may have flare-ups during pregnancy.

 EVIDENCE-BASED MEDICINE

- None of the drugs used for the treatment of SLE are absolutely safe during pregnancy. The use of medicines must be decided after careful assessment of the risks and benefits in consultation with the patient and her partner. Nevertheless, most of the drugs must be avoided during the first trimester.[6]
- Women should be counselled regarding the importance of using contraception while taking drugs for SLE treatment such as methotrexate, leflunomide, cyclophosphamide and mycophenolate. Since some of the drugs have long half-life, they need to be discontinued for several months before the planned conception.[6]
- Women with anti-Ro or anti-La antibodies are at an increased risk of having pregnancies complicated by congenital foetal heart block. Such patients may benefit from serial foetal echocardiographic monitoring.[3]

ANTIPHOSPHOLIPID SYNDROME

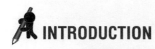 **INTRODUCTION**

Antiphospholipid antibody syndrome, also known as Hughes syndrome, is an autoimmune condition that may manifest with recurrent foetal loss, thrombosis (both arterial and venous) and/or autoimmune thrombocytopenia. APS has emerged as the most important treatable cause of recurrent miscarriage, early onset pre-eclampsia, preterm labour, low-birth-weight-babies and intrauterine growth restriction (IUGR). This disease causes miscarriage by forming antibodies against the body's own tissues and placenta, resulting in thrombosis of vessels and placental infarction.

Classification of Antiphospholipid Syndrome

Definite or classic antiphospholipid syndrome: This category includes patients with LA or medium-to-high levels of IgG or IgM aCL antibodies and those with foetal death, recurrent pre-embryonic or embryonic pregnancy loss, thrombosis, or neonatal death after delivery due to severe pre-eclampsia or foetal distress.

Familial antiphospholipid syndrome: There is some evidence that familial APS shows dominant or codominant inheritance.

AETIOLOGY

The APS is an autoimmune phenomenon. There are three primary classes of antibodies associated with the APS:
1. Anticardiolipin antibodies (directed against membrane anionic phospholipids)
2. The lupus anticoagulant
3. Antibodies directed against specific molecules including a molecule known as β-2 glycoprotein 1.

Based on the presence or absence of an underlying auto-immune disorder, such as SLE, APS may be classified into two, (1) primary and (2) secondary. If the patient has an underlying autoimmune disorder (e.g. SLE, rheumatoid arthritis or some other connective tissue disorder), the patient is said to have secondary APS. If the patient has no known underlying autoimmune disorder, it is termed as primary APS.

Defect in cellular apoptosis has been postulated as an important hypothesis behind the pathogenesis of APS. This exposes the membrane phospholipids so that they can bind with various plasma proteins, such as β-2 glycoprotein 1. Once bound, a phospholipid-protein complex is formed, which subsequently becomes the target of autoantibodies. There may be production of antibodies against coagulation factors, including prothrombin, protein C, protein S and annexins.

Activation of platelets further enhances adherence capacity of endothelial surface. Activation of vascular endothelium, in turn, facilitates the binding of platelets and monocytes resulting in the damage related to APS. Complement activation has been increasingly recognised to play a significant role in the pathogenesis of APS.

Thrombosis of the blood vessels and placental infarction causes a reduction in the uteroplacental blood flow, which results in IUGR, oligohydramnios, and foetal hypoxia, all of which lead to foetal demise. The exact mechanism by which the antiphospholipid and aCL antibodies induce thrombophilic state is not known. In APS, the homeostatic regulation of blood coagulation is altered. However, the mechanisms of thrombosis have yet not been defined.

DIAGNOSIS

Clinical Presentation

Clinically, the series of events in APS, which can lead to hyper-coagulability and recurrent thrombosis can affect virtually any organ system, as shown in Table 10.1.

Thus, history of any of the following should raise the suspicion for APS in obstetrician's mind:

❖ Thrombosis (e.g. DVT, myocardial infarction, transient ischaemic attack, cerebrovascular accident, etc.). This is especially important if the episodes are recurrent, occur at an earlier age, or in the absence of other known risk factors.
❖ History of recurrent miscarriages (especially late trimester) or premature birth.
❖ History of heart murmur or cardiac-valvular vegetations.
❖ History of haematologic abnormalities, such as thrombocytopenia or haemolytic anaemia.
❖ History of nephropathy.
❖ Non-thrombotic neurologic symptoms, such as migraine, headaches, chorea, seizures, transverse myelitis, Guillain-Barré syndrome, etc.
❖ Unexplained adrenal insufficiency.
❖ Avascular necrosis of bone in the absence of other risk factors
❖ Pulmonary hypertension.

Physical Examination

On physical examination, the features enumerated in Table 10.2 can be observed.

❖ *Diagnosis of antiphospholipid antibody syndrome*: In 2006, revised criteria for the diagnosis of APS were published in an international consensus statement. This is described in Table 10.3.[7] In order to reach the diagnosis of APS, at least one clinical criterion and one laboratory criterion must be present.

Table 10.1: Clinical features of antiphospholipid antibody syndrome depending on the organ system affected

Organ system affected	Symptoms
Peripheral venous system	Deep venous thrombosis
Central nervous system	Cerebrovascular accident, stroke, etc.
Haematologic system	Thrombocytopenia, haemolytic anaemia
Effect on pregnancy	Recurrent pregnancy losses, intrauterine growth restriction, pre-eclampsia, etc.
Pulmonary system	Pulmonary embolism, pulmonary hypertension
Dermatologic effect	Livedo reticularis, purpura, infarcts, ulceration
Cardiovascular system	Libman-Sacks valvulopathy, myocardial infarction
Ocular effects	Amaurosis, retinal thrombosis
Adrenal system	Infarction, haemorrhage, etc.
Musculoskeletal	Avascular necrosis of bone

Investigations

The following laboratory tests should be considered in a patient suspected of having APS:

❖ Anticardiolipin antibodies (IgG, IgM)
❖ Anti-β-2 glycoprotein 1 antibodies (IgG, IgM)
❖ Prolongation of the following clotting assays due to the presence of LA:
  • Kaolin clotting time (KCT)
  • Dilute Russell viper venom time (DRVVT)
  • Activated partial thromboplastin time (APTT).
❖ Serologic test for syphilis (false-positive result)
❖ *Complete blood count (thrombocytopenia, haemolytic anaemia)*: Thrombocytopenia is fairly common in persons with APS.

Lupus anticoagulant: Lupus anticoagulant is directed against plasma coagulation molecules, thereby prolonging the in vitro clotting times of plasma by interfering with assembly of components of the coagulation cascade on a phospholipid template. In vitro, presence of this antibody therefore results in the prolongation of clotting assays, such as APTT, KCT and DRVVT. The presence of LA is confirmed by mixing normal platelet poor plasma with the patient's plasma. If a clotting factor is deficient, the addition of normal plasma corrects the prolonged clotting time.

Anticardiolipin antibodies: Anticardiolipin antibodies react primarily with membrane phospholipids, such as cardiolipin and phosphatidylserine. There are three known isotypes of aCL, i.e. IgG, IgM and IgA. Of these three isotypes of aCL, the values of IgG most strongly correlate with the occurrence of thrombotic events. Cardiolipin is the dominant antigen used in most serologic tests for syphilis; consequently, these patients may have a false-positive test result for syphilis.

Cut-off levels for IgG aCL [in IgG phospholipid (GPL) units] and IgM aCL [in IgM phospholipids (MPL) units] have been presented in guidelines issued by the Association of Clinical Pathologists, with negative results defined as less than 5 GPL units and less than 3 MPL units, low positive results defined as values less than 15 GPL units and less than 6 MPL units, medium levels defined as 15–80 GPL units and 6–50 MPL units and high levels defined as less than 80 GPL units or less than 50 MPL units. In detection of LA, the DRVVT test is more sensitive and specific than either the APTT or the KCT tests. aCL antibodies are detected using a standardized enzyme-linked immunosorbent assay (ELISA).

CHAPTER 10

Table 10.2: Physical features of antiphospholipid antibody syndrome observed on clinical examination

Cutaneous lesions	Venous thrombosis	Arterial thrombosis
Livedo reticularis	Leg swelling (deep vein thrombosis)	Abnormal results on neurological examination
Superficial thrombophlebitis	Ascites (Budd-Chiari syndrome)	Digital ulcers, gangrene of distal extremities
Leg ulcers	Tachypnoea (pulmonary embolism)	Signs of myocardial infarction
Painful purpura	Peripheral oedema (renal vein thrombosis)	Heart murmurs (frequently indicative of aortic or mitral insufficiency and Libman-Sacks endocarditis)
Splinter haemorrhages	Abnormal funduscopic examination results indicate thrombosis of retinal vein	Abnormal funduscopic examination results indicating retinal artery occlusion

Table 10.3: Revised classification criteria for the antiphospholipid syndrome[7]

Clinical criteria	
Vascular thrombosis	One or more clinical episodes of arterial, venous, or small vessel thrombosis in any tissue or organ confirmed by findings from imaging studies, Doppler studies, or histopathology (for histopathologic confirmation, thrombosis should be present without significant evidence of inflammation in the vessel wall) or presence of pregnancy morbidity
Pregnancy morbidity (poor obstetric history)	Unexplained death of a morphologically normal foetus at or beyond 10 weeks. One or more premature deliveries before 34 weeks of gestation because of severe pre-eclampsia/eclampsia or severe IUGR. Three or more unexplained consecutive abortions before 10 weeks of gestation (this is controversial, if no foetal heart has been seen, as some believe that very early abortion is not caused by APS)
Paraclinical/laboratory criteria	• The presence of lupus anticoagulant in plasma on two or more occasions at least 12 weeks apart • Presence of moderate to high levels of anticardiolipin (IgG or IgM) in serum or plasma [i.e. >40 IgG phospholipid units (GPL)/mL or IgM phospholipid units (MPL)/mL or >99th percentile] on two or more occasions at least 12 weeks apart. Presence of moderate to high levels of anti-β-2 glycoprotein 1 antibodies (IgG or IgM) in serum or plasma (>99th percentile) on two or more occasions at least 12 weeks apart

Imaging Studies

❖ Imaging studies are helpful for confirming a thrombotic event, e.g. the use of CT scanning or MRI of the brain (cerebrovascular attack), chest (pulmonary embolism), or abdomen (Budd-Chiari syndrome).

❖ Doppler ultrasound studies are recommended for possible detection of DVT.

❖ Two-dimensional echocardiography may help demonstrate an asymptomatic valve thickening, vegetations or valvular insufficiency. Aortic or mitral insufficiency is the most common valvular defect found in persons with Libman–Sacks endocarditis, commonly encountered in women with APS.

MANAGEMENT

Principles of management are listed in Box 10.2 and are described next.

Prevention of Thrombosis

The prophylactic measures comprise of elimination of various risk factors, such as oral contraceptives, smoking, hypertension or hyperlipidaemia. The following drugs have been tried for the prevention of thrombosis:

❖ *Combination of heparin and low-dose aspirin*: Patients with recurrent pregnancy loss must be administered a prophylactic dose of subcutaneous heparin [preferably low-molecular-weight heparin (LMWH) because it is associated with fewer side effects] and low-dose aspirin. Unfractionated heparin (UFH), if used, can be administered in prophylactic doses of 5,000 IU twice daily. Since long-term use of heparin can cause osteoporosis, patients who require heparin administration throughout pregnancy should also receive calcium and vitamin D supplementation and advised to do skeletal weight-bearing exercises. Another dreaded immune-mediated complication of heparin is heparin-induced thrombocytopenia, which necessitates stopping heparin immediately. Thus, platelet counts must be measured 1 week after commencement of therapy and monthly thereafter in all patients on heparin therapy. Therapy is usually withheld at the time of delivery and

Box 10.2: Principles of management in cases of antiphospholipid antibody syndrome

❑ Prevention of thrombosis (thromboprophylaxis)
❑ Antenatal maternal and foetal surveillance
❑ Peripartum care
❑ Postpartum prophylaxis

is restarted after delivery, continuing for 6–12 weeks postpartum. Most obstetricians prefer to avoid the use of warfarin (Coumadin) during pregnancy as it can cross the placental barrier and produce teratogenic changes in the foetus. LMWH in comparison to UFH has fewer complications and is being more frequently used in pregnancy. LMWH inhibits factor Xa and in addition has an anticoagulant effect through its action on antithrombin III and factor IIa. Thus, bleeding complications with LMWH are few with little alteration of prothrombin time (PT) and APTT.

❖ The RCOG guidelines support the use of LMWH in addition to aspirin for treatment of women with APS having recurrent miscarriages.[8] However, presently the use of combination of aspirin with heparin in women with APS is associated with conflicting evidence. A meta-analysis has indicated that the combination of heparin with aspirin is the only combination therapy, which is likely to cause a significant increase in the rate of live births amongst women with APS. This combination also causes significant reduction in the rate of miscarriages by 54%.[9,10] Though the combination of aspirin and heparin helps in substantially improving the birth rate in women with recurrent miscarriage associated with APS, these pregnancies remain at high risk of complications (including pre-eclampsia, preterm birth, foetal growth restriction, repeated miscarriages, etc.) in all the three trimesters, thereby requiring a careful antenatal surveillance.[11,12]

❖ *Aspirin*: Aspirin helps in improving pregnancy outcome by inhibiting thrombosis and preventing damage to trophoblast. Some retrospective, non-randomised studies have shown the beneficial effect of low-dose aspirin in cases without a previous history of thrombosis.[13] Presently available randomised studies do not show the beneficial effects of aspirin probably because they have included very low risk group of women.

❖ *Corticosteroids/immunoglobulins*: Neither corticosteroids nor immunoglobulins improve the live birth rate of women with recurrent miscarriage.[14] Some researchers have examined the use of combination comprising of aspirin and prednisone during pregnancy. Most of the studies suggest that complications associated with prednisone use usually outweigh the benefits associated. Thus, prednisone must not be used in addition to aspirin. In patients for whom the treatment with aspirin and heparin is not successful, intravenous immunoglobulins can be used. At this time, the studies suggest this may be helpful in refractory cases, but is not recommended for use on a routine basis.

❖ In patients with underlying SLE, hydroxychloroquine, which may have intrinsic antithrombotic properties, can be considered.

❖ Consultations with specialists like rheumatologist, haematologist, neurologist, cardiologist, pulmonologist, hepatologist, ophthalmologist, etc. may be required depending on clinical presentation.

❖ The patient must be educated about anticoagulation therapy and explained the importance of planned pregnancies so that long-term warfarin can be switched to aspirin and heparin before pregnancy is attempted. Thromboprophylaxis regimes in cases of APS are described in Table 10.4.

Antenatal Maternal and Foetal Surveillance

Due to a high frequency of pregnancy complications, especially pre-eclampsia and IUGR, despite treatment, the obstetrician should introduce appropriate surveillance starting right from 32 weeks of gestation. This must comprise of the following steps:

❖ A complete profile of antiphospholipid antibodies: If this has been done in preconception period, these tests need not be repeated during pregnancy.

Table 10.4: Thromboprophylaxis regimes in cases of antiphospholipid antibody syndrome

Situations	Treatment regimen
Antiphospholipid syndrome without previous thrombosis and recurrent early miscarriage	Low-dose aspirin (LDA) alone or LDA + unfractionated heparin 5,000–7,500 IU SC every 12 h or LMWH in usual prophylactic doses
Antiphospholipid syndrome without previous thrombosis and foetal death (>10 week's gestation) or previous early delivery (<34 week's gestation)	LDA + unfractionated heparin, 5,000–10,000 IU SC every 12 h (mid-interval APTT 15 times control) or LMWH in prophylactic doses
Antiphospholipid syndrome with thrombosis	LDA + unfractionated heparin, 7,500–10,000 IU SC every 8–12 h (APTT in therapeutic range) or LMWH (therapeutic dose: for twice-daily administration, the therapeutic range is 0.6–1.0 IU/mL and with once daily administration, the range is 1.0–2.0 IU/mL)*

*Prophylactic dose of LMWH is usually half of therapeutic dose

❖ Frequent antenatal visits, at least every 2–4 weeks before third trimester and every 1–2 weeks thereafter

❖ Close maternal and foetal surveillance in form of monitoring of maternal blood pressure, proteinuria, and other features of pre-eclampsia

❖ Obstetric ultrasound to assess foetal growth and amniotic fluid volume

❖ Uterine and umbilical artery Doppler to detect foetal growth restriction and if detected, appropriate foetal surveillance may be required.

❖ Termination of pregnancy must be considered at 37 completed weeks of gestation.

Peripartum Care

This comprises of the following steps:

❖ Low-to-moderate risk patients on LMWH can be changed over to UFH at 36–37 weeks of gestation.

❖ Heparin should be discontinued once patients go into labour.

❖ In patients undergoing induction of labour or elective caesarean delivery, heparin must be discontinued 12–24 hours before the procedure.

❖ In most of the cases, heparin infusion is restarted 6–8 hours following delivery.

Postpartum Prophylaxis

❖ Antithrombotic coverage during the postpartum period is recommended in all women with APS, with or without previous episode of thrombosis.

❖ In low-risk women, prophylactic dose of heparin or LMWH is continued for 4–6 weeks after delivery, although warfarin can also be used as an option.

❖ Breastfeeding women may be administered the combination of heparin and warfarin. If warfarin therapy is instituted, the patient must be instructed to avoid excessive consumption of foods that contain vitamin K.

COMPLICATIONS

The following complications can occur in association with APS:

❖ Increased risk for thrombosis (particularly at unusual sites such as axillary or retinal veins)

❖ Miscarriages (especially in the second trimester)

❖ Placental abruption

❖ Stillbirths

❖ Intrauterine growth restriction

❖ Early onset pre-eclampsia

❖ Premature births.

EVIDENCE-BASED MEDICINE

❖ Current evidence supports the use of heparin throughout pregnancy in women with APS, who have had previous thrombosis.[8]

CHAPTER 10

❖ Evidence from retrospective and cohort studies supports a role of low-dose aspirin for foetal indications.[13]

❖ Use of LMWH in addition to aspirin for foetal indications is associated with conflicting evidence regarding its effectiveness.[9-12]

REFERENCES

1. Madazli R, Bulut B, Erenel H, Gezer A, Guralp O. Systemic lupus erythematosus and pregnancy. J Obstet Gynaecol. 2010;30(1):17-20.

2. Hochberg MC. Updating the American College of Rheumatology revised criteria for the classification of systemic lupus erythematosus. Arthritis Rheum. 1997;40(9):1725.

3. Izmirly PM, Llanos C, Lee LA, Askanase A, Kim MY, Buyon JP. Cutaneous manifestations of neonatal lupus and risk of subsequent congenital heart block. Arthritis Rheum. 2010; 62(4):1153-7.

4. Gladman DD, Tandon A, Ibañez D, Urowitz MB. The effect of lupus nephritis on pregnancy outcome and fetal and maternal complications. J Rheumatol. 2010;37(4):754-8.

5. Chen CY, Chen YH, Lin HC, Chen SF, Lin HC. Increased risk of adverse pregnancy outcomes for hospitalisation of women with lupus during pregnancy: a nationwide population-based study. Clin Exp Rheumatol. 2010;28(1):49-55.

6. Østensen M, Lockshin M, Doria A, Valesini G, Meroni P, Gordon C, et al. Update on the safety during pregnancy of biological agents and some immunosuppressive anti-rheumatic drugs. Rheumatology (Oxford). 2008;47 Suppl 3:28-31.

7. Lockshin MD, Atsumi T, Branch DW, Brey RL, Cervera R, et al. International consensus statement on an update of the classification criteria for definite antiphospholipid syndrome (APS). J Thromb Haemost. 2006;4(2):295-306.

8. The Royal College of Obstetricians and Gynaecologists. The Investigation and Treatment of Couples with Recurrent First trimester and Second-trimester Miscarriage. [online] RCOG website. Available from https://www.rcog.org.uk/globalassets/documents/guidelines/gtg_17.pdf [Accessed May, 2016].

9. Empson M, Lassere M, Craig J, Scott J. Prevention of recurrent miscarriage for women with antiphospholipid antibody or lupus anticoagulant. Cochrane Database Syst Rev. 2005; (2):CD002859.

10. Laskin CA, Spitzer KA, Clark CA, Crowther MR, Ginsberg JS, Hawker GA, et al. Low molecular weight heparin and aspirin for recurrent pregnancy loss: results from the randomized, controlled HepASATrial. J Rheumatol. 2009;36(2):279-87.

11. Backos M, Rai R, Baxter N, Chilcott IT, Cohen H, Regan L. Pregnancy complications in women with recurrent miscarriage associated with antiphospholipid antibodies treated with low dose aspirin and heparin. Br J Obstet Gynaecol. 1999;106(2):102-7.

12. Branch DW, Silver RM, Blackwell JL, Reading JC, Scott JR. Outcome of treated pregnancies in women with antiphospholipid syndrome: an update of the Utah experience. Obstet Gynecol. 1992;80(4):614-20.

13. Dadhwal V, Sharma AK, Deka D, Gupta B, Mittal S. The obstetric outcome following treatment in a cohort of patients with antiphospholipid antibody syndrome in a tertiary care center. J Postgrad Med. 2011;57(1):16-9.

14. Farquharson RG, Quenby S, Greaves M. Antiphospholipid syndrome in pregnancy: a randomized, controlled trial of treatment. Obstet Gynecol. 2002;100(3):408-13.

Respiratory Diseases in Pregnancy

ASTHMA IN PREGNANCY

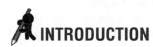 INTRODUCTION

Asthma can be considered as the commonest respiratory disorder encountered during pregnancy, with the prevalence of asthma in pregnancy varying between 1% to 4%. Current evidence indicates that pregnancy outcome is usually good in cases of asthma, specifically the well-controlled cases. In a study by Schatz, there was no increase in the incidence of any obstetric complications amongst the well-controlled asthmatic patients who were pregnant.[1] Poorly controlled asthma in pregnancy (Box 11.1) can be associated with adverse effects such as hypertensive disorders, intrauterine growth restriction (IUGR), premature rupture of membranes (PROM), etc.

AETIOLOGY

Changes in the Respiratory System during Pregnancy

There occurs a state of hyperventilation, resulting in an increase in tidal volume and respiratory minute volume by 40%. At the same time, there is a decrease in total lung capacity, functional residual capacity, expiratory reserve volume and residual volume. This occurs due to the effect of progesterone on respiratory centre and an increase in the sensitivity of respiratory centre to CO_2.

Box 11.1: Signs of inadequately controlled asthma

❑ Chest tightness and wheeziness
❑ Cough
❑ Breathlessness (especially during early morning)

This hyperventilation causes changes in acid-base balance. There is fall in the arterial partial pressure of carbon dioxide ($PaCO_2$) from 38 mmHg to 32 mmHg and a rise in partial pressure of oxygen (PaO_2) from 95 mmHg to 105 mmHg. These changes facilitate the transfer of CO_2 from foetus to the mother and O_2 from mother to the foetus. There is an overall rise in the pH and a base excess of 2 mEq/L. This results in respiratory alkalosis. Increased excretion of bicarbonates by the kidneys results in partial compensation.

There are concerns regarding the safety of radiological examinations during pregnancy. Maximum safe-limit for the exposure to the foetus is 5cGy. Investigations like chest X-rays, venography, ventilation perfusion scanning and pulmonary angiography normally expose the foetus to the levels of radiation lower than this. Moreover, potential benefits of these investigations outweigh the risk. Nevertheless, exposure must be avoided or minimised whenever possible. For example, lateral X-rays carry a greater risk of exposure than the erect anteroposterior (AP) chest films; mobile X-rays carry greater exposure than the departmental films; abdominal shielding should be used wherever possible.

DIAGNOSIS

Clinical Presentation

The following signs and symptoms are required for the diagnosis of asthma:
❖ Episodic symptoms of airflow obstruction (e.g. coughing, wheezing, shortness of breath or chest tightness).
❖ Airflow obstruction that is at least partially reversible.
❖ Absence of alternative diagnoses for explaining the symptoms.

Symptoms of asthma are typically worse during the night and early morning and improve during the daytime.

Table 11.1: Classification of asthma by National Asthma Education Program (NAEP)[2]

Characteristics	Mild asthma	Moderate asthma	Severe asthma
Symptomatic exacerbations	Brief exacerbations (less than 1 hour) occurring with a frequency of less than or equal to twice per week	Symptomatic exacerbations occurring with a frequency of greater than 2 per week	Continuous symptoms or frequent exacerbations limit activity levels
Peak expiratory flow rate (PEFR)	≥80% of the personal best	60–80% of the personal best	Less than 60% of the predicted and may be highly variable
FEV1	≥80% of the predicted when asymptomatic	60–80% of the predicted	Less than 60% of the predicted and may be highly variable
Nocturnal symptoms	None	Nocturnal symptoms may be present	Nocturnal symptoms are present

Box 11.2: Patient's triggers for causing disease exacerbations

❑ Environmental allergens (pollen grains, dust mites, animal danders, moulds, etc.)
❑ Upper respiratory infections
❑ Occupational exposures (industrial chemicals, metal salts, etc.)
❑ Medications [notably aspirin and other non-steroidal anti-inflammatory drugs (NSAIDs), β-blockers, etc.]
❑ Exercise
❑ Emotional stress
❑ Environmental pollutants (e.g. cigarette smoke)

Classification of asthma as described by National Asthma Education Program (NAEP) is described in Table 11.1.[2]

Investigations

A detailed history and physical examination should be performed to make the diagnosis of asthma. The following signs and symptoms must be identified before making the diagnosis of asthma:

❖ Hyperexpansion of the thorax
❖ Expiratory wheezing
❖ Severe rhinitis
❖ Nasal polyps
❖ Atopic dermatitis or eczema.

Additionally, patients with newly diagnosed asthma should undergo spirometric evaluations or pulmonary function tests (PFTs) before and after inhaling β₂ agonists. This would help in demonstrating reversible airway obstruction.

Baseline investigations such as peak flow measurements must be done at the time of booking. Diagnostic evaluation should aim at the identification of the patient's triggers for causing disease exacerbations. Few of such triggers are listed in Box 11.2.

MANAGEMENT

Management of asthma during pregnancy is same as that in non-pregnant women.

Antepartum Period

Management of asthma during the antenatal period comprises of the following steps:

❖ Advising the women to avoid having an exposure to any potential asthma triggers.

❖ Foetal surveillance with regular ultrasound scans and daily foetal movement count.
❖ In case of mild asthma (less than two attacks per week), short-acting β-agonists (albuterol) may be administered for providing symptomatic relief.
❖ In mild persistent cases (≥2 attacks per week), daily-inhaled steroids (budesonide, beclomethasone, fluticasone, etc.) may be administered. Short-acting β-agonists may be administered for short-term relief.
❖ In moderate cases, daily inhaled steroids (in moderate-high dosage) plus long-acting β-agonists (salmeterol) may be given. Short-acting β-agonists may be administered for providing symptomatic relief. Monitoring of peak expiratory flow rate (PEFR) must be done on daily basis.
❖ In case of severe asthmatic attacks, daily administration of inhaled steroids in high dosage may be required. Besides this, daily low-dosage oral steroids (prednisolone) and daily long-acting β-agonists (salmeterol) may also be administered. Regular monitoring of PEFR may be required.
❖ During pregnancy, prednisolone is the oral steroid of choice because nearly 90% gets metabolised by the placenta, thereby limiting foetal exposure. Women being administered prednisolone should be screened for glucose tolerance and in case of impaired glucose tolerance, appropriate steps must be taken.
❖ Step-by-step approach as defined by British Thoracic Society is described in Flow chart 11.1 and Figure 11.1.[3]
❖ Teratogenic risks and possible harmful effects related to maternal systemic steroid administration presently remain controversial. There is no convincing evidence indicating that systemic corticosteroids increase the incidence of congenital anomalies such as cleft lip and palate.[4,5]

Intrapartum Period

Management of asthma during labour comprises of the following steps:
❖ Maternal oxygenation must be well maintained and oxygen saturation must be monitored with pulse oximetry and arterial blood gas determination.
❖ Opiate analgesics must be avoided due to their broncho-constrictor and respiratory depressant effect.
❖ Labetalol must also be avoided due to its risk of precipitating asthma.

Flow chart 11.1: Management of asthma based on the severity of symptoms during pregnancy

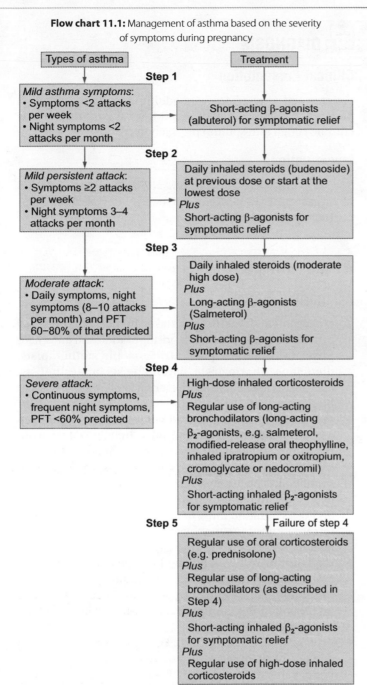

Abbreviations: PFT, pulmonary function tests; PEFR, peak expiratory flow rate

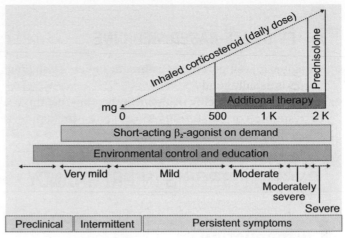

Fig. 11.1: Treatment of asthma during pregnancy

Postpartum Period

Breastfeeding is not contraindicated with the use of any kind of medication. However, use of oral steroids (>40 mg/day) may be associated with an increased risk of neonatal adrenal suppression.

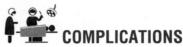

COMPLICATIONS

The recent-most evidence suggests that most women with asthma are likely to have an uneventful pregnancy course.[6-8] For women with well-controlled asthma, pregnancy outcomes are similar to those of women without asthma. Poorly controlled asthma in pregnancy can be associated with the following complications:[9]

❖ Hypertensive disorders, pre-eclampsia, etc.
❖ Intrauterine growth restriction
❖ Premature rupture of membranes
❖ Gestational diabetes
❖ Small for gestational age (SGA) babies
❖ Premature delivery
❖ Increased rate of caesarean delivery.

CLINICAL PEARLS

❖ In order to minimise the radiological exposure to the foetus at the time of radiological examinations, especially X-rays, abdominal shielding should be used wherever possible.
❖ Effects of asthma during pregnancy remain erratic. Approximately one-third of women with asthma may experience improvement in the asthmatic attacks during their pregnancy; one-third may experience worsening of the symptoms and in the remaining one-third, symptoms remain about the same.
❖ Better the control of asthma prior to pregnancy, better are the woman's chances of experiencing few or no asthma symptoms during her pregnancy.

❖ Use of syntocinon is preferred over ergometrine due to the bronchoconstrictor effect of the latter. Use of carboprost [prostaglandin F2α (PGF$_{2\alpha}$)] should be avoided due to the risk of bronchospasm. On the other hand, prostaglandin E1 (PG$_{E1}$) and prostaglandin E2 (PG$_{E2}$) compounds can be used locally for induction of labour or abortion.
❖ Induction of labour and caesarean delivery is limited to obstetric indications. However, delivery may need to be expedited in the most severe cases.
❖ Epidural anaesthesia is preferred over general anaesthesia.
❖ Drugs such as ergometrine, PGF$_{2\alpha}$, aspirin and other non-steroidal anti-inflammatory drugs (NSAIDs) should be avoided as these drugs have been reported to cause bronchospasm.

CHAPTER 11

EVIDENCE-BASED MEDICINE

❖ Outcome in well-controlled asthmatic patients with pregnancy is usually good.[1]
❖ There is no convincing evidence indicating that the use of systemic corticosteroids increase the incidence of congenital anomalies.[4,5]

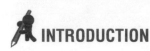

CYSTIC FIBROSIS IN PREGNANCY

INTRODUCTION

Cystic fibrosis is an autosomal recessive disorder resulting from a mutation of a single gene on chromosome 7. Cystic fibrosis during pregnancy is associated with further decline in the functioning of lungs. This could be related to anatomical and physiological changes in cardiorespiratory function, resulting in impaired clearance of mucus, increased atelectasis and predisposition to pulmonary infections.[10]

AETIOLOGY

Cystic fibrosis is a genetic disorder, characterised by exocrine gland dysfunction, with the primary organs, which are affected being the lungs and pancreas. The pulmonary disease consists of chronic, recurrent infections, bronchiectasis and airway obstruction. With improved treatment, patients may well survive into the reproductive age group and even conceive. Patients with mild disease and good nutritional status are likely to tolerate pregnancy well. However, those having more advanced disease and evidence of cor pulmonale, hypoxemia, severe obstructive lung disease and malnutrition should be advised against pregnancy. Many patients lie between these two extremes and the advisability of pregnancy should be based on disease stability.

Risk Factors

Predictors of maternal and foetal outcome in pregnancies complicated by cystic fibrosis are as follows:[11]
❖ Absolute pre-pregnancy pulmonary function tests
❖ Stability of pre-pregnancy pulmonary function tests
❖ Colonisation with *Burkholderia cepacia*
❖ Presence of pulmonary hypertension
❖ Degree of pancreatic insufficiency
❖ Glucose intolerance or diabetes (predating pregnancy or gestational diabetes)
❖ Body mass index
❖ Degree of pancreatic insufficiency
❖ Maternal weight gain during pregnancy
❖ Presence of hepatic disease and portal hypertension.

PART II

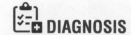

DIAGNOSIS

Clinical Presentation

Patients with cystic fibrosis in adulthood may present with pancreatic insufficiency or respiratory symptoms such as chronic cough and sputum production.

Investigations

Special pulmonary function tests: Spirometry and arterial blood gases must be performed at regular intervals throughout pregnancy.

MANAGEMENT

Antepartum Period

❖ Management should be undertaken in specialist centres by a multidisciplinary team comprising of adult and transplant physicians, nurses, paediatricians, physiotherapists, dieticians, pharmacists, psychologists, anaesthetists, and obstetricians with the experience of cystic fibrosis in pregnancy.
❖ *Pre-pregnancy counselling*: Patients with poor lung function or pulmonary hypertension must be advised to avoid pregnancy. Per cent forced expiratory volume in 1 second (FEV1) less than 50% is often considered as a poor relative contraindication for pregnancy. Also, presence of pulmonary hypertension may be associated with grave consequences and consideration must be given in these cases towards termination of pregnancy to prevent right-sided heart failure. [12]
❖ Vigilance must be maintained for the complications of cystic fibrosis: haemoptysis, pneumothorax, atelectasis, respiratory failure and cor pulmonale. There should be no hesitation in performing chest X-rays, where deemed necessary.
❖ Average weight gain of 10–12 kg during pregnancy puts a demand of an extra calorie requirement of 300 kilocalories per day. In cases of cystic fibrosis, increasing nutritional intake during pregnancy may be difficult. Since pancreatic insufficiency is common in cases of cystic fibrosis, pancreatic enzyme supplements are required during pregnancy to aid digestion. Advice from a dietician may be essential to maintain appropriate calorie intake.
❖ Caesarean section is required only in cases of obstetric indication in women with mild or moderate cystic fibrosis. In severe cases, caesarean section may be employed for patients with deteriorating lung function. General anaesthesia must be avoided as far as possible. Rate of instrumental delivery does not appear to be increased in these cases. Instrumental delivery may be required in cases of prolonged maternal exhaustion.
❖ Careful surveillance for signs of chest infection is important during pregnancy due to complications of pneumonia

during pregnancy. *Pseudomonas aeruginosa* is the most common cause of chest infection in cystic fibrosis. Penicillin, cephalosporins and aminoglycosides are the most commonly used antibiotics (through IV, oral and intramuscular routes). All antibiotics including gentamicin are considered safe during pregnancy. Risk of foetal toxicity can be minimised by ensuring that the maternal serum levels of gentamicin do not exceed recommended levels. Doses of some antibiotics need to be adjusted based on haemodilution and enhanced renal elimination in pregnancy.

❖ Cardiovascular status must be observed by echocardiography during pregnancy.

Intrapartum Period

❖ Facial oxygen may be required in labour.

COMPLICATIONS

Cystic fibrosis can be associated with the following complications during pregnancy:[13,14]

❖ Gestational diabetes
❖ Prematurity
❖ Maternal death within 5 years of delivery (usually in cases with poor pre-pregnancy lung function tests, pancreatic insufficiency, lung colonisation with *Burkholderia cepacia* species), etc.

EVIDENCE-BASED MEDICINE

❖ Pregnancy accelerates the loss of respiratory function in severe cases of cystic fibrosis.[12]
❖ Patients with a severe form of the disease or those showing significant decline in pulmonary function over a short time period or those with frequent infectious exacerbations must be best advised against pregnancy.[13,14]

TUBERCULOSIS IN PREGNANCY

INTRODUCTION

Infection with tuberculosis most commonly presents in African and Indian ethnic groups, especially in the new immigrant population. Human immunodeficiency virus (HIV) infection could be another predisposing factor and may be associated with an increasing incidence of tuberculosis.[15] Treatment is safe and effective during pregnancy and the outcome is usually good. Failure to diagnose the condition and patient's non-compliance with the medication regimens may put the woman and her newborn child at an increased risk.

AETIOLOGY

Infection with the bacterium, *Mycobacterium tuberculosis*, is the most common cause of tuberculosis in the humans worldwide. Infection with this bacterium can result in latent or active infection.[16] Depending on the body organ infected by tubercular infection, the infection can present as pulmonary (lungs are primarily affected) or extrapulmonary (affects larynx, the lymph nodes, the pleura, the brain, the kidneys, or the bones and joints) tuberculosis.

DIAGNOSIS

Clinical Presentation

Pulmonary tuberculosis usually presents with low-grade fever (with late afternoon peak), cough, haemoptysis, weight loss, night sweats, malaise, chest pain, dyspnoea, etc.

Investigations

❖ Diagnostic tools for latent tuberculosis include tuberculin skin testing and interferon-gamma release assays (IGRAs).[17,18]
❖ Patients with positive screening results for latent tuberculosis must undergo clinical evaluation to rule out active tuberculosis. This includes evaluation for symptoms (e.g. fever, cough, weight loss) and radiographic examination of the chest (with appropriate shielding).

MANAGEMENT

❖ Management of such cases requires a multidisciplinary approach comprising of a respiratory consultant, physician and microbiologists.
❖ Initially drugs like isoniazid, rifampicin and ethambutol are used. Ethambutol can be stopped when the sensitivity tests show the other two drugs to be adequate. The therapy is continued for a period of 9 months in total. The most significant side effect of isoniazid is demyelination that may cause a peripheral neuropathy. This can be prevented by pyridoxine supplementation.
❖ Hepatotoxicity may commonly occur with antitubercular drug therapy. Therefore, liver function tests must be performed on a monthly basis.

Vitamin K supplementation may be required in the third trimester. Hepatic enzyme induction by the antitubercular drugs may cause theoretical deficiency of vitamin K resulting in the haemorrhagic disease of the newborn. Ethambutol can result in foetal ocular toxicity. Pyrazinamide should be preferably avoided in pregnancy. It may be used as a second-line agent. In multidrug resistant cases, drugs such as amikacin, kanamycin, ethionamide may be required. Drugs such as streptomycin, kanamycin, amikacin, or capreomycin are not recommended for treatment of tubercular infection in pregnancy.[19] Streptomycin is a known teratogen that interferes with 8th nerve development and may cause congenital deafness. Kanamycin and amikacin probably share this potential for toxicity. Capreomycin is supposed to be associated with toxicity to the 8th nerve and kidneys.

COMPLICATIONS

❖ Intrauterine growth restriction
❖ Prematurity.

CLINICAL PEARLS

❖ In UK, there is no screening program for tuberculosis in pregnancy. Therefore, the clinicians must remain vigilant regarding the development of signs and symptoms suggestive of the disease especially in the immigrant population.
❖ Vertical transmission of tubercular infection is extremely rare and may occasionally occur in cases where the maternal disease remains undetected or untreated.

EVIDENCE-BASED MEDICINE

❖ Pregnancy is not a risk factor for tuberculosis. It does not influence the pathogenesis of tuberculosis or the likelihood of disease progression from latent infection to active disease. Maternal infection can, however, lead to congenital or neonatal infection.[15]
❖ Routine tuberculin skin testing is not indicated for all pregnant women. It may be required for women at high risk of progression from latent to active disease (e.g. women with underlying HIV infection or those who are significantly immunocompromised).[17,18]

REFERENCES

1. Schatz M, Mosen DM, Kosinski M, Vollmer WM, Magid DJ, O'Connor E, et al. Predictors of asthma control in a random sample of asthmatic patients. J Asthma. 2007;44(4):341-5.
2. National Heart, Lung, and Blood Institute. National Asthma Education and Prevention Program. Expert Panel Report 3: Guidelines for the Diagnosis and Management of Asthma. Bethesda: National Heart, Lung and Blood Institute; 2007.
3. British Thoracic Society. The British guidelines on asthma management. Thorax. 1997;52(Suppl):S1-21.
4. Czeizel AE, Rockenbauer M. Population-based case control study of teratogenic potential of corticosteroids. Teratology. 1997;56(5):335-40.
5. Park-Wyllie L, Mazzotta P, Pastuszak A, Moretti ME, Beique L, Hunnisett L, et al. Birth defects after maternal exposure to corticosteroids, prospective cohort study and metaanalysis of epidemiological studies. Teratology. 2000;62(6):385-92.
6. Alexander S, Dodds L, Armson BA. Perinatal outcome in women with asthma during pregnancy. Obstet Gynecol. 1998;92(3):435-40.
7. Bracken MB, Triche EW, Belanger K, Saftlas A, Beckett WS, Leaderer BP. Asthma symptoms, severity, and drug therapy: a prospective study of effects on 2205 pregnancies. Obstet Gynecol. 2003;102(4):739-52.
8. Dombrowski M. Outcomes of pregnancy in asthmatic women. Immunol Allergy Clin North Am. 2006;26(1):81-92.
9. Triche EW, Saftlas AF, Belanger K, Leaderer BP, Bracken MB. Association of asthma diagnosis, severity, symptoms, and treatment with risk of preeclampsia. Obstet Gynecol. 2004;104(3):585-93.
10. Tsui LC, Buchwald M. Biochemical and molecular genetics of cystic fibrosis. Adv Hum Genet.1991;20:153-266.
11. McMullen AH, Pasta DJ, Frederick PD, Konstan MW, Morgan WJ, Schechter MS, et al. Impact of pregnancy on women with cystic fibrosis. Chest. 2006;129(3):706-11.
12. Nelson-Piercy C, Waldron M, Mooe-Gillon J. Respiratory disease in pregnancy. Br J Hosp Med. 1994;51(8):398-401.
13. Gilljam M, Antoniou M, Shin J, Dupuis A, Corey M, Tullis DE. Pregnancy in cystic fibrosis. Fetal and maternal outcome. Chest. 2000;118(1):85-91.
14. McArdle JR. Pregnancy in cystic fibrosis. Clin Chest Med. 2011;32(1):111-20.
15. Knight M, Kurinczuk JJ, Nelson-Piercy C, Spark P, Brocklehurst P, UKOSS. Tuberculosis in pregnancy in the UK. BJOG. 2009;116(4):584-8.
16. Hamadeh MA, Glassroth J. Tuberculosis and pregnancy. Chest. 1992;101(4):1114-20.
17. Targeted tuberculin testing and treatment of latent tuberculosis infection. American Thoracic Society. MMWR Recomm Rep. 2000;49:1-51.
18. Worjoloh A, Kato-Maeda M, Osmond D, Freyre R, Aziz N, Cohan D. Interferon gamma release assay compared with the tuberculin skin test for latent tuberculosis detection in pregnancy. Obstet Gynecol. 2011;118(6):1363-70.
19. Bothamley G. Drug treatment for tuberculosis during pregnancy: safety considerations. Drug Saf. 2001;24(7):553-65.

CHAPTER **12**

Epilepsy and Other Neurological Disorders

EPILEPSY AND PREGNANCY

 ### INTRODUCTION

Epilepsy is the most common pre-existing neurological condition encountered amongst the pregnant women. It is characterised by the occurrence of recurring seizures and affects nearly 600,000 people in the UK. Various antiepileptic drugs (AEDs) used during pregnancy may affect the foetus in several ways.

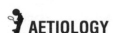 ### AETIOLOGY

Occurrence of epilepsy is primarily related to abnormal patterns of electrical activity in the brain, which may cause the body movements in an uncontrolled manner.

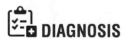 ### DIAGNOSIS

Clinical Presentation

The main symptom of epilepsy is the occurrence of repeated seizures. It can also result in the loss of consciousness for a short period.

Investigations

Diagnosis of epilepsy is mainly based on the findings on history and clinical examination, specifically, the neurological examination. Certain investigations, which may be sometimes required, include electroencephalogram (EEG), computed tomography scan, magnetic resonance imaging, functional magnetic resonance imaging (fMRI), PET, single-photon emission computed tomography (SPECT), etc.

 ### MANAGEMENT

Antepartum Period

❖ Care should be taken by a multidisciplinary team comprising of a specialist having special interest in epilepsy, neurologist, obstetrician, senior neonatologist and specialist nurse.
❖ Genetic counselling should be especially considered in cases where one partner has epilepsy, particularly idiopathic epilepsy and/or a positive family history of epilepsy.
❖ Patients should be taught about airway maintenance and nursing in the 'recovery position'. They should ensure that family, friends and work colleagues are also appropriately trained.
❖ *Screening for congenital anomalies*: The incidence of congenital anomalies is significantly increased amongst the offspring of epileptic mothers. This is most likely due to the AEDs being consumed by the mother. AEDs are prescribed to the mother during pregnancy because the benefits of seizure control during pregnancy outweigh its risks. All women must be screened, especially for those congenital anomalies that are commonly encountered in this group of women. A foetal cardiac scan is warranted at 22 weeks of gestation. Prenatal diagnosis with serum α-fetoprotein levels must be preferably performed at 16 weeks.

　All pregnancies occurring in women on anticonvulsant drugs must be notified to the UK register of AEDs in pregnancy.
❖ *Use of antiepileptic drugs*: All drugs used for treating epilepsy during pregnancy should be regarded as potential teratogens in clinical practice. The main risks associated with these drugs are neural tube defects, facial clefts and cardiac abnormalities.[1] Sodium valproate and carbamazepine are particularly associated with neural tube

Table 12.1: Various abnormalities found in association with foetal anticonvulsant syndrome

Major abnormalities	Minor abnormalities
• Microcephaly	• Distal digital and nail hypoplasia
• Cleft lip and palate	• Flat nasal bridge
• Neural tube defects	• Low set abnormal ears
• Congenital heart defects	• Epicanthal folds
• Intrauterine growth restriction	• Long philtrum
• Developmental delay	

defects, with incidences up to 4% and 1% respectively.[2] There is also the risk of foetal anticonvulsant syndrome (previously known as the foetal hydantoin syndrome), comprising one or lesser abnormalities enlisted in Table 12.1. This syndrome was renamed as foetal anticonvulsant syndrome after realisation of the fact that AEDs other than phenytoin such as carbamazepine, valproate, phenobarbitone, benzodiazepines, etc. can cause a similar collection of symptoms. Now, there are also concerns about intellectual and educational impairment of the foetus.

The patient should be counselled regarding the risk of epilepsy in the offspring. The overall risk of developing epilepsy is about 0.5–1% but may be up to 5% in the children of parents with epilepsy. If a sibling has epilepsy, the risk goes up to 10%. If both parents have epilepsy, the risk is up to 20%.

The greater the number of drugs used to treat the mother, the greater the foetal risk.[3] Polytherapy with more than one AED carries a greater risk to the foetus in comparison to monotherapy. Also, the higher the dosage of the drugs, the greater the risk to the foetus. There is no 'safest drug' to be used during pregnancy, but it is hoped that the newer drugs, gabapentin, levetiracetam and tiagabine, may prove safer.[4] However, the data in humans is largely limited. Lamotrigine appears to carry risks similar to the older drugs. Wherever possible, therapy should be simplified to the use of a single AED in the lowest possible dose to reduce the risk of congenital abnormalities.

Regarding the patient who has had no fits for years, the general advice is that she should be advised to continue with drugs if further fits are likely. If she does stop, she has to be informed of the risks of a further seizure and its consequences. If a fit was to occur, it is most likely that it will be in the first 6 months, so the usual advice is to wait for 6 months before conceiving.

Consideration must be given towards stopping AEDs in women who had been seizure-free for more than 2 years.[5] Cessation of drug therapy in a seizure-free patient should be in consultation with a neurologist, after appropriate counselling related to the risks of further seizures, with an interval of at least 6 months before conception.

❖ *Folic acid supplements*: Folic acid in the dosage of 5 mg daily should be prescribed each day periconceptually, though its efficacy remains unproven. It is likely to reduce the risk of neural tube defects, especially in the women taking valproate and carbamazepine.[6,7]

❖ *Monitoring the blood AED levels*: There is increased drug turnover and some authorities recommend that drug levels be monitored regularly, perhaps monthly. Others take the view that if the woman is fit-free and the levels are not elevated, less frequent monitoring is satisfactory, e.g. once each trimester.[8] There is debate regarding the mode of management in individuals with drug levels below the normal range. If the patient is fit-free, the best policy would be not to interfere with drug dosages. However, in cases where the patient has been experiencing fits, the drug dosage must be adjusted to bring the level within the therapeutic range. The woman should be counselled that her drug levels will be monitored during the pregnancy and that the dosage may need to be increased. The dosage would then be gradually returned to normal after the pregnancy.

Intrapartum Care

❖ Caesarean section is not required because of the epilepsy per se, unless there is status epilepticus or recurrent seizures in labour. In these cases, caesarean delivery is indicated for foetal reasons. Induction of labour and caesarean section are indicated for obstetric indications. In absence of any obstetric indication for caesarean delivery, vaginal delivery is usually indicated.

❖ Delivery should take place in an obstetric unit having facilities for maternal and neonatal resuscitation and treating maternal seizures. During labour, there is a higher risk for seizures due to disruption of sleep, reduced intake and absorption of AEDs, and hyperventilation, which may alter the free levels of AEDs. Every effort must be made to administer anticonvulsants as usual. In these circumstances, intravenous phenytoin can be administered, although it is associated with the risk of arrhythmias.[9]

❖ Seizures during labour are best controlled with intravenous benzodiazepines (e.g. clonazepam or diazepam). Rectal diazepam can be used in cases where there is an absence of intravenous access.

❖ If steroids are prescribed for the usual obstetric indications, women using enzyme-inducing AEDs should be prescribed a total of 48 mg (2 doses of 24 mg dexamethasone, 24 hours apart).

Postpartum Care

❖ *Breastfeeding*: Breastfeeding is acceptable and safe with almost all of the drugs, so the woman should be encouraged to go for it. All women and girls with epilepsy should be encouraged to breastfeed, except in very rare circumstances.[10]

❖ *Administration of vitamin K*: Many of the AEDs induce cytochrome P450 enzymes that reduce vitamin K levels in mother and baby. There is a small risk of neonatal bleeding due to the haemorrhagic disease of the newborn. Most clinicians advise that the mother should be given vitamin K (10 mg daily) in the last month of pregnancy starting from 36 weeks of gestation. All children born to mothers taking enzyme-inducing AEDs should be administered 1 mg of vitamin K parenterally at the time of delivery.

❖ *Advice regarding contraception*: Contraception is an issue, particularly hormonal contraception, which is rendered less effective by AEDs due to the induction of the liver enzymes. Effective contraception, therefore, should be provided.

 COMPLICATIONS

Complications associated with epilepsy in pregnancy are enumerated in Box 12.1.

> **Box 12.1:** Complications associated with epilepsy in pregnancy
> ❑ Foetal malformations (cleft lip/palate, mental retardation, cardiac abnormalities, limb defects, hypoplasia of terminal phalanges, neural tube defects, neonatal haemorrhage, etc.)
> ❑ Intrauterine growth restriction
> ❑ Oligohydramnios
> ❑ Pre-eclampsia
> ❑ Stillbirths

 CLINICAL PEARLS

❖ Three new AEDs have recently been licensed in the UK for the treatment of epilepsy (levetiracetam, zonisamide and pregabalin).

❖ All anticonvulsant drugs interfere with metabolism of folic acid, deficiency of which may result in neural tube defects and other malformations.

 EVIDENCE-BASED MEDICINE

❖ According to the results of a recent large multicentre trial [the SANAD trial (Standard versus New Antiepileptic Drugs)][11] evaluating newer drugs in newly diagnosed cases of epilepsy, sodium valproate should be the drug of choice in generalised and unclassifiable epilepsies, and lamotrigine in focal epilepsies. The available evidence also suggests that lamotrigine may be a clinical and cost-effective alternative to the existing standard drug treatment, carbamazepine, used for treating patients diagnosed as having partial seizures.

❖ There is no clear evidence available regarding the drug, which is safe during pregnancy. The patients with epilepsy planning pregnancy should be managed on the most effective antiseizure drug. Use of monotherapy and lowest possible drug dosage is likely to limit the risk of teratogenicity. The antiseizure drug regimen should be optimized 6 months prior to conception. No changes must be made in the antiseizure drug regimen for the purpose of reducing teratogenic risk in cases of established pregnancy.[3-5]

❖ The present evidence indicates that women taking carbamazepine or valproate or those with a previously affected child must be administered supplementation with folic acid in the dose of 4 mg per day prior to conception for prevention of neural tube defects.[6,7] On the other hand, all the women of childbearing potential must be administered folic acid supplementation in the dose of 0.4–0.8 mg per day during pregnancy.

MULTIPLE SCLEROSIS AND PREGNANCY

 INTRODUCTION

Multiple sclerosis (MS) is a neurological disorder characterised by the presence of inflammation, demyelination and axonal damage due to infiltrating macrophages and lymphocytes. The disease may affect the optic nerve, brain and spinal cord resulting in various neurological deficits, signs and symptoms. Most cases have a relapsing, remitting natural history with slow gradual decline. MS commonly affects young women belonging to the reproductive age groups and is the commonest cause of disability amongst young adults in the UK. Typically, women are affected nearly twice as commonly as men. Incidence of MS is lower in multiparous women in comparison to the nulliparous women.

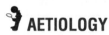 **AETIOLOGY**

Though the exact aetiology of the disease is not clear, some genetic component of the disease does exist. Therefore, risk of developing MS with one affected parent appears to be approximately 4%. This may be as high as 30% if both parents are affected. Infection with a virus can be considered as an important aetiological factor and relapses are more common following non-specific viral illness. Pregnancy does not accelerate course of the disease. In fact, pregnancy may have a protective effect.[12,13] However, relapses are more common in the puerperium.

Pregnancy is associated with a shift from type 1 (pro-inflammatory) to type 2 (anti-inflammatory) T-cell activity. The available evidence suggests that pregnancy itself is associated with a reduction in number of relapses and may even reduce the overall progression of disease in the long run.

DIAGNOSIS

Clinical Presentation

Multiple sclerosis can affect different body parts, thereby causing a range of symptoms such as fatigue, visual problems (temporary loss of vision, colour blindness, eye pain, flashes of light, double vision, involuntary eye movements, etc.), abnormal sensations (e.g. numbness and tingling), muscle spasms, stiffness and weakness, mobility problems, pain, bladder or bowel problems, difficulty in speaking, and/or swallowing, depression, anxiety, cognitive dysfunction, etc.[14]

Investigations

Magnetic resonance imaging has presently become the investigation of choice for the diagnosis and prognosis of MS. Currently, there is no data regarding the safety or otherwise of MRI in pregnancy. Also, there are no reports of associated foetal abnormality due to the use of MRI in pregnancy.

MANAGEMENT

- ❖ Treatment must be based on the individual symptoms and must be requested from a neurologist.
- ❖ Non-pharmacological therapy may be sufficient in some cases.
- ❖ Moderate to severe cases of relapse during pregnancy are treated with high intravenous dose of methylprednisolone followed by a tapering course of oral steroids. Cortico-steroids, however, should be used with caution following discussion related to its risks and benefits. In MS, presently there is no evidence regarding long-term benefit with the use of high-dose corticosteroid in the treatment of relapse.
- ❖ Tricyclic antidepressants, e.g. imipramine may be used for treatment of urinary urgency.
- ❖ Baclofen can be used for treatment of spasticity and paroxysmal pain.
- ❖ Tricyclic antidepressants can be used for treatment of depression and mood changes.
- ❖ Antiepileptic or anticonvulsants can also be used.
- ❖ Cyclophosphamide and azathioprine are commonly used for prophylaxis in cases of MS. Azathioprine is usually not started during pregnancy. β-interferon and glatiramer (a synthetic polymer of amino acid) are more effective. However, none of these drugs must be continued through-out the pregnancy for prophylactic reasons. β-interferon is not licensed for use in pregnancy.[15]
- ❖ Induction of labour and caesarean delivery is reserved for obstetric indications. Vaginal delivery is usually favoured although vaginal delivery may sometimes become imprac-tical in the face of serious disability. Earlier planned delivery may be required if there is exacerbation of urinary symptoms and limb spasm.
- ❖ Epidural anaesthesia is not contraindicated and does not increase the rate of disease progression.

Postpartum Period

- ❖ There is an increased frequency of relapse seen in the puerperium. A mother with MS may be temporarily less able to care for her new child especially if she has a significant relapse. Therefore, there may be a requirement of increased postnatal support during this period.

- ❖ There is no reported evidence to suggest that the children of women with MS are in anyway physically or mentally disadvantaged.
- ❖ Use of intravenous immunoglobulins in the postpartum period is likely to reduce the incidence of postpartum relapse.[16,17]
- ❖ The woman should be advised to breast-feed because relapse rate in the puerperium has been found to be independent of the breastfeeding status. Breastfeeding, however, is not advised while using β-interferons.[18]
- ❖ Due to the increasing use of immunosuppressive agents, the woman must be given appropriate advice regarding contraception.[19]

COMPLICATIONS

Maternal and foetal complications in cases of pregnant women with MS are similar to women without MS. As previously mentioned, the flare-ups of MS tend to decrease during the antepartum period. However, complications commonly encountered in normal pregnancy such as bowel and bladder complications, fatigue and gait-related problems tend to worsen in presence of MS.

CLINICAL PEARLS

- ❖ Pregnancy is not likely to adversely affect the progression of disease.
- ❖ Adequate postnatal support must be planned for a woman with MS due to an increased risk of relapse for 6 months in the postpartum period.
- ❖ There is no evidence to support previously held beliefs that women with MS should not become pregnant.

EVIDENCE-BASED MEDICINE

- ❖ There is weak evidence to suggest that pregnancy may improve the course of MS or delay its onset.[12,13]
- ❖ Though steroids are not contraindicated in pregnancy, they should be used with caution following discussion related to its risks and benefits.[15]

MYASTHENIA GRAVIS AND PREGNANCY

INTRODUCTION

Myasthenia gravis (MG) is a neurological disease characterised by a combination of weakness in ocular, bulbar, limb and respiratory muscles. The disease commonly affects young women and older men. MG may be associated with symptoms such as double vision, difficulty in swallowing, ptosis and failure of respiratory muscles.

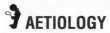

AETIOLOGY

Myasthenia gravis is caused by autoimmune disruption at the neuromuscular junction. It occurs due to abnormal regulation of T cells and production of autoantibodies directed against nicotinic acetylcholine receptors on the neuromuscular endplate of the skeletal muscles. Anti-acetylcholine receptor antibodies can be found in 85–90% patients. Thymic abnormities (hyperplasia or thymomas) are commonly encountered.

DIAGNOSIS

Clinical Presentation

There are two clinical forms of MG: ocular and generalised. In ocular type, weakness is limited to the eyelids and extraocular facial muscles. In generalised type, the weakness involves a variable combination of bulbar, limb, ocular and respiratory muscles. The cardinal clinical feature of the disease is fluctuating muscle weakness often accompanied with true muscle fatigue. Weakness most commonly occurs later in the day or evening or after exercise.

Ocular symptoms typically include ptosis or diplopia. Muscles of jaw closure may be affected resulting in weakness with prolonged chewing. Weakness of oropharyngeal muscles may produce dysarthria and dysphagia.

Investigations

* Initial evaluation in pregnancy involves assessment of baseline motor strength, respiratory status and pulmonary function tests.
* Cardiac evaluation can be through ECG.
* Thyroid function tests must be performed due to association between MG and other autoimmune diseases.
* Diagnosis is mainly established by history and typical findings on clinical examination. Bedside tests such as tensilon test can be performed but are associated with a high false positive rate.

Tensilon test: Administration of edrophonium chloride (short-acting anticholinesterase) transiently causes an improvement in symptoms, typically muscle spasms in patients with MG.

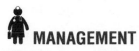

MANAGEMENT

Antepartum Period

* Pregnancy must be managed in conjunction with a neurologist, anaesthetist, paediatrician, nursing specialist, etc.

* Treatment of MG in pregnancy is similar to that in non-pregnant patients.
* Treatment with long-acting acetylcholinesterase inhibitors (neostigmine and pyridostigmine) form the mainstay of treatment. However, dose adjustment may be required in pregnancy due to normal physiological changes of pregnancy such as increased renal clearance, increased maternal blood volume, delayed gastric emptying, frequent emesis, etc.[20]
* Immunosuppressive therapy with corticosteroids, azathioprine, cyclosporine A and methotrexate forms the second-line therapy. These medications have been well studied in pregnancy and have been found to be relatively safe. However, high doses of cyclosporine and azathioprine have been found to be associated with spontaneous abortion, preterm labour, low birthweight, chromosomal damage, haematologic suppression, etc. The risk of continuing these medications in high doses should be weighed against the benefit of controlling myasthenic symptoms.[21]
* Plasmapheresis and intravenous immunoglobulin infusion is used for serious exacerbations.
* Indications for parenteral administration of anticholinesterases during pregnancy include persistent vomiting and prolonged labour (associated with delayed gastric emptying and malabsorption).
* Any infection should be promptly treated.
* Magnesium sulphate, which is commonly administered in clinical practice for management of pre-eclampsia or eclampsia and preterm labour, is contraindicated in patients who have MG since it can precipitate a severe myasthenic crisis. Severe hypertension can be treated with methyldopa or hydralazine, while β-blockers and calcium channel blockers should be preferably avoided.[22,23]
* *Foetal assessment*: The major foetal concern during pregnancy in mothers with MG is related to transplacental passage of IgG anti-acetylcholine receptor antibodies, which can result in the development of foetal abnormalities.

    The patient should be asked to do daily foetal movement count. The perception of foetal movement may be altered in patients with MG. Non-stress test (NST) can be performed in case of abnormalities on DFMC. This may be associated with reduced foetal movements and breathing. Sonographic examination may show abnormal finding such as polyhydramnios due to impaired foetal swallowing. Foetal arthrogryposis multiplex congenita is the most severe finding in the foetuses with neonatal MG. In these cases, lack of generalised foetal movement and diaphragmatic excursion may rarely result in development of joint contractures and pulmonary hypoplasia.

Intrapartum Period

* Myasthenia gravis does not affect the first stage of labour because the uterus is composed of smooth muscle and thereby lacks the postsynaptic acetylcholine receptor.

❖ The second stage of labour may be affected due to weakening of the voluntary striated muscles used during expulsive efforts.[24] This may result in excessive maternal fatigue. Assisted vaginal delivery (vacuum or forceps) in these cases may reduce maternal fatigue and weakness.

❖ An anaesthesiologist must be consulted before labour because patients with myasthenia who undergo general anaesthesia may be at an increased risk for requiring mechanical ventilation. Non-depolarizing muscle relaxants should be avoided in these cases because patients with MG have altered acetylcholinesterase activity.

❖ Anticholinesterase medications should be administered parenterally during labour to avoid complications related to erratic gastrointestinal absorption.

❖ The maternal respiratory status (respiratory rate, pulse oximetry) should be carefully monitored because stress and fatigue associated with labour and delivery may cause worsening of the disease.

Postpartum Period

Breastfeeding: Glucocorticoids can be administered safely during lactation. However, breastfeeding is not recommended for patients with MG taking azathioprine, cyclosporine, and methotrexate because these drugs are likely to cause immunosuppression in the infant and are therefore contra-indicated.

COMPLICATIONS

❖ Preterm labour
❖ High perinatal mortality (especially due to high rate of foetal anomalies).

CLINICAL PEARLS

❖ The second stage of labour may be affected in patients with MG because the voluntary striated muscles used during expulsive efforts may easily weaken. Appropriate steps should be taken to avoid the effects of maternal fatigue on delivery.

❖ All infants of myasthenic mothers should be observed in a special care nursery for the first 2–3 days of life, due to the risk of developing transient neonatal MG which develops in nearly 10–20% of infants born to myasthenic mothers.

EVIDENCE-BASED MEDICINE

❖ Pregnancy has a variable effect on the course of MG. The first trimester and the acute postpartum period are times of highest risk for exacerbation.[24]

❖ Pregnancies complicated by severe pre-eclampsia in patients with MG must not be administered magnesium sulphate.[22,23]

REFERENCES

1. Kaaja E, Kaaja R, Hiilesmaa V. Major malformations in offspring of women with epilepsy. Neurology. 2003;60(4):575-9.

2. Wegner C, Nau H. Alteration of embryonic folate metabolism by valproic acid during organogenesis: implications for mechanism of teratogenesis. Neurology. 1992;42(4 Suppl 5): 17-24.

3. Harden CL, Pennell PB, Koppel BS, Hovinga CA, Gidal B, Meador KJ, et al. Practice parameter update: management issues for women with epilepsy—focus on pregnancy (an evidence-based review): vitamin K, folic acid, blood levels, and breastfeeding: report of the Quality Standards Subcommittee and Therapeutics and Technology Assessment Subcommittee of the American Academy of Neurology and American Epilepsy Society. Neurology. 2009;73(2):142-9.

4. Royal College of Obstetricians and Gynaecologists. Epilepsy in Pregnancy. Green-top Guideline Number 68. London: RCOG Press; 2016.

5. Chadwick D. The discontinuation of AED therapy. In: Pedley TA, Meldrum BS (Eds). Recent Advances in Epilepsy; 1985. p. 111.

6. Morrow JI, Hunt SJ, Russell AJ, Smithson WH, Parsons L, Robertson I , et al. Folic acid use and major congenital malformations in offspring of women with epilepsy: a prospective study from the UK Epilepsy and Pregnancy Register. J Neurol Neurosurg Psychiatry. 2009;80(5):506-11.

7. Ban L, Fleming KM, Doyle P, Smeeth L, Hubbard RB, Fiaschi L, et al. Congenital Anomalies in Children of Mothers Taking Antiepileptic Drugs with and without Periconceptional High Dose Folic Acid Use: A Population-Based Cohort Study. PLoS One. 2015;10(7):e0131130.

8. Yerby MS. Problems and management of the pregnant woman with epilepsy. Epilepsia. 1987;28 Suppl 3:S29-36.

9. Walker SP, Permezel M, Berkovic SF. The management of epilepsy in pregnancy. BJOG. 2009;116(6):758-67.

10. Kaneko S, Sato T, Suzuki K. The levels of anticonvulsants in breast milk. Br J Clin Pharmacol. 1979;7(6):624-7.

11. Marson AG, Appleton R, Baker GA, Chadwick DW, Doughty J, Eaton B, et al. A randomised controlled trial examining the longer-term outcomes of standard versus new antiepileptic drugs. The SANAD trial. Health Technol Assess. 2007;11(37): 1-134.

12. Confavreux C, Hutchinson M, Hours MM, Cortinovis-Tourniaire P, Moreau T. Rate of pregnancy-related relapses in multiple sclerosis. Pregnancy in Multiple Sclerosis Group. N Engl J Med. 1998;339(5):285-91.

13. Runmarker B, Anderson O. Pregnancy is associated with a lower risk of onset and a better prognosis in multiple sclerosis. Brain. 1995;118(Pt 1):253-61.

14. Damek DM, Shuster EA. Pregnancy and multiple sclerosis. Mayo Clin Proc. 1997;72(10):977-89.

15. British Medical Association and the Royal Pharmaceutical Society of Great Britain. British national formulary. London: British Medical Association and the Royal Pharmaceutical Society of Great Britain, 2001. p. 41.

16. Achiron A, Rotstein Z, Noy S, Mashiach S, Dulitzky M, Achiron R, et al. Intravenous immunoglobulin treatment in

PART II

the prevention of childbirth-associated acute exacerbations in multiple sclerosis: a pilot study. J Neurol. 1996;243(1):25-8.

17. Haas J. High dose IVIG in the postpartum period for prevention of exacerbations in MS. Mult Scler. 2000;6(Suppl 2):S18-20.

18. Sadovnick AD, Eisen K, Hashimoto SA, Farquhar R, Yee IM, Hooge J, et al. Pregnancy and multiple sclerosis. Arch Neurol. 1994;51:1120-4.

19. Roullet E, Verdier-Taillefer MH, Amarenco P, Gharbi G, Alperovitch A, Marteau R. Pregnancy and multiple sclerosis: a longitudinal study of 125 remittent patients. J Neurol Neurosurg Psychiatry. 1993;56:1062-5.

20. Plauché WC. Myasthenia gravis in mothers and their newborns. Clin Obstet Gynecol. 1991;34(1):82-99.

21. Varner M. Myasthenia gravis and pregnancy. Clin Obstet Gynecol. 2013;56(2):372-81.

22. Benshushan A, Rojansky N, Weinstein D. Myasthenia gravis and preeclampsia. Isr J Med Sci. 1994;30(3):229-33.

23. Piura B. The association of preeclampsia and myasthenia gravis: double trouble. Isr J Med Sci. 1994;30:243-4.

24. Batocchi AP, Majolini L, Evoli A, Lino MM, Minisci C, Tonali P. Course and treatment of myasthenia gravis during pregnancy. Neurology. 1999;52(3):447-52.

Hepatic and Gastrointestinal Diseases

LIVER DISEASE DURING PREGNANCY

 INTRODUCTION

Acute viral hepatitis is the most common cause of jaundice during pregnancy, the second being intrahepatic cholestasis. Other causes of jaundice specific to pregnancy include severe pre-eclampsia, eclampsia, haemolysis, HELLP syndrome, acute fatty liver, severe hyperemesis gravidarum (HG), endotoxic shock [disseminated intravascular coagulation (DIC)], etc. Course of most viral hepatitis is not altered by pregnancy. Pregnant women may have similar clinical features and mode of acquiring infection as the non-pregnant women.[1]

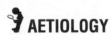 **AETIOLOGY**

The causative organisms for various types of hepatitis include hepatitis virus A, B, C, D and E.

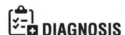 **DIAGNOSIS**

Clinical Presentation

❖ Generalised pruritus
❖ Weakness, nausea and vomiting
❖ *Jaundice*: This is evident as the yellowing of sclera, nail beds and the palmer creases of hands.

Investigations

❖ *Increased serum bilirubin levels*: Serum bilirubin levels greater than 2 mg%
❖ *Liver function tests*: Increased levels of liver enzymes, such as aspartate transaminase (AST), alanine transaminase (ALT) and alkaline phosphatase

❖ *Liver biopsy*: Liver biopsy may show evidence of intrahepatic cholestasis. However, there is no evidence of hepatic necrosis.

 MANAGEMENT

❖ General measures for prevention of hepatitis include precautions, such as provision of safe drinking water and improved sanitation; adequate care of personal hygiene; use of disposable syringes for blood collection and screening of the blood donors for hepatitis B surface antigen (HBsAg).
❖ Infants of HBsAg-positive mothers should receive hepatitis B immune globulins (dosage 0.06 mg/kg, intramuscular). These infants must also receive immunoprophylaxis at birth with hepatitis B vaccine (1 mL, 3 doses) at 1 week, 1 month and 6 months after birth. Immunization is 85–95% effective in preventing both hepatitis B virus infection and the chronic carrier state.
❖ The rate of vertical transmission of the neonatal hepatitis B infection is greatest when the maternal infection occurs during the third trimester or the immediate postpartum period.
❖ Diphenhydramine is used for intense pruritus. Cholestyramine or ursodeoxycholic acid (UDCA) is also used for itching [2]
❖ There is no specific treatment for viral hepatitis; it is usually supportive and comprises of steps such as hospitalisation and bed rest; patient isolation and prescription of diet rich in proteins and carbohydrates.

 COMPLICATIONS

❖ Preterm labour, low-birth-weight babies
❖ Meconium-stained liquor

❖ Intrauterine death
❖ Postpartum haemorrhage (PPH).

 CLINICAL PEARLS

❖ Pre-eclampsia may be associated with hepatic complications, such as HELLP syndrome, acute fatty liver of pregnancy, hepatic infarction and rupture
❖ The course of most viral hepatitis infections, e.g. hepatitis A, B, C and D except for hepatitis E and disseminated herpes simplex virus remains unaltered by pregnancy.

 EVIDENCE-BASED MEDICINE

❖ The patients with hepatitis C infection are at a significant risk (60–80%) of developing cirrhosis over a period of 10–30 years. Detection of hepatitis C virus antibody indicates persistent infection rather than immunity.[1]
❖ Women with hepatitis C infection are at an increased risk of developing obstetric cholestasis (OC) during their pregnancies.[3]

OBSTETRIC CHOLESTASIS

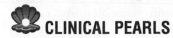 **INTRODUCTION**

There is no agreed definition for OC. It can be generally defined as presence of pruritus and abnormal liver function tests (LFTs) that resolve during the puerperium. Though pruritus affects the whole body, it typically affects the palms and soles in cases of OC. It shows a wide geographic variation, being the most common in Chile, Scandinavia and Southeast Asia. Araucanian women have the world's highest incidence of OC (approximately 5%). The prevalence of OC in UK is about 0.7%.[4]

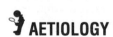 **AETIOLOGY**

The exact aetiology of OC is unknown. It probably results due to an oestrogenic effect, which shows genetic predisposition. The incidence of OC is highest in third trimester (around 30–32 weeks of gestation), because oestrogen levels peak during this time. There is also a risk of recurrence on oestrogen-containing contraception. Nearly one-third of the patients have a positive family history.

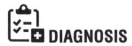 **DIAGNOSIS**

Clinical Presentation

Intense pruritus often occurs on the palms and soles. Usually, there is no rash, unless one inflicted by scratching. If there is a rash, a dermatological opinion must be taken.

Investigations

Liver function tests are typically deranged in cases of OC. Liver enzymes such as ALT and AST are elevated in most women with OC. A small proportion of women may also have raised levels of gamma-glutamyl transaminase and elevated bile acids. Elevated bile acid is a parameter widely used for the diagnosis of OC in the UK.[5] However, it is not mandatory for the diagnosis. The diagnosis of OC is made, once other causes of pruritus and abnormal LFTs have been excluded out. Also, pregnancy-specific reference ranges for LFTs should be used.

Obstetric cholestasis is diagnosed through exclusion. Various differential diagnoses include extrahepatic bile duct obstruction with gallstones, acute or chronic viral hepatitis, primary biliary cirrhosis and chronic active hepatitis. To rule out these conditions, the following investigations are required: hepatic ultrasound, serology for hepatitis A, B, C, Epstein-Barr virus and cytomegalovirus. Levels of hepatic autoantibodies also need to be measured. Absence of antimitochondrial antibodies helps in ruling out primary biliary cirrhosis and anti-smooth muscle antibodies help in excluding chronic active hepatitis.

 MANAGEMENT

The most important complication of OC is intrauterine deaths in late gestation. Steps need to be taken to prevent this. Presently, there is no way of identifying the "at-risk baby" and no proven effective treatment is available. According to Royal College of Obstetricians and Gynaecologists, there is no evidence to support early delivery (prior to 37 weeks of gestation) and it is reasonable to prescribe vitamin K, 10 mg daily, from the time of diagnosis. It has further advised that 'the timing and risks of delivery should be discussed on an individual basis'. Delivery is rarely indicated before 37 weeks. Most commonly used management strategy suggests foetal surveillance and elective early delivery by 38 weeks. Though this practice may be associated with reduced foetal mortality, it may be associated with increased rates of induction of labour, caesarean section, prematurity and admission to neonatal intensive care units.[6,7]

Symptoms can be controlled with a combination of antihistaminics or emollients. UDCA and dexamethasone possibly have a beneficial effect. Use of UDCA improves the symptoms and LFTs.[8] However, it does not cause a reduction in foetal risk. Presently, there is insufficient research to support their routine use.[8,9]

 COMPLICATIONS

Obstetric cholestasis is likely to cause the following complications:
❖ Premature delivery (particularly iatrogenic)
❖ Late gestation foetal death in utero

❖ Postpartum haemorrhage (secondary to vitamin K deficiency due to fat malabsorption)
❖ Meconium-stained liquor
❖ Foetal distress (cardiotocographic abnormalities in labour).

CLINICAL PEARLS

❖ Vitamin K (in the dosage of 10 mg orally daily) must be administered to the mother from the time of diagnosis to reduce the risk of PPH.
❖ No specific method of foetal surveillance can be recommended to predict foetal complications in mothers with OC.

EVIDENCE-BASED MEDICINE

❖ Present evidence supports the use of active management strategy with elective delivery at 38 weeks of gestation. However, the clinician needs to strike a balance between the reduced rate of foetal mortality and increased rates of caesarean delivery and prematurity.[6,7]
❖ Present evidence supports the requirement for a high index of clinical suspicion and serial measurement of LFTs prior to making the diagnosis of OC in women with onset of pruritus predominantly affecting the palms and soles in the third trimester.[9]

MORNING SICKNESS/HYPEREMESIS GRAVIDARUM

INTRODUCTION

Nausea and vomiting of pregnancy, commonly known as 'morning sickness', affects approximately 75–85% of pregnant women.[10] The exact pathology behind morning sickness remains unknown, however many theories have been proposed. The most important of them being the relaxation of gastrointestinal smooth muscles caused by the hormonal changes taking place during pregnancy, especially due to hormones like oestrogen and relaxin. Recent research has also indicated the role of the bacteria, *Helicobacter pylori* in the pathogenesis of more severe form of morning sickness called hyperemesis gravidarum (HG).[11] Morning sickness is generally a mild, self-limited condition, commonly encountered between 4th and 7th week of pregnancy, peaking at approximately 9th week and diminishing greatly in intensity by 14–16 weeks of pregnancy. It may be controlled with conservative measures, usually subsiding or greatly diminishing in intensity by the time the woman approaches the second trimester.[12]

Though mild amount of nausea and vomiting is a common symptom in early pregnancy, a small percentage of women experiences severe nausea and vomiting. This is known as HG.

It is characterised by severe persistent vomiting, dehydration, ketosis, electrolyte disturbances, and weight loss (more than 5% of body weight). The incidence of HG is approximately 0.5–1.5% of live births, commonly associated with certain pregnancy-related conditions like multiple pregnancies, hydatidiform mole and other conditions associated with increased levels of pregnancy hormones.[13]

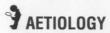

AETIOLOGY

Both the aetiology and pathogenesis of HG remain unknown. Probable aetiology of morning sickness has been described previously in the text.

On one hand, the morning sickness usually has no negative maternal or foetal consequences; HG on the other hand, may have negative implications for maternal and foetal health.[14] Thus, it is the responsibility of the obstetrician to carefully assess the patients with non-resolving or worsening symptoms of nausea and vomiting to rule out the most common pregnancy-related problems, which can be associated with severe vomiting. The obstetrician must also rule out other non-pregnancy-related causes of vomiting which can occur during pregnancy. Severe uncontrolled vomiting during pregnancy can result in complications like Wernicke's encephalopathy and vitamin K deficiency.

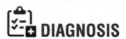

DIAGNOSIS

Clinical Presentation

The woman may present with the following signs and symptoms:
❖ Marked weight loss
❖ Muscle wasting
❖ Ketonuria
❖ Dehydration and electrolyte disturbances including hypokalaemia, and metabolic hypochloraemic alkalosis
❖ *Ptyalism*: A commonly associated symptom, which can be described as the inability to swallow saliva, resulting in the accumulation of excessive saliva in the mouth.

Investigations

Investigations required in cases of HG are listed in Table 13.1.

MANAGEMENT

Management of morning sickness is described in Flow chart 13.1 and comprises of the following:

Table 13.1: Investigations required in cases of hyperemesis gravidarum

Investigation	Abnormalities
Thyroid function test	Raised free thyroxine (T_4) and suppressed TSH levels
Liver function tests	Raised transaminases
Ultrasound scan	Exclusion of H. mole and multiple pregnancy

Flow chart 13.1: Evaluation and management of women with nausea and vomiting during pregnancy

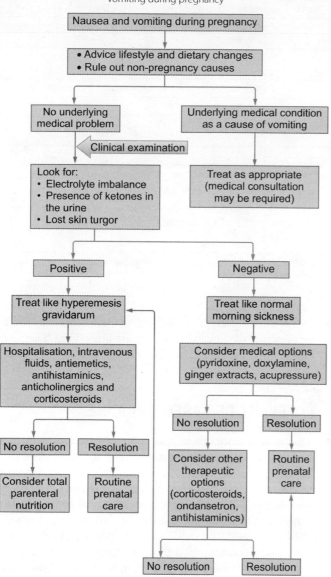

❖ *Exclusion of other causes of nausea and vomiting*: It is important to exclude whether vomiting is pregnancy-related or due to non-pregnancy-related causes (urinary tract infection and thyrotoxicosis, etc.), (Table 13.2). Once other pathologic causes have been ruled out, treatment is individualised and mainly comprises of conservative approach which involves dietary changes, emotional support, etc.

❖ *Assessment of severity on clinical examination*: This is important because assessment of severity on clinical examination helps in determining the management regimen. For example, presence of ketones in the urine, loss of skin turgor, electrolyte imbalance, etc. is a sign indicative of a severe condition (HG). Rehydration (intravenous or oral) and antiemetic therapy are used for severe cases showing presence of ketones in their urine.

❖ *Dietary and lifestyle changes*: The obstetrician must advise the dietary and lifestyle changes (as enumerated in Box 13.1) to the women in order to reduce the discomfort associated with morning sickness.

❖ *Medicines*: Various medicinal substances, which have been implicated in reducing the symptoms of morning sickness, have been listed in Table 13.3. Medications that can be used for obtaining relief from morning sickness include:
- *Herbal medications*: Ginger extract
- Non-conventional pharmacological medications like pyridoxine and doxylamine
- *Antiemetic drugs*: Chlorpromazine (thorazine), pro-chlorperazine (compazine), promethazine (phenergan), trimethobenzamide (tigan), ondansetron (zofran), droperidol (inapsine)
- *Antihistamines and anticholinergic drugs*: Diphen-hydramine (benadryl), meclizine (antivert), dimen-hydrinate (dramamine)
- *Intestinal motility reducing drugs*: Metoclopramide (reglan)
- Non-pharmacological therapy like acupressure.[15,16]

Antiemetic drugs are considered safe in pregnancy. Women with severe hyperemesis may require parenteral dose of more than one antiemetic drug to control their symptoms.

CHAPTER 13

Table 13.2: Differential diagnosis of severe vomiting during pregnancy[12]

Common pregnancy related causes of hyperemesis gravidarum	Common non-pregnancy-related causes of severe vomiting
• Gestational trophoblastic disease • Triploidy, Trisomy 21 (Down's syndrome) • Hydrops foetalis • Multiple pregnancy	• Gastrointestinal disorders (gastroenteritis, hepatitis, peptic ulcer disease) • Genitourinary tract disorders (urinary tract infections, pyelonephritis, uraemia, kidney stones) • Metabolic disorders (diabetic ketoacidosis, hyperthyroidism) • Neurological disorders (pseudotumour cerebri, CNS tumours) • History of hyperemesis gravidarum in previous pregnancy

Box 13.1: Lifestyle and dietary changes to reduce the symptoms of morning sickness

❑ Chewing a piece of dry food (toasted bread, etc.) before getting out of bed
❑ Avoiding fatty and spicy foods
❑ Consuming five portions of fresh foods and vegetables and drinking eight glasses of water daily
❑ Eating small meals multiple times a day
❑ Eating a protein rich snack at bed-time
❑ Sucking on some candy, a piece of lemon, etc. in between meals
❑ She should stop working and lie down whenever she feels nauseated
❑ Emotional and psychological support: Although no underlying psychological abnormality causing morning sickness has been identified, emotional support from family, especially the spouse helps the women in effectively dealing with the condition

Table 13.3: Commonly prescribed therapeutic options for morning sickness[12,15,16]

Drug	Dosage	Route
Pyridoxine (vitamin B$_6$)	25 mg 3 times/day (or 75 mg/day)	Oral
Metoclopramide (antimotility drug)	5–10 mg 3–4 times/day	Oral
Prochlorperazine	25 mg 2 times/day or 50 mg/day	Rectal
Promethazine (Phenergan)	25 mg every 4 hourly or 150 mg/day	Orally or rectally
Prednisolone (corticosteroids)	40–60 mg/day reducing by half every 3 days followed by tapering over 2 weeks	Oral
Ondansetron (Zofran)	4–8 mg 2–3 times/day	Oral
Doxylamine	25 mg single dose of doxylamine at night or can be administered in combination with pyridoxine in the dose of 25 mg TDS	Oral
Ginger	1 g/day (powdered ginger) in divided doses	Can be used in the following forms: biscuits, ginger crystals, powder, tablets, capsules, fresh ginger, teas, preserves, ginger ale, etc.
Acupressure	The most common location for acupressure is the Neiguan point, which is located three finger-breadths above the wrist on the volar surface	Physical pressure application over acupuncture points

PART II

❖ *Adequate hydration*: Adequate hydration must be ensured preferably with normal saline and added potassium chloride. This helps in correcting tachycardia, hypotension and ketonuria, and helps in returning electrolyte levels back to normal. Very severe cases may require nasogastric or parenteral nutrition.

❖ *Thiamine supplementation*: For severe, prolonged hyperemesis, consideration should be given for intravenous thiamine supplementation (100 mg/day) to prevent Wernicke-Korsakoff syndrome, which results from the deficiency of thiamine (vitamin B$_1$) and shows the symptoms of both Wernicke's encephalopathy and Korsakoff's syndrome.[13] Wernicke's encephalopathy is characterised by ophthalmic symptoms like nystagmus, ophthalmoplegia, anisocoria, sluggish pupillary reflexes, and ataxia followed by coma and death, if left untreated. Korsakoff's psychosis on the other hand is characterised by confusion, amnesia (both anterograde and retrograde) and confabulation.

❖ *Corticosteroids*: For women with severe hyperemesis who do not respond to conventional treatment with IV fluids, electrolytes and regular antiemetic drugs, a trial of corticosteroids may be useful.

COMPLICATIONS

Presence of HG during pregnancy can be associated with the following complications:
❖ Foetal growth restriction
❖ Maternal hyponatraemia.

CLINICAL PEARLS

❖ Iron supplements may further induce nausea and vomiting and therefore they should be preferably withheld until the symptoms resolve.

❖ Out of the various pharmacological medications shown to be effective, pyridoxine has the least side effects. The most commonly prescribed drug is metoclopramide.[14]

EVIDENCE-BASED MEDICINE

❖ The present evidence supports the safety of conventional antiemetic drugs during pregnancy including the first trimester. There is sufficient evidence in the literature to support the safety of antiemetics, antacids, sucralfate, histamine 2 (H$_2$)-receptor blockers and proton pump inhibitors in pregnancy. Evidence from observational studies suggests no evidence of teratogenicity from any of the above-mentioned treatment options used for HG or morning sickness.[15,16] However, well-controlled safety and effectiveness trials in patients with morning sickness are lacking for acupressure.

❖ Several RCTs also support the beneficial effect of corticosteroids.[17]

CONSTIPATION DURING PREGNANCY

INTRODUCTION

Constipation is defined as having a bowel movement fewer than 3 times per week. Chronic constipation is a highly prevalent problem, especially in women at the time of pregnancy.

AETIOLOGY

Probable causes of constipation in pregnancy are as follows:
❖ Increase in the levels of circulating progesterone, a smooth muscle relaxant, is responsible for increase in transit

time of gastrointestinal contents through the intestines, especially in the mid and late pregnancy.

❖ Decreased physical activity

❖ In the later stages of pregnancy, the enlarged uterus may also press upon rectum resulting in constipation.

MANAGEMENT

Management of constipation during pregnancy is described in Flow chart 13.2[18,19] and involves the following:

❖ *Dietary modifications*: Dietary modifications for dealing with constipation are enlisted in Box 13.2. The patient must be advised to take a high-fibre diet. Some of the sources of fibre in the diet are enumerated in Box 13.3. The recommended

Flow chart 13.2: Management of constipation during the antenatal period

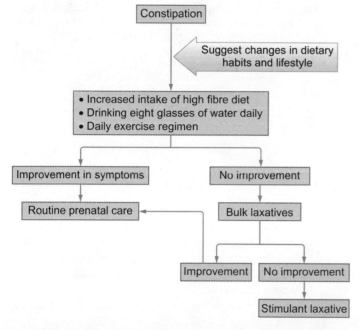

Box 13.2: Dietary modifications for dealing with constipation[20,21]

❑ *High-fibre diet*: Whole grain breakfast cereals and breads, whole-wheat pasta, brown rice, jacket potatoes, peas, beans and lentils

❑ Consumption of food rich in raw fruits and vegetables (five portions of fruits and vegetables daily), legumes, nuts and edible seeds, whole-grain breads, cereals and flour)

❑ Drinking at least eight glasses of water (2 L) daily

Box 13.3: Sources of fibre in the diet

❑ Whole grain containing breads, buns, muffins, etc.

❑ Fruits, including both fresh and dried fruits. Dried fruits include apricots, dates, prunes, raisins, berries like blackberries, raspberries, strawberries, etc. Fresh fruits include fruits like apples, oranges, kiwi fruits, mangoes, pears, etc.

❑ Vegetables like broccoli, green leafy vegetables (spinach, etc.), green peas, etc. are also rich sources of fibre

❑ Another source of fibre is dried peas and beans (kidney beans, black-eyed beans), chickpeas, lentils, seeds and nut

dietary fibre intake during pregnancy is about 28 of fibre every day. It is important to introduce fibre-rich foods gradually in order to avoid excessive bloating and flatulence, which might be present if fibres are introduced suddenly in the diet. These changes are expected to bring about an increase in the number of bowel movements and make the stool consistency softer. Dietary supplements of fibre in the form of bran or wheat fibre are also likely to help the women.

❖ *Laxatives*: If the problem fails to resolve with above-mentioned dietary and lifestyle modifications, laxatives need to be prescribed. Initially, the women should be prescribed milder laxative, followed by stronger ones if the condition does not improve. Initially, the bulk laxatives, which are the safest, like cellulose and hemi-cellulose, psyllium seed, flax seed, ispaghula or osmotic laxatives like lactose, etc. can be advised. Bulk laxatives must be taken with water or they can cause obstruction. Use of magnesium hydroxide is usually discouraged in pregnancy, as alkalis should be avoided in pregnant woman. If bulk laxatives do not appear to be useful and the woman's constipation keeps worsening, stimulant laxatives may be prescribed.[18]

CLINICAL PEARLS

Use of iron supplements during pregnancy is likely to exacerbate the problem of constipation. Short-term interruption of therapy with iron tablets may prove to be useful.

EVIDENCE-BASED MEDICINE

Osmotic laxatives (e.g. lactulose and magnesium hydro-chloride) and stimulant laxatives (glycerol suppositories, senna, etc.) are safe to be used in pregnancy.[18]

REFERENCES

1. Kametas N, Nelson Piercy C. Hyperemesis gravidarum, gastro-intestinal and liver disease in pregnancy. Obstet Gynaecol Reprod Med. 2008;18:69-75.

2. Nelson-Percy C. Liver disease. In: Handbook of Obstetric Medicine, 2nd edition. London: Martin Dunitz; 2001. pp. 199-217.

3. Locatelli A, Roncaglia N, Arreghini A, Bellini P, Vergani P, Ghidini A. Hepatitis C virus infection is associated with a higher incidence of cholestasis of pregnancy. Br J Obstet Gynaecol. 1999;106(5):498-500.

4. Kenyon AP, Girling JC. Obstetric cholestasis. In: Studd J (Ed). Progress in Obstetrics and Gynaecology. Edinburgh: Churchill Livingstone; 2005. pp. 37-56.

5. Royal College of Obstetricians and Gynecologists (RCOG). (2006). Obstetric cholestasis. RCOG Guideline No. 43. [online] RCOG website. Available from www.rcog.org.uk/en/guidelines-research-services/guidelines/gtg43 [Accessed June, 2016].

6. Kenyon AP, Piercy CN, Girling J, Williamson C, Tribe RM, Shennan AH. Obstetric cholestasis, outcome with active management: a series of 70 cases. BJOG. 2002;109(3):282-8.

7. Roncaglia N, Arreghini A, Locatelli A, Bellini P, Andreotti C, Ghidini A. Obstetric cholestasis: outcome with active management. Eur J Obstet Gynecol Reprod Biol. 2002;100(2): 167-70.

8. Chappell LC, Gurung V, Seed PT, Chambers J, Williamson C, Thornton JG. Ursodeoxycholic acid versus placebo, and early term delivery versus expectant management, in women with intrahepatic cholestasis of pregnancy: semifactorial randomised clinical trial. BMJ. 2012;344:e3799.

9. Gurung V, Middleton P, Milan SJ, Hague W, Thornton JG. Interventions for treating cholestasis in pregnancy. Cochrane Database Syst Rev. 2013;6:CD000493.

10. Gadsby R, Barnie-Adshead AM, Jagger C. A prospective study of nausea and vomiting during pregnancy. Br J Gen Pract. 1993;43(371):245-8.

11. Penney DS. Helicobacter pylori and severe nausea and vomiting during pregnancy. J Midwifery Womens Health. 2005;50(5): 418-22.

12. Quinlan JD, Hill DA. Nausea and vomiting of pregnancy. Am Fam Physician 2003;68(1):121-8.

13. Verberg MF, Gillott DJ, Al-Fardan N, Grudzinskas JG. Hyperemesis gravidarum, a literature review. Hum Reprod Update. 2005;11(5):527-39.

14. Sheehan P. Hyperemesis gravidarum—assessment and management. Aust Fam Physician. 2007;36(9):698-701.

15. Jewell D, Young G. Interventions for nausea and vomiting in early pregnancy. Cochrane Database Syst Rev. 2002;(1): CD000145.

16. Mazzotta P, Magee LA. A risk-benefit assessment of pharmacological and nonpharmacological treatments for nausea and vomiting of pregnancy. Drugs. 2000;59(4):781-800.

17. Nelson-Piercy C, Fayers P, de Swiet M. Randomised placebo control trial of corticosteroids for hyperemesis gravidarum. BJOG. 2001;108(1):9-15.

18. Rungsiprakarn P, Laopaiboon M, Sangkomkamhang US, Lumbiganon P, Pratt JJ. Interventions for treating constipation in pregnancy. Cochrane Database Syst Rev. 2015;9:CD011448.

19. Anderson AS, Whichelow MJ. Constipation during pregnancy: Dietary fibre intake and the effect of fibre supplementation. Hum Nutr Appl Nutr. 1985;39(3):202-7.

20. Anderson AS. Dietary factors in the aetiology and treatment of constipation during pregnancy. Br J Obstet Gynaecol. 1986;93(3):245-9.

21. Thompson WG, Longstreth GF, Drossman DA, Heaton KW, Irvine EJ, Muller-Lissner SA. Functional bowel disorders and functional abdominal pain. Gut. 1999;45(Suppl 2):II43-7.

PART II

Anaemia and Other Haematological Abnormalities

IRON DEFICIENCY ANAEMIA

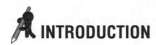

INTRODUCTION

The World Health Organization (WHO) defines anaemia as presence of haemoglobin of less than 11 g/dL and haematocrit of less than 0.33 g/dL.[1] Centre of Disease Control (CDC, 1990) has defined anaemia as haemoglobin levels below 11 g/dL in the pregnant woman in first and third trimester and less than 10.5 g/dL in second trimester. Anaemia may develop in nearly 30–50% of women during pregnancy. Based on the findings of the peripheral smear and the results of various blood indices, anaemia can be classified into three types which have been shown in Table 14.1. Of the various types of anaemia, iron deficiency anaemia is responsible for more than 90% of cases during pregnancy. On the other hand, deficiency of folate may be responsible for another 5% of cases of anaemia during pregnancy. Moreover, the deficiency of folate is almost always the cause of megaloblastic anaemia during pregnancy.

Table 14.1: Classification of anaemia based on the blood values

Types	Laboratory values	Causes
Macrocytic, normochromic anaemia	Increased MCV, normal MCHC (MCV >100 fL; MCHC 34 g%)	Vitamin B_{12} deficiency; folate deficiency anaemia
Microcytic hypochromic anaemia	Low MCHC; low MCV; (MCV <80 fL; MCHC <30 g%)	Thalassaemia; iron deficiency anaemia; anaemia of chronic disease (rare cases)
Normocytic normochromic anaemia	Normal MCHC; normal MCV (MCV >80–99 fL; MCHC 34 g%)	Physiological anaemia of pregnancy, anaemia due to chronic disease, anaemia due to acute haemorrhage; aplastic anaemia; haemolytic anaemia

Abbreviations: MCV, mean corpuscular volume; MCHC, mean corpuscular haemoglobin concentration

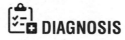

AETIOLOGY

Various causes of iron deficiency anaemia are listed in Box 14.1.

DIAGNOSIS

Clinical Presentation

With mild anaemia, the woman may present with vague complaints of ill health, fatigue and diminished capability to perform hard labour, loss of appetite, digestive upset, breathlessness, palpitation, dyspnoea on exertion, easy fatigability, fainting, light-headedness, tinnitus, exhaustion, nocturnal leg cramps, headache, paraesthesia and numbness in the extremities; oral and nasopharyngeal symptoms; pica; hair loss, etc.

General Physical Examination

❖ *Pallor*: There may be pallor in lower palpebral conjunctiva, pale nails, pale palmar surface of hands, pale tongue, lips, nail beds, etc.
❖ *Epithelial changes*: The epithelial tissues of nails, tongue, mouth, hypopharynx and stomach are affected resulting in development of nail changes (thinning, flattening and finally development of concave 'spoon-shaped nails'

Box 14.1: Causes of iron deficiency anaemia

Nutritional causes
❑ Iron deficiency anaemia (60%)
❑ Dimorphic anaemia both due to deficiency of iron and folic acid
Haemolytic anaemia
❑ Haemoglobinopathies
Anaemia due to blood loss
❑ *Acute*: Antepartum haemorrhage, postpartum haemorrhage
❑ *Chronic*: Hookworm infestation, bleeding piles and malarial infestation

or koilonychias), glossitis, angular stomatitis, atrophic gastritis, etc.

❖ *Pedal oedema*: In severe anaemic cases, there may be pedal oedema.

❖ *Abdominal examination*: Splenomegaly may occur with severe, persistent, untreated iron deficiency anaemia.

Investigations

❖ *Haemoglobin and haematocrit*: Haemoglobin is less than 11 g/dL and haematocrit is less than 0.33 g/dL.

❖ *Blood cellular indices*: Abnormalities in various blood indices with iron deficiency anaemia are described in Table 14.2.

❖ *Peripheral smear in iron deficiency anaemia*: Peripheral smear of blood shows microcytic and hypochromic (Fig. 14.1) cells. There may be anisocytosis (abnormal size of cells) in the form of microcytosis and/or poikilocytosis (abnormal shape of cells) in the form of pencil cells and

Table 14.2: Abnormalities in blood indices with iron deficiency anaemia

Blood indices	Normal values	Values in iron deficiency anaemia
MCH	26.7–33.7 pg/cell (average 30.6 pg/cell)	<26.7 pg/cell
MCHC	32–36 g% (average 33.9 g%)	<30 g%
MCV	83–97 fL (average 90 fL)	<76 fL
Haemoglobin	12.1–14.1 g/dL	<11 g/dL in first and third trimesters and less than 10.5 g/dL in second trimester
Haematocrit	36.1–44.3%	<36.1%
Red cell count	3.9–5.0 × 10^6 cells/µL or (average 4.42 × 10^6 cells/µL)	<3.9 × 10^6 cells/µL
Red cell distribution index	31–36%	<31%

Abbreviations: MCV, mean corpuscular volume; MCH, mean corpuscular haemoglobin; MCHC, mean corpuscular haemoglobin concentration

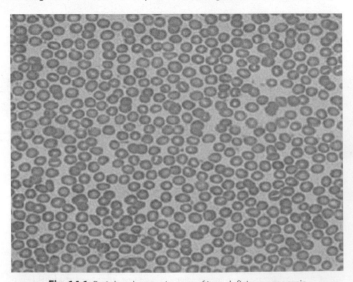

Fig. 14.1: Peripheral smear in case of iron deficiency anaemia

(For colour version, see Plate 1)

Table 14.3: Changes in serum iron studies with iron deficiency anaemia

Blood parameters	Normal values	Values in iron deficiency anaemia
Serum transferrin levels	200–360 mg/dL	>360 mg/dL
Serum iron concentration	60–175 µg/dL	<60 µg/dL
Transferrin saturation	25–60%	<25%
Ferritin levels	50–145 ng/mL	<20 ng/mL
Serum protoporphyrin	30–70 µg/dL	>70 µg/dL

target cells. There may be presence of ring or pessary cells with central hypochromia.

❖ *Osmotic fragility*: Red blood cell osmotic fragility is slightly reduced.

❖ *Serum iron studies*: Changes in the various serum iron parameters are described in Table 14.3. The diagnostic test for iron deficiency during pregnancy is the concentration of ferritin. This is not affected by pregnancy, and a concentration of less than 12 ng/mL is diagnostic.

❖ *Stool examination*: This helps in excluding out parasitic infestation as a cause of anaemia.

❖ *Urine routine or microscopy*: Urine routine or microscopy helps in detecting the presence of pus cells or occult blood or schistosomes.

❖ *Haemoglobin electrophoresis*: Haemoglobin electrophoresis and measurement of haemoglobin A2 and foetal haemoglobin are useful in establishing either β-thalassaemia or haemoglobin C or D as the aetiology of the microcytic anaemia.

❖ *Bone marrow examination*: A bone marrow aspirate stained for iron (Perl's stain) can be diagnostic of iron deficiency.

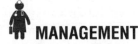

MANAGEMENT

Antenatal Period

Antenatal Visits

Full blood count should be assessed at the time of booking and then again at 28 weeks.

Dietary Changes

Eating a healthy and a well-balanced diet during pregnancy helps in maintaining the iron stores.

Iron Supplements

Treatment of the patient diagnosed with iron deficiency basically depends on the period of gestation as described in Flow chart 14.1.

Oral iron supplements: If the period of gestation is less than 30 completed weeks, oral iron supplements (containing 120–240 mg of elemental iron) must be prescribed in divided doses. In the UK, routine iron supplementation for all women during pregnancy is not recommended. According to the British

PART II

Flow chart 14.1: Treatment of iron deficiency anaemia in pregnancy

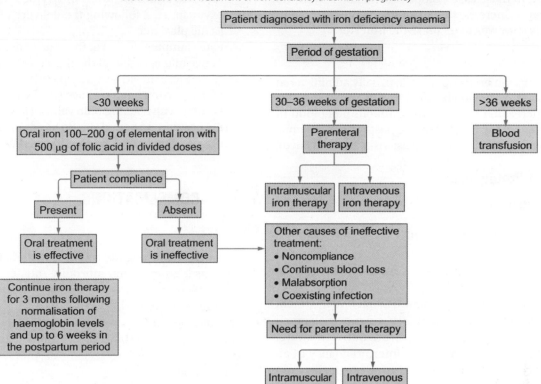

Society for Haematology (2012), oral supplements must be offered only if the ferritin levels are less than 30 µg/L.[2] Women with established iron deficiency can be prescribed elemental iron daily in the dose of 100–200 mg/day. Once haemoglobin value comes in the normal range, supplementation should continue for 3 months and until 6 weeks postpartum to replenish the iron stores.

The main problems associated with the use of oral iron supplements are occurrence of side effects including anorexia, diarrhoea, epigastric discomfort, nausea, etc. Absorption of ferrous salts is better than that of the ferric salts and is therefore preferred. In case of complications such as nausea and epigastric discomfort with a particular iron formulation, preparations with lower iron content should be tried. Slow release and enteric-coated formulations should be preferably avoided.

Parenteral iron therapy: Sometimes parenteral iron therapy (by intramuscular or intravenous routes) is started in cases where there is intolerance to oral form of iron; when iron deficiency is not correctable with oral treatment; there is non-compliance on part of the patient; the patient is unable to absorb iron orally; there are severe gastrointestinal side effects, continuous blood loss or the patient is near term. The two most commonly used parenteral iron preparations include iron sorbitol citric acid complex (Jectofer) and iron dextran (Imferon®).

Intramuscular iron: The iron preparation commonly used for intramuscular administration is iron sorbitol. It has a low-molecular-weight preparation and thus involves rapid absorption from the site of injection. This iron formulation is not suitable for IV use and is administered by a deep intramuscular injection. This may be associated with pain at the time of injection and the tattooing of the skin. The dose of iron sorbitol required for intramuscular injection is calculated based on the degree of iron deficiency and the patient's weight. Repeated injections are frequently required, which are usually administered over the course of 2 weeks.

Intravenous iron: The most common iron preparation previously used for IV administration was iron dextran. It is a slightly viscous sterile liquid complex composed of ferric hydroxide and is administered both intravenously and intra-muscularly. Iron dextran is now withdrawn from clinical practice due to high incidence of anaphylaxis. Various other IV iron preparations (e.g. ferric carboxymaltose) are available which are associated with fewer side effects in comparison to iron dextran. Newer preparations are associated with a greater and more rapid rise in haemoglobin concentration along with fewer side effects. Iron sucrose (Cosmofer) is the oldest IV iron preparation, which is being used as the first-line IV iron of choice in the treatment of patients with chronic kidney disease (whether or not on dialysis) who have iron deficiency anaemia. In some obstetric units in the UK, it is also licensed for total dose replacement in the second and third trimester. It is usually administered in form of a single infusion and takes 4–6 hours for completion.

Blood Transfusion

This may be required towards the end of pregnancy when enough time may not be available to achieve a reasonable haemoglobin level before delivery, for example, patient presents with severe anaemia beyond 36 weeks; there is acute blood loss or associated infections and anaemia is refractory to iron therapy. In these cases, blood transfusion may be the most rapid way to increase the haemoglobin concentration and a relatively slow way to increase the iron stores.

Erythropoietin

Recombinant human erythropoietin is usually administered in cases of anaemia due to chronic renal failure. It can also be used for increasing autologous production of blood in normal individuals (e.g. cases of severe postpartum anaemia, Jehovah's witnesses where blood transfusion has been declined).

Prevention or Prophylaxis

The following steps can be taken for the prevention of iron deficiency:

❖ *Dietary advice*: Iron deficiency (in the absence of an on-going blood loss) can be prevented with a well-balanced diet rich in iron. Appropriate nutritional advice can be provided by a midwife.

❖ *Treatment of iron deficiency*: Identification and treatment of iron deficiency prior to pregnancy can prevent women from becoming pregnant in an iron-deficient state. Nevertheless, many women may enter pregnancy in an iron-deficient state or become so during pregnancy. Iron supplementation during pregnancy is likely to prevent this. Presently, there is not enough data to evaluate that the routine supplementation with iron alone or in combination with folic acid has substantial benefit or adverse effects on maternal and foetal health.[3] Nevertheless, the meta-analysis by Reveiz et al. (2011), which evaluated 23 trials, involving 3,198 women concluded that there was a clear evidence of improvement in haematological indices in women who received iron supplementation during pregnancy.[4]

Intrapartum Period

Patients with anaemia should be preferably delivered in a hospital. According to the British Society for Haematology (2011), the suggested cut-off of haemoglobin for hospitalised delivery is less than 100 g/L and less than 95 g/L for delivery in an obstetrician-led unit.[2]

❖ *First stage of labour*: The following need to be done:
  • Patient's blood grouping and cross-matching
  • Venous access must be available
  • Adequate pain relief must be provided
  • Oxygen inhalation through face mask must be provided
  • Digitalisation may be required, especially if the patient shows a potential to develop congestive heart failure
  • Antibiotic prophylaxis must be given as the anaemic women are prone to develop infections.

❖ *Second stage of labour*: In order to shorten the duration of second stage of labour, forceps or vacuum can be applied prophylactically.

❖ *At the time of delivery*: The precautions that must be taken during the time of delivery in order to reduce the amount of blood loss are described next.

• Routine administration of oxytocic (Methergine®, oxytocin, etc.) following the delivery of baby, as well as the placenta
• Late clamping of cord at the time of delivery
• Active management of the third stage of labour
• Obstetrician must be well prepared for the management of postpartum haemorrhage (PPH) in these cases.
• Women with haemoglobin value of less than 100 g/L in the postpartum period should be administered 100–200 mg elemental iron for 3 months post-delivery.

COMPLICATIONS

Maternal

❖ *Throughout the pregnancy*: These include complications such as high maternal mortality rate, cerebral anoxia, cardiac failure, increased susceptibility to develop infection, abortions, preterm labour, etc.

❖ *During antenatal period*: Poor weight gain, preterm labour, pregnancy-induced hypertension (PIH), placenta praevia, accidental haemorrhage, eclampsia, premature rupture of membranes, etc.

❖ *During intranatal period*: Dysfunctional labour, intranatal haemorrhage, shock, anaesthesia risk, cardiac failure, etc.

❖ *During postnatal period*: Postnatal sepsis, subinvolution, and embolism.

Foetal

❖ Preterm birth, low-birthweight and intrauterine growth restricted babies
❖ Foetal distress and neonatal distress requiring prolonged resuscitation
❖ Impaired neurological and mental development
❖ Tendency of the infants to develop conditions, such as iron deficiency anaemia, failure to thrive, poor intellectual development, delayed milestones and other morbidities later in life.

CLINICAL PEARLS

❖ Out of the various blood indices used, mean corpuscular volume (MCV) and mean corpuscular haemoglobin (MCH) concentration are the two most sensitive indices of iron deficiency.
❖ The earliest haematological response to treatment is reticulocytosis.
❖ The WHO recommends universal iron supplementation comprising of 60 mg elemental iron and 400 µg of folic acid once or twice daily for 6 months in pregnancy, in countries with prevalence of anaemia less than 40% and an additional 3 months postpartum in countries where prevalence is greater than 40%.[1]

PART II

EVIDENCE-BASED MEDICINE

❖ In the UK, treatment of choice for iron deficiency anaemia during pregnancy is oral therapy with ferrous salts.[2] Present evidence indicates that administration of IV iron is most effective in improving the haematological indices. This is followed by the intramuscular administration. Oral therapy is least effective in improving the haematological indices. The mode of administration of iron therapy needs to be decided by balancing the efficacy of therapy against the invasiveness of the procedure and the possible adverse effects, which are the mildest with oral supplementation and most severe with IV route. With parenteral therapy, there are concerns about possible important adverse effects, e.g. venous thrombosis and allergic reactions (with IV treatment) and side effects such as pain, discolouration and allergic reactions (with intramuscular treatment).

❖ Vitamin C helps in the absorption of iron, but presently there is no evidence to support the use of combined preparations.[2]

❖ There is no evidence against the policy of routine iron supplementation in pregnancy.[3,4]

MEGALOBLASTIC ANAEMIA

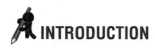

INTRODUCTION

Megaloblastic anaemia is characterised by the presence of megaloblasts, which are large cells having an increased nuclear to cytoplasmic ratio with delayed nuclear maturation and more advanced cytoplasmic maturation. There is a defect in DNA synthesis amongst the rapidly dividing cells. RNA and protein synthesis are also impaired to a certain extent. This results from the production of abnormal precursors called megaloblasts in the bone marrow.[5]

AETIOLOGY

❖ *Isolated deficiency of vitamin B_{12} or folate*: Isolated deficiency of folate is the commonest cause of megaloblastic anaemia during pregnancy. There is a significant increase in folate requirements during pregnancy due to increased red cell replication in the foetus, uterus and bone marrow. Plasma folate concentration decreases throughout pregnancy reaching almost half the non-pregnancy levels by term. The incidence of folate deficiency is higher amongst individuals with multiple pregnancies. In many parts of the world, the deficiency of folate is likely to be due to poor diet. In the UK, many food products have folate supplements added to them due to which it is easier to achieve the daily recommended requirement of 800 µg.

Isolated deficiency of vitamin B_{12} is extremely uncommon during pregnancy because its deficiency in the reproductive age groups is often associated with infertility. Absorption of vitamin B_{12} remains unchanged during pregnancy and it is actively transported across the placenta to the foetus.[6] All diets containing animal products are likely to supply enough B_{12} during pregnancy. Deficiency can develop in strict vegetarians.

❖ *Combined deficiency of both vitamin B_{12} and folate*: Chronic tropical sprue can cause deficiency of both folate and vitamin B_{12} in pregnancy resulting in megaloblastic anaemia.

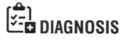

DIAGNOSIS

Clinical Presentation

These are same as those described in the section of iron deficiency anaemia. Some symptoms specific to megaloblastic anaemia include memory loss, depression, personality changes, psychosis, peripheral neuropathy, etc.

General Physical Examination

❖ Pallor
❖ Ulceration in mouth (glossitis) and tongue
❖ Haemorrhagic patches under the skin and conjunctiva
❖ Enlarged liver and spleen.

Investigations

❖ *Complete blood count, haemoglobin and haematocrit*: Haemoglobin is less than 11 g/dL and haematocrit is less than 0.33 g/dL. There may be associated leucopenia and thrombocytopenia.

❖ *Peripheral smear*: This may reveal the presence of macrocytes and megaloblasts; hypersegmentation of neutrophils (showing five lobes or more) (Fig. 14.2); fully haemoglobinised RBCs and Howell-Jolly bodies.

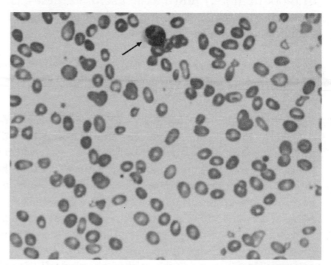

Fig. 14.2: Peripheral smear in case of megaloblastic anaemia (the arrow points towards hypersegmented neutrophil) *(For colour version, see Plate 1)*

❖ *Blood indices*: Mean corpuscular volume and MCH are both increased to values greater than 100 mm³ and 33 pg respectively.

❖ *Serum iron studies*: Serum iron is normal or high, and iron binding capacity is low.

❖ *Serum folate and B₁₂ levels*: Serum folate levels may be less than 3 ng/mL, and B₁₂ levels less than 90 pg/mL.

❖ *Bone marrow studies*: Examination of bone marrow may show megaloblastic erythropoiesis.

MANAGEMENT

❖ Prescription of diet rich in folic acid

❖ *Folate supplements*: This should be in the form of daily administration of folic acid in the dosage of 4 mg orally, continued until 4 weeks following delivery.[7,8]

❖ In case of B₁₂ deficiency, intramuscular injections of vitamin B₁₂ in the dosage of 100 μg daily can be given.

COMPLICATIONS

These are similar to those described previously in the segment of iron deficiency anaemia. Some complications specific to megaloblastic anaemia include abortion, IUGR, prematurity, abruptio placentae, foetal malformations (cleft lip, neural tube defects, etc.).

CLINICAL PEARLS

❖ In cases of severe folate deficiency, 5 mg of oral polyglutamic acid daily or parenteral folate may be administered.

❖ Red cell indices are usually not very useful for diagnosis of megaloblastic anaemia during pregnancy due to the presence of co-existing iron deficiency. Examination of blood film may prove to be useful in these cases. However, the diagnosis during pregnancy often requires examination of the bone aspirate.

EVIDENCE-BASED MEDICINE

❖ Periconceptual folate deficiency can cause serious neural tube defects and other developmental anomalies. Due to this, it is presently advised that all women planning pregnancy must be administered folic acid daily in the dose of 400 μg per day, 1 month prior to conception and continue taking this until first 12 weeks of gestation.[7,8]

❖ Other situations where routine prophylaxis with folic acid may be required throughout pregnancy include women taking anticonvulsant drugs and those with haemolytic anaemia. In these cases, the routine prophylactic dose is 5 mg/day throughout pregnancy.[7]

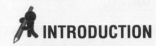

THALASSAEMIAS IN PREGNANCY

INTRODUCTION

Haemoglobinopathies are one of the most common inherited disorders and are associated with an abnormality in one of the globin chains of haemoglobin molecule. They are commonly autosomal recessive disorders. Haemoglobinopathies commonly encountered in clinical practice include thalassaemia and sickle cell syndromes. Thalassaemia is a genetic defect caused by quantitative defect in the production of globin chains. Each year, more than 70,000 babies are born with thalassaemia worldwide.[9] On the other hand, sickle cell syndrome is associated with a qualitative defect of the globin gene. As a result, the structure of the globin chain is abnormal rather than its production.

AETIOLOGY

The thalassaemia syndromes are characterised by a basic defect in the synthesis of globin chains. As a result, there is inadequate haemoglobin content in the resultant red cells. Since damaged red cells are released into the peripheral circulation due to ineffective erythropoiesis, there occurs extravascular haemolysis.[10]

Each haemoglobin molecule has two pairs of globin chains. Haemoglobin A (the most abundant human haemoglobin) has one pair of α-globin chain and one pair of β-globin chain. Production of α-globin chain is under the control of four genes, two inherited from the mother and two from the father. On the other hand, production of β-globin chain is under the control of two genes, one inherited from the father and the other inherited from the mother.

Reduced production of β chains result in β-thalassaemia whereas reduced production of α chains results in α-thalassaemia. Both the thalassaemia disorders can be of different types depending on the number of genes affected.

In case of α-thalassaemia, various types of disorders, which can result depending upon the number of genes affected, are listed in Table 14.4.

In case of β-thalassaemia, one defective β-globin gene (from either parent) results in β-thalassaemia minor. This heterozygous state, also known as β-thalassaemia trait causes mild to moderate microcytic anaemia with no significant detrimental effect on overall health. On the other hand, β-thalassaemia major (homozygous β-thalassaemia) results from the inheritance of a defective β-globin gene from each parent. This results in a severe transfusion-dependent anaemia. Thalassaemia major (homozygous β thalassaemia) results from the inheritance of a defective β globin gene from each parent. This results in a severe transfusion-dependent anaemia.

PART II

Table 14.4: Various types of disorders, which can result depending upon the number of α-globin genes affected

No. of affected genes	Type of α-thalassaemia disorder
Four defective α-globin genes	Hb Bart's hydrops (incompatible with survival). Foetuses with this condition die either in utero or shortly after birth because of severe anaemia
Three defective α-globin genes (two defective genes from one parent and one defective gene from the other parent)	Haemoglobin H disease (causing moderate haemolytic anaemia)
Two defective α-globin genes	• α-thalassaemia⁺ trait (one defective gene from each parent) • α-thalassaemia⁰ trait (both defective genes from one parent)
One defective α-globin genes	α-thalassaemia⁺ trait or α-thalassaemia minima or α (+) thalassaemia minor

Table 14.5: Symptoms associated with the various types of α-thalassaemia disorders

Types of α-thalassaemia disorders	Clinical features
Four defective α-globin genes (Hb Bart's hydrops)	This condition is incompatible with extra uterine life. Foetuses with this condition die either in utero or shortly after birth due to severe anaemia
Three defective α-globin genes (Haemoglobin H disease)	Such patients have severe anaemia and a defect in the oxygen-carrying capacity. Erythroid hyperplasia can result in typical structural bone abnormalities with marrow hyperplasia, bone thinning, maxillary hyperplasia, and pathologic fractures
Two defective α-globin genes: • α-thalassaemia⁺ trait (one defective gene from each parent) • α-thalassaemia⁰ trait (both defective genes from one parent)	The affected individuals are clinically normal but frequently have minimal anaemia and reduced MCV and MCH. RBC count is usually increased, typically exceeding 5.5×10^{12}/L
One defective α-globin genes α-thalassaemia⁺ trait or α-thalassaemia minima or α (+) thalassaemia minor or silent carrier	The affected individuals exhibit no clinical abnormalities and may be haematologically normal or have mild reductions in RBC, MCV and MCH

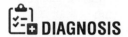

DIAGNOSIS

Clinical Presentation

Individuals with a carrier status (β-thalassaemia trait) are usually asymptomatic or may have mild or moderate symptoms related to anaemia. This anaemia may resemble iron deficiency anaemia. On the other hand, patients with β-thalassaemia major have a major illness. They may have severe anaemia, which may only respond to blood transfusion. Anaemia begins to develop within the first 2 months after birth. It becomes progressively more and more severe. It may be associated with symptoms such as failure to thrive, problems with feeding due to easy fatigability, bouts of fever, diarrhoea and other intestinal problems, etc. Multiple blood transfusions are likely to cause iron overload. This may result in hepatic, cardiac and endocrine dysfunction. Since the anterior pituitary is quite sensitive to iron overload, evidence of dysfunction is commonly observed. Symptoms associated with the various types of α-thalassaemia disorders are listed in Table 14.5.

Investigations

Since many people who are the salient carriers of the condition are likely to be completely unaware of the condition, neonatal screening has now been incorporated into universal spot screening because early diagnosis and prophylactic treatment is likely to cause a significant reduction in the disease-related mortality and morbidity.[11] Screening for thalassaemia is by examining the red cell indices and measurement of the HbA₂ levels. Thalassaemia traits are associated with a reduced MCV, reduced MCH and a normal to near normal MCHC. Of all these various markers, the most accurate marker is the MCH. Additionally, β-thalassaemia is associated with elevated HbA₂ levels (>3.5 g%). In α-thalassaemia trait, the changes may be minimal. DNA analysis may be required in these cases to confirm the diagnosis.

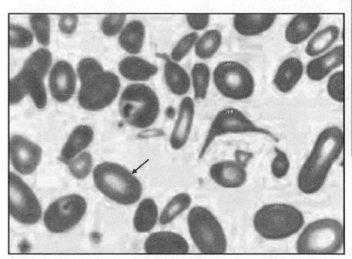

Fig. 14.3: Peripheral smear in case of thalassaemia
(Target cell is indicated by the arrow) *(For colour version, see Plate 1)*

Peripheral Smear

Peripheral smear in case of thalassaemia is shown in Figure 14.3. In thalassaemia, there is presence of polychromatic, stippled and target cells.

Screening and Counselling Prepregnancy

If a woman is found to be carrier of a particular haemoglobinopathy, the partner needs to be screened as soon as possible. If there is a risk of the foetus having a major haemoglobinopathy, urgent expert counselling must be provided to the couple to enable them to make an informed choice regarding the prenatal diagnosis and termination of pregnancy. Ideally, this screening must be done prior to conception.

MANAGEMENT

Women with unknown haemoglobinopathy status with a normocytic or microcytic anaemia, should start a trial of oral iron and haemoglobinopathy screening should be commenced without delay in accordance with the National Health Service (NHS) sickle cell and thalassaemia screening programme.

Periconceptional Care

❖ The mainstay of modern treatment in cases of β-thalassaemia is blood transfusion and iron chelation therapy.[12]

❖ *Iron chelation therapy*: Aggressive chelation in the preconception stage can reduce and optimise the body iron burden, thereby reducing the end-organ damage, particularly diabetes and cardiomyopathy.[13-17] Due to lack of safety data, all chelation therapy should be regarded as potentially teratogenic in the first trimester. Desferrioxamine is the only chelating agent which can be used in the second and third trimester. Iron chelators such as deferasirox and deferiprone must be ideally discontinued 3 months before conception and women converted to desferrioxamine iron chelation. Desferrioxamine has a short half-life and is safe for infusion during ovulation induction therapy. Desferrioxamine, however, should be avoided in the first trimester owing to lack of safety data. It has been used safely after 20 weeks of gestation at low doses.[18] All bisphosphonates are contraindicated in pregnancy and should ideally be discontinued 3 months prior to conception.

❖ *Glycaemic control*: Diabetes is common in women with thalassaemia. Women with diabetes should be referred to a diabetologist. Good glycaemic control is essential in the prepregnancy period. Women with established diabetes mellitus should preferably have serum fructosamine concentrations less than 300 nmol/L for at least 3 months prior to conception. This is equivalent to an HbA1c of 43 mmol/mol.

❖ *Thyroid function tests*: Since hypothyroidism is frequently found in patients with thalassaemia, thyroid function should be determined to ensure that the woman is in the euthyroid state prepregnancy. Untreated hypothyroidism can result in an increased maternal morbidity, as well as perinatal morbidity and mortality.

❖ *Cardiovascular assessment*: All women should be assessed by a cardiologist prior to conception. An echocardiogram, electrocardiogram and T2 star (T2*) cardiac MRI must be preferably performed.

❖ *Liver iron concentration assessment*: Women should be assessed for liver iron concentration using a FerriScan®. Ideally, the liver iron should be less than 7 mg/g [dry weight (dw)]. Ultrasound of liver and gall bladder (and spleen if present) should be performed to detect cholelithiasis and evidence of liver cirrhosis due to iron overload or transfusion-related viral hepatitis.

❖ *Bone density scan*: Osteoporosis is a common finding in adults with thalassaemia. This could be related to a variety of factors including underlying thalassaemic bone disease, chelation of calcium by chelation drugs, hypogonadism and vitamin D deficiency. Therefore, all women should be offered a bone density scan prepregnancy to assess pre-existing osteoporosis. The woman may be prescribed vitamin D supplements if required.

❖ *Red cell antibodies*: Alloimmunity occurs in nearly 16.5% of individuals with thalassaemia. Therefore, ABO and complete blood group genotype and antibody titres should be measured in women with thalassaemia during the prepregnancy period. Red cell antibodies may indicate a risk of haemolytic disease of the foetus and newborn. Moreover, if antibodies are present, there may be challenges in obtaining suitable blood for transfusion.

❖ *Immunisation and antibiotic prophylaxis*: Hepatitis B vaccination is recommended in HBsAg negative women who are transfused or may be transfused. Hepatitis C status should be determined. All women who have undergone a splenectomy should be given penicillin prophylaxis or equivalent. All women who have undergone a splenectomy should be vaccinated for pneumococcus and *Haemophilus influenzae* type b if this has not been done previously.

❖ *Folic acid supplementation*: Folic acid in the dosage of 5 mg/day is recommended preconceptually to all women to prevent neural tube defects. This should be commenced at least 3 months prior to conception.

Antenatal Care

❖ *Multidisciplinary team approach*: Women with thalassaemia are best cared for in a multidisciplinary team setting, including an obstetrician with expertise in managing high-risk pregnancies and a haematologist. This team should provide prepregnancy counselling so that the woman is fully informed about the effect of thalassaemia on pregnancy and vice versa. This team should also provide routine as well as specialist antenatal care. The initial antenatal assessment should include optimisation of thalassaemia management and screening for end-organ damage. The pattern of care should be individualised depending on the degree of end-organ damage.

❖ *Antenatal assessment*: Women with thalassaemia should be reviewed on a monthly basis until 28 weeks of gestation and fortnightly thereafter.

❖ *Diabetic assessment*: Women with both thalassaemia and diabetes should have monthly assessment of serum fructosamine concentrations. They should be regularly reviewed in the specialist diabetic pregnancy clinic.

❖ *Cardiac assessment*: All women with thalassaemia major should undergo specialist cardiac assessment at 28 weeks of gestation and thereafter as appropriate.

PART II

❖ *Thyroid function test*: Thyroid function should be monitored regularly during pregnancy in hypothyroid patients.

❖ *Ultrasound scanning*: Women with thalassaemia often require fertility treatment with ovulation induction to achieve pregnancy. Such women, therefore, should be offered an early scan at 7–9 weeks of gestation to determine viability as well as the presence of a multiple pregnancy. In addition to the routine first trimester scan (11–14 weeks of gestation) and a detailed anomaly scan at 18–20^{+6} weeks of gestation, women should be offered serial foetal biometry scans at every 4-week interval from 24 weeks of gestation due to an increased risk of foetal growth restriction (FGR). Women with both thalassaemia and diabetes are also at an increased risk of early pregnancy loss.

❖ *Transfusion regimen*: All women with thalassaemia major should receive blood transfusions on a regular basis aiming for pretransfusion haemoglobin levels of 100 g/L. Initially, a 2–3 unit transfusion should be administered. Additional top-up transfusion, if required, may be administered the following week until the haemoglobin reaches 120 g/L. The haemoglobin levels should be monitored at every 2–3-week intervals and a 2-unit transfusion is administered if the haemoglobin has fallen below 100 g/L.

❖ *Oral iron therapy*: Women with known haemoglobinopathy should have serum ferritin levels checked and offered oral iron supplements if their ferritin level is less than 30 μg/L. Parenteral iron must never be prescribed in these cases.

❖ *Folic acid supplementation*: Individuals with thalassaemia must be prescribed folic acid in the dosage of 5 mg/day.

Intrapartum Care

❖ Timing of delivery should be in line with national guidance.

❖ Senior midwifery, obstetric, anaesthetic and haematology staff should be informed as soon as the woman is admitted to the delivery suite.

❖ In the presence of red cell antibodies, blood should be cross-matched for delivery in advance since this may delay the availability of blood.

❖ In women with thalassaemia major, IV desferrioxamine in the dosage of 2 g over 24 hours should be administered for the duration of labour.

❖ Continuous intrapartum electronic foetal monitoring should be instituted.

❖ Thalassaemia in itself is not an indication for caesarean section. Caesarean delivery is required in case of obstetric indication.

Postpartum Care

❖ Active management of the third stage of labour is recommended to minimise the amount of blood loss.

❖ Women with thalassaemia should be considered at high risk for venous thromboembolism due to the presence of abnormal red cells in the circulation. Such women should receive low-molecular-weight heparin prophylaxis in the postpartum period while in hospital.[19-21] Additionally, low-molecular-weight heparin should be administered for 7 days post-discharge following vaginal delivery or for 6 weeks following caesarean section.[21]

❖ *Breastfeeding*: Breastfeeding is safe and should be encouraged. In women with thalassaemia major, desferrioxamine should be restarted in the postpartum period as soon as the initial 24-hour infusion of IV desferrioxamine finishes. Though desferrioxamine is secreted in breast milk, it is not orally absorbed and therefore not harmful to the newborn. Presently, minimal safety data is available regarding the use of other iron chelators at the time of breastfeeding.

❖ *Contraception*: There is no contraindication to the use of hormonal methods of contraception such as the combined oral contraceptive pill, the progestogen-only pill, hormonal implants and the Mirena® intrauterine system in women with thalassaemia.[22]

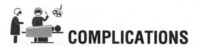

COMPLICATIONS

Thalassaemia is associated with an increased risk to both mother and baby.

Maternal

In particular, there are the issues surrounding cardiomyopathy in the mother due to iron overload. Women with thalassaemia major may also develop new endocrinopathies, mainly, diabetes mellitus, hypothyroidism and hypoparathyroidism due to the increasing iron burden. In case of Hb Bart's hydrops, maternal complications may include early-onset severe pre-eclampsia. Intrapartum problems could be related to the delivery of a grossly hydropic foetus and placenta. Primary PPH is a common occurrence post-delivery.

Foetal

The foetus may be at an increased risk of FGR.

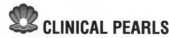

CLINICAL PEARLS

❖ Thalassaemias are inherited disorders of haemoglobin synthesis.

❖ Pregnancy was previously rare in cases of transfusion-dependent β-thalassaemia major. However, nowadays with aggressive iron chelation therapy, the rate of pregnancy in women with thalassaemia major is increasing.

❖ In all cases of β-thalassaemia major, iron overload is a major concern, particularly in terms of cardiac dys-function.

EVIDENCE-BASED MEDICINE

❖ Screening is by examining the red cell indices and the measurement of HbA$_2$ levels. In the individuals with thalassaemia trait, there is reduced MCV, reduced MCH and a normal or a near normal MCHC levels.[11]

❖ The present evidence indicates that optimising body iron in cases of thalassaemias is likely to reduce the end-organ damage, thereby reducing the incidence of endo-crinopathies or cardiac problems.[13-17]

SICKLE CELL ANAEMIA

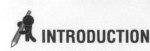

INTRODUCTION

Sickle cell disease (SCD) is a group of genetic single-gene autosomal recessive disorders caused by the 'sickle' gene, which affects haemoglobin structure. This includes sickle cell anaemia (HbSS) and the heterozygous conditions of haemoglobin S and other clinically abnormal haemoglobins, e.g. combination with haemoglobin C (giving HbSC); combination with β-thalassaemia (giving HbSB thalassaemia) and combination with haemoglobin D, E or O-Arab. All of these genotypes will result in a nearly similar clinical phenotype of varying severity. Sickle cell trait (HbAS) is more common than the homozygous condition (HbSS).

Sickle cell disease is most prevalent in individuals of African descent as well as in the Caribbean, Middle East, parts of India, the Mediterranean, and South and Central America. Therefore, this disease is typically prevalent amongst the immigrant population in the UK.[23-26]

AETIOLOGY

Sickle cell disease is characterised by an abnormality in the structure of globin chain rather than its production. The most common and clinically most important form is HbS, where there is a single amino acid substitution (from glutamic acid to valine) in the β-globin chain. This makes the haemoglobin molecule unstable in the deoxygenated state. This results in the polymerisation of the abnormal haemoglobin in low-oxygen conditions, leading to the formation of rigid and fragile sickle-shaped red cells. These cells are liable to an increased breakdown, which causes haemolytic anaemia, and vaso-occlusion in the small blood vessels. These are responsible for most of the complications of SCD, including acute painful crises, stroke, pulmonary hypertension, renal dysfunction, retinal disease, leg ulcers, cholelithiasis and avascular necrosis (which commonly affects the femoral head and may necessitate hip replacement). Though previously SCD was associated with a high rate of early mortality, nowadays majority of children born with SCD in the UK have an average life expectancy of about mid-50s. Thus, the women with SCD are likely to live till the reproductive age group and, conceive and become pregnant.

Box 14.2: Clinical features of sickle cell syndrome

❑ Chronic haemolytic anaemia
❑ Painful crisis
❑ Hyposplenism
❑ Increased risk of infection
❑ Avascular bone necrosis
❑ Increased risk of cerebrovascular accident

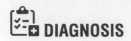

DIAGNOSIS

Clinical Presentation

Clinical features of sickle cell syndrome are enumerated in Box 14.2.

Investigations

The following tests should be performed for the assessment of chronic disease complications in the pregnant patient during preconceptual period:[27]

❖ *Screening for pulmonary hypertension with echocardiography*: The incidence of pulmonary hypertension is increased in patients with SCD and is associated with an increased mortality. A tricuspid regurgitant jet velocity of more than 2.5 m/s across the tricuspid valve is associated with a high risk of pulmonary hypertension.

❖ *Screening for pre-eclampsia*: Measurement of blood pressure and urinalysis (for proteinuria) should be performed to identify women with pre-eclampsia. Renal and liver function tests should be performed annually to identify sickle nephropathy and/or deranged hepatic function.

❖ *Retinal screening*: Proliferative retinopathy is common in patients with SCD, especially patients with HbSC, and can lead to loss of vision.

❖ *Screening for iron overload*: In women who have been transfused several times in the past or those who have a high ferritin level, T2* cardiac magnetic resonance imaging must be performed to assess body iron load. Aggressive iron chelation before conception is advisable in women with significant iron overload.

❖ *Screening for red cell antibodies*: Presence of red cell antibodies may indicate an increased risk of haemolytic disease of the newborn.

Neonatal Disease Screening

Screening for sickle cell variants in the neonates in the intrapartum period is carried out by high performance liquid chromatography or electrophoresis.[28]

Peripheral Smear

Peripheral smear in case of sickle cell anaemia shows presence of crescent-shaped target cells. There may be presence of characteristic sickle-shaped cells (Fig. 14.4). If the person is asplenic, there may be presence of RBCs containing nuclear material (Howell-Jolly bodies).

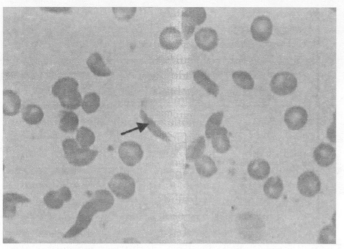

Fig. 14.4: Peripheral smear in case of sickle cell anaemia (Arrow indicates sickle-shaped cell) *(For colour version, see Plate 1)*

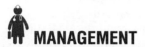

MANAGEMENT

Preconceptual Care

It is usual to diagnose SCD during pregnancy because a vast majority of infected individuals are aware of the diagnosis right from the childhood. Milder forms of the disease (e.g. HbSC) may be diagnosed for the first time during pregnancy or just prior to conception.

❖ *Prepregnancy counselling*: Women with SCD should be seen preconceptually by a sickle specialist for optimisation of management and screening for end-organ damage. Primary care physicians have a significant role in preconceptual screening, including the provision of contraceptive advice. Women with SCD should not only receive the general preconceptual care, which is provided to all women but also additional advice related to vaccinations, medications and avoidance of sickling crisis. She should be counselled regarding the role of dehydration, cold, hypoxia, overexertion and stress in precipitating the sickle cell crises. She should also be advised regarding the risk of worsening anaemia, the increased risk of sickling crises, acute chest syndrome (ACS), and the risk of increased infection (especially urinary tract infection) during pregnancy.

❖ *Genetic screening*: Haemoglobinopathy status of the partners of men and women with SCD should be determined before they get on with their pregnancy. If a partner is identified as a carrier of, or affected by, a major haemoglobinopathy, as per National Screening Committee Guidance, they should receive counselling and advice regarding reproductive options. Sperm donors should also be screened for haemoglobinopathies for couples considering in vitro fertilisation.

❖ *Supplementation with folic acid*: Folic acid in the dosage of 5 mg daily should be prescribed both preconceptually and throughout pregnancy. This is required because haemolytic anaemia in these patients is likely to put them at increased risk of folate deficiency.

❖ *Hydroxycarbamide*: The drug hydroxycarbamide has been demonstrated to decrease the incidence of complications such as acute painful crises and ACS in individuals with SCD. Hydroxycarbamide (hydroxyurea) should be stopped at least 3 months before conception in lieu of its teratogenic effects. If the woman conceives while taking this drug, it should be stopped and a level 3 ultrasound performed to look for any structural abnormality. Surgical termination of pregnancy is not indicated based on exposure to hydroxycarbamide alone.

❖ *Angiotensin-converting enzyme inhibitors and angiotensin receptor blockers*: Renal dysfunction, proteinuria and micro albuminuria are common in patients with SCD. Drugs such as angiotensin-converting enzyme inhibitors or angiotensin receptor blockers are routinely used in patients with SCD with significant proteinuria (protein-creatinine ratio of more than 50 mg/mmol). These drugs should be stopped before conception.

Antenatal Period

❖ *Multidisciplinary team approach*: Antenatal care should be provided by a multidisciplinary team including an obstetrician and midwife with experience of high-risk antenatal care and a haematologist with an interest in SCD. Women with SCD should undergo medical review by the haematologist and be screened for end-organ damage in the antenatal period in case this has not been undertaken preconceptually.

❖ *Vaccination*: The influenza vaccine should be recommended if it has not been administered in the previous year. Live attenuated vaccines should be deferred until after delivery. Additionally, women should be given *H. influenza* type b and the conjugated meningococcal C vaccine as a single dose if they have not received it as part of primary vaccination. The pneumococcal vaccine (Pneumovax®) should be administered at every 5-year interval.[29] Hepatitis B vaccination is also recommended and the woman's immune status should be determined preconceptually. Women with SCD should be advised to receive the influenza and 'swine flu' vaccine annually. Penicillin prophylaxis and vaccinations, which are usually monitored and administered in primary care during the non-pregnant state, should be reviewed by the specialist haematologist or obstetrician during pregnancy.

❖ *Antenatal haemoglobinopathy screening*: If the woman has not been seen preconceptually, she should be offered partner testing. If the partner is a carrier, appropriate counselling should be offered as early as possible in pregnancy. This should be ideally performed by 10 weeks of gestation so that the woman can be offered the option of first trimester diagnosis and surgical termination of pregnancy if the woman so desires.

❖ *Medications*: If women have not undergone a preconceptual review, they should be advised to take daily folic acid and prophylactic antibiotics (if not contraindicated). Drugs that are unsafe in pregnancy (as described before in the text) should be stopped immediately. Iron supplementation should be given only if there is laboratory evidence of iron deficiency. Low-dose aspirin in the dosage of 75 mg once daily must be prescribed from 12 weeks of gestation in order to reduce the risk for development of pre-eclampsia. Women with SCD should be advised to receive prophylactic low-molecular-weight heparin during antenatal hospital admissions. Non-steroidal anti-inflammatory drugs should be prescribed only between 12 weeks to 28 weeks of gestation due to concerns regarding adverse effects on foetal development.

❖ *Monitoring for pre-eclampsia*: Blood pressure and urinalysis should be performed during each consultation. Midstream urine for culture and sensitivity must be performed on monthly basis to rule out infection.

❖ *Ultrasound scanning*: Women should be offered a viability scan at 7–9 weeks of gestation. Women should be offered the routine first trimester scan (11–14 weeks of gestation) and a detailed anomaly scan at 20 weeks of gestation. In addition, women should be offered serial foetal biometry scans every 4 weeks from 24 weeks of gestation.

❖ *Prophylactic transfusion*: Routine prophylactic transfusion is not recommended during pregnancy for women with SCD. Top-up transfusion is indicated for women with acute anaemia.

❖ *Management of iron overload*: Ferritin levels must be checked and if found to be elevated or if there is a previous history of iron overload, the woman must be offered the following investigations: echocardiography or cardiac assessment (to rule out cardiomyopathy); and regular assessment of renal and hepatic functions.

❖ *Folic acid supplementation*: Folic acid in the dose of 5 mg per day must be administered throughout the pregnancy. Levels of Hb and HbS must also be regularly assessed.

❖ *Alloimmunisation*: Alloimmunisation (the formation of antibodies to red cell antigens) is common in SCD and can occur in approximately 18–36% of patients. Alloimmunisation is clinically important as it can lead to delayed haemolytic transfusion reactions or haemolytic disease of the newborn and can render the patients untransfusable. The risk of alloimmunisation is significantly reduced by giving red cells matched for the C, E and Kell antigens. This should be standard practice not only for pregnant patient but also for all patients with SCD even if they are non-pregnant.

❖ *Management of acute painful crisis*: Sickle cell crisis must be ruled out as a matter of urgency in women with SCD who become unwell. The pregnant women presenting with acute painful crisis must be promptly evaluated by the multidisciplinary team and appropriate analgesia should be administered. Primary care physicians should have a low threshold for referring women to secondary care. All women, in whom the pain does not settle with simple analgesic drugs, women who are febrile, have atypical pain or chest pain or symptoms of shortness of breath should be urgently referred to hospital. The management of pain must be done using the WHO analgesic ladder, starting with paracetamol, rest and oral fluids for mild pain. NSAIDs can be used for mild to moderate pain between 12 weeks to 28 weeks of gestation. Weak opioids such as co-dydramol, co-codamol or dihydrocodeine can be used for moderate pain, and stronger opiates such as morphine can be used for severe pain. Morphine or diamorphine can be administered by the oral, subcutaneous, intramuscular or IV route depending on the woman's preference and local expertise. Parenteral opiates can be given by intermittent bolus or patient-controlled administration systems. Opiates are not associated with teratogenicity or congenital malformation but may be associated with transient suppression of foetal movement and a reduced baseline variability of the foetal heart rate. Where a mother has received prolonged administration of opiates in late pregnancy, the neonate should be observed for signs of opioid withdrawal. Pethidine should be avoided because of the risk of toxicity and pethidine-associated seizures in patients with SCD. Outlines for the management of acute pain in cases of SCD are described in Box 14.3.[30] Thromboprophylaxis should also be provided to women with SCD who are admitted to hospital with painful crises.

❖ *Fluid intake*: Fluid intake of at least 60 mL/kg/24 h should be ensured. This can be administered either orally or intravenously if the woman is not able to accept adequate fluids orally.

❖ *Oxygen saturation*: Oxygen saturations should be monitored and facial oxygen should be prescribed if oxygen saturation falls below the woman's baseline or below 95%. The clinician should resort to intensive care therapy in early stages itself if satisfactory oxygen saturation cannot be maintained by oxygen administration through facial or nasal route.

❖ *Assessment for infection*: The woman should be assessed for infection. Therapeutic antibiotics should be prescribed if the woman is febrile or there is a high clinical suspicion of

---

Box 14.3: Outlines for the management of acute pain

❑ Quick clinical assessment
❑ In case of mild to moderate pain, rest, oral fluids and paracetamol can be administered
❑ If pain is severe and paracetamol is not effective, strong opioids (e.g. morphine) must be administered. In these cases, adjuvant non-opioid analgesic drugs can be administered, e.g. paracetamol, NSAID, etc.
❑ NSAIDs must be administered during 12–28 weeks of gestation
❑ Laxatives, antipruritics and antiemetics may be prescribed if required
❑ Initially, the patient must be monitored every 20–30 minutes for parameters such as vital signs, respiratory rate, oxygen saturation and pain. This can be later increased to either hourly or two hourly intervals based on the patient's clinical condition
❑ Rescue doses of analgesia can be administered if required
❑ If respiratory rate is less than 10/minute, maintenance analgesia must be omitted and administration of naloxone be considered
❑ Parenteral administration of analgesic drugs must be changed to oral administration after 2–3 days
❑ The woman must be discharged when pain is controlled and improving without analgesia or on acceptable doses of oral analgesia
❑ Adequate home care and outpatient follow-up appointment must be arranged

infection. White blood cell counts are often raised in cases of SCD and may not necessarily indicate infection.

❖ All patients, carers, medical and nursing staff should be aware of the other acute complications of SCD, including ACS, acute stroke and acute anaemia.

❖ *Management of ACS*: Each hospital should have a protocol in place for the management of ACS in pregnancy, including the use of transfusion therapy. Early recognition of ACS is important. ACS is characterised by the presence of respiratory symptoms such as tachypnoea, chest pain, cough and shortness of breath. There may be the presence of a new infiltrates on the chest X-ray. In these cases, pneumonia and acute severe infection with the H1N1 virus must be ruled out due to an overlap in symptoms. Similar to the non-pregnant women, treatment in these cases is with IV antibiotics, oxygen and blood transfusion.

❖ *Management of acute anaemia*: Acute anaemia in women with SCD may be caused by erythrovirus infection, which may cause a red cell maturation arrest and an aplastic crisis characterised by reticulocytopenia. Therefore, a reticulocyte count should be requested in any woman presenting with an acute anaemia. Treatment is with blood transfusion and the woman must be isolated. There is also an added risk of vertical transmission of erythrovirus infection to the foetus, resulting in hydrops foetalis. Hence, a review by a foetal medicine specialist is indicated.

Intrapartum Care

❖ Women with SCD should be advised to give birth in hospitals that are able to manage both the complications of SCD and high-risk pregnancies.

❖ The relevant multidisciplinary team (senior midwife in charge, senior obstetrician, anaesthetist and haematologist) should be informed as soon as the labour is confirmed.

❖ Vital signs must be observed on an hourly basis. Investigations must be undertaken in case the temperature is raised over 37.5°C.

❖ Women should be kept warm and adequate hydration (either through oral or IV route) be maintained during labour.

❖ There is an increased demand for oxygen during the intrapartum period. Pulse oximetry must be used to detect hypoxia in the mother during labour. Arterial blood gas analysis should be performed and oxygen therapy instituted if oxygen saturation is equal to or less than 94%.

❖ Routine antibiotic prophylaxis in labour is presently not supported by the available evidence.[31,32] The clinician should, however, have a low threshold to initiate broad-spectrum antibiotics.

❖ Blood should be cross-matched for delivery if there is a presence of atypical antibodies present because this may delay the availability of blood. Otherwise, a 'group and save' proves to be sufficient.

❖ In women who have hip replacements due to avascular necrosis, it is important to discuss suitable positions for delivery.

❖ Women with SCD should be offered anaesthetic assessment in the third trimester of pregnancy. Use of pethidine must be avoided. However, other opiates can be used. Regional analgesia is recommended for caesarean delivery. Use of general anaesthesia should be avoided.

❖ Pregnant women with SCD with a normally growing foetus should be offered elective birth through induction of labour, or by elective caesarean section (in presence of obstetric or medical indications) after 38[+0] weeks of gestation.

❖ Sickle cell disease should not in itself be considered a contraindication for attempting vaginal delivery or vaginal birth after caesarean section.

❖ Continuous intrapartum electronic foetal heart rate monitoring is recommended due to an increased risk of foetal distress, which may require an operative delivery.

Postpartum Period

❖ In pregnant women where the baby is at high risk of SCD (i.e. the partner is a carrier or affected), early testing for SCD should be offered.

❖ Maternal oxygen saturation must be maintained above 94%. Adequate hydration must also be maintained.

❖ Low-molecular-weight heparin should be administered to the patient while in hospital and 7 days post-discharge following vaginal delivery or for a period of 6 weeks following caesarean delivery.

❖ The same level of care and vigilance should be maintained as has been described for antenatal care, since acute crisis and other complications of SCD may also develop in the puerperium.

❖ *Advice related to contraception*: Progestogen-containing contraceptives such as the progesterone only pill (Cerazette®), injectable contraceptives (Depo-Provera®) and the levonorgestrel intrauterine system (Mirena®) are safe and effective in SCD. Oestrogen-containing contraceptives should be used as the second-line agents.

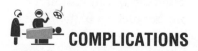

COMPLICATIONS

Maternal

An increase in the incidence of following events can occur during pregnancy:

❖ Acute painful crises
❖ Spontaneous miscarriage
❖ Antenatal hospitalisation
❖ Delivery by caesarean section
❖ Infection
❖ Thromboembolic events[27]
❖ Antepartum haemorrhage
❖ An increased risk of pre-eclampsia and PIH
❖ Peripartum cardiomyopathy
❖ Increased maternal mortality and morbidity.

Foetal

❖ An increased incidence of perinatal mortality
❖ Premature babies
❖ Foetal growth restriction
❖ Foetal distress (which may necessitate induction of labour or operative delivery).

 CLINICAL PEARLS

❖ Prepregnancy counselling remains the gold standard in cases of SCD. However, if that is not possible, further screening and counselling regarding the prenatal diagnosis is required.
❖ Folic acid supplementation (in the dosage of 5 mg/day) and penicillin prophylaxis should be continued for the duration of pregnancy.

 EVIDENCE-BASED MEDICINE

❖ Universal antenatal and neonatal screening for the inherited haemoglobinopathies is being considered because selective screening is not effective.[28]
❖ Neonatal screening for inherited haemoglobinopathies reduces morbidity and mortality by early diagnosis and prompt treatment.[28]

THROMBOEMBOLIC DISORDERS IN PREGNANCY

DEEP VEIN THROMBOSIS

 INTRODUCTION

Extension of puerperal infection along venous route can result in thrombosis and thrombophlebitis of the affected vein. Thrombosis usually originates as an aggregation of platelets and fibrin on the valves in the veins of the lower extremities (especially calf veins). Most cases of deep vein thrombosis (DVT) tend to occur in the left leg and involve the iliofemoral vein. The thrombus can either break-off and embolise to other veins or cause total occlusion of the veins.

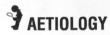 **AETIOLOGY**

Virchow has postulated that three factors are important in the development of thrombosis, which include the following:
1. Impairment of blood flow (stasis)
2. Vascular injury
3. Alterations of the blood coagulability (hypercoagulability).

Causes of Deep Vein Thrombosis during Pregnancy

Increased risk of DVT during pregnancy occurs due to the following factors:
❖ *Thrombogenic state of pregnancy*: Pregnancy is known to be a procoagulant state which is associated with an increase in numerous clotting factors including factor VIII, fibrinogen, factors VII, IX, X, and XII. This acts as body's physiologic adaptation to limit blood loss at delivery.
❖ *Venous stasis*: Reduced venous drainage due to the gravid uterus and/or reduced mobility may be associated with venous stasis and an increased risk for DVT.[33,34]
❖ *Endothelial injury*: Injury to the vascular endothelium at the time of obstetric surgical interventions is another factor which may increase the risk of DVT.

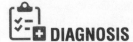 **DIAGNOSIS**

Clinical Presentation

❖ Symptoms of DVT include the following:
  - Swelling of the leg
  - Warmth and redness of the leg
  - Pain that is noticeable, or worse when standing or walking
  - Sometimes, there may be no symptoms and the patient may be asymptomatic.
❖ Signs of DVT include the following:
  - Oedema in the leg
  - Erythema
  - Increased warmth
  - Palpable cord
  - Tenderness
  - Positive Homan's sign (i.e. pain on dorsiflexion of the foot)
  - Difference in the circumference between the affected and the normal leg may be more than 2 cm.

The 'LEFt' rule or the clinical probability score, which has been recently developed, helps in estimating the probability for development of DVT during pregnancy. This score combines three variables: (1) symptoms in the left leg (L); (2) calf diameter of 2 cm or more (E for oedema); and (3) presentation in the first trimester (Ft).[35]

Investigations

❖ *Doppler ultrasound*: This helps in the diagnosis of thrombus by detecting changes in the velocity of blood flow in the femoral veins.
❖ *Compression duplex ultrasound*: This is highly sensitive and specific method for detection of femoral DVT and can be considered as the primary diagnostic test for DVT. If the diagnosis of DVT is confirmed on compression ultrasonography, no further investigation is necessary and treatment for venous thromboembolism (VTE) can be continued.
❖ *CT or MRI*: MRI is preferred over CT during pregnancy due to reduced risk of exposure to ionising radiation.

PART II

❖ *I125 fibrinogen scanning*: This is not recommended for diagnosis of DVT in pregnancy due to the risk of radiation exposure to the foetus.

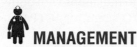

MANAGEMENT

❖ Bed rest with foot elevation above the level of heart
❖ Analgesics can be used to provide pain relief
❖ Antimicrobial therapy must be started
❖ *Anticoagulants*: Anticoagulants, such as heparin, low molecular weight heparin (LMWH) and oral anti-coagulants, such as warfarin can be used. In the post-operative obstetric patients receiving unfractionated heparin, monitoring with platelet count must be performed after every 2–3 days, continuing from days 4 to 14 of heparin therapy or until heparin is stopped. On the other hand, patients receiving LMWH should be monitored using anti-Xa activity. However, monitoring is not required for all the patients. It is mainly required for patients with extremes of weight, those with renal disease, etc. Therapeutic anticoagulant therapy should be continued for the duration of the pregnancy and for at least 6 weeks postnatally and until at least 3 months of treatment has been given in total. Before discontinuing treatment, the continuing risk of thrombosis should be assessed. Consideration can be also given to the use of newer anticoagulants, (e.g. Fondaparinux, Argatroban or r-hirudin) in pregnant women who are unable to tolerate LMWH or unfractionated heparin.[36]
Women who had been receiving long-term anticoagulation with warfarin prior to pregnancy can be converted back to warfarin from LMWH in the postpartum period (usually 5–7 days postdelivery) when the risk of haemorrhage is reduced. Both warfarin and LMWH are safe during breastfeeding.[37]
❖ Graduated elastic compression stockings: Knee-length or thigh-length graduated elastic compression stockings help in reducing the risk of thrombosis. Early ambulation also helps in reducing the risk. Stockings of appropriate size, which provide graduated compression with a calf pressure of 14–15 mmHg, must be preferably used during pregnancy.
❖ Vena cava filters can be used in the cases where anti-coagulant therapy is contraindicated.

COMPLICATIONS

❖ Pulmonary embolism, thrombophlebitis
❖ Varicose ulceration of leg veins
❖ Post-thrombotic syndrome (venous stress disorder).

CLINICAL PEARLS

❖ Warfarin should not be used for VTE treatment in the first trimester because of its likely teratogenic effects on the foetus.

❖ Low molecular weight heparin maintenance therapy should be discontinued 24 hours prior to planned delivery whether by elective caesarean section or induction of labour.
❖ The woman on LMWH maintenance therapy should be advised that once she is in established labour or thinks that she is in labour, she should avoid injecting any further doses of heparin.

EVIDENCE-BASED MEDICINE

❖ Presently, there is insufficient evidence regarding the most appropriate dosage pattern of LMWH: once or twice daily dosage for management of DVT.[38]
❖ Though graduated elastic compression stockings are commonly worn on the affected leg to reduce pain and swelling, the available evidence indicates an unclear role of compression stockings in the prevention of post-thrombotic syndrome.[39,40]

PULMONARY EMBOLISM

INTRODUCTION

Pulmonary embolism (PE) is a condition characterised by partial or complete blockage of pulmonary vessels resulting in acute respiratory and/or haemodynamic compromise. Acute respiratory consequences of PE include increased alveolar dead space, hypoxaemia and hyperventilation. PE can be either acute (embolus is situated centrally within the vascular lumen and is causing its occlusion) or chronic (embolus is eccentric and contiguous with the vessel wall, thereby reducing the arterial diameter by more than 50%).

AETIOLOGY

Pulmonary embolism occurs due to the blockage of the blood vessel carrying blood to the lungs (Fig. 14.5). The most common cause of blockage is a blood clot which has dislodged from one of the deep veins in the legs (DVT). The risk factors related to the development of PE are similar to that of DVT and have been previously described in the text.

DIAGNOSIS

Clinical Presentation

❖ Sudden collapse with acute chest pain and air hunger
❖ Tachypnoea, dyspnoea, haemoptysis
❖ Pleuritic chest pain, cough, tachycardia
❖ Temperature of greater than 37°C.

Investigations

❖ *Chest X-ray*: There may be areas of infarction showing diminished vascular markings, elevation of the dome of

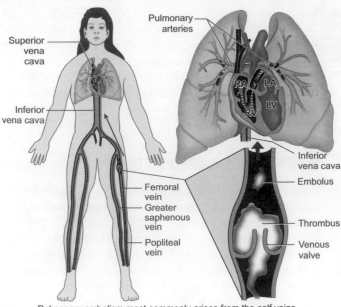

Pulmonary embolism most commonly arises from the calf veins. The venous thromboemboli travel through the right side of the heart to reach the lungs.

Fig. 14.5: Pathogenesis of pulmonary embolism
Abbreviations: RA, right atrium; RV, right ventricle; LA, left atrium; LV, left ventricle

diaphragm and pleural effusion. Other changes such as atelectasis, effusion, focal opacities and pulmonary oedema may also be visualised. In presence of an abnormality on chest X-ray and a clinical suspicion of PE, more definitive investigations such as computerised tomography pulmonary angiography (CTPA) and/or ventilation perfusion scan (V/Q scan) are performed based on the availability and the local protocols.

In case of normal findings on X-ray, bilateral Doppler ultrasound of the legs is performed to confirm or exclude the diagnosis of DVT. If the ultrasound examination does not reveal the presence of DVT, diagnosis of PE can be ruled out.

❖ *Electrocardiogram*: ECG shows tachycardia and signs of right heart strain such as right axis deviation, P-pulmonale, right-bundle branch, etc. An ECG and a chest X-ray must be performed in women presenting with symptoms and signs of an acute PE.

❖ *Arterial blood gases*: There may be reduced PO_2 and oxygen saturation

❖ *Venous perfusion scanning* : There may be diminished perfusion with maintenance of ventilation on V/Q scanning. This investigation is associated with a high negative predictive value. V/Q scan is related with a lower dosage of radiation exposure to the breast tissues and nearly 10-times higher exposure to the foetus. Omitting the ventilation scan can further reduce the dose of radiation.

❖ *Pulmonary angiography*: This can be considered as the most accurate method of diagnosis. It has a better sensitivity and specificity in comparison to V/Q scan. Presently the gold standard investigation of choice for PE is CTPA. Also, CTPA

is useful for diagnosis of other concomitant pathology, e.g. aortic dissection. Ideally, informed consent should be obtained before undertaking either CTPA or V/Q scanning because there is a risk of exposure to radiations with both these methods. In contrast to V/Q scanning, CTPA is associated with a higher dosage of radiation exposure to the breast tissues and a lower exposure to the foetus. Therefore, there is an increase in the future risk of developing breast cancer.

❖ *Doppler ultrasound*: This helps in identifying DVT. If DVT is detected, diagnosis of PE can be assumed in the presence of clinical signs and symptoms.

DIFFERENTIAL DIAGNOSIS

It is important to rule out the presence of respiratory abnormalities such as pneumonia and atelectasis.

MANAGEMENT

❖ *Multidisciplinary team*: The patient should be managed by a multidisciplinary team comprising of senior physicians, obstetricians and radiologists. Management of patients regarding the use of intravenous LMWH/unfractionated heparin, thrombolytic therapy or thoracotomy and surgical embolectomy needs to be individualised.

❖ *Patient resuscitation*: This comprises of cardiac massage and oxygen therapy

❖ *Anticoagulant therapy*: Anticoagulant of choice is usually LMWH (enoxaparin, dalteparin, tinzaparin, etc.). Maternity units should develop guidelines for the administration of LMWH. The available evidence has indicated that LMWH is likely to have an efficacy similar to that of unfractionated heparin (UFH).[38,41,42] At the same time, it is associated with a reduced risk of haemorrhagic complications and an overall reduced mortality rate.

❖ Maintenance of blood pressure using dopamine or adrenaline

❖ Thrombolytic therapy using streptokinase may be administered

❖ Tachycardia can be counteracted using digitalis

❖ *Surgical treatment*: These may include procedures such as vena caval filters, ligation of inferior vena cava and ovarian veins.

COMPLICATIONS

❖ Pulmonary embolism can be considered as the most important cause of maternal death developed nations, only after sudden cardiac arrest. Death usually occurs due to shock and vagal inhibition

❖ Recurrent embolism.

CLINICAL PEARLS

❖ Clinical features are proportional to the size of embolus
❖ Immediate full anticoagulation is mandatory for all patients suspected to have DVT or PE
❖ In case of clinical suspicion of PE, but normal findings on V/Q scan or CTPA, alternative or repeat testing should be carried out
❖ Treatment with anticoagulants should be continued until PE is definitively excluded.

EVIDENCE-BASED MEDICINE

❖ The available evidence does not support the performance of D-dimer testing for establishing a diagnosis of acute VTE during pregnancy.[36]
❖ The present evidence indicates that V/Q scanning in comparison to CTPA may carry a slightly increased risk of childhood cancer. However, it may be associated with a lower risk of maternal breast cancer. Nevertheless, in both the situations, the absolute risk is very small.[37]

REFERENCES

1. World health organization. (2001). Iron deficiency anaemia, assessment, prevention and control: a guide for programme managers. WHO website [online] Available from www.who.int/nutrition/publications/en/ida_assessment_prevention_control.pdf. [Accessed April, 2016].
2. Pavord S, Myers B, Robinson S, Allard S, Strong J, Oppenheimer C. UK guidelines on the management of iron deficiency in pregnancy. Br J Haematol. 2012;156:(5)588-600.
3. Watson F. Routine iron supplementation—is it necessary? Modern midwife. 1997;7:22-6.
4. Reveiz L, Gyte GM, Cuervo LG, Casasbuenas A. Treatment for iron deficiency anaemia in pregnancy. Cochrane Database Syst Rev. 2011;(10):CD003094.
5. Hobbs J, Rodriguez AR. Megaloblastic anemias. Am Fam Physician. 1980;22(6):128-36.
6. Campbell BA. Megaloblastic anemia in pregnancy. Clin Obstet Gynecol. 1995;38(3):455-62.
7. Lumley J, Watson L, Watson M, Bower C. Periconceptual supplementation with folate and/or multivitamins for preventing neural tube defects. Cochrane Database Syst Rev. 2001;3:CD001056.
8. Pena-Rosas JP, Viteri FE. Effects of routine oral iron supplementation with or without folic acid for women during pregnancy. Cochrane Database Syst Rev. 2006;(3):CD004736.
9. Weatherall DJ. The definition and epidemiology of non-transfusion dependent thalassaemia. Blood Rev. 2012;26 Suppl 1:S3-6.
10. Shinar E, Rachmilewitz EA. Oxidative denaturation of red blood cells in thalassaemia. Semin Hematol. 1990;27(1):70-82.
11. Ryan K, Bain BJ, Worthington D, James J, Plews D, Mason A, et al. Significant haemoglobinopathies: guidelines for screening and diagnosis. Br J Haematol. 2010;149(1):35-49.
12. Weatherall DJ. Thalassaemia in the next millennium. Keynote address. Ann N Y Acad Sci. 1998;850:1-9.
13. Alpendurada F, Smith GC, Carpenter JP, Nair SV, Tanner MA, Banya W, et al. Effects of combined deferiprone with deferoxamine on right ventricular function in thalassaemia major. J Cardiovasc Magn Reson. 2012;14:8.
14. Pennell D, Porter JB, Cappellini MD, Li CK, Aydinok Y, Lee CL, et al. Efficacy and safety of deferasirox (Exjade®) in reducing cardiac iron in patients with β-thalassaemia major: results from the cardiac substudy of the EPIC trial [abstract]. Blood. 2008;112 (ASH Annual Meeting Abstracts): Abstract 3873.
15. Barry M, Flynn DM, Letsky EA, Risdon RA. Long-term chelation therapy in thalassaemia major: effect on liver iron concentration, liver histology, and clinical progress. Br Med J. 1974;2(5909):16-20.
16. Davis BA, Porter JB. Long-term outcome of continuous 24-hour deferoxamine infusion via indwelling intravenous catheters in high-risk β-thalassaemia. Blood. 2000;95(4):1229-36.
17. Borgna-Pignatti C, Rugolotto S, De Stefano P, Zhao H, Cappellini MD, Del Vecchio GC, et al. Survival and complications in patients with thalassaemia major treated with transfusion and deferoxamine. Haematologica. 2004;89(10):1187-93.
18. Singer ST, Vichinsky EP. Deferoxamine treatment during pregnancy: is it harmful? Am J Hematol. 1999;60(1):24-6.
19. Eldor A, Rachmilewitz EA. The hypercoagulable state in thalassaemia. Blood. 2002;99(1):36-43.
20. Taher A, Isma'eel H, Mehio G, Bignamini D, Kattamis A, Rachmilewitz EA, et al. Prevalence of thromboembolic events among 8,860 patients with thalassaemia major and intermedia in the Mediterranean area and Iran. Thromb Haemost. 2006;96:(4)488-91.
21. Royal College of Obstetricians and Gynaecologists. Reducing the Risk of Thrombosis and Embolism during Pregnancy and the Puerperium. Green-top Guideline No. 37a. London: RCOG; 2009.
22. Faculty of Reproductive & Sexual Healthcare. UK Medical Eligibility Criteria for Contraceptive Use. London: FRSH; 2009.
23. Chakravarti A, Li CC, Buetow KH. Estimation of the marker gene frequency and linkage disequilibrium from conditional marker data. Am J Hum Genet. 1984;36:177-86.
24. Davies SC, Brozovi M. The presentation, management and prophylaxis of sickle cell disease. Blood Rev. 1989;3:29-44.
25. Serjeant GR. The emerging understanding of sickle cell disease. Br J Haematol. 2001;112:3-18.
26. Streetley A, Latinovic R, Hall K, Henthorn J. Implementation of universal newborn bloodspot screening for sickle cell disease and other clinically significant haemoglobinopathies in England: screening results for 2005-7. J Clin Pathol. 2009;62:26-30.
27. Tuck SM, Studd JW, White JM. Pregnancy in sickle cell disease in the UK. Br J Obstet Gynaecol. 1983;90:112-7.
28. NHS Sickle Cell & Thalassaemia Screening Programme. Standards for the linked antenatal and newborn screening programme. [Online] Available from https://www.gov.uk/government/publications/standards-for-sickle-cell-and-thalassaemia-screening. [Accessed April 2016].
29. Davies EG, Riddington C, Lottenberg R, Dower N. Pneumococcal vaccines for sickle cell disease. Cochrane Database Syst Rev. 2004;(1):CD003885.
30. Rees DC, Olujohungbe AD, Parker NE, Stephens AD, Telfer P, Wright J. Guidelines for the management of acute painful crisis in sickle cell disease. Br J Haematol. 2003;120:744-52.

CHAPTER 14

31. Gaston MH, Verter JI, Woods G, Pegelow C, Kelleher J, Presbury G, et al. Prophylaxis with oral penicillin in children with sickle cell anaemia. A randomized trial. N Engl J Med. 1986;314:1593-9.

32. Working Party of the British Committee for Standards in Haematology Clinical Haematology Task Force. Guidelines for the prevention and treatment of infection in patients with an absent or dysfunctional spleen. BMJ. 1996;312:430-4.

33. Homans J. Thrombosis of the deep leg veins due to prolonged sitting. N Engl J Med. 1954;250(4):148-9.

34. Gertler JP, Perry L, L'Italien G, Chung-Welch N, Cambria RP, Orkin R, et al. Ambient oxygen tension modulates endothelial fibrinolysis. J Vasc Surg. 1993;18(6):939-46.

35. Chan WS, Lee A, Spencer FA, Crowther M, Rodger M, Ramsay T, et al. Predicting deep venous thrombosis in pregnancy: out in "LEFt" field? Ann Intern Med. 2009;151(2):85-92.

36. Royal College of Obstetricians and Gynaecologists (RCOG). (2015). Thromboembolic Disease in Pregnancy and the Puerperium: Acute Management. Green-top Guideline No. 37b. London: RCOG; 2015.

37. Royal College of Obstetricians and Gynaecologists (RCOG). (2015). Reducing the Risk of Venous Thromboembolism during Pregnancy and the Puerperium. Green-top Guideline No. 37a. London: RCOG; 2015.

38. Greer IA, Nelson-Piercy C. Low-molecular weight heparin for thromboprophylaxis and treatment of venous thrombo-embolism in pregnancy: a systematic review of safety and efficacy. Blood. 2005;106(2):401-7.

39. Berntsen CF, Kristiansen A, Akl EA, Sandset PM, Jacobsen EM, Guyatt G, et al. Compression stockings for preventing the postthrombotic syndrome in patients with deep vein thrombosis. Am J Med. 2016;129(4):447.e1-447.e20.

40. Jayaraj A, Meissner M. Impact of graduated compression stockings on the prevention of post-thrombotic syndrome - results of a randomized controlled trial. Phlebology. 2015; 30(8):541-8.

41. Kher A, Bauersachs R, Nielsen JD. The management of thrombosis in pregnancy: role of low-molecular-weight heparin. Thromb Haemost. 2007;97(4):505-13.

42. Eldor A. The use of low-molecular-weight heparin for the management of venous thromboembolism in pregnancy. Eur J Obstet Gynecol Reprod Biol. 2002;104(1):3-13.

Diabetes Mellitus and Gestational Diabetes

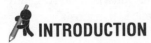 INTRODUCTION

Diabetes mellitus is an endocrine disorder of carbohydrate metabolism resulting from the lack of action of hormone insulin, produced by the pancreatic β-cells in the body. About 2–5% of the total pregnancies may be affected by diabetes. Amongst the pregnancies complicated by diabetes, about 65% cases involve gestational diabetes, whereas 35% cases are associated with pre-existing diabetes, of which 25% of cases may be associated with pre-existing type 1 diabetes and 10% may involve pre-existing type 2 diabetes. The WHO and National Diabetes Data Group (NDDG) have classified diabetic pregnancies as follows:[1,2]

Pre-existing diabetes: Diabetes that antedates pregnancy

❖ Type I: No endogenous insulin, ketosis prone
❖ Type II: Late onset diabetes, associated with obesity, insulin-resistant.

Gestational diabetes: This is defined by WHO as "carbohydrate intolerance resulting in hyperglycaemia of variable severity with onset or first recognition during pregnancy".

❖ *A1*: Euglycaemia achieved with diet and exercise
❖ *A2*: Medications required for achieving euglycaemia.

Gestational diabetes now includes both gestational impaired glucose tolerance and gestational diabetes mellitus (GDM). GDM can be associated with several complications such as increased risk of stillbirths and macrosomia. Diagnosis and management of GDM is important because it can help reduce the rate of complications.

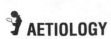 AETIOLOGY

Pathogenesis of GDM is described in Flow chart 15.1. The risk factors, which predispose a woman to develop gestational diabetes, are listed in Box 15.1.[3]

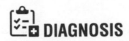 DIAGNOSIS

Clinical Presentation

Clinical signs suggestive of pre-eclampsia may be present as the women with GDM are especially prone to develop pre-eclampsia.

Abdominal Examination

Women with GDM are especially prone to develop polyhydramnios.

Flow chart 15.1: Pathogenesis of gestational diabetes mellitus

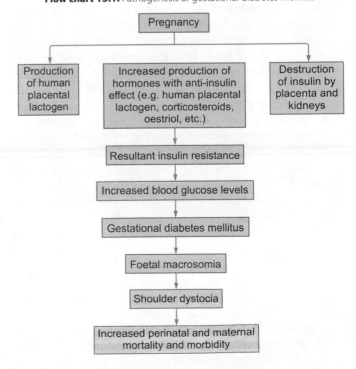

Box 15.1: Risk factors for the development of diabetes[3]

☐ Body mass index above 30 kg/m²
☐ Previous macrosomic baby weighing 4.5 kg or above
☐ Previous history of gestational diabetes
☐ Family history of diabetes (first-degree relative with diabetes)
☐ Minority ethnic origin with a high prevalence of diabetes (e.g. South Asian, Middle Eastern, etc.)

Table 15.1: Diagnostic criteria for gestational diabetes mellitus for the 75 g oral glucose tolerance test

	WHO/NICE (mmol/L)	IADPSG* (mmol/L)
Fasting	≥5.6	≥5.1
1 hour	–	≥10.0
2 hour	≥7.8	≥8.5

Values for venous plasma samples.

*Diagnosis of gestational diabetes mellitus made if this value exceeded at any time point.

Abbreviations: IADPSG, International Association of Diabetes and Pregnancy Study Groups; NICE, National Institute for Health and Clinical Excellence; WHO, World Health Organization

Investigations

Presently, the International Association of Diabetes and Pregnancy Study Groups (IADPSG) consensus panel advocates the use of a single-step approach for the diagnosis of GDM based on the results of Hyperglycaemia and Adverse Pregnancy Outcome (HAPO) study.[4,5] This approach involving the use of 75 g oral glucose tolerance test (OGTT) is being followed in most of the NHS trusts.[6] Women with any one of the risk factors (mentioned in Box 15.1) must be offered testing for gestational diabetes in form of 2-hour 75 g OGTT at 24–28 weeks. Parameters like fasting plasma glucose, random blood glucose, HbA1c, glucose challenge test or urinalysis for glucose are not used for assessing risk of developing gestational diabetes.

Women who have had gestational diabetes in a previous pregnancy must be offered early self-monitoring of blood glucose or a 75 g 2-hour OGTT as soon as possible after booking (whether in the first or second trimester), and a further 75 g 2-hour OGTT at 24–28 weeks if the results of the first OGTT are normal.[7,8]

Gestational diabetes is diagnosed if the woman has either a fasting plasma glucose level of 5.1 mmol/L or above or a 2-hour plasma glucose level of 7.8 mmol/L or above (Table 15.1). Normal fasting levels of blood glucose vary between 3.5 mmol/L and 5.9 mmol/L, whereas 2-hour postprandial blood glucose should be less than 7.8 mmol/L.[9]

MANAGEMENT

Women with GDM should preferably be managed in a joint obstetric or diabetic clinic involving a multidisciplinary approach comprising of the obstetricians, diabetologists, dieticians, specialist nurses, midwives, etc. Women who have been diagnosed with gestational diabetes must be reviewed by the joint diabetes and antenatal clinic within 1 week.

Antenatal Period

❖ *Diabetes education and information*: Education and information regarding diabetes, hypoglycaemia, self-monitoring of blood glucose levels, etc. needs to be provided to the patient.

❖ *Maintenance of blood glucose levels*: This can be done with the help of monthly measurement of the glycosylated haemoglobin levels and self-monitoring of blood glucose levels using a glucose meter. Postprandial blood glucose levels rather than levels of glycosylated HbA1c should be used for monitoring glycaemic control in both the second and third trimester. The pregnant women with any form of diabetes must be advised to maintain their capillary plasma glucose below the following target levels:[9]
  • Fasting: 5.3 mmol/L
  • 1 hour after meals: 7.8 mmol/L
  • 2 hours after meals: 6.4 mmol/L.

❖ Pregnant woman with any form of diabetes, who is unwell or presenting with hyperglycaemia, must be tested urgently for ketonaemia to exclude diabetic ketoacidosis.

❖ In case of women with gestational diabetes, initial control of blood glucose levels must be through exercise and nutritional advice. Women with gestational diabetes must be advised to eat a healthy diet during pregnancy, preferably replacing foods with a high glycaemic index with those having a low glycaemic index. All women with gestational diabetes must be referred to a dietician for obtaining proper nutritional advice.

❖ Women with gestational diabetes must be advised to take regular exercise (such as walking for 30 minutes after a meal) to improve blood glucose control.

❖ If the required blood glucose targets are not achieved through dietary changes and changes in lifestyle within 1–2 weeks, she should be prescribed metformin.[10,11] She can be prescribed insulin instead of metformin if metformin is contraindicated or unacceptable to the woman or if the blood glucose targets are not being achieved with metformin.[11] Glibenclamide can be considered for women with gestational diabetes in whom blood glucose targets are not achieved with metformin, but who decline insulin therapy or who cannot tolerate metformin.[12] Plasma glucose levels must be maintained above 4 mmol/L in women on insulin or glibenclamide.

❖ Women with gestational diabetes, who have fasting plasma glucose level of 7.0 mmol/L or above at the time of diagnosis, must be offered immediate treatment with insulin, with or without metformin, along with dietary changes and exercise. The same treatment must be offered to women with gestational diabetes who have fasting plasma glucose levels between 6.0 mmol/L and 6.9 mmol/L, along with the presence of complications such as macrosomia or hydramnios.

❖ *Maintenance of adequate body weight*: Women with diabetes who are planning to become pregnant and who have a BMI above 27 kg/m² should be offered advice on how to lose weight.[13]

❖ *Regular intake of folic acid*: Women with diabetes who are planning to become pregnant should be advised to take folic acid in the dose of 5 mg/day, starting right from the periconceptional period and extending throughout the period of gestation.

❖ *Insulin therapy*: Insulin therapy may include regular insulin, or rapid-acting insulin analogues (aspart and lispro). Rapid-acting insulin analogues have advantages over regular human insulin during pregnancy and therefore are being considered during pregnancy. During pregnancy, women are usually prescribed four daily insulin injections (three injections of regular insulin to be taken before each meal and one injection of isophane insulin to be taken at night time).

❖ Diabetic women treated with insulin must be counselled about the risks of hypoglycaemia and impaired awareness of hypoglycaemia in pregnancy, particularly in the first trimester. Insulin-treated pregnant women should always have an easy access to a fast-acting form of glucose (for example, dextrose tablets or glucose-containing drinks). Administration of parenteral glucagon may be required in pregnant women with type 1 diabetes having severe hypoglycaemia.

❖ Women with insulin-treated diabetes should be prescribed continuous subcutaneous insulin infusion (insulin pump therapy) during pregnancy if adequate blood glucose control is not obtained by multiple daily injections of insulin without significant disabling hypoglycaemia.

❖ *Foetal monitoring*: An individualised approach must be provided for monitoring foetal growth and well-being for women with diabetes. These include tests such as ultrasound monitoring of foetal growth and amniotic fluid volume every 4 weeks from 28 weeks to 36 weeks onwards. Routine monitoring of foetal well-being (using methods such as foetal umbilical artery Doppler recording, foetal heart rate recording and biophysical profile testing) before 28 weeks is not recommended in pregnant women with diabetes, unless there is a risk of foetal growth restriction.[14]

❖ *Screening for congenital malformations*: First trimester ultrasound scan at 11–13 weeks must be done to look for nuchal translucency, as there is an increased risk of neural tube defects. Maternal serum screening for α-foetal proteins at 16–18 weeks must be done to rule out the risk for neural tube defects. Second trimester ultrasound scan for detailed scanning for foetal congenital anomalies must be performed at 18–20 weeks.[15] A detailed examination of the foetal heart (four chambers, outflow tracts and three vessels) must be also performed at 20 weeks.

❖ Pregnant women with type 1 or type 2 or gestational diabetes who are on a multiple daily insulin injection regimen must be advised to test their fasting, premeal, 1-hour postmeal and bedtime blood glucose levels daily during pregnancy. On the other hand, pregnant women with type 2 diabetes or gestational diabetes on diet and exercise therapy, or oral therapy or a single-dose insulin, must be instructed to test their fasting and 1-hour postmeal blood glucose levels daily.

❖ *Retinal assessment during pregnancy*: Pregnant women with pre-existing diabetes must be offered retinal assessment by digital imaging with mydriasis using tropicamide following their first antenatal clinic appointment (unless they have had a retinal assessment in the last 3 months), and again at 28 weeks. If any diabetic retinopathy is present at booking, an additional retinal assessment must be offered at 16–20 weeks. Women who have preproliferative diabetic retinopathy or any form of referable retinopathy diagnosed during pregnancy must have ophthalmological follow-up for at least 6 months after the birth of the baby. Diabetic retinopathy should not be considered as a contraindication to vaginal birth.

❖ *Renal assessment during pregnancy*: If renal assessment has not been undertaken in the preceding 3 months in women with pre-existing diabetes, it should be done at the time of first antenatal visit during pregnancy. The patient should be referred to a nephrologist in the following cases:
  • Abnormal serum creatinine levels (120 micromol/L or more)
  • The urinary albumin:creatinine ratio is greater than 30 mg/mmol
  • Total protein excretion exceeds 0.5 g/day.

❖ Diabetes should not be considered a contraindication for administration of antenatal steroids for foetal lung maturation or to tocolysis. Women with insulin-treated diabetes, who are receiving steroids for foetal lung maturation, must be administered additional insulin according to an agreed protocol and then be closely monitored. β-mimetic medicines must not be used for tocolysis in women with diabetes.

Management during the Intrapartum Period

❖ *Monitoring the blood glucose levels*: During the time of labour and birth, capillary blood glucose should be monitored on an hourly basis in women with diabetes and maintained at levels between 4 mmol/L to 7 mmol/L by using intravenous dextrose and insulin infusion.[16]

❖ *Timing and mode of birth*: Diabetes per se is not an indication for caesarean delivery. Women with gestational diabetes can be considered for normal vaginal birth unless there is some other obstetric indication for vaginal delivery. In women with previous history of caesarean birth, diabetes should not in itself be considered a contra-indication for attempting vaginal birth after caesarean delivery (VBAC). Timing of delivery must be planned as follows:
  • *Low risk patients*: These women may be allowed to develop spontaneous labour and to deliver by 38–40 weeks of gestation. In case these patients do not go spontaneously in labour, they must have an elective birth by induction of labour, or by elective caesarean section if indicated, between 37[+0] weeks and 38[+6] weeks of pregnancy. Women with gestational diabetes must preferably be delivered no later than 40[+6] weeks if required by induction of labour or caesarean section.
  • *High-risk patients*: These include women with type 1 or type 2 diabetes in presence of any metabolic,

maternal or foetal complications. Elective birth may be considered before 37^{+0} weeks for these patients depending upon the severity of problem. High-risk gestational diabetic patients should definitely have their labour induced when they reach 38 weeks of gestation.

❖ *General anaesthesia*: If general anaesthesia is used for the birth in women with diabetes, blood glucose levels must be monitored at every 30-minute interval from induction of general anaesthesia until after the baby is born and the woman is fully conscious.

Neonatal Care

❖ Women with diabetes must be advised to give birth in hospitals where skills for advanced neonatal resuscitation are available 24 hours a day.

❖ Babies of women with diabetes should stay with their mothers unless there is a clinical complication or there are abnormal clinical signs that warrant admission to an intensive or a special care unit.

❖ Women with diabetes should feed their babies as soon as possible after birth, preferably within first 30 minutes of delivery. Thereafter, the baby must be frequently fed; preferably at the intervals of every 2–3 hours until prefeed capillary plasma glucose levels reach a minimum of 2.0 mmol/L.

❖ After birth, blood glucose testing must be carried out routinely at every 2–4 hours in babies of women with diabetes. Blood tests for polycythaemia, hyperbilirubinaemia, hypocalcaemia and hypomagnesaemia must be done in babies showing clinical signs suggestive of these conditions.

❖ An echocardiogram must be performed for babies of women with diabetes if they show clinical signs associated with congenital heart disease or cardiomyopathy, including heart murmur.

Postnatal Care

❖ Immediately after birth, the insulin requirements may fall; therefore, insulin doses must be reduced immediately to prepregnancy levels, in order to avoid hypoglycaemia. Women with gestational diabetes whose blood glucose levels have returned to normal after the birth must be offered lifestyle advice (including weight control, diet and exercise). Fasting plasma glucose levels must be tested 6–13 weeks after the birth to exclude diabetes.

❖ Women with pre-existing diabetes who were being treated with insulin should be advised to reduce their insulin levels immediately after birth and should monitor their blood glucose levels carefully to establish the appropriate dose. Such women are also at an increased risk of developing hypoglycaemia in the postnatal period, especially when breastfeeding. They should be advised to have a meal or snack before or during feeds.

❖ Women with pre-existing type 2 diabetes who are breast-feeding can resume or continue to take metformin and glibenclamide immediately after birth. However, they should avoid taking other oral blood glucose-lowering agents while breastfeeding.

❖ Women with pre-existing diabetes must be referred back to their routine diabetes care arrangements.

❖ Women with diabetes must be counselled regarding the importance of contraception and the requirement for preconception care when planning future pregnancies.

❖ Women who were diagnosed with gestational diabetes must be explained about the risks of gestational diabetes in future pregnancies, and be advised to get themselves tested for diabetes when planning future pregnancies.

COMPLICATIONS

Diabetes in pregnancy is associated with numerous risks to the mother and the developing foetus, which are enumerated in Table 15.2.

Effect of Diabetes on the Foetus

Foetal hyperinsulinaemia is likely to result in complications mentioned in Table 15.3 and include the following:

❖ An overgrowth of insulin-sensitive tissues such as adipose tissues, especially around the chest, shoulders and abdomen, which increases the risk of shoulder dystocia.

❖ Increased risk for perinatal death, birth trauma and rates of caesarean section.

❖ Neonatal metabolic complications such as hypoglycaemia.

❖ Foetal hypoxia which may increase the risk of intrauterine foetal death.

❖ Foetal polycythaemia, hyperbilirubinaemia and renal vein thrombosis.

❖ An increased long-term risk of obesity and diabetes in the child.

Table 15.2: Maternal and foetal complications related to gestational diabetes

Maternal complications	Foetal complications
• Miscarriage	• Foetal distress and birth asphyxia
• Pre-eclampsia	• Brachial plexus injuries
• Preterm labour	• Macrosomia or foetal birthweight more than 4 kg (Flow chart 15.2)
• Prolonged labour	
• Polyhydramnios (could be associated with foetal polyuria)	• Increased risk for perinatal death, birth trauma and rates of caesarean section
• Shoulder dystocia	• Cephalohematoma, resulting in more pronounced neonatal jaundice
• 35–50% risk of developing type II diabetes later in the life[17]	• Stillbirth, congenital malformations, birth injury, perinatal mortality
• Increased risk of traumatic damage during labour	• Hypoxia and sudden intrauterine death after 36 weeks' gestation
• Increased risk of shoulder dystocia	• Congenital malformations
	• Foetal/neonatal hypoglycaemia, polycythaemia, hyperbilirubinaemia and renal vein thrombosis
• Diabetic retinopathy and nephropathy can worsen rapidly during pregnancy	• Stillbirths
	• An increased long-term risk of obesity and diabetes in the child

Flow chart 15.2: Pathogenesis of foetal macrosomia

Macrosomia can be defined as birthweight more than 4,000 g or birthweight ≥90 percentile for the particular gestational age. These foetuses are also referred to as large for gestational age

Maternal hyperglycaemia

↓

Increased blood glucose levels

↓

Extra glucose crosses the placenta

↓

Stimulation of foetal pancreas

↓

Increased insulin production by foetal pancreas

↓

Stimulation of baby's growth | Foetal hypoglycaemia at birth

↓

Foetal macrosomia

↓

• Increased incidence of operative deliveries
• Shoulder dystocia

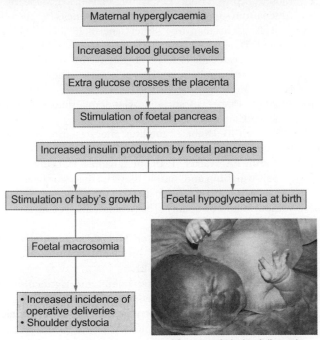

Macrosomic baby delivered by caesarean section

Table 15.3: Foetal problems related to maternal hyperglycaemia in the three trimesters of pregnancy

First trimester	Second trimester	Third trimester
• Foetal congenital malformations • Growth restriction • Recurrent miscarriage	• Hypertrophic cardiomyopathy • Polyhydramnios • Placental insufficiency	• Hypoglycaemia • Hypocalcaemia • Hyperbilirubinaemia • Respiratory distress syndrome • Macrosomia • Hypomagnesaemia • Intrauterine death • Low intelligence quotient in the newborn

❖ *Congenital malformations:* Infants of women with established type I diabetes have more than 10 times the risk in comparison to the general population for development of congenital malformations. They also have five times the risk for stillbirth. If hyperglycaemia is present during the first trimester of pregnancy when organogenesis is taking place, congenital malformations may occur. Some of the congenital abnormalities commonly encountered in the babies of diabetic mothers are listed in Box 15.2.

 CLINICAL PEARLS

❖ Diabetes should not in itself be considered a contraindication for attempting VBAC. Care should be

Box 15.2: Various types of congenital malformations associated with gestational diabetes

❑ Caudal regression sequence
❑ Congenital heart disease: Ventricular septal defect, coarctation of the aorta and transposition of the great arteries, situs inversus, etc.
❑ Congenital microcolon
❑ Renal defects: Agenesis, cystic kidney, duplex ureter, etc.
❑ Neural tube defects: Anencephaly, spina bifida, hydrocephaly, etc.
❑ Cystic fibrosis, in association with meconium ileus
❑ Gastrointestinal abnormalities: Ileal atresia, rectal/ anal atresia, Hirschsprung's disease, etc.

individualised based on the glycaemic control and development of macrosomia.
❖ Early feeding of the neonate is recommended for reducing the risk of neonatal hypoglycaemia.

 EVIDENCE-BASED MEDICINE

❖ Women at risk must be tested with 2-hour, 75 g OGTT at 24–28 weeks of gestation.[8]
❖ A diabetic woman should be offered delivery by 38–39 weeks of gestation. Present evidence indicates that this reduces the risk of shoulder dystocia with vaginal delivery.[18] The shoulder dystocia is more likely when vaginal delivery occurs after 39 weeks of gestation in presence of macrosomia.[19]
❖ The ACOG recommends an elective caesarean section in women with sonographically estimated foetal weight of 4.5 kg.[20]
❖ Hypoglycaemic treatment during pregnancy can either comprise of hypoglycaemic drugs or insulin.[11]
❖ Umbilical artery velocimetry is of no proven value for foetal surveillance. Presently, there is no good evidence indicating that antepartum surveillance strategies for monitoring foetal growth can help reduce the risk of macrosomia and stillbirths.[14]

REFERENCES

1. Alberti KG, Zimmet PZ. Definition, diagnosis and classification of diabetes mellitus and its complications. Part 1: diagnosis and classification of diabetes mellitus provisional report of a WHO consultation. Diabet Med. 1998;15(7):539-53.
2. National Diabetes Data Group. Classification and diagnosis of diabetes mellitus and other categories of glucose intolerance. Diabetes. 1979;28:1039-57.
3. National Institute for Health and Clinical Excellence (NICE). (2010). National Institute for Health and Clinical Excellence guideline for diabetes in pregnancy. Management of diabetes—a national clinical guideline. National clinical guideline 116. [online]. NICE website. Available from www.sign.ac.uk/pdf/sign116.pdf. [Accessed June, 2016].
4. Metzger BE, Lowe LP, Dyer AR, Trimble ER, Chaovarindr U, Coustan DR, et al. Hyperglycemia and adverse pregnancy outcomes. N Engl J Med. 2008;358(19):1991-2002.

CHAPTER 15

5. Metzger BE, Gabbe SG, Persson B, Buchanan TA, Catalano PA, Damm P, et al. International association of diabetes and pregnancy study group's recommendations on the diagnosis and classification of hyperglycemia in pregnancy. Diabetes Care. 2010;33(3):676-82.

6. National Institute for Health and Clinical Excellence. NICE clinical guideline 63: Diabetes in pregnancy: Management from preconception to the postnatal period. London: NICE; 2015. [online] Available from https://www.nice.org.uk/guidance/ng3. [Accessed March 2016].

7. HAPO Study Cooperative Research Group. Hyperglycemia and Adverse Pregnancy Outcome (HAPO) Study: associations with neonatal anthropometrics. Diabetes. 2009;58:453-9.

8. Sacks DA, Greenspoon JS, Abu-Fadil S, Henry HM, Wolde-Tsadik G, Yao JF. Toward universal criteria for gestational diabetes: the 75-gram glucose tolerance test in pregnancy. Am J Obstet Gynecol. 1995;172(2 Pt 1):607-14.

9. Royal College of Obstetricians and Gynaecologists (RCOG). (2011). Diagnosis and treatment of gestational diabetes. [online] RCOG website. Available from www.rcog.org.uk/globalassets/documents/guidelines/sip_no_23.pdf. [Accessed June 2016].

10. Landon MB, Spong CY, Thom E, Carpenter MW, Ramin SM, Casey B, et al. A multicenter, randomized trial of treatment for mild gestational diabetes. N Engl J Med. 2009;361(14): 1339-48.

11. Rowan JA, Hague WM, Gao W, Battin MR, Moore MP; MiG Trial Investigators. Metformin versus insulin for the treatment of gestational diabetes. N Engl J Med. 2008;358(19):2003-15.

12. Langer O, Conway DL, Berkus MD, Xenakis EM, Gonzales O. A comparison of glyburide and insulin in women with gestational diabetes mellitus. N Engl J Med. 2000;343(16):1134-8.

13. Scottish Intercollegiate Guidelines Network (SIGN). (2010). National clinical guideline 116: Management of diabetes. [online] SIGN website. Available from www.sign.ac.uk/pdf/sign116.pdf. [Accessed June, 2016].

14. Kjos SL, Leung A, Henry OA, Victor MR, Paul RH, Medearis AL. Antepartum surveillance in diabetic pregnancies. Predictors of fetal distress in labor. Am J Obstet Gynecol. 1995;173(5):1532-9.

15. Miller E, Hare JW, Cloherty JP, Dunn PJ, Gleason RE, Soeldner JS, et al. Elevated maternal hemoglobin A1c in early pregnancy and major congenital anomalies in infants of diabetic mothers. N Engl J Med. 1981;304(22):1331-4.

16. American Diabetes Association. Gestational diabetes mellitus. Diabetes Care. 2001;24(Suppl 2):S77-9.

17. O'Sullivan JB. Diabetes mellitus after gestational diabetes mellitus. Diabetes. 1991;29(Suppl 2):131-5.

18. McCarthy EA, Walker SP, Ugoni A, Lappas M, Leong O, Shub A. Self-weighing and simple dietary advice for overweight and obese pregnant women to reduce obstetric complications without impact on quality of life: a randomised controlled trial. BJOG. 2016;123(6):965-73.

19. Ben-Haroush A, Yogev Y, Hod M. Fetal weight estimation in diabetic pregnancies and suspected fetal macrosomia. J Perinat Med. 2004;32(2):113-21.

20. American College of Obstetricians and Gynecologists. Committee on Practice Bulletins–Obstetrics. ACOG Practice Bulletin. Clinical management guidelines for obstetrician-gynecologists. Number 30, September 2001 (replaces Technical Bulletin Number 200, December 1994) Gestational diabetes. Obstet Gynecol. 2001;98(3):525-38.

Abdominal Pain during Pregnancy

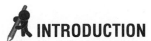 INTRODUCTION

Abdominal pain during pregnancy may present additional challenges for the obstetrician because he/she needs to consider physiologic or anatomic alterations related to pregnancy, gestational age and foetal well-being. Moreover, the causes of acute abdomen that may be more commonly related to the pregnant state or to the obstetrical complications.[1]

During pregnancy, the aetiology of abdominal pain may be related to pregnancy and therefore may directly or indirectly affect the foetus as well.

Mild to moderate abdominal discomfort is a common and usually temporary complaint in normal pregnancy. It can be due to a number of normal physiological causes, such as the enlarging uterus, constipation, changes in foetal position or movement, Braxton-Hicks uterine contractions, the round ligaments pain (due to the stretching of round ligaments), etc.

On the other hand, pain which is severe, sudden, constant, associated with other symptoms (e.g. nausea, vomiting, vaginal bleeding), or in the upper abdomen suggests a disease process unrelated to pregnancy or could be related to a specific pregnancy related complication, e.g. ectopic pregnancy, placental abruption, miscarriage, urinary tract infection, pre-eclampsia, etc.[2]

AETIOLOGY

Various causes of abdominal pain during pregnancy are listed in Table 16.1.[3-8]

DIAGNOSIS

Clinical Presentation

❖ At the time of taking history, a complete medical and surgical history must be taken. The pregnant women should also be enquired about their past and current obstetrical history. They should also be asked if they have experienced symptoms such as vaginal bleeding or leaking fluid (suggestive of rupture of the foetal membranes).

Table 16.1: Differential diagnosis for various causes of abdominal pain in pregnant women

Pregnancy-related causes	
First half of pregnancy	*Second half of pregnancy*
• Miscarriage • Ectopic pregnancy	• Labour (term or preterm) • Placental abruption • Uterine rupture • Pregnancy-related liver disease • Severe pre-eclampsia • HELLP syndrome • Acute fatty liver • Intra-amniotic infection

Non-pregnancy-related causes	
Pain in the upper abdomen	*Pain in the lower abdomen*
• Gastroesophageal reflux • Gallbladder disease • Acute hepatitis • Pancreatic diseases • Pneumonia • Bowel obstruction	• Acute appendicitis • Nephrolithiasis • Inflammatory bowel disease • Diverticulitis

Diffuse abdominal pain or pain in variable locations
• Sickle cell crisis • Trauma • Mesenteric venous thrombosis • Iliopsoas abscess

Gynaecologic causes
• Ovarian torsion • Fallopian tube torsion • Ruptured or haemorrhagic ovarian cyst • Fibroid degeneration or torsion • Pelvic inflammatory disease • Postpartum abdominal pain (endometritis, incisional complications, etc.)

> **Box 16.1:** Symptoms present in association with abdominal pain requiring immediate medical supervision
>
> ❏ Severe or persistent pain
> ❏ Spotting or bleeding
> ❏ Fever
> ❏ Chills
> ❏ Vaginal discharge
> ❏ Light-headedness
> ❏ Discomfort while urinating
> ❏ Nausea and vomiting
> ❏ Peritoneal signs (rebound tenderness, abdominal guarding)

❖ The abdominal pain may vary in intensity depending upon the underlying cause. Pain is usually mild to moderate in association with the normal physiological changes of pregnancy. However, it may be intense or severe in presence of underlying pregnancy-related pathology.

❖ In presence of an underlying obstetric complication, the patient may also experience some other symptoms mentioned in Box 16.1. The patient should immediately contact their health care provider if she experiences any of these symptoms.

❖ The presence of peritoneal signs (rebound tenderness, abdominal guarding) is never normal in pregnancy. Presence of these signs mandates prompt maternal-foetal evaluation.[9]

Abdominal Examination

The abdominal and per vaginal examination should include evaluation of the uterine size, tone and tenderness. The uterus is non-tender and soft in a normal pregnant patient. In the second half of pregnancy, the frequency of uterine contractions must also be assessed on the abdominal examination. Rupture of membranes and cervical dilation or effacement should be assessed on the vaginal examination. Both obstetric and non-obstetric disorders may cause uterine contractions, which may result in cervical changes resembling those of labour. Uterine tenderness or rigidity is abnormal and may be due to conditions such as labour, abruptio-placenta, uterine rupture or intrauterine infection.

Investigations

In general, the following investigations are done:
❖ Complete blood count (inclusive of differential count)
❖ Urinalysis
❖ Liver and pancreatic function tests (aminotransferases, bilirubin, amylase, lipase)[10]
❖ Blood and urine cultures in the presence of fever or unstable vital signs
❖ Coagulation studies, and blood type and cross-match (women with haemodynamic instability)
❖ Serum electrolyte level and renal function tests (women who are vomiting or anorectic)
❖ *Imaging modalities*: Ultrasound examination can be typically considered as the first-line modality for diagnostic imaging of the abdomen in pregnant women.[11] Moreover,

this investigation modality is widely available, portable, does not expose to non-ionising radiations, and has a high degree of diagnostic accuracy. When ultrasound findings are non-conclusive, the choice of the second-line modality depends on the probable differential diagnosis and should take into account availability, diagnostic performance and foetal radiation exposure. When indicated, use of MRI is preferable to CT because it avoids exposure to ionising radiation.[12,13]

❖ *Laparoscopy*: Laparoscopy is sometimes indicated in the evaluation of acute pelvic or abdominal pain, especially when the diagnosis is not clear from the result of less invasive evaluations and there is a suspicion of a potentially life-threatening or an organ-threatening disorder. Laparoscopic examination is usually performed in the first, second, and early third trimester and can be considered largely safe in pregnancy.

MANAGEMENT

❖ The management principles for abdominal pain and the acute abdomen in pregnancy are similar to that in the non-pregnant state.

❖ The most important principle of management is to identify those individuals who have a serious or even life-threatening aetiology for their symptoms and require urgent intervention.

❖ The foetal heart rate must be documented where possible, especially in case of women having severe pain. Continuous foetal heart rate monitoring is usually appropriate in pregnancies that have attained a gestational age of 23–24 weeks.

❖ When evaluating pregnant women with abdominal pain, the clinician needs to consider the normal physiologic or anatomic alterations associated with pregnancy, gestational age and foetal well-being, and causes of abdominal pain or acute abdomen that may be more common due to the pregnant state or related to obstetrical complications.

❖ A thorough history, a complete physical examination and laboratory investigations should be obtained to taper down the differential diagnosis.

❖ Symptoms such as abdominal discomfort, nausea, vomiting and constipation can be a normal part of pregnancy. However, the presence of peritoneal signs (rebound tenderness, abdominal guarding) is never normal in pregnant women and requires immediate maternal-foetal evaluation. Nausea and vomiting when present with symptoms such as abdominal pain, fever, diarrhoea, headache, or localised abdominal findings cannot be considered as normal physiological changes of pregnancy.

❖ Appropriate diagnostic imaging and interventions should be performed as indicated because delay in diagnosis and treatment can increase maternal and foetal or newborn morbidity and mortality.

❖ Abdominal and pelvic ultrasound examinations can be considered as the most useful tests for evaluation of abdominal pain in pregnant women. These examinations can be considered safe from the point of view of the mother and the foetus. When indicated, chest and abdominal plain X-ray films result in very low foetal absorption of ionising radiation and are unlikely to be associated with significant short-term or long-term adverse effects. MRI does not involve ionising radiation and thus is preferable to CT, which exposes the foetus to higher doses of ionising radiation than plain films.

❖ When surgery is planned, the appropriate consultations between the obstetrics, general surgery, anaesthesia, and paediatric departments must be made. Surgical management of pregnant women undergoing surgery may require modifications to the general approach used in non-pregnant women.

CLINICAL PEARLS

❖ Concerns about the possible foetal effects of ionising radiation should not prevent the obstetrician from undertaking the medically indicated diagnostic procedures during pregnancy because delay in the diagnosis can increase the risk of an adverse maternal and/or foetal outcome.

❖ When procedures requiring ionising radiation are necessary, various techniques can be employed to minimise the foetal exposure to ionising radiation dose by adhering to the ALARA principle: 'As Low as Reasonably Achieved' (e.g. use of abdominal shielding before understanding radiological imaging in pregnant women). For further details, kindly refer to Chapter 17 (Malignancy during Pregnancy).[14]

❖ Almost all diagnostic radiological procedures are associated with exposures that are below the threshold for causing adverse foetal effects such as congenital malformations, growth restriction or developmental delay.

EVIDENCE-BASED MEDICINE

❖ Based on the evidence collected from the retrospective studies, laparoscopic surgery for evaluation of pelvic or abdominal pain in pregnancy appears to be as safe as laparotomy.[15-17]

❖ Chest and abdominal radiographs are commonly used in evaluation of adults with abdominal pain. The available evidence indicates that the estimated foetal absorption per chest X-ray is <0.01 mGy (<0.001 rad), which is the dose, well below the doses that are likely to be associated with any short- or long-term adverse effects.[14]

❖ The estimated foetal absorption for abdominal X-rays is 1–4.2 mGy (0.1–0.42 rad), which is also below doses that are likely to be associated with any short- or long-term adverse effects.[14]

REFERENCES

1. Kilpatrick CC, Monga M. Approach to the acute abdomen in pregnancy. Obstet Gynecol Clin North Am. 2007;34(3):389-402.
2. Kilpatrick CC, Orejuela FJ. Management of the acute abdomen in pregnancy: a review. Curr Opin Obstet Gynecol. 2008;20(6):534-9.
3. Neiger R, Sonek JD, Croom CS, Ventolini G. Pregnancy-related changes in the size of uterine leiomyomas. J Reprod Med. 2006;51(9):671-4.
4. Murray A, Holdcroft A. Incidence and intensity of postpartum lower abdominal pain. BMJ. 1989;298(6688):1619.
5. Cook KE, Jenkins SM. Pathologic uterine torsion associated with placental abruption, maternal shock, and intrauterine fetal demise. Am J Obstet Gynecol. 2005;192(6):2082-3.
6. Guié P, Adjobi R, N'guessan E, Anongba S, Kouakou F, Boua N, et al. Uterine torsion with maternal death: our experience and literature review. Clin Exp Obstet Gynecol. 2005;32(4):245-6.
7. Hasson J, Tsafrir Z, Azem F, Bar-On S, Almog B, Mashiach R, et al. Comparison of adnexal torsion between pregnant and nonpregnant women. Am J Obstet Gynecol. 2010;202(6):536.e1-6.
8. Smorgick N, Pansky M, Feingold M, Herman A, Halperin R, Maymon R. The clinical characteristics and sonographic findings of maternal ovarian torsion in pregnancy. Fertil Steril. 2009;92(6):1983-7.
9. Parangi S, Levine D, Henry A, Isakovich N, Pories S. Surgical gastrointestinal disorders during pregnancy. Am J Surg. 2007;193(2):223-32.
10. Kaiser R, Berk JE, Fridhandler L. Serum amylase changes during pregnancy. Am J Obstet Gynecol. 1975;122(3):283-6.
11. Spalluto LB, Woodfield CA, DeBenedectis CM, Lazarus E. MR imaging evaluation of abdominal pain during pregnancy: appendicitis and other nonobstetric causes. Radiographics. 2012;32(2):317-34.
12. Baron KT, Arleo EK, Robinson C, Sanelli PC. Comparing the diagnostic performance of MRI versus CT in the evaluation of acute nontraumatic abdominal pain during pregnancy. Emerg Radiol. 2012;19(6):519-25.
13. Beddy P, Keogan MT, Sala E, Griffin N. Magnetic resonance imaging for the evaluation of acute abdominal pain in pregnancy. Semin Ultrasound CT MR. 2010;31(5):433-41.
14. Groen RS, Bae JY, Lim KJ. Fear of the unknown: ionizing radiation exposure during pregnancy. Am J Obstet Gynecol. 2012;206(6):456-62.
15. Soriano D, Yefet Y, Seidman DS, Goldenberg M, Mashiach S, Oelsner G. Laparoscopy versus laparotomy in the management of adnexal masses during pregnancy. Fertil Steril. 1999;71(5):955-60.
16. Reedy MB, Källén B, Kuehl TJ. Laparoscopy during pregnancy: a study of five fetal outcome parameters with use of the Swedish Health Registry. Am J Obstet Gynecol. 1997;177(3):673-9.
17. Pearl J, Price R, Richardson W, Fanelli R, Society of American Gastrointestinal Endoscopic Surgeons. Guidelines for diagnosis, treatment, and use of laparoscopy for surgical problems during pregnancy. Surg Endosc. 2011;25(11):3479-92.

CHAPTER 16

Malignancy during Pregnancy

GENERAL MALIGNANCY DURING PREGNANCY

 INTRODUCTION

During a woman's reproductive years, malignancy can be considered as the second leading cause of death. The incidence of cancers during pregnancy is generally reported to be 1 for every 1,000 maternities.[1-3] Pregnancy-associated cancer refers to cases in which the initial diagnosis of cancer is made during pregnancy or within 12 months of delivery. The validations for including cancers that are diagnosed after pregnancy include the following:

❖ Woman and her obstetrician may erroneously attribute cancer-related symptoms to be due to the physiological changes of pregnancy.
❖ There may be unwillingness to perform radiographs or invasive procedures during pregnancy, leading to delayed diagnosis.
❖ Less aggressive tumours are more likely to remain undetected until after delivery.

Recently, there has been a rise in the incidence of pregnancy-associated cancers. This increase can be partially explained by the increasing maternal age. Moreover, pregnancy is likely to increase the woman's contact with health services and therefore result in higher possibility for diagnosis.[4]

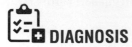 **DIAGNOSIS**

Clinical Presentation

Although pregnancy is not likely to alter the course of the malignancy, the diagnosis of malignancy may be sometimes delayed because symptoms of malignancy may be at times confused with the symptoms of normal pregnancy, e.g. nausea, anorexia, vomiting, weakness, constipation, etc.

Investigations

❖ *Blood investigations*: Routine blood investigations can be carried out depending on the type of underlying malignancy.
❖ *Imaging*: Before undertaking radiological imaging investigations, especially which may expose the foetus to ionising radiations, (e.g. X-ray) appropriate shielding of the mother is essential. Imaging investigating such as ultrasonography and MRI are considered relatively safe during pregnancy. CT scan is usually contraindicated during pregnancy due to the risk of foetal exposure to ionising radiations.
❖ *Histopathological analysis*: Biopsy and tissue analysis for histopathology can be performed based on the clinical circumstances and the type of underlying malignancy.

 MANAGEMENT

❖ Management of malignancy during pregnancy requires a multidisciplinary approach comprising of an obstetrician, an oncologist, paediatrician, oncology nurse, counsellors, etc.
❖ *Psychological counselling*: Pregnant women with malignancy require counselling services through involvement of mental health nurse because fears of limited life expectancy might be preventing them to make future plans regarding the expected children. Her fears regarding the effect of the disease on the foetus also need to be addressed.[5]
❖ Both investigations and treatment for malignancy during the pregnancy may carry risk to the foetus. Therefore, a balance needs to be maintained between administration of the treatment to the mother, and limiting harm to the foetus. Moreover, the side effects due to chemotherapy and radiotherapy may limit the maternal aspects of childbearing in the future.

Effect of Radiotherapy during Pregnancy

❖ *Preventing the foetal radiation exposure during pregnancy*: Appropriate shielding of the mother before undertaking radiological imaging in pregnant women is likely to reduce the foetal exposure by as much as 50%. The period of gestation at which the exposure occurs is also important. Radiosensitivity of the foetal tissues may be altered during different periods of gestation. Also, with the increasing period of gestation, it may become difficult to shield a larger foetus.

❖ *Critical period*: The period of 8–15 weeks of gestation is the critical period for foetal growth and neurological development. During this period, which corresponds to the stage of cortical formation and organisation, the foetus is at the highest risk of damage.[6] After 25 weeks, the risk appears to be minimum. Exposure very early during gestation may either result in complete miscarriage or may cause the pregnancy to continue unaffected. The risk of developing malignancy later in life is increased amongst such children.[7] Risks related to radiation exposure during different periods of gestation is summarised in Table 17.1.

❖ *Dose of radiation*: Lower dosage of radiation (e.g. 10cGy) is responsible for causing intrauterine death and miscarriage early in gestation in comparison to higher dosage (>1 Gy) later, towards term. This implies that the radiation dosage, which induces lethal changes in the embryo, increases from 0.1 Gy at day 1 to nearly 1 Gy after the first trimester.

❖ *Use of radiotherapy during pregnancy*: Use of radiotherapy to the pelvis is absolutely contraindicated during the pregnancy due to the likely damage to the foetus, which cannot be shielded. Cancers where the use of radio-therapy forms a vital treatment option, e.g. breast cancer, lymphomas, etc. shielding of the pelvis prevents sufficient exposure to the foetus.

Effect of Chemotherapy during Pregnancy

❖ *Period of exposure*: Prior to implantation, the blastocyst is immune to the effects of chemotherapy. The period of organogenesis between 5 to 10 weeks is a critically sensitive period because exposure during this period can result in the development of congenital malformations in nearly 10–20% cases. After 12 weeks of gestation, these malformations are less common. However, growth and neurological development may be affected throughout pregnancy. Exposure during the first trimester is likely to be associated with a greater risk to the foetus in compari-

Table 17.1: Risks related to radiation exposure during different periods of gestation

Period of gestation	Likely complications
0–2 weeks	Miscarriage
3–7 weeks	Congenital malformations
Exposure throughout radiation	Generalised growth and neurological abnormalities
At any gestational age	Predisposition to malignancy in future

Table 17.2: Complications likely to be associated with different chemotherapeutic agents

Chemotherapeutic agents	Likely complications
Antimetabolites (e.g. aminopterin, methotrexate, etc.)	Miscarriage, neural tube defects, skeletal and cleft lip abnormalities
Alkylating agents (e.g. cyclophosphamide)	Nearly 15% risk of congenital anomalies in the first trimester. This risk falls to background levels during the second and third trimesters.
Antibiotics such as doxorubicin and bleomycin	No clearly defined teratogenic side effects: Use should be avoided in the first trimester.
Vinca alkaloids: vincristine and vinblastine	Harmful effect in animal pregnancies. Harmful effect is not clearly observed in the human pregnancies.

son to the exposure during the second or third trimesters of pregnancy. Use of combination drugs is further likely to increase this risk. While the exposure to chemotherapeutic drugs during the first trimester is likely to result in teratogenicity, exposure during the second or third trimester is unlikely to produce teratogenic side effects. Nevertheless, exposure during this time can result in adverse effects such as growth restriction, prematurity and stillbirths.

❖ *Type of chemotherapeutic agent*: The development of a specific congenital malformation is also dependent on the type of agent used (Table 17.2).[8] Most cytotoxic chemotherapeutic agents are capable of crossing the placenta and thereby reaching the foetal circulation. The risk to pregnancy due the first trimester is highest with antimetabolites. Therefore, their use should be definitely avoided in the first trimester and later in pregnancy whenever possible. Use of myelosuppressive agents must be preferably avoided 3 weeks prior to delivery due to the possible risk of bone marrow suppression. Fortunately, this is a rare event and is rarely of any clinical significance.

❖ *Effect of chemotherapeutic agents on breastfeeding*: Though the use of chemotherapy during the second or third trimester is unlikely to be associated with any major side effect, breastfeeding is usually discouraged if the treatment continues into the puerperium.

Symptomatic Management

The drugs described in Table 17.3 can be used for symptomatic management of common symptoms related to the presence of malignancy in the pregnant patients.

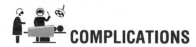

COMPLICATIONS

Exposure of the foetus to radiation and chemotherapeutic agents is likely to result in the following complications:

❖ Congenital malformations (e.g. microcephaly)
❖ Developmental disorders

Table 17.3: Drugs used for symptomatic management in pregnant patients with malignancy

Symptoms	Drugs
Pain	Paracetamol and opiates (NSAIDs should be avoided preferably in the third trimester)
Neuropathic pain	Tricyclic antidepressants (except carbamazepine)
Nausea	Metoclopramide, prochlorperazine, ondansetron, cyclizine, haloperidol and prednisolone (if required)
Constipation	Docusate, magnesium hydroxide, senna

❖ Growth restriction
❖ Severe mental retardation
❖ Increased risk of childhood malignancy
❖ Infertility in the offspring.

 CLINICAL PEARLS

❖ Melanoma in pregnancy is likely to metastasise to the placenta and foetus. However, this rarely occurs. Nevertheless, the placenta in the patient with melanoma must be examined at the time of delivery and sent for histopathological examination.
❖ Treatment for Hodgkin's lymphoma and chronic myeloid leukaemia can be delayed until after pregnancy. However, acute leukaemia and Hodgkin's lymphoma must be treated immediately as the risk to the woman and her pregnancy due to haemorrhage, anaemia and sepsis outweigh the possible foetal harm related to chemotherapy even in the first trimester.

 EVIDENCE-BASED MEDICINE

❖ Delayed complications related to the long-term exposure of the foetus to chemotherapeutic agents presently remains unclear. The present evidence does not suggest any significant adverse effect on fertility, neurological or intellectual development of the exposed individuals. [9]
❖ The current evidence does not suggest any increase in the rate of childhood malignancies in those subjected to chemotherapy in utero.[9]

BREAST MALIGNANCY DURING PREGNANCY

 INTRODUCTION

Breast cancer is the most common cancer in females, accounting for nearly one-fourth of malignancies diagnosed during pregnancy. The lifetime risk of breast cancer is 1 in every 9 women in the UK. It is the leading cause of death in women aged 35–54 years. 15% cases of breast cancer are diagnosed before the age of 45 years. Thus, breast cancer

affects nearly 5,000 women belonging to the reproductive age in the UK annually.[10,11] Treatment success rates in the UK are good and are continually improving, with 5-year survival rates currently being around 80% for the under 50s age group.

Pregnancy itself does not appear to worsen the prognosis for women diagnosed in pregnancy in comparison with non-pregnant controls matched for age and stage.[12] Young pregnant women with breast cancer may have a poor prognosis because younger population may have features, which are associated with a high risk of metastases such as high-grade tumours and oestrogen receptor negative tumours.

AETIOLOGY

The exact cause of breast cancer presently remains unknown. However, some factors, which are likely to be associated with an increased risk for breast cancer, are as follows:
❖ *Female sex*: Females in comparison to males are more likely to develop breast cancer.
❖ *Increasing age*: Most invasive breast malignancies occur in the women at the age of 55 years or above.
❖ *A personal history or family history of breast cancer*: History of cancer in one breast is likely to increase the risk for development of cancer in the other breast. Also, family history of breast cancer, especially in first degree relative (mother, sister or daughter) is associated with an increased risk.
❖ *Presence of inherited genes*: The most common gene mutations which may be associated with an increased risk for breast cancer include the BRCA1 and BRCA2 genes.
❖ *Exposure to radiation*: Exposure of radiation treatment to the chest, especially at the young age.
❖ *Obesity*: Increased body mass index may be associated with higher risk.
❖ *Early menarche and late menopause*: History of menarche at a younger age [less than 12 years and late menopause (>55 years)] is associated with an increased risk.
❖ *Giving birth to the first child at an older age*: History of having first child after the age of 35 years may be associated with an increased risk.
❖ *Nulliparity*: Women who have never been pregnant are at an increased risk of developing breast cancer.
❖ *Breastfeeding*: Breastfeeding is likely to lower the woman's risk of developing breast cancer.
❖ *Postmenopausal HRT*: Women who have taken HRT, especially that containing oestrogen and progesterone are at an increased risk of developing breast cancer.
❖ Drinking alcohol.

DIAGNOSIS

Clinical Presentation

Most common clinical signs and symptoms in case of a breast malignancy have been described next.
❖ *Lump*: The most common presentation of a breast malignancy is a lump in breast. Lump in the axilla may

also be present in case the axillary lymph nodes have become involved.

- ❖ *Skin changes over the breast*: There may be thickening, dimpling or ulceration of the skin.
- ❖ *Nipple changes*: Inversion of the nipple, ulceration, discharge from the nipples (bloodstained or clear).

Investigations

- ❖ *Ultrasound*: Ultrasound examination is the investigation, which is firstly used for assessing the discrete lump.
- ❖ *Ultrasound-guided biopsy*: Tissue diagnosis is with ultrasound-guided biopsy for histology rather than cytology because proliferative changes during pregnancy render cytology inconclusive in many women.
- ❖ *Mammography*: If cancer is confirmed, mammography is necessary (with foetal shielding) to assess the extent of disease and for evaluating the contralateral breast.
- ❖ *Staging for metastatic disease*: Staging for metastases is conducted only if there is high clinical suspicion and consists of chest X-ray (with abdominal shielding) and hepatic ultrasound if possible. Ultrasonography and MRI have largely replaced CT scan for the evaluation of metastasis. Gadolinium-enhanced magnetic resonance imaging is usually not recommended. Tumour markers such as CA15-3, CEA and CA-125 are also not used in early breast cancer and may be misleading in pregnancy. Therefore, their use is not recommended. Investigations such as bone scanning, pelvic X-ray and CT are not recommended because of the possible effect of irradiation on the foetus. If there is concern about bone involvement, a plain film of the relevant area and/or MRI to minimise foetal radiation exposure may be carried out.

MANAGEMENT

- ❖ The management of pregnancy in relation to breast cancer should be by a multidisciplinary team, comprising of obstetricians and gynaecologists, fertility specialists and midwives as well as oncologists and breast care nurses, with inclusion of the obstetric team as core members.
- ❖ The most common surgical management option for breast cancer in the non-pregnant women is lumpectomy followed by postoperative chest wall radiotherapy to reduce the risk of local recurrence. In case of pregnant women, surgical treatment including loco-regional clearance can be undertaken in all trimesters. However, radiotherapy is associated with radiation dosage of 50 cGy. Even with appropriate abdominal shielding, this may result in foetal exposure of 4 cGy early in gestation and exposure of nearly 14–18 cGy in the second trimester when the uterus has increased in size. This dosage is above the accepted threshold for safety and therefore, postoperative radiotherapy should not be advised during pregnancy. A modified radical mastectomy, which does not require postoperative radiotherapy, can be advised at certain times. Conservative breast surgery can be performed in the third trimester with administration of radiotherapy until after the puerperium. Occasionally, a decision may be made to offer neoadjuvant chemotherapy before surgery to allow downstaging of the tumour to facilitate surgery.

- ❖ Breast reconstruction following mastectomy should be preferably delayed until the puerperium to avoid the risk of prolonged anaesthesia related to the reconstructive surgery during pregnancy. Delay would also enable breasts of the pregnant patient to attain optimal symmetry following delivery.
- ❖ Sentinel node biopsy is indicated in women who have a negative result from a preoperative axillary ultrasound and needle biopsy. If the axilla is positive, axillary clearance is indicated.
- ❖ As previously described, radiotherapy is contraindicated until delivery unless it is lifesaving or is used for preservation of organ function (e.g. spinal cord compression).
- ❖ Systemic chemotherapy is contraindicated in the first trimester because of a high risk of foetal congenital abnormalities. However, administration of chemotherapy during the second or third trimester is not associated with an obvious harm to the foetus. Use of chemotherapy during the second or third trimester is not associated with an increased rate of second-trimester miscarriage, foetal growth restriction, organ dysfunction or long-term adverse outcomes.[13,14] Anthracycline regimens are safe. On the other hand, fewer studies are available regarding the safety of taxanes.[14-16] Therefore, use of taxanes should be reserved for high-risk (node-positive) or metastatic disease. Wherever possible, the last dose of chemotherapy must be administered 3 weeks prior to the delivery to limit the effects of foetal bone marrow suppression.
- ❖ Standard antiemetic drugs such as $5HT_3$ serotonin antagonists and dexamethasone can be used during pregnancy. There is no data regarding the use of neurokinin receptor antagonist having very high efficacy in the treatment of chemotherapy-induced emesis.
- ❖ The use of tamoxifen and trastuzumab, a monoclonal antibody targeted against the human epidermal growth factor receptor 2 (HER2)/neu receptor, is presently contraindicated during pregnancy and these drugs should not be used.[17,18] Tamoxifen is not used until after delivery. Due to the long half-life of the drug, women on tamoxifen are advised to stop this treatment 3 months before trying to conceive.
- ❖ *Foetal surveillance*: Although no clear link of chemotherapy with perinatal growth restriction has been established, foetal surveillance through regular growth scanning is performed.
- ❖ *Timing of delivery*: The birth of the baby should be timed after discussion with the woman and the multidisciplinary team. Most women can go to full term of pregnancy and have a normal or induced delivery. Some authors suggest delivery of the baby at 34 weeks of gestation to limit foetal exposure to chemotherapeutic agents. In these cases, consideration must be given towards the use of corticosteroids for attaining foetal lung maturity. However, birth should be preferably timed more than

2–3 weeks after the last session of chemotherapy to allow recovery of maternal bone marrow and to limit the effects of foetal bone marrow suppression, thereby minimising problems related with foetal neutropenia. Neonatal blood sampling is also required to rule out clinically relevant pancytopenia.

❖ *Lactation*: Women should not breastfeed when taking trastuzumab or tamoxifen, because it is unknown whether these drugs are transmitted in breast milk. The woman's ability to breastfeed may depend on the type of surgery and whether major ducts have been excised. The woman should be counselled not to breastfeed while on chemotherapy because these drugs can cross into breast milk, thereby causing neonatal leucopenia with a risk of infection. The woman should be advised to maintain a time interval of at least 14 days or more from the last session of chemotherapy to the start of breastfeeding to allow drug clearance from breast milk.[19]

❖ *Contraceptive advice after treatment of breast cancer*: Hormonal method of contraception is contraindicated in women with current or recent breast cancer (World Health Organization/UK medical eligibility category 4).[20] Non-hormonal contraceptive methods are usually recommended.

❖ *Impact of pregnancy on risk of recurrence*: Women can be reassured that long-term survival after breast cancer is not adversely affected by pregnancy.

❖ *Time interval before pregnancy*: Advice regarding postponement of pregnancy should be individualised and based on the individual patient's treatment and prognosis over time. Most women should wait for at least 2 years after treatment because this is the time when the risk of cancer recurrence is highest.

Management of Pregnancy Following Treatment for Breast Cancer

❖ Increasing numbers of young women who have been treated for breast cancer are now going on to have babies. Therefore, management of pregnancy in such patients has gained importance. Pregnancy following breast cancer should be jointly supervised by the obstetrician, oncologist and breast surgeon.

❖ Left ventricular dysfunction and cardiomyopathy is a rare complication related to the use of chemotherapy agents, anthracyclines (doxorubicin, epirubicin). Echocardiography should be performed during pregnancy in women at risk to detect cardiomyopathy through resting left ventricular ejection fraction or echocardiographic fractional shortening.

❖ During pregnancy, a breast treated by surgery or radiotherapy may not undergo hormonal changes and the woman may require a temporary prosthesis.

❖ If imaging of breast is required, an ultrasound examination is usually preferred.

❖ Metastatic relapse may be harder to detect during pregnancy and common complaints in pregnancy such as backache can be difficult to assess.

❖ *Effect of breast cancer treatment on the woman's fertility*: Infertility after treatment is a major concern for young women with breast cancer.[21-24] The effect of treatment on fertility should be discussed with all women of reproductive age diagnosed with breast cancer. Referral to a fertility specialist should be available, who should provide specialist counselling. Written information should also be provided to the patient and her family.

According to the recommendations of joint working party of the Royal Colleges of Physicians, Radiologists, Obstetricians and Gynaecologists in the UK, people with cancer should be fully informed about the potential gonadotoxicity before treatment. Specialist psychological support and counselling services should also be available for such patients.[25]

• *GnRH analogues*: Use of GnRH analogues have therapeutic role in hormone-sensitive breast cancer, because they induce ovarian suppression and create a low-oestrogen state, thereby protecting the oocyte pool from depletion. Presently, there is insufficient evidence to support the routine use of GnRH analogues for ovarian protection in oestrogen receptor positive breast cancer.[26-29]

• *Cryopreservation*: Established options of cryopreservation for women include embryo and oocyte cryopreservation, both of which have been associated with variable rates of success. Both the treatment options require ovarian stimulation which may not be possible or appropriate in some instances. Modified stimulation regimes should be considered for women with oestrogen-sensitive breast cancer.

🐚 CLINICAL PEARLS

❖ For women diagnosed with breast cancer whilst pregnant, treatment usually begins straight away and is offered according to the type and extent of the cancer in consultation with a multidisciplinary team.

❖ Women with metastatic disease should be advised against having a further pregnancy as life expectancy is limited in these cases, and treatment of metastatic disease would be compromised.

❖ Women who are known to be carriers of breast cancer gene (*BRCA*) may wish to consider preimplantation genetic diagnosis, which is now available in the UK.

EVIDENCE-BASED MEDICINE

❖ Stage-by-stage outcome of breast cancer in pregnancy is no different from that outside pregnancy. Continuing pregnancy in such cases is unlikely to have an adverse outcome on pregnancy, and termination of pregnancy is usually not indicated.[12,18]

❖ *Outcome of pregnancy*: The majority of pregnancies after breast cancer proceed to live birth. There is little evidence to indicate an increased risk of miscarriage or congenital malformations in children conceived after treatment for breast cancer.[30-33]

CERVICAL MALIGNANCY DURING PREGNANCY

 INTRODUCTION

Cervical cancer is one of the most common malignancies in pregnancy, with an estimated incidence of 0.8–1.5 cases per 10,000 births.[34-37] Most cases are identified as a result of cervical cancer screening programmes. In developed countries, most of the patients are diagnosed at an early stage due to routine prenatal screening. For details related to the cervical cancer in non-pregnant women, kindly refer to Chapter 86 (Invasive Cervical Cancer).

AETIOLOGY

The factors, which are associated with an increased risk of cervical cancer, include the following:

Age: Cancer of the cervix can occur at any age. It is found most often in women older than 40 years, but can occur in younger women. However, it rarely occurs in women younger than 21 years. The average age for occurrence of carcinoma cervix is 47 years. The distribution of cases of cervical cancer is usually bimodal with the peak occurring at two points, first between 35 years to 39 years and second between 60 years to 64 years of age.

Obstetric history: Women who give birth to babies at young age, particularly the women who have their first delivery before the age of 20 years are at an increased risk. Multiparous women with poor spacing between pregnancies are also at an increased risk.

Sexual history: The factors in the sexual history, which are associated with an increased risk of cervical cancer, include the following:

❖ Promiscuity or history of having multiple sexual partners.
❖ History of having a male sexual partner who has had sexual intercourse with more than one person (the more partners the person has, the greater is the risk).
❖ Young age (less than 18) at the time of first sexual intercourse.
❖ Having a male sexual partner who has had a sexual partner with cervical cancer.

> These factors can increase the woman's risk for developing cancer of the cervix, because they increase the chances of acquiring human papilloma virus (HPV) infection, which can lead to dysplasia.

❖ Women who have had sexually transmitted diseases in the past including the diseases like HIV infection, herpes simplex 2 virus infection, HPV infection, etc. are also at an increased risk of developing cancer of the cervix.
❖ *Infection with HPV*: The initiating event in cervical dysplasia and carcinogenesis is infection with HPV. There are 100 different types of HPV, out of which nearly 14 are the high risk types. Of these, type 16 and 18 are most commonly found in cases of squamous cell carcinoma.

Personal history: Smoking is associated with an increased risk for development of cancer of cervix. Women who do not come for regular health checkups and Pap tests are also at an increased risk.

Reduced immunity: Women with reduced immunity are at an increased risk of developing cervical cancer. Some of the conditions associated with reduced immunity include the following:

❖ HIV infection
❖ Organ (especially kidney) transplant
❖ Hodgkin's disease

Previous history of cancerous lesions in the cervix: The woman is at a high risk of developing cancer cervix if she has a previous history of high-grade squamous intraepithelial lesions (HSIL); history of cancer of the cervix, vagina, or vulva or has not been getting routine Pap tests done in the past. Pap smear is associated with false-negative rate of up to 50%. Therefore, negative Pap smear should not be relied upon in a symptomatic patient.

Previous vaccination against cervical cancer: Two HPV vaccines, quadrivalent Gardasil® and bivalent Cervarix® have been approved by the US Food and Drug Administration for protection against the HPV subtypes 16 and 18.

Socioeconomic status: Individuals belonging to low socio-economic classes or low-income groups have been found to be at a high risk of developing cervical cancer. This could be probably due to the fact that poor women may not be able to afford good health care such as having regular Pap tests.

Treatment history: History of intake of medicines like diethyl-stilbestrol (DES), OCPs, etc. may be associated with an increased risk of breast cancer.

The daughters of women who consumed DES at the time of their pregnancy are at a slightly higher risk of developing cancer of the vagina and cervix. Long-term use of the contraceptive pills for more than 10 years can slightly increase the woman's risk of developing cervical cancer.

Dietary history: Diets low in fruits and vegetables are linked to an increased risk of cervical and other cancers. Also, women who are overweight are at an increased risk of developing cervical cancer in the future.

Family history: Cervical cancer may run in some families. If the woman's mother or sister had cervical cancer, her chances of getting the disease in future are increased.

DIAGNOSIS

Clinical Presentation

❖ Signs and symptoms of cervical malignancy during pregnancy are dependent on the clinical stage and the size of lesion.

❖ Abnormal vaginal bleeding and discharge is the most common presentation of cervical cancer during pregnancy.

❖ Patients in the more advanced stages of the disease can present with pelvic pain, sciatica type pain, pain in the flanks, chronic anaemia and shortness of breath.

❖ A gross lesion on the cervix can be palpated or visualised.

Physical Examination

Physical examination is important for the process of clinical staging and includes assessment of the primary tumour, uterus and vagina, parametrium, groin, right upper quadrant of the abdomen and supraclavicular nodes.

Investigations

❖ *Screening test (cervical cytology)*: Cervical cancer is first suspected when the screening test for the disease is abnormal. Cervical cytology (Pap smear) for exclusion of cervical malignancy is performed as a part of diagnostic evaluation for abnormal vaginal bleeding in pregnancy.

❖ *Biopsy of the gross lesion*: Women with the pathological confirmation of cervical cancer should be referred to a gynaecological oncologist for staging.

❖ *Colposcopic evaluation*: Only colposcopists who have experience with pregnancy-related changes in cervical appearance should undertake colposcopic evaluation of the cervix during pregnancy. Colposcopy-directed biopsies can be performed during pregnancy. Colposcopy-directed biopsy is required in cases where the lesions are suspicious for cervical intraepithelial neoplasia (CIN) (II or III) or cancer. However, endocervical curettage should not be performed.

❖ *Diagnostic conisation*: Diagnostic conisation is only indicated during pregnancy if confirmation of invasive disease is likely to change either the timing or mode of delivery. Otherwise, diagnostic conisation must be preferably postponed until the postpartum period to avoid potential disruption of pregnancy.

❖ *Investigations for clinical staging of cervical cancer*: Staging examinations are modified in pregnant women to limit foetal exposure to ionising radiation. Some investigations, which may be required for clinical staging of cervical cancer in non-pregnant women, include chest X-ray, cystoscopy, urogram, fluorine-18-labelled fluorodeoxyglucose PET, CT scanning or MRI. PET or CT scanning is usually not recommended during pregnancy because foetal absorption of isotope exceeds the recommended dosage. MRI is the investigation of choice for pelvic imaging during pregnancy. Chest X-ray should be taken after appropriate abdominal shielding. Ultrasound or MRI can be used for the evaluation of urinary tract or liver.

MANAGEMENT

❖ *Multidisciplinary approach*: A multidisciplinary team approach comprising of an oncologist, radiologist and a senior obstetrician is essential for dealing with the complex care issues being faced by a pregnant patient with cervical cancer. An individualised treatment plan should be determined by the multidisciplinary team (having an obstetrician as the core element) in consultation with the patient and her family.

❖ Management in cases of pregnancy with cervical cancer is summarised in Flow chart 17.1 and Table 17.4.[38-40]

❖ Immediate definitive treatment regardless of the gestational age is required in the situations tabulated in Box 17.1.

Management of Preinvasive Lesions

For patients in whom preinvasive cervical cancer is diagnosed, definitive treatment should be postponed until the postpartum period. If a Pap smear taken during pregnancy revealed a low-grade CIN lesion and this is confirmed by colposcopic examination, these women should be managed by a repeat colposcopy in each trimester with a further evaluation in the postpartum period.[41]

In case the results of Pap smear examination and colposcopy both revealed a high-grade CIN lesion, it is important to rule out the presence of microinvasive and invasive lesions. Treatment of CIN II and III should be delayed until after the postpartum period. However, colposcopy should be advised after every 8 weeks in the antenatal period to monitor the disease progression. If microinvasive or invasive disease is suspected, conisation or a large loop excision should be done early in pregnancy. Evaluation in the postpartum period is extremely essential in these cases because the lesion may revert, continue or progress. Therefore, the diagnosis made during pregnancy may require to be upgraded.

Management of Invasive Disease

Management of women with invasive cervical cancer should be decided after taking into consideration the wishes of the patient and her family regarding preservation of the pregnancy and future fertility, the foetal gestational age, and clinical stage of the disease in mother. Patients, who are diagnosed with cervical cancer and continue their pregnancy, should be closely followed until delivery. The definitive treatment for women diagnosed with more advanced disease during pregnancy in whom treatment has been delayed until after delivery is similar to that of the non-pregnant patient. When controlled for stage of cervical cancer, the course of disease and prognosis of cervical cancer in pregnant women is similar to those of non-pregnant women.

Gestational Age at or before 16 Weeks

❖ Immediate treatment must be commenced for patients diagnosed with cervical cancer at or before 16 weeks of gestation, irrespective of stage.

❖ In the early stages, cervical cancer is treated surgically. In more advanced stages of cervical cancer, chemoradiotherapy is administered. This treatment is likely to affect the ovarian, bladder, bowel and sexual functions.

Flow chart 17.1: Algorithm for management of pregnant patients with cervical cancer

Pregnancy with carcinoma cervix

- Carcinoma in situ
  - Periodic cytologic and colposcopic evaluation
    - No contraindication for vaginal delivery

- Micro-invasive disease
  - Cone biopsy
    - Conisation margin is negative
      - Stage 1A1
        - No further treatment, provided there is no evidence of disease on follow-up
      - Stage 1A2
        - Conservative management until delivery
          - Postpartum evaluation
            - Surgical treatment with a simple trachelectomy or large conisation
    - Conisation margin is positive
      - Delivery by classical caesarean section
        - Repeat conisation 6–8 weeks postpartum to rule out invasive disease

- Early invasive cancer (Stage IB, IIA)
  - Treatment to be individualised based on the gestational age, tumour stage, metastatic evaluation and wishes of the patient and her family to continue pregnancy
    - Patient does not desire to continue her pregnancy
      - Management is same as that in non-pregnant patient
    - Patient desires to continue her pregnancy
      - First trimester: Neoadjuvant chemotherapy can be administered if no evidence of lymph node involvement on lymphadenectomy
      - Third trimester: Radical hysterectomy and pelvic lymphadenectomy after classical caesarean delivery

- Advanced invasive disease (Stage III and IV)
  - First trimester
    - Chemotherapy along with external beam radiation
      - Spontaneous abortion or uterine evacuation
        - Brachytherapy
  - Second/third trimester
    - Classical caesarean delivery
      - Neoadjuvant chemotherapy and irradiation (external beam therapy and brachytherapy)

Table 17.4: Treatment based on whether or not woman desires to preserve her future fertility

Cancer stage	Treatment
Women desiring to preserve their fertility	
Stage IA1 disease	No further treatment is warranted if the women desire to preserve their fertility. If the margins of cone biopsy are clear, the pregnancy is allowed to continue with vaginal delivery
Stage IA2 disease or a tumour up to 4 cm in size	A radical trachelectomy can be performed 6–8 weeks after delivery. A lymphadenectomy should also be performed if not done previously
Women who do not desire to preserve their fertility	
Stage IA1 disease	Extrafascial hysterectomy rather than a radical hysterectomy provided there is no evidence of lymphovascular space invasion (LVSI). This can be concomitant with a caesarean delivery
Stage IA1 disease with LVSI, IA2, or IB1 tumours <2 cm	Definitive treatment with a radical hysterectomy rather than chemoradiation. This can be done at the time of caesarean delivery or as a second surgical procedure

Box 17.1: Indications for immediate definitive treatment in cases of carcinoma cervix during pregnancy

❑ Documented metastasis of the lymph nodes

❑ Progression of the disease during pregnancy

❑ Patient chooses for termination of pregnancy

❖ *FIGO stage IA and IB1 (<2 cm)*: In such women with early stage cervical cancer, simple trachelectomy or large conisation appear to be appropriate treatment strategies. Kindly refer to Table 17.4 and Flow chart 17.1 for details.

❖ *FIGO stage IB1 (>2 cm) or greater*: In these cases, neo-adjuvant chemotherapy can be administered if there is no evidence of lymph node involvement on lympha-denectomy.

Gestational Age of More Than 16 Weeks

❖ *Early stage disease*: For pregnant women with early stage disease (FIGO IA1, IA2, IB1 <2 cm) diagnosed after 16 weeks of gestation, treatment may be delayed to allow foetal maturity to occur, provided the tumour size is less than 2 cm. In these cases, steroids can be administered to the mother for promoting foetal lung maturity. With present advances in the care of preterm baby, delivery at 32–34 weeks of gestation can now be justified.

For women with stage IA1 cervical cancer, vaginal delivery is acceptable provided they had negative margins at the time of their diagnostic conisation. However, caesarean delivery should be performed for women with other higher stages of disease due to concerns regarding haemorrhage from cervical lesions and increased dissemination of malignant cells with vaginal delivery. Further evaluation may be required during the postpartum period in women with stage IA1 cervical cancer with positive margins on diagnostic conisation.

❖ *Late stage disease*: For women presenting with late stage disease (FIGO stage IB2 and greater) after 16 weeks of gestation, there is no good evidence supporting the delay of treatment to allow foetal maturity. Some oncologists suggest that treatment should not be postponed for tumour exceeding 4 cm in size or those with positive lymph nodes. However, if the patient does not want an early delivery, administration of neoadjuvant chemotherapy until delivery can prove to be useful.

In these cases, consideration should be given towards the use of neoadjuvant chemotherapy in the second and third trimesters of pregnancy. However, presently there is limited evidence regarding the safety of these drugs. For patients treated with neoadjuvant chemotherapy during pregnancy for locally advanced disease or node-positive disease, the clinician must proceed with a radical hysterectomy, which can be done at the time of caesarean delivery or as a second surgical procedure. However, other oncologists prefer termination of pregnancy and initiation of definitive treatment for these patients because of the high risk of recurrence.

❖ Radiotherapy is employed for more advanced lesions (stage IIB and above). It is usually administered in form of external beam therapy and intracavitary brachytherapy. This is likely to result in exposure of about 40–50 Gy. With such high doses, most pregnancies are likely to abort with 5 weeks. Radiation therapy, therefore, should not be administered to women with invasive cervical cancer who desire preservation of their pregnancy because radiotherapy is likely to result in foetal loss or other harm.

❖ In cases of advanced lesions, the maternal prognosis is poor. The woman may prefer to compromise her own treatment if this could help reduce the risk to her foetus. Careful sensitive counselling by the clinician may be required in these cases.

COMPLICATIONS

Complications associated with cervical cancer in pregnancy are as follows:[42,43]

❖ Miscarriage
❖ Premature labour, premature rupture of membranes, preterm births
❖ Secondary cervical dystocia
❖ Traumatic postpartum haemorrhage (due to injury to the cervix and lower segment)
❖ Lochiometra and pyometra
❖ Uterine sepsis.

CLINICAL PEARLS

❖ Caesarean section is the preferred mode of delivery in all stages of cervical cancer except those with stage IA1 disease with negative margins on diagnostic conisation. Vaginal delivery may be associated with increased dissemination of malignant cells. There is risk of local recurrence within the episiotomy sites.
❖ Radical hysterectomy at the time of caesarean delivery is associated with a greater amount of blood loss. However, the rate of other complications is not increased.

EVIDENCE-BASED MEDICINE

❖ No evidence has been identified, which suggests that pregnancy accelerates the natural history of cervical cancer. The available evidence indicates that the choice of therapeutic modality for pregnancy with cervical cancer should be decided in the same manner as for non-pregnant patients.[38-40]
❖ The available evidence indicates that cervical biopsies can be performed during pregnancy without any increased risk of bleeding. Bleeding, if encountered at the time of biopsy, can be controlled with the application of Monsel's solution or sutures.[44]
❖ Endocervical curettage is not performed during pregnancy because of the concerns that it may disrupt the pregnancy. However, there is no definitive evidence to indicate this.[38]
❖ Cervical conisation during pregnancy is associated with an increased risk of complications such as haemorrhage and spontaneous miscarriage.[45,46] Therefore, diagnostic conisation is only indicated during pregnancy if confirmation of the invasive disease may alter the timing or mode of delivery. Otherwise, it is better to postpone conisation until the postpartum period to avoid disrupting the pregnancy.

OVARIAN TUMOURS DURING PREGNANCY

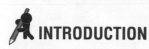

INTRODUCTION

The incidence of ovarian tumours in pregnancy is approximately 1:1,000 deliveries. However, the occurrence of ovarian cancer per se is a rare occurrence in pregnancy. The overall incidence of a symptomatic ovarian cyst in a premenopausal female being malignant is approximately 1:1,000. This risk may increase to 3:1,000 by the age of 50 years. Regarding ovarian cancer during pregnancy, germ cell tumours and epithelial cell cancers each account for 30–40% cases. The remainder are sex-cord stromal cell tumours. Nearly two-thirds of epithelial cell cancers in pregnancy are of 'low malignant potential'. Dysgerminomas are the most common malignant tumours in pregnancy.

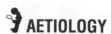

AETIOLOGY

Various adnexal masses, which can be encountered during pregnancy, are enumerated in Box 17.2. Malignancy accounts for nearly 3–6% of the tumours in the ovaries. Various non-neoplastic lesions of the ovary, which may resolve spontaneously after deliveries include luteoma of pregnancy, follicular cysts of pregnancy, hyperreactio luteinalis, granulosa cell proliferations, hilus cell hyperplasia, etc.

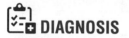

DIAGNOSIS

Clinical Presentation

A thorough medical history should be taken from the woman with specific attention to various reproductive or endocrine

Box 17.2: Types of adnexal masses

Benign ovarian cysts
- Functional cysts
- Endometrioma
- Serous cystadenoma
- Mucinous cystadenoma
- Mature teratoma (dermoid)

Benign non-ovarian cysts
- Paratubal cyst
- Hydrosalpinges
- Tubo-ovarian abscess
- Peritoneal pseudocysts
- Appendiceal abscess
- Diverticular abscess
- Pelvic kidney

Primary malignant ovarian tumours
- Germ cell tumour
- Epithelial carcinoma
- Sex-cord tumour

Secondary malignant ovarian tumours
- Predominantly breast and gastrointestinal carcinoma

Table 17.5: Various reproductive and endocrine factors affecting the risk of ovarian cancer

Factors decreasing the risk of ovarian cancer	Factors increasing the risk of ovarian cancer
• Pregnancy/multiparity • Use of the oral contraceptive pill • Breastfeeding • Tubal ligation or hysterectomy.	• Infertility (nulliparity) • Endometriosis/polycystic ovarian syndrome • Hormone replacement therapy/fertility treatment (role is still doubtful) • Early menarche (before the age of 12 years) and late age at menopause (after the age of 52 years).

Table 17.6: Clinical presentation in cases of epithelial ovarian cancer

Acute presentation	Subacute presentation
• *Pleural effusion*: Shortness of breath • *Bowel obstruction*: Severe nausea and vomiting • Venous thrombo-embolism	• *Adnexal mass*: Discovered on a routine pelvic examination or an imaging study performed for another indication • *Pelvic and abdominal symptoms*: Bloating, urinary urgency or frequency, difficulty in eating or early satiety, pelvic or abdominal pain

factors affecting the risk for ovarian malignancy (Table 17.5) and a family history of ovarian or breast cancer. Symptoms suggestive of endometriosis should be specifically considered. Also, symptoms suggestive of possible ovarian malignancy, e.g. persistent abdominal distension, change in appetite including increased satiety, pelvic or abdominal pain, increased urinary urgency and/or frequency must also be enquired.[47,48] Acute and chronic presentation in cases of epithelial ovarian cancer is described in Table 17.6.

A careful physical examination of the woman is essential and should include abdominal and vaginal examination, and the presence or absence of enlarged lymph nodes.

Investigations

Serum CA-125 Levels

CA-125 is a surface glycoprotein found on the surface of ovarian cancer cells and on some normal tissues. A high CA-125 level could be a sign of cancer or other conditions. The CA-125 test should not be used as a standalone test to diagnose ovarian cancer. The FDA has approved this test for monitoring a woman's response to ovarian cancer treatment and for detecting its return following treatment. Values of CA-125 greater than 35 IU/mL are found in over 80% of cases with non-mucinous epithelial ovarian cancers. In cases of elevated serum CA-125 levels, serial monitoring of CA-125 may be helpful because rapidly rising levels are more likely to be associated with malignancy in comparison to the high levels, which remain static.[49] If serum CA-125 levels are raised but less than 200 units/mL, further investigation may be required to exclude or treat the common causes of adnexal mass.

In case, the serum CA-125 levels are more than 200 units/mL, there are high chances of malignancy. In these cases, discussion with a gynaecological oncologist is recommended.

Estimation of CA-125 levels is associated with low specificity because it can also be raised in presence of benign conditions like endometriosis, tuberculosis, leiomyomas, liver or kidney disease, pelvic inflammatory disease, etc. A serum CA-125 assay does not need to be undertaken in all premenopausal women when an ultrasonographic diagnosis of a simple ovarian cyst has been made.[50-52] In case the adnexal mass does not show any feature of malignancy (i.e. the mass is freely mobile, cystic in consistency and of regular contour), a period of observation of no more than 2 months can be allowed during which hormonal suppression with OCPs can be used. A benign mass would regress, while a malignant mass would be persistent and mandates surgical removal.

Other serum markers: Other serum markers such as lactate dehydrogenase, α-fetoprotein (α-FP) and hCG should be measured in all women under the age of 40 years with a complex ovarian mass because of the possibility of germ cell tumours.

Ultrasonography

Pelvic ultrasound is the single most effective way for evaluating an ovarian mass. Transvaginal ultrasonography is usually preferred over transabdominal ultrasound due to its increased sensitivity.[49] Increased diagnostic accuracy is not likely to occur with the use of colour flow Doppler.[50-52] In complex cases, the combined use of the transvaginal ultrasound examination with colour flow mapping and 3D imaging is likely to improve sensitivity.[53,54] Nevertheless, there is no single ultrasound finding which clearly differentiates between benign and malignant ovarian masses.

Computed Tomography and Magnetic Resonance Imaging

Presently, the routine use of CT and MRI for assessment of ovarian masses is not likely to improve the sensitivity or specificity obtained by transvaginal ultrasonography in the detection of ovarian malignancy. These imaging modalities are likely to have a place in the evaluation of more complex lesions.

Estimation of the Risk of Malignancy

An estimation of the risk of malignancy is essential for the assessment of an ovarian mass. At present, the most widely used index, Risk of Malignancy Index-I (RMI-I) for evaluation of malignancy is described in Box 17.3. However, recent studies have shown that a specific model comprising of the ultrasound parameters, derived from the International Ovarian Tumour Analysis (IOTA) Group (Table 17.7),[55,56] is likely to be associated with increased sensitivity and specificity.[57] On the other hand, a systematic review of diagnostic studies has shown that the RMI-I is likely to be most effective for women with suspected ovarian malignancy.[58] According to the recommendations by the NICE guideline on ovarian cancer,[59] RMI score should be calculated for all women with suspected ovarian malignancy and should be used for guiding the woman's management.

Box 17.3: Risk of Malignancy Index I

Definition
Combination of three presurgical features:
1. Serum CA-125 (CA-125)
2. Menopausal status (M)
3. Ultrasound score (U)

Calculation
RMI = U × M × CA-125

Note: U=ultrasound score. The ultrasound result is scored 1 point for each of the following characteristics: multilocular cysts, solid areas, metastases, ascites and bilateral lesions.
U = 0 (for an ultrasound score of 0), U = 1 (for an ultrasound score of 1), U = 3 (for an ultrasound score of 2–5). The menopausal status is scored as 1 = premenopausal and 3 = postmenopausal; serum CA-125 is measured in IU/mL and can vary from 0 to 100 or even 1,000 of units.

Table 17.7: IOTA Group ultrasound 'rules' for classification of masses as benign or malignant[55,56]

Characteristics	B-rules (Benign)	M-rules (Malignant)
Consistency: Cystic/solid	Unilocular cysts	Irregular solid tumour
Presence of solid components	The largest solid component <7 mm	Solid components >7 mm
Ascites	Absent	Present
Presence of acoustic shadowing	Present	Absent
Papillary structures	Less than four papillary structures	Four or more papillary structures
Surface: smooth/irregular	Smooth	Irregular
Tumour diameter	Largest diameter <100 mm	Largest diameter ≥100 mm
Blood flow	No blood flow	Very strong blood flow

Abbreviation: IOTA, international ovarian tumour analysis

MANAGEMENT

The rationale of management is based on principles summarised in Box 17.4.
- Immediate surgical removal may be required for symptomatic adnexal lesions.
- Many asymptomatic ovarian masses in the premenopausal woman can be managed conservatively, e.g. functional or simple ovarian cysts (thin-walled cysts without internal structures), which are less than 6 cm in maximum diameter. These functional cysts may resolve over 2–3 menstrual cycles without requirement for any intervention. A repeat ultrasound can be performed after 16 weeks to confirm their absence.[60] Ovarian cysts that persist or increase in size are unlikely to be functional and may necessitate surgical management.
- According to the consensus statement by the Society of Radiologists in Ultrasound, asymptomatic simple cysts

CHAPTER 17

Box 17.4: The rationale of management to minimise morbidity in case of adnexal masses encountered during pregnancy

❑ Adoption of conservative management where possible
❑ Use of laparoscopic techniques where appropriate, thus avoiding laparotomy as far as possible
❑ Referral to a gynaecological oncologist where appropriate

30–50 mm in diameter do not require follow-up; cysts 50–70 mm require follow-up, and cysts more than 70 mm in diameter should be considered for either further management in terms of imaging (MRI) or surgical intervention.[61]

❖ If surgery is indicated, a laparoscopic approach is generally considered to be the gold standard for the management of benign ovarian masses.[62-64] Laparotomy may be rarely required for persistent complex ovarian masses.[65,66] Surgery in these cases is performed via a lower midline incision, which allows surgical access with minimal uterine manipulation.

❖ Elevated levels of tumour markers such as CA-125, α-FP and hCG are helpful for management of ovarian masses in non-pregnant women. However, these markers are anyway elevated in a normal pregnancy. Therefore, their measurement does not prove useful for management of adnexal masses in the antenatal period. However, extremely high levels of these markers may be a pointer towards an underlying ovarian tumour.

❖ Wherever possible, a simple cystectomy with ovarian conservation is attempted at the time of surgery. Other-wise, a unilateral salpingo-oophorectomy may be performed. As far as possible, bilateral oophorectomy must be avoided. Peritoneal washings and omental and peritoneal biopsies must be collected at the time of surgery. Frozen sections obtained from the contralateral ovary can help in intraoperative management. Para-aortic lymph node sampling and debulking surgery can be considered in complex cases. Surgical management is usually undertaken after preoperative assessment using RMI-I or ultrasound rules (IOTA Group).

❖ The benign ovarian masses should be preferably removed via the umbilical laparoscopic port due to reduced post-operative pain and a quicker retrieval time than when using lateral ports of the same size.

❖ Spillage of cyst contents should be avoided as far as possible during surgery because preoperative and intra-operative assessments are unable to absolutely rule out malignancy. Consideration should be given towards the use of a tissue bag to avoid spillage of cystic contents into the peritoneal cavity, especially in cases of malignancy. In case there is some inadvertent spillage of the contents of the cyst, meticulous peritoneal lavage of the peritoneal cavity should be performed using large amounts of warmed saline.

❖ Surgical treatment is enough for early stage malignancy such as stage I epithelial cell cancers, tumours of low-grade malignant potential and stage Ia dysgerminomas. Adjunctive treatment is not required in these cases. On the other hand, other forms of germ cell tumours and more advanced epithelial cell cancers require adjunctive treatment with chemotherapy following surgery. In these cases, drugs such as bleomycin, etoposide, cisplatin, vincristine and vinblastine have been tried postoperatively beyond the first trimester.

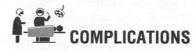

COMPLICATIONS

Recognition of adnexal masses has increased in pregnancy due to the extensive use of ultrasound. Although most adnexal masses remain asymptomatic, 10–15% may rupture, bleed or may be associated with adnexal torsion. These adverse events are likely to increase the risk of adverse events such as miscarriage or preterm labour. Occasionally, a hormone producing adnexal mass may cause virilisation. Ovarian masses may sometimes also cause dystocia during labour.

CLINICAL PEARLS

❖ Aspiration of ovarian cysts through any route, either vaginal or laparoscopic, is usually not effective and is associated with a high rate of recurrence.
❖ Pregnancy does not alter the course of cancer but may cause delay in its diagnosis.

EVIDENCE-BASED MEDICINE

❖ Although clinical examination has poor sensitivity in the detection of ovarian masses (15–51%), it is important in the evaluation of mass tenderness, mobility, nodularity and ascites.[48,67]
❖ The available evidence indicates that the use of chemo-therapy in the first trimester is associated with an increased risk of foetal abnormalities. Treatment during the second and third trimester would appear safer, but the data is limited.[68]

REFERENCES

1. Pavlidis NA. Coexistence of pregnancy and malignancy. Oncologist. 2002;7(4):279-87.
2. Pentheroudakis G, Pavlidis N. Cancer and pregnancy: poena magna, not anymore. Eur J Cancer. 2006;42(2):126-40.
3. Hoellen F, Reibke R, Hornemann K, Thill M, Lueddders DW, Kelling K, et al. Cancer in pregnancy. Part I: basic diagnostic and therapeutic principles and treatment of gynecological malignancies. Arch Gynecol Obstet. 2012;285(1):195-205.
4. Lee YY, Roberts CL, Dobbins T, Stavrou E, Black K, Morris J, et al. Incidence and outcomes of pregnancy-associated cancer in Australia, 1994-2008: a population-based linkage study. BJOG. 2012;119(13):1572-82.
5. Schover LR. Psychosocial issues associated with cancer in pregnancy. Semin Oncol. 2000;27(6):699-703.

6. Fattibene P, Mazzei F, Nuccetelli C, Risica S. Prenatal exposure to ionizing radiation: sources, effects and regulatory aspects. Acta Paediatr. 1999;88(7):693-702.

7. Muirhead CR, Kneale GW. Prenatal irradiation and childhood cancer. J Radiol Prot. 1989;9:209.

8. Doll DC, Ringenberg QS, Yarbro JW. Antineoplastic agents and pregnancy. Semin Oncol. 1989;16(5):337-46.

9. Partridge AH, Garber JE. Long-term outcomes of children exposed to antineoplastic agents in utero. Semin Oncol. 2000; 27(6):712-26.

10. Smith LH, Danielsen B, Allen ME, Cress R. Cancer associated with obstetric delivery: results of linkage with the California cancer registry. Am J Obstet Gynecol. 2003;189(4):1128-35.

11. Andersson TM, Johansson AL, Hsieh CC, Cnattingius S, Lambe M. Increasing incidence of pregnancy-associated breast cancer in Sweden. Obstet Gynecol. 2009;114(3):568-72.

12. Beadle BM, Woodward WA, Middleton LP, Tereffe W, Strom EA, Litton JK, et al. The impact of pregnancy on breast cancer outcomes in women ≤35 years. Cancer. 2009;115(6):1174-84.

13. Hahn KM, Johnson PH, Gordon N, Kuerer H, Middleton L, Ramirez M, et al. Treatment of pregnant breast cancer patients and outcomes of children exposed to chemotherapy in utero. Cancer. 2006;107(6):1219-26.

14. Gwyn K. Children exposed to chemotherapy in utero. J Natl Cancer Inst Monogr. 2005;(34):69-71.

15. Giacalone PL, Laffargue F, Bénos P. Chemotherapy for breast carcinoma during pregnancy: a French national survey. Cancer. 1999;86(11):2266-72.

16. Ring AE, Smith IE, Jones A, Shannon C, Galani E, Ellis PA. Chemotherapy for breast cancer during pregnancy: an 18-year experience from five London teaching hospitals. J Clin Oncol. 2005;23(18):4192-7.

17. Watson WJ. Herceptin (trastuzumab) therapy during pregnancy: association with reversible anhydramnios. Obstet Gynecol. 2005;105(3):642-3.

18. Mir O, Berveiller P, Ropert S, Goffinet F, Pons G, Treluyer JM, et al. Emerging therapeutic options for breast cancer chemotherapy during pregnancy. Ann Oncol. 2008;19(4): 607-13.

19. Egan PC, Costanza ME, Dodion P, Egorin MJ, Bachur NR. Doxorubicin and cisplatin excretion into human milk. Cancer Treat Rep. 1985;69(12):1387-9.

20. Gaffield ME, Culwell KR. (2010). New recommendations on the safety of contraceptive methods for women with medical conditions. World Health Organization's Medical eligibility criteria for contraceptive use, 4th edition. IPPF Medical Bulletin. [online] IPPF website. Available from www.ippf.org/ NR/rdonlyres/D67E0B0E-39C9-4A0A-99E744AD870C5058/0/ MedBullEnglishMar2010.pdf [Accessed July, 2016]

21. Partridge AH, Gelber S, Peppercorn J, Sampson E, Knudsen K, Laufer M, et al. Web-based survey of fertility issues in young women with breast cancer. J Clin Oncol. 2004;22(20):4174-83.

22. Braun M, Hasson-Ohayon I, Perry S, Kaufman B, Uziely B. Motivation for giving birth after breast cancer. Psychooncology. 2005;14(4):282-96.

23. Connell S, Patterson C, Newman B. A qualitative analysis of reproductive issues raised by young Australian women with breast cancer. Health Care Women Int. 2006;27(1):94-110.

24. Peate M, Meiser B, Hickey M, Friedlander M. The fertility related concerns, needs and preferences of younger women with breast cancer: a systematic review. Breast Cancer Res Treat. 2009;116(2):215-23.

25. Royal College of Physicians, The Royal College of Radiologists, Royal College of Obstetricians and Gynaecologists. (2007). The effects of cancer treatment on reproductive functions. Guidance on management. [online] Available from www. bookshop.rcplondon.ac.uk/contents/pub238-5e88e6e4-d9d0-4e99-a2f9-b1bea2daf562.pdf [Accessed July, 2016].

26. Maltaris T, Weigel M, Mueller A, Schmidt M, Seufert R, Fischl F, et al. Cancer and fertility preservation: fertility preservation in breast cancer patients. Breast Cancer Res. 2008;10(2):206.

27. Recchia F, Saggio G, Amiconi G, Di Blasio A, Cesta A, Candeloro G, et al. Gonadotropin-releasing hormone analogues added to adjuvant chemotherapy protect ovarian function and improve clinical outcomes in young women with early breast carcinoma. Cancer. 2006;106(3):514-23.

28. Maisano R, Caristi N, Mare M, Bottari M, Adamo V, Mafodda A, et al. Protective effect of leuprolide on ovarian function in young women treated with adjuvant chemotherapy for early breast cancer: a multicenter phase II study. J Chemother. 2008;20(6):740-3.

29. Badawy A, Elnashar A, El-Ashry M, Shahat M. Gonadotropin releasing hormone agonists for prevention of chemotherapy-induced ovarian damage: prospective randomized study. Fertil Steril. 2009;91(3):694-7.

30. Ives A, Saunders C, Bulsara M, Semmens J. Pregnancy after breast cancer: population based study. BMJ. 2007;334 (7586): 194.

31. Blakely LJ, Buzdar AU, Lozada JA, Shullaih SA, Hoy E, Smith TL, et al. Effects of pregnancy after treatment for breast carcinoma on survival and risk of recurrence. Cancer. 2004;100(3):465-9.

32. Sutton R, Buzdar AU, Hortobagyi GN. Pregnancy and offspring after adjuvant chemotherapy in breast cancer patients. Cancer. 1990;65(4):847-50.

33. Langagergaard V, Gislum M, Skriver MV, Nørgård B, Lash TL, Rothman KJ, et al. Birth outcome in women with breast cancer. Br J Cancer. 2006;94(1):142-6.

34. Smith LH, Dalrymple JL, Leiserowitz GS, Danielsen B, Gilbert WM. Obstetrical deliveries associated with maternal malignancy in California, 1992 through 1997. Am J Obstet Gynecol. 2001;184(7):1504-12.

35. Smith LH, Danielsen B, Allen ME, Cress R. Cancer associated with obstetric delivery: results of linkage with the California cancer registry. Am J Obstet Gynecol. 2003;189(4):1128-35.

36. Demeter A, Sziller I, Csapó Z, Szánthó A, Papp Z. Outcome of pregnancies after cold-knife conization of the uterine cervix during pregnancy. Eur J Gynaecol Oncol. 2002;23(3):207-10.

37. Duggan B, Muderspach LI, Roman LD, Curtin JP, d'Ablaing G, Morrow CP. Cervical cancer in pregnancy: reporting on planned delay in therapy. Obstet Gynecol. 1993;82(4 Pt 1): 598-602.

38. Van Calsteren K, Vergote I, Amant F. Cervical neoplasia during pregnancy: diagnosis, management and prognosis. Best Pract Res Clin Obstet Gynaecol. 2005;19(4):611-30.

39. Hopkins MP, Morley GW. The prognosis and management of cervical cancer associated with pregnancy. Obstet Gynecol. 1992;80(1):9-13.

40. Method MW, Brost BC. Management of cervical cancer in pregnancy. Semin Surg Oncol. 1999;16(3):251-60.

41. Massad LS, Einstein MH, Huh WK, Katki HA, Kinney WK, Schiffman M, et al. 2012 updated consensus guidelines for the management of abnormal cervical cancer screening tests and cancer precursors. Obstet Gynecol. 2013;121(4):829-46.

42. Lee JM, Lee KB, Kim YT, Ryu HS, Kim YT, Cho CH, et al. Cervical cancer associated with pregnancy: results of a

multicenter retrospective Korean study (KGOG-1006). Am J Obstet Gynecol. 2008;198(1):92.e1-6.

43. Zemlickis D, Lishner M, Degendorfer P, Panzarella T, Sutcliffe SB, Koren G. Maternal and fetal outcome after invasive cervical cancer in pregnancy. J Clin Oncol. 1991;9(11):1956-61.

44. Economos K, Perez Veridiano N, Delke I, Collado ML, Tancer ML. Abnormal cervical cytology in pregnancy: a 17-year experience. Obstet Gynecol. 1993;81(6):915-8.

45. Averette HE, Nasser N, Yankow SL, Little WA. Cervical conization in pregnancy. Analysis of 180 operations. Am J Obstet Gynecol. 1970;106(4):543-9.

46. Hannigan EV, Whitehouse HH, Atkinson WD, Becker SN. Cone biopsy during pregnancy. Obstet Gynecol. 1982;60(4):450-5.

47. Department of Health. (2009). Key messages for ovarian cancer for health professionals. [online] Available from www.dh.gov.uk/en/Publicationsandstatistics/publications/publicationspolicyandguidance/DH_110534 [Accessed July, 2016].

48. Ueland FR, Depriest PD, Desimone CP, Pavlik EJ, Lele SM, Kryscio RJ, et al. The accuracy of examination under anesthesia and transvaginal sonography in evaluating ovarian size. Gynecol Oncol. 2005;99(2):400-3.

49. American College of Obstetricians and Gynecologists. Management of Adnexal Masses. ACOG Practice Bulletin No. 83. Washington DC: ACOG; 2007.

50. Sassone AM, Timor-Tritsch IE, Artner A, Westhoff C, Warren WB. Transvaginal sonographic characterization of ovarian disease: evaluation of a new scoring system to predict ovarian malignancy. Obstet Gynecol. 1991;78(1):70-6.

51. Vuento MH, Pirhonen JP, Mäkinen JI, Laippala PJ, Grönroos M, Salmi TA. Evaluation of ovarian findings in asymptomatic postmenopausal women with color Doppler ultrasound. Cancer. 1995;76(7):1214-8.

52. Stein SM, Laifer-Narin S, Johnson MB, Roman LD, Muderspach LI, Tyszka JM, et al. Differentiation of benign and malignant adnexal masses: relative value of gray-scale, color Doppler, and spectral Doppler sonography. AJR Am J Roentgenol. 1995;164(2):381-6.

53. Dai SY, Hata K, Inubashiri E, Kanenishi K, Shiota A, Ohno M, et al. Does three-dimensional power Doppler ultrasound improve the diagnostic accuracy for the prediction of adnexal malignancy? J Obstet Gynaecol Res. 2008;34(3):364-70.

54. Guerriero S, Ajossa S, Piras S, Gerada M, Floris S, Garau N, et al. Three-dimensional quantification of tumor vascularity as a tertiary test after B-mode and power Doppler evaluation for detection of ovarian cancer. J Ultrasound Med. 2007;26(10):1271-8.

55. Timmerman D, Testa AC, Bourne T, Ferrazzi E, Ameye L, Konstantinovic ML, et al. Logistic regression model to distinguish between the benign and malignant adnexal mass before surgery: a multicenter study by the International Ovarian Tumor Analysis Group. J Clin Oncol. 2005;23:8794-801.

56. Timmerman D, Valentin L, Bourne TH, Collins WP, Verrelst H, Vergote I; International Ovarian Tumor Analysis (IOTA) Group. Terms, definitions and measurements to describe the sonographic features of adnexal tumors: a consensus opinion from the International Ovarian Tumor Analysis (IOTA) Group. Ultrasound Obstet Gynecol. 2000;16:500-5.

57. Timmerman D, Testa AC, Bourne T, Ameye L, Jurkovic D, Van Holsbeke C, et al. Simple ultrasound-based rules for the diagnosis of ovarian cancer. Ultrasound Obstet Gynecol. 2008;31(6):681-90.

58. Geomini P, Kruitwagen R, Bremer GL, Cnossen J, Mol BW. The accuracy of risk scores in predicting ovarian malignancy: a systematic review. Obstet Gynecol. 2009;113 (2 Pt 1):384-94.

59. National Institute for Health and Clinical Excellence. Ovarian cancer: The Recognition and Initial Management of Ovarian Cancer. NICE clinical guideline 122. London: NICE; 2011.

60. MacKenna A, Fabres C, Alam V, Morales V. Clinical management of functional ovarian cysts: a prospective and randomized study. Hum Reprod. 2000;15(12):2567-9.

61. Levine D, Brown DL, Andreotti RF, Benacerraf B, Benson CB, Brewster WR, et al. Management of asymptomatic ovarian and other adnexal cysts imaged at US: Society of Radiologists in Ultrasound Consensus Conference Statement. Radiology. 2010;256(3):943-54.

62. Canis M, Botchorishvili R, Manhes H, Wattiez A, Mage G, Pouly JL, et al. Management of adnexal masses: role and risk of laparoscopy. Semin Surg Oncol. 2000;19(1):28-35.

63. Mais V, Ajossa S, Mallarini G, Guerriero S, Oggiano MP, Melis GB. No recurrence of mature ovarian teratomas after laparoscopic cystectomy. BJOG. 2003;110(6):624-6.

64. Yuen PM, Yu KM, Yip SK, Lau WC, Rogers MS, Chang A. A randomized prospective study of laparoscopy and laparotomy in the management of benign ovarian masses. Am J Obstet Gynecol. 1997;177(1):109-14.

65. Panici PB, Muzii L, Palaia I, Manci N, Bellati F, Plotti F, et al. Minilaparotomy versus laparoscopy in the treatment of benign adnexal cysts: a randomized clinical study. Eur J Obstet Gynecol Reprod Biol. 2007;133(2):218-22.

66. Fanfani F, Fagotti A, Ercoli A, Bifulco G, Longo R, Mancuso S, et al. A prospective randomised study of laparoscopy and minilaparotomy in the management of benign adnexal masses. Hum Reprod. 2004;19(10):2367-71.

67. Padilla LA, Radosevich DM, Milad MP. Accuracy of the pelvic examination in detecting adnexal masses. Obstet Gynecol. 2000;96(4):593-8.

68. Cardonick E, Iacobucci A. Use of chemotherapy during human pregnancy. Lancet Oncol. 2004;5(5):283-91.

CHAPTER 17

Dermatological Disorders during Pregnancy

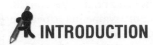

INTRODUCTION

Pregnancy is characterised by many skin changes, which can be divided into three categories: (1) hormone-related, (2) pre-existing, and (3) pregnancy-specific conditions. Normal hormone-related changes during pregnancy may cause benign skin conditions including striae gravidarum (stretch marks); hyperpigmentation (e.g. melasma); and hair, nail and vascular changes. Pre-existing skin conditions may either improve or exacerbate in pregnancy due to immunological changes in pregnancy such as depressed cell-mediated immunity. These include conditions such as atopic dermatitis, psoriasis, fungal infections, cutaneous tumours, etc. There are, however, few severely pruritic inflammatory skin dermatoses that are specific to pregnancy and are observed only during pregnancy. Approximately 30–50% of women may present with one of the specific dermatoses of pregnancy. Although most of these skin dermatoses are benign and resolve in postpartum period, a few can act as a threat to the foetus, thereby requiring antenatal surveillance.

AETIOLOGY

Profound changes occur in the woman's immune system during pregnancy to prevent rejection of the foetus and placenta. A shift occurs from a predominantly T helper 1 lymphocyte profile to a T-helper 2 profile during pregnancy. This transition alters the cytokines that are produced by the placenta. As a result, levels of interleukin 12 and γ-interferon are reduced and those of interleukin 4 and 10 are increased. These changes reduce cell-mediated immunity, thereby increasing the woman's susceptibility to develop skin disease, and increasing the risk of autoimmune diseases and skin infections. Diseases such as psoriasis that are driven by the T helper 1 immune response tend to improve, whereas those driven by the T helper 2 immune response, such as

atopic eczema and systemic lupus erythematosus, may be exacerbated.[1]

The most recent classification of dermatoses proposed by Ambros-Rudolph et al.[2] in 2006 has presented four main conditions:
1. Atopic eruption of pregnancy (AEP)
2. Polymorphic eruption of pregnancy (PEP)
3. Pemphigoid gestationis (PG)
4. Intrahepatic cholestasis (ICP).

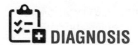

DIAGNOSIS

Clinical Presentation and Investigations

Clinical presentation and investigations of various pregnancy-specific dermatologic disorders are described in Table 18.1. Diagnosis of these conditions is based on clinical history and presentation. In cases of ICP of pregnancy, diagnosis is based on the presence of clinical symptoms such as pruritus with or without jaundice, no primary skin lesions, and laboratory markers of cholestasis. While AEP presents significantly earlier in pregnancy, PEP, PG and ICP present in late pregnancy.

MANAGEMENT

❖ Atopic eruption of pregnancy and PEP are benign skin conditions and are usually not associated with any foetal or maternal risk. Patients with PG and ICP of pregnancy carry foetal risk and require specific treatment. These lesions usually resolve in early postpartum period.
❖ During pregnancy, lesions such as a AEP and PEP respond well to topical emollients and moderately potent steroids in combination with oral antihistaminic agents.
❖ Antepartum surveillance is recommended for patients with ICP of pregnancy, impetigo herpetiformis and PG.

Table 18.1: Clinical presentations and investigations of pregnancy-specific dermatologic disorders

Conditions	Rash presentation	Pregnancy risk
Polymorphic eruption of pregnancy[3,4]		
Also known as pruritic urticarial papules and plaques of pregnancy (PUPPP), it occurs with an incidence of one in 160 pregnancies and is the second most common skin dermatosis in pregnancy after atopic eczema. It is associated with multiple gestation and increased maternal weight gain. It usually occurs in primigravidas in the third trimester and usually does not recur in subsequent pregnancies. The exact aetiology is not known. It has been proposed that stretching of the skin damages the connective tissue causing subsequent conversion of non-antigenic molecules to antigenic ones, resulting in development of skin eruptions.	The eruption begins over the abdomen, commonly involving striae gravidarum. The periumbilical region is usually spared. Skin lesions, which are commonly observed, include polymorphous, erythematous, non-follicular papules, plaques, and sometimes vesicles. The eruption may spread to the breasts, upper thighs and arms. The face, palms, soles and mucosal surfaces are usually spared. The eruption may first appear in postpartum period. PUPPP has a marked pruritic component and the onset of pruritus coincides with the skin lesions.	The lesions resolve near term or in the early postpartum period. The maternal and foetal prognosis is excellent and no adverse effects have been identified.
Prurigo of pregnancy[5]		
This condition occurs approximately one in every 300 pregnancies. The aetiology and pathogenesis is not known, although there may be a history of atopy at times.	Erythematous papules and nodules are present on the extensor surfaces of the legs and upper arms. Sometimes the papules may also be present on the abdomen.	The time of onset is variable and can occur in all the three trimesters. No adverse effects for the mother or the foetus have been identified.
Intrahepatic cholestasis of pregnancy[6,7]		
This condition is also known as pruritus gravidarum because its classic presentation is severe pruritus in the third trimester. The aetiology of intrahepatic cholestasis remains controversial. A family history of the condition is common, and there is an association with the presence of human leukocyte antigen-A31 (HLA-A31) and HLA-B8. There may be a family history of cholelithiasis and a high risk of gallstones. Laboratory investigations suggestive of ICP include elevated serum bile acid levels (10 μmol per L or more) and alkaline phosphatase levels with or without elevated bilirubin levels. Aspartate and alanine transaminase levels and other liver function tests may be mildly abnormal. The condition tends to recur in subsequent pregnancies.	This disorder is characterised by pruritus with or without jaundice, absence of primary skin lesions, and with laboratory markers of cholestasis. The skin lesions are usually secondary linear excoriations and excoriated papules, which are caused by scratching and are localised on the extensor surfaces of the limbs, abdomen and back. The severity of skin lesions relates with the duration of pruritus.	There is a risk of premature delivery, meconium-stained amniotic fluid, intrauterine foetal demise due to anoxia caused by reduced foetal elimination of toxic bile acids. Cholestasis and jaundice in patients with severe or prolonged intrahepatic cholestasis of pregnancy may cause vitamin K deficiency and coagulopathy. Therefore, early diagnosis, prompt treatment, and close obstetric surveillance become obligatory in cases of ICP.
Pemphigoid gestationis[8,9]		
This is a rare autoimmune disorder occurring in approximately one in 50,000 pregnancies. The condition has been linked to the presence of HLA-DR3 and HLA-DR4 and has a rare association with molar pregnancies and choriocarcinoma. The condition usually begins in the second or third trimester and may resolve late in pregnancy. However, the condition may classically flare up again at delivery.	There may be pruritic papules, plaques, and vesicles evolving into generalised vesicles or bullae. Initial periumbilical lesions may sometimes generalise to involve other body parts. However, the face, scalp, and mucous membranes are usually not affected.	Newborns may have urticarial, vesicular, or bullous lesions. There is a risk of premature deliveries and birth of small for gestational age infants as a result of placental failure. Therefore, antenatal surveillance is advised in these cases.
Impetigo herpetiformis[10,11]		
It is a form of severe pustular psoriasis occurring during pregnancy. This condition usually response to steroids.	This disorder is characterised by the presence of round, arched, or polycyclic patches covered with small painful pustules in a herpetiform pattern. Most commonly affected regions are thighs and groin. Sometimes, the rash may coalesce and spread to the trunk and extremities. Mucous membranes may also be involved. Regions such as face, hands and feet are usually not affected.	There are reports of increased foetal morbidity.
Pruritic folliculitis of pregnancy[12,13]		
This rare dermatosis occurs in the second and third trimester of pregnancy and affects approximately one in every 3,000 pregnancies. The skin lesions usually resolve spontaneously 1–2 months following delivery.	The disorder is characterised by presence of an acneiform eruption comprising of multiple, pruritic, 2–4 mm, follicular papules or pustules typically on the abdomen, arms, chest, shoulders and upper back. Pruritus is not a major feature and it may be mistaken for acne or microbial folliculitis.[8,9] The diagnosis is made clinically after excluding other, more common rashes.	No maternal or foetal adverse effects have been identified.
Atopic eruption of pregnancy[14]		
The eruption is more likely to occur in primigravida with single gestation pregnancy.	The skin eruption is likely to affect all parts of the body, including face, palms, and soles. The skin lesions are likely to begin early in pregnancy during the first and second trimester.	

Flow chart 18.1: Algorithm for management of the specific dermatoses of pregnancy

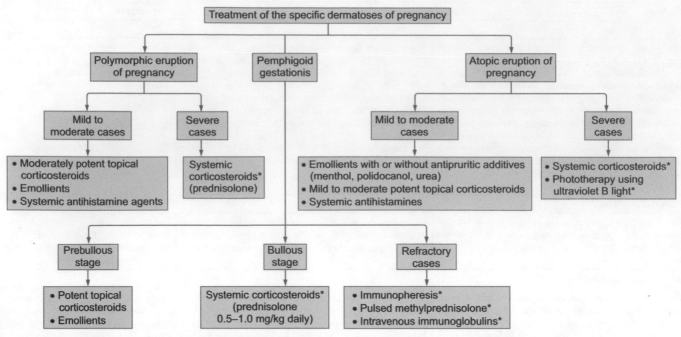

Note: *Management in secondary care under specialist supervision

❖ Treatment options in various dermatoses are summarised in Flow chart 18.1 and are described below:

- *Pruritic folliculitis of pregnancy:* Topical corticosteroids, topical benzoyl peroxide (Benzac) or narrowband (TL-01) ultraviolet B light therapy[15]
- *Impetigo herpetiformis:* Systemic corticosteroids; antibiotics for secondarily infected lesions
- *Pemphigoid gestationis:* Oral antihistamines and topical corticosteroids are used for mild cases. Systemic oral corticosteroids may be used for severe cases. In these cases, prednisolone is usually started in a dose of 0.5–1 mg/kg/day.[16] High-dose intravenous immunoglobulins may be required in cases, which are refractory to conventional therapy.[17]
- *Intrahepatic cholestasis of pregnancy:* Patients with mild pruritus may be treated with oral antihistamines. Patients with more severe cases require ursodeoxycholic acid (UDCA). UDCA helps in providing relief against pruritus and improving cholestasis while reducing adverse foetal outcomes.[18] Patients should receive increased antenatal surveillance at the time of diagnosis, and some authorities recommend delivery by 38 weeks of gestation. The impact of early delivery on reducing perinatal complications is not completely clear.
- *Prurigo of pregnancy:* Mid-potency topical corticosteroids and oral antihistamines.
- *Pruritic urticarial papules and plaques of pregnancy:* Oral antihistamines and topical corticosteroids can be used for pruritus. Systemic steroids may be used for severe cases of PUPPP.

COMPLICATIONS

There may be increased foetal morbidity due to the following causes:

❖ Prematurity
❖ Intrauterine growth restriction
❖ Foetal distress due to meconium-stained amniotic fluid
❖ Intrauterine foetal demise
❖ Coagulopathy due to vitamin K deficiency.

CLINICAL PEARLS

❖ Treatment of the specific dermatoses of pregnancy depends on the stage and severity of the disease.
❖ The aim of management in these cases is to control pruritus and skin lesions.
❖ In severe cases of dermatoses during early pregnancy, ultraviolet B phototherapy is a safe additional tool that can be used under specialist supervision.

EVIDENCE-BASED MEDICINE

❖ Ursodeoxycholic acid is considered to be the drug of choice in cases of ICP of pregnancy because this therapy helps in reducing both maternal pruritus and foetal mortality.[18]
❖ Current evidence does not support treatment with S-adenosylmethionine, anion exchange resins [e.g.

PART II

cholestyramine (Questran)], or corticosteroids in cases of ICP of pregnancy.[19]

REFERENCES

1. Vaughan Jones SA, Black MM. Pregnancy dermatoses. J Am Acad Dermatol. 1999;40(2 Pt 1):233-41.
2. Ambros-Rudolph CM, Mullegger RR, Vaughan-Jones SA, Kerl H, Black MM. The specific dermatoses of pregnancy revisited and reclassified: Results of a retrospective two-center study on 505 pregnant patients. J Am Acad Dermatol. 2006;54:395-404.
3. Matz H, Orion E, Wolf R. Pruritic urticarial papules and plaques of pregnancy: Polymorphic eruption of pregnancy (PUPPP). Clin Dermatol. 2006;24(2):105-8.
4. Brzoza Z, Kasperska-Zajac A, Oles E, Rogala B. Pruritic urticarial papules and plaques of pregnancy. J Midwifery Womens Health. 2007;52(1):44-8.
5. Vaughan Jones S, Ambros-Rudolph C, Nelson-Piercy C. Skin disease in pregnancy. BMJ. 2014;348:g3489.
6. Lammert F, Marschall HU, Glantz A, Matern S. Intrahepatic cholestasis of pregnancy: Molecular pathogenesis, diagnosis and management. J Hepatol. 2000;33(6):1012-21.
7. Glantz A, Marschall HU, Mattsson LA. Intrahepatic cholestasis of pregnancy: Relationships between bile acid levels and fetal complication rates. Hepatology. 2004;40(2):467-74.
8. Shimanovich I, Brocker EB, Zillikens D. Pemphigoid gestationis: New insights into pathogenesis lead to novel diagnostic tools. BJOG. 2002;109(9):970-6.
9. Engineer L, Bhol K, Ahmed AR. Pemphigoid gestationis: A review. Am J Obstet Gynecol. 2000;183(2):483-91.
10. Kroumpouzos G, Cohen LM. Specific dermatoses of pregnancy: An evidenced-based systematic review. Am J Obstet Gynecol. 2003;188(4):1083-92.
11. Kaaja RJ, Greer IA. Manifestations of chronic disease during pregnancy. JAMA. 2005;294(21):2751-7.
12. Fox GN. Pruritic folliculitis of pregnancy. Am Fam Physician. 1989;39(3):189-93.
13. Zoberman E, Farmer ER. Pruritic folliculitis of pregnancy. Arch Dermatol.1981;117(1):20-2.
14. Ambros-Rudolph CM, Vaughan Jones S. Atopic eruption of pregnancy. In: Black MM, Ambros-Rudolph CM, Edwards L, Lynch P (Eds). Obstetric and Gynecologic Dermatology, 3rd edition. Maryland Heights: Elsevier; 2008. pp. 65-72.
15. Reed J, George S. Pruritic folliculitis of pregnancy treated with narrowband (TL-01) ultraviolet B phototherapy.Br J Dermatol.1999;141(1):177-9.
16. Jenkins RE, Black MM. Pemphigoid (herpes) gestationis. In: Black MM, Ambros-Rudolph CM, Edwards L, Lynch P (Eds). Obstetric and Gynecologic Dermatology, 3rd edition. Maryland Heights: Elsevier; 2008. pp. 37-47.
17. Rodrigues Cdos S, Filipe P, Solana Mdel M, de Almeida LS, de Castro JC, Gomes MM. Persistent herpes gestationis treated with high-dose intravenous immunoglobulin. Acta Derm Venereol. 2007;87(2):184-6.
18. Palma J, Reyes H, Ribalta J, Hernandez I, Sandoval L, Almuna R, et al. Ursodeoxycholic acid in the treatment of cholestasis of pregnancy: A randomized, double-blind study controlled with placebo. J Hepatol.1997;27(6):1022-8.
19. Kroumpouzos G, Cohen LM. Dermatoses of pregnancy. J Am Acad Dermatol. 2001;45(1):1-19.

CHAPTER 18

Renal Disease during Pregnancy

ASYMPTOMATIC BACTERIURIA AND ACUTE PYELONEPHRITIS

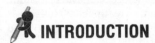 **INTRODUCTION**

The most commonly encountered renal infections during pregnancy are asymptomatic bacteriuria and acute pyelonephritis. Incidence of asymptomatic bacteriuria in pregnancy is about 4–7%. Asymptomatic bacteriuria, if left untreated, may develop into symptomatic urinary tract infection including acute pyelonephritis in 25–40% cases.[1]

AETIOLOGY

Most commonly involved pathogenic organism is *Escherichia coli* in both asymptomatic bacteriuria and acute pyelonephritis. Various physiological changes in pregnancy (Box 19.1) which can predispose to infection include shortened, dilated urethra; relative urinary stasis and reduced emptying; glycosuria; dilatation of upper renal tract, etc.

Risk Factors

Various risk factors for development of these conditions are enumerated in Box 19.2.

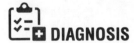 **DIAGNOSIS**

Clinical Presentation

❖ Malaise, nausea, vomiting, fatigue
❖ Fever with or without chills and rigors
❖ Back pain (localised in the upper lumbar area), with or without uterine contractions
❖ Fever, dehydration

Box 19.1: Changes occurring in the renal system during pregnancy

Anatomical changes
❑ Dilatation of ureters and renal calyces
Glomerular filtration rate and renal plasma flow
❑ There is an increase in GFR by 50% and RPF by 50–75% by 16 weeks of pregnancy and is maintained until 34 weeks. While the GFR remains elevated throughout pregnancy, RPF falls after 34 weeks of pregnancy.
❑ This is associated with an increase in urinary protein excretion and creatinine clearance. The upper limit of proteinuria during pregnancy is 300 mg/24 hours.
❑ As a result, there is reduction in maternal plasma levels of creatinine, blood urea, uric acid, etc. The upper limit for serum creatinine decreases to about 65 μmol/L (mean of 54 μmol/L).
❑ There is failure of complete absorption of substances, such as glucose, uric acid, amino acid, etc., from the renal tubules, resulting in an increased excretion of proteins, amino acids and glucose.
❑ Serum creatinine levels decrease during normal gestation to greater than 0.8 mg/dL.
Acid-base balance
❑ There is decreased bicarbonate threshold, and progesterone stimulates the respiratory centre. Therefore, serum bicarbonate decreases by 4–5 mEq/L.
Plasma osmolality
❑ Serum osmolality decreases by 10 mOsm/L during normal gestation. Increased placental metabolism of vasopressin may cause transient diabetes insipidus during pregnancy.

Box 19.2: Risk factors for the development of asymptomatic bacteriuria and acute pyelonephritis

❑ Previous history of urinary tract infection
❑ Diabetes
❑ Immunosuppression
❑ Receiving steroids
❑ Polycystic kidneys
❑ Reflux nephropathy
❑ Congenital abnormalities of renal tract (duplex kidney)
❑ Neuropathic bladder (spina bifida, multiple sclerosis, etc.)
❑ Urinary tract calculi

❖ Tachycardia, hypotension (in severe cases of pyelonephritis)
❖ Costovertebral angle tenderness.

Investigations

❖ *Haemogram*: Haemtocrit including a CBC must be done.
❖ *Urine analysis*: There may be presence of red cells, white cell casts, and bacteria on microscopic examination. Diagnosis of asymptomatic bacteriuria is made if upon culturing the urine sample (collected by midstream catch technique), there is a growth of greater than 10^5 colony-forming units (CFUs). Urine culture and sensitivity may also be done.
❖ *Tests of renal function*: There may be elevated serum BUN and creatinine levels and an abnormally low creatinine clearance.
❖ *Histological examination*: Histological examination shows infiltration of the renal interstitium and tubules by polymorphonuclear leukocytes in cases of acute pyelonephritis.
❖ *Serum electrolyte levels*: Abnormal serum electrolyte levels may be indicative of renal dysfunction.
❖ *Blood culture*: Blood culture must be obtained when the patient has chills or rigors or temperature elevation.
❖ *Ultrasound examination*: Ultrasound examination of the renal tract is indicated in those with pyelonephritis or two or more episodes of urinary tract infection to exclude hydronephrosis, congenital renal anomalies, renal calculi, etc.

DIFFERENTIAL DIAGNOSIS

❖ Acute appendicitis or cholecystitis
❖ Chorioamnionitis or abruptio placentae
❖ Red degeneration of fibroid.

MANAGEMENT

Asymptomatic Bacteriuria

All kinds of bacteriuria in pregnancy require treatment for the prevention of pyelonephritis and preterm delivery. A 3-day course of antibiotics is usually useful for treating the episode of asymptomatic bacteriuria.[2] The choice of antibiotic depends upon the results of culture and sensitivity. The most commonly used antibiotics during pregnancy are penicillin and cephalosporins. Augmentin (co-amoxiclav) should be preferably avoided during pregnancy due to the risk of necrotising enterocolitis in the neonate. The dosages of some commonly used antibiotics are as follows:

❖ Cefadroxil in the dosage of 500 mg twice daily for 3 days proves to be effective against majority of urinary pathogens.
❖ Nitrofurantoin, 100 mg can be given orally twice daily for 3–7 days. Use of nitrofurantoin should be preferably avoided in the third trimester due to the risk of haemolytic anaemia in the neonate.
❖ Trimethoprim-sulfamethoxazole (one single or double-strength tablet, orally twice a day for 3 days). Use of trimethoprim should be avoided in the first trimester due to its antifolate activity.
❖ Amoxycillin (500 mg orally twice a day for 3–7 days)
❖ Cephalexin (500 mg orally twice a day for 3–7 days).

Regular urine cultures can be taken to ensure that the organism is completely eradicated. Nearly 15% of the patients may experience recurrent bacteriuria, requiring a second course of antibiotics.

Acute Pyelonephritis

Aggressive treatment is required in order to avoid disease progression and occurrence of complications. In case of suspected pyelonephritis, treatment should preferably begin before the results of culture become available. For acute cystitis, antibiotics are recommended for 7 days, while in case of pyelonephritis, antibiotics must be prescribed for 10–14 days.[3] In cases of acute pyelonephritis, immediate management comprises of the following steps:

❖ Admission to the hospital
❖ Careful monitoring of the patient's vital signs every 4 hourly
❖ Maintenance of adequate hydration through administration of IV fluids
❖ Treatment with IV antibiotics (cefazolin in the dosage of 2 g at every 8 hourly intervals) in case of pyrexia and vomiting.

COMPLICATIONS

❖ Pre-eclampsia, preterm labour and prematurity
❖ Miscarriage, intrauterine foetal death.

CLINICAL PEARLS

❖ Women with renal disease should be offered low-dose aspirin as prophylaxis against pre-eclampsia, commencing within the first trimester.
❖ The characteristic renal pathology in pre-eclampsia is glomeruloendotheliosis.
❖ Screening for asymptomatic bacteriuria must occur at the time of first prenatal visit.
❖ Acute pyelonephritis is associated with a reduction in glomerular filtration rate, which can be reversed with the treatment of the underlying infection.

EVIDENCE-BASED MEDICINE

Increasing serum creatinine levels are likely to increase the risk of temporary and permanent deterioration of renal function.[4]

RENAL IMPAIRMENT IN PREGNANCY

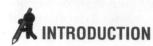

INTRODUCTION

Chronic kidney disease (CKD) can be diagnosed in all individuals if there is a presence of one of the following on at least two occasions for a period of at least 3 months, irrespective of the underlying cause:

❖ An estimated or measured glomerular filtration rate of less than 60 mL/min/1.73 m² and/or
❖ Evidence of kidney damage, albuminuria, proteinuria, haematuria after exclusion of the urological causes or structural abnormalities on kidney imaging tests.

AETIOLOGY

The most important common causes for chronic renal impairment in women of childbearing age groups include reflux nephropathy, diabetes, SLE,[5] glomerulonephritis, adult polycystic kidney disease, etc. Classification of CKD is based on the degree of renal impairment (Table 19.1).[4]

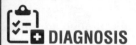

DIAGNOSIS

Clinical Presentation

This may include clinical features such as hypertension, proteinuria and/or haematuria in early pregnancy.

Investigations

In these cases, the following investigations need to be performed:

❖ *Blood tests*: Serum creatinine, uric acid, blood glucose (in diabetic patients), antinuclear antibodies (SLE)
❖ *Urine tests*: Total urinary protein, albumin levels
❖ *Renal tract ultrasound*: This is important for ruling out renal abnormalities such as polycystic kidneys, hydronephrosis, etc.

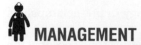

MANAGEMENT

❖ Management should be by a multidisciplinary team comprising of an obstetrician, nephrologist, etc. Pre-pregnancy counselling should be preferably provided to the woman before she plans her pregnancy.
❖ All steps must be taken to control hypertension to minimise the risk of deterioration in the renal function. Blood pressure should be preferably maintained below 140/90 mmHg.[6,7]
❖ Use of ACE inhibitors or ARBs should be discontinued during pregnancy because these drugs are likely to be teratogenic.[8]

Table 19.1: Stages of chronic renal disease[4]

Stages	GFR* (mL/min)	Descriptions
1	>90	The kidney function is normal but there might be abnormalities in renal structure, urine findings or genetic trait, which might point towards a kidney disease.
2	60–89	Mildly reduced kidney function, and other findings (as for stage 1) point to kidney disease.
3A	45–59	Moderately reduced kidney function
3B	30–44	
4	15–29	Severely reduced kidney function
5	<15 or on dialysis	Very severe, or end-stage kidney failure

Note: *All GFR values are normalised to an average surface area (size) of 1.73 m²

❖ Diuretics are usually discontinued during pregnancy except in case of severe hypoalbuminaemia or severe pulmonary oedema.
❖ Clinician must remember that the women with renal disease are at an increased risk of pre-eclampsia. However, it may become difficult to diagnose this condition in the presence of pre-existing hypertension and proteinuria.
❖ Patients should be preferably admitted to the hospital in case of worsening hypertension, increasing serum creatinine levels and increase in proteinuria.[9]
❖ Prophylactic low-dose aspirin can be appropriately used to reduce the risk of pre-eclampsia in those with renal impairment and hypertension.[10]
❖ Serial ultrasound scans for monitoring foetal growth and liquor volume
❖ Serial haematology and biochemistry measurements are essential for monitoring these pregnancies.
❖ During the postpartum period, continued close monitoring is required to ensure that the renal function returns to prepregnancy levels.
❖ Angiotensin-converting enzyme inhibitors can be safely used during breastfeeding.
❖ Referral to the nephrologist must be considered in case of those with newly diagnosed renal disease.

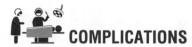

COMPLICATIONS

There could be an increased risk of following complications such as:[11]

❖ Pre-eclampsia
❖ Foetal growth restriction
❖ Iatrogenic preterm delivery (due to rapidly declining renal function)
❖ Polyhydramnios (due to foetal polyuria in response to high maternal osmotic load due to increased maternal urea levels)
❖ Risk of cord prolapse
❖ *Pulmonary oedema and venous thrombosis*: These complications can develop in individuals with nephrotic

syndrome and heavy proteinuria who develop hypoalbuminaemia.

CLINICAL PEARLS

❖ Patients with severe renal impairment (>250 µmol/L) are usually advised against pregnancy.[12]
❖ Renal disease in pregnancy can serve as a predisposing factor for pre-eclampsia and foetal growth restriction.

EVIDENCE-BASED MEDICINE

With increasing baseline serum creatinine levels, risk of obstetric complications such as pre-eclampsia, foetal growth restriction and iatrogenic preterm delivery are likely to increase. Therefore, with increasing serum creatinine levels, chances of successful pregnancy are likely to decrease.[13]

REFERENCES

1. Katz AI, Davison JM, Hayslett JP, Singson E, Lindheimer MD. Pregnancy in women with kidney disease. Kidney Int. 1980;18(2):192-206.
2. Cattell WR. Urinary tract infection in women. J R Coll Physicians Lond. 1997;31(2):130-3.
3. Edipidis K. Pregnancy in women with renal disease. Yes or no? Hippokratia. 2011;15(Suppl 1):8-12.
4. Epstein FH. Pregnancy and renal disease. N Engl J Med. 1996;335(4):277-8.
5. Germain S, Nelson-Piercy C. Lupus nephritis and renal disease in pregnancy. Lupus. 2006;15(3):148-55.
6. Krane NK, Hamrahian M. Pregnancy: kidney diseases and hypertension. Am J Kidney Dis. 2007;49(2):336-45.
7. Lindheimer MD, Taler SJ, Cunningham FG. Hypertension in pregnancy. J Am Soc Hypertens. 2010;4(2):68-78.
8. Cooper WO, Hernandez-Diaz S, Arbogast PG, Dudley JA, Dyer S, Gideon PS, et al. Major congenital malformations after first trimester exposure to ACE inhibitors. N Engl J Med. 2006;354(23):2443-51.
9. Krane NK. Acute renal failure in pregnancy. Arch Intern Med. 1988;148(11):2347-57.
10. Ramin SM, Vidaeff AC, Yeomans ER, Gilstrap LC 3rd. Chronic renal disease in pregnancy. Obstet Gynecol. 2006;108(6): 1531-9.
11. Jones DC, Hayslett JP. Outcome of pregnancy in women with moderate or severe renal insufficiency. N Engl J Med. 1996;335(4):226-32.
12. Hou S. Pregnancy in chronic renal insufficiency and end-stage renal disease. Am J Kidney Dis. 1999;33(2):235-52.
13. Williams D, Davison J. Chronic kidney disease in pregnancy. BMJ. 2008;336(7637):211-5.

CHAPTER 19

Infection during Pregnancy

CHICKEN POX IN PREGNANCY

INTRODUCTION

Varicella or chicken pox is a highly contagious disease caused by the primary infection with varicella-zoster virus (VZV). Chickenpox is a disease commonly occurring in the childhood and causes a mild infection. In England and Wales, nearly 90% of individuals over the age of 15 years are seropositive for VZV immunoglobulin G (IgG) antibody.[1] Therefore, despite of common contact with chickenpox during pregnancy, especially in women with young children, primary VZV infection during pregnancy remains uncommon. It has been estimated to complicate about 3 in every 1,000 pregnancies.[2] Women from tropical and subtropical areas are more likely to be seronegative for VZV IgG and are therefore more likely to develop chickenpox during pregnancy.[3] If VZV infection occurs in pregnant women, it may result in serious maternal morbidity or mortality. It may also cause foetal varicella syndrome (FVS) and varicella infection of the newborn, which includes congenital varicella syndrome and neonatal varicella.

AETIOLOGY

As previously described, chicken pox is caused by VZV, a DNA virus belonging to the herpes family (human herpesvirus 3). VZV causes two distinct diseases: varicella (chicken pox) and herpes zoster (shingles). Both the diseases are contagious and the virus is transmitted by respiratory droplets and by direct personal contact with vesicle fluid or indirectly via fomites (e.g. skin cells, hair, clothing and bedding). The virus enters through the mucosa of the upper respiratory tract and remains latent in the sensory and motor nerve cells. The incubation period of the virus varies from 14 days to 21 days.

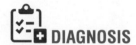

DIAGNOSIS

Clinical Presentation

Chicken pox is characterised by the presence of symptoms such as fever, malaise and a pruritic rash. The rash soon develops into the crops of maculopapules, which become vesicular and crust over before healing. The disease is infectious 48 hours before the appearance of rash and continues to be infectious until the vesicles crust over. The vesicles usually crust over within 5 days. The rash is most extensive on the face and trunk, and is minimal over the extremities.

Following the primary infection, the virus remains dormant in sensory nerve root ganglia. It can, however, be reactivated to cause a vesicular erythematous skin rash in a dermatomal distribution known as herpes zoster, also called 'zoster' or 'shingles'. Shingles present with painful and pruritic vesicles along a single sensory or motor nerve.

Investigations

Laboratory tests help in measuring the levels of IgM and IgG anti-varicella antibodies.

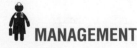

MANAGEMENT

Antepartum Period

❖ Appropriate treatment should be decided in consultation with a multidisciplinary team that includes an obstetrician or a foetal medicine specialist, a virologist and a neonatologist.
❖ At the time of booking for ANC, women should be asked about the previous history of chickenpox or shingles

infection. Women who have not had chickenpox, or are known to be seronegative for chickenpox, should be advised to avoid contact with chickenpox and shingles during pregnancy and to inform healthcare workers of a potential exposure without delay.

❖ *Exposure of a non-immunised woman with VZV*: When a previously non-immunised woman is exposed to chickenpox or shingles, a careful history must be taken to confirm the significance of the contact and the susceptibility of the patient.

- Pregnant non-immunised women or those suspected to be non-immunised or those who come from tropical or subtropical countries, and have been exposed to VZV infection during pregnancy, should have a blood test to determine their VZV IgG antibody immune status. This test should be preferably performed within 24–48 hours.[4]

- If a previously non-immunised pregnant woman has had a significant exposure, she should be offered varicella-zoster immunoglobulin (VZIG) as soon as possible. VZIG is effective when given up to 10 days after contact (from the appearance of the rash in the index case). A second dose of VZIG may be required if a further exposure is reported and 3 weeks have elapsed since the last dose. Women who have had exposure to chickenpox or shingles (regardless of the fact whether or not they have received VZIG) should be asked to notify their doctor or midwife as soon as a rash develops. VZIG has no therapeutic benefit once chickenpox has developed and should therefore not be used in pregnant women who have developed a chickenpox rash.

❖ *Varicella-zoster virus infection during pregnancy*: In women who develop VZV infection during pregnancy, symptomatic treatment and maintenance of hygiene is advised to prevent development of secondary bacterial infection of the lesions. Antipruritic and antipyretic medicines can be prescribed for symptomatic treatment. Oral aciclovir should be prescribed for pregnant women with 20^{+0} weeks of gestation or beyond, having chickenpox if they present within 24 hours of the onset of the rash. Use of aciclovir before 20^{+0} weeks should also be considered.[4] It is prescribed in the dosage of 800 mg five times a day for 7 days. Aciclovir is a synthetic nucleoside analogue that inhibits replication of the VZV. It is not licensed for use in pregnancy. Therefore, before prescribing this drug, the risks and benefits of its use should be discussed with the woman. Pregnant women with severe chickenpox may require IV aciclovir infusion. IV aciclovir infusion may be required in cases of varicella pneumonia, those over 36 weeks of gestation and patients showing clinical deterioration after day 6 of the rash.[5-10] Antibiotics may be required in case of secondary infection of the vesicles. VZIG has no therapeutic benefit once chickenpox has developed and should therefore not be used in pregnant women who have developed a chickenpox rash.

- A pregnant woman who develops a chickenpox rash should immediately contact her general practitioner.

She should be isolated from other pregnant women when she attends a general practice surgery or a hospital for assessment. She should also avoid contact with potentially susceptible individuals, e.g. other pregnant women and neonates, until the lesions have crusted over. This usually occurs about 5 days after the onset of the rash.

- If the pregnant woman develops varicella or shows serological conversion in the first 28 weeks of pregnancy, she should be informed about a small risk of developing FVS.

❖ *Referral to the hospital*: Women, who develop the symptoms or signs of severe chickenpox, e.g. respiratory symptoms or any significant deterioration in their condition, should be immediately referred to the hospital. A hospital assessment should be considered in a woman at high risk of severe or complicated chickenpox even in the absence of concerning symptoms or signs. Women hospitalised with varicella should be nursed in isolation from babies, potentially susceptible pregnant women or non-immune staff.

❖ Women who develop chickenpox in pregnancy should be referred to a foetal medicine specialist, at 16–20 weeks or 5 weeks after infection regarding prenatal diagnosis of varicella infection. A discussion and detailed ultrasound examination should be done during this period.

❖ Women who develop varicella infection during pregnancy should be counselled about the risks versus benefits of amniocentesis to detect varicella DNA by PCR. Amniocentesis has a strong negative predictive value but a poor positive predictive value in detecting foetal damage. Amniocentesis, if undertaken, should not be performed before the skin lesions have completely healed.

Intrapartum Period

❖ The timing and mode of delivery of the pregnant woman with chickenpox must be individualised.

❖ If maternal infection occurs in the last 4 weeks of a woman's pregnancy or delivery is likely to occur during the viraemic period, there is a significant risk of varicella infection of the newborn. In these cases, treatment with aciclovir is recommended and a planned delivery should normally be avoided for at least 7 days after the onset of the maternal rash. At the same time, the obstetrician must make sure that continuing the pregnancy does not pose any additional risks for the mother or baby. This extra time allows for the passive transfer of antibodies from mother to child. Delaying delivery is also likely to reduce the risk of maternal complications such as bleeding, thrombocytopenia and DIC.

❖ A neonatologist should be informed about the birth of all babies born to women who have developed chickenpox at any gestation during pregnancy.

❖ If the woman with chicken pox is administered epidural or spinal anaesthesia, a skin site free of cutaneous lesions should be chosen for the placement of needle.

❖ The neonate must be administered VZIG if the birth occurs within 7 days following the onset of maternal rash or if the mother develops the rash of chicken pox within 7 days period after birth.

Postpartum Period

❖ Varicella vaccination in the postpartum period can be considered for women who are found to be seronegative for VZV IgG.
❖ Women with chickenpox should breastfeed if they wish to do so.
❖ While universal serological antenatal testing is not recommended in the UK, seronegative women identified in pregnancy could be offered postpartum immunisation. Women who are vaccinated postpartum can be reassured that it is safe to breastfeed.

COMPLICATIONS

Maternal

Clinicians should be aware of the increased morbidity associated with varicella infection in adults, including pneumonia, hepatitis and encephalitis.[11,12] Rarely, it may result in death.[13] Chickenpox infection in the first trimester is not associated with an increased risk of spontaneous miscarriage.

Foetal

Foetal varicella syndrome or FVS is characterised by one or more of the following features: scarring of the skin in a dermatomal distribution; eye defects (microphthalmia, chorioretinitis or cataracts); hypoplasia of the limbs; and neurological abnormalities (microcephaly, cortical atrophy, mental retardation or dysfunction of bowel and bladder sphincters).[14,15] FVS has been reported to complicate maternal chickenpox occurring as early as 3 weeks of gestation to as late as 28 weeks of gestation and affects only a minority of infected foetuses.[15]

Neonatal

If maternal infection occurs in the last 4 weeks of a woman's pregnancy, there is a significant risk of varicella infection of the newborn. Varicella infection of the newborn includes congenital varicella syndrome and neonatal varicella. A planned delivery should normally be avoided for at least 7 days after the onset of the maternal rash to allow for the passive transfer of antibodies from mother to child, provided that continuing the pregnancy does not pose any additional risks to the mother or baby.

CLINICAL PEARLS

❖ Chickenpox may be infectious for 2 days before the appearance of the rash and for the duration of the illness while the skin lesions are active. The lesion stops being infectious when it has crusted over.

❖ Varicella vaccine contains live attenuated viral strain and is administered in two separate doses 4–8 weeks apart. Two varicella vaccines are licensed for use in the UK for the prevention of chickenpox: Varivax® and Varilrix®.
❖ Varicella-zoster virus vaccination is not routinely used in the UK. Vaccination in the prepregnancy or postpartum period can be considered as an option for women who are seronegative for VZIG prior to pregnancy or in the postpartum period.
❖ If a woman of reproductive age is vaccinated, she should be advised to avoid pregnancy for 1 month after completion of the two-dose vaccine schedule. She should also be asked to avoid contact with susceptible pregnant women because of the occurrence of postvaccination rash in some cases.

EVIDENCE-BASED MEDICINE

❖ Presently, there is insufficient evidence to support antenatal screening for susceptibility to varicella-zoster infection because presently there is unavailability of reliable information regarding the true incidence of VZV infection in pregnancy and on the outcomes following treatment.[16]
❖ The available evidence has shown that oral aciclovir administered in the dosage of 800 mg five times a day for 7 days helps in reducing the duration of symptoms related to varicella infection in immunocompetent adults if commenced within 24 hours of developing the rash in comparison to placebo. However, its role in the prevention of the serious complications of chickenpox is yet not known.[17] Its use is also not associated with a significant increase in the risk of major foetal malformations during pregnancy.[18-20]

GENITAL HERPES IN PREGNANCY

INTRODUCTION

Genital herpes is one of the most common sexually transmitted diseases worldwide and is caused by HSV type 1 or 2. Transmission occurs during close contact with a person who is shedding the virus. Asymptomatic infection can rarely occur. Women, who acquire primary genital herpes during pregnancy, particularly in the third trimester, may transmit the infection to the baby at the time of delivery. Direct contact with infected maternal secretions in pregnant women with genital herpes may result in neonatal herpes. Neonatal herpes can be caused by HSV type 1 or 2 and occurs rarely in the UK. However, it is a serious viral infection associated with a significantly high rate of morbidity and mortality.[21] Depending on the site of infection in the infant, it can be classified into three subtypes: (1) disease localised to skin, eye and/or mouth; (2) local CNS disease (encephalitis alone); and (3) disseminated infection with multiple organ involvement.

AETIOLOGY

Herpes simplex belongs to the Herpesviridae family of viruses, which is a double-stranded (ds) DNA virus. HSV-1 causes superficial lesions of the face, mouth, pharynx and cornea including infections such as acute herpetic gingivostomatitis, acute herpetic pharyngotonsillitis, herpes labialis, herpes encephalitis, eczema herpeticum and herpetic whitlow. The virus can remain latent in the trigeminal ganglion and dorsal root ganglion and may reactivate as cold sores. HSV-2 is sexually transmitted and can cause infections such as genital herpes, neonatal infection and aseptic meningitis.

DIAGNOSIS

Investigations

❖ Swabs from genital areas
❖ *Herpes simplex virus antibody testing*: For women presenting with first episode of genital herpes in the third trimester, particularly within 6 weeks of expected delivery, type specific HSV antibody testing (IgG antibodies to HSV-1 and HSV-2) is advisable. The result of this testing is likely to influence the advice given regarding mode of delivery and risk of neonatal herpes infection. The presence of antibodies of the same type as the HSV antibodies isolated from genital swabs would confirm this episode to be a recurrence rather than a primary infection and elective caesarean section would not be indicated to prevent neonatal transmission.

MANAGEMENT

❖ Women with suspected genital herpes, who are being managed by the midwife, should be referred for review by a genitourinary medicine physician as well as the obstetrician. Genitourinary medicine physician would help in confirming or disproving the diagnosis by viral PCR.
❖ Paracetamol and topical lidocaine 2% gel can be offered for symptomatic relief in cases of genital herpes infection. There is no evidence indicating that the use of either of them in standard doses is harmful during pregnancy.
❖ Following maternal acquisition of infection in the first or second trimester, aciclovir must be administered in the dosage of 400 mg three times daily from 36 weeks of gestation. This strategy helps in reducing HSV lesions at term and hence the requirement for delivery by caesarean section.[22-27] It has also been shown to reduce asymptomatic viral shedding. In these cases, pregnancy should be managed expectantly and vaginal delivery anticipated, provided that the delivery is not likely to occur within the next 6 weeks.

❖ Following acquisition of infection in the third trimester, treatment should not be delayed. Management of the woman should be based upon her clinical condition and usually involves the use of oral aciclovir in the standard dosage of 400 mg three times daily, usually for 5 days. In the third trimester, treatment should continue with daily suppressive aciclovir in the dosage of 400 mg three times daily until delivery.
❖ Caesarean section should be the recommended mode of delivery for all women developing first episode genital herpes in the third trimester, particularly those developing symptoms within 6 weeks of the date of expected delivery, because the risk of neonatal transmission of HSV in these cases may as high as 41%.[21,28-30]
❖ *Management of pregnant women with recurrent genital herpes*: Women with recurrent genital herpes should be informed that the risk of neonatal herpes in these cases is low even if lesions are present at the time of delivery (0–3% for vaginal delivery). The majority of recurrent episodes of genital herpes are short-lasting and resolve within 7–10 days without requirement for antiviral therapy. Supportive treatment measures using saline bathing and analgesia with standard doses of paracetamol alone are usually sufficient. Vaginal delivery should be anticipated in the absence of any obstetric indications for caesarean section.[31] Daily suppressive aciclovir in the dosage of 400 mg 3 times daily should be considered from 36 weeks of gestation. Presently, there is no evidence to guide the management of women with spontaneous rupture of membranes at term. Most clinicians advise expediting the delivery in an attempt to minimise the duration of potential exposure of the foetus to HSV.

Intrapartum Management

❖ Management of women with primary or recurrent genital lesions at the onset of labour is usually based on clinical assessment, as there will not be any time for performing confirmatory laboratory testing. The clinician must take a history in order to determine whether this is a primary or recurrent episode. A viral swab from the lesion(s) should be taken, because the result may influence management of the neonate.[31]
❖ Vulva and cervix should be carefully examined for the presence of herpetic lesions.
❖ In case of women presenting with primary episode of genital herpes lesions at the time of delivery or within 6 weeks of the expected date of delivery, caesarean section should be recommended. This would help reduce exposure of the foetus to HSV which may be present in maternal genital secretions.[32]
❖ The neonatologist should be informed at the time of delivery.
❖ In the intrapartum period, IV aciclovir must be administered to the mother in the dosage of 5 mg/kg every 8 hours. Subsequently, the administration of IV aciclovir in the dosage of 20 mg/kg at every 8 hourly interval must be considered in the neonate of the mothers opting for

PART II

vaginal delivery.[33,34] It is presently unknown whether intrapartum aciclovir reduces the risk of neonatal HSV infection.

❖ Although vaginal delivery should be avoided as far as possible, in women who deliver vaginally in the presence of primary genital herpes lesions, following precautions must be taken:
  • Invasive procedures (application of foetal scalp electrodes, foetal blood sampling, etc.) must be avoided as far as possible.
  • Rupture of membranes should be avoided.
  • Instrumental deliveries should also be avoided in these cases.

Postpartum Period

❖ In case of presence of orofacial lesions in the mother, she should refrain from close contact with the baby in that region.
❖ Breastfeeding is recommended unless the mother has lesions around the nipples.
❖ Aciclovir can be administered to the mother in the postpartum period, if required. Though aciclovir is excreted in the breast milk, its use is not associated with any adverse effects on the infant.

Management of the Neonate

❖ In all cases, the neonatal team should be informed.
❖ Babies born by caesarean section in mothers with primary HSV infection in the third trimester are at low risk of vertically transmitted HSV infection, so conservative management is recommended. It comprises of the following steps:
  • No active treatment is required for the baby. Also, there is no need to take swabs from the neonate.
  • Normal postnatal care of the baby is advised with a neonatal examination at 24 hours of age, after which the baby can be discharged from the hospital if well and feeding is established.
  • Parents should be educated regarding maintenance of good hand hygiene to reduce the risk of postnatal infection.
  • Parents should be advised to seek medical help if they have concerns regarding their baby. They should be especially advised to look for signs such as lesions in the skin, eye and mucous membrane, and symptoms such as lethargy/irritability, poor feeding, etc.
❖ Babies born by spontaneous vaginal delivery in mothers with a primary HSV infection within the previous 6 weeks are at high risk of vertically transmitted HSV infection. The following steps must be taken in these cases for the prevention of neonatal infection:
  • Neonatal team should be involved in the baby's care.
  • If the baby is doing well, swabs of the skin, conjunctiva, oropharynx and rectum should be sent for herpes simplex PCR.
  • A lumbar puncture is not routinely required.

• Empirical treatment with IV aciclovir (20 mg/kg every 8 hours) should be initiated until evidence of active infection has been ruled out.
• Strict infection control procedures should be put in place for both mother and baby.
• Parents should be advised to immediately report any early signs of infection such as poor feeding, lethargy, fever or any suspicious lesions.
❖ If the baby is unwell or presents with skin lesions, swabs of the skin, lesions, conjunctiva, oropharynx and rectum, should be sent for herpes simplex PCR. A lumbar puncture should also be performed even if CNS features are not present.
❖ In case of babies born to mothers with recurrent HSV infection in pregnancy with or without active lesions at delivery, maternal IgG will be protective for the baby and hence the risk of infection is low. Conservative management of the neonate (as previously described) is appropriate in these cases.[35]

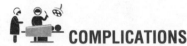

COMPLICATIONS

Primary HSV infection is associated with complications such as spontaneous miscarriage, stillbirths and increased perinatal morbidity (due to preterm labour, foetal growth restriction and low birthweight).[21,36] There is a risk of vertical transmission of the HSV infection to the neonates born by spontaneous vaginal delivery in the mothers who had acquired the primary HSV infection within the previous 6 weeks.

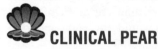

CLINICAL PEARLS

❖ There is no evidence of an increased risk of birth defects with aciclovir, famciclovir or valaciclovir if used in the first trimester.[19]
❖ In case of vaginal delivery in patients with primary episode of genital herpes lesions present at the time of delivery, the risk of neonatal herpes is estimated to be 41%.

EVIDENCE-BASED MEDICINE

❖ Aciclovir is not licensed for use in pregnancy. However, its use during pregnancy can be considered to be safe and the available evidence has not shown any clinically significant adverse maternal or neonatal effects with the use of aciclovir except for few cases of transient neonatal neutropenia.[18,19,37,38]
❖ There is no evidence that HSV infection acquired during pregnancy is associated with an increased incidence of congenital abnormalities.[34]
❖ Presently, there is insufficient evidence to suggest an association between HSV and stillbirth as a cause of foetal death.[39,40]

❖ There is some evidence to suggest that if the membranes have been ruptured for greater than 4 hours, the benefit of caesarean section reduces.[41] However, there may be some benefit in performing a caesarean section even after this time interval.

HIV IN PREGNANCY

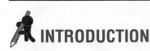 ## INTRODUCTION

Acquired immune deficiency syndrome is caused by infection with HIV, a retrovirus. HIV shows two distinct antigenic types: HIV-1 and HIV-2. The virus affects the normal immune cells in the body, thereby resulting in reduced immunity. This may result in the development of unusual opportunistic infections due to various bacteria and viruses.

AETIOLOGY

Infection with HIV occurs through sexual contact and contact with infected blood. Women in comparison to men are more likely to be infected through sexual contact. Risk factors for HIV infection include unprotected sexual intercourse, promiscuous behaviour, IV drug abuse, etc.

Human immunodeficiency virus infection can also occur as a result of vertical transmission of virus from the mother to child. In the western world, the risk of mother-to-child (MTC) transmission of HIV is of the order of 15%. Perinatal transmission can occur in utero, in the intrapartum period or at the time of breastfeeding. Majority of transmission (>80%) takes place after 36 weeks, mainly during labour and delivery. Less than 2% of transmissions occur during the first and second trimesters. Risk factors for MTC transmission are described in Box 20.1. Currently, there is insufficient evidence for a plasma viral load threshold below which transmission never occurs. However, viral load titres less than 1,000 copies/mL is associated with a relatively lower risk.

In the developing world, the MTC risk is much greater, perhaps due to breastfeeding. In the UK, the rate of transmission is less than 2%.[42] It is now thought that the risk of HIV transmission in the UK can be reduced to less than 1% with the use of various strategies such as aggressive antiviral therapy, elective caesarean section and avoidance of breastfeeding.

Screening for HIV Infection

If screening has been refused in early pregnancy, screening should be offered again at a later stage in pregnancy. Some women, who are at particular risk of HIV infection, especially targeted for screening, include the following:
- ❖ Women who have arrived in the UK as refugees or asylum seekers from high prevalence countries
- ❖ Those with a history of injecting drug use
- ❖ Commercial sex workers.

Box 20.1: Risk factors for mother-to-child transmission[42]

Maternal factors
- ❑ Advanced maternal disease
- ❑ High maternal viral load
- ❑ Resistant strain of the virus
- ❑ Low maternal CD4 count
- ❑ Malnutrition, especially vitamin A deficiency
- ❑ Smoking and use of illicit drugs
- ❑ Maternal obesity
- ❑ Other sexually transmitted diseases, particularly ulcerative.

Obstetric risk factors
- ❑ Prolonged duration of ruptured membranes
- ❑ Chorioamnionitis
- ❑ Preterm delivery—especially <34 weeks
- ❑ Vaginal delivery
- ❑ Use of scalp electrodes
- ❑ Episiotomy
- ❑ Perineal tears and lacerations
- ❑ Breastfeeding
- ❑ Prolonged labour
- ❑ Active genital ulcer disease

DIAGNOSIS

Investigations

The following investigations need to be carried out in HIV positive pregnant women:
- ❖ Liver function tests and a baseline fundoscopic examination must be done in all HIV positive patients.
- ❖ HIV viral load and CD4 lymphocyte count should be measured at the time of initial visit. It should then be repeated in each trimester to monitor the response to therapy.
- ❖ Screening blood test for syphilis, hepatitis B and rubella at the time of booking antenatal visit (keeping up with recommendations for the general population).
- ❖ Additional blood tests, which are recommended for HIV positive pregnant women, include hepatitis C, varicella zoster, measles and toxoplasma.
- ❖ HIV positive pregnant women taking highly active anti-retroviral therapy (HAART) at the time of booking should be screened for gestational diabetes.

 ## MANAGEMENT

Consideration should be given in the third trimester for rescreening women who have continuing high risk of HIV acquisition. In certain situations, it is beneficial to test both the pregnant mother and her partner for HIV. If the pregnant mother is negative but her partner is positive, advice can be given about avoiding transmission of HIV during pregnancy.

Antenatal Period

Voluntary testing for HIV forms an integral part of ANC in the UK and must be offered and recommended to all women irrespective of their risk factors. The following steps need to be taken amongst the pregnant women diagnosed positive for HIV infection:[43]

❖ *Multidisciplinary management*: Women diagnosed as HIV positive during pregnancy should be managed by a multidisciplinary team including an HIV physician, an obstetrician, a midwife, a paediatrician, as well as social support workers. Confidentiality regarding HIV status must be maintained at all times. An early assessment of the social circumstances of all women who are newly diagnosed with HIV positive infection should be done. Women should be encouraged to reveal their HIV status to their partner and must be given appropriate support.

❖ *Initial booking visit*: During this visit, a thorough history must be taken and a complete physical examination must be performed. The patient must also be counselled about the perinatal transmission of the virus and importance of compliance with the antiretroviral regimens. The patient should also be advised that by taking appropriate precautions (e.g. use of antiretroviral therapy, caesarean delivery and avoidance of breastfeeding), the risk of MTC transmission of the virus can be reduced from 25–30% to less than 2%. If required, the patient can be referred for drug treatment and/or detoxification programmes.

❖ *Prenatal diagnostic tests*: The risk of MTC transmission due to prenatal diagnostic procedures such as amniocentesis or CVS is presently uncertain. Advice of a foetal medicine specialist and HIV physician must be sought by the obstetrician if contemplating to perform any of the prenatal diagnostic procedures. Prophylactic therapy with HAART should be considered before carrying out any invasive procedures (amniocentesis, CVS, etc.).

❖ *Screening for genital infections*: All pregnant women who are HIV positive should be screened and treated for genital infections early in pregnancy. This should be repeated during the third trimester. Chlamydia, gonorrhoea, bacterial vaginosis and genital ulceration should especially be looked for. All these genital infections are associated with a greater risk of HIV disease. Additionally, bacterial vaginosis is also associated with preterm labour. Routine antenatal serological screening for hepatitis B and syphilis should also be carried out. Syphilis serology should be repeated in the third trimester. All HIV positive pregnant women should also be tested for hepatitis C virus (HCV).

❖ *Screening for foetal anomalies*: Screening for Down's syndrome and foetal anomalies should be carried out according to national guidelines. A detailed ultrasound scan for foetal anomalies should be carried out at 21 weeks gestation if antiretroviral therapy or prophylaxis for *Pneumocystis carinii* pneumonia (PCP) with folate antagonists [e.g. Septran (cotrimoxazole)] has been used during the first trimester.

❖ *Immunisation*: Immunisation for infections such as hepatitis B, pneumococcus and influenza is recommended for all individuals who are HIV positive. These immunisations can be safely administered in pregnancy. On the other hand, vaccines for injections such as varicella zoster, measles, mumps and rubella are contraindicated during pregnancy. Postpartum immunisation should be considered for women who test negative for IgG antibodies for these infections, depending on their CD4 count.

❖ *Monitoring for drug toxicity*: Pregnant women with HIV should be monitored regularly for drug toxicity. Signs of toxicity due to the use of antiretroviral drugs include pre-eclampsia, liver dysfunction, lactic acidosis, glucose intolerance, diabetes, rashes, etc. Zidovudine (ZDV) is the antiretroviral for which the most extensive safety data is available regarding use in pregnancy.

❖ *Antiretroviral therapy during pregnancy*: Prescription of antiretroviral therapy may be required to reduce the risk of HIV transmission to the foetus. Women, who do not require antiretrovirals to control disease, need to be given these drugs to prevent MTC transmission. In these cases, HAART should be initiated between 20 weeks to 28 weeks and must be discontinued at delivery. The risk of HIV transmission needs to be balanced with the risk of the therapy-related toxicities. ZDV monotherapy is an option for the woman with low levels of HIV viraemia (less than 10,000 copies/mL) and with a sensitive strain. It is also an option if she does not require HAART for her own health or who does not wish to take HAART during pregnancy and is prepared to be delivered by elective caesarean section.[44] ZDV monotherapy must be initiated between 20 weeks to 28 weeks in the dosage 250 mg twice orally daily. It must be administered intravenously at delivery and discontinued immediately thereafter. Presently, HAART has become the standard of care for all individuals who are HIV positive requiring antiretroviral therapy for their own health. Due to concerns about resistance related to the use of single-drug agents, ZDV monotherapy is less commonly used during pregnancy.

Women with HIV, who require antiretroviral therapy to control disease, should be prescribed the same regimes as if they were not pregnant. These drugs should be continued throughout pregnancy and postpartum period.

However, certain combinations of drugs should be avoided during pregnancy. These include dual non-reverse transcriptase inhibitors (NRTI), combination of stavudine with didanosine (due to the risk of lactic acidosis), etc. Women taking HAART are at risk of premature labour. Till date, there is no evidence of any increase in congenital malformations in humans with first trimester exposure to any antiretroviral therapy. However, there is inadequate data to exclude the teratogenic risk for most drugs. Mitochondrial depletion and haematological effects have been noted in infants exposed to antiretroviral therapy. Nevertheless, the use of HAART during pregnancy should be postponed if possible until after the first trimester.

❖ *Prophylaxis of opportunistic infection*: Various opportunistic infections, which can occur in HIV positive women, include

Box 20.2: Indications for caesarean delivery in HIV positive pregnant women

❏ Women taking HAART who have plasma viral load of > 50 copies/mL
❏ Women taking ZDV monotherapy as an alternative to HAART
❏ Women with HIV and hepatitis C virus co-infection
❏ Obstetric indication for caesarean delivery

Abbreviations: HAART, highly active antiretroviral therapy; ZDV, zidovudine

PCP, *Mycobacterium avium*, toxoplasmosis, tuberculosis, herpes simplex, etc. Prophylaxis of opportunistic infection during pregnancy should be based on the criteria similar to those for non-pregnant women with HIV.

Intrapartum Period

❖ *Mode of delivery*: A plan regarding mode of delivery should be made at about 36 weeks of gestation following detailed discussion with the mother. Indications for caesarean delivery in HIV positive pregnant women are given in Box 20.2. A planned caesarean section should be offered to all HIV positive women in the cases, where there is a detectable plasma viral load and/or the woman is taking HAART at approximately 38 weeks of gestation. Planned caesarean delivery in these cases helps in reducing the risk of MCT.[45,46] For women who are HIV positive but not taking HAART and/or have detectable plasma viral load, delivery should be by elective caesarean section because it significantly helps in reducing the risk of MTC transmission.

❖ Value of a caesarean delivery is reduced if there are more than 4 hours between rupture of membranes and delivery because there is an increased risk of vertical transmission if the membranes have been ruptured for more than 4 hours. ZDV infusion must be started 4 hours before beginning caesarean delivery, and it should continue until umbilical cord has been clamped.

❖ Planned caesarean section is also advised if there is co-infection with hepatitis B or C. Risks and benefits of caesarean section need to be considered in each individual case.

❖ Delivery by elective caesarean section for obstetric indications or maternal request should be delayed until after 39 completed weeks of gestation in women with plasma viral loads of less than 50 copies/mL to reduce the risk of transient tachypnoea of the newborn.

❖ The option of vaginal delivery can be considered for women with plasma viral loads of less than 50 copies/mL.[44,47]

❖ *Precautions during caesarean delivery*: Consideration should be given towards using IV ZDV prophylaxis during delivery. In case ZDV is being administered to a woman having a planned section, ZDV infusion should be commenced 4 hours prior to the surgery and this should be continued until the cord is clamped. IV ZDV prophylaxis is not usually indicated for mothers who were not previously on ZDV treatment or for mothers on HAART with less than 50 HIV RNA copies/mL plasma. HAART regimen must be continued throughout labour in these cases.
  • The surgical field should be kept as haemostatic as possible.
  • Care should be taken to try to avoid rupturing the membranes until the foetal head has delivered through the surgical incision.
  • A maternal sample for plasma viral load and CD4 lymphocyte count should be taken at delivery.
  • The cord should be clamped and the baby should be bathed as soon as possible after delivery.

❖ *Precautions during vaginal delivery*: In case a vaginal delivery is planned, the following precautions must be taken:
  • The use of foetal scalp electrodes and foetal blood sampling should be avoided.
  • Membranes should be left intact as far as possible.
  • If instrumental delivery is indicated, the use of forceps is preferable to ventouse due to the lower risk of traumatic injury to the baby.
  • Human immunodeficiency virus infection per se is not an indication for continuous electronic foetal monitoring.
  • Amniotomy and possible use of oxytocin may be considered for augmentation of labour in some cases.

❖ Perioperative antibiotics should be given for all caesarean section deliveries and immediately if membranes rupture during the first stage of labour.

❖ Corticosteroids should be given for threatened preterm delivery.

Postpartum Period

❖ *Breastfeeding*: All women in the UK who are HIV positive should be advised not to breastfeed because breastfeeding is likely to increase the overall rate of MTC HIV transmission.[48]

❖ *Advice related to contraception*: All HIV positive women should receive guidance about contraception in the immediate postpartum period. Use of hormonal contraception is best avoided due to its probable interaction with HAART. Barrier contraception appears to be a safe option in these patients.

Care of the Newborn

❖ *Treatment of the neonate*: All neonates born to HIV positive women should be treated with antiretroviral therapy within 4 hours of birth. ZDV is usually administered twice daily orally for 4 weeks to all neonates of mothers with HIV. An alternative suitable monotherapy may be given to the infant in case of maternal resistance to ZDV. HAART is given to infants at high risk of HIV infection (e.g. infants of untreated mothers or mothers who have plasma viraemia greater than 50 copies/mL despite HAART).

❖ *Prophylaxis against PCP*: This is recommended only for those infants who are born to mothers at high risk of transmission.

❖ *Testing for HIV*: Infants should be tested for HIV infection at day 1, 6 weeks and 12 weeks of age. A confirmatory HIV antibody test may be performed at around 18 months of age. The gold-standard test for diagnosis of HIV infection in infancy is HIV DNA PCR on peripheral blood lymphocytes.[49] Children infected with HIV and those born to HIV infected women must be reported to the National Study of HIV in Pregnancy and Childhood.

COMPLICATIONS

Human immunodeficiency virus infection during pregnancy can be associated with the following complications described next.

Maternal

❖ *Increased risk of opportunistic infections*: There is an increased risk of opportunistic infections in the HIV positive pregnant patients, especially PCP. Symptoms of PCP include fever, dry cough and shortness of breath, and patients are typically hypoxic.
❖ *Complications due to HAART regimens*: These may include side effects such as gastrointestinal disturbances, skin rashes, hepatotoxicity, etc. Lactic acidosis has been reported in pregnant women taking HAART, most commonly with the antiretrovirals such as stavudine and didanosine.
  • Increased risk of preterm delivery.

Foetal

❖ Risk of vertical transmission of the HIV infection
❖ Miscarriage
❖ Intrauterine growth restriction
❖ Stillbirth.

CLINICAL PEARLS

Prophylactic therapy against PCP must be administered to HIV positive pregnant women with CD4 lymphocyte counts less than 200×10^6/L because they are at an increased risk of opportunistic infections.

EVIDENCE-BASED MEDICINE

❖ According to the present British HIV Association (BHIVA) recommendations, HAART must be initiated for pregnant women with symptomatic HIV infection and/or a falling or low CD4 lymphocyte count (less than 350×10^6/L).[42]
❖ The first-line agent for prophylactic therapy against *P. carnii* pneumonia is cotrimoxazole.[50]
❖ The present evidence indicates that ZDV monotherapy is the only antiretroviral agent that is likely to significantly reduce the risk of MTC transmission.[51]

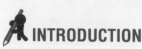

MALARIA IN PREGNANCY

INTRODUCTION

Malaria is the most important parasitic infection in humans and is a disease most commonly encountered in the tropics and subtropics. The disease is most commonly imported into the UK through the immigrants and the second- and third-generation relatives returning home assuming they are immune from malaria. Approximately, 75% of cases are caused by *Plasmodium falciparum* and are associated with the mortality rate of approximately 0.5–1.0%.[52]

AETIOLOGY

Malaria is caused by the protozoan, *Plasmodium*, commonly known as the malaria parasite. The various plasmodium species responsible for causing malaria include *P. falciparum*, *P. vivax*, *P. malariae* and *P. ovale*.[53] Malaria caused by *P. falciparum* is likely to be associated with greater morbidity and mortality in comparison to the non-falciparum infections.[54-58]

Malarial parasite is transmitted by the bite of a sporozoite-bearing female anopheline mosquito. Following the mosquito-bite, initially there is a period of pre-erythrocytic phase in the liver. Following this, the erythrocytic stage of infection occurs, which causes disease manifestations. During this stage, invasion of the erythrocyte by the parasite results in the consumption of haemoglobin and alteration of the red cell membrane. This causes *P. falciparum* infected erythrocytes to cytoadhere inside the small blood vessels of brain, kidneys and other affected organs. There also occurs rosetting, which can be defined as the adherence of uninfected RBCs. Both of these processes, cytoadherence and rosetting interfere with microcirculatory flow and metabolism of vital organs. Another hallmark of falciparum malaria in pregnancy is the sequestration of parasites in the placenta. Sequestered parasites escape host defence mechanisms such as splenic processing and filtration. Sequestration is not known to occur in the benign malarias due to *P. vivax*, *P. ovale* and *P. malariae*.

In pregnancy, the adverse effects of malaria infection result from the systemic infection, comparable to the effects of any severe febrile illness in pregnancy. This can be associated with increased maternal and foetal mortality, miscarriage, stillbirth and premature birth. Malarial infection causes placental reaction by clogging the placental intervillous spaces with *Plasmodium*-infected RBCs, and macrophages, especially during the second half of pregnancy. As a result, the malaria-infected placenta is unable to carry out its main function, i.e. provision of nutrients to the foetus. In a normal woman, the transplacental passive immunity, due to the passage of IgG through the placenta helps in protecting the newborns against infection. This immunity is also deficient in foetuses of malaria-infected woman.

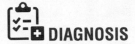

DIAGNOSIS

Clinical Presentation

There are no specific symptoms or signs associated with malarial infection, and the patient may present with a flu-like illness. A pregnant woman with pyrexia of unknown origin should be enquired about history of travel to a malaria-endemic area. Severity of malaria in the pregnant woman should be assessed and documented in the patient's clinical notes because this is likely to help in its management. The severity of malaria helps in determining the course of treatment and predicting the case fatality rate. Uncomplicated malaria in the UK is defined as presence of fewer than 2% parasitised RBCs in a woman with no signs of severity or presence of any complicating features. Complicated malaria, on the other hand, is defined as the presence of 2% or more parasitised red blood. Case fatality rates are low, approximately 0.1% in uncomplicated cases of malaria. In cases of severe malaria during pregnancy, fatality rates can be as high as 50%.[59] Clinical features encountered in cases of severe or complicated malaria in adults are listed in Box 20.3.[60]

Investigations

❖ *Blood film*: In case of clinical suspicion of malaria, diagnosis must be confirmed by performing the microscopic examination of thick and thin blood films for parasites. This is the current gold standard. Rapid diagnostic tests, which help in detecting the specific parasite antigen or enzyme, can also be used. However, these tests are less sensitive than the malaria blood film.[61,62] In a febrile patient, three negative malaria smears 12–24 hours apart helps in ruling out the diagnosis of malaria.

❖ Other laboratory investigations, which may be required in severe cases of malaria, are listed in Box 20.4.

MANAGEMENT

❖ Malaria during pregnancy must be managed as an emergency situation, preferably by a multidisciplinary team comprising of an intensive care specialist, infectious disease specialist, obstetrician, neonatologist, etc.

❖ In the UK, pregnant women with uncomplicated malaria must be admitted to the hospital, whereas pregnant women with severe and complicated malaria must be admitted to an intensive care unit because the clinical condition can deteriorate in these patients. Non-falciparum malaria can be sometimes managed on an outpatient basis depending upon the clinical situation.

❖ Treatment of choice for severe falciparum malaria is IV artesunate. IV quinine may be used if artesunate is not available. Blood films must be monitored at every 24 hourly interval. However, the blood film must be repeated in case of clinical deterioration. Patient's hospitalisation is important for ensuring compliance to therapy. The 7-day course of quinine may be associated with significant adverse effects, principally cinchonism, which may include signs and symptoms such as tinnitus, headache, nausea, diarrhoea, altered auditory acuity and blurred vision. This may be frequently a cause of non-compliance, which may eventually result in the failure of therapy.[60,63-66]

❖ Uncomplicated *P. falciparum* (or mixed infections, such as *P. falciparum* and *P. vivax*) can be treated with drugs such as quinine and clindamycin. Chloroquine can be used for treating infection with *P. vivax*, *P. ovale* or *P. malariae*. Primaquine should not be preferably used during pregnancy. The clinician should switch to IV therapy in case of persistent vomiting.

❖ Antipyretics (paracetamol in standard doses) must be used for the treatment of fever. Prompt treatment of fever in malaria is necessary because it has been found to be associated with complications such as premature labour and foetal distress. Paracetamol should be prescribed in the dosage of 1 g every 4–6 hours (to a maximum of 4 g/day).

❖ Women with malaria must be screened for anaemia and treated appropriately.

❖ Woman who are recovering from an episode of malaria during pregnancy are advised to have regular ANC, including assessment of maternal haemoglobin, platelet and glucose levels, and foetal growth scans.

❖ Women should be advised about the risk of recurrence of malaria, and a suitable follow-up plan must be devised. This may involve repeating the blood film in case the

---

Box 20.3: Clinical presentation in case of severe or complicated malaria in adults[60]

❑ Prostration
❑ Impaired consciousness
❑ Respiratory distress (acidotic breathing, acute respiratory distress syndrome)*
❑ Pulmonary oedema (including radiological evidence)*
❑ Multiple convulsions
❑ Circulatory collapse, shock (blood pressure <90/60 mmHg)
❑ Abnormal bleeding, DIC
❑ Jaundice
❑ Haemoglobinuria (without G6PD deficiency)

Abbreviation: G6PD, glucose-6-phosphate dehydrogenase
Note: * Common feature in pregnant women with severe or complicated malaria

---

Box 20.4: Laboratory findings in cases of severe or complicated malaria in adults

❑ Severe anaemia (haemoglobin <8.0 g/dL)
❑ Thrombocytopenia
❑ Hypoglycaemia (<2.2 mmol/L)*
❑ Acidosis (pH <7.3)
❑ Renal impairment (oliguria <0.4 mL/kg body weight/hour or creatinine >265 µmol/L)
❑ Hyperlactataemia (correlates with mortality)
❑ Hyperparasitaemia (>2% parasitised red blood cells)
❑ 'Algid malaria'—gram-negative septicaemia*
❑ Lumbar puncture to exclude meningitis

Note: *Common features in pregnant women with severe or complicated malaria

symptoms or fever returns. Infections, which recur following treatment, are likely to be intrinsically less sensitive to the drugs that have been previously used against them. The options for treatment of recurrent infection in pregnancy in the UK are limited. However, if quinine and clindamycin have failed as first-line treatment, an alternative should be considered. Atovaquone-proguanil-artesunate and dihydroartemisinin-piperaquine have been effectively used in pregnant women with multiple recurrent infections.[67] The WHO has recommended a 7-day regimen of artesunate in the dosage of 2 mg/kg/day or 100 mg daily for 7 days and clindamycin in the dosage 450 mg three times daily for 7 days.

❖ The general rule of thumb is that the consequences of malaria are more harmful to the woman and her baby in comparison to the side effects related to the use of antimalarial medications.

Intrapartum Period

❖ Uncomplicated malaria in pregnancy per se is not an indication for induction of labour.

❖ In cases of severe malaria, particularly in presence of fever, cardiotocograph monitoring during labour is required. Electronic foetal monitoring may reveal abnormalities such as foetal tachycardia, bradycardia or late decelerations. In cases where the woman is being administered quinine, it is important to exclude maternal hypoglycaemia as the cause of foetal distress. Management of foetal distress is similar to that in normal obstetric cases.

❖ If the patient is being administered IV quinine, the mother's blood glucose levels must be frequently checked. A paediatrician must be alerted well in advance in these cases.

❖ Tocolytic therapy and prophylactic steroid therapy can be administered in the usual obstetric doses provided there are no obstetric contraindications.

❖ The woman must be informed about the risk of vertical transmission of malarial infection. Vertical transmission of malaria takes place when malarial parasites cross the placenta, either during pregnancy or at the time of birth. Vertical transmission to the foetus can occur, particularly when there is infection at the time of birth, and the placenta and cord are blood film positive for malaria.

❖ In cases of peripartum malaria, at the time of baby's birth placental specimen must be sent for histopathological examination. Blood films from the cord and baby's blood must be investigated to detect congenital malaria at an early stage. Though the presence of positive placental blood films and fever in the infant is indicative of congenital malaria, a blood film from the baby is required for confirmation.

❖ All neonates, whose mothers developed malaria in pregnancy, should be screened for malaria with standard microscopy of thick and thin blood films at birth. Blood films should be then taken at weekly intervals for 28 days.

COMPLICATIONS

❖ *Maternal complications*: Malarial infection during pregnancy can have numerous adverse effects on both mother and foetus,[68,69] including general decline in immunity, maternal anaemia (due to increased haemolysis and sequestration of infected RBCs into the reticuloendothelial system), miscarriage, stillbirths, intrauterine death, premature delivery, IUGR, and delivery of low birthweight infants (<2,500 g or <5.5 pounds), foetal heart rate abnormalities, pulmonary oedema, acute respiratory distress syndrome, hypoglycaemia, severe anaemia, secondary bacterial infection, principally gram-negative septicaemia, etc. Secondary bacterial infection should be suspected if the patient becomes hypotensive. These complications are likely to result in an overall increase in maternal and foetal mortality and morbidity. Another problem related to the presence of malarial infection in pregnancy is the widespread concerns regarding the safety of various medications used for treatment and prophylaxis.

❖ *Congenital malaria*: Congenital malaria in the very young infant or newborn results from the passage of parasites or the infected RBCs from the mother to the newborn while in utero or during delivery.

CLINICAL PEARLS

❖ Prompt and effective antimalarial treatment helps in preventing stillbirths and premature delivery due to malaria in pregnancy.

❖ There is usually no requirement for pregnant women with malaria to receive thromboprophylaxis.

❖ Pregnant patients with malaria should be regularly monitored for hypoglycaemia because malarial infection during pregnancy can result in profound and persistent hypoglycaemia, which can be exacerbated by quinine.

❖ Abnormalities in foetal and placental circulation (e.g. increased umbilical artery resistance index with cerebral redistribution, abnormalities in uterine artery flow velocity waveforms, etc.) have been noted on Doppler studies.

EVIDENCE-BASED MEDICINE

❖ The present evidence indicates that the drugs such as atovaquone-proguanil-artesunate and dihydro-artemisinin-piperaquine can be effectively used in pregnant women with multiple recurrent malarial infections, where first-line therapy with quinine and clindamycin has failed.[67] Atovaquone-proguanil is available in the UK.

PART II

❖ Vomiting, which can commonly occur as a symptom of malaria, is a known adverse effect of quinine. It can also occur in association with antimalarial treatment failure.[70-72] Presently, there is no evidence regarding the efficacy of using antiemetic agents for treatment of malaria-associated vomiting during pregnancy. However, in clinical practice, use of metoclopramide is considered safe, even during the first trimester.[73]

HEPATITIS VIRUS INFECTION IN PREGNANCY

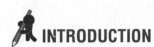

INTRODUCTION

The most common cause for hepatitis in pregnancy is acute viral hepatitis. The course of viral infection is not affected by pregnancy. Hepatitis caused by the hepatitis viruses A, B, C, D, E and G would be primarily discussed in this chapter.

Hepatitis A: Hepatitis A virus (HAV) is an RNA virus, which causes a mild and self-limiting illness.

Hepatitis B: Hepatitis B virus (HBV) is a double-walled spherical structure and measures 42 nm in diameter (Dane particle). The outer surface or envelope of virus contains hepatitis B surface antigen (HBsAg). Two other structural antigens present are core antigen (HBcAg) and e antigen (HBeAg). This is an extremely infectious virus, with its prevalence being as high as 1% in the UK.[74]

Hepatitis C: The HCV is a single-stranded, enveloped RNA flavivirus. It is structurally similar to the flaviviruses, 30–38 nm in size, having a genome of 9379–9481 base pairs.

Hepatitis D virus: The hepatitis D virus (HDV) is an unusual, single-stranded, circular RNA virus and is unique in being an incomplete virus that requires hepadnavirus (particularly hepatitis B virus) helper functions for propagation in hepatocytes.

Hepatitis E virus: Hepatitis E virus (HEV) is the primary cause of enterically transmitted non-A, non-B hepatitis.

Hepatitis G virus: This is a recently discovered flavivirus, which is probably similar to hepatitis C. Clinical features of this virus are presently under evaluation. It probably has a predilection for chronic hepatitis disease.

AETIOLOGY

Hepatitis A: This virus spreads via faecal-oral route and has an incubation period of 15–40 days.

Hepatitis B: Hepatitis B is a DNA virus, which is blood-borne. There are three important modes of transmission: (1) parenteral transmission, (2) perinatal transmission (vertical transmission from the mother to the child) and (3) sexual transmission. It is usually transmitted through the inoculation of blood products (e.g. transfusion, sharing of contaminated needles by the drug addicts, etc.).[75] Persons handling blood or those working in the haemodialysis units are at a special risk.

Hepatitis C: Whilst both HBV and HCV are transmitted through blood and blood products, HBV is a DNA virus and hepatitis C is an RNA flavivirus. HCV is mainly transmitted by IV drug use and blood products. Screening of blood donors and blood products has reduced the associated risks, so IV drug use is now the biggest risk factor.

Hepatitis D: Transmission of HDV occurs parenterally. Spread is via coinfection or superinfection with hepatitis B.

Hepatitis E: Spread of hepatitis E infection occurs via faecal-oral route.

Hepatitis G: Hepatitis G virus (HGV) is a parenterally transmitted infection. There is some evidence for sexual transmission based on the high detection rates of HGV amongst prostitutes and individuals with multiple sexual partners.

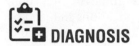

DIAGNOSIS

Clinical Presentation

Hepatitis A: Hepatitis A is generally a self-limiting infection and usually lasts for about 3–6 weeks. This infection is not associated with a carrier state. Most infected children under the age of 6 years are asymptomatic. Clinical presentation in older children and adults may vary from a mild, non-specific, anicteric infection to fulminant hepatic failure. Symptoms such as fever, malaise, anorexia, nausea, vomiting, abdominal discomfort, jaundice, dark urine and hepatomegaly may be present.

Hepatitis B: Non-specific signs and symptoms of hepatitis B infection include nausea, vomiting, fatigue, malaise, photophobia, diarrhoea, headache, right upper quadrant abdominal pain, etc. No abnormality is usually revealed on physical examination although abnormalities such as hepatomegaly, splenomegaly and/or lymphadenopathy may be present in a few cases. Infection with hepatitis B is often asymptomatic except in cases of IV drug users, where nearly 30% of the patients would develop jaundice.

Infection with hepatitis B virus may cause acute or chronic hepatitis. Chances of becoming chronically infected vary with age. Infected neonates and young children are more likely to develop chronic infection. Acute hepatitis B infection is usually a self-limiting illness and most of the patients are likely to show complete clearance of the virus. Clinical outcomes in case of acute hepatitis B infection are described in Flow chart 20.1. Fulminant hepatic failure is likely to develop in nearly 1% cases. All cases of fulminant hepatitis must be notified, and sexual and close household contacts must be screened and vaccinated. Although the majority of patients recover completely from hepatitis B, some patients may go on to

Flow chart 20.1: Clinical outcomes of acute hepatitis B infection

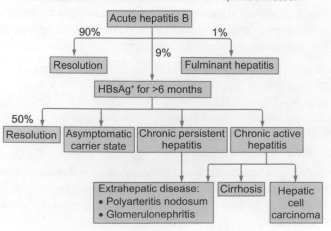

develop hepatocellular carcinoma or cirrhosis. Less than 50% of patients will progress to chronic liver disease.

Hepatitis C: Hepatitis C virus (incubation period of 30–60 days) can cause acute HCV infection, chronic HCV infection, cirrhosis, hepatoma and other complications induced by hepatitis. Clinical features of hepatitis C are non-specific. It is asymptomatic in nearly 75% cases. It can establish a long-term carrier state in nearly 80% of infected individuals. Cirrhosis may develop in approximately 20–40% patients, whereas hepatocellular carcinoma may develop in nearly 3% patients.

Individuals with HCV are at increased risk of other viral infections, such as HIV and hepatitis B. When coexisting HIV infection is also present, the risk of transmitting one or both viruses is much higher. Until recently, HCV was the most likely cause of post-transfusion hepatitis.[75] It accounts for most cases of viral hepatitis previously designated as non-A, non-B viral hepatitis. Blood or blood products and the organs of infected patients are the major sources of infection. Sexual and mother-to-baby transmission can sometimes occur. The risk of sexual transmission from an infected to a non-infected partner is less than 5%.

Hepatitis D: Double infection with hepatitis B and hepatitis D is particularly severe and carriers of both are at a risk of developing rapidly progressive cirrhosis.

Hepatitis E: It usually causes an acute, self-limiting disease similar to HAV. Infection with hepatitis E is not common in the UK. The infection with HEV can be particularly severe in pregnancy with a mortality rate of about 30% and nearly 15% risk of fulminant hepatic failure.

Hepatitis G: Most patients remain asymptomatic and do not require specific treatment.

Investigations

Hepatitis A: On liver function tests, serum alanine trans-aminase levels may be raised. HAV can be demonstrated in the stools by immunoelectron microscopy. Enzyme-linked immunosorbent assay (ELISA) is the method of choice for detection of IgM and IgG antibodies in the serum.

Hepatitis B: Diagnosis of hepatitis B is based on the presence of the following tests:

❖ *Serological tests*: Specific diagnosis of hepatitis B rests on serological demonstration of the viral markers and can be carried out by detection of HBsAg, anti-HBs, HBeAg, anti-HBe, IgM anti-HBc, IgG anti-HBc and HBV DNA in the serum. The sequence of appearance of viral markers in the blood is important. Presence of the HBsAg in the serum of these patients indicates that the infection is active and is associated with viral shedding. Presence of HBeAg is also associated with high infectivity. Appearance of antibodies to these antigens is associated with reduced infectivity and disease resolution. Complete resolution of the disease is associated with the disappearance of HbsAg and appearance of the surface antibodies.

Presence of these serological markers can be detected by sensitive and specific tests like ELISA and RIA (radio-immune assay). HBV DNA is also an indicator of viral replication and infectivity. Molecular methods such as DNA hybridization and PCR are used for HBV. Figure 20.1 shows hepatitis antigens, antibodies and DNA in a patient recovering from acute HBV infection.

❖ *Haematological tests*: Haematological tests may show presence of leucopenia, anaemia and/or thrombocyto-penia.

❖ *Liver function tests*: Liver function tests may reveal elevated levels of the enzyme aminotransferase.

Hepatitis C: Antibodies to hepatitis C appear relatively later in the course of illness. Therefore, in presence of high clinical suspicion for diagnosis of hepatitis C infection, antibody to HCV antigen can be detected by ELISA. The HCV RNA can be amplified by reverse transcription-PCR.

Hepatitis E: Specific diagnostic tests for infection due to HEV include PCR to detect HEV RNA, and ELISA, which detects both IgG and IgM anti-HEV antibodies.

Hepatitis G: The basic marker for the diagnosis of HGV infection is the presence of RNA diagnosed by real-time polymerase chain reaction (RT-PCR) amplification. HGV

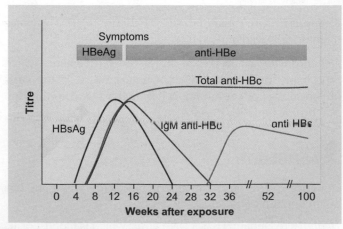

Fig. 20.1: Hepatitis antigens, antibodies and DNA in a patient recovering from acute hepatitis B virus infection

Abbreviations: HBsAg, hepatitis B surface antigen; HBeAg, hepatitis B e antigen; anti-HBc, anti-hepatitis B core antigen

infection also results in the development of antibodies against the E1 and E2 envelope proteins. The antibodies can be detected by an enzyme immunoassay. Presence of antibodies is a marker of previous infection, whereas presence of HGV RNA is an indicator of ongoing infection.

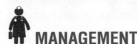

MANAGEMENT

Hepatitis A

❖ Advice to the pregnant women travelling to areas where HAV is endemic must be available.

❖ Hepatitis A virus can be prevented by use of vaccines containing formalin-inactivated HAV. The vaccine is likely to provide protection for nearly 10 years. The safety of this vaccine has yet not been determined during pregnancy. However, the probable risk to the foetus from an inactivated vaccine appears to be low.

❖ Prophylaxis with hepatitis A immunoglobulin can be administered to the contacts within 2 weeks of exposure. It provides protection against hepatitis A by either preventing infection or by attenuating the symptoms. Protection is short-limited, so the immunoglobulin injection needs to be repeated after every 3–6 months.

❖ Treatment is supportive and complete recovery usually occurs with no long-term sequelae.

Hepatitis B

General Management

❖ *Serological monitoring*: Patient should be monitored to ensure that the fulminant hepatic disease does not develop. Serological testing should be done 3 months after infection to ensure that the virus has cleared from the blood. However, HBsAg may test positive in 5–10% of the patients even after 3 months. A smaller proportion of the patients would continue to have ongoing viral replication. A follow-up with the hepatologist is required in these cases.

❖ *General prophylaxis*: This consists of avoiding risky practices like promiscuous sex, injectable drug abuse and direct or indirect contact with blood, semen or other body fluids of patients and carriers.

❖ *Immunisation*: Both passive and active methods of immunisation are available.

• *Passive immunisation*: Hyperimmune hepatitis B immune globulin (HBIG) administered IM in a dose of 300–500 IU soon after exposure to infection provides passive immunity. It may not prevent infection but protects against chronic illness and the carrier state. HBIG must be administered as soon as possible after an accident and preferably within 48 hours.[76] If the victim has not been previously vaccinated, a course of active immunisation is started along with the administration of HBIG. The two substances must be injected into different body sites.

• *Active immunisation*: Active immunisation is more effective in comparison to passive immunisation. Older vaccines were made from the plasma of hepatitis B carriers, obtained by plasmapheresis. Vaccine currently used is a recombinant yeast hepatitis B vaccine prepared through genetic engineering and comprises of non-glycosylated HBsAg particles. Three doses given at 0, 1 and 6 months administered via IM injection into the deltoid muscle (in adults) or into the anterolateral aspect of the thigh (in infants), constitute the full course. Other hepatitis B vaccines, which have also been successfully used, include recombinant Chinese hamster ovary cell hepatitis vaccine, synthetic peptide vaccines and hybrid virus vaccine.

Antepartum Period

❖ All pregnant women must be routinely offered testing for hepatitis B antibodies during their antenatal booking visit.

❖ If the patient has tested positive for the first time, serological tests must be done to determine the infectious state of the patient. The woman's partner must also be tested for HbsAg. Both the partners must also be tested for HIV, hepatitis C and other sexually transmitted diseases. A baseline liver function tests must also be performed for the patient.

Intrapartum Period

❖ Invasive procedures such as use of scalp electrodes and foetal blood sampling must be avoided.

❖ Use of forceps rather than vacuum has been suggested as a more useful mode of instrumental delivery because it is considered less traumatic. This strategy, however, is not supported by adequate evidence.

Postpartum Period

❖ Infants of HBsAg positive mothers who are HBeAg negative should receive active vaccination after delivery, i.e. the infant should receive a vaccine based on HBsAg.

❖ Infants of HBsAg positive mothers who are also HBeAg positive should receive both active and passive vaccination after delivery, i.e. the infant should receive a vaccine based on HBsAg as well as hepatitis B immunoglobulin.

❖ Arrangements must be made to complete the vaccination schedule when the mother and the baby are transferred to primary care.

❖ Once the babies are immunised, the mothers can breastfeed the baby.[77]

The available evidence suggests that various strategies such as use of hepatitis B vaccine alone; hepatitis B immuno-globulins alone; and the combination of hepatitis B vaccine and hepatitis B immunoglobulin, all reduce the risk of perinatal transmission of hepatitis B in newborn infants of HBsAg positive mothers who are also positive for HBeAg. However, the optimal treatment regimen presently remains unclear.[78]

Hepatitis C and Pregnancy

Antepartum Period

❖ Systematic screening of all pregnant women for HCV infection is not indicated. Screening, however, may be indicated in high-risk groups or cases where tests for HBV or HIV are positive.

❖ A multidisciplinary team approach comprising of an obstetrician, a physician having an interest in hepatitis C virus and a neonatologist is required.

❖ Women who test positive for HCV should be counselled about the risk of giving birth to an infected newborn. Determination of HCV RNA can be important in these cases because if this comes out to be negative, the patients can be counselled about the lower risk of transmission.

❖ Hepatitis C virus positive women are more at risk of obstetric cholestasis. For further information related to this, kindly refer to Chapter 13 (Hepatic and Gastrointestinal Diseases). Treatment with interferon and the drug ribavirin have been shown to be effective in the non-pregnant women. Early treatment with α-interferon is likely to reduce the risk of chronic infection. Ribavirin is contraindicated in pregnancy.

Intrapartum Period

❖ Management in the intrapartum period is similar to that in hepatitis B infection. Further research is required regarding whether the delivery by caesarean section is likely to reduce the risk of transmission.

Postpartum Period

❖ Infection with HCV per se is not a contraindication for breastfeeding.[77] However, many HCV-infected mothers have other coexisting problems (e.g. HIV infection, cracked nipples, etc.), which disallow breastfeeding.

❖ No neonatal immunoprophylaxis is available to prevent MTC transmission.

❖ *Foetal infection*: The main risk to the baby is infection with HCV. However, vertical transmission from mother to child is reckoned to occur in about 10–15% of cases. The risk is highest for mothers with detectable virus in their blood or those having a high titre of hepatitis C RNA. The woman whose partner has both HCV and HIV is at a much higher risk of infection. If a woman is both HCV and HIV positive, the risk of vertical transmission to her baby is much increased. The long-term implications of perinatal infection are unknown. There is no evidence that pregnancy has an adverse effect on the course of the woman's infection.

Hepatitis D

❖ Presently, there is no antiviral therapy found to be effective against acute or chronic HDV infection.

❖ Long-term use of α-interferon and pegylated α-interferon has been shown to bring about disease remission with reduced viral replication in non-pregnant women.

❖ Use of antiviral agents such as aciclovir, ribavirin, lamivudine, etc. are ineffective against the virus. Immunosuppressive agents are also ineffective.

❖ Immunisation against HBV prevents HDV infection amongst individuals who were previously HBV negative. However, administration of immunoglobulins and HBV immunisation in HBV carriers does not protect against HDV infection.

Hepatitis E

❖ General measures for preventing HEV infection include improving the standards of sanitation and chlorination of water.

❖ A vaccine may soon be available.

Hepatitis G

❖ Supportive therapy is useful in symptomatic patients.

❖ Screening for HGV infection in the pregnant population is not justified.

❖ Transmission of HGV may occur during the intrapartum or postnatal period. Intrapartum transmission at the time of delivery appears to be significantly reduced by use of caesarean delivery in comparison to the vaginal delivery.

COMPLICATIONS

Hepatitis A: No long-term adverse maternal or foetal consequences have been observed.

Hepatitis B: There is a risk of vertical transmission of HBV infection to the foetus.

Hepatitis C: There is a risk of vertical transmission of HCV infection to the foetus. There is an increased maternal risk of obstetric cholestasis.

Hepatitis E: Hepatitis E virus infection especially during the third trimester of pregnancy may result in fulminant HEV disease and maternal mortality in nearly 20% of patients. Other complications associated with HEV infection include increased risk of premature deliveries with high infant mortality, gestational hypertension, pre-eclampsia, proteinuria, oedema and kidney disease.

Hepatitis G: There is increased risk of vertical transmission of infection. Although perinatal transmission of HGV occurs, it is not likely to cause clinical disease in the newborns.

CLINICAL PEARLS

❖ Vertical transmission of hepatitis infection is more likely to occur at the time of delivery. It occurs at a rate of 95% in the mothers who test positive for both HbsAg as well as HbeAg antigens.

❖ During labour, the obstetrician must aim at keeping the membranes intact for as long period as possible.

EVIDENCE-BASED MEDICINE

❖ There is limited evidence regarding the appropriate mode of delivery (vaginal versus caesarean) in these cases.[76]
❖ Breastfeeding is permitted in case of maternal hepatitis infection.[77]

REFERENCES

1. Vyse AJ, Gay NJ, Hesketh LM, Morgan-Capner P, Miller E. Seroprevalence of antibody to varicella zoster virus in England and Wales in children and young adults. Epidemiol Infect. 2004;132(6):1129-34.
2. Miller E, Marshall R, Vurdien JE. Epidemiology, outcome and control of varicella-zoster infection. Rev Med Microbiol. 1993;4:222-30.
3. Lee BW. Review of varicella zoster seroepidemiology in India and South-east Asia. Trop Med Int Health. 1998;3(11):886-90.
4. Royal College of Obstetricians and Gynaecologists.(RCOG) (2015). Chickenpox in pregnancy. Green-top guideline no. 13. [online] RCOG website. Available from www.rcog.org.uk/en/guidelines-research-services/guidelines/gtg13/. [Accessed June, 2016].
5. Daley AJ, Thorpe S, Garland SM. Varicella and the pregnant woman: prevention and management. Aust N Z J Obstet Gynaecol. 2008;48(1):26-33.
6. Lamont RF, Sobel JD, Carrington D, Mazaki-Tovi S, Kusanovic JP, Vaisbuch E, et al. Varicella-zoster virus (chickenpox) infection in pregnancy. BJOG. 2011;118(10):1155-62.
7. Gardella C, Brown ZA. Managing varicella zoster infection in pregnancy. Cleve Clin J Med. 2007;74(4):290-6.
8. Kempf W, Meylan P, Gerber S, Aebi C, Agosti R, Büchner S, et al. Swiss recommendations for the management of varicella zoster virus infections. Swiss Med Wkly. 2007;137(17-18):239-51.
9. Shrim A, Koren G, Yudin MH, Farine D; Maternal Fetal Medicine Committee. Management of varicella infection (chickenpox) in pregnancy. J Obstet Gynaecol Can. 2012;34(3):287-92.
10. Nathwani D, Maclean A, Conway S, Carrington D. Varicella infections in pregnancy and the newborn. A review prepared for the UK Advisory Group on Chickenpox on behalf of the British Society for the Study of Infection. J Infect. 1998;36 (Suppl 1):59-71.
11. Tan MP, Koren G. Chickenpox in pregnancy: revisited. Reprod Toxicol. 2006;21(4):410-20.
12. Harger JH, Ernest JM, Thurnau GR, Moawad A, Momirova V, Landon MB, et al. Risk factors and outcome of varicella-zoster virus pneumonia in pregnant women. J Infect Dis. 2002;185(4):422-7.
13. Rawson H, Crampin A, Noah N. Deaths from chickenpox in England and Wales 1995-7: analysis of routine mortality data. BMJ. 2001;323(7321):1091-3.
14. Health Protection Agency. (2011) Guidance on Viral Rash in Pregnancy: Investigation, Diagnosis and Management of Viral Rash Illness, or Exposure to Viral Rash Illness, in Pregnancy. [online] Available from www.gov.uk/government/publications/viral-rash-in-pregnancy. [Accessed June, 2016]
15. Enders G, Miller E, Cradock-Watson J, Bolley I, Ridehalgh M. Consequences of varicella and herpes zoster in pregnancy: prospective study of 1739 cases. Lancet. 1994;343(8912):1548-51.
16. Manikkavasagan G, Bedford H, Peckham C, Dezateux C. Antenatal Screening for Susceptibility to Varicella Zoster Virus (VZV) in the United Kingdom: A review commissioned by the National Screening Committee. London: MRC Centre of Epidemiology for Child Health; 2009. pp. 1-53.
17. Wallace MR, Bowler WA, Murray NB, Brodine SK, Oldfield EC 3rd. Treatment of adult varicella with oral acyclovir. A randomized, placebo-controlled trial. Ann Intern Med. 1992;117(5):358-63.
18. Stone KM, Reiff-Eldridge R, White AD, Cordero JF, Brown Z, Alexander ER, et al. Pregnancy outcomes following systemic prenatal acyclovir exposure: Conclusions from the international acyclovir pregnancy registry, 1984–99. Birth Defects Res A Clin Mol Teratol. 2004;70(4):201-7.
19. Pasternak B, Hviid A. Use of acyclovir, valacyclovir and famcyclovir in the first trimester of pregnancy and the risk of birth defects. JAMA. 2010;304(8):859-66.
20. Mills JL, Carter TC. Acyclovir exposure and birth defects: an important advance, but more are needed. JAMA. 2010;304(8):905-6.
21. Brown ZA, Selke S, Zeh J, Kopelman J, Maslow A, Ashley RL, et al. The acquisition of herpes simplex virus during pregnancy. N Engl J Med. 1997;337(8):509-15.
22. Sheffield JS, Hollier LM, Hill JB, Stuart GS, Wendel GD. Acyclovir prophylaxis to prevent herpes simplex virus recurrence at delivery: a systematic review. Obstet Gynecol. 2003;102(6):1396-403.
23. Watts DH, Brown ZA, Money D, Selke S, Huang ML, Sacks SL, et al. A double-blind, randomized, placebo-controlled trial of acyclovir in late pregnancy for the reduction of herpes simplex virus shedding and cesarean delivery. Am J Obstet Gynecol. 2003;188(3):836-43.
24. Scott LL, Hollier LM, McIntire D, Sanchez PJ, Jackson GL, Wendel GD. Acyclovir suppression to prevent recurrent genital herpes at delivery. Infect Dis Obstet Gynecol. 2002;10:71-7.
25. Brocklehurst P, Kinghorn G, Carney O, Helsen K, Ross E, Ellis E, et al. A randomised placebo controlled trial of suppressive acyclovir in late pregnancy in women with recurrent genital herpes infection. Br J Obstet Gynaecol. 1998;105(3):275-80.
26. Scott LL, Sanchez PJ, Jackson GL, Zeray F, Wendel GD. Acyclovir suppression to prevent cesarean delivery after first-episode genital herpes. Obstet Gynecol. 1996;87:69-73.
27. Braig S, Luton D, Sibony O, Edlinger C, Boissinot C, Blot P, et al. Acyclovir prophylaxis in late pregnancy prevents recurrent genital herpes and viral shedding. Eur J Obstet Gynecol Reprod Biol. 2001;96(1):55-8.
28. Brown ZA, Vontver LA, Benedetti J, Critchlow CW, Sells CJ, Berry S, et al. Effects on infants of a first episode of genital herpes during pregnancy. N Engl J Med. 1987;317(20):1246-51.
29. Prober CG, Sullender WM, Yasukawa LL, Au DS, Yeager AS, Arvin AM. Low risk of herpes simplex virus infections in neonates exposed to the virus at the time of vaginal delivery to mothers with recurrent genital herpes simplex virus infections. N Engl J Med. 1987;316(5):240-4.
30. Brown ZA, Benedetti J, Ashley R, Burchett S, Selke S, Berry S, et al. Neonatal herpes simplex virus infection in relation to asymptomatic maternal infection at the time of labor. N Engl J Med. 1991;324(18):1247-52.
31. Royal College of Obstetricians and Gynaecologists.(RCOG) (2014). British Association for sexual health and HIV. Management of Genital Herpes in Pregnancy. [online] RCOG website. Available from www.rcog.org.uk/en/guidelines-research-services/guidelines/genital-herpes. [Accessed June, 2016].

CHAPTER 20

32. Brown ZA, Wald A, Morrow RA, Selke S, Zeh J, Corey L. Effect of serologic status and cesarean delivery on transmission rates of herpes simplex virus from mother to infant. JAMA. 2003;289(2):203-9.

33. Nahmias AJ. Neonatal HSV infection Part 1: continuing challenges. Herpes. 2004;11(2):33-7.

34. Ács N, Bánhidy F, Puhó E, Czeizel AE. No association between maternal recurrent genital herpes in pregnancy and higher risk for congenital abnormalities. Acta Obstet Gynecol Scand. 2008;87(3):292-9.

35. Drake AL, John-Stewart GC, Wald A, Mbori-Ngacha DA, Bosire R, Wamalwa DC, et al. Herpes simplex virus type 2 and risk of intrapartum human immunodeficiency virus transmission. Obstet Gynecol. 2007;109:403-9.

36. Brown ZA, Benedetti J, Selke S, Ashley R, Watts DH, Corey L. Asymptomatic maternal shedding of herpes simplex virus at the onset of labor: relationship to preterm labor. Obstet Gynecol. 1996;87(4):483-8.

37. Andrews WW, Kimberlin DF, Whitley R, Cliver S, Ramsey PS, Deeter R. Valacyclovir therapy to reduce recurrent genital herpes in pregnant women. Am J Obstet Gynecol. 2006;194(3):774-81.

38. Ratanajamit C, Vinther Skriver M, Jepsen P, Chongsuvivatwong V, Olsen J, Sørensen HT. Adverse pregnancy outcome in women exposed to acyclovir during pregnancy: a population-based observational study. Scand J Infect Dis. 2003;35(4):255-9.

39. Syridou G, Spanakis N, Konstantinidou A, Piperaki ET, Kafetzis D, Patsouris E, et al. Detection of cytomegalovirus, parvovirus B19 and herpes simplex viruses in cases of intrauterine fetal death: association with pathological findings. J Med Virol. 2008;80(10):1776-82.

40. Eskild A, Jeansson S, Stray-Pedersen B, Jenum PA. Herpes simplex virus type-2 infection in pregnancy: no risk of fetal death: results from a nested case-control study within 35,940 women. BJOG. 2002;109(9):1030-5.

41. Nahmias AJ, Josey WE, Naib ZM, Freeman MG, Fernandez RJ, Wheeler JH. Perinatal risk associated with maternal genital herpes simplex virus infection. Am J Obstet Gynecol. 1971;110(6):825-37.

42. British HIV Association. British HIV Association guidelines for the management of HIV infection in pregnant women 2012 (2014 interim review). HIV Med. 2014;15 (Suppl 4):1-77.

43. Royal College of Obstetrician and Gynaecologists. Management of HIV in Pregnancy. Green-top Guideline No. 39. London: RCOG; 2010.

44. Townsend CL, Cortina-Borja M, Peckham CS, de Ruiter A, Lyall H, Tookey PA. Low rates of mother-to-child transmission of HIV following effective pregnancy interventions in the United Kingdom and Ireland, 2000-2006. AIDS. 2008;22(8):973-81.

45. European Mode of Delivery Collaboration. Elective caesarean section versus vaginal delivery in prevention of vertical HIV-1 transmission: a randomised clinical trial. Lancet. 1999;353(9158):1035-9.

46. International Perinatal HIV Group. The mode of delivery and the risk of vertical transmission of human immunodeficiency virus type 1--a meta-analysis of 15 prospective cohort studies. N Engl J Med. 1999;340(13):977-87.

47. Warszawski J, Tubiana R, Le Chenadec J. Mother-to-child HIV transmission despite antiretroviral therapy in the ANRS French Perinatal Cohort. AIDS. 2008;22(2):289-99.

48. Dunn DT, Newell ML, Ades AE, Peckham CS. Risk of human immunodeficiency virus type 1 transmission through breastfeeding. Lancet. 1992;340(8819):585-8.

49. Owens DK, Holodniy M, Garber AM, Scott J, Sonnad S, Moses L, et al. Polymerase chain reaction for the diagnosis of HIV infection in adults. A meta-analysis with recommendations for clinical practice and study design. Ann Intern Med. 1996;124(9):803-15.

50. Gazzard BG, Anderson J, Babiker A, Boffito M, Brook G, Brough G, et alBritish HIV Association Guidelines for the treatment of HIV-1-infected adults with antiretroviral therapy 2008. HIV Med. 2008;9(8):563-608.

51. Connor EM, Sperling RS, Gelber R, Kiselev P, Scott G, O'Sullivan MJ, et al. Reduction of maternal-infant transmission of human immunodeficiency virus type 1 with zidovudine treatment. Pediatric AIDS Clinical Trials Group Protocol 076 Study Group. N Engl J Med. 1994;331(18):1173-80.

52. Lalloo DG, Shingadia D, Pasvol G, Chiodini PL, Whitty CJ, Beeching NJ, et al. UK malaria treatment guidelines. J Infect. 2007;54:111-21.

53. Nosten F, McGready R, Mutabingwa T. Case management of malaria in pregnancy. Lancet Infect Dis. 2007;7(2):118-25.

54. Dondorp A, Nosten F, Stepniewska K, Day N, White N. Artesunate versus quinine for treatment of severe falciparum malaria: a randomised trial. Lancet. 2005;366(9487):717-25.

55. Davis TM, Suputtamongkol Y, Spencer JL, Wilson SG, Mekhton S, Croft KD, et al. Glucose turnover in pregnant women with acute malaria. Clin Sci (Lond). 1994;86(1):83-90.

56. Dellicour S, Hall S, Chandramohan D, Greenwood B. The safety of artemisinins during pregnancy: a pressing question. Malar J. 2007;6:15.

57. ter Kuile F, White NJ, Holloway P, Pasvol G, Krishna S. Plasmodium falciparum: in vitro studies of the pharmacodynamic properties of drugs used for the treatment of severe malaria. Exp Parasitol. 1993;76(1):85-95.

58. Jelinek T. Intravenous artesunate for treatment of patients with severe malaria: position statement of TropNetEurop. Euro Surveill. 2005;10(11):E051124.5.

59. Nosten F, McGready R, d'Alessandro U, Bonell A, Verhoeff F, Menendez C, et al. Antimalarial drugs in pregnancy: a review. Curr Drug Saf. 2006;1(1):1-15.

60. Dilling JW, Gemmell AA. A preliminary investigation of fetal deaths following quinine induction. J Obstet Gynecol. 1929;36:352-66.

61. Poespoprodjo JR, Fobia W, Kenangalem E, Lampah DA, Warikar N, Seal A, et al. Adverse pregnancy outcomes in an area where multidrug-resistant plasmodium vivax and Plasmodium falciparum infections are endemic. Clin Infect Dis. 2008;46(9):1374-81.

62. McGready R, Cho T, Keo NK, Thwai KL, Villegas L, Looare-esuwan S, et al. Artemisinin antimalarials in pregnancy: a prospective treatment study of 539 episodes of multidrug resistant Plasmodium falciparum. Clin Infect Dis. 2001;33(12):2009-16.

63. van Vugt M, Leonardi E, Phaipun L, Slight T, Thway KL, McGready R, et al. Treatment of uncomplicated multidrug resistant falciparum malaria with artesunate-atovaquone-proguanil. Clin Infect Dis. 2002;35(12):1498-504.

64. Royal College of Obstetricians and Gynaecologists. Preventing Malaria in Pregnancy. Green-top Guideline No. 54A. London: RCOG; 2010.

65. Tarning J, McGready R, Lindegardh N, Ashley EA, Pimanpanarak M, Kamanikom B, et al. Population pharma-cokinetics of lumefantrine in pregnant women treated with artemetherlumefantrine for uncomplicated Plasmodium falciparum malaria. Antimicrob Agents Chemother. 2009; 53:3837-46.

66. Novartis Pharmaceuticals UK Ltd. 2009. Riamet 20/120 mg tablets. Summary of Product Characteristics. Electronic Medicines Compendium. [online] Available from www.emc. medicines.org.uk/medicine/9196/SPC/Riamet+20+120mg+t ablets/#PREGNANCY [Accessed June, 2016]

67. Royal College of Obstetricians and Gynaecologists. (RCOG). The diagnosis and treatment of malaria in pregnancy. Green-top Guideline No. 54B. London: RCOG; 2010.

68. Meira DA. Plasmodium falciparum infection and pregnancy. Case reports. Rev Soc Bras Med Trop. 1989;22(2):99-101.

69. Bounyasong S. Randomized trial of artesunate and mefloquine in comparison with quinine sulfate to treat P. falciparum malaria pregnant women. J Med Assoc Thai. 2001;84(9):1289-9.

70. Tagbor H, Bruce J, Browne E, Randal A, Greenwood B, Chandramohan D. Efficacy, safety, and tolerability of amodiaquine plus sulphadoxine-pyrimethamine used alone or in combination for malaria treatment in pregnancy: a randomised trial. Lancet. 2006;368 (9544):1349-56.

71. Arnold J, Alving AS, Hockwald RS, Clayman CB, Dern RJ, Beutler E, et al. The effect of continuous and intermittent primaquine therapy on the relapse rate of Chesson strain vivax malaria. J Lab Clin Med. 1954;44(3):429-38.

72. Doherty JF, Day JH, Warhurst DC, Chiodini PL. Treatment of Plasmodium vivax malaria: time for a change? Trans R Soc Trop Med Hyg. 1997;91(1):76.

73. Fryauff DJ, Baird JK, Basri H, Sumawinata I, Purnomo, Richie TL, et al. Randomised placebo-controlled trial of primaquine for prophylaxis of falciparum and vivax malaria. Lancet. 1995;346(8984):1190-3.

74. Chisari FV, Ferrari C. Viral hepatitis. In: Nathanson N, Ahmed R, Gonzalez-Scarano F, et al (Eds). Viral Pathogenesis. Philadelphia: Lippincott-Raven; 1997. pp. 745-78.

75. Marik PE. The hazards of blood transfusion. Br J Hosp Med (Lond). 2009;70(1):12-5.

76. American Academy of Pediatrics. Breastfeeding and the use of human milk. Work Group on Breastfeeding. Pediatrics. 1997;100(6):1035-9.

77. ACOG Practice Bulletin No. 86: Viral hepatitis in pregnancy. Obstet Gynecol. 2007;110(4):941-56.

78. Lee C, Gong Y, Brok J, Boxall EH, Gluud C. Hepatitis B immunisation for newborn infants of hepatitis B surface antigen-positive mothers. Cochrane Database Syst Rev. 2006;(2):CD004790.

CHAPTER 20

Smoking during Pregnancy

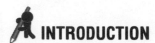

INTRODUCTION

While men are known to consume more tobacco than women, a sizeable number of the women are also consuming tobacco and that too during reproductive age and pregnancy. The prevalence of domestic environmental tobacco smoke (ETS) exposure and maternal smoking during pregnancy was shown to be high in the UK as well.[1] In the study by Ward et al., in the UK, nearly 13% of infants were exposed to ETS and 36% to maternal smoking during the antenatal period.

Exposure to tobacco smoke can result in numerous adverse effects for the general population as well as the pregnant woman and her baby. Smoking is the most common exogenous factor responsible for producing low-birthweight babies. Besides this, smoking during pregnancy can result in numerous adverse maternal, foetal and neonatal outcomes resulting in an increased maternal and neonatal morbidity and mortality. Cigarette smoking by the mother is equally harmful to the foetus as the exposure to second-hand smoke. The primary aim of the obstetrician is to help women quit smoking either through use of behaviour modification or pharmacotherapies.

AETIOLOGY

Mcohanism of Effect of Cigarette Smoke

Cigarette smoke consists of numerous toxic, poisonous and carcinogenic substances, which can be harmful to the foetus and placenta. Some of them are as follows:[2,3]

❖ Substances like tar, arsenic, cadmium and nickel, vinyl chloride, creosote, formaldehyde, etc. present in cigarette smoke are potentially carcinogenic in nature.
❖ Smoking during pregnancy, by raising the level of CO in blood, results in a physiological response, interfering with delivery of oxygen to the foetus. CO reduces the oxygen carrying capacity of blood and induces adaptive changes in the placenta in order to maintain the oxygen supply. Compensatory changes cause the placenta to become larger for the given gestational age and result in increased placental ratio (ratio of placental diameter to the thickness). Though placenta is thinner in the women smoking tobacco, their diameter is larger. The other changes, which can occur in the placenta, include placenta praevia, abruptio placentae, premature ageing, etc.
❖ The nicotine present in cigarette smoke may first stimulate and then depress the autonomic nervous system through the release of epinephrine from adrenal medulla, thereby resulting in decreased responsiveness of the foetal cardio-vascular system to external stresses of labour, impairing foetal development.

Effects of Nicotine on the Body

It is a well-known fact that tobacco consumption is hazardous to the health. Tobacco smoke contains numerous chemicals, which can produce acute and chronic adverse health outcomes.[2,3]

❖ *Acute risks*: These include shortness of breath, exacerbation of asthma, impotence, infertility, and increased serum CO levels.
❖ *Long-term risks*: Heart attacks, strokes, chronic obstructive pulmonary diseases (bronchitis and emphysema), cancers (lung cancer, cancer of larynx, oral cavity, pharynx, oeso-phagus, pancreas, bladder, cervix, etc. to name a few), etc.
❖ *Risk during pregnancy*: It is now also apparent that tobacco smoking is deleterious to both the pregnancy and prenatal outcome, some of which are described later in the text.
❖ *Risk due to second-hand smoke*: Even if the woman does not herself smoke during pregnancy, her foetus can be harmed as a result of exposure to the second-hand smoke from the environment. The exposure to environmental tobacco smoke can result in the following risks:
  • *Risk to the mother*: Pregnant women who are exposed to second-hand smoke have a 20% higher risk of giving

birth to a low-birthweight baby than women who are not exposed to second-hand smoke during pregnancy. Inhalation of environmental tobacco smoke by the pregnant woman is an important cause of lung cancer.[4]

- *Risk to the baby*: Children who are exposed to second-hand smoke are at an increased risk for bronchitis, pneumonia, middle ear infections, severe asthma, respiratory symptoms, and reduced pulmonary growth and development.[5,6] Parental smoking and prone sleep positioning are recognised causal factors for sudden infant death. When there is a pregnant woman in the household, there is a need for interventions to reduce environmental tobacco smoke exposure in utero to the foetus and other young children in the household by educating the parents and adolescents.

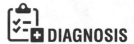

DIAGNOSIS

History and Clinical Presentation

Diagnosis is usually based on the history. From the first antenatal appointment, the midwife needs to enquire from the patient whether she or any other member of the household smokes. This is important so that the appropriate support and help can be provided to her and her family to help her stop smoking as soon as possible. The frequency of smoking and the number of cigarettes smoked per day also needs to be asked.

Investigations

Carbon Monoxide Test

A CO test is an immediate and non-invasive biochemical method for assessing whether or not someone smokes. However, the best cut-off point for determining smoking status is presently unclear. Some suggest a CO level as low as 3 parts per million (ppm), others use a cut-off point of 6–10 ppm.[7] When trying to identify pregnant women who smoke, it is best to use a low cut-off point. The midwife performs this test at the first antenatal appointment to measure the woman's level of exposure to CO. CO levels are higher in women who smoke and in passive smokers than in women who do not.

All pregnant women are advised to have the test whether they smoke or not because CO levels may also be high if the women have faulty gas appliances at home. If the woman doesn't smoke and she is not exposed to tobacco smoke but still her CO levels are high, she should contact the free Health and Safety Executive Gas Safety Advice Line on 0800- 300-363. CO levels may also be raised if she is exposed to high levels of pollution or if she is suffering from lactose intolerance.

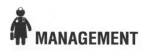

MANAGEMENT

The various recommendations by NICE guidelines are tabulated in Table 21.1. According to the first recommendation by the NICE guidelines, midwives must identify the pregnant

Table 21.1: Recommendations by NICE guidelines[7]

Recommendations	Specifications
Recommendation 1	Action for midwives—identifying pregnant women who smoke and referring them to NHS Stop Smoking Services
Recommendation 2	Action for others in the public, community and voluntary sectors (GPs, practice nurses, health visitors, family nurses, obstetricians, paediatricians, sonographers and other members of the maternity team other than the midwives)—identifying pregnant women who smoke and referring them to NHS Stop Smoking Services
Recommendation 3	Stop Smoking Services—contacting referrals (NHS Stop Smoking Services specialist advisers should contact all referrals on telephone)
Recommendation 4	Stop Smoking Services—initial and ongoing support to be provided by the NHS Stop Smoking Services specialist advisers. This involves offering women the following interventions to help them quit smoking: cognitive behaviour therapy, motivational interviewing and structured self-help and support from NHS Stop Smoking Services.
Recommendation 5	Use of NRT and other pharmacological support
Recommendation 6	NHS Stop Smoking Services—meeting the needs of disadvantaged pregnant women who smoke
Recommendation 7	Meeting the needs of partners and others in the household who smoke
Recommendation 8	Training to deliver interventions

Abbreviations: GPs, general practitioners; NHS, National Health Service; NRT, nicotine replacement therapy

women who smoke and refer them to NHS Stop Smoking Services.[7]

The Stop Smoking Service team offers one-to-one appointments to the woman and also helps suggest ways to help her cope up with her cravings and withdrawal symptoms, which may occur once she stops smoking. The length of time for which the woman may require support would vary for each woman and may depend on her circumstances. Typically, a 12-week programme is likely to be useful to most women through their initial period. The referral pathway from maternity services to NHS Stop Smoking Services is illustrated in Flow chart 21.1.[7]

Reducing tobacco use among women at the time of pregnancy forms one of the topmost public health priorities in the UK. The two main methods of helping the woman give up smoking include behavioural modification and pharmacotherapy. Though the harmful effects of medicines, which help in giving up smoking, have not been demonstrated in well-designed clinical studies, pregnant women are more reluctant to use cessation medications.[8,9] In practice, behavioural modification and counselling are commonly used as the first-line treatment. Heavy smokers who do not respond to a behavioural intervention may benefit from pharmacotherapy.

Nicotine Replacement Therapy

Nicotine is the addictive chemical present in the cigarettes. Use of nicotine replacement therapy (NRT) helps prevent nicotine withdrawal symptoms when the woman quits, and

Flow chart 21.1: The referral pathway from maternity services to NHS Stop Smoking Services[7]

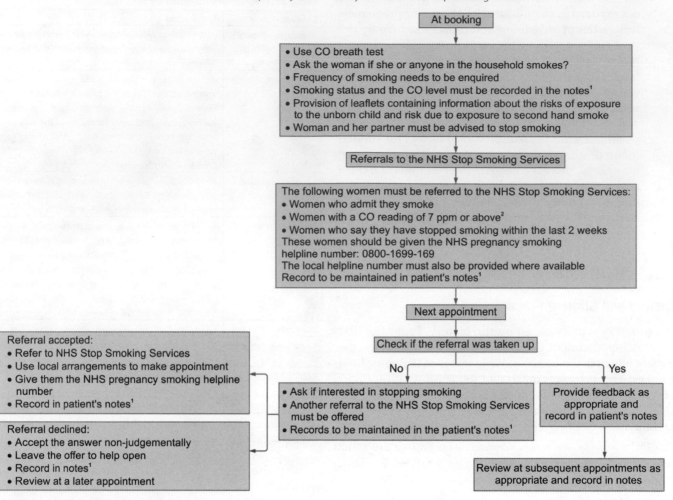

Notes: [1]Preferably the patient's handheld records; [2]Lower levels (e.g. 3 ppm) may apply for light or infrequent smokers

PART II

does not contain harmful substances such as tar or CO.[10] NRT is available in different delivery methods: oral products, spray, patches, inhalers, etc. Oral products, such as chewing gum, mouth sprays and lozenges, which are available over-the-counter, are considered as the safer option, because they provide short bursts of nicotine. A pregnant patient, however, may be feeling too nauseous to use oral forms of nicotine. In these cases, a patch serves as a good option.

According to the ACOG, 'Smoking cessation during pregnancy education Bulletin of September 2000', the use of nicotine replacement products or other pharmaceuticals substances, which help the pregnant patient in giving up her smoking habit during pregnancy, have not been sufficiently evaluated (in form of level A evidence) to determine its efficacy or safety.[8] Thus, prescribing any medication or encouraging the use of non-prescription medicines during pregnancy is a matter of individual clinical judgement. Risks and benefits of each therapeutic option must be evaluated and shared with the pregnant woman.

Presently, there is conflicting evidence regarding the effectiveness of NRT in helping women to stop smoking during pregnancy. No evidence regarding the efficacy of NRT or its effect on the child's birthweight has been found even in the most vigorous trials till date. In addition, there is insufficient data to form a judgement about whether or not NRT has any impact on the likelihood of a child requiring special care or being stillborn.

The NHS Stop Smoking Services advisors must discuss the risks and benefits of NRT with pregnant women who smoke, particularly those who are interested in using NRT. Use of NRT must be advised only if smoking cessation without the use of NRT has failed. The obstetricians must use their own professional judgement when deciding whether to offer a prescription for NRT or not.[11]

Nicotine replacement therapy should be only prescribed, once the woman has stopped smoking. Initially, NRT must be prescribed only for 2 weeks from the day the woman has agreed to stop smoking. Subsequent prescriptions must be given only to the women who have demonstrated that they are still not smoking on reassessment. Pregnant women who are using nicotine patches must be advised to remove them before going to bed.[11] Non-nicotine medications, such as varenicline or bupropion should not be offered to pregnant or breastfeeding women.[12]

Electronic cigarettes are becoming a popular alternative to tobacco smoking. They have been found to contain some harmful substances as well as nicotine. Presently, their use is not recommended during pregnancy because the long-term risks on the baby due to their use remain unknown.[4]

 COMPLICATIONS

Various maternal and foetal complications related to smoking during pregnancy are enumerated in Table 21.2 and are described next in details.

Maternal Effects

Pre-eclampsia

A negative correlation between maternal smoking and pre-eclampsia has been reported. Gestational cigarette smoking, which is widely accepted to be harmful to both the mother and foetus, is believed to be protective against pre-eclampsia by reducing the inflammatory reaction associated with aberrant cytokine production.[13,14] In a study by Dowling et al., nicotine and other cholinergic agonists were shown to significantly suppress placental cytokine production, via NFKβ pathway, a critical regulator of inflammation, thereby producing a protective response against pre-eclampsia.[14] However, cigarette smoking is associated with an increased risk of perinatal mortality if pre-eclampsia or hypertension does develop in a smoker. Women who smoke are much less likely to nurse their babies than the non-smoker. There is requirement of further research in the future to clarify the negative correlation between smoking and pre-eclampsia.

Abruptio Placentae

Many studies have shown significant relationship between tobacco consumption and higher incidence of abruptio placentae and other types of bleeding commonly encountered during pregnancy.[10,15] The authors have emphasised the importance of simple strategies like patient education, smoking cessation programs, and early prenatal care in the prevention of placental abruption.

Table 21.2: Adverse effects of smoking

Maternal	Foetal
• Pre-eclampsia and abruptio placentae	• Stillbirths
• Ectopic pregnancy	• Low-birthweight babies (preterm and intrauterine growth restriction)
• Miscarriage	• Risk of congenital anomalies (e.g. cleft lip and palate)
• Abnormal placental attachment resulting in placenta praevia	• Developmental and behavioural abnormities in the child
• Vaginal bleeding	• Poor performance in school
• Suppression of lactation	• Short attention span and hyperactivity
	• Reduced IQ and cognitive performance
	• Sudden infant death syndrome
	• Asthma, chest and ear infections, and pneumonia

Abbreviation: IQ, intelligence quotient

Increased Incidence of Spontaneous Abortions and Ectopic Pregnancy

Smoking during pregnancy is associated with increased risk of spontaneous abortions and ectopic pregnancy during early gestation.[16,17]

Adverse Effect of Smoking on Lactation

Maternal high levels of nicotine have been shown to reach the infant through the breast milk, especially if the mother smokes 20 or more cigarettes per day. If the maternal smoking exceeds 20–30 cigarettes per day, milk yield may significantly decrease and nicotine present in the milk may cause nausea, vomiting, abdominal cramping and diarrhoea in the infants.[18] Studies have also suggested that smoking during pregnancy and postpartum period significantly reduced the prevalence of breastfeeding among smokers, but there was no significant reduction among non-smokers. Since the rate of breastfeeding decreases with smoking, smoking should be discouraged, particularly in developing countries where breastfeeding is an important practice to ensure supply of adequate nutrition to the child.

Foetal Effects

Risk of Low-birthweight Babies, Prematurity and IUGR

In developed countries, the most important risk factor for low birthweight has been found to be cigarette smoking, followed by poor nutrition during pregnancy and low prepregnancy weight. Smoking accounts for 20–30% of all low-birthweight babies born and can be considered as the single most important preventable cause of low birthweight in developed countries.[19] Maternal smoking during pregnancy has also been shown to impair foetal growth, resulting in IUGR babies,[20-24] and shortens the period of gestation resulting in PROM and premature delivery. These are important factors associated with significant foetal and infant mortality and morbidity. Women who smoke have approximately double the risk of premature delivery. This is principally due to spontaneous preterm delivery but can also increase the risk of need for iatrogenic delivery due to association of smoking with placenta praevia and abruption. The greater the duration of smoking during the period of pregnancy, the greater would be her risk of complications. For example, if a pregnant woman stops smoking during the first half of her pregnancy, her baby will most likely be of normal weight. If she continues to smoke throughout the pregnancy, she will probably have a low-birthweight baby. So if the woman who had been smoking through the first half of pregnancy has not been successful in quitting smoking in the first half of pregnancy, she should still be encouraged to continue trying or at the very least cutting down on the number of cigarettes she smokes per day as it can still benefit her and her baby. This foetal growth restriction due to smoking is followed by an accelerated 'catch up' growth rate in the early months following birth (Strauss and Dietz, 1998).[25]

Congenital Anomalies

Components of tobacco like tar, nicotine, CO, nitrosamine, etc. are known carcinogens and mutagens. However, presently the overall relation between malformations and maternal smoking during pregnancy is uncertain. Study by Kallen reported a protective effect of maternal smoking in reducing the incidence of neural tube defects, which was not statistically significant.[26]

Some of the congenital malformations, which have been reported in association with smoking, include oral clefts (cleft lip and palate),[27,28] limb reduction defects,[29,30] and kidney malformations.[31,32] Maternal smoking has been found to be one of most important exogenous factors involved in the aetiology of cleft lip and cleft palate in humans.

Maternal smoking has been found to be associated with increased prevalence of hydrocephalus, microcephaly, omphalocele, gastroschisis, cleft lip/palate, clubfoot, polydactyly, syndactyly, adactyly, etc.[33] However, the exact relationship between the maternal tobacco smoking during pregnancy and presence of congenital anomalies largely remains unknown as the various studies have presented with inconsistent and conflicting results.

Neonatal Effects

As previously mentioned, these include increased incidence of sudden infant death syndrome, pneumonia, bronchitis, middle ear infections, respiratory symptoms, etc.

Problems Related to Cessation of Smoking

Addiction to Smoking

According to Diagnostic and Statistical Manual of Mental Disorders: revised fourth edition (DSM-IV-R)[34] (2000), nicotine dependence is defined as compulsive use of nicotine despite development of severe and devastating negative consequences and is associated with three (or more) of the following symptoms occurring at any time in the same 12-month period:

1. Development of tolerance towards the drug, which is being used
2. Development of withdrawal symptoms when tobacco smoking is stopped. Smoking tobacco helps in obtaining relief from withdrawal symptoms.
3. The substance is consumed in either larger amounts or for longer duration of time than intended; the person has made numerous unsuccessful efforts to control substance use; great deal of time is spent on drug-related activities (e.g. procuring, using or recovering from effects of drugs); important social and occupational activities are given up because of the time spent on substance use and the person continues to use substance despite the knowledge regarding its possible physical or psychological harms.

CLINICAL PEARLS

❖ Babies who are exposed to passive smoking in utero are likely to have a higher than normal risk of complications such as stillbirths, prematurity, small for gestational age, etc. Their growth and health after birth may also be adversely affected.

❖ E-cigarettes are currently not recommended for use during pregnancy.

EVIDENCE-BASED MEDICINE

❖ The present evidence presents with mixed results regarding the effectiveness of NRT in helping women to stop smoking during pregnancy.[10,11]

❖ Non-nicotine medications are usually not prescribed to pregnant or breastfeeding women.[7,8]

REFERENCES

1. Ward C, Lewis S, Coleman T. Prevalence of maternal smoking and environmental tobacco smoke exposure during pregnancy and impact on birth weight: retrospective study using Millennium Cohort. BMC Public Health. 2007;7:81
2. Law MR, Hackshaw AK. Environmental tobacco smoke. Br Med Bull. 1996;52(1):22-34.
3. Frieden TR, Blakeman DE. The dirty dozen: 12 myths that undermine tobacco control. Am J Public Health. 2005;95(9):1500-5.
4. Hackshaw AW, Law MR, Wald NJ. The accumulated evidence on lung cancer and environmental tobacco smoke. BMJ. 1997;315(7114): 980-8.
5. Cook DG, Strachan DP. Health effects of passive smoking-10: summary of effects of parental smoking on the respiratory health of children and implications for research. Thorax. 1999;54(4):357-66.
6. Anderson ME, Johnson DC, Batal HA. Sudden infant death syndrome and prenatal maternal smoking: rising attributed risk in the back to sleep era. BMC Med. 2005;11:3-4.
7. National Institute of Clinical Excellence. (NICE) (2010). Smoking: stopping in pregnancy and after childbirth: public health guideline. [online] NICE website. Available from www.nice.org.uk/guidance/ph26 [Accessed June, 2016].
8. West R, Mc Neill A, Raw M. Smoking cessation guidelines for health professionals: an update. Health Education Authority. Thorax. 2000;55(12):987-99.
9. American College of Obstetricians and Gynecologists. (ACOG), (2000). "Smoking cessation during pregnancy." ACOG educational bulletin 260 [online]. ACOG website. Available from www.acog.org/Resources-And-Publications/Committee-Opinions/Committee-on-Health-Care-for-Underserved-Women/Smoking-Cessation-During-Pregnancy [Accessed June, 2016].
10. Ananth CV, Savitz DA, Bowes WA Jr, Luther ER. Influence of hypertensive disorders and cigarette smoking on placental abruption and uterine bleeding during pregnancy. Br J Obstet Gynaecol. 1997;104(5):572-8.
11. Fang WL, Goldstein AO, Butzen AY, Hartsock SA, Hartmann KE, Helton M, et al. Smoking cessation in pregnancy: a review of postpartum relapse prevention strategies. J Am Board Fam Pract. 2004;17(4):264-75.
12. French GM, Groner JA, Wewers ME, Ahijevych K. Staying smoke free: an intervention to prevent postpartum relapse. Nicotine Tob Res. 2007;9(6):663-70.
13. Takahashi HK, Iwagaki H, Hamano R, Yoshino T, Tanaka N, Nishibori M. Effect of nicotine on IL-18-initiated immune response in human monocytes. J Leukoc Biol. 2006;80(6): 1388-94.

14. Dowling O, Rochelson B, Way K, Al-Abed Y, Metz CN. Nicotine inhibits cytokine production by placenta cells via NFkappa B: potential role in pregnancy-induced hypertension. Mol Med. 2007;13(11-12):576-83.

15. Ananth CV, Smulian JC, Vintzleos AM. Incidence of placental abruption in relation to cigarette smoking and hypertensive disorders during pregnancy: a meta-analysis of observational studies. Obstet Gynecol. 1999;93(4):622-8.

16. Habib P. What are the consequences of smoking on pregnancy and delivery. J Gynecol Obstet Biol Reprod (Paris). 2005;34 Spec No 1:3S353-69.

17. Dekeyser-Boccara J, Millien J. Smoking and ectopic pregnancy: is there a causal relationship? J Gynecol Obstet Biol Reprod (Paris). 2005;34 Spec No 1:3S119-23.

18. Najdawi F, Faouri M. Maternal smoking and breastfeeding. East Mediterr Health J. 1999;5(3):450-6.

19. Kramer MS. Determinants of low birth weight: methodological assessment and meta-analysis. Bull World Health Organ. 1987;65(5):663-737.

20. Robinson JS, Moore VM, Owens JA, McMillen IC. Origins of fetal growth restriction. Eur J Obstet Gynecol Reprod Biol. 2000;92:13-9.

21. Sadler L, Belanger K, Saftlas A, Leaderer B, Hellenbrand K, McSharry JE, et al. Environmental tobacco smoke exposure and small-for-gestational-age birth. Am J Epidemiol. 1999; 150(7):695-705.

22. Jaakkola JJ, Jaakkola N, Zahlsen K. Fetal growth and length of gestation in relation to prenatal exposure to environmental tobacco smoke assessed by hair nicotine concentration. Environ Health Perspect. 2001;109(6):557-61.

23. Conter V, Cortinovis I, Rogari P, Riva L. Weight growth in infants born to mothers who smoked during pregnancy. BMJ. 1995;310(6982):768-71.

24. Fox NL, Sexton M, Hebel RJ. Prenatal exposure to tobacco. Effects on physical growth at age three. Int J Epidemiol. 1990;19(1):66-71.

25. Strauss RS, Dietz WH. Growth and development of term children born with low birth weight: effects of genetic and environmental factors. J Pediatr. 1998;133(1):67-72.

26. Kallen K. Maternal smoking, body mass index, and neural tube defects. Am J Epidemiol. 1998;147(12):1103-11.

27. Ericson A, Kalian B, Westerholm P. Cigarette smoking as an etiologic factor in cleft lip and palate. Am J Obstet Gynecol. 1979;135(3):348-51.

28. Khoury MJ, Weinstein A, Panny S, Holtzman NA, Lindsay PK, Farrel K, et al. Maternal cigarette smoking and oral clefts: a population-based study. Am J Public Health. 1987;77(5):623-5.

29. Aro T. Incidence, secular trends and risk indicators of reduction limb defects. Health Services Research by the National Board of Health in Finland. Helsinki: National Board of Health; 1984.

30. Czeizel A, Kodaj I, Lenz W. Smoking during pregnancy and congenital limb deficiency. BMJ. 1994;308:1473-6.

31. Li DK, Mueller BA, Hickok DE, Daling JR, Fantel AG, Checkoway H, et al. Maternal smoking during pregnancy and the risk of congenital urinary tract anomalies. Am J Public Health. 1996;86:249-53.

32. Kallen K. Maternal smoking and urinary organ malformations. Int J Epidemiol. 1997;26:571-4.

33. Honein MA, Paulozzi LJ, Watkins ML. Maternal smoking and birth defects. Validity of birth certificate data for effect estimation. Public Health Reports. 2001;116:327-35.

34. American Psychiatric Association. (2000). Diagnostic and Statistical Manual of Mental Disorders, 4th edition (DSM-IV R). [online] Available from www.behavenet.com/capsules/disorders/subdep.html. [Accessed June, 2016].

Alcohol and Drug Usage during Pregnancy

ALCOHOL USAGE DURING PREGNANCY

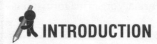 INTRODUCTION

Prevalence of alcohol consumption amongst pregnant women has been growing. The consumption of alcohol by the pregnant woman has not been observed to have any beneficial effects on foetal and neonatal outcome, rather alcohol has been observed to be both teratogenic and foetotoxic in the humans.[1] Alcohol passes freely across the placenta to the foetus, and both alcohol and its primary metabolite, acetaldehyde, have been found to be teratogenic. Underreporting of alcohol consumption is thought to be widespread, such that adverse effects in the offspring may not always be recognised. It is important for general practitioners, obstetricians and midwives to be aware of this problem and devise ways of identifying women who may suffer from problem drinking, during or before any pregnancy and in the early gestational period so that potentially beneficial interventions can be offered in order to improve foetal outcomes.

Furthermore, there is considerable doubt as to whether infrequent and low levels of alcohol consumption during pregnancy convey any long-term harm, particularly after the first trimester of pregnancy. It is important that long-term prospective RCTs be conducted in future in order to address these issues. Multidisciplinary approaches encompassing basic laboratory animal research, human clinical research, and well-designed epidemiological studies are required in order to devise practical approaches for preventing and treating foetal alcohol syndrome (FAS), alcohol-related neurodevelopmental disorders (ARND), and alcohol-related birth defects (ARBD). Although great strides have been made in identifying and characterising the physical and neurobehavioral problems of FAS and ARND, further research is needed to clinically recognise women at risk of drinking behaviour before and during pregnancy, devising more effective interventions to modify their drinking behaviour during pregnancy, and developing in utero approaches to prevent or minimise alcohol-induced prenatal injury. Development of more effective ways to identify FAS and ARND across the life span, especially in infants and children and strategies to address the neurodevelopmental and learning problems of children with FAS and ARND, including the use of appropriate behavioural and cognitive therapies, medications, and special education programs is required in the future.

AETIOLOGY

Alcohol is a teratogen that results in dysmorphia through interference with nerve cell development and functioning, alterations in the ability of cells to grow and survive, increased formation of cell-damaging free radicals, altered pathways of biochemical signals within cells, and altered expression of certain genes and genetic information. Dysmorphic features in FAS occur as the result of disturbances of cellular migration during organogenesis along the midline of the face.[2]

Safe Drinking Limit during Pregnancy

There is an increasing body of evidence suggesting harm to the foetus from alcohol consumption during pregnancy. However, presently there is considerable doubt regarding the safe upper limit for alcohol consumption during pregnancy. It is not known for certain whether even low levels of alcohol consumption during pregnancy would result in long-term foetal harm. The safest approach for the obstetrician therefore would be to advise the patient to absolutely avoid any alcohol intake during pregnancy. However, this may not be a practical option in every case. Presently, there is insufficient evidence to show that low levels of alcohol consumption, defined as no more than one or two units of alcohol, consumed once or twice a week may be equally toxic as consumption of large quantities of alcohol. The RCOG (2006) and the NICE guidelines (2008) recommend a safe limit of one or two units of alcohol, once or twice per week.[3,4]

Alcoholic women ingesting eight or more drinks daily throughout pregnancy have a 30–50% risk of having a child with all features of FAS. Women at high risk are those who chronically ingest large quantities or those who engage in binge drinking.

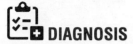

DIAGNOSIS

History and Clinical Presentation

History taking has been recognised as one of the most difficult issues in the identification of this disorder. The woman may not always be point-blank about their history of alcohol intake. Also most of the times, they may not be able to recall accurately the precise timing and severity of many different kinds of events from their past.

Investigations

There are blood tests, which could be used to screen for alcohol abuse such as gamma glutamyl transpeptidase and carbohydrate-deficient transferrin. The most commonly used screening tool for detecting alcohol abuse in antenatal clinics is T-ACE questionnaire, though at some places CAGE questionnaire is also used. Both the questionnaires are acronyms for a set of four questions, which must be enquired from the patient for alcohol screening. These questionnaires, T-ACE and CAGE, are described respectively in Tables 22.1 and 22.2.[6]

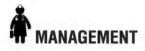

MANAGEMENT

Prevention

The RCOG and the NICE (UK) recommend that women who are trying to become pregnant or are at any stage of pregnancy should not drink more than 1–2 units of alcohol once or twice a week and should avoid episodes of intoxication or binge drinking.[3,4]

Units are a simple way of expressing the amount of pure alcohol in a drink. One unit can be considered to be equal to 10 mL or 8 g of pure alcohol. Each of the following is considered to constitute one 'unit' of alcohol: a single measure of spirits, one small glass of wine, and a half pint of ordinary strength beer, lager or cider (Table 22.3). Women can be reassured that light infrequent alcohol consumption constitutes no risk to their baby. Though the most vulnerable period for the foetus is the first trimester (especially 4–10 weeks of gestation), alcohol-related damage may occur throughout pregnancy. Thus, benefit to the infant can be obtained if alcohol is withdrawn at any stage of gestation. It is recommended that women avoid alcohol during the first trimester and then limit their intake to 1–2 units once or twice a week for the remainder of their pregnancy.[5]

Table 22.1: T-ACE questionnaire for alcohol screening[6]

1. How many drinks does it take to make you feel high? 0. Less than or equal to 2 drinks 1. More than 2 drinks	Tolerance
2. Have people annoyed you by criticising your drinking? 0. No 1. Yes	Annoyance
3. Have you felt you ought to cut down on your drinking? 0. No 1. Yes	Cut Down
4. Have you ever had a drink first thing in the morning to steady your nerves or to get rid of a hangover? 0. No 1. Yes	Eye Opener
Total Score = _____	

The T-ACE score has a range of 0–5. The value of each answer to the four questions is totalled to determine the final T-ACE score. A total score of 2 or greater is considered to be clinically significant.

Table 22.2: CAGE questionnaire for alcohol screening[6]

1. Have you ever felt you needed to cut down on your drinking? 0. No 1. Yes	Cut
2. Have people annoyed you by criticising your drinking?	Annoyance
0. No	
1. Yes	
3. Have you ever felt guilty about drinking?	Guilty
0. No	
1. Yes	
4. Have you ever had a drink first thing in the morning to steady your nerves or to get rid of a hangover?	Eye Opener
0. No	
1. Yes	
Total Score = _____	

The CAGE score has a range of 0–5. The value of each answer to the four questions is totalled to determine the final CAGE score. A total score of 2 or greater is considered to be clinically significant.

Assisting People Born with Foetal Alcohol Syndrome and Alcohol-related Neurodevelopmental Disorders

Children born with FAS and ARND are in critical need of interventions that can reduce the effect of their neurocognitive and behavioural deficits.[2,7] In a review of the literature on adolescents and adults, Streissguth and O Malley (2000) found that alcohol use during pregnancy is associated with numerous neurocognitive problems in the child including mental health problems, school problems, legal difficulties, and problems with alcohol and other drugs.[8] However, they also found that people who receive appropriate supportive services get along better with respect to secondary disabilities and life functioning than those who do not receive such services. Multiple approaches are needed, including social support, special education, behavioural and cognitive therapy, and medications.

Table 22.3: Strength of various alcoholic drinks

Alcoholic drink	Amount	Alcohol by volume (ABV) strength (%)	Units
Small glass of white/red/rosé wine	125 mL	12	1.5
Standard glass of white/red/rosé wine	175 mL	12	2.1
Large glass of white/red/rosé wine	250 mL	12	3
Higher strength lager/beer/cider	1 pint	5.2	3
Lower strength lager/beer/cider	1 pint	3.6	2
Can of lager/beer/cider	440 mL	4.5	2
Alcopop	275 mL	5.5	1.5
Single small shot of spirits (e.g. gin, rum, whisky, vodka, tequila, sambuca)	25 mL	40	1
Single large shot of spirits	35 mL	40	1.4

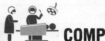

COMPLICATIONS

Adverse Outcomes of Alcohol Consumption on the Reproductive Process

Alcohol may exert toxic effects throughout the woman's reproductive process resulting in spectrum of disorders ranging from infertility through miscarriage, aneuploidy, structural congenital anomalies, disordered foetal growth, perinatal death, growth developmental delay and increased susceptibility to diseases in adult life. Though alcohol has been shown to adversely affect female fertility, its dose-dependent effects on male fertility and human spermatogenesis are presently not well known.

Relationship between Alcohol Consumption and Infertility

Even moderate alcohol consumption, corresponding to a weekly alcohol intake of five or fewer drinks, has been shown to have a significant adverse effect on fecundability.[9,10] In experimental animals, alcohol consumption is known to decrease concentrations of sex hormones, inhibit ovulation, and interfere with the transportation of sperms through the fallopian tube.[11] Thus, it seems reasonable to encourage women to avoid intake of alcohol when they are trying to become pregnant. In a study by Jensen et al., the OR (odd's ratio) for fecundability decreased as the alcohol consumption increased; the OR decreased from 0.61 (95% CI, 0.40–0.93) among women who consumed 1–5 drinks a week to 0.55 (95% CI, 0.36–0.85) among those consuming 6–10 drinks a week to 0.34 (95% CI, 0.22–0.52) amongst women consuming 11–15 drinks a week.[12] No dose-response relationship was found in male partners after adjustment for the same confounding factors. Exposure to alcohol has also been considered to be responsible for reducing male fertility by deteriorating the semen quality; however, there is absence of strong evidence supporting this fact.

Table 22.4: Maternal and foetal complications associated with alcohol consumption during pregnancy

Maternal effects	Foetal effects
• Miscarriage • Preterm labour	• Foetal alcohol spectrum disorders • Foetal alcohol syndrome • Growth restriction/stillbirths • Neurodevelopmental anomalies • More prone to illness during infancy and childhood, and as an adult

Adverse Effect of Alcohol in Pregnancy

Prenatal alcohol exposure increases the risk of pregnancy-related maternal and foetal complications (Table 22.4).

Maternal Effects

Miscarriage: Alcohol consumption is associated with an increased rate of miscarriage. Alcohol may harm human foetuses not only when it is consumed excessively, but also when taken in moderation.

Preterm labour: Increased rates of preterm delivery, a major reason behind increased perinatal morbidity and mortality, have been associated with prenatal alcohol exposure, although results reported by various studies have been inconsistent. For every unit increase in alcohol exposure, risk of extreme preterm delivery has been found to increase significantly (OR 34.8).[13,14] Eliminating alcohol use during pregnancy helps in substantially reducing the risk of preterm delivery.

Foetal Effects

Teratogenic effect of alcohol: Human studies by Streissguth et al. have shown alcohol to be a potent teratogen, which can cause FASD.[8]

FOETAL ALCOHOL SPECTRUM DISORDERS

Streissguth and O' Malley (2000) proposed the term FASD for inclusion in the Diagnostic and Statistical Manual of Mental Disorders (DSM-IV).[8] Prenatal alcohol exposure can result in a whole spectrum of CNS sequel that persists throughout the life span and manifests in form of a spectrum (ranging from mild to severe) of structural anomalies, behavioural and neurocognitive disabilities in the foetus.[8] Children at the severe end of the spectrum have been defined as having the most serious form of the disorder, also termed as FAS. The IOM (Institute of Medicine) (1996) developed five diagnostic categories (Box 22.1) for classifying alcohol-related disorders.[5]

Category 1: Foetal Alcohol Syndrome with Confirmed Maternal Alcohol Exposure

Historically, FAS has been defined by growth deficiency, a pattern of facial anomalies, and presence of brain dysfunction

PART II

Box 22.1: IOM-recommended diagnostic criteria for foetal alcohol spectrum disorders[5]

Category 1: FAS with confirmed maternal alcohol exposure
☐ Confirmed maternal alcohol exposure
☐ Characteristic pattern of facial anomalies, including short palpebral fissures, and abnormalities of the premaxillary zone (e.g. flat upper lip, flattened philtrum, flat midface)
☐ Growth restriction, such as low birthweight, lack of weight gain over time, disproportional low weight to height
☐ Neurodevelopmental abnormalities of the CNS, such as microcephaly at birth; structural brain abnormalities with age-appropriate neurological hard or soft signs (e.g. impaired fine motor skills, neurosensory hearing loss, poor tandem gait, poor eye-hand coordination)

Category 2: FAS without confirmed maternal alcohol exposure
☐ No exposure to alcohol, rest of the features are same as category 1.

Category 3: Partial FAS with confirmed maternal alcohol exposure
☐ Confirmed maternal alcohol exposure
☐ Characteristic pattern of facial anomalies (all anomalies may not be present)
☐ Growth restriction
☐ Neurodevelopmental abnormalities of the CNS
☐ Complex pattern of behavioural or cognitive abnormalities inconsistent with developmental level and unexplained by genetic background or environmental conditions (e.g. learning difficulties; deficits in school performance; poor impulse control; problems in social perception; language deficits; poor capacity for abstraction; specific deficits in mathematical skills; and problems in memory, attention, or judgement)

Category 4: Alcohol-related birth defects
☐ Confirmed maternal alcohol exposure
☐ One or more congenital defects, including malformations and dysplasia of the heart, bone, kidney, vision, or hearing systems.

Category 5: Alcohol-related neurodevelopmental disorder
☐ Confirmed maternal alcohol exposure
☐ CNS neurodevelopmental abnormalities as in Category 1 and/or complex pattern of behavioural or cognitive deficits as in Category 3

Abbreviations: IOM, Institute of Medicine; FAS, foetal alcohol syndrome; CNS, central nervous system

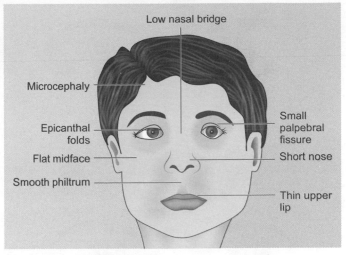

Fig. 22.1: Foetal alcohol syndrome

Lip-philtrum guide	ABC-score*	Upper lip circularity
	C	178
	C	80
	B	65
	A	50
	A	35

Fig. 22.2: Lip-philtrum guide[17]

Note: *ABC Score: A (score of 1 or 2) >10th centile; B (score of 3) >3rd and ≤10th centile; C (score of 4 or 5) ≤3rd centile

CHAPTER 22

(Fig. 22.1). Controversy still occurs regarding the measurement of each of these components and the importance to be given to each of them. Each of the craniofacial features can vary from being characteristically distinctive to being close to the normal range.

The diagnostic criteria for FAS can be defined as follows:
❖ *Maternal alcohol exposure*: This is defined as a pattern of excessive alcohol intake characterised by substantial, regular intake or a heavy episodic (i.e. binge) drinking. This pattern of drinking may be associated with the signs of alcohol dependence. Establishing the foetal alcohol exposure may be cumbersome for the clinician. Presently, there is no validated objective biological marker to confirm maternal drinking during pregnancy or alcohol exposure of the foetus.
❖ *Dysmorphia:* Human congenital malformations are referred to as dysmorphic features or dysmorphia. The individual to be diagnosed with FAS must exhibit all three characteristic facial dysmorhic features: smooth philtrum,

thin vermillion upper lip border, and small palpebral fissures.[15-17]

These features can be described as follows:
• Smooth philtrum is defined as a measurement equivalent to 4 or 5 on Lip-philtrum guide (Fig. 22.2).
• Thin vermilion border (upper lip) is defined as a measurement equivalent to 4 or 5 on Lip-philtrum guide.[17]
• Small palpebral fissures are defined as measurement of less than 10th percentile or less according to age and racial norms.[17]

Although the three above-mentioned dysmorphic features must definitely be present for the diagnosis of FAS, other additional dysmorphic features like microcephaly, short nose, flattened nasal bridge, micrognathia, maxillary hypoplasia

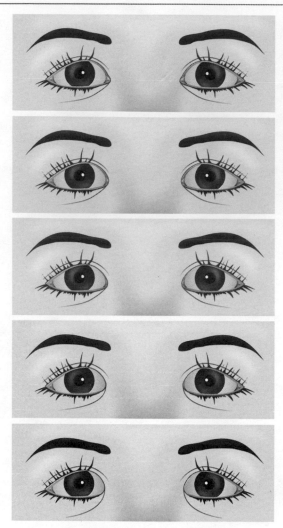

Fig. 22.3: Epicanthal fold severity guide

(with prognathism), presence of epicanthal folds (Fig. 22.3), altered palmar flexional crease patterns (i.e. hockeystick crease), cardiac anomalies, joint disability, overlapping fingers, ear anomalies, haemangiomas, ptosis, hypoplastic nails, pectus deformities, cleft lip, micrognathia, protruding auricles, short or webbed neck, vertebra and rib anomalies, short metacarpal bones, meningomyelocele, hydrocephalus, hypoplastic labia majora, etc. may also be present. After puberty, the characteristic facial features associated with FAS can become more difficult to detect. Epicanthal fold is the lateral extension of the skin of nasal bridge along the medial canthus of the eye. These folds can be unilateral or bilateral. The set of uppermost pair of eyes in Figure 22.3 are normal eyes having no epicanthal fold. As we move downwards, the severity and extension of epicanthal folds gradually increases with the lowermost pair of eyes showing the most prominent epicanthal folds bilaterally.

Category 2: Foetal Alcohol Syndrome without Confirmed Maternal Alcohol Exposure

If it is not known for sure that there was alcohol exposure during pregnancy, even then a diagnosis of FAS can be made if the affected person appears to have all the signs of FAS.

Category 3: Partial Foetal Alcohol Syndrome

Category 3 includes partial FAS with confirmed maternal alcohol exposure. In other words, for diagnosis of this category, some, but not all, of the facial characteristics required for diagnosis of FAS must be present as well as there should be a confirmed evidence of maternal alcohol exposure. In addition, at least one of the three following indicators also must be present: growth deficits normally characteristic of FAS, neurodevelopmental abnormalities, or behavioural and cognitive problems consistent with those observed in FAS. The cognitive abnormalities could be in the form of complex pattern of deficits in learning, school performance, impulse control, behavioural pattern, etc.

Category 4: Alcohol-related Birth Defects

Category 4 encompasses ARBD and includes people who had been prenatally exposed to alcohol and were diagnosed with heart, bone, kidney, visual or hearing defects. Although these anomalies may not be consistently observed, they are not uncommon either.

Category 5: Alcohol-related Neurodevelopmental Disorder

Category 5 is defined when the individual shows behavioural and cognitive problems similar to those seen in FAS and partial FAS, but the facial features are normal. Evidence of CNS neurodevelopmental abnormalities is believed to be there if at least one of the following is present:

❖ Decreased cranial size at birth, with specific reduction in the size of the caudate nucleus, thinning or agenesis of the corpus callosum and reduced size of the hippocampus and cerebellum.
❖ Structural brain abnormalities (e.g. microcephaly, partial or complete agenesis of the corpus callosum, cerebellar hypoplasia, etc.)
❖ Age appropriate neurological hard or soft signs such as impaired fine motor skills, neurosensory hearing loss, poor tandem gait, poor eye-hand coordination, etc.

Variety of behavioural and cognitive features have been proposed as indicators of brain dysfunction in FAS. Some of these include poor performance on tests of intelligence and educational achievement, impaired language development, poor impulse control, and problems with memory and judgement. At present, however, no consensus has been achieved as to which features are most appropriate for the diagnosis of FAS.

These features too are considered to be on a spectrum, ranging from near normal to severely impaired. They are also influenced by other factors such as parental intelligence, educational experience and various social (impoverished postnatal environment) and cultural influences. Furthermore, these cognitive and behavioural features are less specific to FAS than are the physical features. Not only these features tend to change with time, they also tend to occur in association with a wide range of other childhood neurodevelopmental and psychiatric conditions, attention-deficit hyperactivity disorders, etc.

❖ *Foetal behavioural studies*: Maternal alcohol consumption may also have an effect on spontaneous movements, startle reaction and habituation of the foetus at 18, 27 and 36 weeks of gestation.

❖ *Attention and hyperactivity problem*: Attention problems are often noted for children with FAS, with many children receiving a diagnosis of attention-deficit hyperactivity disorder (ADHD).

 ## CLINICAL PEARLS

❖ Drinking too much alcohol during pregnancy can affect the way the baby develops and grows; the baby's health at birth; and the child's ability to learn (learning difficulties).

❖ Presently, there is no proven safe amount of alcohol that the woman can drink during pregnancy. The only way the woman can be certain that her baby is not harmed by alcohol is by not drinking at all during pregnancy or while breastfeeding.

❖ Besides the adverse effects of alcohol per se, excessive alcohol intake also leads to reduced blood folate levels. This could have implications for the developing foetus. Therefore, it is important to ensure that women take folic acid supplements in the dosage up to 5 mg daily.

 ## EVIDENCE-BASED MEDICINE

❖ It is recommended that the pregnant woman should not consume any alcohol during the first 3 months of pregnancy. She can drink small amounts of alcohol after this time because it does not appear to be harmful for the unborn baby. However, she should preferably avoid this. In any case, she should not drink more than one or two units, more than once or twice per week. Binge drink (consuming six units or more of alcohol on any one occasion) is strictly prohibited during pregnancy.[3,4,6]

❖ If a couple is planning a pregnancy, it is recommended that both the partners should not consume any alcohol during the preconception period.[6]

❖ If the woman is breastfeeding, she should not drink more than one or two units, more than once or twice a week.[3,4,6]

DRUG USAGE DURING PREGNANCY

 ## INTRODUCTION

Drug use or abuse by the today's youth is one of the most difficult social problems, which is being faced by our society at present. According to the British Crime Survey (2005), 33% of men and 21% of women amongst the group of young people between the age of 16–24 years, in England and Wales were reported to be taking illicit drugs. Commonly, these drugs are

used by the young people either in a manner or a quantity, which is different from what is directed by the physician.[18] When drugs are used in this manner for illegitimate purposes, it is known as drug abuse [Diagnostic and Statistical Manual of Mental Disorders, 4th edition (DSM-IV), 1994]. Drugs being used in this manner include either illicit drugs, which are forbidden by law or use of prescription or over-the-counter drugs, which are medically used for different purposes.[19] Excessive drug abuse in the long run can result in development of drug dependence or addiction.

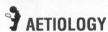 ## AETIOLOGY

Most Common Drugs

National Institute on Drug Abuse (NIDA) 2007 has classified the most commonly used drugs (controlled substances) into five major categories, namely central nervous stimulants, CNS depressants, hallucinogens, opiates and narcotics, and drugs in which the main ingredient is tetrahydrocannabinol. All these drugs have the ability to affect the mood, feelings and thinking process of an individual. All these five categories of drugs are capable of being abused as all of them are able to alter the person's mood, disconnect him or her from reality and make him or her feel good or relaxed (NIDA, 2007). Each of the five categories of drugs, including some examples of the commonly used drugs in each category is shown in Table 22.5.[20]

Cocaine

Cocaine is one of the most powerful stimulant drug which can result in devastating situation due to its highly addictive nature.[21] Pure cocaine is obtained from the leaves of cocoa plant and is usually consumed in form of a white chalk-like powdered salt of cocaine called cocaine hydrochloride. The white powder of cocaine hydrochloride can be dissolved in water and injected intravenously.[22] Cocaine hydrochloride powder is also commonly snorted (inhalation through the nose) or smoked. Frequent snorting of cocaine can result in the development of chronic nasal irritation. Crack is a commonly used street name for cocaine (in its basic form) and is derived from cocaine hydrochloride. During the process of manufacture of crack, firstly cocaine hydrochloride is processed with the help of chemicals like ammonia or sodium bicarbonate (baking soda) and water. This is followed by heating of the mixture. The heating results in production of crackling sounds that led to the nomenclature of the word 'crack'. The crack cocaine in form of a rock crystal is in a ready-to-smoke form.[22]

Narcotics and Opiates

Narcotics are drugs that have been used legally as painkillers since a long time. Opiate drugs like codeine and morphine are commonly used as analgesic agents in medicine, whereas narcotic drugs like diacetylmorphine (heroin) are commonly used as illicit drugs. These drugs are usually derived from the opium (poppy) plant [US Department of Justice (USDOJ), 2011].[23] These drugs can be consumed in a number of ways

Table 22.5: Classification of various commonly used drugs depending on their chemical composition and action produced[20]

Drug categories	Examples	Main effect produced
Central nervous stimulants	Amphetamines, cocaine, dextroamphetamine, methamphetamine, and methylphenidate (Ritalin) system	These drugs have a stimulating effect over the central nervous system.
Central nervous system depressants	Barbiturates (amobarbital, pentobarbital, secobarbital), benzodiazepine (Valium, Ativan, Xanax), chloral hydrate, alcohol, gamma-hydroxybutyric acid (GHB), etc.	These substances depress the central nervous system resulting in sedation (drowsiness) and reduction of anxiety.
Hallucinogens	Lysergic acid diethylamide (LSD), psilocybin and psilocin 'magic mushrooms', and ecstasy	These drugs have hallucinogenic properties and result in hallucinations.
Opiates and narcotics	Heroin, opium, codeine, meperidine (Demerol), hydromorphone (Dilaudid), oxycodone, etc.	These drugs are powerful painkillers that have sedative action and produce a feeling of well-being and elation.
Tetrahydrocannabinol	Cannabis, marijuana and hashish	They mainly produce relaxation. However, they can also produce some anxiety and paranoid behaviour.

including oral ingestion (suppositories), IV injections, transdermally through skin patches, intranasally (snorting) or smoking. If consumed in high doses, narcotic drugs can result in death by causing respiratory depression.

Heroin: Heroin (diacetylmorphine) is an opium (poppy) derived drug, which is consumed by a small proportion of individuals in the UK.[24] Although initially introduced into the field of medicine as a respiratory stimulant, it was later discovered to be a respiratory depressant. Nowadays, heroin is used in the UK as a strong analgesic and is highly effective in the treatment of pain. Illicit heroin can be available in various grades, mainly the smokeable and injectable grades. Although heroin is mainly injected intravenously, it can also be smoked by the people abusing this drug. The smokeable grade is pinkish brownish form of heroin, which is basic in nature and evaporates without forming any residue on being heated. On the other hand, the injectable grade is heroin hydrochloride, which is available in form of a white water soluble powder. While smoking, the smokeable grade of heroin is kept on an aluminium foil and heated (not burnt). The resultant fumes are inhaled with help of a tube.

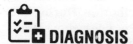 **DIAGNOSIS**

Clinical Presentation

Typical clinical features associated with some commonly used drugs of abuse are as follows:

❖ *Cocaine:* Consumption of cocaine results in an increase in the heart rate and blood pressure, loss of appetite, wakefulness and other sleep disturbances, mental confusion, anxiety, paranoid behaviour, hallucinations, etc. This drug can also cause stimulation of cardiovascular system and cerebrovascular system resulting in development of heart attack or stroke respectively. Use of cocaine, commonly, results in rapid development of addiction, which soon progresses towards dependence. Development of dependence or tolerance in the long run can result in

destructive consequences and social deterioration. Cocaine withdrawal symptoms are characteristically associated with cocaine craving.

❖ *Narcotics and opiates:* Narcotic drugs produce a sense of well-being by reducing tension, anxiety and pain. Other signs of narcotic overdose include constriction of pupils, cold clammy skin, confusion, convulsions, severe drowsiness, etc. Use of narcotics can also result in drowsiness, inability to concentrate, apathy, reduced level of physical activity, constriction of the pupils, constipation, nausea, vomiting, etc. Long-term use of narcotics can result in the development of tolerance and both physical and psychological dependence to the drug (USDOJ, 2005). Some symptoms associated with early stages of withdrawal reaction include watery eyes, runny nose, yawning, sweating, etc. In later stages, this can result in restlessness, irritability, loss of appetite, nausea, tremors, vomiting, depression, bone pains and muscle spasms.

❖ *Heroin:* When abused, heroin produces a feeling of well-being and drowsiness resulting in a 'trance-like' sedative state. Side effects associated with heroin abuse include nausea, dry mouth, decreased appetite, constipation, menstrual disorders, etc. Prolonged use can result in both psychological and physical forms of dependence. When drug consumption is suddenly stopped or markedly reduced, withdrawal symptoms are produced. These include flu-like symptoms (like fever, watery nose and eyes), sleep disorders, muscular pain, diarrhoea, etc. The amount of problems caused by heroin use is related to the method in which heroin is consumed. Injecting heroin is more dangerous than smoking it. Injecting heroin intravenously is also associated with the risk of transmission of blood-borne infections like HIV, hepatitis B, hepatitis C, etc.

Investigations

Investigations to be done in the pregnant women abusing drugs during the antenatal period are listed in Box 22.2.

CHAPTER 22

Box 22.2: Investigations to be done in antenatal period

- ❏ Screening for hepatitis B and C, HIV and bacterial vaginosis
- ❏ First trimester ultrasound for accurate gestational dating
- ❏ Regular antenatal foetal monitoring (foetal heart rate monitoring, ultrasonography, cardiotocography, etc.)
- ❏ Multidisciplinary team (involving communication with the anaesthetic and paediatric services)

Box 22.3: Points that should be taken into consideration in the history

- ❏ Does her partner use drugs?
- ❏ Has she been in legal trouble due to substance abuse?
- ❏ Has she ever tried quitting drugs previously?
- ❏ Does she practice safe sex?
- ❏ Does she inject herself with drugs?
- ❏ Does she use clean needle or does she use shared needles?
- ❏ Does she use multiple drugs, alcohol or cigarettes?
- ❏ Detailed socio-economic history

 ## MANAGEMENT

Antenatal Care

History

As previously discussed, the foetal outcome can be considerably improved if the woman can stop taking drugs as soon as possible, in early gestation. To be able to achieve this, the obstetrician needs to diagnose the problem of substance abuse in the woman. The obstetrician needs to take a detailed history from the patient, highlighting the points enumerated in Box 22.3. Based on the woman's history and clinical examination, the clinician needs to devise an ANC programme centred around the individual woman's needs and requirements.[25] After taking a detailed history from the patient, the clinician should counsel the patient regarding the adverse effects of substance abuse on neonatal and foetal outcome. Communication with the anaesthetic and paediatric services is important because cocaine and opiate abuses may pose particular problems for obstetricians, anaesthetists and admission to a special baby care unit (SBCU) may be very likely.

Clinical Tests

During the antenatal period, the obstetrician needs to conduct certain clinical tests listed in Box 22.2. The women abusing drugs commonly share infected needles for injecting drugs. Also, the woman abusing drugs might be commonly involved in unsafe sexual practices, commonly with partners who themselves might be abusing drug. Thus, it is important to screen these patients for blood-borne infections like hepatitis B, hepatitis C, HIV and bacterial vaginosis.

The clinician needs to promote the concept of harm reduction as advocated by the 'Drug strategy 2010 (UK)'. The approach of harm reduction aims at taking steps in order to minimise the potential harms to health, which can be caused due to illicit use of drugs. For example, sharing of needles during the IV abuse of drugs can result in transmission of blood-borne infections like HIV, hepatitis B, etc. IV injection of drugs through dirty needles can also result in development of abscesses, etc. Drug abuse is often associated with prostitution and increased frequency of sexual intercourse with partners who themselves abuse drugs. This can result in further transmission of sexually transmitted diseases and HIV. Through the policy of harm reduction, the UK government aims at reducing health-related risks by making use of simple strategies like syringe exchange programmes, provision of condoms, methadone maintenance therapy, etc.[26]

An early first trimester ultrasound is required for accurate gestational dating and a second trimester ultrasound for detailed foetal anomaly scanning. Multidisciplinary team approach involving communication with the anaesthetic and paediatric services is required as substance abuse by the woman during pregnancy may pose particular problems for the obstetrician, anaesthetists and paediatrician involved in patient care.

Counselling

Counselling the pregnant woman aims to help and support the individuals by helping them to take control of their lives, improve their social relationships and take control of their drugs habits.[27] The various types of counselling strategies, which can be used to control the drug problem, include 'person-centred counselling', cognitive behavioural therapy and motivational interviewing. Motivational interviewing helps the individuals in identifying their drug problem and also helps them recognise a motivational factor that would help them in maintaining remission. Cognitive behavioural therapy is believed to motivate the patient to remain abstinent, helps them in fighting against the withdrawal symptoms and preventing relapse.

Intrapartum Care

The clinician must take care of the following in the intrapartum period:

- ❖ The clinician must do continuous foetal monitoring in form of continuous cardiotocographic trace (CTG monitoring) as there is increased risk of placental compromise, which may result in foetal compromise.
- ❖ The clinician must be aware that opiates may influence CTG and therefore the interpretation may become more difficult.
- ❖ Avoid as far as possible, foetal blood sampling, use of foetal scalp electrodes and other invasive tests to reduce the risk of the vertical transmission of HIV and hepatitis.
- ❖ Maintenance dose of methadone must be administered in order to prevent withdrawal. This however will not have an analgesic action; therefore, extra analgesia needs to be provided in addition.
- ❖ Administration of systematic opiates must be avoided in those women who have undergone supervised withdrawal from the opiates during the antenatal period. Nitrous oxide must not be given to opiate-dependent mothers or their offsprings as severe withdrawal may occur.

❖ In cocaine users, ephedrine may be less effective in reversing hypotension secondary to regional analgesia. Phenylephrine is a useful alternative.

Postnatal Period

❖ If baby seems well, it should be transferred to the postnatal ward with the mother. Neonatal abstinence syndrome (NAS) in infants whose mother had been receiving opiates during pregnancy is usually present in the first 2 days, and the baby must be closely observed for signs of this. Methadone withdrawal may take a little longer but will usually begin by 4 days (the minimum time period for which the women are advised to stay in hospital). If the infant is demonstrating the withdrawal symptoms, it would require special care facilities.

❖ Breastfeeding is encouraged in most women, even on methadone. Infant weaning should occur gradually. The exception to this is the women who are HIV positive, and those using large quantities of benzodiazepines or cocaine.

❖ Babies born to hepatitis B mothers should be immunised and advised accordingly.

❖ Advice regarding contraception and safe sexual practices should be given on discharge.

Pharmacotherapy for Drug Abuse

Methadone Maintenance Treatment

Drug abuse results in numerous problems including physical, psychological and social. Thus, numerous treatment modalities are available to people with drug problems. These include pharmacotherapy, psychological help and social support.[28] Substitute treatment, i.e. prescribing a substitute drug like methadone forms the mainstay of treatment for those abusing opiates. Women using street narcotics and opiates should be offered methadone maintenance treatment (MMT).[29] Methadone is a long-acting synthetic opiate drug, which produces same actions on the brain as that of opiate drugs that are derived naturally from opium. Methadone is chemically similar to the opioid drugs; therefore, it combines with the same receptors in the brain where the illicit drug also combines. Thus, the substitute drug is able to prevent the emergence of withdrawal symptoms associated with physical dependence on drugs. As a result, the woman does not experience much physical discomfort when she reduces her dosage of drugs and is able to maintain remission. Methadone has a larger half-life than heroin and as a result, its blood levels remain more stable. The clinician needs to consider a gradual withdrawal, e.g. a reduction in dose of 2–2.5 mg every 7–10 days. The best time for initiating MMT is in the second trimester. Starting it earlier may increase the risk for spontaneous abortions, whereas starting it later in the third trimester may increase the risk for preterm labour. Safety of methadone maintenance therapy during pregnancy has not been established with certainty. Methadone therapy to the pregnant woman is associated with potentially serious neonatal withdrawal syndrome.

Box 22.4: Symptoms of newborn opiate withdrawal

❑ Tremulousness, trembling (exclude hypocalcaemia or hyperglycaemia)
❑ Tachypnoea (respiratory alkalosis)
❑ Irritability (hyperactive reflexes, sleep disturbance, excessive crying)
❑ Vomiting, diarrhoea and dehydration
❑ Shrill and high-pitched foetal crying
❑ Thermal instability resulting in fever
❑ Sweating, yawning, stuffy nose
❑ Increase in muscular tone
❑ Seizures (late findings)

Newborn Opiate Withdrawal

Tremulousness is the first sign of withdrawal and can be elicited by suddenly surprising the infant or by using minimum tactile stimulation. Use of opiates (commonly prescribed methadone or illicit heroin) by pregnant women may result in a withdrawal syndrome in their newborn infants, some of the symptoms of which are listed in Box 22.4.

In severely affected infants undergoing withdrawal, tremulousness occurs even without provoking the infant. Before attributing the tremors to withdrawal symptoms, it is necessary to exclude hypocalcaemia and hyperglycaemia, which are two common causes for tremors in the newborns. If the symptoms are attributed to neonatal withdrawal syndrome, there is a requirement for careful reduction of the maternal methadone dosage during pregnancy under intensive medical and psychosocial surveillance so as to minimise the amount of harm that can be caused to the drug-exposed newborn infant.[30-32] Methadone exposure to the foetus prenatally may be potentially neurotoxic to the developing brain. In a study by Hans and Jeremy, it was shown that prenatal opiate exposure had small but consistent effects on mental and psychomotor function throughout infancy. Also, children exposed to methadone prenatally exhibited smaller subcortical volumes and associated neurocognitive deficits.[33] These preliminary findings suggest that prenatal methadone exposure may be neurotoxic to the developing brain. Thus, there is a need for further research regarding the safety of use of maternal methadone maintenance therapy on neonatal outcomes.

 COMPLICATIONS

Complications due to drug abuse during pregnancy are enumerated in Table 22.6.

Presently, the teratogenic, cognitive or behavioural effects associated with prenatal exposure to marijuana, cigarettes, cocaine or opiates have not been well established. The most convincing finding related to prenatal exposure to such substances is IUGR. Impaired foetal growth, especially of brain, may indirectly mediate adverse effects on cognition.

Medical complications encountered in pregnancy due to addiction include: anaemia, bacteraemia, endocarditis (valvular heart disease), cellulitis, poor dental hygiene

Table 22.6: Complications due to drug abuse during pregnancy

Maternal complications	Foetal complications
• Miscarriage (opiates, cocaine, CNS stimulants) • Preterm rupture of membranes • Preterm labour • Chorioamnionitis • Pre-eclampsia, abruption	• Intrauterine growth restriction, intrauterine death • Breech presentation • Neural tube defects

(periodontitis), oedema and woody subcutaneous tissues, hepatitis (acute and chronic) pelvic inflammatory disease, phlebitis, pneumonia, septicaemia, tetanus, tuberculosis, urinary tract infection (cystitis and urethritis), venereal infection, etc.

Effect of Abuse of Opiates and Narcotics

In order to determine the perinatal impacts of heroin and amphetamine on both mothers and infants, a retrospective study on the influence of amphetamine and heroin on pregnant women and their newborn infants was conducted by Thaithumyanon et al. Poor obstetric history were noted in the groups of women consuming heroin and amphetamine. The results of this study showed a lack of prenatal care in 74.9%, a high incidence of previous abortion in 22.3%, positive HIV serological test in 11.1%, pre-eclampsia in 5.2%, infection in 3.3% and antepartum haemorrhage in 1.9% subjects.[34] The incidence of prematurity, low birthweight, IUGR and microcephaly was not statistically different between both groups of infants, and there was no statistical difference in terms of mean birthweight, gestational age, length, head circumference and APGAR score between the groups of amphetamine and heroin-exposed infants.

It is the duty of the clinician to increase the awareness and understanding regarding the harmful effects of drug abuse among pregnant women. Prenatal exposure of the foetus to opiate drugs is associated with an increased risk of regulatory dysfunction and neuropsychological difficulties.[35-38] This relationship between the maternal drug abuse and presence of neuropsychological abnormalities in the child can be partly attributed to the environmental and social risks factors, including factors like, poverty, stress, maternal psychopathology, disruptions in maternal care, poor interaction with the primary care provider, etc.[35]

Cocaine Use during Pregnancy

Cocaine currently is one of the most widely abused drugs in the US. The risk for specific congenital anomalies accompanying maternal cocaine abuse during an individual pregnancy is unknown. Adverse effects result from vasoconstriction and hypertensive effects. Research suggests that, possibly through mechanisms initiated by vasoconstriction leading to vessel thrombosis or embolism, cocaine causes vascular disruption defects. Frequent cocaine use during early pregnancy could disrupt multiple organ systems in the foetus. Abruptio placentae is the most common abnormality encountered. Neurodevelopmental problems in the infant especially in

the neonatal period have been reported. Cocaine-induced bilateral asymmetric upper limb amputation defects have also been reported.[39,40] Numerous studies have suggested that foetal vascular disruption accompanying maternal cocaine abuse may lead to cavitary CNS lesions, including skull defects, cutis aplasia, porencephaly, subependymal and periventricular cysts, and genitourinary anomalies including ileal atresia, visceral infarcts, urinary tube defects, prune belly syndrome etc.[41-43] Thus, evidence from the available literature suggest that the obstetrician must counsel the pregnant women concerning cocaine use and should warn her about the possibility of potential embryonic, vascular disruption or limb reduction defects in the foetus. Adverse neonatal effects associated with foetal cocaine exposure follow a linear dose-response relationship; newborns with higher levels of prenatal cocaine exposure show higher rates of impairments in foetal head growth and abnormalities of muscle tone, movements, and posture.[12] Review of the literature suggests strongly that the popular belief about the relative safety of cocaine is unfounded and that maternal cocaine abuse during pregnancy may be associated with increased perinatal morbidity and mortality.[44]

CLINICAL PEARLS

❖ Abruptio placentae is the most common abnormality encountered with cocaine abuse during pregnancy.
❖ Invasive tests such as foetal blood sampling, use of foetal scalp electrodes and other invasive tests must be avoided as far as possible to reduce the risk of the vertical transmission of HIV and hepatitis.

EVIDENCE-BASED MEDICINE

❖ It is important to screen these patients for blood-borne infections like hepatitis B, hepatitis C, HIV and bacterial vaginosis because these women may be commonly sharing infected needles for injecting drugs.[26] Also, the woman abusing drugs might be commonly involved in unsafe sexual practices, commonly with partners who themselves might be abusing drug.
❖ Methadone therapy is usually prescribed for those individuals who abuse either illicit opioid drugs (like heroin), or prescription opioids like codeine.[28,29]
❖ There is no clear evidence regarding the probable reasons for increased likelihood of the opiate withdrawal effects in the newborn child. Until the studies in future are clearly able to show absence of any correlation between maternal methadone dose and severity of foetal withdrawal symptoms, the maternal methadone dosage during pregnancy must be carefully reduced under intensive medical and psychosocial surveillance so as to minimise the amount of harm that can be caused to the drug-exposed newborn infant.[30-32]

CHAPTER 22

REFERENCES

1. Kaufman MH. The teratogenic effects of alcohol following exposure during pregnancy, and its influence on the chromosome constitution of the pre-ovulatory egg. Alcohol Alcohol. 1997;32(2);113-28.

2. Warren KR, Foudin LL. Alcohol-related birth defects—the past, present, and future. Alcohol Res Health. 2001;25(3):153-8.

3. Royal College of Obstetricians and Gynaecologists (RCOG). (2006). Alcohol consumption and the outcomes of pregnancy. RCOG Statement No. 5.[online] RCOG website. Available from www.rcog.org.uk/en/guidelines-research-services/guidelines/alcohol-consumption-and-the-outcomes-of-pregnancy-rcog-statement-5 [Accessed July, 2016]

4. National Institute of Clinical Excellence. (2008) (NICE guideline). Antenatal care: routine care for the healthy pregnant woman. [online] NICE website. Available from www.nice.org.uk/guidance/cg62/documents/antenatal-care-nice-guideline2 [Accessed May, 2016].

5. Nykjaer C, Alwan NA, Greenwood DC, Simpson NA, Hay AW, White KL, et al. Maternal alcohol intake prior to and during pregnancy and risk of adverse birth outcomes: evidence from a British cohort. J Epidemiol Community Health. 2014;68(6): 542-9.

6. Robert JS. Finding the risk drinker in your clinical practice. In: Robinson G, Armstrong R (Eds). Alcohol and Child/Family Health: Proceedings of a Conference with Particular Reference to the Prevention of Alcohol-Related Birth Defects. Vancouver: B.C. FAS Resource Group; 1988.

7. Warren KR, Bast RJ. Alcohol-related birth defects: an update. Public Health Rep. 1988;103(6):638-42.

8. Streissguth AP, O Malley K. Neuro-psychiatric implications and long-term consequences of foetal alcohol spectrum disorders. Semin Clin Neuropsychiatry. 2000;5(3):177-90.

9. Olsen J, Rachootin P, Schicdt AV, Damsbo N. Tobacco use, alcohol consumption and infertility. Int J Epidemiol. 1983; 12(2):179-84.

10. Olsen J, Bolumar F, Boldsen J, Bisanti L. The European study group of infertility and subfecundity. Does moderate alcohol intake reduce fecundability? A European multicenter study on infertility and subfecundity. Alcohol Clin Exp Res. 1997; 21(2):206-12.

11. Sharma SC, Chaudhury RR. Studies on mating. II. The effect of ethanol on sperm transport and ovulation in successfully mated rabbits. Indian J Med Res. 1970;58(4):501-4.

12. Jensen TK, Hjollund NH, Henriksen TB, Scheike T, Kolstad H, Giwercman A, et al. Does moderate alcohol consumption affect fertility? Follow up study among couples planning first pregnancy. BMJ. 1998;317(7157):505-10.

13. Sokol RJ, Janisse JJ, Louis JM, Bailey BN, Ager J, Jacobson SW, et al. Extreme prematurity: an alcohol-related birth effect. Alcohol Clin Exp Res. 2007;31(6):1031-7.

14. Kesmodel U, Oslen SF, Secher NJ. Does alcohol increase the risk of preterm delivery? Ugeskr Laeger. 2001;163(34):4578-82.

15. Astley SJ, Clarren SK. Measuring the facial phenotype of individuals with prenatal alcohol exposure: correlations with brain dysfunction. Alcohol Alcohol. 2001;36(2):147-59.

16. Hoyme HE, May PA, Kalberg WO, Kodituwakku P, Gossage JP, Trujillo PM, et al. A practical clinical approach to diagnosis of foetal alcohol spectrum disorders: clarification of the 1996 institute of medicine criteria. Pediatrics. 2005;115(1):39-47.

17. Astley SJ, Clarren SK. Diagnosing the full spectrum of foetal alcohol-exposed individuals: introducing the 4-digit diagnostic code. Alcohol Alcohol. 2000:35(4);400-10.

18. Crime survey. (2005). Facts and figures related to drug use among youth in UK. [online] UK youth website. Available from www.ukyouth.org [Accessed July, 2016].

19. DSM. (2000). Diagnostic and statistical manual of mental disorders, text revision (DSM-IV R), 4th edition. American Psychiatric Association. [online] Available from www.behavenet.com/capsules/disorders/subdep.htm. [Accessed July, 2016].

20. US National Institute on Drug Abuse. (NIDA). (2007). Commonly abused drugs. [online] Available from www.nida.nih.gov/DrugPages/DrugsofAbuse.html. [Accessed July, 2016].

21. Smith DE, Schwartz RH, Martin DM. Heavy cocaine use by adolescents. Paediatrics. 1989;83(4):539-42.

22. Warner EA. Cocaine abuse. Ann Intern Med. 1993;119(3):226-35.

23. US Department of Justice (USDOJ). (2011). Drugs of abuse. [online] Available from www.dea.gov/docs/drugs_of_abuse_2011.pdf. [Accessed July, 2016].

24. Stimson GV, Metrebian N. (2003). Prescribing heroin: What is the evidence? Joseph Rowntree Foundation. [online] Available from www.jrf.org.uk/report/prescribing-heroin-what-evidence. [Accessed July, 2016].

25. Luesley DM. Drugs in pregnancy. In: Luesley DM, Beker PN, Drife J (Eds). Obstetrics and Gynaecology. An Evidence Based Text for MRCOG. Philadelphia: Hodder Arnold; 2004.

26. Home Office. (2010). Drug strategy: consultation paper—a response by the Social Security Advisory Committee. [online] Available from www.gov.uk/government/uploads/system/uploads/attachment_data/file/324309/ssac-drug-strategy-response.pdf. [Accessed July, 2016].

27. McGovern MP, Wrisley BR, Drake RE. Relapse of substance use disorder and its prevention among persons with co-occurring disorders. Psychiatr Serv. 2005;56(10):1270-3.

28. Leshner AI. US National Institute on Drug Abuse. (1999). Principles of drug addiction treatment—a research based guide. [online] NIDA website. Available from www.nida.nih.gov/PODAT/PODATIndex.html. [Accessed July, 2016].

29. Farrell M, Ward J, Mattick R, Hall W, Stimson GV, des Jarlais D, et al. Methadone maintenance in opiate dependence: a review. BMJ. 1994;309(6960):997-1001.

30. Doberczak TM, Kandall SR, Friedmann P. Relationship between maternal methadone dosage, maternal-neonatal methadone levels, and neonatal withdrawal. Obstet Gynecol. 1993;81(6):936-40.

31. Malpas TJ, Darlow BA, Lennox R, Horwood LJ. Maternal methadone dosage and neonatal withdrawal. Aust N Z J Obstet Gynaecol. 1995;35(2):175-7.

32. Berghella V, Lim PJ, Hill MK, Cherpes J, Chennat J, Kaltenbach K. Maternal methadone dose and neonatal withdrawal. Am J Obstet Gynecol. 2003;189(2):312-7.

33. Hans SL, Jeremy RJ. Postneonatal mental and motor development of infants exposed in utero to opioid drugs. Infant Mental Health Journal. 2001;22:300-15.

34. Thaithumyanon P, Limpongsanurak S, Praisuwanna P, Punnahitanon S. Perinatal effects of amphetamine and heroin use during pregnancy on the mother and infant. J Med Assoc Thai. 2005;88(11):1506-13.

35. Suess PE, Newlin DB, Porges SW. Motivation, sustained attention, and autonomic regulation in school-age boys exposed in utero to opiates and alcohol. Exp Clin Psychopharmacol. 1997;5(4):375-87.

PART II

36. Moe V, Slinning K. Prenatal drug exposure and the conceptualization of long-term effects. Scand J Psychol. 2002;43(1):41-7.

37. Moe V. Foster-placed and adopted children exposed in utero to opiates and other substances: prediction and outcome at four and a half years. J Dev Behav Pediatr. 2002;23(5):330-9.

38. Slinning K. Foster placed children prenatally exposed to polysubstances—attention-related problems at ages 2 and 41/2. Eur Child Adolesc Psychiatry. 2004;13(1):19-27.

39. Hannig VL, Philips JA. Maternal cocaine abuse and foetal anomalies: evidence for teratogenic effects of cocaine. South Med J. 1991;84(4):498-9.

40. Behnke M, Eyler FD. The consequences of prenatal substance use for the developing foetus, newborn, young child. Int J Addict. 1993;28(13):1341-91.

41. Hoyme HE, Jones KL, Dixon SD, Jewett T, Hanson JW, Robinson LK, et al. Prenatal cocaine exposure and foetal vascular disruption. Pediatrics. 1990;85(5):743-7.

42. Jones KL. Developmental pathogenesis of defects associated with prenatal cocaine exposure: foetal vascular disruption. Clin Perinatol. 1991;18(1):139-46.

43. Martin ML, Khoury MJ, Cordero JF, Waters GD. Trends in rates of multiple vascular disruption defects, Atlanta, 1968-1989: Is there evidence of a cocaine teratogenic epidemic? Teratology. 1992;45(6):647-53.

44. Roland EH, Volpe JJ. Effect of maternal cocaine use on the foetus and newborn: review of the literature. Pediatr Neurosci. 1989;15(2):88-94.

SECTION 4

Complications Specific to Pregnancy

OBSTETRICS

Multifoetal Gestation

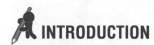 INTRODUCTION

Development of two or more embryos simultaneously in a pregnant uterus is termed as multifoetal gestation. Development of two foetuses (whether through monozygotic or dizygotic fertilisation) simultaneously is known as twin gestation; development of three foetuses simultaneously as triplets; four foetuses as quadruplets; five foetuses as quintuplets and so on.

Due to an increase in the use of assisted reproductive technology (ART) to attain pregnancy, there had been an increase in the incidence of multiple pregnancy in the beginning of the century. However, now with an increasing number of embryo transfers occurring at the blastocyst stage and more women opting to have only one embryo transferred at a time, there has been a decline in the overall rate of multiple pregnancies. In 2013, one in six pregnancies was a multiple pregnancy, compared with one in four in 2008 [Human Fertilisation and Embryology Authority (HFEA), 2013].[1]

AETIOLOGY

The risk factors, which are most likely to result in multifoetal gestation, include the following:
* Increased maternal age and parity
* Previous history of twin gestation
* Family history of twin gestation (especially on maternal side)
* Conception following a long period of infertility
* Pregnancy attained through the use of ART (in vitro fertilisation or use of clomiphene citrate)
* Racial origin (twin gestation is more common amongst the women of West African ancestry)
* History of using progestational agents or combined oral contraceptives, which may cause reduction in the tubal mobility
* Previous history of twin gestation.

Types of Twin Gestation

Multifoetal gestation occurs due to the presence of more than one embryo. This could be due to division of a fertilised ovum or fertilisation of more than one ova by sperms. Based on the likely aetiology, multifoetal twin gestation can be of two types: monozygotic (Fig. 23.1) twins and dizygotic twins (Fig. 23.2). The differences between these two are described in Table 23.1 and Figure 23.3. In monozygotic multiple pregnancies, different types can result depending on the timing of the division of the ovum (Fig. 23.4).[2]

Different Types of Monozygotic Twins

Diamniotic dichorionic monozygotic twin pregnancy (Fig. 23.5A): The embryo splits at or before 3 days of gestation. This results in development of two chorions and two amnions. There is development of two distinct placentae or a single fused placenta. This type of monozygotic twin accounts for nearly 8% of all twin gestations.

Diamniotic monochorionic monozygotic twin pregnancy (Fig. 23.5B): The cleavage division is delayed until the formation of inner cell mass and the embryo splits between 4 and 7 days of

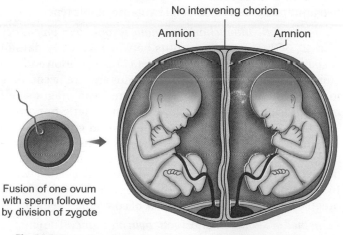

Fusion of one ovum with sperm followed by division of zygote

Fig. 23.1: Formation of monozygotic twins (monochorionic diamniotic)

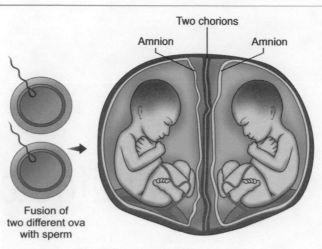

Two chorions
Amnion   Amnion

Fusion of
two different ova
with sperm

Fig. 23.2: Formation of dizygotic twins

Table 23.1: Difference between monozygotic and dizygotic twins

Parameters	Monozygotic twins (identical twins)	Dizygotic twins (non-identical or fraternal twins)
Aetiology	Division of a fertilised ovum into two	Fertilisation of two or more ova by sperms
Sex	Same	Can be different
Placenta	Single	Each foetus has a separate placenta
Communication between foetal vessels	Present	Absent
Genetic features (DNA fingerprinting)	Same	Different
Blood group	Same	Different
Skin grafting	Acceptance by the other twin	Rejection by the twin
Intervening membrane between the two foetuses	Composed of 0–3 layers: (a fused chorion in the middle surrounded by amnion on two sides) depending on the type of monozygotic twin	Composed of four layers: two chorions in the middle surrounded by amnion on two sides
Foetal growth and congenital malformations	More common	Less common
Incidence	Comprises of one-third of total cases of twins	Comprises of two-thirds of total cases of twins
Frequency	The frequency of monozygotic twin births is relatively constant worldwide and is approximately one set per 250 live births	Variable
Influence of various factors	Though the occurrence of monozygotic twins is largely independent of factors such as race, heredity, age, and parity, there is now increasing evidence that assisted reproductive technology increases the incidence of zygotic splitting	The incidence of dizygotic twinning is greatly influenced by factors such as race, heredity, maternal age, parity, nutrition and fertility treatment

gestation. This results in development of a single chorion and two amnions. Nearly 20% of all twins are of this type.

Monoamniotic monochorionic monozygotic twin pregnancy (Fig. 23.5C): The embryo splits between 8 and 12 days of gestation. This results in development of one chorion and one amnion. Such types of monozygotic twins are rare, accounting for less than 1% of all twin gestations. The diagnosis of monochorionic (MC) pregnancy is particularly important because it can be associated with several complications specific to the MC pregnancies such as twin-to-twin transfusion syndrome (TTTS), the consequences to foetal death of the co-twin and the discordant growth between the twins. In addition, MC monoamniotic pregnancies (1% of twin pregnancies) carry a very high risk of cord entanglement.

Conjoined or Siamese monozygotic twin pregnancy: The embryo splits at or after 13 days of gestation, resulting in development

of conjoined twins, which share a particular body part with each other. Development of such type of monozygotic twins is extremely rare. Joining of the twins can begin at either pole and may be dorsal, ventral and lateral. Different types of conjoined twins are enlisted in Table 23.2.

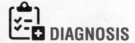

DIAGNOSIS

Clinical Presentation

Abdominal Examination

❖ On inspection, there may be abdominal overdistension or barrel-shaped abdomen.
❖ The uterus may be palpable abdominally, earlier than 12 weeks of gestation.

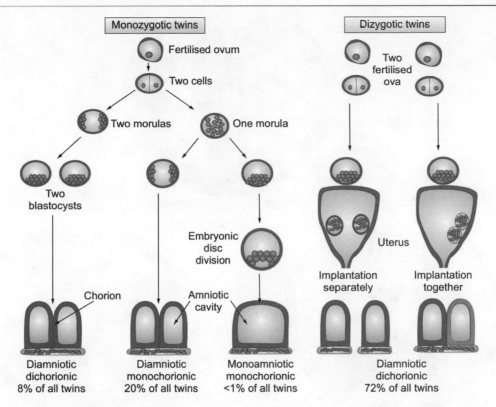

Fig. 23.3: Difference between the monozygotic and dizygotic twins

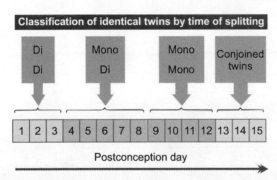

Fig. 23.4: Formation of different types of monozygotic twins
Abbreviations: Di Di, diamniotic dichorionic; Mono Di, monochorionic diamniotic; Mono Mono, monoamniotic monochorionic

❖ Height of the uterus is greater than period of amenorrhoea (fundal height is typically 5 cm greater than the period of amenorrhoea in the second trimester).
❖ Abdominal girth at the level of umbilicus is greater than the normal abdominal girth at term.
❖ Multiple foetal parts may be palpable (e.g. palpation of two foetal heads).
❖ Hydramnios may be present.
❖ Two foetal heart sound (FHS) can be auscultated, located at two separate spots separated by a silent area in between.

Investigations

Ultrasound examination: Ultrasound examination at 10–13 weeks of gestation helps in assessment of foetal viability, number of foetuses, chorionicity, major congenital malformations and nuchal translucency (NT). There may be presence of two or more foetuses or gestational sacs (Figs 23.6A and B; Fig. 23.7). There may be two or more placentas lying close to one another or presence of a single large placenta with a thick dividing membrane. Due to the presence of excessive congenital anomalies in these cases, detailed ultrasound examination is also important in the second trimester to rule out the presence of congenital anomalies. Increased ultrasound surveillance is also warranted in case of triplet (Fig. 23.7) and other higher-order pregnancies that include a MC pair due to higher risk of foetal loss and TTTS.

DIFFERENTIAL DIAGNOSIS

❖ Hydramnios
❖ Wrong dates
❖ Hydatidiform mole
❖ Uterine fibroids
❖ Adnexal masses
❖ Foetal macrosomia.

MANAGEMENT

Antenatal Period

❖ *Steps for prevention of preterm labour*: Some of these include bed rest, administration of tocolytic agents, regular monitoring of uterine activity (if possible using external cardiotocography), prophylactic cervical cerclage, etc.

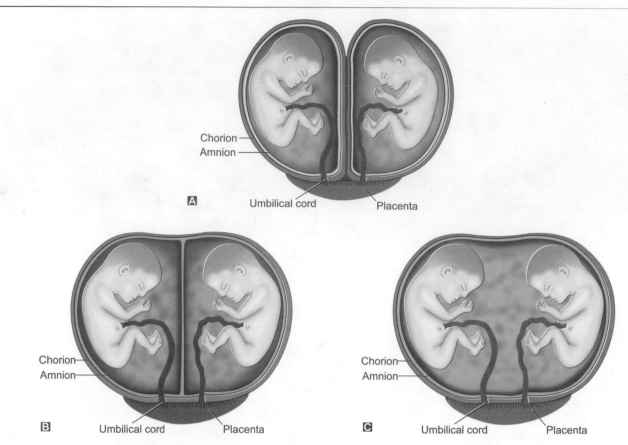

Figs 23.5A to C: (A) Diamniotic dichorionic monozygotic twin pregnancy; (B) Diamniotic monochorionic monozygotic twin pregnancy; (C) Monoamniotic monochorionic monozygotic twin pregnancy

PART II

Table 23.2: Different types of Siamese twins

Types of Siamese twin	Description
Thoracopagus	Joined at the chest
Omphalopagus	Joined at the anterior abdominal wall
Craniopagus	Joined at the head
Pyopagus	Joined at the buttocks
Ischiopagus	Joined at the ischium

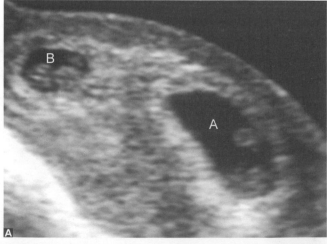

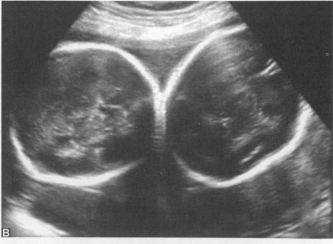

Figs 23.6 A and B: (A) Presence of two gestational sacs on ultrasound, with sac A = 7.6 weeks and sac B = 5.7 weeks; (B) Ultrasound of the same patient at 30 weeks of gestation showing two foetal heads

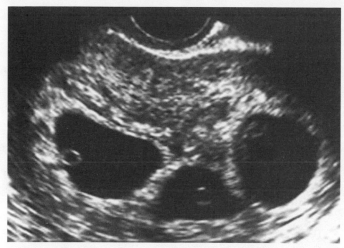

Fig. 23.7: Transvaginal ultrasound of triplets at 7 weeks of gestation showing three separate gestational sacs

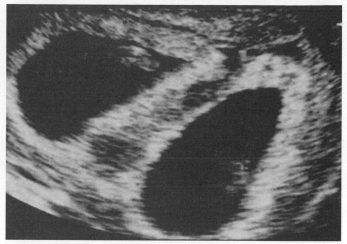

Fig. 23.8: Diamniotic dichorionic twins at 7 weeks of gestation. There are two separate chorionic sacs surrounding each of the two amniotic sacs, with each sac containing an embryo. The intervening membrane between the twins is composed of four layers: two layers of chorion in the middle surrounded by a layer of amnion on either side (*For colour version, see Plate 1*)

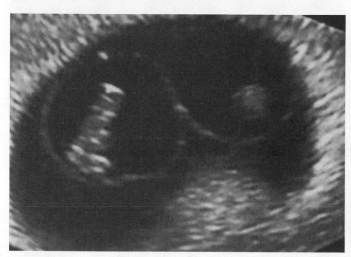

Fig. 23.9: Monochorionic diamniotic twins. In this case, each embryo is surrounded by a separate amniotic sac. There is common chorionic sac which surrounds the two amniotic sacs. Therefore, the intervening membrane between the two twins comprises of two layers of amnion

❖ *Increased daily requirement for dietary calories, proteins and mineral supplements*: There is an additional calorie requirement to the extent of 300 kcal/day above that required for a normal singleton gestation. Moreover, there is a requirement for increased iron, calcium and folic acid supplements in order to meet the demands of multifoetal pregnancy. Iron requirement must be increased to the extent of 60–100 mg/day and folic acid to 1 mg/day.

❖ *Increased frequency of antenatal visits*: The patient should be advised to visit the antenatal clinic every 2 weeks, especially if some problem is anticipated. Clinical care for women with multifoetal gestation must be co-ordinated in such a way as to minimise the number of hospital visits and provide care as close to the woman's home as possible. Continuity of care must be provided within and between hospitals and the community.

❖ *Screening for foetal aneuploidy*: Patients with MC gestation who wish to have screening for foetal aneuploidy must be offered measurements of NT. Since screening for aneuploidies through serum biochemical screening is not as effective as that in singleton pregnancies, a combined screening method [NT scan along with biochemical tests, pregnancy-associated plasma protein-A (PAPP-A) and β-hCG] can be employed in the first trimester to calculate the risk for each foetus). The available evidence regarding the role of NT measurements in predicting TTTS presents with unclear results.[3-5]

❖ *Karyotyping*: The procedure of amniocentesis can be carried out in multifoetal gestation and is associated with a similar rate of pregnancy loss as in singletons. Chorionic villus sampling is also possible in cases of multifoetal gestation. It can be carried out at an earlier period of gestation. However, it is associated with a higher rate of foetal loss. Moreover, this procedure may be less reliable than amniocentesis due to the risk of co-twin contamination. Both the procedures, however, must be undertaken after careful ultrasound mapping of the placentae and gestational sacs.

❖ *Determination of chorionicity*: Determination of chorionicity of twins with help of ultrasound examination must be done at 10–13 weeks of gestation (Figs 23.8 to 23.10). This should be preferably performed before 14 weeks of gestation because chorionicity can be determined with nearly 100% accuracy in the first trimester. On the other hand, determination of chorionicity in the second trimester is associated with an accuracy of 80–90%. Presence of two placentae or two foetuses with different genders is most likely indicative of dichorionic (DC) gestation. Visualisation of twin peak or lambda sign (Fig. 23.11) is also indicative of DC gestation. However, absence of this sign does not confirm monochorionicity.

❖ *Increased foetal surveillance*: Foetal monitoring can be done with the help of serial ultrasound examination, BPP, NST, amniotic fluid index (AFI) and Doppler ultrasound examinations.

CHAPTER 23

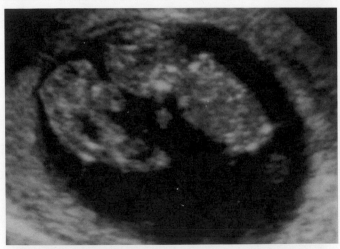

Fig. 23.10: Monochorionic monoamniotic twins. There is absence of any intervening membrane between the two twins, in this case

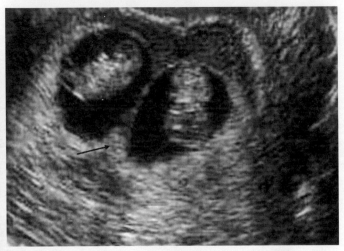

Fig. 23.11: Twin peak sign (indicated by the λ sign as shown by the arrow)

❖ *Monitoring of foetal growth:* Serial foetal growth scans must be performed to evaluate foetal growth velocity, amniotic fluid volume and abnormalities in umbilical artery Doppler waveform analysis. In case of DC twins, four weekly scans must be performed preferably from 24 weeks of gestation to identify foetal growth restriction. More frequent scans may be required in case of suboptimal growth. According to the RCOG guidelines (2009), monitoring of MC pregnancies must be preferably done at every 2-week interval from 16 weeks of gestation.[6]

❖ *Antenatal steroids:* NICE guidelines (2011) recommend the course of antenatal corticosteroids in cases where preterm delivery appears likely. Steroids should also be offered to MC twins as part of planned delivery after 36 weeks and in triplets as part of planned delivery after 35 weeks.[7]

❖ *Multifoetal pregnancy reduction:* Since triplets and quadruplets are associated with higher rates of adverse outcomes, especially preterm delivery, there is a consensus that multifoetal pregnancy reduction must be offered to the woman with triplets and other higher-order pregnancies at approximately 12 weeks of gestation. This is likely to bring about a significant improvement in foetal outcome by reducing the risk of preterm labour, thereby increasing the chances of a healthy baby.[8]

Intrapartum Period

The following precautions need to be observed in the intrapartum period:

❖ Blood to be arranged and kept cross-matched
❖ Paediatrician or anaesthesiologist needs to be informed.
❖ Patient should be advised to stay in bed as far as possible in order to prevent PROM.
❖ Labour should be monitored with the help of a partogram and the heart rate of both the foetuses must be monitored, preferably using a cardiotocogram.
❖ Prophylactic administration of corticosteroids for attaining pulmonary maturity in cases of anticipated preterm deliveries may be required.
❖ IV access in the mother must be established.
❖ Careful foetal monitoring is required.
❖ Vaginal examination must be performed soon after the rupture of membranes (ROM) to exclude cord prolapse and to confirm the presentation of first twin.
❖ *Monochorionic twins:* In case of both MC and DC twins, it is suitable to aim for vaginal birth of MC twins unless there is presence of an accepted, specific, clinical indication for caesarean section, e.g. the first twin lying in non-vertex presentation. Delivery should be preferably planned for 36–37 weeks of gestation, unless there is an indication for an earlier delivery.
❖ Most MC, monoamniotic twins are best delivered at 32 weeks by an elective caesarean delivery, following a course of corticosteroids due to the risk of cord entanglement.

Time of Delivery

In both types of twins (MC and DC), continuing pregnancy beyond 38[+0] weeks of gestation may be associated with an increased risk of foetal death. Therefore, in case of uncomplicated DC twins, elective delivery must be considered at 37[+0] weeks and at 36[+0] weeks in case of uncomplicated MC twins (following a course of corticosteroids). Triplet pregnancies continuing beyond 36[+0] weeks of gestation may also be associated with an increased risk of foetal death.[6] These patients should be offered elective birth at 35[+0] weeks of gestation (following a course of corticosteroids). In presence of complications such as TTTS, timing of delivery must be individualised.

Delivery of the First Baby

❖ Delivery of the first baby should be conducted according to guidelines for normal pregnancy (Flow chart 23.1).
❖ Ergometrine is not to be given at the birth of the first baby.
❖ Cord of the first baby should be clamped and cut to prevent exsanguination of the second twin in case the communicating blood vessels between the twins exist.

Delivery of Second Baby

❖ After the delivery of the first baby, an abdominal and vaginal examination should be performed to confirm the lie, presentation and FHS of the second baby.

❖ External version can be attempted at the time of abdominal examination, in case the lie is transverse.

❖ Vaginal examination also helps in diagnosing cord prolapse, if present. According to the ACOG (1998), the interval between the deliveries of twins is not critical in determining the outcome of twins delivered.

❖ Depending on the presentation of second twin, various options can be adopted as shown in Flow chart 23.2.

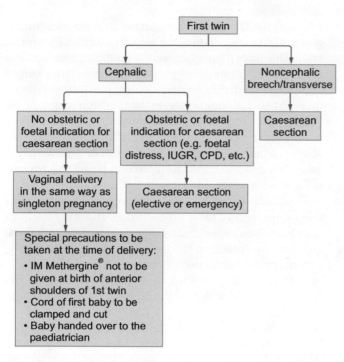

Flow chart 23.1: Intrapartum management of first twin

Abbreviation: CPD, cephalopelvic disproportion

Mode of Delivery

Mode of delivery is usually based on the presentation of first twin (Table 23.3). In case of both the twins in vertex presentation, vaginal delivery is preferred. In case of first twin presenting as vertex and second twin presenting as non-vertex, the presently available evidence provides support for both caesarean section and normal vaginal delivery based on clinical circumstances.[9] Caesarean delivery is usually preferred in cases of first twin in non-vertex presentation. Though caesarean delivery is also preferred in cases of triplets and other higher-order pregnancies, some authors suggest that they can be also safely delivered vaginally.[10] Other indications for caesarean delivery in case of multifoetal gestation are enumerated in Table 23.4.

Table 23.3: Mode of delivery in case of twin gestation

Type of twins	Mode of delivery
Both cephalic	Vaginal delivery
First twin cephalic, second twin non-cephalic	The obstetrician needs to decide between vaginal delivery and caesarean delivery
First twin non-cephalic, second twin cephalic	Caesarean section
Both twins non-cephalic	Caesarean section

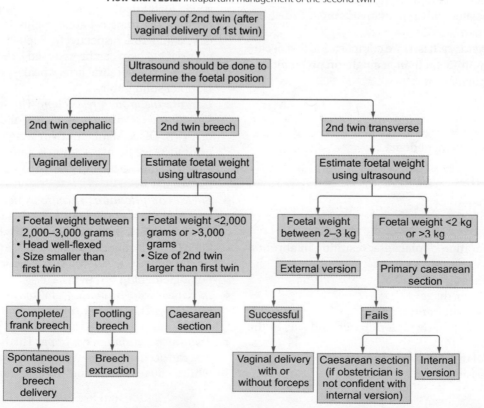

Flow chart 23.2: Intrapartum management of the second twin

CHAPTER 23

Table 23.4: Indication for caesarean section in cases of multiple pregnancies

Obstetric indications	Foetal indications	Indications specific to twin gestation
• Placenta praevia • Previous caesarean section • Contracted pelvis	• Twin with IUGR • First twin non-cephalic, second twin cephalic	• First foetus with non-cephalic presentation • Both twins non-cephalic • MC twins with TTTS • Locking of twins • Conjoined twins

COMPLICATIONS

Maternal

Antenatal Period

❖ Spontaneous abortion
❖ *Anaemia*: Due to increased iron requirement by two foetuses, early appearance of anaemia is a common complication.
❖ *Preterm labour*: Preterm labour and delivery is the most important cause for adverse perinatal outcomes in case of multiple pregnancy. Cervical length assessment has been suggested as the method for estimating the risk of preterm labour. The mean cervical length in twin pregnancy is similar to that in a singleton and measures approximately 4 cm. In singleton pregnancy, cervical length of 15 mm is predictive of preterm labour. However, in case of twin gestation, cervical length of 25 mm prior to 30 weeks of gestation is associated with a spontaneous preterm delivery rate of approximately 80%.
❖ *Fatty liver of pregnancy*: It is a rare complication that occurs more often in multifoetal than in singleton pregnancies.
❖ Hyperemesis gravidarum
❖ Polyhydramnios
❖ Pre-eclampsia
❖ Antepartum haemorrhage
❖ Varicosities, dependent oedema.

Labour

❖ Foetal malpresentation
❖ Vasa praevia
❖ Cord prolapse
❖ Premature separation of placenta, resulting in abruptio placentae
❖ Cord entanglement
❖ Postpartum haemorrhage
❖ Dysfunctional uterine contractions
❖ Increased rate of operative interference and stay in the hospital
❖ Increased risk of problems with breastfeeding
❖ Postnatal depression.

Puerperium

❖ Subinvolution
❖ Infection
❖ Failure of lactation.

Foetal

❖ Miscarriage
❖ *Prematurity*: The most frequent neonatal complications of preterm birth are hypothermia, respiratory difficulties, intra-cranial bleeding, hypoglycaemia, necrotising enterocolitis, infections retinopathy of prematurity, low-birth weight babies, etc. The risk of prematurity is approximately 5 times more in twins in comparison to the singleton pregnancies. Delivery prior to 32 weeks is nearly twice as common in MC twins as in the DC twins. Nearly one-fourth of triplets are also born before 32 weeks. Discordance in twin weight is another factor associated with preterm births and adverse neonatal outcomes.
❖ *Congenital anomalies*: These can especially occur with the monozygotic twin pregnancies and may include malformations such as neural tube defects, cardiac defects, cleft lip abnormalities, lesions such as hydranencephaly, porencephaly, small bowel atresia, etc. Maldevelopmental anomalies such as talipes, congenital dysplasia of the hip, etc. can occur due to the constraints of sharing the uterine cavity.
❖ *Single intrauterine foetal death*: This may occur either early in gestation or later with the progress of pregnancy. Foetal death after 24 weeks of gestation is relatively uncommon. Morbidity and mortality of the surviving foetus largely depends upon the chorionicity of pregnancy, with the risk being higher with MC than the DC twins. Following single foetal death in case of MC pregnancy, the risk of death or neurological abnormality in the surviving twin is 12% and 18% respectively. Foetal anaemia in the case of surviving twin can be assessed by measurement of the foetal middle cerebral artery peak systolic velocity using Doppler sonography.
❖ *Intrauterine growth restriction*: The incidence is similar for MC and DC twin pregnancies following the exclusion of TTTS. Discordance in twin weight of more than 4% prior to 32 weeks of gestation is another important factor which is associated with growth restriction, specifically of the second twin.
❖ *Foetal complications specific to twin gestation*: These may include complications such as discordant growth, TTTS, acardiac twin or twin reversed arterial perfusion (TRAP) syndrome, conjoined twins, interlocking of twins, umbilical cord accidents such as cord prolapse or cord entanglement in MC twins, etc.
❖ *Increased rate of perinatal, foetal and neonatal mortality and morbidity*: This is more common in MC than in DC twins mainly due to increased incidence of TTTS in MC twins.
❖ *Twin-twin transfusion syndrome*: This is a rare complication that can occur in monozygotic twins (sharing the placenta), which causes the blood to pass from one twin to the

PART II

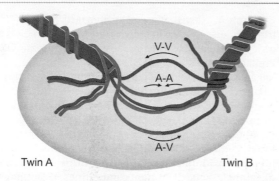

Fig. 23.12: Diagrammatic representation of placenta showing arteriovenous anastomosis

CHAPTER 23

Box 23.1: Ultrasound criteria for the diagnosis of TTTS[11]

- ❑ Monochorionic twins
- ❑ Twins having same gender
- ❑ Presence of hydramnios (defined as the largest vertical pocket >8 cm) in one twin and oligohydramnios (defined as the largest vertical pocket is <2 cm) in the other twin
- ❑ Discrepancy in the size of umbilical cord between the two twins
- ❑ Cardiac dysfunction in the recipient twin along with the presence of hydramnios
- ❑ Abnormal findings on the Doppler velocimetry of umbilical vessels or ductus venosus
- ❑ Discordant bladder appearance: The donor's bladder may not be visualised, whereas the recipient's bladder may be enlarged.
- ❑ Significant discordance of growth amongst the twins

Table 23.5: The Quintero classification system[15]

Stages	Classifications
I	There is a discrepancy in amniotic fluid volume with oligo-hydramnios of a maximum vertical pocket (MVP) ≤2 cm in one sac and polyhydramnios in other sac (MVP ≥8 cm). The bladder of the donor twin is visible and Doppler studies are normal
II	The bladder of the donor twin is not visible (during length of examination, usually around 1 hour) but Doppler studies are not critically abnormal
III	Doppler studies are critically abnormal in either twin and are characterised as abnormal or reversed end-diastolic velocities in the umbilical artery, reverse flow in the ductus venosus or pulsatile umbilical venous flow
IV	Ascites, pericardial or pleural effusion, scalp oedema or overt hydrops are present
V	One or both babies are dead

other. TTTS complicates approximately 10–15% of MC pregnancies. TTTS usually occurs due to the presence of placental vascular communication. The placental vascular anastomoses responsible for the development of TTTS could be from artery-to-artery (A-A), artery-to-vein (A-V), or from vein-to-vein (V-V) (Fig. 23.12). As a result of the vascular communication, one of the twins, which donates blood (donor twin) becomes thin and undernourished, while the other twin which receives blood (recipient twin) grows at the expense of donor twin. The donor twin in TTTS usually shows poor growth, oliguria, anaemia and hyperproteinaemia, low or absent liquor, resulting in development of oligohydramnios, abnormal umbilical artery waveforms, etc. With the severe disease, the donor may not produce any urine, resulting in oligohydramnios and non-visualisation of urinary bladder on ultrasound examination. In these cases, the twin may become wrapped by its amniotic membrane, resulting in the formation of a 'stuck' twin. On the other hand, the recipient twin shows polyuria, polyhydramnios and an enlarged urinary bladder. In the long run, this twin frequently develops polycythaemia, biventricular cardiac hypertrophy and diastolic dysfunction with tricuspid regurgitation. In untreated cases, the mortality rates are extremely high (>90%). The diagnosis of TTTS is based on ultrasound criteria as described in Box 23.1.[11] The Quintero system of staging TTTS (Table 23.5) having some prognostic value is sometimes used. However, the course of the condition is unpredictable and may involve improvement or rapid deterioration.

Management of TTTS should be in conjunction with regional foetal medicine centres employing specialist expertise. Severe TTTS presenting before 26 weeks of gestation should be preferably treated by laser ablation rather than by amnioreduction or septostomy.[12,13] Laser ablation remains the treatment of choice in these cases because it causes a significant reduction in the long-term neurological morbidity.[14] On the other hand, laser ablation does not cause significant improvement in the foetal survival in comparison to the other modalities of treatment such as amnioreduction or selective reduction. Nevertheless, the procedure of amnioreduction continues to be used at the places in the UK where laser therapy is not available or where TTTS occurs later in pregnancy (>26 weeks).

❖ *Acardiac twin or twin reversed arterial perfusion syndrome*: This is an unusual form of TTTS, occurring in about 1 in 15,000 pregnancies. In these MC twins, one twin develops normally, while the other twin fails to develop a heart as well as other body structures. This abnormal twin, called an acardiac foetus, shows characteristic features in which the cardiac structures are absent or non-functioning and the head, upper body and upper extremities are poorly developed. The lower body and lower extremities are, however, more or less normal. The acardiac twin acts as a recipient and depends on the normal donor (pump) twin for obtaining its blood supply via transplacental anastomoses and retrograde perfusion of the acardiac umbilical cord. Perfusion of the malformed (acardiac) foetus occurs via artery-to-artery and vein-to-vein anastomoses between the foetuses. The perfusion pressure of the donor twin overpowers that in the recipient twin, who thus receives reverse blood flow from its twin sibling. Deoxygenated umbilical arterial blood from the donor, thus, flows into the umbilical artery of the recipient, with its direction reversed. In these pregnancies, the umbilical cord from the acardiac twin branches directly from the umbilical cord of the normal twin. This blood flow is reversed from the normal direction leading to the name for this condition—TRAP syndrome. As a result, there is better perfusion of the lower part of the deformed body. On the other hand, the upper part of the body, showing lack of head, heart and upper extremities remains poorly perfused. Normal twin (donor) eventually develops high output failure because it is responsible for maintaining the circulation of both the twins. Thus, the circulatory load of the donor twin may become extremely large resulting in heart failure. The perinatal mortality of this pump twin is considerably high with death usually occurring through complications of high output cardiac failure leading to hydrops foetalis or polyhydramnios-induced preterm delivery. Treatment options in these cases include cord disruption of the acardiac twin, or ablation of intrafoetal vessels via laser, diathermy or radiofrequency interstitial thermal ablation (RITA).

CLINICAL PEARLS

❖ Caesarean section is not required in routine clinical practice for every case of twin gestation. However, in case of presence of an obstetric or foetal indication, a caesarean delivery may be required.

❖ There are some indications specific to twin gestation for caesarean section, which are as follows: MC twins with TTTS; conjoined twins; locking of twins, etc.

EVIDENCE-BASED MEDICINE

❖ Monochorionic twins are associated with a higher rate of complications and thereby a higher rate of morbidity and mortality in comparison to the DC twins.[16]

❖ Routine use of β-mimetics, cervical cerclage, home uterine monitoring, foetal fibronectin estimation, and bed rest has not been supported by good evidence for the prevention of preterm labour in cases of twin gestation.[17]

REFERENCES

1. Human Fertilisation and Embryology Authority (HFEA). (2013). Fertility trends in 2013: trends and figures. [online] Available from http://www.hfea.gov.uk/docs/HFEA_Fertility_Trends_and_Figures_2013.pdf [Accessed April, 2016].
2. Campbell DM. Multiple pregnancy. Baillieres Clin Obstet Gynaecol. 1990;4(1):109-27.
3. Sperling L. Detection of chromosomal abnormalities, congenital abnormalities and transfusion syndrome in twins. Ultrasound Obstet Gynecol. 2007;29(5):517-26.
4. El Kateb A, Nasr B, Nassar M, Bernard JP, Ville Y. First-trimester discordance in crown-rump length predicts timing of development of twin-twin transfusion syndrome: OP05.02. Prenat Diagn. 2007;27(10):922-5.
5. Kagan KO, Gazzoni A, Sepulveda G, Sotiriadis A, Nicolaides KH. Discordance in nuchal translucency thickness in the prediction of severe twin-to-twin transfusion syndrome. Ultrasound Obstet Gynecol. 2007;29(5):527-32.
6. Royal College of Obstetricians and gynaecologists (2009). RCOG guideline No 57. Management of monochorionic twin pregnancy. [online] Available from https://www.rcog.org.uk/globalassets/documents/guidelines/t51management monochorionictwinpregnancy2008a.pdf. [Accessed April, 2016].
7. National Institute of Clinical Excellence (2011). NICE clinical guidelines 129. Multiple pregnancy: Management of twin and triplet pregnancies in the antenatal period. [online] Available from https://www.nice.org.uk/guidance/cg129/resources/multiple-pregnancy-antenatal-care-for-twin-and-triplet-pregnancies-35109458300869. [Accessed April, 2016].
8. Dodd JM, Crowther CA. Reduction of the number of fetuses for women with a multiple pregnancy. Cochrane Database Syst Rev. 2012;10:CD003932.
9. Schmitz T, Carnavalet Cde C, Azria E, Lopez E, Cabrol D, Goffinet F. Neonatal outcomes of twin pregnancy according to the planned mode of delivery. Obstet Gynecol. 2008; 111(3):695-703.
10. Wimalasundera RC, Trew G, Fisk NM. Reducing the incidence of twins and triplets. Best Pract Res Clin Obstet Gynaecol. 2003;17(2):309-29.
11. Harkness UF, Crombleholme TM. Twin-twin transfusion syndrome: where do we go from here? Semin Perinatol. 2005;29(5):296-304.
12. Senat MV, Deprest J, Boulvain M, Paupe A, Winer N, Ville Y. Endoscopic laser surgery versus serial amnioreduction for severe twin-to-twin transfusion syndrome. N Engl J Med. 2004;351(2):136-44.
13. Moise KJ, Dorman K, Lamvu G, Saade GR, Fisk NM, Dickinson JE, et al. A randomized trial of amnioreduction versus septo-stomy in the treatment of twin-twin transfusion syndrome. Am J Obstet Gynecol. 2005(3 Pt 1);193:701-7.
14. Roberts D, Neilson JP, Kilby MD, Gates S. Interventions for treatment of twin-twin transfusion syndrome. Cochrane Database Syst Rev. 2014;1:CD002073.
15. Quintero RA, Morales WJ, Allen MH, Bornick PW, Johnson PK, Kruger M. Staging of twin-twin transfusion syndrome. J Perinatol. 1999 (8 Pt 1);19:550-5.
16. Hack KE, Derks JB, Elias SG, Franx A, Roos EJ, Voerman SK, et al. Increased perinatal mortality and morbidity in monochorionic versus dichorionic twin pregnancies: clinical implications of a large Dutch cohort study. BJOG. 2008;115(1):58-67.
17. Consensus views arising from the 50th Study Group: Multiple pregnancy. In: Kilby M, Baker P, Critchley H, Field D (Eds). Multiple Pregnancy. London: RCOG Press; 2006. pp. 283-6.

PART II

Preterm Labour and Premature Rupture of Membranes

PRETERM LABOUR

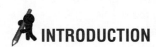 **INTRODUCTION**

Preterm labour is defined as onset of labour (uterine contractions accompanied by cervical dilatation and effacement) before 37 completed weeks of pregnancy (starting from the first day of last menstrual period). In the UK, preterm births are considered between 24^{+0} and 36^{+6} weeks of gestation. The degree of severity of preterm birth is described in Table 24.1.

Babies born before 37 weeks of pregnancy are called premature babies. Premature delivery may be preceded by either uterine contractions or premature rupture of membranes (PROM). When the bag of membranes ruptures before the commencement of labour, this is known as premature or prelabour rupture of membranes. When the rupture of membranes occurs prior to 37 weeks of gestation, it is known as preterm premature rupture of membranes.

AETIOLOGY

The exact cause of preterm labour is presently unknown. Some of the probable causes are as follows:

❖ *Endocrinal causes*: Preterm labour could be related to mechanisms involving increased production of prostaglandins, utcrotonic agents (e.g. oxytocin) and enzymes, which weaken the foetal membranes and degrade the cervical stroma. Early activation of the foetal hypothalamic-pituitary-adrenal axis has also been implicated in the pathogenesis of preterm labour.

❖ *Infection*: Subclinical infection of the choriodecidual space and amniotic fluid has been considered as the most important factor underlying spontaneous preterm labour. Intrauterine infection has been found to be associated with an increased risk of various neonatal morbidities such as periventricular leucomalacia, cerebral palsy, bronchopulmonary dysplasia, etc. Infection is an important aetiological factor in the pathogenesis of preterm labour and can include various causes such as asymptomatic bacteriuria, group B streptococcal colonisation, bacterial vaginosis (BV), *Trichomonas vaginalis*, infection by *Chlamydia trachomatis, Neisseria gonorrhoeae, Ureaplasma urealyticum, Mycoplasma hominis*, etc. Infections such as asymptomatic bacteriuria, pyelonephritis, pneumonia, acute appendicitis, etc. may also be responsible for producing intra-amniotic inflammatory response, which may trigger uterine contractions. Treatment of BV should be with metronidazole and erythromycin, both of which are likely to lower the risk of preterm births by 60%. Oral therapy in standard dosage is administered for 5–7 days.[1] Infections may lead to preterm labour and PROM by the following three mechanisms: (1) maternal inflammatory response; (2) foetal infection; and (3) foetal inflammatory response.

The role of group B *Streptococcus* (GBS) is not clear but is also found to be associated with preterm labour. RCOG presently does not recommend screening for GBS. Treatment with appropriate antibiotics must only be given in the intrapartum period because administration of antenatal antibiotics is not supposed to lower the risk of perinatal transmission. In fact, overaggressive treatment of GBS in the antenatal period can cause an increase in the neonatal infection with penicillin-resistant *Escherichia coli*. The risk of preterm birth due to asymptomatic bacteriuria can be reduced with appropriate antibiotic treatment. Antenatal treatment of chlamydia does not lower the rate of prematurity. It, however,

Table 24.1: Degree of severity of preterm birth

Severity of preterm birth	Period of gestation
Moderate to late preterm births	32^{+0} to 36^{+6} weeks
Very preterm birth	28^{+0} to 31^{+6} weeks
Extreme preterm birth	24^{+0} to 27^{+6} weeks

PART II

Box 24.1: High-risk groups for preterm delivery

❑ Smokers
❑ Women with low BMI
❑ Less than 1-year gap between two consecutive pregnancies
❑ Young maternal age (teenage multipara)
❑ Parity (nulliparity or grandparity)
❑ Low socioeconomic status (low level of education, unemployment, etc.)
❑ Women with previous history of preterm labour
❑ Women with uterine malformations
❑ Women with a previous history of cervical surgery (particularly cone biopsy)

does prevent perinatal transmission. Treatment of both chlamydia and gonococcus must involve contact tracing and treatment of the partner in consultation with GUM clinic.

❖ *Vascular causes*: Increased decidual haemorrhages are likely to be associated with an increase in the haemosiderin deposits, which may be associated with preterm labour.

❖ *Mechanical factors*: Overdistension of the uterus due to multiple pregnancy and polyhydramnios are thought to be associated with preterm labour. Mechanical stretching of the myometrium is likely to result in an increase in oxytocin receptors and formation of prostaglandins.

Risk Factors

Women at high risk for preterm delivery are tabulated in Box 24.1. Some risk factors for preterm labour are as follows:

❖ *Previous history of induced or spontaneous abortion or preterm delivery*: Of the various risk factors for preterm birth, past obstetric history of preterm birth may act as one of the strongest predictors for recurrent preterm birth. If we consider the baseline risk for preterm birth as 10–12%, the risk of recurrent preterm births after 1, 2 and 3 consecutive preterm births may be increased to approximately 15%, 30% and 45%, respectively.

❖ Previous history of pregnancy complications such as pre-eclampsia, antepartum haemorrhage (especially abruptio placenta), unexplained vaginal bleeding, preterm PROM, uterine anomalies such as cervical incompetence, etc.

❖ History of medical and surgical illnesses such as chronic hypertension, acute pyelonephritis, diabetes, renal diseases, acute appendicitis, etc.

❖ Previous history of foetal complications such as congenital malformations and intrauterine death

❖ Previous history of placental complications such as infarction, thrombosis, placenta praevia or abruption

❖ Iatrogenic causes where labour is induced or infant is delivered by a prelabour caesarean section.

❖ Psychological factors, such as depression, anxiety and chronic stress, have also been implicated as the causative factors.

❖ Twins and higher-order multifoetal births

❖ Spontaneous unexplained preterm labour with intact membranes

❖ Idiopathic preterm PROM

❖ Preterm PROM: Nearly 30% of preterm births could be due to preterm PROM. It usually results from intra-amniotic infections (especially BV, *U. urealyticum* and *M. hominis*).

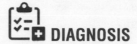 **DIAGNOSIS**

Clinical Presentation

The following are clinical presentations suggestive of preterm labour:

❖ Cervical dilatation of greater than or equal to 1 cm and effacement of 80% or more

❖ Uterine contractions of greater than or equal to 4 per 20 minutes or greater than or equal to 8 per hour, lasting for more than 40 seconds

❖ Cervical length on transvaginal ultrasound scan less than or equal to 2.5 cm and funnelling of internal os

❖ Symptoms such as menstrual cramps, pelvic pressure, backache and/or vaginal discharge or bleeding

❖ Bishop's score may be 4 or greater.

❖ Lower uterine segment may be thinned out and the presenting part may be deep in the pelvis.

Based on the findings of clinical examination, preterm labour can be of two types:

1. *Early preterm labour*: In cases of early preterm labour, cervical effacement is greater than or equal to 80% and cervical dilatation is greater than or equal to 1 cm, but less than 3 cm.

2. *Advanced preterm labour*: In cases of advanced preterm labour, cervical dilatation is greater than or equal to 3 cm.

Abdominal Examination

Abdominal examination may reveal the presence of uterine tenderness suggestive of abruption or chorioamnionitis.

Investigations

Various investigations used for predicting preterm birth are as follows:

❖ *Uterine activity monitoring*: Hospital-based external cardio-tocography has been found to be effective for monitoring uterine contractions for evaluating preterm labour.

❖ *Cervical length measurement*: Presently, transvaginal screening of cervical length with an empty bladder during midgestation (19–24 weeks) is the gold standard test for predicting preterm labour, which must be offered to all pregnant women. The risk of prematurity is inversely proportional to the cervical length. Cervical length of less than 2.5 cm and/or cervical score [cervical score = cervical length (cm) – cervical dilation (cm) at the internal os] of less than 0 in the second trimester is associated with high chances of having preterm birth at less than 35 weeks of gestation.

The patients with a short cervix should be educated regarding the signs and symptoms of preterm labour, especially as the pregnancy approaches potential viability.

Reduction in the length of cervix of greater than 6 mm between two successive ultrasound examinations is also associated with a high risk for preterm labour. Funnelling or change in the diameter of internal os by greater than or equal to 5 mm can also be considered as an independent risk factor for the development of preterm labour. According to RCOG guidelines (2011), sonographic measurement of cervical length must be preferably performed from 14 weeks of gestation for women with previous history of preterm labour or second-trimester losses.

❖ *Measurement of fibronectin levels*: Fibronectin is a glyco-protein, secreted by the chorionic tissue at the maternal-foetal interface, due to which it may be present in the amniotic fluid, placental tissues and decidua basalis. It acts as biological glue that helps in binding blastocyst to endometrium. It is normally present in the cervicovaginal secretions up to 20–22 weeks of gestation. From around 22 weeks, the chorion fuses completely with the underlying decidua. Therefore, this prevents the leakage of fibronectin into the vaginal secretions until at the time of labour when the membranes rupture or the cervix dilates. Therefore, presence of fibronectin in the vaginal secretions between 22 weeks to 34 weeks serves as an important marker of preterm labour. This test is usually performed after 22 weeks of gestation because fibronectin is rarely present in vaginal secretions between 22 weeks and 34 weeks of gestation. Swabs can be taken from the ectocervix or posterior vaginal fornix for collection of cervicovaginal secretions. Prior to this test, digital examination of cervix should not have been performed and lubricating jelly should not have been used. There should not have been any sexual intercourse or vaginal bleeding preferably 24 hours prior to the time of performing the test.

Enzyme-linked immunosorbent assay (ELISA) with FDC-6 monoclonal antibody is used for detecting foetal fibronectin (fFN). A cut-off value of 50 ng/mL is considered positive. Presence of fibronectin is associated with sensitivity of 89% and specificity of 86%. On the other hand, absence of fibronectin from the cervicovaginal secretions is associated with a low risk for preterm delivery. Although a negative test result appears to be useful in ruling out preterm delivery within 2 weeks, a positive fFN has limited value in predicting women who will deliver preterm. Nevertheless, fFN has a predictive value in identifying patients who will or will not deliver within the subsequent 1–2 weeks. The clinical implications of a positive result have not been evaluated fully because no intervention has been shown to decrease the risk of preterm delivery. Presence of fibronectin (values >50 ng/mL) in the cervicovaginal discharge between 24 weeks to 34 weeks of gestation in asymptomatic women, prior to rupture of membrane (ROM), is indicative of preterm labour in nearly 46% patients. Negative test implies that delivery is unlikely to occur within the coming 7 days.[2-4]

❖ *Salivary oestriol levels*: The onset of preterm labour is likely to result in an increase in the maternal salivary oestriol levels.

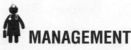

MANAGEMENT

Obstetric Management

Management of patients with preterm labour is described in Flow chart 24.1. For most of the patients, prolonging pregnancy does not offer any benefit because, in a majority of cases, preterm labour serves as a protective mechanism for foetuses threatened by problems such as infection or placental insufficiency. There is no evidence regarding the benefit of bed rest or hospitalisation in women with preterm labour. Preterm labour is often associated with PROM. The management of preterm labour associated with ruptured membranes is described later in the text. The following considerations should be given regarding delivery in women with preterm labour:

❖ For pregnancies less than 34 weeks of gestation in women with no maternal or foetal indication for delivery, expectant management comprising of the following may be used:
  • Close monitoring of uterine contractions
  • *Foetal surveillance and monitoring*: Since the preterm babies are susceptible to the development of foetal hypoxia and acidosis, these foetuses must be carefully monitored for signs of hypoxia during labour, preferably by continuous electronic foetal monitoring.
  • *Steroids*: Corticosteroids may be used for enhancing pulmonary maturity.
  • *Neuroprotection*: Use of magnesium sulphate infusion for 12–24 hours, helps in providing neuroprotection to the foetus.
  • *In utero transfer*: For cases where delivery appears inevitable, the baby should be preferably delivered in a tertiary care setting, with appropriate facilities for the care of preterm baby. In case adequate neonatal intensive care unit (NICU) facilities are not available in the ANC unit where the patient is being treated, consideration should be given towards in utero transfer to a unit with adequate neonatal facilities.
  • *Antibiotic therapy*: Prophylactic therapy for group B streptococcal infection should be administered, especially in the cases where membranes have also ruptured.

Once the episode of preterm labour has been controlled with tocolytic agents, women in early preterm labour should be managed on an outpatient basis with the exception to those who have a positive fibronectin test. In these patients, the risk of preterm delivery is substantial and they should be admitted in the hospital for bed rest.

❖ For pregnancies at 34 weeks or more, women with preterm labour must be monitored for labour progression and foetal well-being. Intrapartum management in these cases comprises of the following steps:
  • *Foetal surveillance*: Foetal surveillance to be performed with continuous electronic foetal monitoring
  • *Mode of delivery*: Delivery must be conducted in presence of an expert neonatologist capable of dealing

Flow chart 24.1: Management of preterm labour

History/clinical examination suggestive of preterm labour

Signs and symptoms
- Lower abdominal cramping
- Pelvic pressure
- Low back pain
- Change in the vaginal discharge
- Painless or painful, but regular uterine activity

Physical examination
- Vital signs
- Abdominal examination
- Per speculum examination
- Foetal heart rate to be evaluated with the help of cardiotocography

Per speculum examination
- Exclude PROM
- Foetal fibronectin (fFN) levels to be estimated
- High vaginal, low vaginal or anorectal swabs to be taken
- Digital vaginal examination to assess cervical dilatation
- Transvaginal cervical length (TVCL) measurement

- No evidence of cervical change on digital examination
- Negative fFN
- TVCL ≥25 mm

→ Low risk of delivery within 7 days

→ Monitor uterine contractions

Infrequent, irregular uterine contractions

Regular uterine contractions

Gradually subside

Persistent contractions

Admit for observation, offer analgesia, reassess after 2 hours

Gradually subside

- Discharge home
- Follow-up in the OPD after 7 days

- Evidence of cervical change on digital examination
- Positive fFN
- TVCL <25 mm

→ High risk of delivery within 7 days

≥34 weeks of gestation

>34 weeks of gestation

Delivery of the patient

- Discharge home
- Follow-up in the OPD after 7 days

- Admit patient and offer analgesia
- Administer steroids
- Commence tocolysis
- Commence antibiotics for GBS
- Continuous foetal cardiotocographic monitoring
- Transfer to tertiary care if required

---

with the complications of prematurity. Ventouse application is contraindicated in preterm deliveries. Caesarean delivery is indicated only in case of obstetrical indications. In case, a caesarean section is performed early in gestation, the lower uterine segment may be poorly formed at that time. Therefore, vertical uterine incision can be given at that time. However, a classical uterine incision is associated with nearly 12% increased risk of uterine rupture. A modified De Lee vertical incision on the lower uterine segment is associated with risk similar to that of a transverse Pfannenstiel incision and is therefore preferred over the classical caesarean scar. The De Lee incision is a modified vertical incision wherein two-third of the incision lies in the lower segment and one-third lies in the upper segment. For

the purpose of intrapartum analgesia, the epidural analgesia is frequently favoured.

In case of a vaginal delivery, at the time of delivery, an episiotomy may be given to facilitate the delivery of foetal head. However, there is no need for routine application of forceps.

Medical Management

The medications prescribed in cases of preterm labour are:
- *Progesterone therapy*: There is increasing evidence that the use of progesterone therapy can help reduce the incidence of preterm birth. Progesterone can be administered vaginally (natural form) or via IM route (synthetic form: 17-α-hydroxyprogesterone). A recent meta-analysis has

shown that the antenatal administration of exogenous progesterone is beneficial in reducing the risk of preterm births and adverse perinatal outcomes.[5] The results of the PREGNANT trial [Vaginal Progesterone bioadhesive gel (prochieve)® Extending Gestation A New Therapy, (2011)] showed that treatment using 100 mg of progestogen gel intravaginally resulted in a 45% reduction in the rate of earlier preterm birth, at less than 33 weeks, along with an improved neonatal outcome.[6] Further studies are required to define the optimum progesterone preparation, its dosage, timing, route of administration and indications. RCOG presently does not recommend the routine use of progesterone in women at an increased risk of preterm labour until its short-term and long-term effects become clear.

❖ *Tocolytic therapy*: There is no clear evidence that tocolytic drugs improve outcomes and therefore it is reasonable not to use them. Use of a tocolytic drug is not associated with a clear reduction in perinatal or neonatal mortality, or neonatal morbidity. Nevertheless, tocolytics are occasionally used in cases of preterm labour for indications described in Box 24.2. Women most likely to benefit from use of a tocolytic drugs are those who are in very preterm labour, those needing transfer to a hospital, which is well equipped with neonatal intensive care facilities and women who have not yet completed a full course of corticosteroids. Prior to the use of tocolytic drugs, the clinician must ensure that there is no contraindication for prolonging the pregnancy, e.g. woman may be in advanced labour. In these cases, the possibility of prolonging the pregnancy may be hazardous for the woman or her baby because of risk of intrauterine infection or placental abruption.

A wide variety of drugs have been recommended for use as tocolytic agents, e.g. β-agonists, calcium channel blockers, oxytocin receptor antagonists, prostaglandin synthetase inhibitors, nitric oxide donors and magnesium sulphate. Use of multiple tocolytic drugs is likely to be associated with an increased risk of adverse effects and therefore should be avoided. Once the decision to use a tocolytic drug has been made, the drug of choice would be the one, which is most effective with the fewest adverse effects, both immediate and long-term. In recent years, there has therefore been considerable interest in identifying a safer alternative. Before prescribing a particular tocolytic agent, the available evidence should be discussed with the woman and her partner and their preferences taken into account while determining the patient care. The various tocolytic drugs used in the clinical practice are described next.

Box 24.2: Indications for the use of tocolysis in cases of preterm labour

❑ Management of intrapartum foetal distress
❑ To facilitate external cephalic version at term
❑ To gain a few days which can be put to good use, such as in utero transfer
❑ To delay delivery for up to 48 hours, thereby buying time to allow the maximum benefit of glucocorticoids in order to reduce the incidence of respiratory distress syndrome.

• *Beta-agonists*: The use of the β-agonists, e.g. ritodrine hydrochloride for tocolysis, which was widespread in the past, has presently declined due to a high incidence of cardiovascular side effects in the mother such as tachycardia, palpitations, hypotension, etc. Maternal deaths due to acute cardiopulmonary compromise have also been reported. Though ritodrine is still licensed for use in the UK, its use has significantly declined.[7,8]

• *Oxytocin antagonist*: An oxytocin antagonist such as atosiban is widely used in the UK. It is the only drug apart from ritodrine, which is licensed for use in the UK because of its reduced frequency of side effects in comparison to β-agonists. However, its efficacy is less than that of β-agonists or calcium channel blockers.[9,10] Moreover, it is a costly drug. Atosiban is administered intravenously in an initial bolus dose of 6.75 mg over 1 minute. This is followed by an infusion of 18 mg/h for 3 hours, then 6 mg/h for up to 45 hours (to a maximum of 330 mg).

• *Calcium channel blockers*: Although the use of nifedipine for preterm labour is an unlicensed indication in the UK, the calcium channel blockers have an advantage of oral administration and lower cost in comparison to atosiban. Moreover, the clinical efficacy of both the drugs in delaying birth for up to 7 days is similar. Nifedipine is administered in an initial oral dose of 20 mg followed by 10–20 mg, three to four times daily, adjusted according to the uterine activity for up to 48 hours. A total dose greater than 60 mg is likely to be associated with an increase in the risk of adverse events such as headache and hypotension.

• *NSAIDs*: Non-steroidal anti-inflammatory drugs such as cyclooxygenase (COX) inhibitors are commonly being used for tocolysis. COX enzymes have a role in the production of prostaglandins, which are important in the onset and maintenance of labour. Inhibitors of these enzymes therefore might be able to cause effective tocolysis with fewer foetal side effects. Their potential side effect is premature closure of ductus arteriosus and consequent pulmonary hypertension. This can be limited by restricting their use to less than 72 hours. Also, they should not be used prior to 30 weeks of gestation. Presently, there is confusing evidence regarding the role of COX-2 inhibitors in reducing the risk of preterm birth.[11]

• *Magnesium sulphate*: Magnesium sulphate is popular for tocolysis in the USA and some other parts of the world, but has rarely been used for this indication in the UK. In the UK, this drug is largely used for the prevention of cerebral palsy.[12] Use of magnesium sulphate is likely to provide neuroprotection, thereby reducing the risk of cerebral palsy. Antenatal administration of magnesium sulphate must be considered when spontaneous or iatrogenic preterm birth is likely within 24 hours.

• *Antibiotics*: The results of the ORACLE II (Overview of the Role of Antibiotics in Curtailing Labor and Early delivery) trial, a RCT has shown that the use of antibiotics in case of uncomplicated preterm labour

PART II

was not associated with any significant improvement in neonatal or perinatal morbidity or mortality in cases of uncomplicated preterm labour. On the other hand, antibiotic prescription was associated with a lower occurrence of maternal infection.[13]

In order to determine the long-term effect on children related to the prescription of antibiotics, a 7-year follow-up study was performed on 4,221 women who had completed the ORACLE II study and were eligible for follow-up. The prescription of erythromycin for women in spontaneous preterm labour with intact membranes was associated with an increase in functional impairment amongst their children at 7 years of age. In fact, there was an increase in the incidence of cerebral palsy in a 7-year follow-up study.[14] On the other hand, significant advantages were obtained when antibiotics were prescribed to the women with preterm PROM without an associated increase in the incidence of cerebral palsy in the long run.[15]

❖ *Corticosteroid therapy*: The administration of glucocorticoids is recommended in patients with preterm labour, whenever the gestational age is between 26 weeks to 34 weeks. The recommended dosage of betamethasone or dexamethasone comprises of two 12 mg doses, administered 24 hours apart. There is no difference between the use of either betamethasone or dexamethasone as long as the total dose of 24 mg of either drug is administered over a 24–48 hour's period.[16] Maximum benefit of steroids is observed when steroids are received more than 24 hours and less than 7 days before delivery. Use of a course of steroids is associated with a marked improvement in neonatal outcome and a significant reduction in the risk of respiratory distress syndrome, neonatal deaths and intraventricular haemorrhage. Courses of steroids received at less than 24 hours and more than 7 days before delivery are not associated with a significant reduction in the risk of respiratory distress syndrome.

There is considerable reassuring evidence regarding the long-term safety of a single course of corticosteroids.[17] However, there is growing concern regarding the adverse outcomes associated with repeated courses.[18,19] These include complications such as increased sepsis in cases of preterm PROM, restricted foetal growth, reduced growth of the brain, adrenal suppression, neonatal deaths, etc.

❖ *Cervical cerclage*: Cerclage remains a commonly performed prophylactic intervention used by most obstetricians. Current RCOG guidelines suggest that women with a history of three or more second-trimester miscarriages or preterm deliveries must be offered cervical cerclage.[20] Cerclage must also be offered to women with history of one or more second-trimester miscarriages or preterm deliveries having cervical length of 25 mm or less prior to 24 weeks of gestation. Presently, the use and efficacy of cerclage in different high-risk groups, e.g. history of multiple pregnancy, uterine anomalies, history of cervical surgery (e.g. conisation), is highly controversial since the present evidence presents with conflicting studies. Furthermore, there is little consensus regarding the

optimal technique for cerclage and the timing of suture placement.

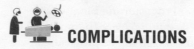

COMPLICATIONS

Maternal

Maternal complications associated with preterm labour include the following:

❖ *Infection*: Infection could be related to acute or chronic chorioamnionitis. There are high chances of ascending infection if ROM is present for greater than 24 hours. Signs and symptoms suggestive of acute choriamnionitis include maternal tachycardia greater than 100 bpm; foetal tachycardia greater than 160 bpm; maternal temperature greater than 37.8°C; uterine tenderness; foul smelling amniotic fluid; maternal leucocytosis greater than 15,000/mm³; and C-reactive protein (CRP) greater than 0.8 ng/mL. Details related to chorioamnionitis are described later in the text.

Children of women suffering from chorioamnionitis are more likely to experience complications such as sepsis, respiratory distress syndrome, early onset seizures, intraventricular haemorrhage, periventricular leucomalacia, etc.

❖ *Premature rupture of membranes*: Premature rupture of membrane is an important cause for preterm labour. In about 80–90% of the cases, labour starts within 24 hours of PROM. Complications related to PROM have been described in details later in the text.

Foetal

Some of the complications, which can occur in preterm infants, include:

❖ *Pulmonary complications*: Respiratory distress, bronchopulmonary dysplasia, etc.

❖ *Gastrointestinal complications*: Hyperbilirubinaemia, necrotising enterocolitis, failure to thrive, etc.

❖ *Central nervous system complications*: Intraventricular haemorrhage, hydrocephalus, cerebral palsy, neurodevelopmental delay and hearing loss

❖ *Ophthalmological complications*: Retinopathy of prematurity, retinal detachment, etc.

❖ *Cardiovascular complications*: Hypotension, patent ductus arteriosus, pulmonary hypertension, etc.

❖ *Renal complications*: Water and electrolyte imbalance, acid-base disturbances

❖ *Haematological complications*: Iatrogenic anaemia, requirement for frequent blood transfusions, anaemia of prematurity, etc.

❖ *Endocrinological complications*: Hypoglycaemia, transiently low thyroxine levels, cortisol deficiency and increased insulin resistance in adulthood.

❖ *Neurodevelopmental impairment*: Disability and handicap.[21]

CLINICAL PEARLS

❖ The present threshold of non-viability for premature births is weight less than 750 g and period of gestation less than 26 weeks.
❖ The main goals of obstetric patient management in preterm labour are provision of prophylactic pharmacologic therapy to prolong the period of gestation and avoiding delivery prior to 34 completed weeks of gestation.
❖ In cases of acute or chronic chorioamnionitis, delivery must be achieved rapidly.

EVIDENCE-BASED MEDICINE

❖ Use of a tocolytic drug is not associated with a clear reduction in perinatal or neonatal mortality or morbidity. The main effect of tocolytic drugs when used for women in preterm labour is to reduce the number of patients who deliver within 48 hours or within 7 days of experiencing signs of preterm labour so as to buy time to maximise the effect of corticosteroid therapy.[22]
❖ Presently, there is no evidence regarding the benefit associated with the use of antibiotics in cases of uncomplicated preterm labour. In fact, the available evidence points to the likely harm associated with the use of antibiotics in uncomplicated cases of preterm labour with intact membranes.[13-15]

PREMATURE RUPTURE OF MEMBRANES

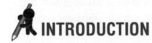

INTRODUCTION

Premature rupture of membranes can be defined as spontaneous ROM beyond 28 weeks of pregnancy, but before the onset of labour. ROM occurring beyond 37 weeks of gestation, but before the onset of labour is known as term PROM. On the other hand, ROM occurring before 37 completed weeks of gestation but before the onset of labour is called preterm PROM. If the ROM is present for more than 24 hours before delivery, it is known as prolonged ROM.

AETIOLOGY

❖ Increased friability and reduced tensile strength of the membranes
❖ Polyhydramnios
❖ Cervical incompetence
❖ Multiple pregnancy
❖ Intrauterine infection such as chorioamnionitis, urinary tract or lower genital tract infection.

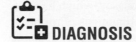

DIAGNOSIS

Clinical Presentation

There may be escape of watery discharge per vaginum either in the form of gush of fluid or slow leakage. The mother gives a typical history of feeling a gush of fluid escaping from the vagina followed by recurrent dampness. The diagnosis of PROM can be confirmed by a sterile per speculum examination after the mother has been supine for about 20–30 minutes following ROM. Normal liquor is a clear-coloured watery fluid. Presence of meconium in the liquor must be noted. Preterm presence of meconium in the intra-amniotic fluid is suggestive of intra-amniotic infection. This, however, is not diagnostic and therefore needs to be confirmed. At term, presence of meconium in liquor contraindicates expectant management. Digital vaginal examination is best avoided in women with PROM unless there is a strong suspicion that the woman may be in labour. Digital examination could cause transportation of microorganisms from the vagina into the cervix, resulting in intrauterine infection, release of prostaglandins and precipitation of preterm labour. Repeated digital examination is supposed to be associated with an increased risk of chrioamnionitis, postpartum endometritis and neonatal infection. Diagnosis of PROM can be confirmed by performing the following tests. The two most commonly used tests include the use of nitrazine paper and ferning:

❖ *Nitrazine paper test*: A per speculum examination must be performed to collect the fluid from posterior fornix (vaginal pool). The pH of the fluid collected from the vaginal fornix must be detected using litmus or nitrazine paper. Since the liquor is normally alkaline in nature (pH 7–7.5), the normally acidic vaginal pH (4.5–5.5) turns alkaline in the presence of PROM, causing the colour of the nitrazine paper to change from yellow to blue.[23,24]
❖ *Ferning*: The liquor smeared slide when examined under the microscope shows appearance of a characteristic ferning pattern. The characteristic ferning of liquor smear slide is related to the crystalline pattern of dried amniotic fluid due to its high content of sodium chloride and protein.[25,26]
❖ *Staining of the centrifuged cells with 0.1% Nile blue sulphate*: There may be orange-blue discolouration of the cells due to presence of exfoliated fat containing cells from sebaceous glands of the foetus.
❖ *Intra-amniotic injection of a coloured dye*: Presence of blue discolouration of the fluid emanating from cervical os, following the injection of 2–3 mL of sterile solution of the dye indigo carmine into the amniotic cavity is indicative of PROM.
❖ *Alpha-foetoproteins*: Presence of α-foetoproteins in the vaginal secretions is indicative of PROM.
❖ *Ultrasound examination*: Ultrasound examination is useful to help confirm the diagnosis of spontaneous PROM in some cases by demonstrating oligohydramnios.[27-30]

CHAPTER 24

❖ *AmniSure®*: This is a rapid immunoassay, which has also been shown to be accurate in the diagnosis of ruptured membranes, having a sensitivity and specificity of 98.9% and 100%, respectively.[31]

Investigations

❖ Full blood count
❖ White cell count
❖ Differential count
❖ Determination of levels of CRP
❖ Urine routine microscopy and culture
❖ *Speculum examination*: This helps in confirming the diagnosis of preterm PROM by obtaining fluid for determining pulmonary maturity and obtaining endo-cervical samples for *Chlamydia* and *N. gonorrhoea*.
❖ Ultrasound for BPP; estimation of gestational age and weight; measurement of cervical length and amniotic fluid volume
❖ Non-stress test.

MANAGEMENT

Main aim of management in case of PROM is to avoid delivery prior to 34 weeks of gestation. Women who need to be delivered irrespective of the period of gestation include the following:

❖ Those with acute chorioamnionitis or subclinical infection/inflammation or those at a high risk of infection
❖ Those with mature lungs or with period of gestation greater than 36 weeks
❖ Foetuses with lethal congenital anomalies having non-reassuring foetal heart sounds.
❖ Women in advanced labour, with cervical effacement of 80% or more and cervical dilatation of 5 cm or more
❖ Caesarean section is not routinely required but may be required in the presence of an obstetric indication.
❖ The tocolytic agent of choice for women with preterm PROM is nifedipine. It is given in the initial dosage of 20–30 mg followed by 10–20 mg at every 6 hourly interval.

After confirmation of diagnosis of PROM, further management is described in the Flow chart 24.2. Delivery should be considered at 34 weeks of gestation. In cases where expectant management is considered beyond 34 weeks of gestation, women should be informed about the increased risk of chorioamnionitis and the reduced risk of respiratory problems in the neonate.

❖ *Preterm premature rupture of membranes*: In these cases, the following steps need to be taken:
  • *Corticosteroids*: A single course of corticosteroids must be administered to reduce the risk of respiratory distress syndrome. A single course of steroids is not associated with an increased risk of complications such as sepsis.[32]
  • *Tocolytics*: Use of tocolytics in cases of PROM is not recommended in the absence of clear evidence that tocolysis improves perinatal or neonatal outcome.[33-35]

• *Antibiotics*: Use of prophylactic antibiotics in such situations is supported by the UK ORACLE I trial.[36] Use of oral erythromycin in the dosage of 250 mg QDS for 10 days has been recommended by the RCOG. Use of erythromycin is associated with a significant reduction in neonatal morbidity and mortality. On the other hand, use of coamoxiclav is associated with a significant increase in the incidence of neonatal necrotising colitis. In these cases, women should be observed for signs of clinical chorioamnionitis. There is no need to perform high vaginal swabs or to carry out maternal full blood count or CRP assessment on a weekly basis. Cardiotocography, however, appears to be a useful investigation because presence of foetal tachycardia could be indicative of clinical chorioamnionitis. BPP score and Doppler velocimetry can also be carried out. However, these tests have limited value in predicting foetal infection.
• *Role of transabdominal amnioinfusion*: Presently, there is insufficient evidence to recommend amnioinfusion in very preterm PROM as a method to prevent pulmonary hypoplasia.
• *Role of fibrin glue in the sealing of chorioamniotic membranes*: There is insufficient evidence to recommend fibrin sealants as a routine treatment for second-trimester oligohydramnios caused by preterm PROM, thereby preventing the occurrence of pulmonary hypoplasia.
• *Amnioinfusion in labour*: The recent Cochrane review[37] does not recommend the use of amnioinfusion during labour in women with preterm ROM in order to prevent the risk of umbilical cord compression.

❖ *Term premature rupture of membranes*: The outcome in patients with term PROM is similar in cases where the labour is induced immediately in comparison to those cases that are managed conservatively. If possible, the women must be offered a choice between conservative management and immediate induction. Induction of labour using oxytocin may be required in cases that are colonised with GBS. Immediate induction is likely to be associated with increased use of epidural analgesia.

COMPLICATIONS

Maternal

❖ *Infection*: Infection could be related to acute or chronic chorioamnionitis. There are high chances of ascending infection if ROM is present for greater than 24 hours. Diagnosis of chorioamnionitis is made in case of maternal temperature greater than 38.0°C (100.0°F) and presence of two out of the five following signs:
1. White blood cell count greater than 15,000 cells/mm³
2. Maternal tachycardia greater than 100 bpm
3. Foetal tachycardia greater than 160 bpm
4. Tender uterus
5. Foul-smelling discharge.

Flow chart 24.2: Management of premature rupture of membranes

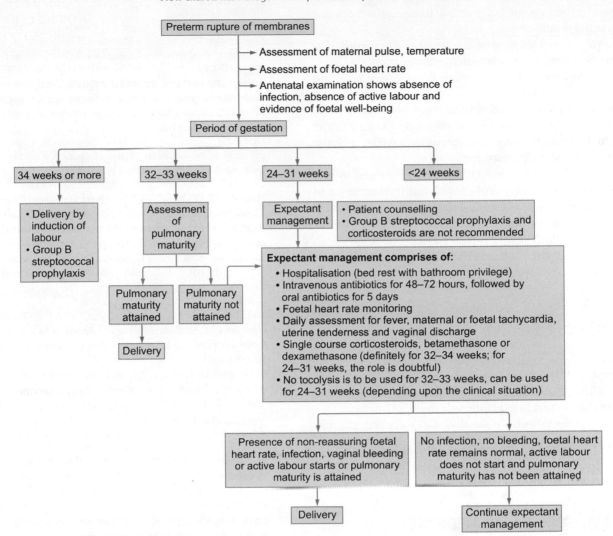

The woman should be regularly examined for such signs of intrauterine infection and presence of an abnormal parameter or a combination of these may indicate intrauterine infection. The measurement of maternal temperature, pulse and foetal heart rate auscultation should be preferably performed between every 4–8 hourly intervals.[27,28,38]

In situations in which the diagnosis remains unclear, an amniocentesis for fluid culture (aerobic or anaerobic bacteria), Gram stain (bacteria present if Gram stain is positive or if WBC count is >50 cells/mm³), glucose level (positive if <15 mg/dL), or leucocyte esterase evaluation may be considered. However, amniocentesis may result in a false-positive fFN test result if the fFN level estimation is performed after amniocentesis.

The available data suggests an association between subclinical intrauterine infection and adverse neonatal outcome. Positive cultures of amniotic fluid cultures is likely to increase the risks of complications such as preterm delivery, neonatal sepsis, respiratory distress syndrome, chronic lung disease, periventricular leucomalacia, intraventricular haemorrhage and cerebral palsy.[39-42] However, presently, there is insufficient evidence to recommend the use of amniocentesis in the diagnosis of intrauterine infection.

❖ *Preterm labour*: Premature rupture of membranes is an important cause for preterm labour.
❖ *Cord prolapse*: Sudden gush of amniotic fluid may be associated with an increased incidence of cord prolapse and/or premature placental separation (placental abruption) and/or oligohydramnios.
❖ *Abruption*: Preterm PROM may be associated with an increased risk of complications such as abruption and requirement for operative delivery.

Foetal/Neonatal

❖ *Respiratory distress syndrome or hyaline membrane disease*: The newborn infant may suffer from severe respiratory distress, thereby requiring ventilatory support after birth.
❖ *Non-reassuring foetal heart rate pattern*: Most common abnormality is variable decelerations associated with umbilical cord compression as a result of oligohydramnios. Moderate or severe variable or late decelerations may be present as a result of placental insufficiency and are indicative of intrapartum foetal distress.

CHAPTER 24

- *Pulmonary hypoplasia*: This condition may be characterised by the presence of multiple pneumothoraces and interstitial emphysema.
- *Cerebral palsy*: This may be the result of intraventricular bleeding, intrapartum foetal acidosis and hypoxia.
- *Foetal deformities*: These may especially include facial and skeletal deformities.
- *Foetal trauma*: This could be related to foetal macrosomia, which may be responsible for producing injury to the brachial plexus, fracture of humerus or clavicle, cephalic hematomas, skull fracture, etc.
- *Postmaturity syndrome*: This is characterised by the presence of wrinkled skin due to reduced amount of subcutaneous fat. These foetuses are small, tolerate labour poorly and may be acidotic at birth.
- *Neonatal deaths*: The three major causes of neonatal death in association with preterm PROM are prematurity, sepsis and pulmonary hypoplasia.

CLINICAL PEARLS

Recommended prophylaxis for group B streptococcal infection may comprise of the following:

- Penicillin G, 5 million units IV initial dose, then 2.5 million units IV at every 4 hourly intervals until delivery, or
- Ampicillin, 2 g IV initial dose, then 1 g IV at every 4 hourly or 2 g at every 6 hourly until delivery, or
- Cefazolin, 2 g IV initial dose, then 1 g IV at every 8 hourly intervals until delivery.

EVIDENCE-BASED MEDICINE

- Although the available data suggests an association between subclinical intrauterine infection and adverse neonatal outcome, the role of amniocentesis in improving neonatal outcome presently remains undetermined. There is insufficient evidence to recommend the use of amniocentesis in the diagnosis of intrauterine infection.[37-39]
- Amnioinfusion during labour is also not recommended in women with preterm ROM in order to prevent the risk of umbilical cord compression.[37]
- Presently, there is insufficient evidence to recommend the use of fibrin sealants in cases of very preterm PROM as a method to prevent pulmonary hypoplasia.[40]

REFERENCES

1. Hauth JC, Goldenberg RL, Andrews WW, DuBard MB, Copper RL. Reduced incidence of preterm delivery with metronidazole and erythromycin in women with bacterial vaginosis. N Engl J Med. 1995;333(26):1732-6.
2. Goldenberg RL, Iams JD, Mercer BM, Meis PJ, Moawad AH, Copper RL, et al. The preterm prediction study: the value of new versus standard risk factors in predicting early and all spontaneous preterm births. Am J Public Health. 1998;88(2):233-8.
3. Iams JD, Casal D, McGregor JA, Goodwin TM, Kreaden US, Lowensohn R, et al. Fetal fibronectin improves the accuracy of diagnosis of preterm labour. Am J Obstet Gynecol. 1995; 173(1):141-5.
4. Abbott DS, Radford SK, Seed PT, Tribe RM, Shennan AH. Evaluation of quantitative fetal fibronectin test for spontaneous preterm birth in symptomatic women. Am J Obstet Gynecol. 2013;208(2):122.e1-6.
5. Dodd JM, Jones L, Flenady V, Cincotta R, Crowther CA. Prenatal administration of progesterone for preventing preterm birth in women considered to be at risk of preterm birth. Cochrane Database Syst Rev. 2013;7:CD004947.
6. Hassan SS, Romero R, Vidyadhari D, Fusey S, Baxter JK, Khandelwal M, et al. Vaginal progesterone reduces the rate of preterm birth in women with a sonographic short cervix: a multicenter, randomized, double-blind, placebo-controlled trial. Ultrasound Obstet Gynecol. 2011;38(1):18-31.
7. Anotayanonth S, Subhedar NV, Neilson JP, Harigopal S. Betamimetics for inhibiting preterm labour. Cochrane Database Syst Rev. 2004;(4):CD004352.
8. de Heus R, Mol BW, Erwich JJ, van Geijn HP, Gyselaers WJ, Hanssens M, et al. Adverse drug reactions to tocolytic treatment for preterm labour: prospective cohort study. BMJ. 2009;338:b744.
9. Papatsonis D, Flenady V, Cole S, Liley H. Oxytocin receptor antagonists for inhibiting preterm labour. Cochrane Database Syst Rev. 2005;(3):CD004452.
10. Coomarasamy A, Knox EM, Gee H, Song F, Khan KS. Effectiveness of nifedipine versus atosiban for tocolysis in preterm labour: a meta-analysis with an indirect comparison of randomised trials. BJOG. 2003;110(12):1045-9.
11. King J, Flenady V, Cole S, Thornton S. Cyclo-oxygenase (COX) inhibitors for treating preterm labour. Cochrane Database Syst Rev. 2005;(2):CD001992.
12. Doyle LW, Crowther CA, Middleton P, Marret S, Rouse D. Magnesium sulphate for women at risk of preterm birth for neuroprotection of the fetus. Cochrane Database Syst Rev. 2009;(1):CD004661.
13. Kenyon SL, Taylor DJ, Tarnow-Mordi W; ORACLE Collaborative Group. Broad spectrum antibiotics for spontaneous preterm labour: the ORACLE II randomised trial. ORACLE Collaborative Group. Lancet. 2001;357(9261):989-94.
14. Kenyon S, Pike K, Jones DR, Brocklehurst P, Marlow N, Salt A, et al. Childhood outcomes after prescription of antibiotics to pregnant women with preterm labour: 7-year follow-up of the ORACLE I trial: 7-year follow-up of the ORACLE I trial. Lancet. 2008;372:1319-27.
15. Kenyon S, Pike K, Jones DR, Brocklehurst P, Marlow N, Salt A, et al. Childhood outcomes after prescription of antibiotics to pregnant women after preterm rupture of membranes 7-year follow-up of the ORACLE I trial. Lancet. 2008;372(9646): 1310-8.
16. Royal College of Obstetricians and Gynaecologists. Antenatal Corticosteroids to Reduce Neonatal Morbidity and Mortality. Green-top Guideline No. 7. London: RCOG; 2010.
17. Wapner RJ, Sorokin Y, Mele L, Johnson F, Dudley DJ, Spong CY, et al. Long term outcomes after repeat dose of antenatal corticosteroids. N Engl J Med. 2007;357:1190-8.
18. Murphy KE, Hannah ME, Willan AR, Hewson SA, Ohlsson A, Kelly EN. Multiple courses of antenatal corticosteroids for preterm births (MACS): a randomised control trial. Multiple

PART II

courses of antenatal corticosteroids for preterm births (MACS): a randomised control trial. Lancet. 372(9656):2143-51.

19. Banks BA, Cnaan A, Morgan MA, Parer JT, Merrill JD, Ballard PL, et al. Multiple courses of antenatal corticosteroids and outcomes of premature neonates. Am J Obstet Gynecol. 1999;181(3):709-17.

20. Royal College of Obstetricians and Gynaecologists. Cervical Cerclage. Green-top Guideline No. 60. London: RCOG; 2011.

21. Wood NS, Marlow N, Costeloe K, Gibson AT, Wilkinson AR. Neurologic and developmental disability after extreme preterm birth. N Engl J Med. 2000;343(6):378-84.

22. Royal College of Obstericians and Gynaecologists. (2006). Preterm Prelabour Rupture of Membranes. Green-top Guideline No. 44. [online] Available from www.rcog.org.uk/globalassets/documents/guidelines/gtg_44.pdf. [Accessed July, 2016].

23. Baptisti A. Chemical test for the determination of ruptured membranes. Am J Obstet Gynecol. 1938;35:688-90.

24. Abe T. The detection of rupture of the fetal membranes with the nitrazine indicator. Am J Obstet Gynecol. 1940;39:400-4.

25. Paavola A. Methods based on the study of crystals and fat staining: use in diagnosing rupture of the membranes. Ann Chir Gynaecol Fenn. 1958;47(1):22-8.

26. Volet B, Morier-Genoud J. The crystallization test in amniotic fluid. Gynaecologia. 1960;149:151-61.

27. Ismail MA, Zinaman MJ, Lowensohn RI, Moawad AH. The significance of C-reactive protein levels in women with premature rupture of membranes. Am J Obstet Gynecol. 1985;151(4):541-4.

28. Carlan SJ, O'Brien WF, Parsons MT, Lense JJ. Preterm premature rupture of membranes: a randomized study of home versus hospital management. Obstet Gynecol. 1993;81(1):61-4.

29. Carroll SG, Papiaoannou S, Nicolaides KH. Assessment of fetal activity and amniotic fluid volume in the prediction of intrauterine infection in preterm prelabor amniorrhexis. Am J Obstet Gynecol. 1995;172(5):1427-35.

30. Combs CA, McCune M, Clark R, Fishman A. Aggressive tocolysis does not prolong pregnancy or reduce neonatal morbidity after preterm premature rupture of the membranes. Am J Obstet Gynecol. 2004;190(6):1723-8.

31. Cousins LM, Smok DP, Lovett SM, Poelter DM. AmniSure placental alpha microglobulin-1 rapid immunoassay versus standard diagnostic methods for detection of rupture of membranes. Am J Perinatol. 2005;22(6):317-20.

32. Harding JE, Pang J, Knight DB, Liggins GC. Do antenatal corticosteroids help in the setting of preterm rupture of membranes? Am J Obstet Gynecol. 2001;184(2):131-9.

33. How HY, Cook CR, Cook VD, Miles DE, Spinnato JA. Preterm premature rupture of membranes: aggressive tocolysis versus expectant management. J Matern Fetal Med. 1998;7(1):8-12.

34. Levy D, Warsof SL. Oral ritodrine and preterm premature rupture of membranes. Obstet Gynecol. 1985;66(5):621-3.

35. Dunlop PD, Crowley PA, Lamont RF, Hawkins DF. Preterm ruptured membranes, no contractions. J Obstet Gynecol. 1986;7:92-6.

36. Kenyon S, Boulvain M, Neilson J. Antibiotics for preterm rupture of membranes. Cochrane Database Syst Rev. 2003;(2): CD001058.

37. Hofmeyr GJ. Amnioinfusion for preterm rupture of membranes. Cochrane Database Syst Rev. 2000;(2):CD000942.

38. Romem Y, Artal R. C-reactive protein as a predictor for chorio-amnionitis in cases of premature rupture of the membranes. Am J Obstet Gynecol. 1984;150 (5 Pt 1):546-50.

39. Yoon BH, Jun JK, Romero R, Park KH, Gomez R, Choi JH, et al. Amniotic fluid inflammatory cytokines (interleukin-6, interleukin-1 beta, and tumor necrosis factor-alpha), neonatal brain white matter lesions, and cerebral palsy. Am J Obstet Gynecol. 1997;177:19-26.

40. Yoon BH, Romero R, Jun JK, Park KH, Park JD, Ghezzi F, et al. Amniotic fluid cytokines (interleukin-6, tumor necrosis factor-alpha, interleukin-1 beta, and interleukin-8) and the risk for the development of bronchopulmonary dysplasia. Am J Obstet Gynecol. 1997;177(4):825-30.

41. Yoon BH, Park CW, Chaiorapongsa T. Intrauterine infection and the development of cerebral palsy. BJOG. 2003;110 (Suppl 20):124-7.

42. Sciscione AC, Manley JS, Pollock M, Maas B, Shlossman PA, Mulla W, et al. Intracervical fibrin sealants: a potential treatment for early preterm premature rupture of the membranes. Am J Obstet Gynecol. 2001;184(3):368-73.

CHAPTER 24

Antepartum Haemorrhage

PLACENTA PRAEVIA

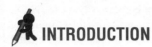

INTRODUCTION

Antepartum haemorrhage (APH) can be defined as the haemorrhage from the genital tract occurring from 24^{+0} weeks of pregnancy, but before the delivery of baby or the onset of labour.[1] It does not include bleeding, which occurs after the delivery of the baby [postpartum haemorrhage (PPH)]. Obstetric haemorrhage on the other hand, includes both antepartum and postpartum bleeding. Worldwide, especially in the developing countries, APH is associated with significant maternal and perinatal morbidity and mortality. In the UK, deaths from obstetric haemorrhage are relatively uncommon. According to the Eighth Report of the CEMDs in the United Kingdom (2006-08), only four deaths were attributed to APH.[2]

In the UK, rates of placenta praevia and placental abruption are rising due to an increase in the rate of caesarean delivery. Placenta praevia is commonly complicated by a condition known as placenta accreta. Rise in the incidence of placenta accreta is also associated with an increasing rate of caesarean delivery. These occur due to the pathological adherence of placenta. Women with placenta praevia who have had a previous caesarean section are at an increased risk of placenta accreta and should be managed as if they have abnormally adherent placenta, with appropriate preparations for surgery made. Abnormally adherent placenta can result in severe bleeding and may often require caesarean hysterectomy. All the conditions associated with morbidly adherent placenta (MAP), i.e. placenta accreta, increta and percreta are described later in the text.

AETIOLOGY

Antepartum haemorrhage can occur due to placental and extraplacental causes (Flow chart 25.1). Besides this,

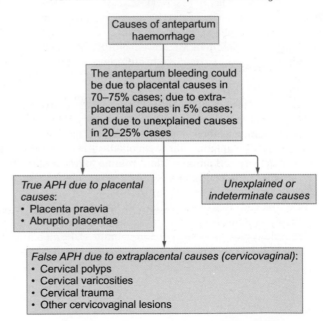

Flow chart 25.1: Causes of antepartum haemorrhage

some cases of APH could be due to unexplained causes (indeterminate APH). The placental causes of bleeding are termed as true APH and can be due to placenta praevia or placental abruption. In the UK, all the maternal deaths due to abruption and placenta praevia need to be reported. These two are most important causes of APH, although these may not be the most common. Clinicians must also remember that domestic violence in pregnancy may result in APH. Placenta praevia can be defined as abnormal implantation of the placenta in the lower uterine segment. Depending on the location of placenta in the relation of cervical os, there can be four degrees of placenta praevia, which are described in Figure 25.1 and are as follows:

❖ *Type 4 placenta praevia*: This is also known as total or central placenta praevia. In total placenta praevia, the placenta completely covers the cervix and is centrally placed.

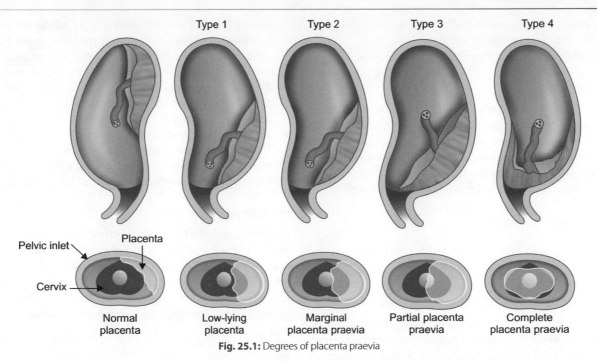

Fig. 25.1: Degrees of placenta praevia

- *Type 3 placenta praevia*: This is also known as partial placenta praevia. In partial placenta praevia, the placenta partly covers the cervical os. Grades 3 and 4 represent the major degree placenta praevia.
- *Type 2 placenta praevia*: This is also known as marginal placenta praevia. In marginal placenta praevia, the placenta does not in any way cover the cervical os, but it approaches the edge of the cervix and the placental edge lies less than or equal to 2.5 cm from the internal cervical os.
- *Type 1 placenta praevia*: This is also known as low-lying placenta. Low-lying placenta is a term used to describe a placenta which is implanted in the lower uterine segment, but is not as close enough to the cervix to qualify as marginal placenta praevia.

    Grades 1 and 2 represent the minor degree placenta praevia.

Risk Factors

Some risk factors, which are associated with an increased incidence of placenta praevia and need to be elicited in the history, include the following:[3-10]

- Multiparity
- *Previous history of caesarean delivery*: History of a single previous caesarean section may increase the incidence of placenta praevia in a subsequent pregnancy to as much as 5%. The risk further increases as the number of previous caesarean deliveries increase. Previous history of suction curettage is associated with an increased risk. Damage to the uterine endometrium as a result of endometritis and manual removal of placenta is also associated with an increased risk.

    It is important to elicit the history of previous uterine surgery because presence of a uterine scar along with placenta praevia may be often associated with placenta accreta, increta or percreta.

- *Advanced maternal age*: The risk of placenta praevia also increases with advancing maternal age, with the risk increasing by 2% after 35 years of age and by 5% after the age of 40 years.
- History of placenta praevia in the previous pregnancy
- History of smoking
- *History of multiple pregnancy*: Multifoetal pregnancy is usually associated with a large placenta that commonly encroaches upon the lower uterine segment.
- Foetal malpresentation and foetal congenital anomalies
- Submucous fibroid
- Assisted conception.

DIAGNOSIS

Clinical Presentation

Bleeding: Placenta praevia is typically associated with sudden, painless, apparently causeless, recurrent and profuse bleeding, which is bright red in colour and occurs after 20 weeks of gestation. The amount of bleeding may range from light to heavy. The patient's physical condition is proportional to the amount of blood loss. Repeated bleeding can result in anaemia, whereas heavy bleeding may cause shock, hypotension and/or tachycardia. Nearly 10% of the patients with placenta praevia have a coexistent abruption also.

Abdominal Examination

- Uterus is soft, relaxed and non-tender.
- Uterine contractions may be palpated.
- Size of the uterus is proportional to the period of gestation.
- The foetal presenting part may be high and cannot be pressed into the pelvic inlet due to the presence of placenta.

❖ There may be abnormal foetal presentation (e.g. breech presentation, transverse lie, etc.)

❖ Foetal heart rate is usually within normal limits.

Vaginal Examination

Vaginal or rectal examination must never be performed in suspected cases of placenta praevia. Instead, an initial inspection must only be performed. On inspection and per speculum examination, the amount and colour of the bleeding must be noted. Any local cause of bleeding per vaginum (e.g. cervical erosions, polyps, etc.) must also be ruled out.

Investigations

Investigations should be performed to assess the extent and physiological consequences of APH.

Maternal Investigations

❖ *Blood tests*: A CBC and coagulation screen must be carried out in all the cases of major haemorrhage. Urea, electrolytes and liver function tests should be assayed. At least four units of blood needs to be cross-matched and arranged. If at any time severe haemorrhage occurs, the patient may require a blood transfusion. In cases of minor haemorrhage, a full blood count and 'group and save' should be performed. A coagulation screen is not indicated unless the platelet count is abnormal.

❖ *Imaging studies*: The main way of confirming the diagnosis of placenta praevia is by imaging studies, both TAS (Fig. 25.2) and TVS (more accurate). Ultrasound scanning is a well-established investigation for determining placental location and diagnosing placenta praevia.[11,12] Colour flow Doppler imaging may also prove to be helpful in these cases.

Transabdominal ultrasound scan at 18–20 weeks may be associated with a false-positive diagnosis regarding a low-lying placenta due to placental migration later in pregnancy. Therefore, a repeat TVS is advised at 20–24 weeks. If the placenta appears to cover the internal os, a rescan is again recommended at 32 weeks because there is a lower chance of migration in these cases. In women with minor placenta praevia, a full assessment must be undertaken at 36 weeks to decide the mode of delivery.

❖ *Magnetic resonance imaging*: This may be required when the images obtained by ultrasound (both TAS and TVS) are unsatisfactory.

❖ *The Kleihauer test*: This should be performed in rhesus D (RhD)-negative women to estimate the amount of foetomaternal haemorrhage in order to measure the dose of anti-D immunoglobulin (anti-D Ig) required.

Foetal Investigation

Cardiotocography: Cardiotocography is usually performed for assessing the foetal heart rate in women presenting with APH, once the mother is stabilised or resuscitation has begun, to help reach a decision regarding the mode of delivery. Ultrasound should be carried out to establish foetal heart pulsation if foetal viability cannot be detected using external auscultation.

OBSTETRIC MANAGEMENT

Management plan in cases of severe and moderate/mild placenta praevia is described in Flow charts 25.2 and 25.3 respectively.

Antepartum Period

❖ *Referral to a hospital-maternity unit*: Women with APH presenting to a midwifery-led maternity unit, a general practitioner or to an accident and emergency (A and E) department should be assessed and stabilised if required. They must then be transferred to a maternity unit in a hospital having facilities for resuscitation

Flow chart 25.2: Management plan in a patient with severe placenta praevia (type 4 and 3)

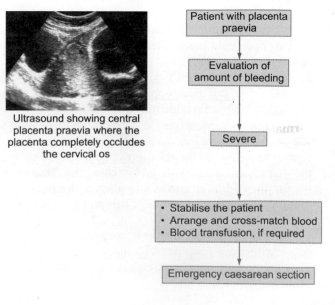

Ultrasound showing central placenta praevia where the placenta completely occludes the cervical os

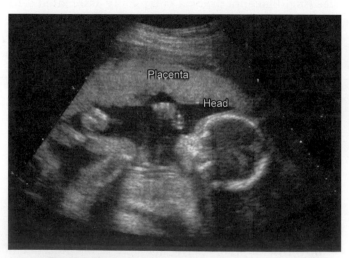

Fig. 25.2: Placental localisation on transabdominal imaging

Flow chart 25.3: Management plan in a patient with moderate/mild placenta praevia (type 2 and 1)

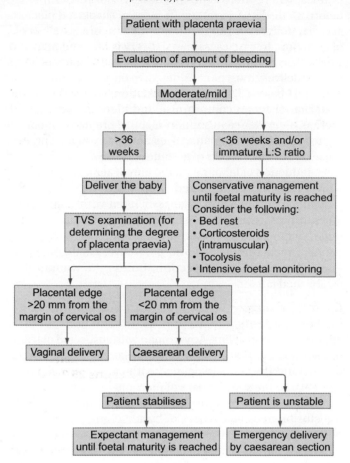

Box 25.1: Factors to be considered before making management decisions

- ☐ Degree of placenta praevia
- ☐ Period of gestation
- ☐ Presence of coexisting risk factors such as scarred uterus
- ☐ Women living in close vicinity of the hospital
- ☐ Presence of an adult at home.

each woman. Currently, there is no evidence to support recommendations regarding duration of inpatient management following APH. Women presenting with spotting, who are no longer bleeding and where placenta praevia has been excluded, can go home after a reassuring initial clinical assessment. All women with APH having bleeding heavier than spotting and those with ongoing bleeding should remain in hospital at least until the bleeding has stopped. For women who have had bleeding, most obstetricians recommend inpatient management from 32 weeks to 34 weeks with a few exceptions, e.g. women with a minor degree of placenta praevia. RCOG recommends inpatient management for women with a major degree placenta praevia who have experienced bleeding from 34 weeks onwards.[13] Various factors to be considered before making management decisions are enlisted in Box 25.1. Such decisions should be preferably made after consultation of the senior obstetrician with the woman and her partner. Discharge from the hospital should be based on availability of a telephone consultation between the woman and the hospital the next day following discharge. Before discharging them home, it is the duty of clinician to make certain they have safety precautions in place. Not only they should have a readily available access to the hospital, there should be an adult available at home to help them in case the need arises. The woman being managed at home should be adequately counselled that she should attend the antenatal clinic immediately in case she experiences any bleeding, contractions or pain.

❖ *Prophylaxis against venous thromboembolism for inpatients*: Prolonged immobility during the inpatient care can be associated with an increased risk of thromboembolism. Therefore, such patients should be encouraged to follow some amount of mobility along with the use of thromboembolic deterrent stockings and maintenance of adequate hydration. The use of anticoagulation in women for thromboprophylaxis is best limited to women at a high risk of thromboembolism.[14]

❖ *Management of patients with severe bleeding*: In case of severe bleeding, the most important step in management is to stabilise the patient; arrange and cross-match at least four units of blood and start blood transfusion, if required. All efforts must be made to shift her to the operating theatre as soon as possible for an emergency caesarean delivery.

❖ *Management of patients with mild-moderate bleeding*: If the period of gestation is between 32 to 36 weeks in patients with mild-moderate bleeding, assessment of foetal lung maturity needs to be done using the L:S ratio. The L:S ratio of greater than or equal to 2 indicates

(such as anaesthetic support and resources for blood transfusion) and performing emergency operative delivery.

❖ *Multidisciplinary care*: Clinical assessment should be preferably provided by a multidisciplinary team comprising of midwifery and obstetric staff, with immediate access to laboratory, operation theatre, neonatal and anaesthetic services.

❖ *Immediate clinical assessment*: A patient presenting with a probable history of APH must undergo clinical assessment on an urgent basis. The role of clinical assessment in women presenting with APH is to establish whether urgent intervention is required to manage maternal or foetal compromise. An assessment of the extent of vaginal bleeding must also be done. In case the cardiovascular condition of the mother and foetal well-being are within normal limits, and bleeding is within control, a detailed history must be taken to assess maternal symptoms such as pain, bleeding, etc. In case of women presenting with a major or massive haemorrhage, or maternal and/or foetal compromise, resuscitation must be started immediately. The mother is the priority in these situations and should be stabilised prior to establishing the foetal condition.

❖ *Duration of hospitalisation*: Each woman must be assessed on an individual basis and sound clinical judgement must be applied based on the individual history of foetal lung maturity, implying that the foetus can be delivered in these cases. If L:S ratio is less than 2, the foetal lungs have yet not attained maturity. In these cases, expectant management comprising of complete bed rest, intramuscular corticosteroid injection, intensive foetal monitoring and use of tocolytic agents to prevent uterine activity, can be undertaken if the patient remains stable for next 24–48 hours.

❖ All Rh-negative women with placenta praevia who bleed must be offered anti-D immunoglobulin injections in order to prevent the risk of Rh isoimmunisation.

Intrapartum Care

Prior to delivery, the obstetrician must have a detailed discussion with the woman having placenta praevia and her partner. This should include provision of information related to the condition, a discussion regarding mode and timing of delivery, indications for blood transfusion and a requirement of hysterectomy if indicated. Any queries or refusals for treatment should be dealt with effectively and clearly documented on the patient's notes.

Mode of delivery: The mode of delivery should be based on clinical judgement supplemented by sonographic information. Caesarean delivery is necessary for most cases of placenta praevia, especially the major degree placenta praevia including Type II (posterior), Type III and Type IV. Indications for immediate delivery by an emergency caesarean section irrespective of the period of gestation or type of placenta praevia are listed in Box 25.2. In case of foetal death, vaginal birth is the recommended mode of delivery for most women (provided the maternal condition is satisfactory). However, caesarean birth may still be required in some cases. In women with minor placenta praevia, an ultrasound assessment must be undertaken at 36 weeks of gestation to decide the mode of delivery. If the placenta is anterior, a vaginal delivery is undertaken when the distance of placenta from the internal os is greater than 2 cm. On the other hand, a woman with a placental edge less than 2 cm from the internal os in the third trimester is likely to require delivery by caesarean section, especially if the placenta is thick.[15,16] If placenta is posterior, the critical distance is considered to be 3 cm. Thickness of placental edge is also important because a thin leading edge is more favourable for vaginal delivery.

Timing of delivery: The optimum timing for delivery of women presenting with unexplained APH and no associated maternal and/or foetal compromise is not established. A senior obstetrician should be involved in determining the timing and mode of birth of these women. According to RCOG,

elective delivery by caesarean section in women with placenta praevia, where there is no bleeding, is not recommended before 37 weeks of gestation. In cases of suspected placenta accreta, delivery is not recommended before 36–37 weeks of gestation. In case caesarean delivery is planned before 37 weeks of gestation, administration of corticosteroids 48 hours prior to delivery must be considered. In the women presenting with APH before 37[+0] weeks of gestation, where there is no maternal or foetal compromise and bleeding has settled, there is no evidence to support elective premature delivery of the foetus. If the woman with established placenta praevia presents after 37[+0] weeks of gestation, in the event of a minor APH, induction of labour with the aim of achieving a vaginal delivery should be considered.

Antepartum haemorrhage associated with maternal or foetal compromise is an obstetric emergency. Such women must be immediately delivered. Stabilisation of the maternal condition remains the first priority. Delivery in this situation is usually by caesarean section, unless the woman is in established labour.

Consent for surgery: Before undertaking caesarean delivery in these patients, it is important to take consent after appropriate counselling. Any woman with suspected placenta praevia accreta giving consent for caesarean section should understand the risks associated with caesarean section in general and the specific risks of placenta praevia in terms of massive obstetric haemorrhage, the requirement for blood transfusion and the chances of hysterectomy. A consultant obstetrician should review her in the antenatal period. The different risks and treatment options should be discussed with the patient and her partner. The plan agreed upon, should be clearly mentioned in the consent form.

Planning a caesarean delivery: The delivery should be performed or supervised by an experienced obstetrician. A consultant obstetrician must be present at the time of surgery in such patients. The most recent CEMACH has emphasised the importance of considering calling in another senior colleague(s) with superior gynaecological surgical skills early during the surgery.[17]

Prior to the caesarean delivery, it is important to rule out the possibility of placenta accreta in these patients. Presence of a previous uterine scar is typically associated with an increased risk of MAP. Placenta praevia with a MAP especially carries the risk of massive obstetric haemorrhage and a requirement for hysterectomy. Management of such patients should, therefore, be carried out in a unit with a blood bank and facilities for high dependency care. Radiological assessment with a view to catheterisation of the internal iliac or uterine vessels (with the opinion of embolisation) must be considered in cases where there is a high suspicion of placenta accreta. Discussion with a urological or surgical team may be required because bladder involvement commonly occurs in cases of MAP. There is a risk of ureteric injury with hysterectomy in these cases. To prevent this risk, placement of a ureteric stent has been suggested prior to caesarean delivery. A detailed ultrasound scan should be preferably performed prior to surgery to plot out the placental extent. This would help the surgeon

---

Box 25.2: Indications for an emergency caesarean section

- ❑ Bleeding is heavy and/or uncontrolled
- ❑ Major degree placenta praevia (Type II posterior, Type III and Type IV)
- ❑ Foetal distress
- ❑ Obstetric factors like cephalopelvic disproportion, foetal malpresentation, etc.

Box 25.3: Six elements essential for good care for suspected placenta accreta

- ❏ Planning and direct supervision of delivery by the consultant obstetrician
- ❏ Planning and direct supervision of the anaesthetic at delivery by the consultant anaesthetist
- ❏ Availability of the blood and its products
- ❏ Preoperative planning by a multidisciplinary team
- ❏ Patient consent and detailed discussion related to the use of possible interventions (e.g. hysterectomy, leaving the placenta in place, cell salvage, intervention radiology, etc.)
- ❏ Local availability of a level 2 critical care bed

Box 25.4: Factors related to technical difficulty of caesarean delivery for cases of placenta praevia

- ❏ Period of gestation
- ❏ Degree of placenta praevia
- ❏ Presence of morbidly adherent placenta
- ❏ Previous history of uterine/abdominal surgery
- ❏ Morbid obesity
- ❏ Sonographic or MRI appearance of the placenta

Box 25.5: Steps for the management of a massive haemorrhage

- ❏ Use of uterotonic agents
- ❏ Use of prostaglandin F2α, misoprostol, intramyometrial vasopressin, etc. for haemostasis
- ❏ Oversewing the individual bleeding sinuses
- ❏ Bimanual uterine compression or aortic compression
- ❏ Packing of uterine cavity and vagina with sterile gauze
- ❏ Balloon tamponade (using an inflated balloon device)
- ❏ The B-Lynch suture
- ❏ Vertical compression sutures
- ❏ Suturing an inverted lip of cervix over the bleeding placenta bed
- ❏ Uterine and internal iliac artery ligation
- ❏ Uterine artery embolisation

correlate the position of placenta in relation to the uterine incision. The care bundle (Box 25.3) for suspected placenta accreta should be applied in all cases where there is a placenta praevia, especially with the history of previous uterine scar. The haematology staff should be alerted when the caesarean is likely to involve significant haemorrhage. Appropriate amount of blood must be kept cross-matched in advance.

Techniques of surgery: The choice of skin and uterine incision during caesarean delivery must be based on the surgeon's discretion so as to avoid the placenta as far as possible based on its location. A low transverse skin incision is usually preferred because it allows access to the lower half of the uterus. This incision also proves to be useful if the upper margin of the anterior aspect of the placenta does not rise into the upper uterine segment. In case of an anterior placenta praevia, the uterine vessels may cover the entire lower segment, and the placenta may be encountered beneath the uterine incision.

If, however, the placenta is anterior and extends towards the level of the umbilicus, a midline skin incision may be required. This would enable the surgeon to give to an incision in the upper uterine segment (classical caesarean delivery). An upper segment uterine incision may also be required in extreme cases of central placenta praevia with a potential for accreta. In these cases, the baby can be delivered through the uterine incision. Placenta can be entirely avoided and left in utero or removed by performing a planned hysterectomy. Cutting straight through the placenta in order to deliver the baby is associated with much bleeding and a high chance of hysterectomy, and therefore it should be avoided. Factors related to technical difficulty of caesarean delivery for cases of placenta praevia are listed in Box 25.4.

Delivery of the baby: The obstetrician can deliver the baby by passing his/her hand around the margins of placenta or by incising the placenta. It may be easier to deliver the baby by bringing down his/her feet and performing breech extraction rather than trying to grasp the foetal head, which is present high up past the placenta. In case the placenta has been cut, the foetal delivery must be expedited due to the risk of foetal exsanguination.

Delivery of the placenta: In cases of suspected placenta praevia accreta, if the placenta separates out on its own, it must be delivered as in normal cases and any haemorrhage that occurs needs to be dealt with in the normal way. If the placenta partially separates, the safest option in these cases is to perform a hysterectomy. Alternatively, the separated portion(s) need to be delivered and any haemorrhage that occurs needs to be dealt with in the normal way. Adherent portions can be left in place. However, blood loss in such circumstances can sometimes become large and massive, and the surgeon needs to remain vigilant in these cases. Steps for management of massive haemorrhage are enlisted in Box 25.5.

If the placenta fails to separate with the usual measures, it can be left in place and the uterus be closed. This can be followed by a hysterectomy, especially if the woman continues to bleed and has completed her family. This approach of leaving the placenta in place and performing a hysterectomy is likely to be associated with significantly reduced short-term morbidity (admission to the ICU, requirement of massive blood transfusion, coagulopathy, urological injury, relaparotomy, etc.) in comparison with the attempts to remove the placenta.[18] The approach of 'elective' hysterectomy would be unacceptable to women desiring uterine preservation. In such cases, placenta can be left in place, which gets automatically expelled out on its own.[19-24] In such cases of placental retention, the woman should be warned about the postoperative risk of bleeding and infection. Administration of prophylactic antibiotics in the immediate postpartum period may help reduce this risk. Use of neither methotrexate nor arterial embolisation reduces these risks and is therefore not recommended routinely. Such women must be followed-up using ultrasound examination and measurement of serum β-human chorionic gonadotropin levels.

Blood products: Blood should be readily available for use during the peripartum period. At least four units of blood should be cross-matched and available. Nevertheless, the amount of blood required needs to be individualised based on the clinical features of each individual case and the availability of the local blood bank services. Even though there is no evidence to support the use of autologous blood transfusion for cases with placenta praevia, cell salvage may be considered in women at high risk of massive haemorrhage and in women who refuse to receive donor blood.[25]

❖ *Foetal monitoring*: Continuous electronic foetal monitoring may be required in the following cases:
   • Women in labour with active vaginal bleeding
   • Women who are in preterm labour whose pregnancies have been complicated by major APH or recurrent minor APH
   • Women with minor APH with evidence of placental insufficiency (e.g. foetal growth restriction, oligo-hydramnios, etc.)
   • There has been clinical suspicion of an abruption.

Intermittent auscultation is appropriate in women who have experienced one episode of minor APH in which there have been no subsequent concerns regarding maternal or foetal well-being.

❖ *Mode of anaesthesia*: Regional anaesthetic is recommended for operative delivery unless there is a specific contra-indication for its use (e.g. maternal cardiovascular instability, coagulopathy, etc.). In a case of APH where maternal or foetal condition is compromised and caesarean section required, a general anaesthetic should be considered. In the case of severe foetal compromise but with a stable mother, it is reasonable to employ general anaesthesia in the foetal interest to expedite rapid delivery. A consultant anaesthetist should be preferably involved in the intrapartum care of women with APH with associated compromise.

❖ *Management of the third stage of labour*: The clinician must particularly remain vigilant regarding the occurrence of PPH in women who have experienced APH. Active management of the third stage of labour is strongly recommended in women with APH due to placental abruption or placenta praevia. Consideration should be given to the use of ergometrine-oxytocin (Syntometrine®) for managing the third stage of labour in such women in the absence of hypertension.

❖ *Administration of anti-D immune globulins*: All non-sensitised RhD-negative women with APH should be administered anti-D immune globulins following any episode of bleeding, irrespective of whether routine antenatal prophylactic anti-D had been administered or not.

   In the event of recurrent vaginal bleeding after 20[+0] weeks of gestation in the non-sensitised RhD-negative woman, anti-D Ig in the dosage of 500 IU should be given at a minimum of 6 weekly intervals. This should be followed by a test to identify foetomaternal haemorrhage greater than 4 mL red blood cells. Additional dose of anti-D immune globulins should be administered if required.

❖ *Antenatal corticosteroids*: Clinicians should offer a single course of antenatal corticosteroids to women at the risk of preterm birth between 24[+0] and 34[+6] weeks of gestation. Antenatal corticosteroids are associated with a significant reduction in rates of neonatal death, respiratory distress syndrome and intraventricular haemorrhage.

❖ *Tocolytic therapy*: A senior obstetrician should make any decision regarding the initiation of tocolysis in the cases of APH. Women most likely to benefit from use of a tocolytic drug are those requiring expectant management, e.g. preterm patients, where L:S ratio is less than 2, those requiring transfer to a hospital that can provide NICU, those who have not yet completed a full course of corticosteroids, etc. Tocolysis should not be used to delay delivery in a woman presenting with a major APH, haemodynamically unstable women, or if there is evidence of foetal compromise. Towers et al. have reported no adverse maternal or foetal effects related to tocolysis.[26] However, a prospective randomised trial is required to determine if the use of tocolytics is associated with any benefits. The tocolytic drug of choice in a woman with a history of APH should have fewest maternal cardiovascular side effects. The calcium antagonist nifedipine has been associated with cases of maternal hypotension and is therefore best avoided.[27] When the use of tocolysis is considered, agents other than β-agonists must be considered due to the risk of cardiovascular side effects. An oxytocin antagonist can be probably considered as the first choice due to the lack of cardiovascular side effects.

COMPLICATIONS

Maternal

❖ *Bleeding*: The bleeding can be heavy enough to cause maternal shock or even death.

❖ *Invasive placenta, morbidly adherent placenta*: Pathological adherence of the placenta is termed as invasive placenta or MAP. In this condition, the trophoblastic invasion occurs beyond the normal boundary established by the Nitabuch's fibrinoid layer. While the term 'accreta' refers to abnormal attachment of the placenta to the uterine surface, the terms 'increta' and 'percreta' refer to much deeper invasion of the placental villi into the uterine musculature (Fig. 25.3).

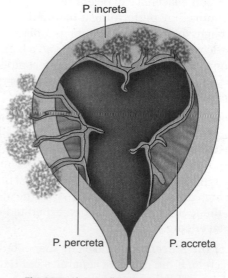

Fig. 25.3: Abnormally adherent placenta
Abbreviation: P, placenta

Sonographic imaging in the antenatal period along with the use of MRI can help distinguish women at special risk of placenta accreta (Figs 25.4 to 25.6). Table 25.1 describes the criteria for diagnosis of placenta accreta.[28]

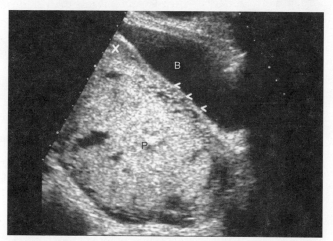

Fig. 25.4: Abdominal sonography at 27 weeks' gestation showing a morbidly adhering placenta
Abbreviations: B, bladder; P, placenta

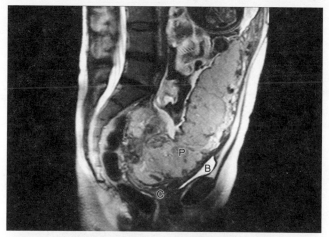

Fig. 25.5: Magnetic resonance imaging of the patient with placenta percreta at 27 weeks of gestation
Abbreviations: P, placenta; C, cervix; B, bladder

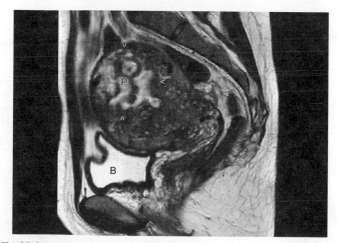

Fig. 25.6: Magnetic resonance imaging of placenta increta at 10 days postpartum
Abbreviations: P, placenta; B, bladder

Table 25.1: Criteria for the diagnosis of placenta accreta[28]

Ultrasound criteria for diagnosis		
Grey scale ultrasound	**Colour Doppler**	**Three-dimensional power Doppler**
• Loss of the retroplacental sonolucent zone • Irregular retroplacental sonolucent zone • Thinning or disruption of the hyperechoic serosa-bladder interface • Presence of focal exophytic masses invading the urinary bladder • Abnormal placental lacunae	• Diffuse or focal lacunar flow • Vascular lakes with turbulent flow (peak systolic velocity >15 cm/s) • Hypervascularity of serosa-bladder interface • Markedly dilated vessels over peripheral subplacental zone	• Numerous coherent vessels involving the whole uterine serosa-bladder junction (basal view) • Hypervascularity (lateral view) • Inseparable cotyledonal and intervillous circulations, chaotic branching, detour vessels (lateral view)
MRI features of placenta accreta		
• Uterine bulging • Heterogeneous signal intensity within the placenta • Dark intraplacental bands on T2-weighted imaging		

❖ *Anaemia and infection*: Excessive blood loss can result in anaemia and increased susceptibility to infections.
❖ Maternal shock
❖ Renal tubular necrosis
❖ Consumptive coagulopathy
❖ Postpartum haemorrhage
❖ Prolonged hospital stay
❖ Psychological sequelae
❖ Complications of blood transfusion.

Foetal

❖ *Premature birth*: Severe bleeding may force the obstetrician to proceed with an emergency preterm caesarean delivery. The babies born are often small for gestational age or growth-restricted.
❖ *Foetal death or foetal distress*: Severe maternal bleeding in cases with placenta praevia is sometimes also responsible for producing foetal distress or hypoxia.

 CLINICAL PEARLS

❖ It is considered good practice to avoid vaginal and rectal examinations in women with placenta praevia because this can sometimes provoke an episode of torrential bleeding. These women must also be advised to avoid penetrative sexual intercourse for similar reasons.
❖ Women having placenta praevia with a previous history of uterine scar are at an increased risk of developing a MAP.

EVIDENCE-BASED MEDICINE

❖ Presently, there is insufficient evidence regarding the use of cervical cerclage for preventing or reducing bleeding and prolonging pregnancy in patients with APH.[11, 29-31]

❖ Presently, there is insufficient evidence regarding the use of prophylactic tocolytics in women with placenta praevia to prevent bleeding.[11]

❖ Clinical suspicion should be expressed in all women with vaginal bleeding after 20 weeks of gestation. Though the definitive diagnosis is usually based on ultrasound imaging, signs such as a high presenting part, an abnormal lie and painless or provoked bleeding, irrespective of the results of previous ultrasound scans are more suggestive of a low-lying placenta. Clinician needs to remain vigilant in these cases.[3-8]

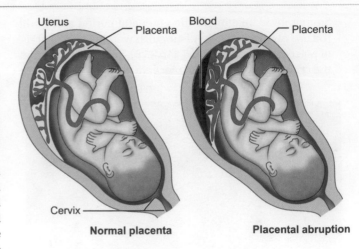

Fig. 25.7: Placental abruption and its comparison with normal placenta

PLACENTAL ABRUPTION

INTRODUCTION

Placental abruption, also known as accidental haemorrhage, can be defined as abnormal, pathological separation of the normally situated placenta from its uterine attachment. As a result, bleeding occurs from the opened sinuses present in the uterine myometrium. Clinical classification of placental abruption is described in Table 25.2.

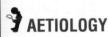

AETIOLOGY

The specific cause of placental abruption is often unknown. Separation of the normally situated placenta results in haemorrhage into decidua basalis (Fig. 25.7). A retroplacental clot develops between the placenta and the decidua basalis, which interferes with the supply of oxygen to the foetus, resulting in the development of foetal distress (Flow chart 25.4). Based on the type of clinical presentation, there can be three types of placental abruption as described next.

Flow chart 25.4: Pathophysiology of abruptio placentae

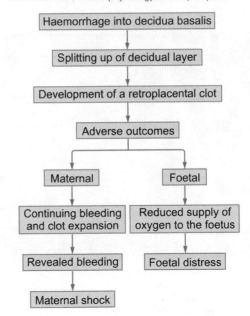

PART II

Table 25.2: Clinical classification of placental abruption

Parameters	Grade 0	Grade 1	Grade 2	Grade 3
External bleeding	Absent	Slight	Mild to moderate	Moderate to severe
Uterine tenderness	Absent	Uterus irritable, uterine tenderness may or may not be present	Uterine tenderness is usually present	Tonic uterine contractions and marked tenderness
Abdominal pain	Absent	Abdominal pain may or may not be present	Abdominal pain is usually present	Severe degree of abdominal pain may be present
Foetal heart sounds	Present	Present	Foetal distress	Foetal death
Maternal shock	Absent	Absent	Generally absent	Present
Perinatal outcome	Good	Good	May be poor	Extremely poor
Complications	Absent	Rare	May be present	Complications like disseminated intravascular coagulation and oliguria
Volume of retroplacental clot	Absent	<200 mL	150–500 mL	>500 mL

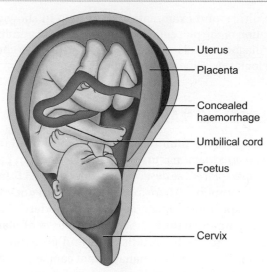

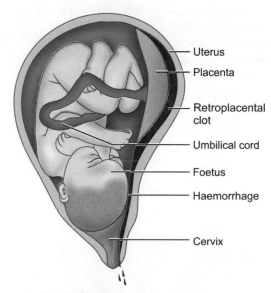

Fig. 25.8: Concealed type of placental abruption

Fig. 25.9: Revealed type of placental abruption

1. *Concealed type*: In this case, the blood loss is not visible because it collects between the foetal membranes and decidua in form of the retroplacental clot (Fig. 25.8).
2. *Revealed type*: In this type, the blood does not collect between the foetal membranes and the decidua but moves out of the cervical canal and is visible externally (Fig. 25.9).
3. *Mixed type*: This is the most common type of placental abruption and is associated with both revealed and concealed haemorrhage.

Risk Factors

Risk factors for abruptio placentae are as follows:[32-35]
- Previous history or family history of placental abruption
- Pre-eclampsia, foetal growth restriction
- Non-vertex presentations
- Polyhydramnios
- Advanced maternal age, multiparity
- Low BMI

- Pregnancy following assisted reproductive techniques
- Intrauterine infection or chorioamnionitis
- Premature rupture of membranes
- Abdominal trauma (both accidental and resulting from domestic violence)
- Smoking and drug misuse (cocaine and amphetamines) during pregnancy
- Maternal thrombophilia (especially women who are heterozygous for factor V Leiden or prothrombin gene)
- First-trimester bleeding increases the risk of abruption later in the pregnancy
- Abnormal placentation
- Rapid uterine decompression (e.g. rupture of membranes with polyhydramnios).

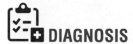 **DIAGNOSIS**

Clinical Presentation

- *Vaginal bleeding*: The most common symptom of placental abruption is dark red vaginal bleeding with pain, usually occurring after 28 weeks of gestation.
- *Abdominal pain*: Abdominal and back pain often begins suddenly.
- Uterine tenderness may be present.
- *Other symptoms*: Some women may experience slightly different symptoms including faintness and collapse, nausea, thirst, reduced foetal movements, etc.
- *Shock*: The patient may be in shock (tachycardia and low blood pressure)
- *Pre-eclampsia*: There may be signs and symptoms suggestive of pre-eclampsia.

Abdominal Examination

- Uterine hypertonicity and frequent uterine contractions are commonly present. It may be difficult to feel the foetal parts due to presence of uterine hypertonicity.
- Severe degree of placental abruption may be associated with foetal bradycardia and other foetal heart rate abnormalities. In extreme cases, foetal demise may even be detected at the time of examination.

Vaginal Examination

Although presence of placental abruption is not a contra-indication for vaginal examination, it should not ideally be performed in patients with history of APH due to the risk of placenta praevia.

Investigations

- The platelet count, if low, may indicate a consumptive process seen in relation to significant abruption; this may be associated with a coagulopathy.
- *Ultrasound examination*: Placental abruption is a clinical diagnosis and there are no sensitive or reliable diagnostic

CHAPTER 25

tests available. Ultrasound has limited sensitivity in the identification of retroplacental haemorrhage (Fig. 25.10).[36] However, when the ultrasound suggests an abruption, the likelihood that there is an abruption is high. Moreover,

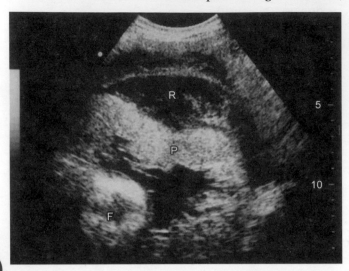

Fig. 25.10: Ultrasound examination in case of placental abruption showing presence of a retroplacental clot
Abbreviations: R, retroplacental clot; P, placenta; F, foetus

the ultrasound examination does help in showing the location of the placenta and thereby making or ruling out the diagnosis of placenta praevia. It also helps in checking the foetal viability and presentation.

OBSTETRIC MANAGEMENT

The management plan depends on grade of placental abruption and foetal maturity. Treatment plans in patients with abruptio placentae described in Flow chart 25.5. In cases with mild abruption, where foetal maturity has not yet been attained, expectant management can be undertaken until the foetus attains maturity. A moderate case of placental abruption requires hospitalisation and constant foetal monitoring. The expectant management can be continued if the mother remains stable. If at any time, maternal or foetal distress appears in these cases or the women present with severe placental abruption, the following steps need to be urgently undertaken:

❖ Urgent admission to the hospital
❖ Insertion of a central venous pressure line, IV line and a urinary catheter

Flow chart 25.5: Treatment plan for the patient with abruptio placentae

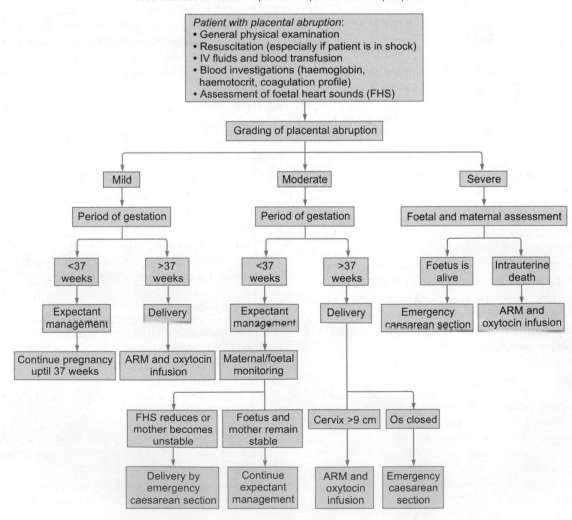

Box 25.6: Indications for emergency caesarean section in case of placental abruction

❏ Appearance of foetal distress
❏ Bleeding continues to occur or there is an abnormal progress of labour despite the artificial rupture of membranes and oxytocin infusion
❏ Foetal malpresentation
❏ Appearance of complications (disseminated intravascular coagulation, oliguria, etc.)
❏ Associated obstetric factors.

❖ Blood to be sent for ABO and Rh typing, cross-matching and CBC
❖ Blood transfusion must be started if signs of shock are present.
❖ Inspection of vaginal pads and monitoring of vitals (pulse, blood pressure, etc.) at every 15–30-minute interval depending upon the severity of bleeding needs to be done.
❖ Blood coagulation profile needs to be done at every 2 hourly interval.
❖ The placental position must be localised using an ultrasound scan.
❖ The foetal heart sounds must be monitored continuously.
❖ Intramuscular corticosteroids need to be administered to the mother in case of foetal prematurity.
❖ Definitive treatment in these cases is the delivery of the baby. In case of severe abruption, delivery should be performed by the fastest possible route. Caesarean delivery needs to be performed for most cases with severe placental abruption. Other indications for an emergency caesarean delivery are listed in Box 25.6.

COMPLICATIONS

Maternal

❖ Maternal shock due to severe bleeding.
❖ *Maternal death*: This may be due to severe bleeding, shock and DIC.
❖ *Renal failure*: Severe shock resulting from Grade 3 placental abruption and/or DIC can be responsible for the development of renal failure.
❖ *Couvelaire uterus or uteroplacental apoplexy*: This condition is characterised by massive intravasation of blood into the uterine musculature up to the level of serosa.
❖ Risk of recurrence of abruption in future pregnancies.
❖ Postpartum uterine atony and PPH.
❖ *Disseminated intravascular coagulation*: Disseminated intravascular coagulation is a syndrome associated with both thrombosis and haemorrhage. It can result in development of hypoxia, ischaemia and necrosis, which ultimately results in end-stage organ damage, especially renal and hepatic failure.

The pathophysiology of DIC is shown in Flow chart 25.6. In DIC, initially there is activation of the coagulation pathways,

both intrinsic and extrinsic, due to thromboplastin released from the decidual fragments and placental separation. As the process of coagulation continues, it results in consumption of various clotting factors and widespread deposition of fibrin. This can result in development of hypoxia, ischaemia and necrosis, which ultimately results in end-stage organ damage, especially renal and hepatic failure. This consumptive coagulopathy and activation of the fibrinolytic system results in development of hypofibrinogenaemia (<150 mg/dL); elevation in the levels of fibrin degradation products (FDPs); increased levels of D-dimers; and variable decrease in the levels of various coagulation factors and platelets. As a result of consumptive coagulopathy and activation of fibrinolytic system, bleeding takes place. Massive bleeding and end stage organ failure in patients with DIC is ultimately responsible for producing death.

Clinical presentation: Most common sign of DIC is bleeding. It can be manifested in form of ecchymosis, petechiae and purpura. There can be oozing or frank bleeding from multiple sites. Extremities may become cool and mottled. Pleural and pericardial involvement may be responsible for producing dyspnoea and chest pain respectively. Haematuria is commonly produced. Bleeding and renal failure are the most important manifestations in cases with DIC.

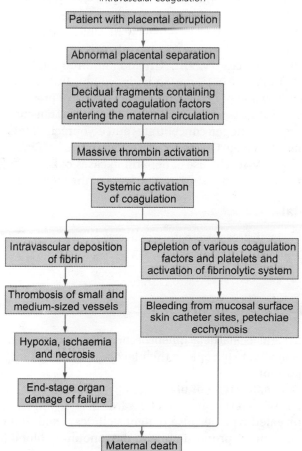

Flow chart 25.6: Pathophysiology of disseminated intravascular coagulation

Table 25.3: Abnormal results of coagulation profile in cases of disseminated intravascular coagulation

Test	Normal	Disseminated intravascular coagulation
Fibrinogen	150–600 mg/dL	Reduced (<150 mg/dL)
Prothrombin time	11–16 seconds	Prolonged
APTT	22–37 seconds	Prolonged
TT	15–25 seconds	Prolonged
Platelet count	1.2–1.5 lakh/mm³	Reduced
D-dimer	<0.5 mg/L	Increased (>0.5 mg/L)
FDP	<10 µg/dL	Increased (>10 µg/dL)

Diagnosis: In the cases of DIC, coagulation profile is mainly affected. Abnormal results of various tests in coagulation profile in patients with DIC are shown in Table 25.3. Fibrinogen levels are reduced; prothrombin time, APTT and thrombin time are prolonged; platelet levels are reduced and levels of D-dimer and FDPs are increased. The findings on peripheral smear in patients with DIC are suggestive of microangiopathic haemolytic anaemia. The peripheral smear shows presence of multiple helmet cells, fragmented red blood cells, microspherocytes and schistocytes and paucity of platelet cells.

Treatment of disseminated intravascular coagulation: Treatment of DIC mainly involves the treatment of the underlying cause. Platelets can be transfused in patients at high risk of bleeding, e.g. those who need to undergo surgery. Replacement therapy with fresh frozen plasma (FFP) may also be administered. FFP is usually administered to maintain fibrinogen levels above 150 mg/dL. FFP usually contains the clotting factors V, VIII, XIII and antithrombin III. Usual dose of FFP is 10–15 mg/kg body weight. Indications for administration of FFP include prolongation of prothrombin time and fibrinogen levels less than 50 mg/dL. Transfusion of platelets, fibrinogen concentrates and cryoprecipitate is also sometimes given. Cryoprecipitate is composed of fibrinogen and factor VIII. The use of heparin in cases of DIC is largely controversial and is supposed to worsen the bleeding.

Foetal

❖ Foetal distress, premature delivery
❖ Stillbirth and foetal death.

CLINICAL PEARLS

❖ Once placental detachment occurs, presently, no treatment is available to replace the placenta back to its original position.
❖ Concealed type of placental abruption carries higher risk of maternal and foetal hazards in comparison to the revealed type because patient's clinical condition may often be disproportionate to the amount of blood loss, especially in cases of concealed haemorrhage.

EVIDENCE-BASED MEDICINE

❖ According to the RCOG Green-top Guideline No. 1b, tocolytic therapy is contraindicated in patients with placental abruption.[37]
❖ Large abruptions may be associated with a high risk of DIC and require a multidisciplinary approach to optimize care.[38]

VASA PRAEVIA

INTRODUCTION

Vasa praevia is an uncommon obstetric complication, which may be associated with a high risk of foetal demise if it is not recognised before rupture of membranes. In vasa praevia, umbilical vessels traverse the membranes in the lower uterine segment in front of the foetal presenting part. Neither the umbilical cord nor the placenta supports the vessels. Due to the absence of Wharton's jelly, the vessels may be easily lacerated at the time the membranes rupture. Also during uterine contractions, foetal vessels can get compressed, resulting in foetal hypoxia and death. The reported incidence of the condition varies between 1 in 2,000 to 1 in 6,000 pregnancies.[39] However, the condition is often under-reported in the literature.

AETIOLOGY

Some risk factors for vasa praevia include the following:
❖ Bilobed and succenturiate lobes of placentas (where the foetal vessels run through the membranes joining the separate lobes together)
❖ Low-lying placentas
❖ Multiple pregnancies
❖ Marginal insertion of the cord
❖ Velamentous insertion of the cord.

DIAGNOSIS

Clinical Presentation

❖ Patients with vasa praevia present with painless, fresh vaginal bleeding at the time of spontaneous rupture of membranes or amniotomy. Since the bleeding occurs from foetal vessels, foetal shock or demise can occur rapidly. The blood is from the foetal circulation and therefore, the foetus can bleed to death.
❖ Foetal heart rate abnormalities such as decelerations, bradycardia, a sinusoidal trace or foetal demise.[40]
❖ *Antepartum period*: During the antenatal period, in the absence of vaginal bleeding, there is no method to diagnose vasa praevia clinically.

PART II

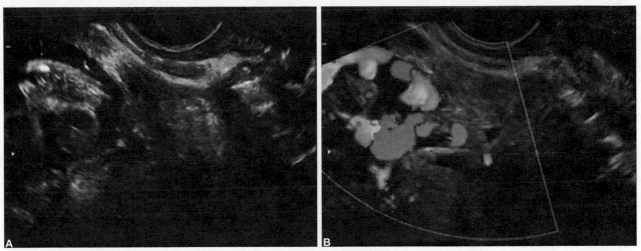

Figs 25.11A and B: Diagnosis of vasa praevia. (A) Transvaginal ultrasound; (B) Doppler ultrasound showing presence of foetal blood vessels in front of the foetal presenting part *(For colour version, see Plate 2)*

❖ *Intrapartum period*: During the intrapartum period, in the absence of vaginal bleeding, vasa praevia can occasionally be diagnosed at the time of vaginal examination by clinically palpating the foetal vessels in the membranes once cervix starts dilating. This can be confirmed by direct visualisation using an amnioscope.

Investigations

❖ Diagnosis of vasa praevia can be made by TVS examination, particularly Doppler ultrasound (Figs 25.11A and B).
❖ The presence of foetal blood can be confirmed by performing the Apt test. In this test, one drop of blood is added to 9 drops of 1% sodium hydroxide in a glass test tube. The colour of the test tube must be checked after 1 minute. If the blood is of foetal origin, the mixture remains pink. However, if the blood is of maternal origin, the mixture turns brown in colour.
❖ In order to differentiate between foetal and maternal bleeding, Lindqvist and Gren[41] have recently described a much simpler bedside test. In this test, 0.14 M sodium hydroxide solution is used which denatures adult haemoglobin, turning it a brownish green colour. On the other hand, foetal haemoglobin is resistant to denaturation and retains its red colour.

MANAGEMENT

❖ Vasa praevia is an important cause for foetal mortality. The most important step for reducing blood loss from vasa praevia is its prenatal diagnosis.
❖ Foetal well-being should be confirmed at the time of any antepartum or intrapartum haemorrhage. This is best achieved through electronic foetal monitoring using the cardiotocograph.
❖ Since the foetal blood volume is around 80–100 mL/kg, the loss of relatively small amount of blood can have major implications for the foetus. Therefore, rapid delivery and aggressive resuscitation including the use of blood transfusion if required are essential.

❖ Presently, there is no definite recommendation regarding the optimal time of delivery in these women. The patient is usually hospitalised at 30–32 weeks and is posted for an elective caesarean delivery at 35–36 weeks' gestation without confirmation of lung maturity by amniocentesis. This strategy helps in reducing the risk related to rupture of membranes before the onset of labour, which may occur in nearly 10% cases and is associated with a high mortality rate.
❖ When the patient with vasa praevia presents for the first time in labour, if the cervix is almost fully dilated, the foetus can be delivered vaginally. If cervix is not completely dilated, an emergency caesarean section must be performed to save the foetus.

COMPLICATIONS

Unlike placenta praevia, vasa praevia carries no major maternal risk but is associated with significant risk to the foetus. When the foetal membranes are ruptured, either spontaneously or artificially, the unprotected foetal vessels are at risk of disruption with consequent foetal haemorrhage and high foetal mortality rates.

CLINICAL PEARLS

❖ Cases of vasa praevia identified in the second trimester should undergo a repeated imaging in the third trimester to confirm its persistence.
❖ Confirmed cases of vasa praevia in the third trimester must be preferably admitted to the hospital unit with appropriate neonatal facilities between 28 to 32 weeks of gestation. This would facilitate quicker intervention in the event of bleeding or labour.
❖ Laser ablation in utero may have a role in the treatment of vasa praevia in future.[42]

CHAPTER 25

EVIDENCE-BASED MEDICINE

❖ If signs of acute foetal compromise are present, delivery should be achieved as soon as possible, usually by caesarean section, to minimise the risk of foetal exsanguination.[43]

❖ In view of the increased risk of preterm delivery, corticosteroids must be administered for accelerating the foetal lung maturity.[44]

REFERENCES

1. Calleja-Agius J, Custo R, Brincat MP, Calleja N. Placental abruption and placenta praevia. Eur Clin Obstet Gynaecol. 2006;2(3):121-7.

2. Cantwell R, Clutton-Brock T, Cooper G, Dawson A, Drife J, Garrod D, et al. Saving Mothers' Lives: Reviewing maternal deaths to make motherhood safer, 2006–08. The Eighth Report of the Confidential Enquiries into Maternal Deaths in the United Kingdom. BJOG. 2011;118:1-203.

3. Parazzini F, Dindelli M, Luchini L, La Rosa M, Potenza MT, Frigerio L, et al. Risk factors for placenta praevia. Placenta. 1994;15(3):321-6.

4. Sheiner E, Shoham-Vardi I, Hallak M, Hershkowitz R, Katz M, Mazor M. Placenta previa: obstetric risk factors and pregnancy outcome. J Matern Fetal Med. 2001;10(6):414-9.

5. Faiz AS, Ananth CV. Etiology and risk factors for placenta previa: an overview and meta-analysis of observational studies. J Matern Fetal Neonatal Med. 2003;13(3):175-90.

6. Healy DL, Breheny S, Halliday J, Jaques A, Rushford D, Garrett C, et al. Prevalence and risk factors for obstetric haemorrhage in 6730 singleton births after assisted reproductive technology in Victoria Australia. Hum Reprod. 2010;25(1): 265-74.

7. Yang Q, Wen SW, Phillips K, Oppenheimer L, Black D, Walker MC. Comparison of maternal risk factors between placental abruption and placenta previa. Am J Perinatol. 2009;26(4):279-86.

8. Rasmussen S, Albrechtsen S, Dalaker K. Obstetric history and the risk of placenta previa. Acta Obstet Gynecol Scand. 2000;79(6):502-7.

9. Ananth CV, Smulian JC, Vintzileos AM. The association of placenta previa with history of cesarean delivery and abortion: a meta-analysis. Am J Obstet Gynecol. 1997;177(5):1071-8.

10. Hendricks MS, Chow YH, Bhagavath B, Singh K. Previous cesarean section and abortion as risk factors for developing placenta previa. J Obstet Gynaecol Res. 1999;25(2):137-42.

11. Royal College of Obstetricians and Gynaecologists. Placenta praevia, placenta praevia accreta and vasa praevia: diagnosis and management. Green-top Guideline No. 27. London: RCOG; 2011.

12. Oyelese Y. Placenta previa: the evolving role of ultrasound. Ultrasound Obstet Gynecol. 2009;34(2):123-6.

13. Royal College of Obstetricians and Gynaecologists. Placenta praevia and placenta accreta: diagnosis and management. Green-top Guideline No. 27. London: RCOG; 2005.

14. Royal College of Obstetricians and Gynaecologists. (2015). Reducing the Risk of Venous Thromboembolism during Pregnancy and the Puerperium. Green-top Guideline No. 37a. [online] Available from www.rcog.org.uk/globalassets/documents/guidelines/gtg-37a.pdf. [Accessed July, 2016].

15. Oppenheimer LW, Farine D, Ritchie JW, Lewinsky RM, Telford J, Fairbanks LA. What is a low-lying placenta? Am J Obstet Gynecol. 1991;165(4 Pt 1):1036-8.

16. Bhide A, Prefumo F, Moore J, Hollis B, Thilaganathan B. Placenta edge to internal os distance in the late third trimester and mode of delivery in placenta praevia. BJOG. 2003;110(9):860-4.

17. Confidential Enquiry into Maternal and Child Health. Saving mothers' lives: reviewing maternal deaths to make motherhood safer—2003–2005. The Seventh Report of the Confidential Enquiries into Maternal Deaths in the UK. London: CEMACH; 2007.

18. Eller AG, Porter TF, Soisson P, Silver RM. Optimal management strategies for placenta accreta. BJOG. 2009;116(5):648-54.

19. Bretelle F, Courbière B, Mazouni C, Agostini A, Cravello L, Boubli L, et al. Management of placenta accreta: morbidity and outcome. Eur J Obstet Gynecol Repro Biol. 2007;133(1):34-9.

20. Chan BC, Lam HS, Yuen JH, Lam TP, Tso WK, Pun TC, et al. Conservative management of placenta praevia with accreta. Hong Kong Med J. 2008;14(6):479-84.

21. Lee PS, Bakelaar R, Fitpatrick CB, Ellestad SC, Havrilesky LJ, Alvarez Secord A. Medical and surgical treatment of placenta percreta to optimize bladder preservation. Obstet Gynecol. 2008;112 (2 Pt 2):421-4.

22. Most OL, Singer T, Buterman I, Monteagudo A, Timor-Tritsch IE. Postpartum management of placenta previa accreta left in situ: role of 3-dimensional angiography. J Ultrasound Med. 2008;27(9):1375-80.

23. Teo SB, Kanagalingam D, Tan HK, Tan LK. Massive postpartum haemorrhage after uterus-conserving surgery in placenta percreta: the danger of the partial placenta percreta. BJOG. 2008;115(6):789-92.

24. Chiang YC, Shih JC, Lee CN. Septic shock after conservative management for placenta accreta. Taiwan J Obstet Gynecol. 2006;45(1):64-6.

25. Royal College of Obstetricians and Gynaecologists. (2008). Blood transfusions in obstetrics. Green-top Guideline No. 47. [online] Available from www.rcog.org.uk/globalassets/documents/guidelines/gtg-47.pdf. [Accessed July, 2016].

26. Towers CV, Pircon RA, Heppard M. Is tocolysis safe in the management of third-trimester bleeding? Am J Obstet Gynecol. 1999;180(6 Pt 1):1572-8.

27. Khan K, Zamora J, Lamont RF, Van Geijn Hp H, Svare J, Santos-Jorge C, et al. Safety concerns for the use of calcium channel blockers in pregnancy for the treatment of spontaneous preterm labour and hypertension: a systematic review and meta-regression analysis. J Matern Fetal Neonatal Med. 2010;23(9):1030-8.

28. Warshak CR, Eskander R, Hull AD, Scioscia AL, Mattrey RF, Benirschke K, et al. Accuracy of ultrasonography and magnetic resonance imaging in the diagnosis of placenta accreta. Obstet Gynecol. 2006;108 (3 Pt 1):573-81.

29. Arias F. Cervical cerclage for the temporary treatment of patients with placenta previa. Obstet Gynecol. 1988;71(4):545-8.

30. Cobo E, Conde-Agudelo A, Delgado J, Canaval H, Congote A. Cervical cerclage: an alternative for the management of placenta praevia? Am J Obstet Gynecol. 1998;179(1):122-5.

31. Derbala Y, Grochal F, Jeanty P. Vasa previa. J Prenat Med. 2007;1(1):2-13.

32. Pariente G, Wiznitzer A, Sergienko R, Mazor M, Holcberg G, Sheiner E. Placental abruption: critical analysis of risk factors and perinatal outcomes. J Matern Fetal Neonatal Med. 2010;24(5):698-702.

33. Rasmussen S, Irgens LM. Occurrence of placental abruption in relatives. BJOG. 2009;116(5):693-9.

34. Tikkanen M. Etiology, clinical manifestations, and prediction of placental abruption. Acta Obstet Gynecol Scand. 2010;89(6): 732-40.

35. Kennare R, Heard A, Chan A. Substance use during pregnancy: risk factors and obstetric and perinatal outcomes in South Australia. Aust N Z J Obstet Gynaecol. 2005;45(3):220-5.

36. Glantz C, Purnell L. Clinical utility of sonography in the diagnosis and treatment of placental abruption. J Ultrasound Med. 2002;21(8):837-40.

37. Royal College of Obstetricians and Gynaecologists. Tocolytic drugs for women in preterm labour. Green-top Guideline No. 1B. London: RCOG; 2011.

38. Sher G, Statland BE. Abruptio placentae with coagulopathy: a rational basis for management. Clin Obstet Gynecol. 1985;28(1):15-23.

39. Catanzarite V, Maida C, Thomas W, Mendoza A, Stanco L, Piacquadio KM. Prenatal sonographic diagnosis of vasa previa: ultrasound findings and obstetric outcome in ten cases. Ultrasound Obstet Gynecol. 2001;18(2):109-15.

40. Oleyese KO, Turner M, Lees C, Campbell S. Vasa previa: an avoidable obstetric tragedy. Obstet Gynecol Surv. 1999;54(2): 138-45.

41. Lindqvist PG, Gren P. An easy-to-use method for detecting fetal hemoglobin—a test to identify bleeding from vasa previa. Eur J Obstet Gynecol Reprod Biol. 2007;131(2):151-3.

42. Quintero RA, Kontopoulos EV, Bornick PW, Allen MH. In utero laser treatment of type II vasa previa. J Matern Fetal Neonatal Med. 2007;20(12):847-51.

43. National Institute for Clinical Excellence. (2011). Clinical Guideline 132: Caesarean section. [online] Available from www.nice.org.uk/guidance/cg132/resources/caesarean-section-35109507009733. [Accessed July, 2016].

44. Royal College of Obstetricians and Gynaecologists. Green-top Guideline No.7: Antenatal corticosteroids to reduce neonatal morbidity and mortality. London: RCOG; 2010.

CHAPTER 25

Rhesus Isoimmunisation

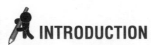 INTRODUCTION

Rhesus (Rh) blood group classification system is the most important blood group system after the ABO blood group system. Although the Rh system contains five main antigens (C, c, D, E and e), antigen D is considered to be the most immunogenic. According to the Rh classification, the blood groups can be classified as Rh positive (those having D antigen) and Rh negative (those not having D antigen).

AETIOLOGY

Rhesus incompatibility occurs due to difference in blood groups between the mother and foetus. It may develop when a woman with Rh-negative blood marries a man with Rh-positive blood and conceives a foetus with Rh-positive blood group (who has inherited Rh factor gene from the father). Rh-positive foetal RBCs from the foetus leak across the placenta and enter the woman's circulation. Throughout the pregnancy, small amounts of foetal blood can enter the maternal circulation (foetomaternal haemorrhage or FMH), with the greatest transfer occurring at the time of delivery or during the third trimester. This transfer stimulates maternal antibody production against the Rh factor, which is called isoimmunisation. The process of sensitisation has no adverse health effects for the mother. During the time of first Rh-positive pregnancy, the production of maternal anti-Rh antibodies is relatively slow and usually does not affect that pregnancy. Therefore, Rh incompatibility is not a factor in the first pregnancy, because few foetal blood cells reach the mother's bloodstream until delivery. The antibodies that form after delivery cannot affect the first child. However, if the mother is exposed to the RhD antigens during subsequent pregnancies, the immune response is quicker and much greater. The anti-D antibodies produced by the mother can cross the placenta and bind to RhD antigen on the surface of foetal RBCs, causing lysis of the foetal RBCs, resulting in development of haemolytic anaemia. Severe anaemia can lead to foetal heart failure, fluid retention, hydrops and intrauterine death. The whole pathogenesis of Rh isoimmunisation is summarised in Flow chart 26.1.

In the UK, the most important cause of anti-D antibodies is immunisation during pregnancy where there has been no explicit sensitising event. Late immunisation, during the third trimester of first pregnancy, is responsible for 18–27% of cases. Immunisation during a second or subsequent pregnancy probably accounts for a similar proportion of cases.[1]

DIAGNOSIS

Clinical Presentation

Clinical manifestations in the neonate can include the following:
❖ Hydrops foetalis, icterus gravis neonatorum and congenital anaemia of the newborn
❖ Haemolysis often results in hyperbilirubinaemia, which may cause kernicterus.

Investigations

❖ Blood grouping (both ABO and Rh)
❖ *Coomb's test*: Alloimmunisation can be defined as the development of antibodies in the mother against the D antigen present on the surface of foetal RBCs. Whether or not the woman has developed antibodies against the foetal RBCs can be assessed with the help of indirect Coomb's test (ICT). The maternal antibody screen in order to detect the presence of the antibodies needs to be carried out at 28 weeks of gestation. ICT aims at measuring the presence of antibodies, which are present unbound in the maternal serum. In the ICT, RhD-positive RBCs are incubated with maternal serum. Any anti-RhD antibody present in the serum will adhere to the RBCs. The RBCs are then washed and suspended in serum containing antihuman globulin

Flow chart 26.1: Pathogenesis of Rh isoimmunisation

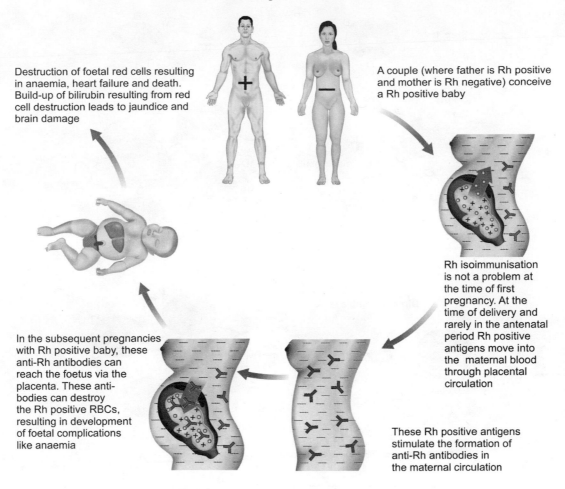

Destruction of foetal red cells resulting in anaemia, heart failure and death. Build-up of bilirubin resulting from red cell destruction leads to jaundice and brain damage

A couple (where father is Rh positive and mother is Rh negative) conceive a Rh positive baby

Rh isoimmunisation is not a problem at the time of first pregnancy. At the time of delivery and rarely in the antenatal period Rh positive antigens move into the maternal blood through placental circulation

In the subsequent pregnancies with Rh positive baby, these anti-Rh antibodies can reach the foetus via the placenta. These antibodies can destroy the Rh positive RBCs, resulting in development of foetal complications like anaemia

These Rh positive antigens stimulate the formation of anti-Rh antibodies in the maternal circulation

(Coomb's serum). Red cells coated with maternal anti-RhD will be agglutinated by the antihuman globulin (positive ICT; Fig. 26.1A).

The direct Coomb's test, on the other hand, aims at detecting the antibodies that are bound to the surface of foetal RBCs. This test is done after birth to detect the presence of maternal antibody on the neonatal RBCs. In the direct Coomb's test, the infant's RBCs are placed in Coomb's serum. If the cells are agglutinated, this indicates the presence of maternal antibody (Fig. 26.1B).

❖ *Kleihauer-Betke test*: This is a blood test for measuring the amount of foetal haemoglobin transferred from the foetal bloodstream to that of the mother due to FMH. This test for quantifying the amount of FMH is recommended in the UK. Approximately 99% of women are likely to have an FMH of less than 4 mL at delivery. A large FMH (>4 mL) is likely to occur in situations tabulated in Box 26.1.

According to the recommendations by the RCOG (2011)[2] and British Committee for Standards in Haematology (BCSH, 2014),[3] an anticoagulated blood sample should be obtained as soon as possible (preferably within 2 hours of birth) from the mother and a Kleihauer screening test must be performed on it. This would help identify the

RhD-negative women with a large FMH who may require an additional dose of anti-D immunoglobulin (Ig).

In some European countries (except the countries such as UK, France and Ireland), a standard postnatal dose of 1,000–1,500 IU anti-D Ig is administered to the mother with no requirement for a routine Kleihauer test.[4] However, this policy is likely to miss approximately 0.3% of women who have an FMH greater than 15 mL. This much amount of haemorrhage is unlikely to be neutralised by the standard dose of 1,500 IU of anti-D Ig. In cases where there is no facility to perform Kleihauer testing to quantify the FMH at delivery, it is reasonable to administer a standard postnatal dose of 1,500 IU anti-D Ig.

Flow cytometry serves as an alternative technique for quantifying the size of FMH.[5] Flow cytometry in comparison to the Kleihauer test is more accurate and reproducible making it particularly helpful in women with high levels of foetal haemoglobin. It is probably best used in cases where a Kleihauer screening test indicates a large FMH, requiring accurate quantitation and follow-up. The rosetting technique is another relatively simple, alternative, serological method, which helps in quantifying FMH of RhD-positive red cells greater than 4 mL.

Indirect Coomb's test

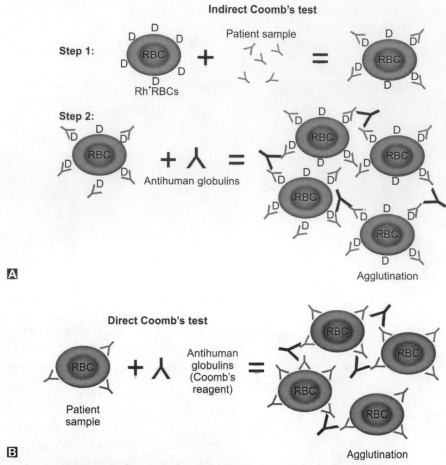

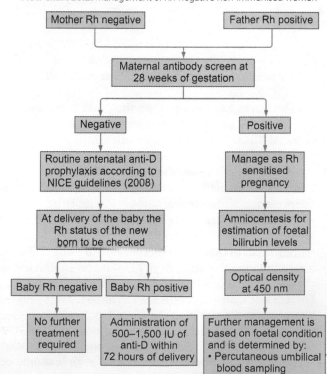

Figs 26.1A and B: Coomb's test. (A) Indirect Coomb's test; (B) Direct Coomb's test

Box 26.1: Situations likely to be associated with a large foetomaternal haemorrhage

❏ Traumatic deliveries including caesarean section and assisted vaginal delivery
❏ Manual removal of the placenta
❏ Stillbirths and foetal deaths
❏ Abdominal trauma during the third trimester
❏ Multiple pregnancy (during the intrapartum period)
❏ Unexplained hydrops foetalis

 MANAGEMENT

Antenatal Period

The Rh-negative women whose husbands are Rh positive can be divided into two groups: (1) Rh-negative non-immunised women and (2) the Rh-negative immunised women.

Rh-negative Non-immunised Women

Management of Rh-negative non-immunised women is summarised in the Flow chart 26.2. As per the recommendations by the BCSH guidelines, a sample should be taken for the routine antenatal 28-week blood group and antibody screen (ICT).[3] According to the recommendations by the NICE (2002–2008), all D-negative pregnant women who

Flow chart 26.2: Management of Rh-negative non-immunised women

Mother Rh negative → Father Rh positive

↓

Maternal antibody screen at 28 weeks of gestation

↓ Negative | ↓ Positive

Negative:
Routine antenatal anti-D prophylaxis according to NICE guidelines (2008)
↓
At delivery of the baby the Rh status of the new born to be checked
↓
Baby Rh negative | Baby Rh positive
↓ | ↓
No further treatment required | Administration of 500–1,500 IU of anti-D within 72 hours of delivery

Positive:
Manage as Rh sensitised pregnancy
↓
Amniocentesis for estimation of foetal bilirubin levels
↓
Optical density at 450 nm
↓
Further management is based on foetal condition and is determined by:
• Percutaneous umbilical blood sampling
• Amniotic fluid analysis
• Dopper ultrasound of middle cerebral artery

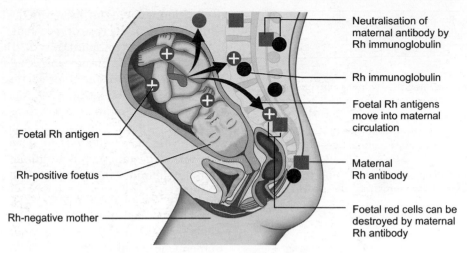

Fig. 26.2: Mechanism of action of anti-D immunoglobulins

do not have immune anti-D, should be offered additional routine antenatal anti-D Ig prophylaxis (RAADP) (Fig. 26.2) during the third trimester of pregnancy (typically 28 weeks of gestation).[6,7] If anti-D is identified in this sample, further investigations should be undertaken to determine whether this is immune or passive (i.e. previous administration of anti-D Ig). Passive anti-D can be detected for up to 8 weeks following administration of anti-D Ig and the levels of passive anti-D are generally less than or equal to 1 IU/mL.

After delivery of the baby, the Rh status of the newborn is to be checked. If the baby is Rh positive, 500 IU of anti-D immunoglobulins must be administered within 72 hours of delivery. In case the maternal antibody screen turns out to be positive, the woman must be further managed as Rh-sensitised pregnancy.

The woman's eligibility for second dose of anti-D Ig needs to be determined at the time of the delivery of the baby (Box 26.2).

Administration of anti-D IgG

Anti-D Ig preparations licensed for use in the UK: Various anti-D Ig preparations, which are licensed for use in the UK, are enumerated in Table 26.1.[6]

Dose of anti-D Ig, which should be administered: An IM dose of 500 IU of anti-D Ig is likely to neutralise an FMH of up to 4 mL. For each millilitre of FMH In excess of 4 mL, a further 125 μg of anti-D Ig is required. Minimum recommended dose of anti-D Ig at less than 20^{+0} weeks of gestation is 250 IU and at more than 20^{+0} weeks of gestation is 500 IU.

Mode of administration of anti-D Ig: For successful immuno-prophylaxis, anti-D Ig should be administered as soon as possible after the potentially sensitising event, preferably within 72 hours. If it is not possible to administer anti-D Ig before 72 hours, every effort should still be made to administer the anti-D Ig, because a dose even administered within 10 days may still provide some protection. Ideally, anti-D Ig should be administered into the deltoid muscle. Injections into the gluteal region should be by far avoided because this may be associated with delayed absorption.

Box 26.2: Criteria for administration of second dose of anti-D immunoglobulins to Rh-negative non-immunised women

☐ The baby born is Rh positive
☐ Direct Coomb's test on the umbilical cord blood is negative.
☐ The cross-match between the anti-D Ig and mother's red cells is compatible.

Table 26.1: Anti-D Ig preparations are available for use in the UK[6]

Anti-D Ig preparations	Mode of administration
D-GAM®: 250 IU, 500 IU, 1,500 IU and 2,500 IU vials	Intramuscular use only
Partobulin SDF: 1,250 IU prefilled syringe	Intramuscular use only
Rhophylac®: 1,500 IU prefilled syringe	Intramuscular or intravenous use
WinRho SDF®: 1,500 IU and 5,000 IU vials	Intramuscular or intravenous use (in the UK, this product is mainly used for the treatment of idiopathic thrombocytopenic purpura)

Subcutaneous or IV route rather than the IM route must be adopted for women who have a bleeding disorder. Prior to the administration of anti-D Ig, consent should be obtained and recorded in their case notes. Women who are already sensitised to RhD should not be given anti-D Ig.

Anti-D Ig prophylaxis following miscarriage, ectopic pregnancy and termination of pregnancy: Indications for the administration of anti-D Ig prophylaxis following miscarriage, ectopic pregnancy and termination of pregnancy are described in Box 26.3. When indicated, anti-D Ig must be administered in a dose of 250 IU up to 19^{+6} weeks of gestation and in a dose of 500 IU thereafter. Size of FMH should be determined when administering anti-D Ig at or after 20^{+0} weeks of gestation.

Prophylaxis with anti-D Ig following sensitising events before delivery: Anti-D Ig should be given to all non-sensitised RhD-negative women after potentially sensitising events during pregnancy as enlisted in Box 26.4. This should be in

Box 26.3: Prophylaxis with anti-D Ig following miscarriage, ectopic pregnancy and termination of pregnancy

Miscarriage
❑ *Administration required*
  – All non-sensitised RhD-negative women who have a spontaneous complete or incomplete miscarriage at or after 12^{+0} weeks of gestation
  – All non-sensitised RhD-negative women undergoing surgical evacuation of the uterus, regardless of the period of gestation
  – All non-sensitised RhD-negative women undergoing medical evacuation of the uterus, regardless of the gestation.
❑ *Administration not required*
  – Anti-D Ig is not required for spontaneous miscarriage before 12^{+0} weeks of gestation, provided there is no instrumentation of the uterus

Threatened miscarriage
❑ *Administration required*
  – All non-sensitised RhD-negative women with a threatened miscarriage after 12^{+0} weeks of gestation
  – Non-sensitised RhD-negative women in whom bleeding continues intermittently after 12^{+0} weeks of gestation, anti-D Ig should be given at 6 weekly intervals
  – Non-sensitised RhD-negative women in whom there is heavy or repeated bleeding or associated abdominal pain as gestation approaches 12^{+0} weeks (The period of gestation should be confirmed by ultrasound)

Ectopic pregnancy
❑ *Administration required*
  – All non-sensitised RhD-negative women who have an ectopic pregnancy, regardless of the mode of management

Therapeutic termination of pregnancy
❑ *Administration required*
  – All non-sensitised RhD-negative women undergoing therapeutic termination of pregnancy, whether by surgical or medical methods, regardless of the gestational age

---

Box 26.4: Sensitising events prior to the delivery requiring anti-D Ig prophylaxis

❑ Invasive prenatal diagnosis (amniocentesis, chorion villus sampling, cordocentesis, intrauterine transfusion)
❑ Other intrauterine procedures (e.g. insertion of shunts, embryo reduction, laser)
❑ Antepartum haemorrhage
❑ External cephalic version of the foetus (including attempted)
❑ Any abdominal trauma (direct/indirect, sharp/blunt, open/closed)
❑ Intrauterine foetal death and stillbirth
❑ Ectopic pregnancy
❑ Evacuation of molar pregnancy
❑ Miscarriage, threatened miscarriage
❑ Therapeutic termination of pregnancy
❑ Delivery—normal, instrumental or caesarean section
❑ Intraoperative cell salvage

addition to any dosage they had already received. A minimum dose of 250 IU is recommended for prophylaxis following sensitising events up to 19^{+6} weeks of gestation. For all the sensitising events, which have occurred at or after 20^{+0} weeks

of gestation, a minimum dosage of 500 IU anti-D Ig should be administered. In the case of recurrent vaginal bleeding after 20^{+0} weeks of gestation, anti-D Ig should be given at a minimum of 6 weekly intervals. An appropriate additional dose of anti-D Ig should be administered for each new sensitising event regardless of the timing or dose of anti-D Ig administered for a previous event. Appropriate tests for FMH should be carried out for all D-negative, previously non-sensitised, pregnant women who have had a potentially sensitising event after 20 weeks of gestation, and additional dose(s) of anti-D Ig should be administered if required.

Routine antenatal anti-D prophylaxis (RAADP programme): Routine antenatal anti-D Ig prophylaxis should be offered to all non-sensitised RhD-negative women. It is not required in women who are RhD-sensitised. It is a completely separate entity from the additional dosage of anti-D Ig required for potentially sensitising events. According to NICE (2008), there are two regimens for providing RAADP:
1. Two doses of 500 IU anti-D Ig can be administered at 28 weeks and 34 weeks of gestation.
2. A single dose of 1,500 IU anti-D can be administered at 28 weeks of gestation. Presently, there is no evidence to indicate that there is a difference in the efficacy of the single-dose or two-dose regimens. According to the recommendations by NICE (2008), the preparation with the lowest associated cost (acquisition plus administration costs) should preferably be used.

Women who are eligible for RAADP should receive written information from their healthcare provider before making an informed decision about opting for treatment. Consent should be obtained in the case notes. In case the patient declines to receive RAADP, this decision should be accepted and documented in the case notes along with the reasons for the decision (Box 26.5). In case the patient declines RAADP, antibody screening should be performed at the time of booking and again at 28 weeks of gestation to identify cases where sensitisation has occurred. Sensitisation occurring in the third trimester is unlikely to cause significant foetal problems in that pregnancy. Routine use of antenatal anti-D Ig prophylaxis should not be altered by previous anti-D Ig prophylaxis administered for a sensitising event, which had occurred earlier in the same pregnancy.

In the women willing for RAADP, the routine 28-week antibody-screening sample must be taken before administration of the first dose of anti-D. RAADP helps in reducing

---

Box 26.5: Causes for women to decline routine antenatal anti-D Ig prophylaxis

❑ Objection on the basis of religious grounds
❑ Women who will be sterilised after the birth
❑ Women who are certain they will have no more children in future
❑ Women who are in a stable relationship with the genetic father of their children and the father is known or found to be RhD-negative

the incidence of rhesus alloimmunisation amongst previously non-sensitised Rh-D negative women who deliver an RhD-positive baby.[8-11] Presently, there is no evidence to suggest that RAADP is associated with any adverse events for the mother or baby. There is a small possibility regarding the transmission of blood-borne infection. However, there are procedures in place to minimise this risk.

Postnatal prophylaxis: Following the delivery of an RhD-positive infant, at least 500 IU of anti-D Ig must be administered to every non-sensitised RhD-negative woman within 72 hours.[12] This includes women with alloantibodies other than anti-D. 500 IU (100 μg) of anti-D Ig administered intramuscularly is normally capable of suppressing immunisation by 4 mL of RhD-positive red cells.

A test to detect FMH greater than 4 mL must also be undertaken so that the additional dose of anti-D Ig can be administered if required. In case the pregnancy is non-viable and no sample can be obtained from the baby, anti-D Ig should be administered to a non-sensitised RhD-negative woman within 72 hours of the diagnosis of IUD, irrespective of the time of subsequent delivery.

Following the baby's birth, cord blood sample should be tested to determine the ABO and RhD type of the baby. If a cord blood sample cannot be collected for any reason, a heel-prick sample should be obtained from the baby as soon as possible (BCSH, 2007). If the baby's blood group cannot be established for some reason, at least 500 IU anti-D Ig should be administered to RhD negative, previously non-sensitised women. A direct antiglobulin test (DAT) is not routinely performed on the cord blood sample because it may be positive in a proportion of cases due to antenatal prophylaxis with anti-D Ig. However, a DAT should be performed if haemolytic disease of the newborn is suspected or anticipated due to a low cord blood haemoglobin concentration and/or the presence of maternal immune red cell antibodies.

In cases where intraoperative cell salvage (ICS) is used at the time of caesarean delivery in D negative, previously non-sensitised women, and where cord blood group is confirmed as D positive (or unknown), a minimum dose of 1,500 IU anti-D Ig should be administered following the reinfusion of salvaged red cells. Maternal samples should also be taken for the estimation of FMH, 30–45 minutes after reinfusion to evaluate the requirement for extra dose of anti-D Ig.

Transfusion of RhD-positive blood to RhD-negative women: Anti-D Ig should be given to RhD-negative women of reproductive capacity who inadvertently receive a transfusion of RhD-positive blood. The dose of anti-D Ig should be calculated on the basis that 500 IU of anti-D Ig is likely to suppress immunisation by 4 mL of RhD-positive red blood cells.

Exchange transfusion may be necessary for large volumes of transfused blood (more than 2 units of RhD-positive blood).

Role of non-invasive assessment of foetal blood type (cell-free foetal DNA): The breakthrough in foetal blood group genotyping has come with the development of cell-free foetal DNA (cffDNA) from maternal plasma. This is a non-invasive technique for disease assessment and progression. This involves the extraction of cffDNA from biofluids such as blood, plasma and urine, which yields very low levels of highly fragmented DNA. Numerous studies have now been published regarding the accuracy of determination of foetal RhD status from cffDNA. A meta-analysis by Geifman-Holtzman et al. (2006) has shown that the use of cffDNA from maternal plasma is associated with an overall diagnostic accuracy of 96.5%.[13] Due to increased efficacy, this technique, besides ascertaining RhD status, can also help identify other rarer antigens including K (Kell), Rh C, c and E.[14] Currently, the use of this technique in the UK is mainly confined to women at high risk of haemolytic disease where the partner has a heterozygous genotype. In this situation, knowledge of the foetal blood type would affect the management of the pregnancy. Soothill et al. (2015) recommend that the policy of offering cffDNA testing to all RhD-negative women at about 16 weeks' gestation must be extended to all UK NHS services. This policy would help avoid anti-D administration to the mother when the foetus is RhD-negative. Presently, in the UK, all RhD-negative women are offered RAADP.[15] The major disadvantage of this policy is that approximately 40% of RhD-negative women, who are carrying an RhD-negative child, receive unnecessary antenatal anti-D Ig, implying that approximately 40,000 women in the UK currently receive unnecessary prophylaxis.[6]

Rh-negative Immunised Women

Management of immunised Rh-negative pregnancy is summarised in Flow charts 26.3A and B.[1] In Rh-negative immunised women, the main objective of the management is to diagnose and treat foetal anaemia as soon as possible. This can be done through one of the following ways: measurement of the peak systolic velocity (PSV) of the foetal middle cerebral artery; Doppler ultrasound; amniocentesis and amniotic fluid analysis; ultrasound examination of the foetus and percutaneous umbilical cord blood sampling (cordocentesis).

With the advancements in foetomaternal medicine, there is a shift towards the use of non-invasive methods for the assessment of foetal anaemia. Use of foetal middle cerebral artery peak systolic velocity (MCA-PSV) for diagnosis of moderate to severe anaemia has therefore emerged as an important non-invasive method for identification of foetal anaemia and helps in avoiding invasive procedures in nearly 70% cases.[16-18] Due to this, MCA-PSV is preferred over amniocentesis.

The use of MCA-PSV is based on the principle that foetal anaemia results in lowering of the blood viscosity, thereby resulting in an increase in the peak flow velocity of the systolic flow in the middle cerebral artery. The risk of foetal anaemia is high in foetuses with PSV of 1.5 times the median or higher. Foetuses with values below 1.5 are unlikely to have any anaemia or may have only mild anaemia. The interval between rescanning for MCA assessments is 1–2 weeks. This is used reliably from 18 weeks of gestation. However, its use is not recommended after 36 weeks due to an increase in the rate of false-positive tests for predicting foetal anaemia.

Flow chart 26.3A: Antenatal management of immunised Rh-negative pregnancy

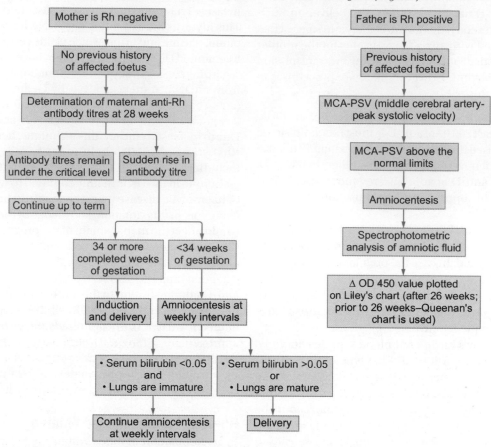

Flow chart 26.3B: Intrapartum management of immunised Rh-negative pregnancy

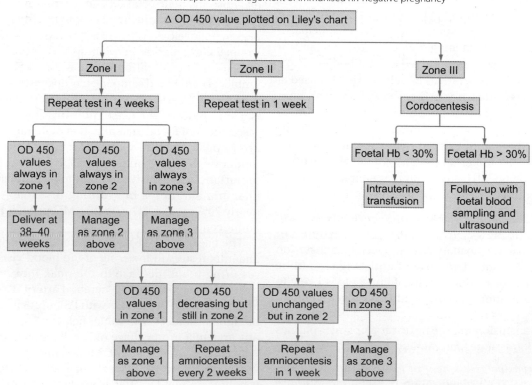

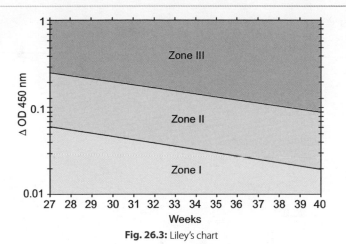

Fig. 26.3: Liley's chart

Amniotic fluid analysis involves determination of bilirubin concentration in the amniotic fluid and spectrophotometric analysis. The OD 450 values are plotted on Liley's chart (Fig. 26.3). Zone 3 on the Liley's curve corresponds to severely affected infants, zone 2 to moderately affected infants and zone 1 to unaffected or mildly affected infants. If bilirubin levels in amniotic fluid remain normal, the pregnancy can be allowed to continue to term and the clinician can await spontaneous labour. If bilirubin levels are elevated, indicating impending intrauterine death, the foetus can be given intrauterine blood transfusions at 10-day to 2-week intervals, generally until 35–36 weeks of gestation, following which the delivery is usually performed by 37–38 weeks. If at any time, the OD 450 value lies in the zone 3 or shows a rising trend, the foetus is in imminent danger of the intrauterine death. In these cases, cordocentesis must be done and foetal haemoglobin values must be determined. If foetal haematocrit values are less than 30%, intrauterine transfusion is indicated. Treatment of foetal anaemia can be in the form of in utero transfusion (intraperitoneal or intravascular) if foetal anaemia is severe, or exchange transfusion after birth.

Intrapartum Management

Precautions to be Taken at the Time of Delivery

Following steps must be taken to minimise the chances of foetomaternal bleeding during the time of delivery:
- Prophylactic ergometrine with the delivery of the anterior shoulder must be withheld.
- If the manual removal of the placenta is required, it should be performed gently.
- Rh-positive blood transfusion must be preferably avoided in Rh-negative woman right from birth until menopause.
- Invasive procedures, like amniocentesis, chorionic villus sampling, etc. should be followed by administration of anti-Rh immunoglobulins in the dosage as previously described.
- Careful foetal monitoring needs to be performed during the time of labour.

- Delivery should be as non-traumatic as possible.
- The clinician should remain vigilant regarding the possibility for the occurrence of PPH.
- Umbilical cord should be clamped as soon as possible to minimise the chances of FMH.
- At the time of caesarean section, all precautions should be taken to prevent any spillage of blood into the peritoneal cavity.

Flow chart 26.4 describes the algorithm for deciding the timing for delivery in Rh-negative women.

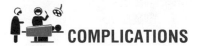

COMPLICATIONS

Various complications as a result of Rh sensitisation are described in Flow chart 26.5 and are as follows:[19]

Foetal

- *Erythroblastosis foetalis*: Clinical manifestations of erythroblastosis foetalis include hydrops foetalis, icterus gravis neonatorum and congenital anaemia of the newborn. Excessive destruction of foetal RBCs results in hyperbilirubinaemia, jaundice and/or kernicterus, which can lead to deafness, speech problems, cerebral palsy or mental retardation.
- *Hydrops foetalis*: This is a condition characterised by an accumulation of fluids within the baby's body, resulting in development of ascites, pleural effusion, pericardial effusion, skin oedema, etc.

Maternal

- Recurrent miscarriages and intrauterine deaths
- Complications, such as abortion and preterm labour, are related to procedures such as foetal cord blood sampling.

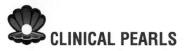

CLINICAL PEARLS

- Routine antenatal anti-D Ig prophylaxis is not an alternative to anti-D Ig for sensitising events and vice versa. It should be given irrespective of whether anti-D Ig has been given at an earlier gestation, e.g. prenatal diagnosis or vaginal bleeding. Similarly, sensitising events that occur after administration of RAADP should be covered with an additional dose of anti-D Ig (500 IU, unless Kleihauer testing indicates that a larger dose is required).
- In case RhD-positive platelets are transfused to RhD-negative women of childbearing age group, prophylaxis against Rh alloimmunisation should be given.[20] 250 IU (50 micrograms) of anti-D Ig should be given following every three adult doses (i.e. derived from up to 18 routine donations) of platelets.

Flow chart 26.4: Deciding the timing for delivery in Rh-negative women

```
┌──────────────────────┐              ┌──────────────────────┐
│ Mother is Rh negative │              │ Father is Rh positive │
└──────────┬───────────┘              └──────────┬───────────┘
           └──────────────┬─────────────────────┘
                ┌───────────────────────┐
                │ Indirect Coomb's test  │
                └───────────┬───────────┘
           ┌────────────────┴─────────────────┐
┌────────────────────┐              ┌────────────────────┐
│ No antibody present │              │  Antibody present  │
└──────────┬─────────┘              └──────────┬─────────┘
┌────────────────────┐              ┌────────────────────┐
│    Rh-negative      │              │    Rh-negative      │
│   non-immunised     │              │     immunised       │
│      women          │              │      women          │
└──────────┬─────────┘              └──────────┬─────────┘
┌────────────────────┐              ┌──────────────────────────┐
│ Pregnancy allowed   │              │ Δ OD 450 values of amniotic fluid │
│   to continue       │              │ plotted on Liley's chart │
└──────────┬─────────┘              └──────────┬───────────────┘
┌────────────────────┐         ┌───────────────┼───────────────────┐
│  Delivery at term   │     ┌────────┐     ┌────────┐        ┌─────────┐
└──────────┬─────────┘     │ Zone I │     │ Zone II│        │Zone III │
                            └────┬───┘     └────┬───┘        └────┬────┘
```

Precautions to be taken at time of delivery
- I/M ergometrine not to be given at delivery of anterior shoulders
- Minimise the chance of foetomaternal haemorrhage
- Foetal cord blood to be sent for lab. analysis (ABO/Rh typing, direct Coomb's test, Hb, bilirubin levels and peripheral smear)

Zone I → Pregnancy allowed to continue → Delivery at term

Zone II / Zone III → Period of gestation → <34 weeks / >34 weeks

>34 weeks → Delivery

<34 weeks → Haematocrit >30% / Haematocrit <30%

Haematocrit >30% → Follow-up with foetal blood sampling and ultrasound at weekly intervals → Decision for delivery based on foetal condition and maturity

Haematocrit <30% → Intrauterine blood transfusion (at 1–2 week intervals) → Delivery at 34–36 weeks

EVIDENCE-BASED MEDICINE

❖ Present evidence indicates that the administration of RAADP helps in reducing the incidence of rhesus alloimmunisation amongst previously non-sensitised RhD negative women who deliver an RhD-positive baby.[2,3]

❖ There is sufficient evidence showing that significant FMH occurs only after curettage to remove products of conception but does not occur after complete spontaneous miscarriages.[21,22] Anti-D Ig should, therefore, be administered when there has been an intervention to evacuate the uterus.

❖ Medically induced evacuation of the uterus with prostaglandins is likely to result in increased uterine contractions and bleeding in comparison with spontaneous miscarriage. There is a lack of evidence to guide the use of anti-D Ig for medical evacuation of the uterus but it seems reasonable to consider anti-D administration in such circumstances. By contrast, the risk of immunisation by spontaneous miscarriage before 12+0 weeks of gestation is negligible when there has been no instrumentation to evacuate the products of conception. Therefore, anti-D Ig is not required in these circumstances.[7-10]

PART II

Flow Chart 26.5: Various foetal complications arising from Rh isoimmunisation

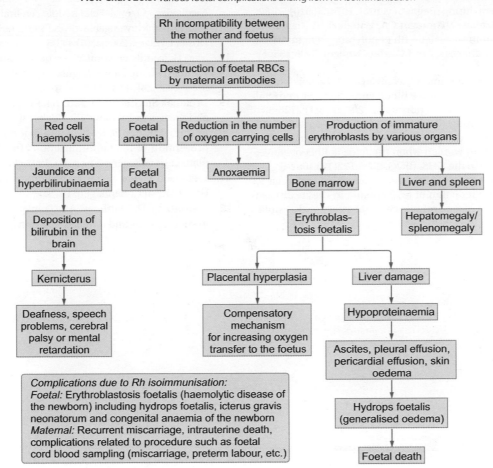

Complicated block:
Complications due to Rh isoimmunisation:
Foetal: Erythroblastosis foetalis (haemolytic disease of the newborn) including hydrops foetalis, icterus gravis neonatorum and congenital anaemia of the newborn
Maternal: Recurrent miscarriage, intrauterine death, complications related to procedure such as foetal cord blood sampling (miscarriage, preterm labour, etc.)

REFERENCES

1. Mollinson PL, Engelfriet CP, Contreras M. Haemolytic disease of the fetus and newborn. In: Mollinson PL (Ed). Blood Transfusion in Clinical Medicine, 10th edition. Oxford: Blackwell Scientific; 1997. p. 414.

2. Royal College of Obstetricians and Gynaecologists, (RCOG): (2011). The Use of Anti-D Immunoglobulin for Rhesus D Prophylaxis. Green-top Guideline No. 22. [online] Available from https://www.rcog.org.uk/en/guidelines-research-services/guidelines/gtg22/. [Accessed May, 2016].

3. Qureshi H, Massey E, Kirwan D, Davies T, Robson S, White J, et al. BCSH guideline for the use of anti-D immunoglobulin for the prevention of haemolytic disease of the fetus and newborn. Transfus Med. 2014;24(1):8-20.

4. Committee for Proprietary Medicine Products. Notes for guidance: core summary of product characteristics for human anti-D immunoglobulin I.M. III/34463/92-EN. Brussels: Co-ordinating European Council; 1994.

5. Johnson PR, Tait RC, Austin EB, Shwe KH, Lee D. Flow cytometry in diagnosis and management of large fetomaternal haemorrhage. J Clin Pathol. 1995;48:1005-8.

6. Lee D, Contreras M, Robson SC, Rodeck CH, Whittle MJ. Recommendations for the use of anti-D immunoglobulin for Rh prophylaxis. British Blood Transfusion Society and the Royal College of Obstetricians and Gynaecologists. Transfus Med. 1999;9(1):93-7.

7. National Institute for Health and Clinical Excellence, (NICE). (2008). Routine antenatal anti-D prophylaxis for women who are rhesus D negative (TA156). [online] Available from www.nice.org.uk/guidance/ta156/resources/routine-antenatal-antid-prophylaxis-for-women-who-are-rhesus-d-negative-82598318102725. [Accessed August, 2016].

8. National Institute for Health and Clinical Excellence (NICE). Full guidance on the use of routine antenatal anti-D prophylaxis for RhD negative women. Technology Appraisal Guidance No. 41. 2002.

9. Pilgrim H, Lloyd-Jones M, Rees A. Routine antenatal anti-D prophylaxis for RhD-negative women: a systematic review and economic evaluation. Health Technol Assess. 2009;13(10):1-103.

10. MacKenzie IZ, Bowell P, Gregory H, Pratt G, Guest C, Entwistle CC. Routine antenatal Rhesus D immunoglobulin prophylaxis: the results of a prospective 10 year study. Br J Obstet Gynaecol. 1999;106(5):492-7.

11. Mayne S, Parker JH, Harden TA, Dodds SD, Beale JA. Rate of RhD sensitisation before and after implementation of a community based antenatal prophylaxis programme. BMJ. 1997;315(7122):1588.

12. Controlled trial of various anti-D dosages in suppression of Rh sensitization following pregnancy. Report to the Medical Research Council by the working party on the use of anti-D

CHAPTER 26

immunoglobulin for the prevention of isoimmunization of Rh-negative women during pregnancy. BMJ. 1974;2(5910):75-80.

13. Geifman-Holtzman O, Grotegut CA, Gaughan JP. Diagnostic accuracy of noninvasive fetal Rh genotyping from maternal blood—a meta-analysis. Am J Obstet Gynecol. 2006;195(4):1163-73.

14. Finning K, Martin P, Summers J, Daniels G. Fetal genotyping for the K (Kell) and Rh C, c, and E blood groups on cell-free fetal DNA in maternal plasma. Transfusion. 2007;47(11):2126-33.

15. Soothill PW, Finning K, Latham T, Wreford-Bush T, Ford J, Daniels G. Use of cffDNA to avoid administration of anti-D to pregnant women when the fetus is RhD-negative: implementation in the NHS. BJOG. 2015;122(12):1682-6.

16. Scheier M, Hernandez-Andrade E, Carmo A, Dezerega V, Nicolaides KH. Prediction of fetal anemia in rhesus disease by measurement of fetal middle cerebral artery peak systolic velocity. Ultrasound Obstet Gynecol. 2004;23(5):432-6.

17. Hernandez-Andrade E, Scheier M, Dezerega V, Carmo A, Nicolaides KH, et al. Fetal middle cerebral artery peak systolic velocity in the investigation of non-immune hydrops. Ultrasound Obstet Gynecol. 2004;23(5):442-5.

18. Mari G. Middle cerebral artery peak systolic velocity: is it the standard of care for the diagnosis of fetal anemia? J Ultrasound Med. 2005;24(5):697-702.

19. Urbaniak SJ, Greiss MA. RhD haemolytic disease of the fetus and the newborn. Blood Rev. 2000;14(1):44-61.

20. Murphy MF, Lee D. Dose of anti-D immunoglobulin for the prevention of RhD immunisation after RhD-incompatible platelet transfusions. Vox Sang. 1993;65(1):73-4.

21. Jorgensen J. Feto-maternal bleeding. MD thesis. Denmark: University of Copenhagen; 1975.

22. Matthews CD, Matthews AE. Transplacental haemorrhage in spontaneous and induced abortion. Lancet. 1969;1:694-5.

PART II

Abnormal Presentation

BREECH PRESENTATION

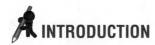 INTRODUCTION

Breech presentation is a type of abnormal presentation where the foetus lies longitudinally with the buttocks presenting in the lower pole of the uterus. The different types of breech presentations, like complete breech, footling breech and frank breech, are shown in Figure 27.1. Frank breech is the most common type of breech presentation (50–70% cases). In these cases, buttocks present first with flexed hips and legs extended on the abdomen. Extended breech is type of breech, which is easiest to be delivered vaginally. Complete breech is present in nearly 5–10% cases. In this, the buttocks present first with flexed hips and flexed knees. Feet are not below the buttocks. In case of footling breech, one or both the baby's feet present as both hips and knees are in extended position. As a result, feet are palpated at a level lower than the buttocks. This type of presentation is present in 10–30% cases. The denominator of breech presentation is considered to be the sacrum. Since most babies in breech presentation spontaneously turn to the cephalic presentation with increasing period of gestation, the incidence of breech presentation decreases from about 20% at 28 weeks of gestation to 3–4% at term. Management of breech presentation acts as a challenge for the obstetricians because it is associated with a higher perinatal mortality and morbidity in comparison to the cephalic presentation. This is principally related to prematurity, congenital malformations and birth asphyxia or trauma.[1,2]

AETIOLOGY

- *Maternal factors*: Maternal risk factors which increase the incidence for breech presentation include factors such as cephalopelvic disproportion; liquor abnormalities (polyhydramnios and oligohydramnios); uterine anomalies (bicornuate or septate uterus); space occupying lesions (e.g. fibroids in the lower uterine segment); placental abnormalities (placenta praevia, cornuofundal attachment of placenta), multiparity (especially grand multiparas); cord abnormalities (very long or very short cord); previous history of breech delivery, etc.
- *Foetal factors*: These include factors such as prematurity; foetal anomalies (e.g. neurological abnormalities, hydrocephalus, anencephaly and meningomyelocele); intrauterine foetal death, etc.

DIAGNOSIS

Clinical Presentation

Women with breech presentation may have complaints such as a hard lump or discomfort under the ribs.

Abdominal Examination

- Foetal lie is longitudinal with foetal head on one side and breech on the other side.
- First Leopold's manoeuvre or fundal grip shows smooth, hard, ballotable structure suggestive of foetal head.

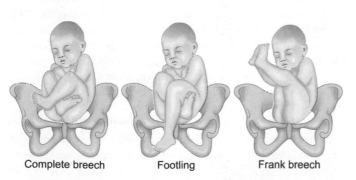

Complete breech   Footling   Frank breech

Fig. 27.1: Different types of breech presentation

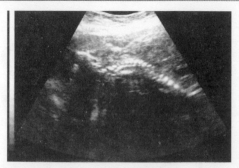

Fig. 27.2: Ultrasound examination in case of breech presentation

PART II

❖ On second Leopold's manoeuvre or lateral grip, there is a firm, smooth board-like foetal back on one side and knob-like structures suggestive of foetal limbs on other side.

❖ On pelvic grips, foetal head cannot be palpated. Instead, there is soft broad irregular mass.

❖ The foetal heart sounds are loudest above the maternal umbilicus.

Vaginal Examination

Following features may be observed on vaginal examination:

❖ Palpation of three bony landmarks of the breech, namely, two ischial tuberosities and a sacral tip

❖ Feet may be felt besides the buttocks in cases of complete breech

❖ Fresh meconium may be found on the examining fingers; presence of thick, dark meconium is a normal finding in cases of breech presentation

❖ Palpation of the male genitalia.

Investigations

Ultrasound examination: Ultrasound helps in confirming the type of breech presentation (Fig. 27.2). Other things, which can be observed on the ultrasound, include the following: Presence of uterine and/or foetal anomalies; foetal maturity; placental location and grading; adequacy of liquor and presence of multiple pregnancy.

OBSTETRIC MANAGEMENT

The management in cases of breech presentation is based on three options: (1) breech vaginal delivery, (2) external cephalic version (ECV) and (3) caesarean delivery, and depends on various parameters listed in Box 27.1.

In cases of breech presentation, obstetrician must enable informed choice to the mother and support her in the decision-making process. Nowadays, shared decision-making partnership between the patient and the clinician helps the patient in making an informed choice. In relation to this, women should be informed about the benefits and risks, both for the current and for future pregnancies, in relation to the various options, i.e. planned caesarean section versus planned vaginal delivery for breech presentation at term. Women should be given an opportunity to make informed decision about their care and treatment in partnership with their healthcare professionals.

Box 27.1: Parameters for deciding the mode of delivery in cases of breech presentation

❑ Timing of diagnosis (antepartum or intrapartum)
❑ Term or preterm baby
❑ Parity
❑ Underlying cause for breech presentation
❑ Cervical dilatation, station of the presenting part
❑ Estimated foetal weight
❑ Placental location
❑ Patient's choice

Women should be informed that there is no evidence that the long-term health of the babies with a breech presentation delivered at term is influenced by the mode of delivery (caesarean or vaginal birth). Women should be assessed carefully before being selected as the probable candidate for vaginal breech birth. Women with unfavourable clinical features for a successful vaginal delivery should be specifically advised that attempting vaginal breech birth is likely to be associated with an increased risk to them as well as their babies. Routine radiological pelvimetry for pelvic assessment in such patients is not necessary.

Diagnosis of breech presentation for the first time during labour should not be a contraindication for vaginal breech birth. Before reaching a particular decision, the benefits of each option need to be weighed against factors such as the mother's preference for vaginal birth and risks such as future pregnancy complications likely to occur in the woman's specific healthcare setting.

Choosing the Route of Delivery for a Woman with Breech Presentation at Term

Vaginal breech deliveries had been routinely used in the past. The question regarding the use of vaginal route or abdominal route for delivery of the foetuses in breech presentation has been associated with much controversy. This controversy was particularly flared up after the declaration of the results of the 'Term Breech Trial (TBT)' (2000), a large multicentric RCT, designed to determine the safest mode of delivery for a term breech foetus.[3] This trial involved 121 centres in 26 countries including the UK. A total of 2,088 women were recruited in this study. Women with extended or flexed breech pregnancies were randomised to delivery either by caesarean or vaginal route. Almost 10% of women, who were randomised to receive a caesarean delivery, actually had a vaginal breech birth. Only 57% of the patients randomised to vaginal breech delivery actually had a vaginal breech birth. This implies that the conversion rates to caesarean delivery in women assigned to receive vaginal delivery was approximately 43%. The women should be made aware of this fact while counselling them for informed choice.

The results of this TBT showed that perinatal mortality and morbidity was significantly lower for women with breech presentation undergoing planned caesarean delivery in comparison to those having planned vaginal delivery. In breech presentation, sudden delivery of foetal head at the time of vaginal birth can cause excessive pressure on the aftercoming head of the breech resulting in a high risk for tentorial tears and intracranial haemorrhage in comparison to the foetuses in cephalic presentation. After the declaration of these results, it was proposed that all breech presentations should be delivered abdominally to reduce the rates of perinatal morbidity and mortality. As a result, there was an abrupt shift in the obstetric clinical practice, and term breech caesarean section rates increased around the world. Following the publication of TBT (2000), both the ACOG and the RCOG guidelines recommended that the best method of delivering a term frank or complete breech singleton is by planned caesarean section (ACOG, 2001, Opinion No. 265; RCOG, 2006).[4,5]

The Cochrane review by Hofmeyr et al. (2015) analysed 2,396 patients from the individual studies up to March 2015.[6] The results have shown a similarity to that of TBT and have revealed a similar reduction in the rate of perinatal and neonatal mortality and morbidity in the group with planned caesarean delivery in the settings with a low national perinatal mortality rate. However, similar findings were not observed in the settings with a high national perinatal mortality rate. Moreover, planned caesarean section was associated with modestly increased short-term maternal morbidity (such as abdominal pain). However, after 3 months of delivery, women allocated to the planned caesarean section group reported less urinary incontinence and perineal pain.

After 2 years, there were no differences in the combined neonatal outcome (death or neurodevelopmental delay) in between the two groups. More infants, who had been allocated to undergo planned caesarean delivery, had medical problems at 2 years. Maternal outcomes at 2 years were also similar. In countries with low perinatal mortality rates, the protocol of planned caesarean section was associated with lower healthcare costs. This however was not inclusive of the future costs, which could be associated with a scarred uterus, e.g. likelihood of a repeat caesarean delivery, risk of uterine rupture, etc.

However, some authorities still favour vaginal route for breech delivery because numerous weaknesses have also been identified since the publication of TBT despite its various strengths. The recommendations for caesarean delivery were made based on the short-term outcomes. However, based on the follow-up data from the past 2 years, assessing the long-term outcomes, there appears to be no evidence to recommend planned caesarean section. The 2-year follow-up study showing no difference in the combined outcome (death and neurodevelopmental delay) was a completely unexpected outcome. This suggested that there was no long-term benefit of caesarean section over vaginal delivery. The higher number of deaths in the group having vaginal births was balanced by the number of neurologically delayed infants in the group undergoing caesarean delivery. These infants had appeared normal at birth and therefore were not counted in the perinatal morbidity figures.

The major study limitation was that some women choose to deliver vaginally and not opt for a planned caesarean section. Furthermore, some labour too quickly even when an elective caesarean delivery has been planned. The second study limitation is that larger sample size is required to report accurately on perinatal and maternal mortality rates. Thirdly, there were difficulties in maintaining standardised management protocols across multitude of sites. Some of these difficulties included variable practitioner experience; requirement of the staff to follow rigid protocols with which they were unfamiliar; unequal access to prenatal diagnosis; electronic FHR monitoring; senior obstetrician was not always present at the time of delivery, etc. Fourthly, less than 10% of women in the trial underwent pelvimetry using plain radiography, CT or MR scanning. Moreover, in more than 30% cases, attitude of foetal head was determined only using clinical methods and not through ultrasound. Approximately 3% of the babies in the trial were actually cephalic. Ultrasound assessment of the baby to rule out foetal growth restriction and macrosomia was also not done. Many women were recruited in active labour and there were large institutional variations in the standard of care. Some breech presentations included in the study were footling; these should have been excluded.

Moreover, in response to the TBT, Goffinet et al. (2006) published the PREMODA study, a multicentric descriptive study four times larger than the TBT. In this study, data was collected from 8,105 women across 174 centres in France and Belgium.[7] The outcomes of PREMODA study were in stark contrast with those of the TBT. There was no difference in the rates of perinatal mortality or serious neonatal morbidity amongst the groups undergoing trial of labour (TOL) or planned caesarean delivery. Years after the analysis of follow-up data from the TBT, ACOG (2006, opinion 340) recommended that decision regarding the mode of delivery depends upon the experience of healthcare provider.[8] Planned vaginal delivery of a singleton breech foetus may be a reasonable option under hospital-specific protocol guidelines. Before deciding the mode of delivery, women should be informed about the benefits and risks, both for the current and for future pregnancies, of planned caesarean section versus planned vaginal delivery for breech presentation at term.[9] Women should be informed that planned caesarean section carries a reduced rate of perinatal mortality and early neonatal morbidity for babies with breech presentation at term compared with planned vaginal birth.

All women should be given information related to external cephalic version, which must be definitely used as an option unless it is contraindicated or woman refuses to give her consent. RCOG guidelines (2006) suggest that women should be informed that there is no evidence that the mode of delivery would influence the long-term health of babies with a breech presentation delivered at term.[5] They should also be counselled regarding the reduced perinatal mortality and early neonatal morbidity for babies with breech presentation undergoing a planned caesarean delivery in comparison to vaginal birth. However, planned caesarean for breech presentation may be associated with a small increase in the risk of immediate complications for the mother (e.g. abdominal pain). Women should be advised that the long-term effects of planned caesarean delivery for breech presentation on them and their babies are uncertain.

Management of Preterm Breech

There is insufficient evidence to support routine caesarean section for preterm breech deliveries.[10,11] Mode of delivery for preterm delivery should be individualised for each woman based on the clinical situation and the wishes of woman and her partner. Similar rates of head entrapment have been described in cases of preterm breech presentation delivered by vaginal or abdominal routes.[12] Poor neonatal outcomes are more likely to be due to the complications of prematurity rather than due to vaginal birth.

It is particularly important for preterm breech vaginal deliveries that the obstetrician confirms the second stage by vaginal examination before the patient starts pushing. If the obstetrician is unable to prevent the patient from pushing before full dilatation of cervix occurs, then an epidural should be encouraged. If there occurs head entrapment during a preterm (or term) breech delivery, administration of lateral incisions to the cervix should be considered. A senior obstetrician and a senior paediatrician must be present at the delivery of all babies with less than 34 weeks of gestation.

Management of Twin Breech

For the first twin presenting as breech, caesarean delivery is likely to improve neonatal APGAR score at 5 minutes. Women should be informed about the benefits of planned caesarean section for breech presentation of the first twin. This includes reduced risk of perinatal mortality both for the current and future pregnancies. Women should also be advised that planned caesarean section for breech presentation is associated with a very small increase in serious immediate complications for them in comparison to the planned vaginal birth of the first twin with breech presentation. A caesarean section for first twin in breech presentation may also prevent the extremely rare complication of 'interlocking' if the second twin is vertex.

Presently, there is insufficient evidence to support the routine delivery of the second twin in breech presentation by caesarean section. Moreover, presentation of the second twin at the time of delivery may not always be predictable. The chances of cephalic delivery may be improved by routinely guiding the head of the second twin towards the pelvis during and immediately after delivery of the first twin. On the other hand, some clinicians prefer to routinely accelerate delivery of the second twin by internal version and breech extraction irrespective of the baby's presentation.

External Cephalic Version

Version can be defined as a procedure, which helps in changing the lie of the foetus so as to bring the favourable foetal pole to the lower pole of the uterus. Version could be external (involving abdominal manipulation) or internal (involving manipulation by introducing a hand through the vagina). If the cephalic pole is brought down to the lower pole of the uterus through abdominal manipulation, it is known as ECV. ECV can be defined as a procedure in which the clinician externally rotates the foetus from a breech presentation into a cephalic presentation.

Women with breech presentation should be counselled that ECV helps in reducing the chance of breech presentation at delivery and therefore helps in lowering their chances of having a caesarean delivery. Review of literature shows that the efficacy of ECV varies between 48% and 77%, with an average of 62%. Spontaneous reversion to breech presentation after successful ECV occurs in less than 5% cases.[13,14]

However, labour with a cephalic presentation following ECV is associated with a higher rate of obstetric intervention in comparison to the cases where ECV had not been required.

If the first attempt at ECV fails, the possibility of a second further attempt should be discussed. Though use of second attempt is likely to lead to a small increase in the overall success rates, use of tocolysis at the time of second attempt is likely to cause a marked increase in the success rate.[15]

Timing of External Cephalic Version

External cephalic version should be offered to all women with breech presentation who donot have any contraindication for ECV from 36 weeks of gestation in nulliparous women and from 37 weeks onwards in multiparous women. ECV performed before 36 weeks of gestation is not associated with a significant reduction in the number of non-cephalic births or caesarean deliveries.[16] Moreover, after 36 weeks of gestation, the rate of spontaneous version is quite less (approximately 8% in nulliparous breeches) and the rate of complications is quite low. Presently, there is no upper time limit regarding the period of appropriate gestation at which ECV can be performed. Success has been reported when ECV has been performed at 42 weeks of gestation and even during early labour, provided the membranes are intact.[13,17]

Complications of External Cephalic Version

Though ECV is largely a safe procedure, it can rarely have some complications. Women undergoing ECV should be alerted about the following potential complications of ECV:

❖ Premature onset of labour
❖ Premature rupture of the membranes
❖ Placental abruption
❖ *A small amount of foetomaternal haemorrhage*: This is especially dangerous in cases of Rh-negative pregnancies as it can result in the development of Rh isoimmunisation. Therefore, in cases of Rh-negative pregnancy, anti-D immunoglobulins must be administered to the mother following the procedure of ECV. Kleihauer testing, however, is unnecessary.
❖ *Foetal distress*: Occurrence of foetal distress may result in an emergency caesarean delivery. At times, there may be transient reduction of FHR, probably due to vagal response related to head compression with ECV.
❖ *Failure of version*: The baby might turn back to the breech position after the ECV is done. ECV is associated with a high rate of spontaneous reversion into breech presentation if performed before 36 weeks of gestation.
❖ *Risk of cord entanglement*: If foetal bradycardia is detected after a successful version, it is recommended that the

infant be returned to its previous breech presentation with the hope of reducing the risk of a tangled cord.

Contraindications to External Cephalic Version

Some absolute and relative contraindications for ECV are listed in Table 27.1. Absolute contraindications for ECV are conditions, which are likely to be associated with increased mortality or morbidity. Relative contraindications are conditions where ECV might be more complicated.

Procedure of External Cephalic Version

Prerequisites for External Cephalic Version

❖ *Counselling*: Women should be counselled that, with a trained operator, about 50% of ECV attempts will be successful but this rate can be individualised for them. Prior to the procedure, the women must also be counselled that ECV can be painful and the procedure may be stopped if they wish so.
❖ *Timing for ECV*: It is preferable to wait until term (37 completed weeks of gestation) before external version is

attempted because of an increased success rate and avoidance of preterm delivery if complications arise
❖ Facilities for an immediate caesarean section and foetal monitoring must be available. Ultrasound facilities to enable FHR visualisation must also be available
❖ Blood grouping and cross-matching should be done
❖ In case the mother is Rh negative, administration of 50 µg of anti-D immunoglobulin is required after the procedure
❖ Anaesthetists must be informed well in advance
❖ Maternal intravenous access must be established
❖ The patient should be NPO for at least 8 hours prior to the procedure
❖ An ultrasound examination must be performed to confirm the foetal presentation, check the rate of foetal growth, amniotic fluid volume and to rule out any associated anomalies
❖ A NST or a BPP must be performed to confirm foetal well-being
❖ A written informed consent must be obtained from the mother
❖ A tocolytic agent, such as terbutaline in a dosage of 0.25 mg, may be administered subcutaneously
❖ The patient is placed in a supine or slight Trendelenburg position for the procedure.

Obstetric Procedure

❖ Ultrasonic gel is applied liberally over the abdomen in order to decrease friction and to reduce the chances of an over-vigorous manipulation
❖ Initially, the degree of engagement of the presenting part should be determined and gentle disengagement of the presenting part be performed, if possible
❖ While performing ECV, the clinician helps in gently manipulating the foetal head towards the pelvis while the breech is brought up cephalad towards the fundus. Two types of manipulation of foetal head can be performed: a forward roll and a backward roll. The clinician must attempt a forward roll (Figs 27.3A to D) first and then a backward roll (Figs 27.4A to C), if the initial attempt is unsuccessful.

Table 27.1: Contraindications for external cephalic version

Absolute contraindications	Relative contraindications
• Cases where there is an absolute indication for caesarean delivery • Multiple pregnancy (except delivery of second twin) • Herpes simplex virus infection • Placenta praevia • Non-reassuring foetal heart tracing • Premature rupture of membranes • Presence of another obstetric indication for caesarean delivery • Major uterine and/or foetal anomalies • Antepartum haemorrhage within the last 7 days or recurrent antepartum haemorrhage during pregnancy	• Amniotic fluid abnormalities (polyhydramnios or oligohydramnios) • Evidence of uteroplacental insufficiency (small for gestational age foetus with abnormal Doppler parameters, pre-eclampsia, etc.) • Maternal cardiac disease • Women with a uterine scar • Unstable lie

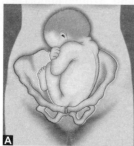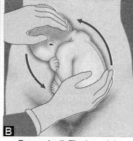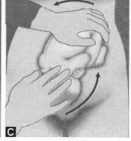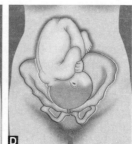

A	B	C	D
Baby in breech presentation	Forward roll: The breech is disengaged and simultaneously pushed upward	The vertex is gently pushed toward the pelvis	Forward roll is completed

Figs 27.3A to D: External cephalic version through forward roll

CHAPTER 27

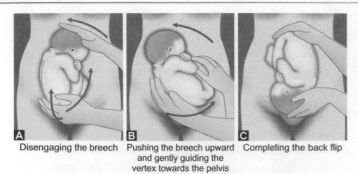

| A | B | C |
| Disengaging the breech | Pushing the breech upward and gently guiding the vertex towards the pelvis | Completing the back flip |

Figs 27.4A to C: Procedure of external cephalic version through back-flip

Post-procedural Care

❖ Whether the process has been successful or has failed, a NST and ultrasound examination must be performed after each attempt of ECV and after the end of the procedure in order to rule out foetal bradycardia and to confirm successful version

❖ Cardiotocography should be performed after the procedure to confirm the foetal well-being

❖ If unsuccessful, the version can be reattempted later.

Elective Caesarean Delivery

Some of the absolute indications for caesarean section in cases of breech presentation are enumerated in Box 27.2. Details regarding caesarean delivery have been described in Chapter 45 (Caesarean Delivery).

Trial of Breech (Vaginal Breech Delivery)

Vaginal delivery in case of breech presentation can be conducted in two ways: breech extraction and assisted breech vaginal delivery. Breech extraction is not routinely used in the UK because breech extraction is likely to cause extension of the arms and head. Although breech vaginal delivery is not routinely used, it may become unavoidable in certain circumstances (Box 27.3). On the other hand, factors regarded as unfavourable for breech vaginal birth are enumerated in Box 27.4.

Intrapartum Care for Patients Undergoing Breech Vaginal Delivery

Intrapartum care for patients undergoing breech vaginal delivery comprises of the following steps:

❖ Vaginal breech birth should take place in a hospital with facilities for emergency caesarean section. Ready access to caesarean section must be available, particularly in case of poor progress in the second stage of labour.

❖ Informed consent must be taken from the patient after explaining that the trial of breech can fail in nearly 20% cases, thereby requiring a caesarean section

❖ Plan for vaginal breech delivery must be clearly documented in the mother's notes

❖ Care should be provided by an experienced obstetrician and midwife. Anaesthetist and paediatrician must also be present. Early assessment by an anaesthetist

---

Box 27.2: Absolute indications for caesarean section in breech presentation

❑ Cephalopelvic disproportion
❑ Placenta praevia
❑ Estimated foetal weight >4 kg
❑ Hyperextension of foetal head
❑ Footling breech (danger of entrapment of head in an incompletely dilated cervix)
❑ Severe intrauterine growth restriction
❑ Clinician not competent with the technique of breech vaginal delivery
❑ A viable preterm foetus in active labour

Box 27.3: Indications for breech vaginal delivery

❑ Estimated foetal weight 2,000–4,000 g
❑ Frank or complete breech presentation
❑ Flexed foetal head, i.e. an extension angle of less than 90°
❑ No major foetal anomalies or placenta praevia on ultrasound
❑ No obstetric contraindication for breech vaginal delivery (e.g. cephalopelvic disproportion, placenta praevia, etc.)
❑ Delivery is imminent
❑ Presence of severe foetal anomaly or foetal death
❑ Mother's preference for vaginal birth

Box 27.4: Factors regarded as unfavourable for breech vaginal birth

❑ Presence of other contraindications to vaginal birth (e.g. placenta praevia, compromised foetal condition)
❑ Clinically inadequate pelvis
❑ Footling or kneeling breech presentation
❑ Large baby (weight more than 3,800 g)
❑ Growth-restricted baby (usually defined as smaller than 2,000 g)
❑ Hyperextended foetal neck in labour (diagnosed with ultrasound or X-ray where ultrasound facilities are not available)
❑ Lack of a clinician trained in vaginal breech delivery
❑ Previous history of caesarean section

---

is recommended. There is no evidence that epidural anaesthesia is essential. Women should be given the choice of analgesia. Ranitidine, 150 mg orally must be administered every 6 hours in case caesarean delivery is required in future.

❖ At the time of labour, the risk factors for presence of breech presentation should be reviewed again (presence of placenta praevia, twins, etc.) and a complete abdominal and vaginal examination needs to be carried out.

❖ According to the eighth Annual Report of the confidential enquiry into stillbirths and deaths in infancy (CESDI), suboptimal care can be considered as the most avoidable factor for causing stillbirths and deaths amongst breech babies.[18] Since both the mother and the foetus are at an increased risk during the course of breech vaginal delivery, increased maternal and foetal surveillance is required in patients undergoing breech vaginal delivery in comparison to those foetuses with cephalic presentation. Close monitoring of maternal vital conditions, uterine contractions and FHR needs to be done. Close surveillance of FHR can be done using internal and external cardiotocographic techniques.

- Maternal IV line must be set up as the mother may require emergency induction of anaesthesia at any time
- Women should be advised to remain in bed to avoid the risk of PROM and cord prolapse. The foetal membranes must be left intact as long as possible; they must not be ruptured artificially, but allowed to rupture on their own in order to prevent the hazard of overt cord prolapse. In case the bag of membranes ruptures spontaneously, a per vaginal examination must be performed immediately to rule out cord prolapse.
- Active management of labour preferably using a partogram needs to be done. A satisfactory progress of labour is indicative of pelvic adequacy.
- In case of suspected foetal acidosis, foetal blood sampling from the buttocks is not advised due to an insufficient evidence base for this technique.
- Following ROM, a vaginal examination needs to be performed to rule out cord prolapse. It is advisable to do continuous FHR recording for 5–10 minutes following ROM to rule out occult cord prolapse.
- Breech presentation should be confirmed by an ultrasound examination in the labour ward
- Use of oxytocin induction and augmentation for breech presentation is controversial. Many clinicians fear that forceful uterine contractions induced by oxytocin could result in an incompletely dilated cervix and an entrapped head. Labour induction for breech presentation may be considered if individual circumstances are favourable. However, labour augmentation is generally not recommended.
- An anaesthesiologist and paediatrician should be present for all vaginal breech deliveries. A paediatrician is needed because of the higher prevalence of neonatal depression and an increased risk for unrecognised foetal anomalies. An anaesthesiologist may be needed if intrapartum complications develop and the patient requires general anaesthesia.
- Mother should be in dorsal lithotomy position for breech vaginal delivery
- Epidural analgesia should not be routinely advised. Women should be given a choice of analgesia during breech labour and birth. Lumbar epidural analgesia may be used to provide pain relief and to prevent voluntary bearing down efforts prior to complete dilatation of cervix. This would help to prevent the slipping of breech through a partially dilated cervix and the arrest of after-coming head of the breech.
- Routine episiotomy for every breech vaginal delivery is not required. However, if the clinician feels that the birth passage is too small, he/she must use his/her own discretion in giving an episiotomy. Episiotomy should be performed when indicated to facilitate delivery. Administration of an episiotomy helps in preventing soft tissue dystocia.
- In case of breech footling presentation, if the foetal feet prolapse through the vagina, treat expectantly as long as the FHR is stable to allow the cervix to completely dilate around the breech.
- Caesarean section should be considered if there is delay in the descent of the breech in the first or second stage of labour. Failure of the presenting part to descend may be a sign of relative foetopelvic disproportion.
- Delivery should be conducted in the operation theatre by 'assisted breech vaginal delivery' and an anaesthetist standby.

Steps for Assisted Breech Vaginal Delivery

During the assisted vaginal delivery, the following steps must be undertaken:

- Once the buttocks have entered the vagina and the cervix is fully dilated, the woman must be advised to bear down with the contractions
- Episiotomy may be performed, if the perineum appears very tight
- *Delivery of buttocks and lower back*: A 'no-touch policy or hands off the breech policy' must be adopted by the clinician until the buttocks and lower back deliver till the level of umbilicus. At this point, the baby's shoulder blades can be seen.
- Sometimes the clinician may have to make use of manoeuvres like Pinard's manoeuvre and groin traction (will be described later), if the legs have not delivered spontaneously.
- The clinician should be extremely careful and should gently hold the baby by wrapping it in a clean cloth in such a way that the baby's trunk is present anteriorly. This will allow the foetal head to enter the pelvis in occipitoanterior position.
- The baby must be held by the hips and not by the flanks or abdomen as this may cause kidney or liver damage. At no point, must the clinician try to pull the baby out; rather the patient must be encouraged to push down.
- In order to avoid compression on the umbilical cord, it should be moved to one side, preferably in the sacral bay.
- *Delivery of foetal shoulders and arm*: Appearance of axilla at the vulval outlet indicates that the time has come for the delivery of foetal shoulders. Two methods can be used:
  1. In the first method, once the scapula is visible at the vulval outlet, the trunk is rotated in clockwise direction by 90° in such a way that the anterior shoulder and arm appears at the vulva (Figs 27.5A to E). It can then be easily released and delivered. The body of the foetus is then rotated similarly in the reverse direction (anticlockwise) to deliver the other arm and shoulder.
  2. Second method is employed if the first method is unsuccessful. In the second method, the posterior shoulder is delivered first (described later in the text). Following the delivery of posterior arm, the body of the foetus is depressed to allow the anterior arm to slip out spontaneously. If this does not work, the obstetrician can use two fingers of right hand to sweep the anterior arm down over the thorax.
- *Nuchal arms*: Sometimes due to inappropriate traction and rotational manoeuvres, the shoulder is extended and elbow is flexed. In these cases, the forearm gets trapped behind the occiput. If the obstetrician tries to

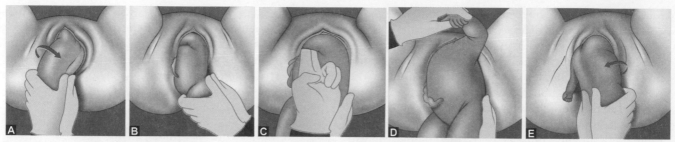

Figs 27.5A to E: Delivery of foetal shoulders and arms. (A) Rotation of foetal pelvis by 90° in clockwise direction; (B to D) Application of gentle traction to deliver the anterior shoulder, arm and forearm; (E) Rotation of the foetal pelvis in anticlockwise direction to deliver the posterior arm and forearm

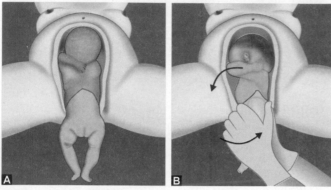

Figs 27.6A and B: Delivery of nuchal arm. (A) Forearm is trapped behind the occiput; (B) Rotation of foetal body in the direction in which the baby's hand is pointing

hook down the trapped arm, there may occur a fracture of the humerus. Therefore, in these cases, the following manoeuvre (Figs 27.6A and B) can be used—the foetus is rotated in the direction in which the baby's hand is pointing. This would cause the occiput to slip past the forearm. Friction of the rotation causes the shoulder to flex and become accessible for delivery.

❖ The obstetrician must wait to deliver the shoulders until axilla is visible. Attempts must not be made to release the arms immediately after the emergence of costal margins.

❖ The clinician must wait for the arms to deliver spontaneously. If arms are felt on chest, the clinician must allow the arms to disengage spontaneously one by one.

❖ Assistance should be provided only if necessary. After spontaneous delivery of the first arm, the buttocks must be lifted towards the mother's abdomen to enable the second arm to deliver spontaneously. If the arm does not spontaneously deliver, place one or two fingers in the elbow and bend the arm, bringing the hand down over the baby's face.

❖ If the arms still do not deliver, the clinician must reach into the vagina to determine their position. If they are flexed in front of the chest, gentle pressure must be applied to the crook of the elbow to straighten the arm and aid delivery.

❖ The same manoeuvre must be repeated with the other arm

❖ The clinician needs to be aware that there are other manoeuvres to deliver the arms and shoulders if needed, including Løvset's manoeuvre (described later)[19] to deliver the extended arms, which are stretched above the baby's head.

❖ Once the shoulders are delivered, the baby's body with the face down must be supported on the clinician's

forearm. The clinician must be careful not to compress the umbilical cord between the infant's body and their arm.

❖ One of the following manoeuvres, which would be described next, can be then used for delivery of after-coming head of the foetus.

Manoeuvres for Delivery of the After-coming Head

Delay in engagement of the after-coming head in the pelvis should be managed by the application of suprapubic pressure by an assistant. This manoeuvre is likely to help assist flexion of the foetal head. Other manoeuvres for assisting engagement of foetal head inside the pelvis, thereby facilitating its delivery include manoeuvres such as the Mauriceau-Smellie-Veit manoeuvre and Burns Marshall technique. Mauriceau-Smellie-Veit manoeuvre helps in displacing the head upwards and rotating it to the oblique diameter to facilitate its engagement. Presently, there is no evidence to indicate the best method that helps in assisting engagement of the foetal head in the pelvis. Concern has been expressed regarding the risks of the Burns-Marshall method if used incorrectly because in these cases, it can result in the overextension of the baby's neck. Delivery by forceps is also sometimes used for facilitating the delivery of foetal head.

If the above-mentioned conservative methods fail, symphysiotomy or caesarean section should be performed to facilitate delivery in case of obstructed after-coming head.

Burns-Marshall technique: Following the delivery of shoulders and both the arms, the baby must be let to hang unsupported from the mother's vulva. This would help in encouraging flexion of foetal head (Fig. 27.7A). The nursing staff must be further advised to apply suprapubic pressure in downward and backward direction in order to encourage further flexion of the baby's head. As the nape of baby's neck appears, efforts must be made by the clinician to deliver the baby's head by grasping the foetal ankles with the finger of right hand between the two.

Then the trunk is swung up forming a wide arc of the circle, while maintaining continuous traction when doing this (Fig. 27.7B). The left hand is used to provide pelvic support and to clear the perineum off successively from the baby's face and brow as the baby's head emerges out.

Mauriceau-Smellie-Veit manoeuvre: This is another commonly used manoeuvre for the delivery of after-coming foetal head and is named after the three clinicians who had described the method of using this grip. This manoeuvre comprises of the following steps:

❖ The baby is placed face down with the length of its body over the supinated left forearm and hand of the clinician.

❖ The clinician must then place the first (index) and second finger (middle finger) of this hand on the baby's cheekbones and the thumb over the baby's chin. This helps in facilitating flexion of the foetal head. In the method originally described by Mauriceau, Smellie and Veit, the index finger of the left hand was placed inside the baby's mouth. This is no longer advocated as placing a finger inside the infant's mouth is supposed to stimulate the vagal reflex. An assistant may provide suprapubic pressure to help the baby's head remain flexed.

❖ The right hand of the clinician is used for grasping the baby's shoulders. The little finger and the ring finger of the clinician's right hand is placed over the baby's right shoulder, the index finger over the baby's left shoulder and the middle finger over the baby's suboccipital region (Figs 27.8A to C). With the fingers of right hand in this position, the baby's head is flexed towards the chest. At

the same time left hand is used for applying downward pressure on the jaw to bring the baby's head down until the hairline is visible.

❖ Thereafter, the baby's trunk is carried in upwards and forward direction towards the maternal abdomen, till the baby's mouth, nose and brow and lastly the vertex and occiput are delivered.

❖ In this manoeuvre, the clinician uses both the arms simultaneously, in synchronisation to exert gentle downwards traction at the same time, both on the foetal neck and maxilla.

Delivery of after-coming head using forceps: Application of forceps (Fig. 27.9) is the technique of choice to ensure safe delivery of baby's head because it provides protection to the foetal head from sudden forces of compression and decompression. Also, the use of forceps helps in better maintenance of flexion of foetal head and helps in transmitting the force to the foetal head rather than the neck. This helps in reducing the risk of foetal injuries. Furthermore, flexion of foetal head helps in reducing the diameter of foetal head, thereby aiding descent. For delivery of foetal head using forceps, the following steps are required:

❖ Ordinary forceps or Piper's forceps (especially designed forceps with absent pelvic curve) or divergent Laufe's forceps can be used.

❖ While the clinician is applying forceps, the baby's body must be wrapped in a cloth or towel and held on one side by the assistant. Suspension of the baby in a towel prior to application of forceps helps in effectively holding the baby's body and keeping the arms out of the way. At the time of application of forceps, the assistant must hold the infant's body at or just above the horizontal plane. Assistant must be instructed not to hold the foetal body higher than this plane because hyperextension of foetal neck can cause injuries such as dislocation of cervical spine, bleeding in the venous plexus around the cervical spine and sometimes even quadriplegia.

❖ Left blade of the forceps is applied first followed by the right blade and the handles are locked.

❖ The forceps are used for both flexing and delivering the baby's head. During the initial descent of foetal head,

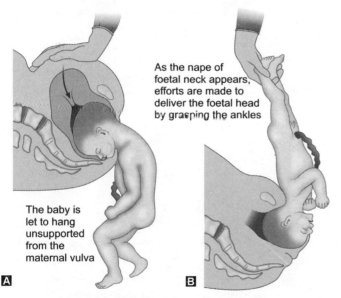

As the nape of foetal neck appears, efforts are made to deliver the foetal head by grasping the ankles

The baby is let to hang unsupported from the maternal vulva

A   **B**

Figs 27.7A and B: Burns-Marshall technique

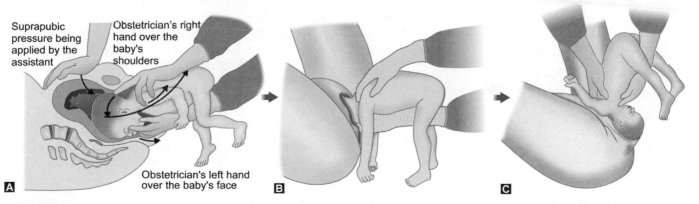

Suprapubic pressure being applied by the assistant

Obstetrician's right hand over the baby's shoulders

Obstetrician's left hand over the baby's face

A   **B**   **C**

Figs 27.8A to C: Mauriceau Smellie Veit manoeuvre. (A) The baby is laid flat over the obstetrician's forearm with the fingers of left hand over the baby's face and right hand over the occiput; (B) The baby's head is gradually flexed; (C) The baby's trunk is carried upwards and forwards to deliver the foetal head

CHAPTER 27

foetal body must remain in horizontal plane. Once the chin and mouth are visible over the perineum, the forceps, body and legs of the foetus are raised to complete the delivery.

❖ The head must be delivered slowly over 1 minute in order to avoid sudden compression or decompression of foetal head, which may be a cause for intracranial haemorrhage.

Delivery of Baby's Shoulders

Reverse Prague's manoeuvre: At times, the back of foetus may fail to rotate anteriorly. In these cases, stronger traction on foetal legs or bony pelvis may be applied to turn the back anterior. If the baby's back still remains posterior, head can be extracted using Mauriceau manoeuvre and delivering the baby with back down. Alternatively, modified Prague's manoeuvre can be used (Fig. 27.10). In this manoeuvre, two fingers of obstetrician's one hand grasp the shoulders of back down foetus from below and exert traction in downward and backward direction. Simultaneously, the other hand draws the feet up over the maternal abdomen to flex the infant and aid the delivery of the occiput.

Løvset's manoeuvre: If the baby's arms are stretched above the head, the manoeuvre called Løvset's manoeuvre is used for delivery of foetal arms. This manoeuvre is based on the principle that due to the curved shape of the birth canal, when the anterior shoulder is above the pubic symphysis, the posterior shoulder would be below the level of pubic symphysis. The manoeuvre should be initiated only when the foetal scapula becomes visible underneath the pubic arch and includes the following steps (Figs 27.11A to C):

❖ First, the baby is lifted slightly to cause lateral flexion of the trunk.

❖ Then the baby, which is held by pelvifemoral grip, is turned by half a circle, keeping the back uppermost. Simultaneously, downward traction is applied so that the arm that was initially posterior and below the level of pubic symphysis now becomes anterior and can be delivered under the pubic arch.

❖ Delivery of the arm can be assisted by placing one or two fingers on the upper part of the arm. Then the arm is gradually drawn down over the chest as the elbow is flexed, with the hand sweeping over the face.

❖ In order to deliver the second arm, the baby is again turned by 180° in the reverse direction, keeping the back

uppermost and applying downward traction and then delivering the second arm in the same way under the pubic arch as the first arm was delivered.

Delivery of the Posterior Shoulder

If the clinician is unable to turn the baby's body to deliver the arm that is anterior first, through Løvset's manoeuvre, then the clinician can deliver the shoulder that is posterior first

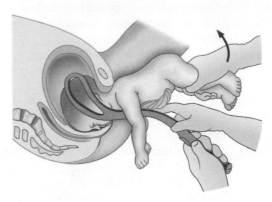

Fig. 27.9: Delivery of after-coming head of the breech using forceps

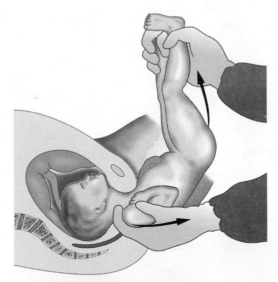

Fig. 27.10: Prague's manoeuvre

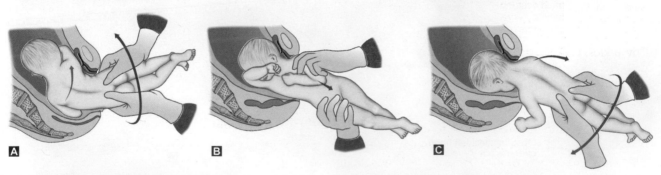

Figs 27.11A to C: Løvset's manoeuvre. (A) Trunk is rotated through 180° keeping the back anterior. This causes the posterior arm to emerge under pubic arch; (B) Posterior arm is hooked out; (C) Trunk is rotated in reverse direction to deliver the anterior shoulder

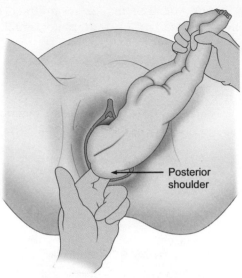

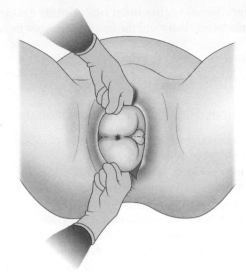

Fig. 27.12: Delivery of posterior shoulder

Fig. 27.13: Groin traction

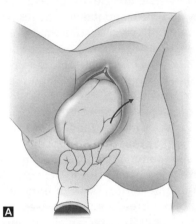

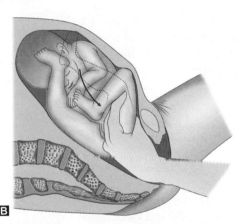

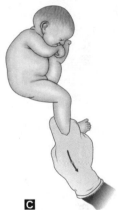

Figs 27.14A to C: Pinard's manoeuvre. (A) Pressure is exerted against the foetal popliteal fossa; (B) Due to application of pressure, the foetal knee gets flexed and abducted; (C) As the foetal leg moves downward, it is pulled out by the clinician

(Fig. 27.12).[19] Delivery of the posterior shoulder involves the following steps:

* The clinician must hold and lift the baby up by the ankles. At the same time, the baby's chest must be moved towards the woman's inner thighs. The clinician must then hook the baby shoulder with fingers of his/her hand. This would help in delivering the shoulder that is posterior, followed by the delivery of arm and hand.
* Then the baby's back should be lowered down, still holding it by ankles. This helps in the delivery of anterior shoulder followed by the arm and hand.

Delivery of Baby's Legs

Groin traction: If the buttocks and hip do not deliver by themselves, the clinician can make use of simple manoeuvres including groin traction or Pinard's manoeuvre to deliver the legs. Groin traction could be of two types: single or double groin traction. In single groin traction, the index finger of one hand is hooked in the groin fold and traction is exerted towards the foetal trunk rather than towards the foetal femur, in accordance with the uterine contractions. In double groin traction, the index fingers of both the hands are hooked in the groin folds and then traction is applied (Fig. 27.13).

Pinard's manoeuvre: In this manoeuvre pressure is exerted against the inner aspect of the knee (popliteal fossa), with help of the middle and index fingers of the clinician (Fig. 27.14A). As the pressure is applied, the knee gets flexed and abducted. This causes the lower leg to move downwards, which is then swept medially and gently pulled out of the vagina (Figs 27.14B and C).

Postdelivery Care

* The baby's mouth and nose must be suctioned.
* The cord must be clamped and cut.
* Active management of the third stage of labour needs to be done.

❖ The cervix and vagina must be carefully examined for presence of any tears and the episiotomy must be repaired.

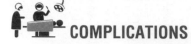 **COMPLICATIONS**

Complications Related to External Cephalic Version

Complications related to ECV are as follows:
❖ Failure of the procedure
❖ Premature onset of labour, PROM
❖ Small amount of foetomaternal haemorrhage, resulting in the development of Rh isoimmunisation
❖ Foetal distress leading to an emergency caesarean delivery
❖ Risk of cord entanglement and transient reduction of the FHR
❖ Forceful attempt at version may result in placental abruption.

Complications Related to Breech Presentation Per se

Foetal Complications

❖ *Low APGAR Scores*: Low APGAR scores, especially at 1 minute of birth are more common with vaginal breech deliveries and could be related to birth asphyxia. Increased risk of birth asphyxia in cases of breech vaginal delivery could be due to the following causes:
  • Cord compression
  • Cord prolapse
  • Premature attempts by the baby to breathe while the head is still inside the uterine cavity
  • Delay in the delivery of the head often due to head entrapment.
❖ *Foetal head entrapment*: Foetal head entrapment may result from an incompletely dilated cervix and foetal head that lacks time to mould to the maternal pelvis. This occurs in 0–8.5% of vaginal breech deliveries. This percentage is higher with preterm foetuses (<32 weeks), when the head is larger in comparison to the rest of the body. In most of the cases, foetal head entrapment is also associated with umbilical cord compression. Therefore, this condition must be dealt with urgently. Sometimes, with gentle traction on the foetal body, the cervix can be manually slipped over the occiput. If this does not work, Dührssen incisions, i.e. 1–3 cm deep cervical incisions made through several portions of the cervical canal (to facilitate delivery of the foetal head) may be necessary to relieve cervical entrapment (Fig. 27.15). However, severe haemorrhage and extension can occur into the lower segment of the uterus.

  Therefore, the operator must be equipped to deal with this complication. Alternatively, 100 µg of IV nitroglycerin can be used to provide cervical relaxation. General anaesthesia can also be used in extreme cases.
❖ *Preterm birth*: Preterm birth (delivery of baby at <28 weeks) commonly occurs in breech presentation. Preterm birth can often result in complications related to prematurity.
❖ *Neonatal trauma/injuries*: Neonatal trauma including brachial plexus injuries, haematomas, fractures, visceral

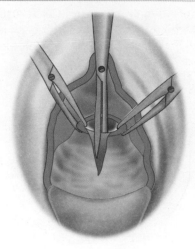

Fig. 27.15: Dührssen incision

injuries, etc. can occur in about 25% of cases. There can be fractures of humerus, clavicle and/or femur. Haematomas of sternocleidomastoid muscle can also commonly occur. However, they disappear spontaneously. Testicular injury resulting in anorchia may also sometimes follow breech vaginal delivery. Pressure on the brachial plexus by the obstetrician's fingers exerting traction may cause the paralysis of upper extremity. Brachial plexus injury can also be caused by overstretching of neck while freeing the arms. This carries a poor prognosis for shoulder function. Risks of foetal injuries may be reduced by avoiding rapid extraction of the infant during delivery of the body. Cervical spine injury is predominantly observed when the foetus has a hyperextended head prior to delivery. Successive compression and decompression of unmoulded after-coming head of the breech and increased risk of head entrapment can result in intracranial haemorrhage and tentorial tears.
❖ *Cord prolapse*: Cord prolapse is a condition associated with abnormal descent of the umbilical cord before the descent of the foetal presenting part. Cord prolapse has been described in details later in this chapter.

Maternal Complications

There may be an increased maternal morbidity and mortality due to higher incidence of operative delivery. There also may be an increased incidence of traumatic injuries to the genital tract.

 CLINICAL PEARLS

❖ Depending on the relationship of the sacrum with the sacroiliac joint, the positions of the breech, which are possible, include the left sacroanterior (LSA) position; right sacroanterior (RSA) position; right sacroposterior (RSP) position and left sacroposterior (LSP) position. Of these various positions, LSA is the most common.
❖ Regular drill and conduct of vaginal breech delivery should be followed in all maternity units across the UK.

PART II

- As per the recommendations by RCOG (2006), all women in the UK with an uncomplicated breech pregnancy at term should be offered ECV, provided there are no contra-indications.
- For taking the decision regarding whether to attempt vaginal delivery or plan an elective caesarean section, current RCOG guidelines suggest that the women should be counselled fully regarding the advantages and disadvantages of each mode of delivery. The final decision should then be based on informed-decision making by the patient in partnership with her healthcare professional and currently available evidence.
- While conducting the breech vaginal delivery, at no point, the clinician must try to pull the baby out; rather the patient must be encouraged to push down.

EVIDENCE-BASED MEDICINE

- The use of tocolysis should be considered where an initial attempt at ECV without tocolysis has failed. The success rate of ECV is likely to be increased with the use of tocolysis with agents such as ritodrine, salbutamol and terbutaline. However, use of glyceryl trinitrate (GTN) either as a patch or sublingually, or nifedipine are not likely to be beneficial.[20,21]
- There is no evidence that the mode of delivery (vaginal delivery vs planned caesarean section) would influence the long-term health of babies with a breech presentation delivered at term.[3]
- The current evidence indicates that the proven benefits to the preterm baby are not related to the mode of delivery, rather to the factors such as the use of antenatal steroids, consideration of maternal magnesium sulphate infusion for foetal neuroprotection, delayed cord clamping, etc.[10,11]
- There is insufficient evidence to support the use of postural management or moxibustion as a method of promoting spontaneous version over ECV.[22,23] Moxibustion is a traditional Chinese therapy involving the rubbing of a dried herb, mugwort (moxa) over certain body points and is not recommended as a method of promoting spontaneous version over ECV.

TRANSVERSE LIE

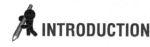

INTRODUCTION

Transverse lie is an abnormal foetal presentation in which the foetus lies transversely with the shoulders presenting in the lower pole of the uterus. As a result, the presenting part becomes the foetal shoulder. The denominator is the foetal back. Depending on whether the position of the foetal back is anterior, posterior, superior or inferior (Fig. 27.16), the following positions are possible: dorsoanterior (foetal

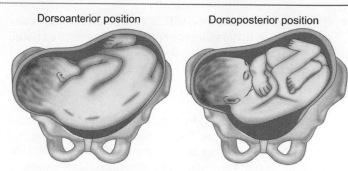

Dorsoanterior position   Dorsoposterior position

Fig. 27.16: Different positions of transverse lie

back is anterior); dorsoposterior (foetal back is posterior); dorsosuperior (foetal back is directed superiorly) and dorso-inferior (foetal back is directed inferiorly).

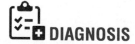

AETIOLOGY

The risk factors for transverse lie are as follows:[24]

- *Maternal*: Maternal risk factors for transverse lie are: cephalopelvic disproportion, contracted maternal pelvis liquor abnormalities (polyhydramnios and oligohydram-nios); uterine anomalies (bicornuate, septate, etc.); presence of pelvic tumours and other space occupying lesions (e.g. fibroids in the lower uterine segment); placental abnormalities (placenta praevia, cornuofundal attachment of placenta); multiparity (especially grand multiparas).
- *Foetal*: Foetal risk factors for transverse lie are: prematurity, twins, hydramnios, intrauterine foetal death, foetal anomalies, etc.

DIAGNOSIS

Clinical Presentation

The findings on examination are as follows:[25]

Abdominal Examination

- Foetal lie is in the horizontal plane with foetal head on one side of the midline and podalic pole on the other.
- The abdomen often appears barrel-shaped and is asymmetrical.
- Fundal height is less than the period of amenorrhoea.
- *First Leopold's manoeuvre or fundal grip*: No foetal pole (either breech or cephalic) is palpable on the fundal grip.
- *Second Leopold's manoeuvre/lateral grip*: Soft, broad, smooth irregular part suggestive of foetal breech is present on one side of the midline, while a smooth hard globular part suggestive of the foetal head is present on the other side of the midline.
- *Third Leopold's manoeuvre*: Pelvic grip appears to be empty during the time of pregnancy. It may be occupied by the shoulder at the time of labour.

❖ *Foetal heart auscultation*: FHR is easily heard much below the umbilicus in dorsoanterior position. On the other hand, in dorsoposterior position, the foetal heart may be located at a much higher level and is often above the umbilicus.

Vaginal Examination

On vaginal examination during the antenatal period, the pelvis appears to be empty. Even if something is felt on vaginal examination, no definite foetal part may be identified. At the time of labour, on vaginal examination, foetal shoulder including scapula, clavicle, humerus and grid-iron feel of foetal ribs can be palpated. Due to ill-fitting foetal part, an elongated bag of membranes may be felt on vaginal examination. If the membranes have ruptured, the foetal shoulder can be identified by feeling the acromion process, scapula, clavicle, axilla, ribs and intercostal spaces. If the arm prolapse has occurred, the foetal arm might be observed lying outside the vagina.

Investigations

Ultrasound examination: Ultrasound helps in confirming the transverse lie (Fig. 27.17). The other things, which can be observed on the ultrasound, include the following: presence of uterine and/or foetal anomalies; foetal maturity; placental location and grading; adequacy of liquor and ruling out the presence of multiple pregnancy.

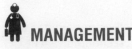

MANAGEMENT

Algorithm for management of transverse lie is described in Flow chart 27.1.[26-28]

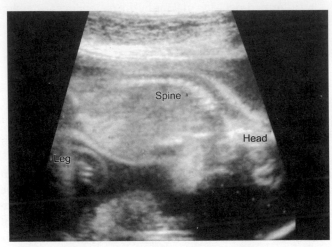

Fig. 27.17: Ultrasound examination at 24 weeks showing transverse lie

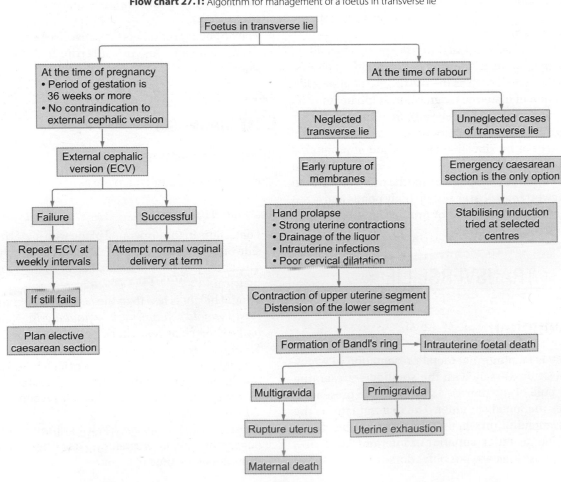

Flow chart 27.1: Algorithm for management of a foetus in transverse lie

Foetus in transverse lie

At the time of pregnancy
• Period of gestation is 36 weeks or more
• No contraindication to external cephalic version

External cephalic version (ECV)

Failure → Repeat ECV at weekly intervals → If still fails → Plan elective caesarean section

Successful → Attempt normal vaginal delivery at term

At the time of labour

Neglected transverse lie → Early rupture of membranes → Hand prolapse
• Strong uterine contractions
• Drainage of the liquor
• Intrauterine infections
• Poor cervical dilatation

Contraction of upper uterine segment
Distension of the lower segment

Formation of Bandl's ring → Intrauterine foetal death

Multigravida → Rupture uterus → Maternal death

Primigravida → Uterine exhaustion

Unneglected cases of transverse lie → Emergency caesarean section is the only option → Stabilising induction tried at selected centres

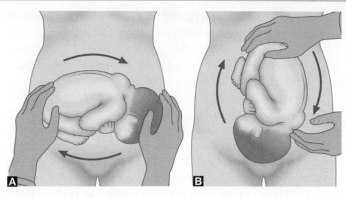

Figs 27.18A and B: Procedure for ECV in case of transverse lie

Management during pregnancy: The management options for transverse lie include ECV during pregnancy (Figs 27.18A and B) or delivery by caesarean section (elective or an emergency). If the version is unsuccessful, the only option for delivering the foetus in transverse lie is performing a caesarean delivery.

Management during labour: If the maternal and foetal conditions are stable, the best option in these cases would be to perform a caesarean section.

At some centres, stabilising induction is used for converting transverse to cephalic presentation at the time of labour. In these cases, the patient is taken to the operation theatre with all facilities available for an emergency caesarean delivery if required. ECV is firstly performed. A clinical pelvimetry is then done to rule out any cephalopelvic disproportion. Foetal membranes are ruptured in a controlled manner. Oxytocin infusion can be started in a controlled manner if the patient is not getting adequate uterine contractions. Continuous electronic foetal monitoring should be done to ensure the foetal well-being.

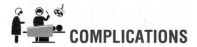

COMPLICATIONS

Complications related to version: These have been previously described.

Foetal arm prolapse: Due to the ill-fitting foetal part, the sudden ROM can result in the escape of large amount of liquor and the prolapse of foetal arm, which is often accompanied by a loop of cord.

Obstructed labour: If the transverse lie with or without a prolapsed arm is left neglected, a serious complication including obstructed labour can occur. If the uterine obstruction is not immediately relieved, uterine inertia or rupture of the uterus can occur in primigravida and multigravida patients respectively.

Long-term complications: Long-term maternal complications include development of genitourinary fistulas, secondary amenorrhoea (related to Sheehan's syndrome associated with PPH), hysterectomy, etc.

Foetal asphyxia: Tonic uterine contractions can interfere with uteroplacental circulation resulting in foetal distress. Other foetal complications may include preterm birth, PROM, intrauterine foetal death and increased foetal mortality.

CLINICAL PEARLS

❖ Ribs and intercostal spaces upon palpation give feeling of grid-iron on vaginal examination.
❖ While doing the ECV, the foetus should be moved gently rather than using forceful movements.
❖ There is no mechanism of labour for a foetus in transverse lie, which remains uncorrected until term. A caesarean section is required to deliver the baby with shoulder presentation.

EVIDENCE-BASED MEDICINE

Caesarean delivery may sometimes become difficult in these cases and consideration must be given towards the administration of a vertical uterine incision. Transverse lie is the commonest indication for classical caesarean delivery (a vertical uterine incision, but a low transverse skin incision).[26,27]

UNSTABLE LIE

INTRODUCTION

Unstable lie can be defined as a condition in which the foetal lie may be oblique or transverse and the foetal presentation may vary at different periods of examination after 38 weeks of gestation.[28]

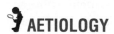

AETIOLOGY

The probable causes for unstable lie are as follows:[29]

Maternal

❖ Grand multipara (progressive laxity of the uterine musculature)
❖ Polyhydramnios
❖ Placenta praevia
❖ Presence of a pelvic tumour
❖ Contracted maternal pelvis.

Foetal Causes

❖ Hydrocephalus
❖ Tumours of the foetal neck or sacrum
❖ Foetal neuromuscular dysfunction.

CHAPTER 27

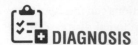

DIAGNOSIS

Clinical Presentation

There is absence of the foetal pole in the pelvis on abdominal or vaginal examination either in the antenatal period or during labour.

Investigations

Ultrasound examination helps in the confirmation of diagnosis, measurement of the liquor volume, evaluation of placental location, foetal anomalies, pelvic tumours, congenital uterine anomalies, etc.

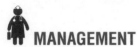

MANAGEMENT

Management options in case of an unstable lie comprise of the following:[30,31]

❖ In presence of an obstructive foetal or uterine pathology, caesarean delivery must be planned at an appropriate period of gestation.

❖ A classical caesarean delivery may be sometimes required based on the extent of the anomaly. The woman should be counselled in advance regarding this possibility. She should also be counselled regarding the increased risk of complications such as cord prolapse and rupture of membranes. She should be advised to immediately report to the hospital in case she experiences any of these complications.

❖ In cases of transverse, oblique or unstable lie, the clinician must discuss elective admission to hospital after 37^{+0} weeks of gestation with the patient due to a small risk of cord prolapse. Two types of management plans can be adopted, conservative or active. The pros and cons of each option must be explained to the patient before she can make a choice regarding the management plan and whether or not she wants to be admitted in the hospital.

  • *Conservative management*: If there are no other contra-indications to vaginal delivery, it is sensible to wait until 41–42 weeks to allow spontaneous version and possible vaginal delivery. In majority of cases, spontaneous version to the longitudinal lie may occur prior to the ROM or the onset of labour. If the foetal lie remains non-longitudinal until term or post-term, the obstetrician must opt for a caesarean delivery.

  • *Active management*: In these cases, an ECV is attempted to convert an unstable lie into a longitudinal one. The patient is then discharged home if the lie continues to remain longitudinal. Recent RCOG guidelines recommend that ECV for unstable lie should be pre-ferably performed with immediate induction, also known as stabilising induction.[16] This, however, may be associated with a significant intrapartum complication

rate. Al-Sibai has reported a success rate of more than 60% for stabilising induction at term in a retrospective study comprising of 1,330 grand multipara.[32] Caesarean delivery may be required if the stabilising induction is unsuccessful. Stabilising induction or caesarean delivery is usually delayed until 39 weeks of gestation to promote foetal lung maturity.

Prior to giving stabilising induction, the clinician must ensure that the cervix is favourable. Facilities for an emergency caesarean delivery must also be available in the event of cord prolapse. If the patient presents early in labour, ECV can be attempted with an early recourse to caesarean section if the attempt at ECV is unsuccessful. ECV should not be attempted if the membranes have ruptured.

COMPLICATIONS

Unstable lie can be associated with the following complications:

❖ Umbilical cord prolapse
❖ Premature rupture of membranes
❖ Increased requirement for operative delivery
❖ Complications associated with ECV (previously described in the text).

EVIDENCE-BASED MEDICINE

A vertical uterine incision (classical caesarean section) is sometimes required because the baby's delivery may be complicated due to the lack of liquor or difficulty in manoeuvring the foetus into a longitudinal lie.[30]

COMPOUND PRESENTATION

INTRODUCTION

In compound presentation, one or two of the foetal extremities enter the pelvis simultaneously with the presenting part. The most common combinations are head-hand (Fig. 27.19), breech-hand and head-arm-foot.

AETIOLOGY

The predisposing factors for the development of compound presentation include the following:

❖ Prematurity
❖ Multiparity
❖ Twin or multiple pregnancy
❖ Pelvic tumours
❖ Cephalopelvic disproportion
❖ Macerated foetus.

PART II

DIAGNOSIS

Clinical Presentation

The diagnosis is confirmed on vaginal examination.

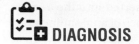 **OBSTETRIC MANAGEMENT**

In most cases, the prolapsed extremity does not cause any interference with the normal progress of labour and vaginal delivery. In most of the cases, the prolapsed limbs spontaneously rise up with the descent of the presenting part. In presence of cephalopelvic disproportion and/or cord prolapse, caesarean section is required.

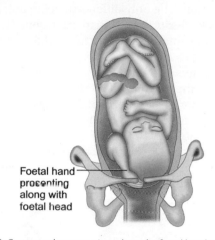

Fig. 27.19: Compound presentation where the foetal hand is seen to be entering the pelvis

 COMPLICATIONS

❖ The most common complication associated with compound presentation is cord prolapse.
❖ Temptation to replace the limb early during labour is associated with an increased maternal and foetal mortality and morbidity.

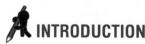 **EVIDENCE-BASED MEDICINE**

❖ Compound presentation involving the presence of limbs alongside the vertex may often resolve and result in vaginal delivery if the progress is satisfactory.[33]
❖ All other compound presentations require delivery via caesarean section if the foetus is alive.[33]

FACE PRESENTATION

INTRODUCTION

This is an abnormal foetal position characterised by an extreme extension of the foetal head so that the foetal face rather than the foetal head becomes the presenting part and the foetal occiput comes in direct contact with the back. Denominator in these cases is mentum or chin. Four positions are possible depending on the position of the chin with left or right sacroiliac joints (Fig. 27.20): (1) right mentoposterior position (deflexed LOA); (2) left mentoposterior position (deflexed

CHAPTER 27

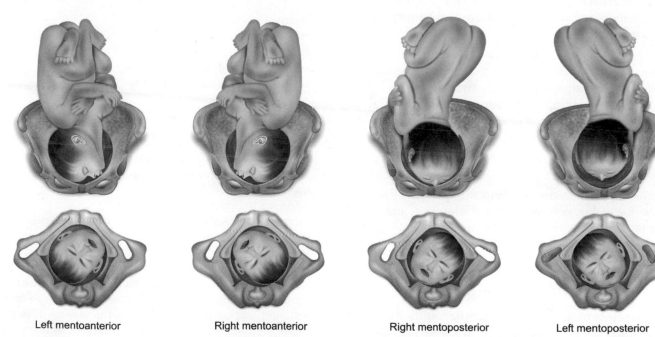

Left mentoanterior   Right mentoanterior   Right mentoposterior   Left mentoposterior

Fig. 27.20: Different positions in face presentation

ROA); (3) left mentoanterior position (deflexed ROP); (4) right mentoanterior position (deflexed LOP). The most common type of face presentation is left mentoanterior position.

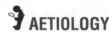

AETIOLOGY

Maternal Causes

❖ Multiparity with pendulous abdomen
❖ Contracted pelvis
❖ Face presentation is likely to be associated with poly-hydramnios and macrosomia and therefore may be commonly encountered amongst diabetic women.

Foetal Causes

❖ Congenital causes (anencephaly, congenital goitre, congenital bronchocele, etc.)
❖ Several twists of cord around foetal neck
❖ Dolichocephalic head (with long anterior-posterior diameter)
❖ Increased tone of extensor group of muscle.

DIAGNOSIS

Clinical Examination

Abdominal examination: In case of mentoanterior positions, the foetal limbs can be palpated anteriorly. Foetal chest is also present anteriorly against the uterine wall. The FHS is thus clearly audible. On abdominal palpation, the groove between the head and neck is not prominent and cephalic prominence lies on the same side as the foetal back. Sometimes on abdominal palpation, a deep depression may be felt between the anterior shoulders and the foetal head, where no foetal part can be felt. On pelvic grip, the head is not engaged. In case of mentoposterior positions, the back is better palpated towards the front.[34]

Vaginal examination: Diagnosis of face presentation is made on vaginal examination. On the vaginal examination, the following structures can be felt: Alveolar margins of the mouth, nose, malar eminences, supraorbital ridges and the mentum. There is absence of meconium staining on the examining fingers, unlike in breech presentation.

Investigations

Ultrasonography: Ultrasonography must be performed in order to assess foetal size, presence of foetal anomalies and to rule out the presence of any bony congenital pelvic malformations.

DIFFERENTIAL DIAGNOSIS

Diagnosis of face presentation can often be confused with that of breech presentation. This can be differentiated from breech presentation with the help of following two rules given next.

1. When the examining finger is inserted into the anus, it offers resistance due to the presence of anal sphincters.
2. Anus is present in line with the ischial tuberosities, whereas the mouth and malar prominences form a triangle.

OBSTETRIC MANAGEMENT

Delivery occurs spontaneously in most of the cases of anterior face presentation. In presence of normal cervical dilatation and descent, there is no need for the health care professional to intervene. Labour will be longer, but if the pelvis is adequate and the head rotates to a mentoanterior position, a vaginal delivery can be expected. It can be assisted with help of forceps and appropriate analgesia. The mechanism of delivery and corresponding body movements in case of anterior face presentations are similar to that of the corresponding occipito-anterior position. The only difference being that delivery of head occurs by flexion rather than extension. The engaging diameter is submentobregmatic in case of a fully extended head. If the head rotates backward to a mentoposterior position, a caesarean section may be required. In case of posterior face presentations, the mechanism of delivery is same as that of occipitoposterior position except that the anterior rotation of the mentum occurs in only 20–30% of the cases.[35] In the remaining 70–80% cases, there may be incomplete anterior rotation, no rotation or short posterior rotation of mentum. There is no possibility of spontaneous vaginal delivery in case of persistent mentoposterior positions. Caesarean section may be required in these cases.

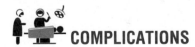

COMPLICATIONS

Maternal

❖ Delayed labour
❖ Risk of perineal injuries or damage to the sphincters
❖ Postpartum haemorrhage
❖ Increased rate of operative deliveries
❖ Second-stage caesarean delivery.

Foetal

❖ Caput formation and moulding
❖ Increased chances of cord prolapse
❖ Foetal cerebral congestion due to poor venous return from head and neck
❖ Neonatal infection
❖ Increased maternal morbidity due to operative delivery and vaginal manipulation
❖ Neglected cases of face presentation may result in obstructed labour and uterine rupture.
❖ Marked caput formation and moulding may distort the entire face. Facial soft tissue trauma in form of facial bruising and oedema can persist for several days and cause difficulty in feeding. This usually subsides within a few days.

CLINICAL PEARLS

❖ On abdominal examination in case of face presentation, head feels big and is often not engaged. Although the engaging diameter of the head in flexed vertex and face presentation is the same [submentobregmatic in face (9.5 cm) and suboccipitobregmatic in case of vertex (9.5 cm)], the clinical course of labour is significantly delayed. This could be due to the ill-fitting face in the lower uterine segment, which results in delayed engagement due to the absence of moulding.

❖ While conducting a normal vaginal delivery, one should wait for spontaneous delivery. Liberal mediolateral episiotomy must be given to protect the perineum against injuries.

❖ Forceps may be applied in case of delay

❖ Indications for an elective caesarean section in case of face presentation include coexisting conditions such as contracted pelvis, large-sized baby or presence of associated complicating factors.

EVIDENCE-BASED MEDICINE

❖ In cases of delayed progress of labour, augmentation is sometimes done. However, this is not recommended and the obstetrician must preferably proceed to a caesarean delivery, which helps in reducing maternal and foetal complications.[35]

❖ Delivery by vacuum is contraindicated in cases of face presentation.[35]

BROW PRESENTATION

INTRODUCTION

This is a type of cephalic presentation where the foetal head is incompletely flexed (Fig. 27.21). The head is short of complete extension, which could have resulted in a face presentation. As a result, presenting part becomes the brow.

AETIOLOGY

The predisposing factors for the brow presentation are similar to that for face presentation.

DIAGNOSIS

Abdominal Examination

Findings on abdominal examination are similar to that of face presentation.

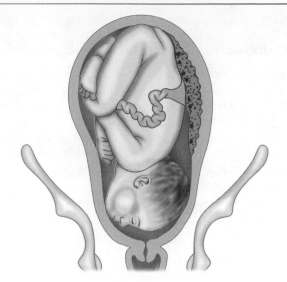

Fig. 27.21: Brow presentation

Vaginal Examination

Brow presentation can be confirmed on vaginal examination due to the presence of supraorbital ridges and anterior fontanelle.

Investigations

Ultrasonography: This helps in ruling out the presence of any congenital malformations.

OBSTETRIC MANAGEMENT

Since the engaging diameter of the head is mentovertical (14 cm), there would be no mechanism of labour with an average-sized baby and a normal pelvis.[36] Vaginal delivery may be the possible option only in cases where there is spontaneous conversion to face or vertex presentation. Therefore, after ruling out the cephalopelvic disproportion and foetal congenital anomalies, the obstetrician must await spontaneous delivery. In cases where this does not occur, caesarean section is the best method of treatment.

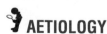

COMPLICATIONS

❖ Obstructed labour and uterine rupture can occur in cases of neglected brow presentation

❖ There can be considerable amount of moulding and caput formation of the foetal skull.

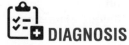

CLINICAL PEARLS

Brow presentation may temporarily persist as it may get converted to either a vertex or face presentation with complete flexion or extension respectively.

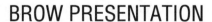

EVIDENCE-BASED MEDICINE

❖ Caesarean delivery is advised in cases where there is a failure to progress in the late first or second stages of labour. Delayed progress of labour should raise the suspicion of abnormal presentation.[36]

❖ Use of syntocinon for either induction or augmentation of labour is not recommended in these cases because it is likely to result in uterine rupture.[37]

OCCIPITOPOSTERIOR POSITION

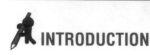

INTRODUCTION

This is a type of abnormal position of the vertex where the occiput is placed over the left sacroiliac joint [left occipito-posterior (LOP) or 4th vertex] or right sacroiliac joint [right occipitoposterior (ROP) or 3rd vertex] (Figs 27.22A and B) or directly over the sacrum [direct occipitoposterior (OP) position]. ROP position is more common than the LOP position as dextrorotation of the uterus favours ROP if the back is on right side. Also, the left oblique diameter is slightly reduced in size due to the presence of sigmoid colon due to which the right oblique diameter is slightly longer than the left oblique diameter. OP position can be considered as an abnormal position of the vertex rather than an abnormal presentation. It can be of two types:

1. *Primary*: Occurrence of the OP position before the onset of labour and during the antenatal period
2. *Secondary*: Occurrence of the OP position during the labour.

Caesarean section is not indicated per se in the cases of OP position. Most of the foetuses in OP position before labour rotate back into occipitoanterior (OA) position in the intrapartum period. Persistence of the OP position is important because it can be associated with labour abnormalities and numerous maternal and neonatal complications (e.g. birth trauma, neonatal acidosis, etc.). The likely outcomes in case of OP position are summarised in Flow chart 27.2.

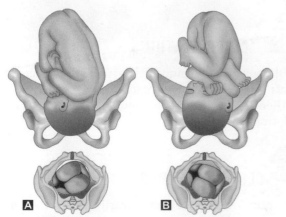

Figs 27.22A and B: (A) Left occipitoanterior position and (B) Left occipitoposterior position

AETIOLOGY

Occipitoposterior position can be related to the following conditions:

❖ Presence of an anthropoid or android pelvis
❖ Marked deflexion of foetal head
❖ High pelvic inclination
❖ Attachment of placenta on the anterior uterine wall
❖ Brachycephaly of foetal head
❖ Abnormal uterine contractions.

DIAGNOSIS

Clinical Presentation

Symptoms suggestive of OP position are as follows:

❖ Early ROMs
❖ Backache which worsens with progress of labour
❖ Frequent filling of the bladder
❖ Prolongation of labour (in nulliparous women, the labour may be prolonged).

Abdominal Examination

The following findings may be observed on abdominal examination:

❖ On abdominal inspection, there is flattening of the abdomen below the umbilicus. The abdominal contour may appear concave (scaphoid).
❖ There may be a depression at or immediately below the umbilicus in the OP position. On the other hand, there is fullness of the abdomen below the umbilicus in OA position.
❖ In OP position, the foetal back is directed posteriorly, whereas the limbs are directed anteriorly. As a result, the abdomen looks flattened due to the absence of round contour of the foetal back.
❖ Foetal limbs are palpated more easily nearly the midline on either side
❖ Foetal back and anterior shoulders are far away from the midline
❖ On pelvic grip, the head is not engaged. The cephalic prominence is not felt as prominently as felt in OA position (Figs 27.23A and B). The FHS is difficult to locate and may be best heard in the flanks.

Vaginal Examination

The following findings may be observed on vaginal examination:

❖ Presence of an elongated bag of membranes
❖ Sagittal sutures occupy any of the oblique diameters of the pelvis
❖ Posterior fontanelle and lambdoid suture are felt near the sacroiliac joint
❖ Anterior fontanelle can be felt more easily due to the deflexed head and at times it may be at a lower level than the posterior one. Anterior fontanelle would be

Flow chart 27.2: Occipitoposterior position and its likely outcomes

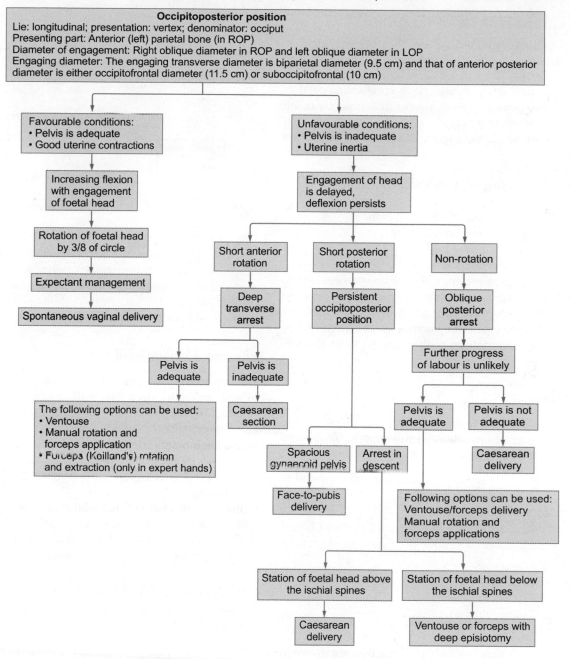

Occipitoposterior position
Lie: longitudinal; presentation: vertex; denominator: occiput
Presenting part: Anterior (left) parietal bone (in ROP)
Diameter of engagement: Right oblique diameter in ROP and left oblique diameter in LOP
Engaging diameter: The engaging transverse diameter is biparietal diameter (9.5 cm) and that of anterior posterior diameter is either occipitofrontal diameter (11.5 cm) or suboccipitofrontal (10 cm)

Favourable conditions:
• Pelvis is adequate
• Good uterine contractions

Unfavourable conditions:
• Pelvis is inadequate
• Uterine inertia

Increasing flexion with engagement of foetal head

Engagement of head is delayed, deflexion persists

Rotation of foetal head by 3/8 of circle

Short anterior rotation

Short posterior rotation

Non-rotation

Expectant management

Deep transverse arrest

Persistent occipitoposterior position

Oblique posterior arrest

Spontaneous vaginal delivery

Pelvis is adequate

Pelvis is inadequate

Further progress of labour is unlikely

The following options can be used:
• Ventouse
• Manual rotation and forceps application
• Forceps (Koilland's) rotation and extraction (only in expert hands)

Caesarean section

Pelvis is adequate

Pelvis is not adequate

Spacious gynaecoid pelvis

Arrest in descent

Caesarean delivery

Face-to-pubis delivery

Following options can be used:
Ventouse/forceps delivery
Manual rotation and forceps applications

Station of foetal head above the ischial spines

Station of foetal head below the ischial spines

Caesarean delivery

Ventouse or forceps with deep episiotomy

CHAPTER 27

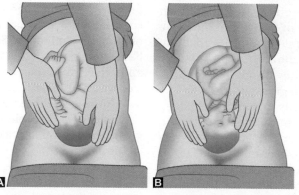

Figs 27.23A and B: Palpation of the foetal head (third pelvic grip): (A) Occipitoanterior position; (B) Occipitoposterior position

felt anteriorly, while the posterior fontanelle would be posterior and hence difficult to feel, especially if the head is deflexed.

❖ Sagittal sutures would be in one of the oblique diameters of maternal pelvis (e.g. right oblique diameter in case of ROP position)

❖ Cervix may not be well applied to the presenting part

❖ With the progress of labour, posterior fontanelle is felt laterally and then anteriorly.

In addition to the above, vaginal examination also shows the following:

❖ Degree of deflexion of foetal head

❖ Degree of moulding of foetal head (presence of caput succedaneum)

❖ Degree of cervical dilatation and effacement

❖ Rupture of membranes and cord prolapse

❖ Direction of the occiput

❖ Exclusion of contracted pelvis.

In late labour, diagnosis may be difficult due to considerable moulding and formation of caput succedaneum over the presenting part, which obliterates the sutures and the fontanelles. In these cases, the occiput can be identified by the direction of the unfolded pinna, which points towards the occiput.

Investigations

Diagnosis of OP position is generally made by digital examination, but in case of uncertainty in diagnosis, ultrasound examination is both useful and accurate.

Ultrasonography: Ultrasound examination can be useful in the following:

❖ Confirmation of the diagnosis

❖ Other parameters such as foetal weight, foetal well-being, placental localisation, amniotic fluid volume, etc. can be determined.

 OBSTETRIC MANAGEMENT

The likely consequences related to OP position are shown in Figure 27.24. In majority of cases, good uterine contractions result in the flexion of foetal head. Descent occurs and the occiput undergoes rotation by three-eighths of the circle to lie behind the pubic symphysis, resulting in an OA position. In a small number of cases, the outcome may be unfavourable, resulting in short anterior rotation, non-rotation and short posterior rotation. In case of short anterior rotation, the occiput rotates through one-eighth of the circle anteriorly so that the sagittal sutures lie in the bispinous diameter. This position is known as the 'deep transverse arrest'. In case of non-rotation of the occiput, sagittal sutures lie in the oblique diameter. Further progress of labour is unlikely and this is known as oblique posterior arrest. In case of short posterior rotation, posterior rotation of the sinciput occurs by one eighth of the circle, putting the occiput in the sacral hollow. This position is known as

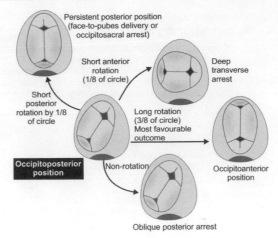

Fig. 27.24: Consequences related to occipitoposterior position

persistent OP position. Under favourable conditions with an average-sized baby, spacious pelvis and good uterine contractions, spontaneous face-to-pubis delivery can occur. If conditions are not favourable, delivery may not occur, resulting in an occipitosacral arrest.

Expectant Management

With expectant management, more than 50% multiparous women and more than 25% nulliparous women with OP foetuses are likely to achieve spontaneous vaginal delivery. Watchful expectancy must be observed for around 1 hour hoping for long anterior rotation of the occiput, which will result in normal delivery in 90% of the cases.

Prerequisites for expectant management of OP position are as follows:

❖ Presence of a reassuring foetal heart rate

❖ Average-sized baby and spacious pelvis

❖ Continued progress in the second stage

❖ Multiparous women with persistent OP foetuses.

Intrapartum Management

Intrapartum management in the cases of OP position comprises the following steps:

First Stage of Labour

Occipitoposterior position may be commonly associated with conditions such as contracted pelvis, cord presentation or cord prolapse. Therefore, pelvis must be assessed for adequacy and cord presentation or prolapse must be ruled out at the time of vaginal examination. Since cases of OP position are more liable to poor and abnormal progress of labour, PROM and abnormal and/or incoordinate uterine action, the following steps must be taken:

❖ Intravenous infusion of ringer lactate must be started in anticipation of prolonged labour.

❖ Due to high chances of PROM, the following steps must be observed:

• Bed rest

• Maternal straining to be avoided even if there is premature urge to bear down

- High enema must be avoided
- Vaginal examination must be minimised

❖ There may be marked backache. Therefore, analgesic drugs in form of pethidine or epidural analgesics may be administered.

❖ Since uterine inertia and prolonged labour are expected, oxytocin infusion must be started unless there is some contraindication present.

Second Stage of Labour and Delivery of the Baby

❖ During the second stage of labour, mother and foetus must be carefully assessed.

❖ Oxytocin can be used to combat inertia unless there is some contraindication to the use of oxytocin.

❖ Liberal episiotomy should be given to prevent perineal tears.

❖ Since in the majority of cases, long anterior rotation of head occurs, delivery occurs spontaneously or with low forceps or ventouse.

❖ In cases of occipitotransverse or oblique OP positions, ventouse application can be done. In cases of POP, under favourable conditions with an average-sized baby, spacious pelvis and good uterine contractions, spontaneous face-to-pubis delivery or vaginal delivery with the aid of forceps or ventouse can occur.

❖ Manual rotation of foetal head or rotation using Kielland's forceps, both of which were previously performed are no longer done nowadays.

❖ Nowadays, caesarean section is the most commonly used mode of delivery in cases of POP (occipitosacral arrest) or deep transverse arrest.

COMPLICATIONS

❖ Prolonged duration of both first and second stages of labour (due to labour dystocia; delayed engagement of the foetal head and abnormal uterine contractions with slow dilatation of cervix)

❖ Early ROM

❖ Extreme degree of moulding of foetal skull can result in tentorial tears

❖ Increased tendency for postpartum haemorrhage

❖ High chances of perineal injuries and trauma including complete perineal tears

❖ High maternal morbidity due to increased rate of operative delivery

❖ Increased perinatal morbidity and mortality due to asphyxia or trauma.

CLINICAL PEARLS

❖ Occipitoposterior position can be considered as an abnormal position of the vertex rather than an abnormal presentation

❖ There are higher chances of perineal injuries with face to pubis delivery because the biparietal diameter stretches

the perineum and occipitofrontal diameter emerges out of the introitus

❖ Caesarean section is not indicated per se in the cases of OP position.

EVIDENCE-BASED MEDICINE

Whether epidural analgesia has a causative role in OP position at delivery remains a matter of controversy. Many studies have demonstrated that the women with OP position had epidural anaesthesia in place.[40-42] It is still not very clear whether the epidural anaesthesia is a cause or effect of OP position. It is possible that under the effect of the epidural anaesthesia, the relaxation of pelvic musculature either promotes foetal rotation of OA position to OP or inhibits rotation from OP to OA position. Alternatively, OP position is associated with more painful and prolonged labours, thereby increasing the requirement of epidural anaesthesia for pain control. The available evidence does not clearly suggest that relaxation of pelvic musculature associated with epidural analgesia is likely to lead to malpositioning of the foetal head. There is insufficient evidence to show that epidural analgesia when the foetal head is still unengaged is likely to be associated with an increased rate of occiput posterior and transverse malpositions during labour.[43]

CORD PRESENTATION/CORD PROLAPSE

INTRODUCTION

Cord prolapse has been defined as descent of the umbilical cord through the cervix alongside the presenting part (occult presentation) or past it (overt presentation) in the presence of ruptured membranes. In occult prolapse, the examiner's fingers cannot feel the cord at the time of vaginal examination. In overt cord prolapse, the cord is found lying inside the vagina or outside the vulva following the ROM (Fig. 27.25). Cord presentation, on the other hand, is the presence of one or more loops of umbilical cord between the foetal presenting part and the cervix, with the membranes being intact (Fig. 27.26).

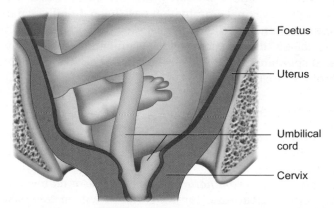

Fig. 27.25: Overt cord prolapse

CHAPTER 27

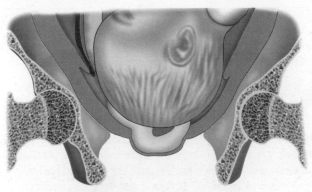

Loop of umbilical cord caught between vaginal wall and foetal head with membrane intact

Fig. 27.26: Cord presentation

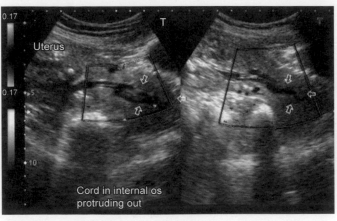

Fig 27.27: Internal os appears dilated with umbilical cord within the cervix; this finding is diagnostic of cord prolapse *(For colour version, see Plate 2)*

Table 27.2: Causes of cord prolapse

General causes	Procedure-related causes
• Multiparity • Low birthweight (<2.5 kg) • Prematurity (<37 weeks) • Foetal congenital anomalies • Breech/shoulder presentation • Second twin • Polyhydramnios • Unengaged presenting part • Low placenta and other abnormal placentation • Cord abnormalities (such as true knots or low content of Wharton's jelly)	• Artificial ROM (particularly with unengaged head) • Vaginal manipulation of foetus with ruptured membranes • External cephalic version • Internal podalic version • Stabilising induction of labour • Application of foetal scalp electrodes or placement of intrauterine catheters

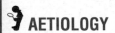

AETIOLOGY

Various probable causes of cord prolapse are listed in Table 27.2.

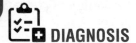

DIAGNOSIS

Clinical Presentation

Speculum and/or digital vaginal examination should be performed whenever the cord prolapse is suspected. Clinical findings on vaginal examination have been described in the 'introduction'. The clinician must exclude cord presentation or prolapse during each vaginal examination in labour and after spontaneous ROM, especially if the risk factors for cord prolapse are present.

Investigations

* *Cardiotocography*: There may be variable decelerations of heart rate pattern on continuous electronic foetal monitoring.
* *Ultrasound examination*: Doppler ultrasound may help in identification of umbilical cord within the cervix (Fig. 27.27).

MANAGEMENT

Suggested management plan in cases of cord prolapse is summarised by the acronym CORD and is shown in Flow chart 27.3.[44] Suspicion of cord prolapse should be considered in the following cases:

Prevention and First Aid

Steps for prevention: Artificial ROM should be avoided whenever possible if the presenting part has yet not engaged or is mobile. In cases where ROM becomes necessary even in such circumstances, this should be performed in an operation theatre with facilities available for an immediate caesarean birth. At the time of vaginal examination, especially in cases of ruptured membranes, the obstetrician must try to keep the upward pressure on the presenting part at a minimum because of the risk of upward displacement of the presenting part and the consequent cord prolapse. ROM should be avoided if the cord is felt below the presenting part at the time of vaginal examination.

First aid: In cases of cord prolapse where immediate vaginal delivery is not possible, assistance should be called immediately; venous access should be obtained, consent taken and immediate preparations be made for an urgent caesarean delivery. The following steps can be followed until facilities for caesarean section are made available:[44]

* To prevent vasospasm, there should be minimal handling of loops of cord lying outside the vagina, which can be covered with surgical packs soaked in warm saline.
* To prevent cord compression, some clinicians recommend that the presenting part must be elevated either manually or by filling the urinary bladder with normal saline. However, presently there is insufficient evidence to recommend manual replacement of the prolapsed cord above the presenting part to allow continuation of labour. This practice is therefore not recommended.
* Cord compression can be further reduced by advising the mother to adopt knee-chest position or head-down tilt (preferably in left lateral position).

PART II

Flow chart 27.3: Management plan in cases of cord prolapse[44]

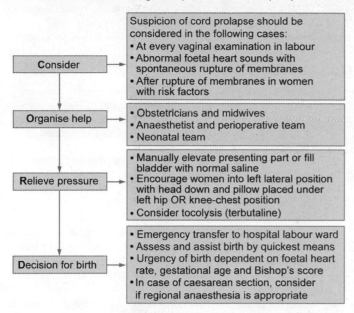

Consider	→	Suspicion of cord prolapse should be considered in the following cases: • At every vaginal examination in labour • Abnormal foetal heart sounds with spontaneous rupture of membranes • After rupture of membranes in women with risk factors
Organise help	→	• Obstetricians and midwives • Anaesthetist and perioperative team • Neonatal team
Relieve pressure	→	• Manually elevate presenting part or fill bladder with normal saline • Encourage women into left lateral position with head down and pillow placed under left hip OR knee-chest position • Consider tocolysis (terbutaline)
Decision for birth	→	• Emergency transfer to hospital labour ward • Assess and assist birth by quickest means • Urgency of birth dependent on foetal heart rate, gestational age and Bishop's score • In case of caesarean section, consider if regional anaesthesia is appropriate

❖ Tocolysis can also be considered to delay the labour especially if there are persistent FHR abnormalities after attempts to prevent compression mechanically. This is particularly important when the caesarean section is likely to be delayed.

Definitive Management

Cord presentation/prolapse is an emergency situation and delivery should occur promptly in these cases. Pressure of the foetal presenting part and bony pelvis may cause occlusion of the cord and obstruction of foetal circulation, resulting in foetal hypoxia. Prolapse of the cord beyond introitus may also result in arterial spasm.

Definitive management of these cases, therefore, comprises of immediate delivery. While the delivery is being expedited, continuous foetal monitoring should be in place. In cases where vaginal delivery is possible, forceps can be applied in cases of cephalic presentation if the head has engaged. In case of breech presentation, breech extraction can be done for example, after internal podalic version for a second twin. In case of transverse lie (especially, second twin), internal version followed by breech extraction must be performed. A caesarean section is the recommended mode of delivery in cases of cord prolapse when vaginal delivery is not imminent. A caesarean section should ideally be performed within 30 minutes or less (from the point of diagnosis to the delivery of the baby).[45] A category 1 caesarean section should be performed if the cord prolapse is associated with a suspicious or pathological FHR pattern, but without compromising maternal safety. Verbal consent is satisfactory for category 1 caesarean section (refer to Chapter 45, Caesarean Delivery).

Category 2 caesarean birth can be considered for women in whom the FHR pattern is normal. Nevertheless, in these cases, continuous assessment of the foetal heart trace is essential. If the cardiotocograph becomes abnormal at any stage, the management should be immediately recategorised to category 1 birth.

Discussion between the obstetrician and the anaesthetist should take place regarding the decision to use the appropriate form of anaesthesia. Decision to use regional anaesthesia can take place following consultation with an experienced anaesthetist.

A practitioner competent in the resuscitation of the newborn should attend all births following cord prolapse. Paired cord blood samples should be taken for the measurement of pH and base excess.

COMPLICATIONS

Maternal: There is an increased maternal morbidity due to greater incidence of operative delivery.

Foetal: Cord compression and umbilical artery vasospasm may cause asphyxia, which may result in hypoxic-ischemic encephalopathy and cerebral palsy.

CLINICAL PEARLS

❖ Incidence of cord prolapse has greatly reduced due to the increased use of elective caesarean deliveries in cases of non-cephalic presentation.
❖ In order to prevent vasospasm of umbilical artery, there should be minimal handling of loops of cord lying outside the vagina.

EVIDENCE-BASED MEDICINE

❖ In cases of cord presentation/prolapse, administration of terbutaline (0.25 mg subcutaneous) should be considered as a tocolytic of choice to minimise cord compression.[46]
❖ Regular dry drills should be conducted to help the clinicians maintain their skills to be able to handle such clinical situations as and when they arise.[46]

REFERENCES

1. Pritchard JA, MacDonald PC. Dystocia caused by abnormalities in presentation, position, or development of the fetus. In: Williams Obstetrics. Norwalk, CT: Appleton-Century-Crofts; 1980. pp. 787-96.
2. Cheng M, Hannah M. Breech delivery at term: a critical review of the literature. Obstet Gynecol. 1993;82(4 Pt 1):605-18.
3. Hannah ME, Hannah WJ, Hewson SA, Hodnett ED, Saigal S, Willan AR. Planned caesarean section versus planned vaginal birth for breech presentation at term: a randomised multicentre trial. Term Breech Trial Collaborative Group. Lancet. 2000;356(9239):1375-83.
4. American College of Obstetricians and Gynecologists (ACOG). Mode of term singleton breech delivery. ACOG Committee Opinion No. 265. Washington: ACOG; 2001.
5. Royal College of Clinicians and Gynaecologists (RCOG). Green-top Guideline No. 20b. The management of breech

presentation.. London (UK): Royal College of Clinicians and Gynaecologists; 2006. pp. 1-13.

6. Hofmeyr GJ, Hannah M, Lawrie TA. Planned caesarean section for term breech delivery. Cochrane Database Syst Rev. 2015;7:CD000166.

7. Goffinet F, Carayol M, Foidart JM, Alexander S, Uzan S, Subtil D, et al. Is planned vaginal delivery for breech presentation at term still an option? Results of an observational prospective survey in France and Belgium. Am J Obstet Gynecol. 2006; 194(4):1002-11.

8. American College of Obstetricians and Gynecologists (ACOG). Mode of term singleton breech delivery. ACOG Committee Opinion No. 340. Washington: ACOG; 2006.

9. Cruikshank DP. Breech presentation. Clin Obstet Gynecol. 1986;29(2):255-63.

10. Penn ZJ, Steer PJ. How obstetricians manage the problem of preterm delivery with special reference to the preterm breech. BJOG. 1991;98(6):531-4.

11. Penn ZJ, Steer PJ. Preterm breech. Contemp Rev Obstet Gynaecol. 1992;4:172-6.

12. Robertson PA, Foran CM, Croughan-Minihane MS, Kilpatrick SJ. Head entrapment and neonatal outcome by mode of delivery in breech deliveries from 28 to 36 weeks of gestation. Am J Obstet Gynecol. 1996;174(6):1742-7.

13. Lumley J. Any room left for disagreement about assisting breech births at term? Lancet. 2000;356(9239):1369-70.

14. Su M, Hannah WJ, Willan A, Ross S, Hannah ME; Term Breech Trial Collaborative Group. Planned caesarean section decreases the risk of adverse perinatal outcome due to both labour and delivery complications in the Term Breech Trial. BJOG. 2004;111(10):1065-74.

15. Doyle NM, Riggs JW, Ramin SM, Sosa MA, Gilstrap LC. Outcomes of term vaginal breech delivery. Am J Perinatol. 2005;22(6):325-8.

16. Royal College of Clinicians and Gynaecologists (RCOG). Green-top Guideline No. 20a External cephalic version and reducing the incidence of breech presentation. London (UK): Royal College of Clinicians and Gynaecologists; 2006. pp. 1-8.

17. Broche DE, Riethmuller D, Vidal C, Sautiere JL, Schaal JP, Maillet R. Obstetric and perinatal outcomes of a disreputable presentation: the nonfrank breech. J Gynecol Obstet Biol Reprod. 2005;34(8):781-8.

18. CEEDI National Advisory Body. Confidential Enquiry into Stillbirths and Deaths in Infancy. 8th Annual Report. London: Maternal and Child Health Research Consortium; 2001.

19. Løvset J. Vaginal operative delivery. Oslo: Scandinavian University Books; 1968.

20. Impey L, Pandit M. Tocolysis for repeat external cephalic version after a failed version for breech presentation at term: a randomised double-blind placebo controlled trial. BJOG. 2005;112(5):627-31.

21. Hofmeyr GJ. Interventions to help external cephalic version for breech presentation at term. Cochrane Database Syst Rev. 2004;(1):CD000184.

22. Hofmeyr GJ, Kulier R. Cephalic version by postural management for breech presentation. Cochrane Database Syst Rev. 2000;(3):CD000051.

23. Cardini F, Weixin H. Moxibustion for correction of breech presentation: a randomised controlled trial. JAMA. 1998; 280(18):1580-4.

24. Gemer O, Segal S. Incidence and contribution of predisposing factors to transverse lie presentation. Int J Gynaecol Obstet. 1994;44(3):219-21.

25. Hankins GD, Hammond TL, Snyder RR, Gilstrap LC. Transverse lie. Am J Perinatol. 1990;7(1):66-70.

26. Phelan JP, Boucher M, Mueller E, McCart D, Horenstein J, Clark SL. The nonlaboring transverse lie. A management dilemma. J Reprod Med. 1986;31(3):184-6.

27. Nicholson JM. Non-cephalic presentation in late pregnancy. BMJ. 2006;333(7568):562-3.

28. Okonofua FE. Management of neglected shoulder presentation. BJOG. 2009;116(13):1695-6.

29. Bancroft-Livingston G, Gordon H. Unstable lie in pregnancy and in labour. Postgrad Med J. 1967;43(496):92-6.

30. Edwards RL, Nicholson HO. The management of the unstable lie in late pregnancy. J Obstet Gynaecol Br Commonw. 1969; 76(8):713-8.

31. Szaboova R, Sankaran S. Diagnosis and management of unstable lie in pregnancy. BJOG. 2013;120:30-1.

32. Al-Sibai MH, Rahman MS, Rahman J. Obstetric problems in the grand multipara: a clinical study of 1330 cases. J Obstet Gynaecol. 1987;8(2):135-8.

33. Cruikshank DP, White CA. Obstetric malpresentations: twenty years' experience. Am J Obstet Gynecol. 1973;116(8):1097-104.

34. Tapisiz OL, Aytan H, Altinbas SK, Arman F, Tuncay G, Besli M, et al. Face presentation at term: a forgotten issue. J Obstet Gynaecol Res. 2014;40(6):1573-7.

35. Depp R. Cesarean delivery. In: Gabbe SG, Niebyl JR, Simpson JL (Eds). Obstetrics: Normal and Problem Pregnancies, 4th edition. New York: Churchill Livingstone; 2002. p. 551.

36. American Academy of Family Physicians. Advanced Life Support in Obstetrics (ALSO) Instructor Manual, 5th edition. Washington, DC: AAFP; 2012.

37. Grady K, Howell C, Cox C (Eds). Managing Obstetric Emergencies and Trauma. The MOET Course Manual, 2nd edition. London: RCOG Press; 2007.

38. Griffin RJ. Management of the occiput posterior. J Ky Med Assoc. 1964;62:860-1.

39. Chou MR, Kreiser D, Taslimi MM, Druzin ML, El-Sayed YY. Vaginal versus ultrasound examination of fetal occiput position during the second stage of labor. Am J Obstet Gynecol. 2004;191(2):521-4.

40. Anim-Somuah M, Smyth RM, Jones L. Epidural versus non-epidural or no analgesia in labour. Cochrane Database Syst Rev. 2011;(12):CD000331.

41. Cheng YW, Shaffer BL, Caughey AB. Associated factors and outcomes of persistent occiput posterior position: A retrospective cohort study from 1976 to 2001. J Matern Fetal Neonatal Med. 2006;19(9):563-8.

42. Lieberman E, Davidson K, Lee-Parritz A, Shearer E. Changes in fetal position during labor and their association with epidural analgesia. Obstet Gynecol. 2005;105(5 Pt 1):974-82.

43. Le Ray C, Carayol M, Jaquemin S, Mignon A, Cabrol D, Goffinet F. Is epidural analgesia a risk factor for occiput posterior or transverse positions during labour? Eur J Obstet Gynecol Reprod Biol. 2005;123(1):22-6

44. Module 10. Cord Prolapse. In: Winter C, Crofts J, Laxton C, Barnfield S, Draycott T (Eds). PROMPT: Practical Obstetric Multi-Professional Training. Practical locally based training for obstetric emergencies. Course Manual, 2nd edition. Cambridge: Cambridge University Press; 2012. pp. 169-78.

45. National Collaborating Centre for Women's and Children's Health. Intrapartum care: care of healthy women and their babies during childbirth. London: RCOG Press; 2007.

46. Royal College of Obstetricians and Gynaecologists, (RCOG). (2014). Green-top guideline 50. Umbilical cord prolapse. [online] RCOG website. Available from www.rcog.org.uk/en/guidelines-research-services/guidelines/gtg50 [Accessed August, 2016].

CHAPTER **28**

Intrauterine Death

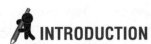 **INTRODUCTION**

According to the Perinatal Mortality Surveillance Report by CEMACH, stillbirth has been defined as 'a baby delivered with no signs of life known to have died after 24 completed weeks of pregnancy'.[1] Intrauterine foetal death (IUFD), on the other hand, refers to babies with no signs of life in utero. Foetal deaths may be divided into two: (1) antepartum IUFD (foetal deaths occurring in the antenatal period) and (2) intrapartum IUFD (foetal deaths occurring during labour). For statistical purposes, intrauterine foetal demise can be defined as the diagnosis of the stillborn infant (with the period of gestation being >24 weeks and foetal weight >350 g). A death that occurs prior to 24 weeks of gestation is classified as a spontaneous abortion. Occurrence of stillbirths is common in the UK, with 1 in every 200 babies being born dead. This is in comparison with one sudden infant death per 10,000 live births. There were 4,037 stillbirths in the UK in 2007, at a rate of 5.2 per 1,000 total births. In addition to any physical effects, stillbirth often has profound emotional, psychiatric and social effects on parents, their relatives and friends.

AETIOLOGY

Various causes of IUFD have been described in Table 28.1.

DIAGNOSIS

Clinical Presentation

Patient with underlying IUFD may present with the following symptoms:

❖ Absence of foetal movement interpretation by the mother for more than a few hours
❖ Retrogression of the positive pregnancy changes (breast changes disappear, fundal height becomes smaller than

Table 28.1: Causes of intrauterine death

Maternal causes	Foetal causes
• Hypertensive disorders • Chromosomal anomalies • Antepartum haemorrhage: Placenta praevia, abruptio placentae, etc. • Pre-existing medical disease such as chronic hypertension, chronic nephritis, diabetes, severe anaemia, hyperpyrexia, syphilis, hepatitis, toxoplasmosis, etc. • Rh incompatibility • Severe anaemia • Hyperpyrexia • External version • Maternal infection • Antiphospholipid syndrome	• Chromosomal anomalies • Foetal infections • Rh incompatibility • Iatrogenic causes such as external version
Placental causes	
• *Placental causes*: Placental insufficiency, antepartum haemorrhage, cord accidents, twin-to-twin transfusion syndrome, etc.	

the period of amenorrhoea, uterine tone diminishes and the uterus becomes flaccid)
❖ No foetal heart sounds can be heard.

General Physical Examination

No specific finding is observed on general physical examination except that there may be retrogression of the positive breast changes (normally seen during pregnancy).

Abdominal Examination

❖ Gradual retrogression of the height of the uterus
❖ Uterine tone is diminished
❖ Foetal movements are not felt during palpation
❖ Foetal heart sounds are not audible
❖ Foetal head shows eggshell cracking feeling upon palpation (late sign).

Investigations

The clinical investigations must be carried out with the aim of assessing maternal well-being (including coagulopathy), determining the cause of death and the probable chance of recurrence, and possible means of avoiding further complications during pregnancy. Parents should be advised that no specific cause may be found in almost half of stillbirths. However, identification of a cause can help prevent adverse outcomes in the future pregnancies. Identification of the cause of death is done following a correlation between blood tests and postmortem examination. Various tests, which need to be done in cases of IUFD to identify the underlying aetiology are listed in Box 28.1. The tests performed in an individual patient are based on the clinical presentation. Some of those, which are commonly performed, include:

Confirmation of Intrauterine Foetal Death

❖ *Absent foetal heart*: Evidence of absent foetal heart sounds is required for confirmation of IUFD. Auscultation, cardiotocography or external Doppler ultrasound should not be used to investigate suspected IUFD. Real-time ultrasonography is essential for the accurate diagnosis of IUFD. Under ideal situations, facilities of real-time ultrasonography should be available at all times. A clinician should seek a second opinion whenever practically possible. Real-time ultrasound allows direct visualisation of the foetal heart. Imaging can be technically difficult, particularly in the presence of conditions such as maternal obesity, abdominal scars and oligohydramnios. However, the real-time view can be often improved by inclusion of colour Doppler examination of the foetal heart and umbilical cord.

Definitive diagnosis of IUFD is made by observing the lack of foetal cardiac motion during a 10-minute period of careful examination with real-time ultrasound. Besides the absence of foetal cardiac activity, other secondary features suggestive of IUFD include collapse of the foetal skull with overlapping bones, hydrops, and maceration resulting in unrecognisable foetal mass.[2] Late signs suggestive of IUFD include oligohydramnios and collapse of cranial bones. Presence of intrafoetal gas, i.e. within the heart, blood vessels and joints is another late feature associated with IUFD that might limit the quality of real-time images.[3,4] Mothers should be counselled regarding the possibility of passive foetal movements. In case, the mother mentions that she has felt passive foetal movement following the scan for the diagnosis of IUFD, a repeat scan should be offered.

❖ *X-ray abdomen*: Abdominal X-ray may show presence of Spalding sign (irregular overlapping of the cranial bones), which usually occurs approximately within 7 days after death; hyperflexion of the spine; and crowding of ribs and appearance of gas shadows in the heart and great vessels (Robert's sign), which usually appears by 12 hours after birth. Spalding sign can also be observed on ultrasound examination (Fig. 28.1).

Other Tests for Investigating the Cause of Intrauterine Foetal Death

❖ *Blood grouping (ABO and Rh) and cross-matching*: Besides the blood group of mother, it is also important to know the baby's blood group (ABO and Rh) status. If blood sample cannot be obtained from the baby or cord, rhesus D (RhD) typing should be undertaken using ffDNA from maternal blood taken shortly after birth. A Kleihauer test should be urgently undertaken in women who are RhD-negative in order to detect large FMH that might have occurred a few days earlier. Anti-RhD gammaglobulin should be administered as soon as possible after presentation. If there has been a large FMH, the dose of anti-RhD gamma globulin should be calculated based on the amount of leakage. The Kleihauer test should be repeated at

Box 28.1: Tests for evaluation of intrauterine foetal death

❑ Foetal autopsy
❑ Placental evaluation
❑ Foetal karyotype
❑ Indirect Coomb's test
❑ Serologic test for syphilis
❑ Testing for foetal-maternal haemorrhage (Kleihauer-Betke or other)
❑ Parvovirus serology
❑ Lupus anticoagulant, anticardiolipin anticoagulant, for antiphospholipid testing
❑ Anti-β$_2$-glycoprotein 1 IgG or IgM antibodies
❑ Diabetes testing using haemoglobin A1c and a fasting blood glucose
❑ Syphilis screening using the VDRL or rapid plasma reagin test
❑ Thyroid function testing (i.e. TSH, FT$_4$)
❑ Urine toxicology screening
❑ Factor V Leiden
❑ Prothrombin mutation
❑ TORCH titres
❑ Protein C, protein S, and antithrombin III deficiency (useful in some circumstances)

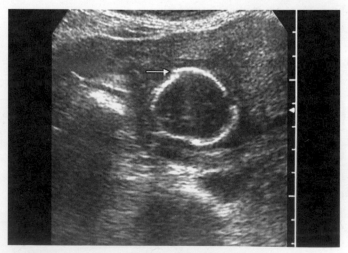

Fig. 28.1: Spalding sign: Showing overlapping of the foetal skull bones (indicated by arrow)

48 hours to ensure the clearance of foetal red cells. Administration of anti-RhD gamma globulins beyond 72 hours, after the sensitising event may be associated with reduced efficacy.[5-7]

❖ *Tests for detecting the underlying cause*: These include investigations such as blood sugar, thyroid function tests, TORCH screening, VDRL, thrombophilia studies, lupus anticoagulant and anticardiolipin antibodies, urine routine microscopy for pus cells and casts, etc.

❖ *Clotting profile*: Tests, such as blood fibrinogen levels and partial thromboplastin time, may especially be required, if the foetus has been retained for more than 2 weeks.

Sexing the Baby

In difficult situations (e.g. extremely preterm, severely macerated or grossly hydropic infants), parents can be counselled regarding the potential difficulty in sexing the baby before the baby's birth. Before deciding the baby's sex in difficult cases, the external genitalia of the infant must be inspected by two experienced healthcare practitioners (midwives, obstetricians, neonatologists or pathologists). This is especially important because errors in foetal sexing may result in severe emotional harm for parents.

In case of any difficulty or doubt where the baby's sex cannot be clinically determined on external physical inspection, the genetic sex can be rapidly determined using the skin or the placental tissue, even in case of macerated or deformed babies. In these cases, rapid karyotyping using quantitative fluorescent polymerase chain reaction (QF-PCR) or fluorescence in situ hybridisation (FISH) can be offered.[8] These tests are likely to provide highly accurate result within two working days. If these techniques also fail, sex can be determined on cell culture or at postmortem, but these methods are likely to take a longer time. If the genital sex is not clear and the parents do not wish for getting the postmortem testing done, they can be advised to judge the sex themselves for registration purposes. This can be perhaps based on the results of an earlier scan, or done in consultation with the midwife or doctor. Some parents may not wish to decide the baby's sex and give a neutral name. Stillborn babies can be registered to be having indeterminate sex.

Cytogenetic Analysis of the Baby

Karyotyping is essential because approximately 6% of stillborn babies will have a chromosomal abnormality, which may be potentially recurrent and may occur in future pregnancies.[9-11] Written consent should be taken before taking any foetal samples for karyotyping. Samples should be preferably taken from multiple tissues. Most commonly used perinatal specimens suitable for karyotyping include skin, cartilage and placenta. More than one cytogenetic technique should be available to increase the chances for obtaining informative results. Culture of tissues provides maximum amount of information related to genetic abnormalities (e.g. trisomies, monosomies, translocations, major deletions and marker chromosomes). Culture fluid should be preferably stored in a refrigerator and thawed thoroughly before use.

In case the culture is not successful, QF-PCR can be performed on extracted DNA.[12,13]

Nowadays, DNA-based methods for routine chromosome analysis are being preferred rather than cell culture. It is an efficient and cheap technique for detection of aneuploidies and is associated with a high rate of success.[14] However, the DNA-based methods provide slightly less-detailed limited genetic information and are unreliable for the detection of translocations and marker chromosomes.

Perinatal Postmortem Examination

Examination of the dead baby and placenta (placental cultures for suspected infection) needs to be done in order to detect the cause of baby's death. Autopsy and chromosomal analysis for detection of foetal anomalies and dysmorphic features need to be done. Postmortem examination of the baby and placenta is associated with a high diagnostic yield amongst all the investigations. Parents should be offered full postmortem examination to explain the cause of an IUFD. Parents should be advised that postmortem examination provides more information than other less invasive tests and this can sometimes be critical for the management of future pregnancy. However, the procedure can be emotionally disturbing for some parents. Therefore, they must not be forcefully persuaded to choose postmortem examination. Individual, cultural and religious beliefs of the parents must be given due respect.

Written consent must be obtained prior to the examination. Parents should be briefly offered a description of the procedure and the likely appearance of the baby afterwards. This should include information regarding the treatment of the baby with dignity and any arrangements for transport. Information leaflets must be provided along with the provision of verbal information. According to the recommendations by 8th CESDI report,[15] all practitioners who discuss postmortem examinations with the parents have a responsibility to understand the process so that a fully informed consent is taken. The consent form should include information regarding the purpose of postmortem examination; the extent of the examination; possible organs or tissues that must be retained and their purpose; the fate of tissues or organs following the postmortem examination; and the relevance of postmortem examination for research and education purposes.[15]

Postmortem examination includes external examination along with the measurement of birthweight, histology of relevant tissues and skeletal X-rays. Whether or not the postmortem examination of the baby is requested, pathological examination of the cord, membranes and placenta should always be undertaken in cases of IUFD.

The examination should preferably be undertaken by a specialist perinatal pathologist.

Parents who are not willing for a full postmortem examination might be offered a limited examination, which spares certain organs. Less invasive procedures such as needle biopsies can also be sometimes offered. However, these alternative procedures are much less informative and reliable in comparison to the conventional postmortem examination. Medical imaging, especially of the brain and spinal cord can act as a useful adjunct to full postmortem examination. The use of MRI is currently being evaluated in the MaRIAS (Magnetic Resonance Imaging Autopsy Study) trial.[16] However, it has not yet been found suitable in clinical practice. Ultrasound has been used to visualise foetal brain, heart, lung and renal development in stillbirths when the patients refuse to give consent for autopsy. Ultrasound and MRI should not yet be offered as a substitute for conventional postmortem examination.[16]

MANAGEMENT

Prevention

Intrauterine death can be prevented by observing the following precautions:

❖ Regular antenatal care
❖ Screening out the high-risk patients to carefully monitor the foetal well-being and to terminate the pregnancy at the earliest evidences of foetal compromise. Regular antepartum surveillance is required in these cases in order to prevent foetal death.

Obstetric Management

Patient Counselling

Reassurance and counselling must be provided to the bereaving parents. If the woman attends the clinic unaccompanied, an immediate offer should be made to call her partner, relatives or friends before breaking the bad news to her. While making decisions related to treatment, discussions between the patients and clinician must be directed to support maternal or parental choice. Parent should be offered written information in form of leaflets to supplement verbal discussions.

Mode of Delivery of the Dead Foetus

Once the foetal death has been diagnosed, the options of expectant or active management must be discussed with the patient.

Expectant management: The following need to be done in case expectant management is planned:

❖ The obstetrician must await spontaneous onset of labour during the coming 4 weeks
❖ The woman must be assured that in 90% of cases the foetus would be expelled spontaneously during the waiting period with no complications.
❖ If platelet levels are found to be decreasing on serial examinations, 4 weeks have passed without onset of spontaneous labour, fibrinogen levels are found to be low, or the woman requests active management, the obstetrician must consider induction of labour.

Induction of labour:

❖ In case induction of labour is planned, cervix must be firstly assessed.

❖ If the cervix is favourable, labour can be induced with oxytocin. If cervix is unfavourable, it must be ripened using vaginal PGE$_2$ or synthetic PGE$_1$ analogue (misoprostol).
❖ The membranes must be preferably not ruptured.

Labour and Delivery

❖ Women should be advised to have labour in the ward having appropriate facilities for emergency care based on individual circumstances, paying special attention towards the woman's emotional and practical needs without compromising on their safety. Care in labour should be preferably provided by an experienced midwife.
❖ In most of the cases, spontaneous expulsion occurs within 2 weeks of death. In cases where spontaneous expulsion does not occur, induction by oxytocin infusion or prostaglandins (PGE$_2$ gel or 25–50 µg of misoprostol) may be required.
❖ First-line intervention for induction of labour in a woman with unscarred uterus is combination of mifepristone with a prostaglandin preparation (usually PGE$_2$ gel). As per the recommendations by NICE (2008), misoprostol can be used in preference to PGE$_2$ because it is associated with equivalent safety and efficacy that too at a lower cost. However, it is to be used at doses lower than those currently marketed in the UK. The currently available 200 µg tablet in the UK can be divided into portions by pharmacists or dissolved in water and administered in form of measured portions.[17] In these cases, mifepristone is administered in the dosage of 200 mg, 24–48 hours prior to induction.
❖ Women should be advised that vaginal misoprostol is as effective as oral therapy, but associated with fewer adverse effects. The dose of misoprostol used for induction in cases of late IUFD should be adjusted according to gestational age (100 µg 6-hourly before 26^{+6} weeks; 25–50 µg 4-hourly at 27^{+0} weeks or more, up to 24 hours).[18]
❖ Women in whom labour is delayed for more than 48 hours should be advised to have testing for DIC twice weekly. This involves the estimation of maternal coagulation time and the fibrinogen levels. Falling fibrinogen levels must be arrested by controlled infusion of heparin.
❖ If a woman returns home before labour, she should be given a 24-hour contact number from where she can obtain appropriate information and support when required.
❖ Women considering prolonged expectant management should be advised that the value of postmortem examination may be reduced and appearance of the baby may deteriorate.
❖ Vaginal birth is the recommended mode of delivery for most women, but caesarean birth might be required in some cases. The woman might herself request for a caesarean delivery because of previous experiences or a wish to avoid vaginal birth of a dead baby.
❖ *Induction of labour in case of scarred uterus:* In case of induction of labour in a woman with the history of single lower segment caesarean section (LSCS), she should be advised that in general, the absolute risk of induction of

labour with prostaglandins in such cases is only a little higher in comparison to women with unscarred uterus. According to the recommendations by the RCOG Green-top Guideline on VBAC, women should be informed that there is a slightly higher risk of uterine rupture in cases of induction of labour with prostaglandins.[19] In the UK, misoprostol can be safely used for induction of labour in women with a single previous LSCS and an IUFD but with lower doses than those currently marketed. Mifepristone can also be used alone to increase the chance of labour significantly within 72 hours, at the same time avoiding the use of prostaglandins. In these cases, mifepristone is used in the dosage of 600 mg once daily for 2 days.[20]

Women with two previous LSCS should be advised that in general, the absolute risk of induction of labour with prostaglandin is only a little higher than for women with a single previous LSCS. Women with more than two LSCS deliveries or atypical scars should be advised that the safety of induction of labour is unknown. VBAC is not ordinarily recommended for women with three previous caesarean sections, previous uterine rupture or upper segment incisions.[19]

Oxytocin augmentation can be used for VBAC, but the decision should be made following discussion by a consultant obstetrician. Women undergoing VBAC should be closely monitored for features of scar rupture. Though it is not possible to monitor the patient for signs of early scar dehiscence using FHR abnormalities in these patients, the patient can be monitored through other clinical features such as maternal tachycardia, atypical pain, vaginal bleeding, haematuria on catheter specimen, maternal collapse, etc.

❖ *Intrapartum antimicrobial therapy*: Intravenous broad-spectrum antibiotic therapy (including antichlamydial agents) must be administered to the women with sepsis. However, there is no requirement for routine antibiotic prophylaxis in all women with IUFD.

❖ *Pain relief in labour*: All usual analgesic modalities should be available to the woman in labour including regional anaesthesia and patient-controlled anaesthesia. Diamorphine should be used in preference to pethidine because it has greater analgesic qualities and longer duration of action. The woman should be assessed for DIC and sepsis before the administration of regional anaesthesia.

❖ *Suppression of lactation*: Suppression of lactation may be required in patients with IUFD following delivery due to the risk of breast engorgement. Suppression of lactation may also be of psychological importance for some women following IUFD. Simple measures such as use of support brassiere, ice packs and analgesics may be useful in some patients. However, nearly one-third of patients may experience severe breast pain with these simple measures.[21] Dopamine agonists can be successfully used for suppressing lactation in a very high proportion of women. In this context, cabergoline is superior to bromocriptine. Dopamine agonists should not be administered to women with hypertension or pre-eclampsia. Oestrogens should not be preferably used for suppressing lactation.

Psychological and Social Aspects of Care

It is important for the obstetrician to remember that the woman and her partner and their children are all at an increased risk of prolonged severe psychological reactions including post-traumatic stress disorder.[22, 23] Perinatal death is also associated with an increased risk of postnatal depression. Clinicians should be aware regarding the possible variations in individual and cultural approaches to death. Moreover, reaction of different family members may be varied. Counselling should be offered to all women and their partners as well as other family members, especially existing children and grandparents. Bereavement officers should be selected to organise the services. Parents should be advised about support groups. Support groups, such as Stillbirth and Neonatal Death Society (SANDS), have been developed to offer help to both partners. Some maternity units in the UK offer debriefing services for parents who have experienced traumatic events in relation to childbirth. In absence of support groups, some parents are likely to develop prolonged psychological problems after stillbirth. Presently, there is a paucity of evidence from randomised trials regarding the benefits and pitfalls of psychological interventions after perinatal death.[24]

Parental Contact with the Dead Baby

Many parents particularly wish to see and hold their dead baby. The parents must not be forcefully persuaded to have contact with their stillborn baby. However, if the parents themselves express such desires, the clinician should strongly support them. Some parents may wish to name their baby, but others may not want to do so. Either option is allowable in law [Births and Deaths Registration Act 1953; amended by the Stillbirth (Definition) Act 1992].[25] Parents who want to name their babies should be counselled that once a name has been registered, it cannot be re-entered or changed again later. If parents do decide to name their baby, obstetricians should use the same name while referring to the baby during the follow-up meetings. If the parents express the desire to retain the artefacts of remembrance of their dead newborn, they must be supported by the obstetrician. Maternity units should have the facilities for producing photographs, palm and footprints and locks of hair of the stillborn child with presentation frames. If the parents do not wish to have mementos, the staff of the maternity unit should stock them securely in the maternal case records so that they can be accessed in future if required. There is no definite evidence to show that keeping mementoes of the dead baby is associated with any adverse outcomes. [26-28]

Legal Requirements for Medical Certification of Stillbirth

The current law on stillbirth registration is set out in the Births and Deaths Registration Act 1953 [amended by the Stillbirth (Definition) Act 1992].[25] The following practice guidance is derived from this act and the code of practice. The law holds the parents responsible for registering the birth but they can delegate the task to a healthcare professional, including a midwife or doctor present at the birth or a bereavement support officer. The registration should be normally done within 42 days (21 days in Scotland), but with a final limit of 3 months for exceptional circumstances. Stillbirth must be medically certified by a fully registered doctor or midwife; the doctor or midwife must have been present at the birth or should have examined the baby after birth. The cause and sequence of medical events leading to the IUFD should be described in as much detail as possible. Certification should not be delayed for the results of the postmortem.

In case of doubt regarding the status of birth, HM coroner must be contacted. In case of suspicion of deliberate action to cause stillbirth, the police should be contacted. Dead foetuses, which are delivered later than 24 weeks, but in cases where the death had clearly occurred before the end of the 24th week, need not be certified or registered. If the baby's sex cannot be clearly determined, the baby can be registered as indeterminate sex, awaiting further tests.

The birth is entered onto the Stillbirth Register. This is separate from the standard Register of Births. The parents are then issued with a Certificate of Stillbirth and the documentation for burial or cremation. Before the registration of stillbirth, a certificate for cremation cannot be issued. The legal responsibility for the child's body rests with the parents but can be they can delegate it to hospital services.

Maternity units should have arrangements with religious elders or spiritual leaders of all common faiths and nonreligious spiritual organisations so that the parents can obtain spiritual guidance and support regarding the child's burial, cremation and remembrance ceremonies. Funeral options including burial and cremation should be discussed with parents, taking into account religious and cultural considerations. Parents should be allowed to choose freely about the individuals who would be attending the funeral service. They should be provided with a leaflet containing information related to the available options. Maternity units should provide a book of remembrance for parents, relatives and friends. The parents should be provided with the option of leaving toys, pictures and messages in the coffin.

COMPLICATIONS

❖ Psychological upset
❖ Infection (typically with anaerobic infections such as *Clostridium welchii*)
❖ Blood coagulation disorder (DIC)
❖ *During labour*: Uterine inertia, retained placenta and postpartum haemorrhage.

CLINICAL PEARLS

❖ The obstetricians must remain vigilant regarding the development of postpartum depression in women with

a previous IUFD. The clinician should be aware that maternal bonding during future pregnancies could be adversely affected.
❖ Women with a previous unexplained IUFD should be recommended to have obstetric antenatal care during their future pregnancies. Such women should also be recommended to have screening for gestational diabetes.
❖ For women in whom the stillborn baby had shown evidence of being small for gestational age, in subsequent pregnancies, serial assessment of growth by ultrasound biometry should be recommended.

EVIDENCE-BASED MEDICINE

❖ Psychological problems are more likely to occur in cases of IUFD in absence of introduction of the bereaved parents to the support groups. Presently, there is insufficient evidence regarding the benefits and pitfalls of psychological interventions following perinatal death.[24]
❖ There is no definite evidence to show that keeping mementoes of the dead baby is associated with any adverse outcomes.[26-28]

REFERENCES

1. Confidential Enquiry into Maternal and Child Health (CEMACH). Perinatal Mortality 2007: United Kingdom. London: CEMACH; 2009.
2. Zeit RM. Sonographic demonstration of fetal death in the absence of radiographic abnormality. Obstet Gynecol. 1976;48(1 Suppl):49S-52S.
3. Weinstein BJ, Platt LD. The ultrasonic appearance of intravascular gas in fetal death. J Ultrasound Med. 1983;2(10):451-4.
4. McCully JG. Gas in the fetal joints: a sign of intrauterine death. Obstet Gynecol. 1970;36(3):433-6.
5. Royal College of Obstetricians and Gynaecologists (2002). Green-top Guideline No. 22. Anti-D immunoglobulin for Rh prophylaxis. [online] Available from www.rcog.org.uk/en/guidelines-research-services/guidelines/gtg22 [Accessed August, 2016].
6. Lee D, Contreras M, Robson SC, Rodeck CH, Whittle MJ. Recommendations for the use of anti-D immunoglobulin for Rh prophylaxis. British Blood Transfusion Society and the Royal College of Obstetricians and Gynaecologists. Transfus Med. 1999;9(1):93-7.
7. The estimation of fetomaternal haemorrhage. BCSH Blood Transfusion and Haematology Task Forces. Transfus Med. 1999;9(1):87-92.
8. Derom C, Vlietinck R, Derom R, Boklage C, Thiery M, Van den Berghe H. Genotyping of macerated stillborn fetuses. Am J Obstet Gynecol. 1991;164(3):797-800.
9. Genest DR. Estimating the time of death in stillborn fetuses: II. Histologic evaluation of the placenta; a study of 71 stillborns. Obstet Gynecol. 1992;80(4):585-92.
10. Genest DR, Singer DB. Estimating the time of death in stillborn fetuses: III. External fetal examination; a study of 86 stillborns. Obstet Gynecol. 1992;80(4):593-600.

11. Genest DR, Williams MA, Greene MF. Estimating the time of death in stillborn fetuses: I. Histologic evaluation of fetal organs; an autopsy study of 150 stillborns. Obstet Gynecol. 1992;80(4):575-84.

12. Diego-Alvarez D, Garcia-Hoyos M, Trujillo MJ, Gonzalez Gonzalez C, Rodriguez de Alba M, Ayuso C, et al. Application of quantitative fluorescent PCR with short tandem repeat markers to the study of aneuploidies in spontaneous miscarriages. Hum Reprod. 2005;20(5):1235-43.

13. Zou G, Zhang J, Li XW, He L, He G, Duan T. Quantitative fluorescent polymerase chain reaction to detect chromosomal anomalies in spontaneous abortion. Int J Gynaecol Obstet. 2008;103(3):237-40.

14. Cirigliano V, Voglino G, Cañadas MP, Marongiu A, Ejarque M, Ordoñez E, et al. Rapid prenatal diagnosis of common chromosome aneuploidies by QF-PCR. Assessment on 18000 consecutive clinical samples. Mol Hum Reprod. 2004;10(11): 839-46.

15. Confidential Enquiry into Stillbirths and Deaths in Infancy. 8th Annual Report. London: Maternal and Child Health Research Consortium; 2001.

16. Furness ME, Weckert RC, Parker SA, Knowles S. Ultrasound in the perinatal necropsy. J Med Genet. 1989;26(6):368-72.

17. Misoprostol Organisation: Safe Usage guide for obstetrics and Gynaecology. (2009). How to dilute 200 mcg of misoprostol in 200 ml water. Misoprostol.org website [online] Available from www.misoprostol.org/dilute-200-mcg-misoprostol-200 ml-water. [Accessed August, 2016].

18. Gómez Ponce de León R, Wing D, Fiala C. Misoprostol for intrauterine fetal death. Int J Gynaecol Obstet. 2007;99 (Suppl 2):S190-3.

19. Royal College of Obstetricians and Gynaecologists. (RCOG), (2015). Green-top Guideline No. 45: Birth after previous caesarean birth. [online] Available from www.rcog.org.uk/globalassets/documents/guidelines/gtg_45.pdf. [Accessed August, 2015],

20. British Medical Association and Royal Pharmaceutical Society of Great Britain. British National Formulary (BNF) 58. London: BMJ Publishing Group Ltd and RPS Publishing; 2009.

21. Buckman R. Communications and emotions. BMJ. 2002;325 (7366):672.

22. Hughes P, Turton P, McGauley GA, Fonagy P. Factors that predict infant disorganization in mothers classified as U in pregnancy. Attach Hum Dev. 2006;8:113-22.

23. Turton P, Hughes P, Evans CD, Fainman D. Incidence, correlates and predictors of post-traumatic stress disorder in the pregnancy after stillbirth. Br J Psychiatry. 2001;178:556-60.

24. Flenady V, Wilson T. Support for mothers, fathers and families after perinatal death. Cochrane Database Syst Rev. 2008;(1): CD000452.

25. Royal College of Obstetricians and Gynaecologists. (2005). Good Practice Guideline No. 4: Registration of stillbirths and certification for pregnancy loss before 24 weeks of gestation. [online] Available from www.rcog.org.uk/globalassets/documents/guidelines/goodpractice4registrationstillbirth2005.pdf. [Accessed August, 2016].

26. Hughes P, Turton P, Hopper E, Evans CD. Assessment of guidelines for good practice in psychosocial care of mothers after stillbirth: a cohort study. Lancet. 2002;360(9327):114-8.

27. Rådestad I, Steineck G, Nordin C, Sjögren B. Psychological complications after stillbirth—influence of memories and immediate management: population based study. BMJ. 1996;312:1505-8.

28. Samuelsson M, Rådestad I, Segesten K. A waste of life: fathers' experience of losing a child before birth. Birth. 2001;28:124-30.

CHAPTER 28

Recurrent Miscarriage

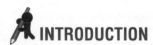 INTRODUCTION

Miscarriage is defined as the spontaneous loss of pregnancy before the foetal viability is attained. This term encompasses all pregnancy losses from the time of conception until 24 weeks of gestation. RCOG (2011)[1] has defined recurrent miscarriage as the clinically recognised loss of three or more consecutive pregnancies with the same partner before 24 weeks of gestation. However, due to advances in neonatal care, a small number of babies are also able to survive before 24 weeks of gestation. Recurrent miscarriage affects nearly 1% of couples trying to conceive.[2] It has been estimated that approximately 1–2% of second-trimester pregnancies are likely to miscarry before 24 weeks of gestation.[3]

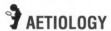 AETIOLOGY

In most cases, the causes remain undetermined. Some important causes of recurrent miscarriage are enlisted in Box 29.1 and are described here in details:

Genetic Causes

Parental Chromosomal Abnormalities

Presence of chromosomal abnormality in either of the parents is responsible for a high proportion of early first-trimester miscarriages. All couples with a history of recurrent miscarriage should have peripheral blood karyotyping performed. Chromosomal abnormalities of the conceptus account for more than half of sporadic (pre) embryonic losses

---

Box 29.1: Causes of recurrent pregnancy loss

❑ *Genetic*
  - Chromosomal abnormalities in the embryo or foetus
  - Parental chromosomal abnormalities
  - Inherited thrombophilias (mutation in prothrombin gene, hyperhomocystinaemia, deficiencies in antithrombin III, protein S, C, etc.). These cause microthrombi/thrombosis/infarction of the placental vessels.
❑ *Anatomical*
  - Congenital uterine malformations (e.g. unicornuate uterus, uterine didelphys, septate uterus, etc.)
  - Leiomyomas: Submucous
  - Intrauterine adhesions
❑ *Immunological*
  - Autoimmune: SLE and APLA
  - Alloimmune: Abnormal maternal response to foetal or placental antigens (due to maternal cytotoxic antibodies, absent maternal blocking antibodies and/or disturbances in the natural killer cell function and distribution)
❑ *Endocrine*
  - Thyroid disease, diabetes, PCOS, and luteal phase deficiency
❑ *Infectious causes* (e.g. *Chlamydia, Ureaplasma, Mycoplasma*, toxoplasmosis, *Listeria, Campylobacter*, Herpes, Cytomegalovirus, bacterial vaginosis)
❑ *Environmental*
  - Smoking, alcohol, and heavy coffee consumption
❑ *Epidemiological factors*
  - Advancing maternal age and number of previous miscarriages
❑ *Unexplained factors*

and in many cases, a visible embryo never forms. The most common types of parental chromosomal abnormalities are balanced reciprocal or Robertsonian translocations.[4-7] These translocations are commonly associated with advanced maternal age and premature ovarian failure. Although the carriers of a balanced translocation are usually phenotypically normal, their pregnancies are at increased risk of miscarriage. The live births in such cases may be associated with multiple congenital malformations and/or mental disability due to an unbalanced chromosomal arrangement. The risk of miscarriage is influenced by the size and the genetic content of the rearranged chromosomal segments.

Single gene defects and skewed inactivation of X chromosome are other emerging causes of recurrent miscarriage. As the number of miscarriages increases, the possibility of miscarriage due to the presence of chromosomal abnormality decreases and the chance of miscarriage due to the presence of recurring maternal cause increases. Genetic factors are the most important cause for sporadic miscarriage. If an abnormal parental karyotype is identified, the patient in any case must be referred to a clinical geneticist and offered genetic counselling, familial chromosomal studies and appropriate prenatal diagnosis in future pregnancies. In all couples with a previous history of recurrent miscarriage, cytogenetic analysis of the products of conception should be performed if the next pregnancy fails.

Approximately 50–70% of genetic pregnancy losses are due to chromosomal aneuploidies, the most common amongst which are monosomy X and other autosomal trisomies like trisomy 16, 13, 18 and 21.

Embryonic Chromosomal Abnormalities

In couples with recurrent miscarriage, nearly 30-57% cases could be as a result of the chromosomal abnormalities of the embryo.[8] The risk of miscarriage occurring as a result of the chromosomal abnormalities of the embryo increases with advancing maternal age.

Inherited thrombophilias including factor V Leiden (FVL) mutation, prothrombin G20210A mutations, deficiency of protein C and S, and hyperhomocysteinaemia are considered as established causes of systemic thrombosis. In addition, inherited thrombophilias have been implicated as a possible cause of recurrent miscarriage and late pregnancy complications with probable mechanism being thrombosis of the uteroplacental circulation.

Factor V Leiden and prothrombin G20210A mutations are common genetic mutations that predispose the carriers to develop venous thromboembolism. FVL is the most common cause of primary and recurrent venous thromboembolism in pregnancy. FVL carriage has also consistently been shown to increase the risk of early onset gestational hypertension, HELLP syndrome, severe placental abruption and foetal gsyndrome rowth restriction.

Endocrine Factors

Hormonal factors have been proposed to contribute to recurrent miscarriage in 10–20% of patients. Hormonal aberrations may result from problems with certain endocrine glands, such as the pituitary, thyroid, adrenal or ovaries.

Luteal Phase Defect

Progesterone, a hormone produced by the ovary during the secretory stage, is necessary for maintenance of a healthy pregnancy. Low progesterone levels, often called luteal phase defect (LPD), has been thought to be a cause of spontaneous abortions. LPD has been found to be associated with poor follicular phase oocyte development, which may result in disordered oestrogen secretion and subsequent dysfunction of the corpus luteum.

Polycystic Ovary Syndrome

Polycystic ovary syndrome has been considered as a cause of a variety of menstrual disorders ranging from amenorrhoea to dysfunctional uterine bleeding, hirsutism and infertility. Hypersecretion of luteinising hormone (LH) in PCOS, resulting in the elevation of LH:FSH ratio, is thought to be responsible for causing recurrent miscarriages. However, the exact mechanism behind miscarriage still remains unclear. Polycystic ovarian morphology, elevated levels of serum luteinising hormone or elevated serum testosterone levels do not predict an increased risk of future pregnancy loss among ovulatory women with a history of recurrent miscarriage who conceive spontaneously.[9] The increased risk of miscarriage in women with PCOS has been recently attributed to causes such as insulin resistance, hyperinsulinaemia and hyperandrogenaemia. An elevated free androgen index also appears to be a prognostic factor for a subsequent miscarriage in women with recurrent miscarriage.[10]

Hypothyroidism

Maternal hypothyroidism may place the mother at an increased risk of adverse obstetric outcomes. Thyroid disease may cause ovulatory dysfunction and LPDs. Presence of antithyroid antibodies has also been found to be associated with recurrent miscarriage. Treated thyroid dysfunction, however, is not a risk factor for recurrent miscarriage. Untreated hypothyroidism, on the other hand, can result in an increased risk for pre-eclampsia, placental abruption, miscarriage and perinatal mortality. Maternal hypothyroidism in the second trimester has been found to be associated with an increased rate of foetal death after 16 weeks of gestation.

Diabetes Mellitus

Women with diabetes who have high haemoglobin A1c (glycosylated haemoglobin) levels in the first trimester are at an increased risk of miscarriage and foetal malformations. However, neither well-controlled diabetes mellitus nor treated thyroid diseases have been observed to be the risk factors for recurrent miscarriage.[11,12]

Hyperprolactinaemia

Hyperprolactinaemia may adversely affect corpus luteal function. However, presently there is insufficient evidence to assess the effect of hyperprolactinaemia as a risk factor for recurrent miscarriage.

Maternal Infection

Any severe infection that leads to bacteraemia or viraemia can cause sporadic miscarriage. The role of infection in recurrent miscarriage is unclear. Role of infective agents as a cause of recurrent miscarriage is presently considered controversial in developed countries. An infection can be implicated in the aetiology of repeated pregnancy loss, only if it is capable of persisting in the genital tract, without being detected early or without causing sufficient symptoms, which could disturb the women. Some infections, which have been implicated in the causation of recurrent miscarriage, include TORCH, bacterial vaginosis, *L. monocytogenes, M. hominis, Herpes virus, C. trachomatis,* Cytomegalovirus, Group B streptococci, Ureaplasma, etc.

TORCH Group of Infections

Infections caused by TORCH complex are thought to be important causes for bad obstetric history, which is treatable, especially in the developing countries. The association between TORCH group of infections and recurrent miscarriage is not yet clear. The RCOG (2011) recommends that routine TORCH screening should be abandoned. TORCH infections are generally mild in the mother but can prove disastrous to the foetus. The degree of severity is dependent on the gestational age of the foetus when infected, the virulence of the organism, the damage to the placenta and the severity of maternal disease. Infections by TORCH agents in women are usually asymptomatic and chronic.

Bacterial Vaginosis

Bacterial vaginosis has been found to be strongly associated with late miscarriage, preterm ROM and preterm labour. However, the evidence for its association with first trimester miscarriage is inconsistent.[13,14] The standard antibiotic regime recommended for treatment of bacterial vaginosis in pregnancy is metronidazole 400 mg, 12 hourly for 5–7 days. In order to reduce systemic side effects, intravaginal 2% clindamycin cream or 0.75% metronidazole gel may also be used. Single-dose therapy in the form of 2 g metronidazole or tinidazole 2 g has also been found to be effective in pregnancy. Long-term treatment with probiotics may play a role in re-establishing normal vaginal flora. Presently, there is no evidence to assess the role of antibiotic therapy in women with a previous second-trimester miscarriage.

Syphilis

Syphilis, a sexually transmitted disease, has been implicated as the cause for second-trimester miscarriages, stillbirths, preterm labour, growth restriction, neonatal infections, etc.

Chronic Endometritis

Chronic endometritis may be due to organisms such as *Chlamydia, Mycobacterium tuberculosis,* etc. PCR-based testing for *M. tuberculosis* and *Chlamydia* can be performed on endometrial aspirates. Hysteroscopic diagnosis using chromohysteroscopy with methylene blue has been suggested as a diagnostic procedure.

Environmental Factors

This may include factors such as previous radiation exposure, occupational hazards, addictions, cigarette smoking, alcohol consumption, etc. Cigarette smoking by the mother and caffeine consumption has been associated with an increased risk of spontaneous miscarriage in a dose-dependent manner. However, presently, there is insufficient evidence to confirm this association.[15,16] Heavy alcohol consumption is toxic to the embryo and the foetus. Even moderate consumption of alcohol in the dosage of five or more units per week may increase the risk of sporadic miscarriage. Maternal obesity is also likely to increase the risk of both sporadic and recurrent miscarriage.[17-19]

Immune Causes

The immune factors associated with pregnancy loss can be classified as autoimmune and alloimmune factors.

Autoimmune Factors

The autoimmune factors include the synthesis of autoantibodies, e.g. antiphospholipid antibodies (APS), antinuclear antibodies, antithyroid antibodies, etc.

Antiphospholipid antibodies: The main types of anti-phospholipid antibodies are lupus anticoagulant (LA) and anticardiolipin (aCL) antibodies (IgG and IgM). The association between antiphospholipid antibodies and recurrent miscarriage is referred to as antiphospholipid syndrome. APS is the most important treatable cause of recurrent miscarriage.[20,21] Presence of antiphospholipid antibodies in the blood may result in an increase in the blood viscosity. This may result in the development of thrombosis inside the placental blood vessels, which may be responsible for producing placental insufficiency and/or miscarriage. Adverse pregnancy outcomes in these cases may include one of the following:

❖ Three or more consecutive miscarriages before 10 weeks of gestation
❖ One or more morphologically normal foetal losses after the 10th week of gestation
❖ One or more preterm births before the 34th week of gestation owing to placental disease

The mechanisms by which antiphospholipid antibodies cause pregnancy-related morbidity are listed in Box 29.2.[22-27]

Box 29.2: Mechanisms by which antiphospholipid antibodies cause pregnancy-related morbidity[22-27]

❑ Inhibition of trophoblastic function and differentiation
❑ Activation of complement pathways at the maternal-foetal interface resulting in a local inflammatory response
❑ Thrombosis of the uteroplacental vasculature later in pregnancy

Alloimmune Factors

Blocking antibodies: Under normal circumstances, the maternal immune system recognises implanting embryo as foreign body and produces 'blocking antibodies', thereby protecting the embryo from rejection. These blocking antibodies coat the placental cells, thereby preventing their destruction by maternal lymphocytes. In recurrent miscarriages, there is absence of these blocking antibodies due to failure of recognition of cross-reactive antigens of trophoblast lymphocyte by the mother. Alloimmune traits such as immunologic differences between reproductive partners have been proposed as the factor responsible for this. There is no clear evidence to support the hypothesis that the incompatibility related to HLA antigens between couples, the absence of maternal leucocytotoxic antibodies or the absence of maternal blocking antibodies is responsible for causing recurrent miscarriages. Hence, these tests for HLA type and antipaternal cytotoxic antibody should not be routinely offered at the time of investigation of couples with recurrent miscarriage.

Natural killer cells: Uterine natural killer (NK) cells are likely to play an important role in trophoblastic invasion and angiogenesis, besides being an important component of the local maternal immune response to pathogens. There is no clear evidence that altered peripheral blood or uterine natural killer cells are related to recurrent miscarriage.[28,29] Therefore, testing for peripheral blood or uterine NK cells as a surrogate marker of the events at the maternal-foetal interface is inappropriate and should not be offered routinely in the investigation of couples with recurrent miscarriage.

Cytokines: Cytokines are immune molecules that control both immune as well as other cells. Abnormal cytokine response may be another cause for recurrent miscarriage. It has been suggested that normal pregnancy might be the result of a predominant T-helper-2 cytokine response, whereas women with recurrent miscarriage may have an exaggerated T-helper-1 cytokine response. Available evidence does not suggest that routine cytokine tests should be introduced into clinical practice for evaluation of cases with recurrent miscarriage.[30]

Anatomical Causes

Anatomical defects of the reproductive system could be one of the most common causes of recurrent miscarriage. Uterine malformations, either congenital or acquired, could be responsible for approximately 12–15% cases of recurrent abortion. History of uterine malformations is often associated with late miscarriages. Congenital uterine anomalies include Müllerian duct abnormalities, presence of uterine septum and uterine or cervical anomalies. Acquired uterine anomalies leading to foetal loss include leiomyomas and endometriosis. Uterine abnormalities could result in impaired vascularisation of pregnancy and limited space for the growing foetus due to distortion of the uterine cavity. Hysterosalpingography (HSG) helps in diagnosing uterine anomalies. However, the routine use of HSG as a screening test for uterine anomalies in women with recurrent miscarriage, is questionable.

The exact role of congenital uterine anomalies in the pathogenesis of recurrent miscarriage presently remains unclear. The prevalence of uterine malformations appears to be higher in women with second-trimester miscarriages in comparison to those who suffer first-trimester miscarriages. However, this could be due to the cervical weakness that frequently occurs in association with uterine malformation.[31]

Uterine Malformations

Uterine malformations such as Müllerian anomalies could result in an abnormal or an irregularly shaped uterus, which could result in improper implantation and/or growth of the embryo, thereby resulting in recurrent miscarriages. The various Müllerian anomalies, which can be implicated as a cause of recurrent miscarriage, include septate uterus (50–60%), unicornuate uterus (34–44%), etc. Presence of a uterine anomaly such as uterine septum is a potentially treatable cause for recurrent miscarriage or infertility. However, not all patients with uterine anomalies experience repeated pregnancy losses. For example, patients with bicornuate uterus and uterus didelphys are not associated with recurrent miscarriage. It is yet not explained why some patients with uterine anomalies have normal reproductive function, while others experience recurrent miscarriages.

Uterine septum: Presence of a uterine septum results in repeated pregnancy losses due to the following factors:

❖ Reduced intrauterine space for foetal growth
❖ Placental implantation on a poorly vascularised uterine septum
❖ Associated cervical incompetence, luteal phase insufficiency and distortion of the uterine milieu.

Removal of the uterine septum or metroplasty is best performed using operative hysteroscopy. Patients with septate uterus are likely to show an improved pregnancy outcome following hysteroscopic septum resection.

Asherman's Syndrome

In addition to Müllerian anomalies, an acquired anatomical cause of recurrent abortions is Asherman's syndrome, which is characterised by development of intrauterine adhesions, occurring in women who have had several dilatation and curettage procedures. The pathogenesis of intrauterine adhesions and Asherman's syndrome is most often related to endometrial trauma. These adhesions may cause amenorrhoea, repeated miscarriages and infertility. Diagnosis of Asherman's syndrome can be reached by doing tests like hysteroscopy and TVS examination. Treatment involves hysteroscopic surgery to cut and remove the adhesions or scar tissue. After the removal of scar tissue, the uterine cavity must be kept open. Over the years, many surgical adjuncts have been tested in an attempt to prevent the reformation of adhesions. Some of these surgical adjuncts include intrauterine devices (inert), intrauterine Foley catheters, antiadhesion barriers, amnion grafts, hormonal therapy, antibiotic therapy, etc. Postoperative evaluation for reformation of adhesion in form of HSG or hysteroscopy should be considered mandatory.

Uterine Fibroids

Uterine fibroids, most commonly those that are submucosal, may distort the endometrial cavity, thereby resulting in recurrent pregnancy losses. No association with recurrent miscarriage could be established for either intramural or subserosal fibroids.

Endometrial Polyps

Endometrial polyps are frequently associated with infertility. Most experts feel that polypectomy should be performed with hysteroscopic guidance. Polypectomy can be performed by grasping and avulsing the stalk with ring forceps or sharply severing the base with electrosurgical instruments.

Cervical Incompetence

Cervical incompetence is a medical condition in which the pregnant woman's cervix starts dilating and effacing before her pregnancy has reached term, usually between 16 to 28 weeks of gestation, without any associated pain or uterine contractions. As a result, cervical incompetence may cause second and third-trimester miscarriages and preterm births. Though cervical incompetence is a recognised cause of second-trimester miscarriage, its true incidence remains unknown, because the diagnosis is essentially a clinical one. Currently, there is no satisfactory objective test that can identify women with cervical weakness in the non-pregnant state. The diagnosis is usually based on a history of second-trimester miscarriage preceded by spontaneous ROM or painless cervical dilatation. The women often give history of recurrent second-trimester pregnancy losses, occurring earlier in gestation in successive pregnancies and present with a significant cervical dilatation of 2 cm or more in the early pregnancy. However, usually there is absence of any other symptoms. In the second trimester, cervix may dilate up to 4 cm in association with active uterine contractions. This may be associated with rupture of the membranes resulting in the spontaneous expulsion of the foetus. Cervical incompetence could be due to congenital or acquired causes. The most common acquired cause of cervical incompetence is a history of cervical trauma or the previous history of cervical lacerations. Therefore, history of any cervical procedure including cervical conisation, loop electrosurgical excision procedure (LEEP), instrumental vaginal delivery or forceful cervical dilatation during previous miscarriage needs to be elicited. History of any cervical cerclage performed at the time of previous pregnancy also needs to be elicited. Some of the risk factors for development of cervical incompetence are listed in Box 29.3.

Box 29.3: Risk factors for development of cervical incompetence

❏ Diagnosis of cervical incompetence in a previous pregnancy
❏ Previous history of preterm premature rupture of membranes
❏ History of diethylstilbestrol exposure, which can cause anatomical defects in uterus and cervix
❏ History of previously having received trauma to the cervix

Epidemiological Factors

Advancing maternal age and number of previous miscarriages can be considered as two independent risk factors for further miscarriages.[32,33] Advancing maternal age is likely to result in a decline in both the number and quality of the remaining oocytes. Previous reproductive history is another independent predictor for future pregnancy outcomes because the risk of further miscarriages increases after each successive pregnancy loss, reaching approximately 40% after three consecutive pregnancy losses. However, history of a previous live birth does not prevent a woman from developing recurrent miscarriages in the future.[34]

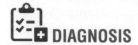 **DIAGNOSIS**

Clinical Presentation

Bad obstetric history could be related to recurrent miscarriages or a history of previous unfavourable foetal outcome in terms of two or more consecutive spontaneous abortions, early neonatal deaths, stillbirths, IUDs, congenital anomalies, etc.

Investigations

Women with recurrent first-trimester and second-trimester miscarriage should be attended by a health professional having necessary skills and expertise, preferably in a recurrent miscarriage clinic. The loss of pregnancy at any stage can be a distressing experience for both the parents. Therefore, particular sensitivity is required on the part of clinician while assessing and counselling the couples with recurrent miscarriage. Ideally, both the partners should be counselled together and provided accurate information for facilitating the decision-making process related to future pregnancies. They should be provided with clearly written patient-leaflets, which the couple can take home. The following tests need to be performed:

❖ *Cytogenetic analysis and parental karyotype*: Cytogenetic analysis should be performed on products of conception of the third and subsequent consecutive miscarriage(s). In cases where testing of products of conception reveals an unbalanced structural chromosomal abnormality, parental peripheral blood karyotyping of both partners should be performed. Selective parental karyotyping appears to be an appropriate option because it is associated with reduced healthcare costs.

Knowledge regarding the karyotype of the products of conception allows the clinician to provide an informed prognosis regarding future pregnancy outcomes. While a sporadic foetal chromosome abnormality is the most common cause of any single miscarriage, the risk of miscarriage as a result of foetal aneuploidy decreases with an increasing number of pregnancy losses.[35] If the karyotype of the miscarried pregnancy is abnormal, next pregnancy is likely to be associated with a better prognosis.[36]

PART II

❖ Thyroid function test
❖ Serum prolactin levels
❖ Blood glucose levels
❖ Blood grouping
❖ VDRL test for syphilis
❖ TORCH test
❖ High vaginal swab for detection of infections
❖ *Ultrasound examination*: This must be done for evaluation of the anatomical abnormalities of the uterine cavity and cervix. A pelvic ultrasound examination for the assessment of uterine anatomy must be performed in all women with recurrent first-trimester miscarriage and all women with one or more second-trimester miscarriages. In case of suspected uterine anomalies, further investigations such as hysteroscopy, laparoscopy or three-dimensional pelvic ultrasound may be done to confirm the diagnosis. Combined examination with hysteroscopy and laparoscopy and possibly three-dimensional ultrasound scanning can be used for establishing the definitive diagnosis. The value of MRI scanning in these cases remains undetermined.
❖ *Antiphospholipid antibodies such as lupus anticoagulant and anticardiolipin antibodies (IgG or IgM)*: For the diagnosis of antiphospholipid syndrome, it is mandatory that the woman has two positive tests at least 12 weeks apart either for LA or aCL antibodies of immunoglobulin G and/or immunoglobulin M class present in a medium or high titre over 40 g/L or above the 99th percentile.

   For the detection of LA, the dilute Russell's viper venom time test together with a platelet neutralisation procedure is more sensitive and specific than either the activated partial thromboplastin time test or the kaolin clotting time test. Anticardiolipin antibodies, on the other hand, can be detected using a standardised ELISA.
❖ Thrombophilia screening for FVL, factor II (prothrombin) gene mutation and protein S.
❖ Tests for cervical incompetence: This can be done using ultrasound examination and passage of No. 6–8 Hegars dilator through the internal os without any pain or resistance, especially in the premenstrual period.

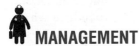

MANAGEMENT

Management of women with recurrent miscarriage should be in a specialist clinic and must comprise of the following steps depending upon the aetiology.

Psychological Support

It is important to alleviate patient's anxiety and to provide psychological support. About 40–50% of the total cases of recurrent abortion remain unexplained. For these cases, tender loving care (TLC) especially by the family and the partner, reassurance and supportive care are all that are usually required. However, presently there are no RCTs in support of TLC. All obstetricians should be aware of the psychological sequel associated with miscarriage and should provide adequate psychological support and follow-up,

as well as access to formal counselling when required. The obstetrician must remain vigilant until the delivery in these cases.

Genetic Counselling

Genetic abnormalities require referral to a clinical geneticist. In case of detection of a chromosomal anomaly, strategies such as genetic counselling, familial chromosomal studies, and appropriate prenatal diagnosis in future pregnancies provide the couple with a good prognosis for future pregnancies. These couples should also be offered the options of preimplantation genetic diagnosis, IVF, donor gametes, adoption, etc. Preimplantation genetic diagnosis or prenatal diagnosis (amniocentesis and chorionic villus sampling) helps in identifying embryos having or not having chromosomal abnormalities.

Preimplantation genetic diagnosis has been proposed as a treatment option for the individuals who are carriers of a translocation defect.[37] However, such patients should be informed that they have a nearly 50–70% higher chance of giving birth to a healthy newborn in future untreated pregnancies following natural conception than is achieved after preimplantation genetic diagnosis/IVF.[38-40] Furthermore, preimplantation genetic screening with IVF treatment in women with unexplained recurrent miscarriage does not improve live birth rates.

Various IVF procedures, which can be considered in different cases of recurrent miscarriage, are enlisted in Table 29.1.

Control of Diabetes and Thyroid Dysfunction

Prepregnancy glycaemic control is particularly important for women with overt diabetes mellitus. Replacement with thyroid hormone analogues may be required in hypothyroid women.

Table 29.1: Indications for in vitro fertilisation in cases of recurrent miscarriage

Indications	IVF procedure
Balanced chromosomal translocation and advanced maternal age	IVF with donor oocytes
Premature ovarian failure	IVF donor oocytes
Male factors (i.e. reduced capacitation or reduced fertilisation potential) responsible for reduced fertility	Intracytoplasmic sperm injection
Uncorrectable uterine factors	Surrogate mother
Recurrent implantation failure	Blastocyst culture with assisted hatching
Immunological causes	IVF with multiple embryo replacement
Patients undergoing pre-implantation genetic screening	Selection, and intrauterine transfer of normal embryos
Irreversible endometrial damage (e.g. Asherman's syndrome)	IVF with surrogacy

CHAPTER 29

Operative Hysteroscopy

Operative hysteroscopy can help in treatment of the following anomalies:

❖ Removal of submucous leiomyomas
❖ Resection of intrauterine adhesions
❖ Resection of intrauterine septa: Presently, there is insufficient evidence to indicate that the surgical correction of uterine anomalies (e.g. uterine septum resection) is beneficial for prevention of further miscarriages in women with previous history of recurrent miscarriages.

Treatment of Endocrine Problems

Luteal Phase Defects

Treatment of LPD is done using micronised progesterone in the dosage of 100 mg daily. Progesterone supplementation must continue until 10–12 weeks following gestation.

Progesterone Supplementation

Presently, there is insufficient evidence to evaluate the effect of progesterone supplementation during pregnancy to prevent a miscarriage in women with recurrent miscarriage.[41] Progesterone is crucial for successful implantation and maintenance of pregnancy. Progesterone induces a pregnancy-protective shift from proinflammatory T-helper-1 cytokine responses to a more favourable anti-inflammatory T-helper-2 cytokine response. A large multicentre study [Progesterone in Recurrent Miscarriage (PROMISE)] is currently under way to assess the beneficial effect of progesterone supplementation in women with unexplained recurrent miscarriage.

Supplementation with Human Chorionic Gonadotrophin

Presently, there is insufficient evidence to evaluate the effect of supplementation with hCG in pregnant women to prevent recurrent miscarriage.[42]

Polycystic Ovarian Disease

Suppression of high levels of luteinising hormone: Hypersecretion of luteinising hormone is a common feature of PCOS and has been reported as a risk factor for early pregnancy loss. However, prepregnancy pituitary suppression of high levels of luteinising hormone amongst ovulatory women with recurrent miscarriage and polycystic ovaries is not likely to improve the rate of live birth.[43] Moreover, the outcome of pregnancy without pituitary suppression is likely to be similar to that of women without raised levels of luteinising hormone.

Metformin supplementation: Polycystic ovary syndrome is likely to result in an increased risk of recurrent miscarriage due to insulin resistance and hyperinsulinaemia. Presently, there is insufficient evidence regarding the beneficial effect of metformin (an insulin sensitising agent) supplementation during pregnancy to prevent a miscarriage in women with recurrent miscarriage.[44]

Antiphospholipid Antibody Syndrome

Patients with positive antiphospholipid antibodies and thrombophilias must be treated with aspirin in the dosage of 50 mg daily. In case of a thrombotic event, subcutaneous heparin in the dosage of 5,000 IU BD should also be administered. LMWH may also prove to be useful. A Cochrane review[45] has shown that the treatment combination comprising of aspirin plus unfractionated heparin is likely to result in a significant increase in the rate of live births amongst women with APS. This treatment combination is likely to cause a significant reduction in the rate of miscarriage rate by 54%. LMWH is as safe as unfractionated heparin and has potential advantages during pregnancy, because it is associated with a reduced incidence of side effects such as heparin-induced thrombocytopenia and heparin-induced osteoporosis.[46] For details related to the treatment of APS, kindly refer to Chapter 10 [Connective Tissue Disorders (Autoimmune Disorders)].

Cervical Incompetence

Various surgical procedures for cervical incompetence are described as follows:

❖ *McDonald's procedure*: The most commonly used trans-vaginal cervical cerclage procedure in clinical practice is the McDonald's procedure (Fig. 29.1). In this procedure, a 5-mm band of permanent purse string suture using 4–5 bites is placed high on the cervix. It is usually removed at 37 weeks, unless there is a reason (e.g. infection, preterm labour, preterm ROM, etc.) for an earlier removal
❖ *Shirodkar's procedure*: Shirodkar's procedure (Figs 29.2A and B) is another commonly used cerlarge procedure. In this procedure a permanent purse string suture, which would remain intact for life, is applied. As a result, the patient requires to be delivered via caesarean section. The suture is placed submucosally as close to the internal cervical os as possible by giving incisions both over the mucosa on the anterior and posterior aspects of the cervix. This procedure also requires bladder dissection in comparison to the McDonald's procedure where no bladder dissection is required. Other advantages of

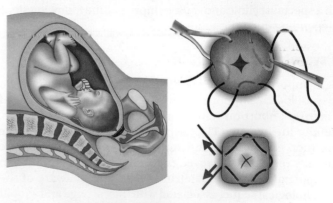

Fig. 29.1: McDonald's procedure

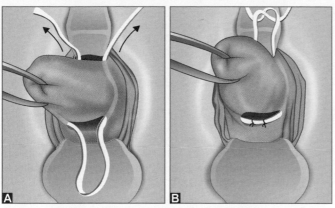

Figs 29.2A and B: Shirodkar's procedure

McDonald's procedure over Shirodkar's procedure include the following:
- Simplicity of the procedure (does not involve bladder dissection or complete burial of the sutures)
- Ease of removal at the time of delivery
- The stitch can also be applied when the cervix is effaced or the foetal membranes are bulging.

The disadvantage of the McDonald's procedure is the occurrence of excessive vaginal discharge with the exposed suture material.

Cervical cerclage is associated with potential risks related to the surgery and the danger of stimulating uterine contractions and therefore should be considered only in women who are likely to benefit from it. Women with a history of second-trimester miscarriage and suspected cervical weakness in whom cerclage has not been done may be offered serial cervical sonographic surveillance. An ultrasound-indicated cerclage can be offered if cervical length of 25 mm or less is detected by TVS performed before 24 weeks of gestation in women with a singleton pregnancy and a history of one second-trimester miscarriage attributable to cervical factors. A meta-analysis[47] has found no conclusive evidence that use of prophylactic cerclage helps in reducing the risk of pregnancy loss and preterm delivery in women at risk of preterm birth or mid-trimester recurrent miscarriage due to cervical factors. Furthermore, the procedure has also been found to be associated with a high risk of minor, but no serious morbidity.

A short cervical length (less than 25 mm) on TVS during pregnancy may be useful in predicting preterm birth in some cases of suspected cervical weakness.[48] Transabdominal cerclage has been suggested as a treatment option for second-trimester miscarriage and the prevention of early preterm labour in selected women with a previous failed transvaginal cerclage and/or a very short and scarred cervix.[49,50]

Immunotherapy

Various options for immunotherapy such as paternal cell immunisation, third-party donor leucocytes, trophoblast membranes and IV immunoglobulin in women with previous unexplained recurrent miscarriage have not been shown to improve the rate of live birth.[51] Moreover, immunotherapy is expensive and has potentially serious adverse effects such as transfusion reaction, anaphylactic shock and hepatitis. Therefore, immunotherapy should no longer be offered as a therapeutic option in women with unexplained recurrent miscarriage. Also, there is no published data regarding the use of anti-TNF agents to improve pregnancy outcome in women with recurrent miscarriage. Furthermore, anti-TNF agents are likely to cause potentially serious morbidity such as lymphoma, granulomatous disease such as tuberculosis, demyelinating diseases, congestive heart failure, etc. Therefore, immune treatments should not be offered routinely to women with recurrent miscarriage outside formal research studies.

Inherited Thrombophilia

Women with known heritable thrombophilia are at an increased risk of venous thromboembolism. Presently, there is insufficient evidence regarding the beneficial effect of heparin for prevention of miscarriage in women with recurrent first-trimester miscarriage associated with inherited thrombophilia.[52] Heparin therapy during pregnancy may, however, improve the rate of live birth in women with recurrent second-trimester miscarriage associated with inherited thrombophilias.

Use of LMWH (enoxaparin) is found to be effective in improving the rate of live births for the treatment of women, carrying the FVL or prothrombin gene mutation or those having protein S deficiency, with a history of a single late miscarriage after 10 weeks of gestation.[53]

Unexplained Recurrent Miscarriage

Women with unexplained recurrent miscarriage usually have an excellent prognosis for future pregnancy outcome if offered only supportive care in the setting of a dedicated early pregnancy assessment unit. They usually do not require any pharmacological intervention.[54,55] However, the prognosis is likely to deteriorate with increasing maternal age and the number of previous miscarriages. It has also been shown that the use of empirical treatment (in any form) in women with unexplained recurrent miscarriage is unnecessary and the clinician must refrain from instituting any such therapy.

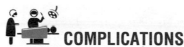

COMPLICATIONS

- ❖ Recurrent foetal loss, IUD
- ❖ Intrauterine growth restriction
- ❖ Severe pre-eclampsia/eclampsia/HELLP syndrome
- ❖ Placental abruption
- ❖ Recurrent thrombotic events, thrombocytopenia.

CLINICAL PEARLS

- ❖ If the cause of miscarriage remains undetermined, constant vigilance followed by hospitalisation during the early and later months of pregnancy usually works.

❖ If a mishap occurs in two subsequent pregnancies, it is likely to occur in the third pregnancy as well. Therefore, the obstetrician must remain vigilant regarding the same.

EVIDENCE-BASED MEDICINE

❖ The presently available evidence shows that working with or using video display terminals is not associated with an increased risk of miscarriage.[56]

❖ Recent retrospective studies have reported that maternal obesity is likely to increase the risk of both sporadic and recurrent miscarriage.[18-20]

❖ Testing for uterine and peripheral blood natural killer cells should not be routinely offered in the investigation of recurrent miscarriage.[28-29]

REFERENCES

1. Royal College of obstetricians and gynaecologists. (2011). The investigation and treatment of couples with Recurrent First trimester and Second-trimester miscarriage. Green-top Guideline No. 17. [online] Available from www.rcog.org.uk/globalassets/documents/guidelines/gtg_17.pdf. [Accessed July, 2016].

2. Stirrat GM. Recurrent miscarriage. Lancet. 1990;336(8716):673-5.

3. Wyatt PR, Owolabi T, Meier C, Huang T. Age-specific risk of fetal loss observed in a second trimester serum screening population. Am J Obstet Gynecol. 2005;192(1):240-6.

4. de Braekeleer M, Dao TN. Cytogenetic studies in couples experiencing repeated pregnancy losses. Hum Reprod. 1990;5(5):519-28.

5. Clifford K, Rai R, Watson H, Regan L. An informative protocol for the investigation of recurrent miscarriage: preliminary experience of 500 consecutive cases. Hum Reprod. 1994; 9(7):1328-32.

6. Stephenson MD, Sierra S. Reproductive outcomes in recurrent pregnancy loss associated with a parental carrier of a structural chromosome rearrangement. Hum Reprod. 2006;21(4): 1076-82.

7. Franssen MT, Korevaar JC, van der Veen F, Leschot NJ, Bossuyt PM, Goddijn M. Reproductive outcome after chromosome analysis in couples with two or more miscarriages: index [corrected]-control study. BMJ. 2006;332(7544):759-63.

8. Carp H, Toder V, Aviram A, Daniely M, Mashiach S, Barkai G. Karyotype of the abortus in recurrent miscarriage. Fertil Steril. 2001;75:678-82.

9. Rai R, Backos M, Rushworth F, Regan L. Polycystic ovaries and recurrent miscarriage—a reappraisal. Hum Reprod. 2000;15(3):612-5.

10. Cocksedge KA, Saravelos SH, Wang Q, Tuckerman E, Laird SM, Li TC. Does free androgen index predict subsequent pregnancy outcome in women with recurrent miscarriage? Hum Reprod. 2008;23(4):797-802.

11. Mills JL, Simpson JL, Driscoll SG, Jovanovic-Peterson L, Van Allen M, Aarons JH, et al. Incidence of spontaneous abortion among normal women and insulin-dependent diabetic women whose pregnancies were identified within 21 days of conception. N Engl J Med. 1988;319(25):1617-23.

12. Abalovich M, Gutierrez S, Alcaraz G, Maccallini G, Garcia A, Levalle O. Overt and subclinical hypothyroidism complicating pregnancy. Thyroid. 2002;12(1):63-8.

13. Hay PE, Lamont RF, Taylor-Robinson D, Morgan DJ, Ison C, Pearson J. Abnormal bacterial colonisation of the genital tract and subsequent preterm delivery and late miscarriage. BMJ. 1994;308(6924):295-8.

14. Leitich H, Kiss H. Asymptomatic bacterial vaginosis and intermediate flora as risk factors for adverse pregnancy outcome. Best Pract Res Clin Obstet Gynaecol. 2007;21(3):375-90.

15. Lindbohm ML, Sallmén M, Taskinen H. Effects of exposure to environmental tobacco smoke on reproductive health. Scand J Work Environ Health. 2002;28 Suppl 2:84-96.

16. Rasch V. Cigarette, alcohol, and caffeine consumption: risk factors for spontaneous abortion. Acta Obstet Gynecol Scand. 2003;82(2):182-8.

17. Lashen H, Fear K, Sturdee DW. Obesity is associated with increased risk of first trimester and recurrent miscarriage: matched case-control study. Hum Reprod. 2004;19(7):1644-6.

18. Metwally M, Ong KJ, Ledger WL, Li TC. Does high body mass index increase the risk of miscarriage after spontaneous and assisted conception? A meta-analysis of the evidence. Fertil Steril. 2008;90(3):714-26.

19. Metwally M, Saravelos SH, LedgerWL, Li TC. Body mass index and risk of miscarriage in women with recurrent miscarriage. Fertil Steril. 2010;94(1):290-5.

20. Wilson WA, Gharavi AE, Koike T, Lockshin MD, Branch DW, Piette JC, et al. International consensus statement on preliminary classification criteria for definite antiphospholipid syndrome: report of an international workshop. Arthritis Rheum. 1999;42(7):1309-11.

21. Miyakis S, Lockshin MD, Atsumi T, Branch DW, Brey RL, Cervera R, et al. International consensus statement on an update of the classification criteria for definite antiphospho-lipid syndrome (APS). J Thromb Haemost. 2006;4(2):295-306.

22. Di Simon N, De Carolis S, Lanzone A, Ronsisvalle E, Giannice R, Caruso A. In vitro effect of antiphospholipid antibody-containing sera on basal and gonadotrophin releasing hormone-dependent human chorionic gonadotrophin release by cultured trophoblast cells. Placenta. 1995;16(1):75-83.

23. Sthoeger ZM, Mozes E, Tartakovsky B. Anti-cardiolipin antibodies induce pregnancy failure by impairing embryonic implantation. Proc Natl Acad Sci U S A. 1993;90(14):6464-7.

24. Katsuragawa H, Kanzaki H, Inoue T, Hirano T, Mori T, Rote NS. Monoclonal antibody against phosphatidylserine inhibits in vitro human trophoblastic hormone production and invasion. Biol Reprod. 1997;56(1):50-8.

25. Bose P, Black S, Kadyrov M, Weissenborn U, Neulen J, Regan L, et al. Heparin and aspirin attenuate placental apoptosis in vitro: implications for early pregnancy failure. Am J Obstet Gynecol. 2005;102(1):23-30.

26. Salmon JE, Girardi G, Holers VM. Activation of complement mediates antiphospholipid antibody-induced pregnancy loss. Lupus. 2003;12(7):535-8.

27. DeWolf F, Carreras LO, Moerman P, Vermylen J, Van Assche A, Renaer M. Decidual vasculopathy and extensive placental infarction in a patient with repeated thromboembolic accidents, recurrent fetal loss, and a lupus anticoagulant. Am J Obstet Gynecol. 1982;142(7):829-34.

28. Wold AS, Arici A. Natural killer cells and reproductive failure. Curr Opin Obstet Gynecol. 2005;17(3):237-41.

29. Tuckerman E, Laird SM, Prakash A, Li TC. Prognostic value of the measurement of uterine natural killer cells in the

PART II

endometrium of women with recurrent miscarriage. Hum Reprod. 2007;22(8):2208-13.

30. Bombell S, McGuire W. Cytokine polymorphisms in women with recurrent pregnancy loss: meta-analysis. Aust N Z J Obstet Gynaecol. 2008;48(2):147-54.

31. Acién P. Incidence of Müllerian defects in fertile and infertile women. Hum Reprod. 1997;12(7):1372-6.

32. Nybo Anderson AM, Wohlfahrt J, Christens P, Olsen J, Melbye M. Maternal age and fetal loss: population based register linkage study. BMJ. 2000;320(7251):1708-12.

33. Regan L, Braude PR, Trembath PL. Influence of past reproductive performance on risk of spontaneous abortion. BMJ. 1989;299(6698):541-5.

34. Clifford K, Rai R, Regan L. Future pregnancy outcome in unexplained recurrent first trimester miscarriage. Hum Reprod. 1997;12(2):387-9.

35. Ogasawara M, Aoki K, Okada S, Suzumori K. Embryonic karyotype of abortuses in relation to the number of previous miscarriages. Fertil Steril. 2000;73(2):300-4.

36. Carp H, Toder V, AviramA, Daniely M, Mashiach S, Barkai G. Karyotype of the abortus in recurrent miscarriage. Fertil Steril. 2001;75(4):678-82.

37. Scriven PN, Flinter FA, Braude PR, Ogilvie CM. Robertsonian translocations—reproductive risks and indications for preimplantation genetic diagnosis. Hum Reprod. 2001;16(11):2267-73.

38. Stephenson MD, Sierra S. Reproductive outcomes in recurrent pregnancy loss associated with a parental carrier of a structural chromosome rearrangement. Hum Reprod. 2006;21(4):1076-82.

39. Regan L, Rai R, Backos M, El Gaddal S. Recurrent miscarriage and parental karyotype abnormalities: prevalence and future pregnancy outcome. Abstracts of the 17th Annual Meeting of the ESHRE, Lausanne, Switzerland 2001. Hum Reprod. 2001;16 Suppl 1:177-8.

40. Lalioti MD. Can preimplantation genetic diagnosis overcome recurrent pregnancy failure? Curr Opin Obstet Gynecol. 2008;20(3):199-204.

41. Haas DM, Ramsey PS. Progestogen for preventing miscarriage. Cochrane Database Syst Rev. 2008;(2):CD003511.

42. Harrison RF. Human chorionic gonadotrophin (hCG) in the management of recurrent abortion; results of a multi-centre placebo-controlled study. Eur J Obstet Gynecol Reprod Biol. 1992;47(3):175-9.

43. Clifford K, Rai R, Watson H, Franks S, Regan L. Does suppressing luteinising hormone secretion reduce the miscarriage rate? Results of a randomised controlled trial. BMJ. 1996;312(7045):1508-11.

44. Palomba S, Falbo A, Orio F, Zullo F. Effect of preconceptional metformin on abortion risk in polycystic ovary syndrome: a systematic review and meta-analysis of randomized controlled trials. Fertil Steril. 2009;92(5):1646-58.

45. Empson M, Lassere M, Craig J, Scott J. Prevention of recurrent miscarriage for women with antiphospholipid antibody or lupus anticoagulant. Cochrane Database Syst Rev. 2005;(2):CD002859.

46. Greer IA, Nelson-Piercy C. Low-molecular-weight heparins for thromboprophylaxis and treatment of venous thrombo-embolism in pregnancy: a systematic review of safety and efficacy. Blood. 2005;106(2):401-7.

47. Drakeley AJ, Roberts D, Alfirevic Z. Cervical cerclage for prevention of preterm delivery: meta-analysis of randomized trials. Obstet Gynecol. 2003;102:621(23)-7.

48. Berghella V, Odibo AO, To MS, Rust OA, Althuisius SM. Cerclage for short cervix on ultrasonography: meta-analysis of trials using individual patient-level data. Obstet Gynecol. 2005;106(1):181-9.

49. Gibb DM, Salaria DA. Transabdominal cervicoisthmic cerclage in the management of recurrent second trimester miscarriage and preterm delivery. Br J Obstet Gynaecol. 1995;102(10):802-6.

50. Anthony GS, Walker RG, Cameron AD, Price JL, Walker JJ, Calder AA. Transabdominal cervico-isthmic cerclage in the management of cervical incompetence. Eur J Obstet Gynecol Reprod Biol. 1997;72(2):127-30.

51. Porter TF, LaCoursiere Y, Scott JR. Immunotherapy for recurrent miscarriage. Cochrane Database Syst Rev. 2006;(2):CD000112.

52. Royal College of Obstetricians and Gynaecologists (2009). Reducing the risk of thrombosis and embolism during pregnancy and the puerperium. Green-top Guideline No. 37a. [online] Available from www.rcog.org.uk/womens-health/clinical-guidance/reducing-risk-of-thrombosis-greentop37a. [Accessed August 2016]

53. Gris JC, Mercier E, Quéré I, Lavigne-Lissalde G, Cochery-Nouvellon E, Hoffet M, et al. Low-molecular weight heparin versus low-dose aspirin in women with one fetal loss and constitutional thrombophilic disorder. Blood. 2004;103(10):3695-9.

54. Brigham SA, Conlon C, Farquharson RG. A longitudinal study of pregnancy outcome following idiopathic recurrent miscarriage. Hum Reprod. 1999;14(11):2868-71.

55. Liddell HS, Pattison NS, Zanderigo A. Recurrent miscarriage—outcome after supportive care in early pregnancy. Aust N Z J Obstet Gynaecol. 1991;31(4):320-2.

56. Marcus M, McChesney R, Golden A, Landrigan P. Video display terminals and miscarriage. J Am Med Womens Assoc. 2000;55(2):84-8, 105.

CHAPTER 29

Pregnancy after Previous Caesarean Delivery

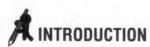 **INTRODUCTION**

With the increasing incidence of operative abdominal deliveries (caesarean births), the number of patients with the previous history of one or more previous caesarean births being encountered in clinical practice, is progressively on rise. As a result, the obstetrician must be well versed in dealing with the complications related to previous caesarean birth.

DIAGNOSIS

Clinical Presentation

A complete history of previous caesarean births must be taken including the type of the scar given (classical or the lower segment); any technical difficulties encountered during the procedure; the reason for which the caesarean birth was performed; and whether there was any history of complications during the surgery. For details related to caesarean delivery per se, kindly refer to Chapter 45 (Caesarean Delivery).

General Physical Examination

The obstetrician must be particularly vigilant regarding the detection of signs of impending scar rupture, which include the following:

* Dull suprapubic pain or severe abdominal pain, especially, if persisting in between the uterine contractions
* Slight vaginal bleeding or haematuria
* Bladder tenesmus or frequent desire to pass urine
* Unexplained maternal tachycardia
* Maternal hypotension
* Chest pain, shoulder tip pain or sudden onset of shortness of breath.

Abdominal Examination

* Besides the routine obstetric abdominal examination, careful examination of the abdominal scar and elicitation of scar tenderness is important.
* Abnormal FHR pattern may be observed on external CTG.

Investigations

Routine ANC investigations including blood grouping (ABO and Rh typing):

* Complete blood count
* Ultrasound examination.

 MANAGEMENT

In the past, management of the patient with a history of caesarean scar was considered as 'once a caesarean, always a caesarean'. This dictum has now been changed to 'once a caesarean, always hospitalisation'. Presently, the two most commonly used options for delivery in these patients comprise of VBAC and ERCS. Planned VBAC is an appropriate option that may be offered to the majority of women with a singleton pregnancy of cephalic presentation at 37^{+0} weeks or beyond, and those who have had a single previous lower segment caesarean delivery, with or without a history of previous vaginal birth. This is likely to be associated with a planned VBAC success rate of 85–90%.[1] The criteria for VBAC are described in Box 30.1.

Antepartum Period

Antenatal Counselling

Antenatal counselling must be provided to women with the previous history of one or more caesarean deliveries

(Box 30.2). This also needs to be documented in their cases notes. This would help ensure taking informed consent and making shared decisions in women undergoing VBAC. A patient information leaflet should be provided along with the consultation. The final decision regarding mode of birth (VBAC vs ERCS) should be agreed upon following the consultation between the woman and member(s) of the maternity team before the expected or planned date of delivery. The benefits and risks of each option (VBAC vs ERCS) must be discussed with the mother (Table 30.1). Since rupture of the previous scar is the major dreaded complication likely to be associated with VBAC, the obstetrician must remain vigilant regarding the factors (Box 30.3), which are likely to increase the risk of scar rupture. In the majority of cases where there is no contraindication (Box 30.4) for planned VBAC, counselling for mode of delivery could be

---

Box 30.1: Criteria for VBAC

- ❑ Previous history of one uncomplicated lower segment transverse caesarean section
- ❑ Low transverse incision on the uterus
- ❑ Pelvis is adequate
- ❑ Patient is willing for VBAC
- ❑ Facilities for continuous foetal monitoring during labour are available
- ❑ No other contraindications for caesarean section
- ❑ Previous history of vaginal birth, particularly VBAC
- ❑ VBAC should be undertaken in settings where facilities for emergency caesarean section are present

---

Box 30.2: Points to be taken into consideration while counselling women with previous history of caesarean delivery

Vaginal birth after caesarean
- ❑ Women should be made aware that successful VBAC is associated with the lowest rate of complications, and therefore, while choosing the mode of delivery it is important to estimate the success and failure rates of VBAC in each case
- ❑ Trial of VBAC resulting in emergency caesarean delivery is associated with the greatest risk of adverse outcomes
- ❑ Planned VBAC is associated with ~1 in 200 (0.5%) risk of uterine rupture
- ❑ VBAC is associated with an extremely low absolute risk of birth-related perinatal deaths, which is comparable to that of nulliparous women in labour
- ❑ The success rate of planned VBAC varies between 72% and 75%.
- ❑ Women with one or more previous vaginal births should be informed that the history of previous vaginal delivery, particularly previous VBAC, acts as the most important predictor for successful VBAC. This is associated with a planned VBAC success rate of 85–90%.

Elective repeat caesarean section
- ❑ When a date for ERCS is being decided upon, a plan for the event of labour, starting before the scheduled date should be documented in the patient's case notes
- ❑ Women should be informed that ERCS is associated with a small increased risk of complications such as placenta praevia and/or accreta and/or pelvic adhesions in the future pregnancies
- ❑ The risk of perinatal death with ERCS is extremely low. However, there is a small increase in neonatal respiratory morbidity when ERCS is performed before 39^{+0} weeks of gestation

CHAPTER 30

Table 30.1: Risks and benefits of planned VBAC versus ERCS from 39^{+0} weeks of gestation

Benefits	Risks
Vaginal birth after caesarean	
• VBAC is associated with the fewest complications • The absolute risk of birth-related perinatal death associated with VBAC is extremely low and comparable to the risk for nulliparous women in labour • Chances of VBAC being successful are 72–75% • If successful, VBAC is associated with a shorter duration of hospital stay and recovery period • VBAC increases the likelihood of future vaginal births • Risk of maternal death with VBAC is lower than that with ERCS • VBAC is associated with 2–3% risk of transient respiratory morbidity, which is lower than that with ERCS.	• Greatest risk of adverse outcome occurs in a trial of VBAC resulting in emergency caesarean delivery • Risk of uterine rupture associated with VBAC is ~0.5%. If occurs, it is associated with significant maternal morbidity and foetal morbidity/mortality • Risk of anal sphincter injury in women undergoing VBAC is 5% • VBAC is associated with an increased risk of instrumental delivery • VBAC is associated with an increased risk (0.08%) of hypoxic-ischaemic encephalopathy (HIE) • Associated with 4 per 10,000 (0.04%) risk of delivery-related perinatal death • The rates of hysterectomy, thromboembolic disease, transfusion and endometritis do not differ significantly between planned VBAC and ERCS.
Elective repeat caesarean section	
• May be possible to plan a known delivery date in selected patients • Practically avoids the risk of uterine rupture (actual risk is extremely low: less than 0.02%) • Associated with a reduced risk of pelvic organ prolapse and urinary incontinence • Offers the option for permanent sterilisation if fertility is no longer desired • Less than 1 per 10,000 (<0.01%) risk of delivery-related perinatal death or HIE.	• ERCS is associated with a small increased risk of placenta praevia and/or accreta in future pregnancies and of pelvic adhesions complicating any future abdominopelvic surgery • The risk of perinatal death with ERCS is extremely low, but there is a small increase in neonatal respiratory morbidity when ERCS is performed before 39^{+0} weeks of gestation • It is associated with a longer recovery period • Future pregnancies—likely to require caesarean delivery, increased risk of placenta praevia or accreta and adhesions with successive caesarean deliveries or abdominal surgery • Risk of maternal death with ERCS is higher than that with VBAC • Risk of transient respiratory morbidity of 4–5% (higher than that with VBAC)

conducted by a member of the maternity team soon after the woman's mid-trimester ultrasound. In presence of some complication, e.g. the woman has contraindications that make VBAC unacceptable, she is uncertain about the mode of delivery, she has specifically requested ERCS, the woman requires induction of labour (e.g. >41^{+0} weeks of gestation) or she has developed specific pregnancy complications (e.g. pre-eclampsia, breech presentation, foetal growth restriction, macrosomia), an obstetrician should be involved. In case of women with relative contraindication for VBAC, caution should be implemented and the senior obstetrician should make decisions on a case-by-case basis.

Prior to taking any decision in such women, the obstetrician must also remember that previous vaginal delivery is also independently associated with a reduced risk of uterine rupture. Successful VBAC is also more likely amongst women with previous caesarean for foetal malpresentation (84%) in comparison to women with previous caesarean for indications such as labour dystocia (64%) or foetal distress (73%).[2,3] History of having an emergency caesarean delivery in their first birth is also associated with a lower VBAC success rate. This particularly includes those individuals who underwent emergency caesarean delivery due to failed induction of labour as a result of occiput posterior position or prolonged second stage.

Many models for predicting the success rate of VBAC have been developed by several authors. However, further research is required to predict the VBAC success using these models, although initial results appeared to be promising. Some authors have used a VBAC score to predict the success of women attempting VBAC. Schoorel et al. created the retrospective VBAC score using five features: (1) Bishop score at the time of admission; (2) maternal age; (3) indication for previous caesarean delivery; (4) BMI and (5) previous vaginal birth. Higher VBAC score is likely to be associated with a higher success rate. Women with a VBAC score of more than 16 were associated with a success rate of greater than 85%. On the other hand, those with a VBAC score of 10 were only associated with a success rate of approximately 50%.[4,5] Some factors which are associated with an increased likelihood of successful VBAC are tabulated in Box 30.5. Obstetrician needs to remain vigilant regarding the presence of underlying complications, such as postdated pregnancy, twin gestation, foetal macrosomia, antepartum stillbirth or maternal age of 40 years or more, etc., which act as relative contraindication for VBAC.

Twin gestation: The National Institute of Child Health and Human Development (NICHD) studies have reported similar success rates of VBAC with twin pregnancies in comparison to singleton pregnancies.[6]

Suspected foetal macrosomia: Birthweight of 4 kg or more in cases of VBAC is associated with an increased risk of complications, such as uterine rupture, unsuccessful VBAC, shoulder dystocia and third- and fourth-degree perineal laceration.[7]

In most cases, the decision regarding mode of delivery should be finalised by 36^{+0} weeks of gestation. The ANC schedule in these women should be in accordance with the ANC guideline, recommended by NICE.[8]

Box 30.3: Factors which are likely to be associated with an increased risk of uterine rupture in women undergoing VBAC

- ❑ Short interdelivery interval (<12 months since last delivery)
- ❑ Postdated pregnancy
- ❑ Maternal age of 40 years or more
- ❑ Obesity
- ❑ Lower prelabour Bishop score
- ❑ Foetal macrosomia
- ❑ Decreased ultrasonographic lower segment myometrial thickness[9]

Box 30.4: Contraindications to VBAC

Absolute contraindications
- ❑ Women with a history of previous uterine rupture
- ❑ Previous classical caesarean scar[10]
- ❑ Women who have any absolute contraindication to vaginal birth which is applicable irrespective of the presence or absence of a scar (e.g. major placenta praevia)[11]

Relative contraindications
- ❑ Type of previous uterine incision (previous inverted T or J incisions, low vertical uterine incisions or significant inadvertent uterine extension at the time of primary caesarean)
- ❑ Previous history of uterine surgery (e.g. hysteroscopic resection of uterine septum, laparoscopic or abdominal myomectomy, especially where the uterine cavity has been penetrated)[12,13]
- ❑ Presence of underlying complications such as postdated pregnancy, twin gestation, foetal macrosomia, antepartum stillbirth or maternal age of 40 years or more, etc.

Box 30.5: Factors associated with an increased likelihood of successful VBAC

- ❑ Greater maternal height
- ❑ Maternal age <40 years
- ❑ BMI <30 kg/m^2
- ❑ Gestational age of <40 weeks
- ❑ Infant birthweight <4 kg
- ❑ Spontaneous onset of labour
- ❑ Vertex presentation
- ❑ Foetal head engagement or presence at a lower station
- ❑ Higher admission Bishop score

Women with History of Two or More Prior Caesareans

Women who have had two or more prior lower segment caesarean deliveries may be offered VBAC after counselling by a senior obstetrician. This should include the risk of uterine rupture and maternal morbidity, and the individual likelihood of successful VBAC (e.g. given a history of prior vaginal delivery). Women with two previous caesarean deliveries who are considering VBAC should be counselled that these cases are associated with success rate of approximately 70% and the uterine rupture rate of 1.36%. Maternal morbidity in these cases is comparable to that associated with the repeat caesarean delivery option.[14] The rates of hysterectomy and transfusion are also likely to be higher in women undergoing VBAC after two previous caesarean births compared with one previous caesarean birth.[14] Labour in these cases should be preferably conducted in a centre by an obstetrician with

Table 30.2: Risk of placenta praevia and placenta accreta in the subsequent pregnancies based on the number of previous caesarean deliveries[15]

Number of previous caesarean deliveries	Risk of placenta praevia (%)	Risk of placenta accreta (%)
1	1	11–14
2	1.7	23–40
3 or more	2.8	Up to 67

suitable expertise having an alternative of immediate surgical delivery if required. Women who plan to have multiple (e.g. 3 or more) pregnancies in the future should be counselled that opting for ERCS may result in greater surgical risks for future pregnancies due to the risk of complications, such as placenta praevia, placenta accreta and hysterectomy (Table 30.2). Therefore, preference should be given towards VBAC in such patients. An individualised assessment regarding the suitability for VBAC should be made in women keeping into consideration those factors which are likely to increase the risk of uterine rupture (Box 30.3).

Intrapartum Period

Vaginal Birth after Caesarean

With VBAC, the following steps must be observed during the intrapartum period:

❖ One-to-one supportive care should preferably be provided to the patients undergoing VBAC, with regular monitoring of maternal sign and symptoms and assessment of their cervicometric progress in labour (at no less than 4-hourly intervals).
❖ Blood should be sent for grouping, cross-matching and CBC (including haemoglobin and haematocrit levels). Blood should be preferably arranged.
❖ Intravenous access must be established and Ringer's lactate to be started.
❖ Clinical monitoring of the mother for the signs of scar dehiscence needs to be done (Box 30.6).
❖ Careful monitoring of FHR, preferably using continuous external CTG.
❖ The use of prostaglandins for induction of labour in women with the previous history of caesarean section must be best avoided.
❖ Epidural analgesia can be safely given at the time of labour. However, if there is an increasing requirement for pain relief in labour, the clinician must become vigilant regarding the possibility of an impending uterine rupture.
❖ The labour should be continuously monitored in these patients to be able to promptly identify the signs of maternal or foetal compromise, labour dystocia and/or uterine scar rupture.
❖ Intrapartum monitoring regarding the progress of labour must be done using a partogram.
❖ Second stage of labour can be cut short by using prophylactic forceps or ventouse.

❖ Preterm women who are considering the options for VBAC should be informed that planned preterm VBAC has success rates similar to that of planned term VBAC. However, planned preterm VBAC is associated with a lower risk of uterine rupture.
❖ Routine uterine exploration following VBAC is not recommended. If the patient shows signs of uterine rupture, uterine exploration may be done. Laparotomy may be required if a uterine rent is found on the uterine exploration.
❖ Resources should also be available for immediate caesarean delivery and advanced neonatal resuscitation in case attempt at VBAC fails.

Induction of labour: Although induction and augmentation is not contraindicated in women with previous caesarean delivery, use of induction and augmentation in such patients presently remains controversial. The decision to induce or augment labour during VBAC should be determined following careful obstetric assessment and be made by senior obstetricians in consultation with the woman and her partner. An informed consent should be taken from the woman prior to induction. Before taking consent, women should be made aware of the increased risks of complications such as uterine rupture and emergency caesarean delivery associated with induction and/or augmentation of VBAC labour. Probable complications associated with the alternative option of ERCS also need to be deliberated. The senior obstetrician needs to discuss the following with the woman: the decision to induce labour, the proposed method of induction and different modes of induction (oxytocin, prostaglandins or mechanical means). The senior obstetrician also needs to decide the time intervals for serial vaginal examination. The nursing staff should be well acquainted with the particular parameters (e.g. scar tenderness) for monitoring progress of labour which may require discontinuing VBAC.

Box 30.6: The clinical features associated with uterine scar rupture or impending scar rupture

❑ Abnormal CTG trace
❑ Dull suprapubic pain or severe abdominal pain, especially if persisting between contractions
❑ Acute onset of scar tenderness
❑ Abnormal vaginal bleeding
❑ Haematuria
❑ Cessation of previously efficient uterine activity
❑ Unexplained maternal tachycardia, hypotension, fainting or shock
❑ Chest pain or shoulder tip pain or sudden onset of shortness of breath
❑ Onset of unexpected antepartum or PPH
❑ On vaginal examination, there may be loss of station of the presenting part
❑ There may be a failure of normal descent of the presenting part, and the presenting part may remain high up on vaginal examination
❑ Change in abdominal contour
❑ Inability to pick up FHR at the old transducer site
❑ Bladder tenesmus or frequent desire to pass urine

CHAPTER 30

Sweeping of membranes is recommended for induction of labour in such women after 40 weeks of gestation. Augmentation with oxytocin is associated with an increased risk of scar rupture.[16] Obstetrician should be aware that induction of labour using mechanical methods (amniotomy or Foley's catheter) is associated with a lower risk of scar rupture in comparison with induction using prostaglandins. Induction (especially in women with an unfavourable cervix or through the use of prostaglandins method) or augmentation of VBAC labour is associated with a twofold to threefold increased risk of uterine rupture. It is also associated with approximately 1.5-fold increased risk of caesarean delivery compared with spontaneous labour in cases of VBAC. Before considering induction of labour, all steps to optimise the progress of labour must be undertaken.

Women who are contemplating many future pregnancies must be counselled about the potential long-term surgical risks associated with multiple repeat caesarean deliveries. Instead, they should be advised to accept the additional risks associated with induction and/or augmentation.

Presently, there is insufficient evidence from RCTs to determine the method of induction of labour which is associated with lowest risk in cases of previous caesarean delivery.[17]

Elective Repeat Caesarean Section

Planning and conducting ERCS: For the physician, ERCS may be associated with some advantages such as saving of time and reduced fear of legal litigation in case of complications with VBAC. Management of these cases comprises of the following steps:

❖ The management of women undergoing ERCS should be done by a multidisciplinary approach.

❖ Informed consent must be taken from the patient prior to undertaking surgery.

❖ Elective repeat caesarean section should preferably be planned after 39[+0] weeks of gestation in case of the previous history of lower segment uterine scar. In case of previous history of classical scar, the woman must preferably be hospitalised at 36 weeks and posted for an elective caesarean section at 38 weeks.

❖ Women considering ERCS should be counselled that delaying delivery by 1 week from 38[+0] to 39[+0] weeks is likely to result in a 5% reduction in the risk of respiratory morbidity (particularly transient tachypnoea of the newborn).[18-20] However, this delay may be associated with a 5 per 10,000 (0.05%) increase in the risk of antepartum stillbirth.[21] In case ERCS is required prior to 39 weeks of gestation, consideration should be given towards administering corticosteroids to the mother. However, the current RCOG Green-top guideline on administration of antenatal corticosteroids[22] raises a concern that presently there is an absence of evidence regarding the safety of antenatal corticosteroids administration to the babies born after 36[+0] weeks of gestation.

❖ Antibiotics should be administered prior to the skin incision in women undergoing ERCS to help achieve a reduction in the risk of maternal infection. This is not likely to cause any detrimental effects on the baby. Ideally, the chosen antibiotic should protect against endometritis and urinary tract and wound infections, e.g. cefuroxime and metronidazole.[23]

❖ All women undergoing ERCS should receive thromboprophylaxis according to existing RCOG guidelines.

❖ Since ERCS is associated with a high risk of placenta praevia, early recognition of the complication can help prevent future morbidity and mortality.

❖ The planning and conduction of ERCS should be as per the recommendations provided in the NICE guidelines for caesarean section.[21]

COMPLICATIONS

❖ If VBAC turns out to be unsuccessful, an emergency caesarean section may be required.

❖ *Uterine rupture:* There is a risk of the scar dehiscence and rupture, which may be associated with increased maternal and perinatal mortality. Since this is the most dreaded complication of VBAC, it is described next in details under a separate heading.

❖ Pelvic floor dysfunction

❖ Elective repeat caesarean section may be associated with difficult surgery due to the presence of adhesions.

Uterine Rupture

Disintegration of the scar, also known as scar rupture is one of the most disastrous complications associated with VBAC. In a patient with a previous caesarean delivery, vaginal delivery may cause the previous uterine scar to separate. The risk of uterine rupture in an unscarred uterus is extremely rare and occurs at the rate of 2 per 10,000 (0.02%) deliveries. In case of unscarred uterus, this risk is mainly restricted to multiparous women in labour.[24,25] On the other hand, the risk of uterine rupture in cases of planned VBAC is approximately 20–50 per 10,000 (0.2–0.5%). In contrast, in cases of ERCS, the risk of uterine rupture is 2 per 10,000 (0.02%).[26-28] The exact risk of scar rupture following VBAC depends upon the type of uterine incision given at the time of previous caesarean delivery. The weakest type of scar that may give way at the time of VBAC is the previous classical incision in the upper segment of the uterus.

Uterine rupture can result in complete extrusion of the foetus into the maternal abdominal cavity. In other cases, rupture is associated with foetal distress or severe haemorrhage from the rupture site. Abnormal CTG is the most reliable finding in cases of uterine rupture and may be present in 60–80% of these cases. Though uterine rupture is often associated with foetal bradycardia, there is no specific FHR pattern which indicates the onset of uterine rupture. Variable and/or late decelerations often occur before the onset of foetal bradycardia. However, nearly 50% of such cases present with a combination of findings (most often abnormal CTG and abdominal pain). The diagnosis of uterine rupture is made during emergency caesarean delivery or postpartum laparotomy. Another important clinical finding which is indicative of uterine rupture is the onset of unexpected antepartum haemorrhage or PPH. Various signs and symptoms suggestive of uterine rupture are tabulated in Box 30.6. The classical triad associated with scar rupture includes abdominal pain, abnormal vaginal bleeding and abnormal CTG. More than 90% of the uterine ruptures occur during labour, with the peak incidence at the cervical dilatation of 4–5 cm.[24]

Types of Uterine Rupture

Uterine rupture is defined as a disruption of the uterine muscle extending to and involving the uterine serosa. The uterine rupture can be of two types: (1) complete rupture and (2) incomplete rupture.

1. *Complete rupture*: It describes a full-thickness defect of the uterine wall and serosa resulting in direct communication between the uterine and the peritoneal cavity.
2. *Incomplete rupture*: Incomplete rupture, also known as uterine dehiscence, describes a defect of the uterine wall that is contained by the visceral peritoneum or broad ligament.

Obstetrician must remain vigilant regarding the early diagnosis of uterine scar dehiscence or rupture so that they can initiate prompt laparotomy and neonatal resuscitation to reduce associated morbidity and mortality.

Assessment of Scar Integrity

In order to identify the previous caesarean scars, which are likely to give way during VBAC, the following investigations can be done:

❖ *Hysterogram*: Radiographic imaging of the uterus, which shows uterine defect in the lateral view
❖ *Ultrasound imaging*: Ultrasound examination for visualisation of scar defects and measurement of scar thickness
❖ *Manual exploration*: Manual exploration of placenta to check scar integrity is especially useful in case of continuing PPH and in case of other third-stage problems.

Ultrasound Imaging for Visualisation of Scar Defects and Measurement of Scar Thickness

Ultrasound measurement of scar thickness at 37 weeks of gestation is based on the fact that the risk of a defective scar is directly related to the degree of thinning of the lower uterine segment at around 37 weeks of pregnancy. According to the largest study by Rozenberg et al. (1997),[25] cut-off value of 3.5 mm on ultrasound measurement of scar thickness at 36 weeks was observed to show negative predictive value of 99.3% for scar rupture. The high negative predictive value of this method may encourage the obstetricians to offer a trial of labour to patients with a thickness value of 3.5 mm or greater. Different studies show different cut-off values for estimating the strength of the scar. Therefore, presently there is no clear-cut value of scar thickness to indicate the strength of the scar.[29] Transvaginal ultrasound seems to be more accurate than transabdominal ultrasound, yet it is not commonly used.[30]

Management of Rupture Uterus

When uterine rupture is diagnosed or strongly suspected, surgery is necessary. While in the previous days, most cases of uterine rupture were managed with hysterectomy, nowadays they are managed by controlling the bleeding surgically and repairing the defect. A decision must be made regarding, whether to perform hysterectomy or to repair the rupture site. If future fertility is desirable and the rent in the uterus appears to be repairable (straight-cut scar, rupture in the body of uterus, pelvic blood vessels are intact), repair of the rupture site must be performed. If future fertility is not desirable or the uterine rent appears to be unrepairable (multiple rents with ragged margins, injury to the iliac vessels, etc.), hysterectomy should be performed. Typically, longitudinal tears, especially those in a lateral position, should be treated by hysterectomy, whereas low transverse tears may be repaired. A lower segment rupture can cause transection of the uterine vessels. Therefore, the obstetrician must make special efforts to localise the site of bleeding, before placing clamps at the time of hysterectomy, in order to avoid injury to the ureter and iliac vessels. Bladder rupture must also be ruled out at the time of laparotomy by clearly mobilising and inspecting the bladder to ensure that it is intact. Though steps must be taken to resuscitate the patient, surgery should not be delayed owing to hypovolemic shock because it may not be easily reversible, until the haemorrhage from uterine rupture has been controlled. Uterine rupture may be associated with massive PPH. Therefore upon laparotomy, various steps such as application of aortic compression, administration of oxytocics (oxytocin, ergot alkaloids, carboprost, misoprostol, etc.) and surgical options, like ligation of the hypogastric artery, uterine artery or ovarian arteries can be taken to reduce the amount of bleeding. Due to the risk of rupture recurrence in a subsequent pregnancy, women with previously repaired uterine ruptures are advised not to attempt labour in the future. In case of future pregnancy, a repeat caesarean section should be performed prior to the onset of uterine contractions in these cases.

CLINICAL PEARLS

❖ The patient with previous caesarean section must be considered as high risk and frequent antenatal check-ups are required.
❖ The identification or suspicion of uterine rupture is a medical emergency and must be followed by an immediate and urgent response from the obstetrician. An emergency laparotomy is usually required to save the patient's life.

EVIDENCE-BASED MEDICINE

❖ The present evidence indicates that planned VBAC is a safe and appropriate mode of delivery for the majority of pregnant women with a single previous lower segment caesarean delivery.[1,31,32]

CHAPTER 30

❖ According to recommendations by RCOG (2007), women with history of previous two or more uncomplicated low transverse caesarean sections can also be considered for the planned VBAC. Present evidence indicates that there is no significant difference in the rates of uterine rupture in VBAC with two or more previous caesarean births in comparison with a single previous caesarean birth.[33-35]

REFERENCES

1. Royal College of Obstetricians and Gynaecologists (RCOG). (2015). Birth after previous caesarean birth. Green-top Guideline No. 45. [online]. Available from www.rcog.org.uk/en/guidelines-research-services/guidelines/gtg45/. [Accessed June, 2016].

2. Landon MB, Hauth JC, Leveno KJ, Spong CY, Leindecker S, Varner MW, et al. Maternal and perinatal outcomes associated with a trial of labor after prior cesarean delivery. N Engl J Med. 2004;351(25):2581-9.

3. Landon MB, Leindecker S, Spong CY, Hauth JC, Bloom S, Varner MW, et al. The MFMU Cesarean Registry: factors affecting the success of trial of labor after previous cesarean delivery. Am J Obstet Gynecol. 2005;193(3 Pt 2):1016-23.

4. Schoorel EN, Melman S, van Kuijk SM, Grobman WA, Kwee A, Mol BW, et al. Predicting successful intended vaginal delivery after previous caesarean section: external validation of two predictive models in a Dutch nationwide registration-based cohort with a high intended vaginal delivery rate. BJOG. 2014;121(7):840-7.

5. Schoorel EN, van Kuijk SM, Melman S, Nijhuis JG, Smits LJ, Aardenburg R, et al. Vaginal birth after a caesarean section: the development of a Western European population-based prediction model for deliveries at term. BJOG. 2014;121(2):194-201.

6. Grobman WA, Gersnoviez R, Landon MB, Spong CY, Leveno KJ, Rouse DJ, et al. Pregnancy outcomes for women with placenta previa in relation to the number of prior cesarean deliveries. Obstet Gynecol. 2007;110(6):1249-55.

7. Jastrow N, Roberge S, Gauthier RJ, Laroche L, Duperron L, Brassard N, et al. Effect of birth weight on adverse obstetric outcomes in vaginal birth after cesarean delivery. Obstet Gynecol. 2010;115(2 Pt 1):338-43.

8. National Institute for Health and Care Excellence (NICE). (2008). Antenatal care for uncomplicated pregnancies. NICE clinical guideline 62. [online]. Available from www.nice.org.uk/guidance/cg62. [Accessed June, 2016].

9. Kok N, Wiersma IC, Opmeer BC, de Graaf IM, Mol BW, Pajkrt E. Sonographic measurement of lower uterine segment thickness to predict uterine rupture during a trial of labor in women with previous Cesarean section: a meta-analysis. Ultrasound Obstet Gynecol. 2013;42(2):132-9.

10. Greene RA, Fitzpatrick C, Turner MJ. What are the maternal implications of a classical caesarean section? J Obstet Gynaecol. 1998;18(4):345-7.

11. Royal College of Obstetricians and Gynaecologists (RCOG). (2011). Placenta Praevia, Placenta Praevia Accreta and Vasa Praevia: Diagnosis and Management. Green-top Guideline No. 27. [online]. Available from www.rcog.org.uk/en/guidelines-research-services/guidelines/gtg27/ [Accessed June, 2016].

12. Shokeir T, Abdelshaheed M, El-Shafie M, Sherif L, Badawy A. Determinants of fertility and reproductive success after hysteroscopic septoplasty for women with unexplained primary infertility: a prospective analysis of 88 cases. Eur J Obstet Gynecol Reprod Biol. 2011;155(1):54-7.

13. Nouri K, Ott J, Huber JC, Fischer EM, Stögbauer L, Tempfer CB. Reproductive outcome after hysteroscopic septoplasty in patients with septate uterus—a retrospective cohort study and systematic review of the literature. Reprod Biol Endocrinol. 2010;8:52.

14. Tahseen S, Griffiths M. Vaginal birth after two caesarean sections (VBAC-2)—a systematic review with meta-analysis of success rate and adverse outcomes of VBAC-2 versus VBAC1 and repeat (third) caesarean sections. BJOG. 2010;117(1):5-19.

15. Gurol-Urganci I, Cromwell DA, Edozien LC, Smith GC, Onwere C, Mahmood TA, et al. Risk of placenta previa in second birth after first birth cesarean section: a population based study and meta-analysis. BMC Pregnancy Childbirth. 2011;11:95.

16. Landon MB, Hauth JC, Leveno KJ, Spong CY, Leindecker S, Varner MW, et al. Maternal and perinatal outcomes associated with trial of labour after prior caesearn delivery. N Engl J Med. 2004;351(25):2581-9

17. Jozwiak M, Dodd JM. Methods of term labour induction for women with a previous caesarean section. Cochrane Database Syst Rev. 2013;(3):CD009792.

18. Go MD, Emeis C, Guise JM, Schelonka RL. Fetal and neonatal morbidity and mortality following delivery after previous cesarean. Clin Perinatol. 2011;38(2):311-9.

19. Kamath BD, Todd JK, Glazner JE, Lezotte D, Lynch AM. Neonatal outcomes after elective cesarean delivery. Obstet Gynecol. 2009;113(6):1231-8.

20. Richardson BS, Czikk MJ, daSilva O, Natale R. The impact of labor at term on measures of neonatal outcome. Am J Obstet Gynecol. 2005;192(1):219-26.

21. Smith GC, Pell JP, Dobbie R. Caesarean section and risk of unexplained stillbirth in subsequent pregnancy. Lancet. 2003;362(9398):1779-84.

22. Royal College of Obstetricians and Gynaecologists (RCOG). (2010). Antenatal corticosteroids to reduce neonatal morbidity and mortality. Green-top Guideline No. 7. [online]. Available from www.rcog.org.uk/en/guidelines-research-services/guidelines/gtg7/. [Accessed June, 2016].

23. National Institute for Health and Clinical Excellence (NICE). (2011). Caesarean section. NICE clinical guideline 132. [online]. Available from www.nice.org.uk/guidance/cg132. [Accessed June, 2016].

24. Zwart JJ, Richters JM, Ory F, de Vries JI, Bloemenkamp KW, van Roosmalen J. Uterine rupture in The Netherlands: a nationwide population-based cohort study. BJOG. 2009;116(8):1069-70.

25. Rozenberg P, Goffinet F, Phillippe HJ, Nisand I. Ultrasonographic measurement of lower uterine segment to assess risk of defects of scarred uterus. Lancet. 1996;347(8997):281-4.

26. Naji O, Abdallah Y, Bij De Vaate AJ, Smith A, Pexsters A, Stalder C, et al. Standardized approach for imaging and measuring Cesarean section scars using ultrasonography. Ultrasound Obstet Gynecol. 2012;39(3):252-9.

27. Ofir K, Sheiner E, Levy A, Katz M, Mazor M. Uterine rupture: differences between a scarred and an unscarred uterus. Am J Obstet Gynecol. 2004;191(2):425-9.

28. Guise JM, Eden K, Emeis C, Denman MA, Marshall N, Fu RR, et al. Vaginal birth after cesarean: new insights. Evid Rep Technol Assess (Full Rep). 2010;(191):1-397.

29. Fitzpatrick KE, Kurinczuk JJ, Alfirevic Z, Spark P, Brocklehurst P, Knight M. Uterine rupture by intended mode of delivery in the UK: a national case-control study. PLoS Med. 2012;9(3): e1001184.

30. Dekker GA, Chan A, Luke CG, Priest K, Riley M, Halliday J, et al. Risk of uterine rupture in Australian women attempting vaginal birth after one prior caesarean section: a retrospective population-based cohort study. BJOG. 2010; 117(11):1358-65.

31. Dodd JM, Crowther CA, Huertas E, Guise JM, Horey D. Planned elective repeat caesarean section versus planned vaginal birth for women with a previous caesarean birth. Cochrane Database Syst Rev. 2004;(4):CD004224.

32. Dodd JM, Crowther CA. Elective repeat caesarean section versus induction of labour for women with a previous caesarean birth. Cochrane Database Syst Rev. 2012;(5):CD004906.

33. Landon MB, Spong CY, Thom E, Hauth JC, Bloom SL, Varner MW, et al. Risk of uterine rupture with a trial of labor in women with multiple and single prior cesarean delivery. Obstet Gynecol. 2006;108(1):12-20.

34. Macones GA, Cahill A, Pare E, Stamilio DM, Ratcliffe S, Stevens E, et al. Obstetric outcomes in women with two prior cesarean deliveries: is vaginal birth after cesarean delivery a viable option? Am J Obstet Gynecol. 2005;192(4):1223-8.

35. Miller DA, Diaz FG, Paul RH. Vaginal birth after cesarean: a 10-year experience. Obstet Gynecol. 1994;84(2):255-8.

Post-term Pregnancy (Prolonged Pregnancy)

INTRODUCTION

Post-term or postmature pregnancy can be defined as any pregnancy continuing beyond 2 weeks of the expected date of delivery (>294 days). The gestational age should have been established on ultrasound examination in the first trimester or preferably prior to 16 weeks of gestation. Prolonged pregnancy and post-term pregnancy are used to denote the same condition and is likely to occur in 5–10% cases.[1]

AETIOLOGY

Although the exact causes of postdated pregnancy remain unknown, some likely causative factors are as follows:

* *Wrong dates*: This can be considered as the most common cause of postmaturity.[2,3] In these cases, use of ultrasonography helps in determining the accurate estimation of gestational age.
* *Maternal factors*: These include factors such as primiparity, previous history of prolonged pregnancy, sedentary habits and elderly multipara.
* *Foetal congenital anomalies*: Foetal congenital anomalies such as anencephaly and adrenal hypoplasia may be implicated in the causation of postmaturity.
* *Placental factors*: Placental factors such as sulfatase deficiency (a rare X-linked recessive disorder) may be involved.

DIAGNOSIS

Clinical Presentation

* *Maternal weight record*: Stationary or falling maternal weight

* *Abdominal girth*: Gradually diminishing abdominal girth due to gradually reducing liquor volume
* *False labour pains*: Appearance of labour pains which quickly subside
* *Abdominal palpation*: The uterus may feel 'full of foetus' due to the diminishing volume of the liquor
* *Internal vaginal examination*: Ripe cervix could be suggestive of foetal maturity. Hard skull bones may be felt through the cervix or vaginal fornix, thereby suggesting foetal maturity.

Investigations

* *Ultrasonography*: Ultrasound parameters, such as crown-rump length (CRL), biparietal diameter (BPD) and femur length (FL), help in the assessment of gestational age. Ultrasound scans performed early in gestation are more helpful in the accurate assessment of gestational age. Amniotic fluid pocket of less than 2 cm and amniotic fluid index (AFI) less than or equal to 5 cm on ultrasound examination is an indication for induction of labour or delivery. Absent end-diastolic flow on umbilical artery Doppler is another indicator of foetal jeopardy.
* *Tests for foetal well-being*: These include tests, such as NST, BPP and ultrasound assessment of the amniotic fluid volume, which may be performed on a bi-weekly basis.

MANAGEMENT

The obstetric management is based on two principles; the first being determination of accurate gestational age and second being increased foetal surveillance. Management of post-term pregnancy has been described in the Flow chart 31.1. To reduce perinatal morbidity, induction of labour at 41 completed weeks of gestation and beyond is favoured. The review by Gülmezoglu et al. has shown that this strategy is likely to reduce the risk of perinatal morbidity.[4] However, this strategy

Flow chart 31.1: Management of post-term pregnancies

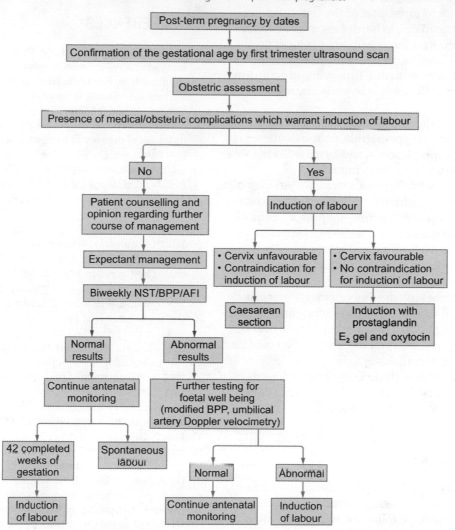

did not result in reduction in the rate of operative deliveries in comparison to the conservative management. On the other hand, the RCT by Hannah et al.[5] has demonstrated a lower rate of caesarean section in the group where the labour was induced in comparison to the group undergoing conservative management. SOGC and ACOG also recommend induction of labour at 41–42 weeks of gestation.[6,7] Current guidance regarding the management of prolonged pregnancy in the United Kingdom is based on NICE guidelines on induction of labour and antenatal care. These guidelines also offer induction of labour from 41[+0] weeks of gestation.

Though induction of labour at 41 completed weeks of gestation is likely to reduce the perinatal mortality rate, some women would opt for conservative management with foetal surveillance because they may visualise induction as an interference with the natural process of childbirth. Therefore, treatment of every patient must be individualised. After appropriate counselling, she should be allowed to make her own decision regarding induction. As per the recommendations by NICE, management of post-term pregnancy beyond 42 completed weeks should comprise of at least twice per weekly cardiotocographic monitoring and ultrasound-assisted measurement of the maximum

amniotic pool depth.[8,9] No proven benefit of cardiotocographic monitoring has been demonstrated till date. This is recommended mainly on the basis of observational data. It is thought that computerized cardiotocography may be superior to conventional tocography. However, this has yet not been tested in the clinical trials. The use of Doppler analysis for the various foetal arterial systems, which has been advocated in the management of post-term pregnancies, has also not been evaluated by randomised trials. The use of umbilical arterial Doppler is likely to be useful in these situations. Presently, there is no good evidence which supports the hypothesis that foetal monitoring can help reduce perinatal mortality in post-term pregnancies. However, this has been suggested as a good practice by the NICE guidelines.

COMPLICATIONS

❖ *Foetal distress*: Diminished placental function and oligohydramnios due to PROM may result in foetal hypoxia and distress
❖ *Macrosomia*: This is associated with an increased incidence of shoulder dystocia and operative delivery

❖ *Birth trauma*: There is an increased incidence of traumatic birth deliveries due to large size of the baby and non-moulding of foetal head due to hardening of skull bones

❖ *Respiratory distress*: Respiratory distress can occur due to chemical pneumonitis, atelectasis and pulmonary hypertension. This may occur following meconium aspiration and eventually result in hypoxia and respiratory failure.

❖ *Neonatal problems*: After birth, many neonatal complications can arise, such as hypothermia, poor subcutaneous fat, hypoglycaemia, hypocalcaemia, and increased incidence of injuries, such as brachial plexus injuries.

❖ *Increased perinatal mortality and morbidity*: An overall increase in the rate of perinatal morbidity and mortality could be related to complications such as meconium aspiration, neonatal acidaemia, low APGAR (Appearance, Pulse, Grimace, Activity, Respiration) scores, foetal macrosomia, shoulder dystocia with resultant orthopaedic or neurological injury, etc.

❖ *Postmaturity syndrome*: Prolonged labour may be associated with an increased risk of postmaturity syndrome, IUGR, meconium-stained liquor, oligohydramnios, foetal distress, loss of subcutaneous fat, and cracked skin. These could be the signs of placental insufficiency.

❖ *Maternal risk*: This can include complications such as increased risk of operative delivery, infection, haemorrhage, considerable psychological morbidity, etc.

CLINICAL PEARLS

❖ In uncomplicated cases of post-term pregnancy, where foetal maturity has been attained, expectant attitude may be extended for 7–10 days, following which the labour is induced

❖ Prolonged labour must be expected due to a large baby and poor moulding of the foetal head

❖ Expectant management is appropriate between 40 weeks to 41 weeks of gestation

❖ Delivery becomes mandatory when the period of gestation reaches 42 weeks, because the risk of antepartum stillbirths and maternal complications is significant enough.

EVIDENCE-BASED MEDICINE

❖ The available evidence has shown that the use of ultrasound in the early pregnancy for precise dating is likely to reduce the number of prolonged pregnancies compared to the dating based on last menstrual period or the second trimester ultrasound.[10-13]

❖ Sweeping of membranes (also known as stripping of membranes) is an evidence-based intervention, which is likely to reduce the incidence of prolonged pregnancy. There is presently insufficient evidence regarding the use of other techniques such as nipple stimulation, sexual intercourse or acupuncture for reducing the occurrence of prolonged pregnancy.[14,15]

REFERENCES

1. Shea KM, Wilcox AJ, Little RE. Postterm delivery: a challenge for epidemiologic research. Epidemiology. 1998;9(2):199-204.
2. Whitworth M, Bricker L, Neilson JP, Dowswell T. Ultrasound for fetal assessment in early pregnancy. Cochrane Database Syst Rev. 2010;(4):CD007058.
3. Crowley P. Interventions for preventing or improving the outcome of delivery at or beyond term. Cochrane Database Syst Rev. 2000;(2):CD000170.
4. Gülmezoglu AM, Crowther CA, Middleton P, Heatley E. Induction of labour for improving birth outcomes for women at or beyond term. Cochrane Database Syst Rev. 2012;(6): CD004945.
5. Hannah ME, Hannah WJ, Hellmann J, Hewson S, Milner R, Willan A. Induction of labor as compared with serial antenatal monitoring in post-term pregnancy. A randomized controlled trial. The Canadian Multicenter Post-term Pregnancy Trial Group. N Engl J Med. 1992;326(24):1587-92.
6. SOGC Clinical Practice Guidelines. (2008) Guidelines for the management of pregnancy at 41+0 to 42+0 weeks. No. 214. [online] Available from http://sogc.org/wp-content/ uploads/2013/01/gui214CPG0809.pdf [Accessed July, 2016].
7. American College of Obstericians and Gynaecologists (ACOG). (2004). Management of post-term pregnancy. ACOG Practice Bulletin No 55. [online] Available from http://residents. fammed.org/Block%20Curriculum/G1/FMS%20B%20G1%20 articles/ACOG_Management_of_Postterm.52.pdf [Accessed July, 2016].
8. National Collaborating Centre for Women's and Children's Health; National Institute for Health and Clinical Excellence: Guidance. NICE Guidelines 62. Antenatal Care. Routine Care for Healthy Pregnant Women. London: RCOG Press; 2008.
9. National Collaborating Centre for Women's and Children's Health; National Institute for Health and Clinical Excellence: Guidance. NICE guidelines 70. Induction of labour. National collaborating centre for women and children health. London: RCOG Press; 2008.
10. Tunón K, Eik-Nes SH, Grøttum P. A comparison between ultrasound and a reliable last menstrual period as the predictors of the day of delivery in 15,000 examinations. Ultrasound Obstet Gynecol. 1996;8(3):178-85.
11. Doherty L, Norwitz ER. Prolonged pregnancy: when should we intervene? Curr Opin Obstet Gynecol. 2008;20(6):519-27.
12. Clinical Practice Obstetrics Committee; Maternal Fetal Medicine Committee, Delaney M, Roggensack A, Leduc DC, Ballermann C, et al. Guidelines for management of pregnancy at 41+0 to 42+0 weeks. J Obstet Gynaecol Can. 2008;30(9): 800-23.
13. Bennett KA, Crane JM, O'shea P, Lacelle J, Hutchens D, Copel JA. First trimester ultrasound screening is effective in reducing postterm labour induction rates: a randomised controlled trial. Am J Obstet Gynecol. 2004;190(4):1077-81.
14. Boulvain M, Irion O, Marcoux S, Fraser W. Sweeping of the membranes to prevent post-term pregnancy and to induce labour: a systematic review. Br J Obstet Gynaecol. 1999;106(5): 481-5.
15. de Miranda E, van der Bom JG, Bonsel GJ, Bleker OP, Rosendaal FR. Membrane sweeping and prevention of post-term pregnancy in low-risk pregnancies: a randomised controlled trial. BJOG. 2006;113(4):402-8.

PART II

Liquor Abnormalities

OLIGOHYDRAMNIOS

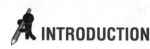 **INTRODUCTION**

Oligohydramnios can be defined as having less than 200 mL of amniotic fluid at term or an amniotic fluid index (AFI) of less than 5 cm or presence of deepest vertical pool (DVP) which does not measure more than 2 cm at its largest diameter.[1]

AETIOLOGY

Known causes of oligohydramnios include the following:

* *Preterm premature rupture of the membranes*: Preterm PROM (PPROM) is the most common cause for oligohydramnios
* *Idiopathic*: The majority of women with mild oligohydramnios may have no identifiable cause
* *Birth defects*: Birth defects, especially those involving the kidneys and urinary tract, e.g. renal agenesis, renal dysplasia or obstruction of the urinary tract (posterior urethral valves or atresia)
* Post-term pregnancy (>40 weeks)
* *Placental dysfunction*: Presence of amnion nodosum (squamous metaplasia of amnion) on the placenta, placental thrombosis or infarction, abruptio placentae, twin-to-twin transfusion (i.e. twin polyhydramnios-oligohydramnios sequence)
* *Maternal health conditions*: Gestational diabetes mellitus, pre-eclampsia, chronic hypertension, collagen vascular disease, nephropathy, thrombophilia, etc.
* *Certain medications*: Medications including ACE inhibitors, prostaglandin inhibitors (aspirin, etc.) can cause oligohydramnios
* Foetal chromosomal abnormalities
* *Intrauterine growth restriction associated with placental insufficiency*: In these cases, the following features may be present; abdominal circumference below 10th percentile for gestational age, poor growth velocity and abnormal umbilical artery waveform velocimetry. When foetal growth restriction is present in association with an oligohydramnios, it is associated with an increased perinatal mortality.

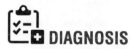 **DIAGNOSIS**

Clinical Presentation

* The patient may give a history of experiencing reduced foetal movements
* Fundal height is less than that estimated on the basis of last menstrual period
* Uterus appears full of foetus
* Evidence of IUGR may be present.

Investigations

* *Ultrasound examination*: Ultrasound can help establish the diagnosis of oligohydramnios by measuring the AFI or DVP (Fig. 32.1). Ultrasound examination may reveal IUGR. A combination of biophysical studies and Doppler waveform analysis (of umbilical and uterine vessels) also helps in the evaluation of foetal well-being in cases of IUGR.[2,3]
* *Other investigations*: Based on clinical circumstances, additional tests, e.g. karyotype analysis to reveal chromosomal abnormalities (e.g. Trisomy 13 and triploidy) and instillation of dye (for evaluation of the amniotic fluid volume), can be used.

 OBSTETRIC MANAGEMENT

* The main principle of management is to confirm the aetiology of oligohydramnios and to define its prognosis.

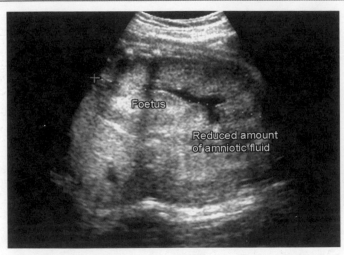

Fig. 32.1: Ultrasound scan of 26-week-old foetus showing oligohydramnios

❖ Women with otherwise normal pregnancies, who develop oligohydramnios near term probably need no treatment because in most of these cases of oligohydramnios would resolve itself without treatment.[4]

❖ There is no effective long-term treatment of oligohydramnios. In cases of idiopathic oligohydramnios, maternal treatment can comprise of the following: IV isotonic solution, oral hydration, or amnioinfusion. These procedures often result in short-term treatment.

❖ Hospitalisation may also be sometimes required in severe cases.

❖ *Reduced physical activity*: Many providers advise women to observe bed rest.

❖ *Maternal hydration*: Simple maternal hydration has been suggested as a way of increasing amniotic fluid volume (AFV).

❖ *Amnioinfusion*: This method involves infusion of sterile water through the cervix into the uterine cavity. This treatment may help to reduce complications during labour and delivery and also reduce the requirement for caesarean section.[5,6]

❖ *Foetal surveillance*: In the third trimester, there exists an inverse relationship between AFV and the incidence of adverse pregnancy outcomes. Adverse pregnancy outcomes in these cases may be related to abnormalities, such as umbilical cord compression, uteroplacental insufficiency and meconium aspiration. Close foetal surveillance of these patients is therefore required. An NST and AFI (or BPP) can be performed once or twice weekly until delivery. If one of these tests shows abnormality, early delivery by fastest route may be required even if the foetus is preterm.

❖ For women with idiopathic oligohydramnios, delivery is usually suggested at 37–38 completed weeks of gestation rather than observing an expectant management. Though induction of an unfavourable cervix in cases of idiopathic oligohydramnios may be associated with an increased risk of caesarean delivery, there is insufficient evidence to show that conservative management of idiopathic oligohydramnios at term is associated with a perinatal outcome similar to that with induced delivery.[7-9]

COMPLICATIONS

Oligohydramnios can be associated with the following complications:[10]

❖ *Complications during early pregnancy*:
  • Restriction of the amount of free space inside the uterine cavity
  • Amniotic adhesions causing deformities or constriction of the umbilical cord
  • Pressure deformities such as clubfeet.

❖ *Complications during the late pregnancy*:
  • Foetal distress, IUGR
  • Cord compression, resulting in foetal hypoxia and asphyxia
  • Prolonged rupture of membranes, chorioamnionitis subsequent to PPROM
  • Foetal malformations (renal agenesis, polycystic kidneys, urethral obstruction, etc.)
  • Postmaturity syndrome
  • Birth defects [compression of foetal organs, resulting in lung defects (pulmonary hypoplasia, etc.) and limb defects]
  • Potter's syndrome (sequela of oligohydramnios characterised by flattened facies, postural deformities and pulmonary hypoplasia)
  • Miscarriage, premature birth, stillbirth
  • Increased risk of meconium aspiration syndrome
  • Increased requirement for operative delivery
  • Overall increased perinatal morbidity.

CLINICAL PEARLS

❖ Premature rupture of the membranes and preterm labour early in pregnancy is commonly associated with oligohydramnios and developmental pulmonary hypoplasia.

❖ Reduced amniotic fluid in the first trimester appears to be an ominous finding and is associated with a poor prognosis.

EVIDENCE-BASED MEDICINE

❖ The available evidence indicates a strong association between early-onset oligohydramnios and perinatal mortality.[9]

❖ Increased concentration of maternal serum alpha foetoprotein (MSAFP) levels has been found to be associated with the second trimester oligohydramnios, with or without an anomalous foetus. This combination (elevated MSAFP levels and oligohydramnios) carries an extremely poor prognosis: foetal growth restriction, foetal death, preterm delivery and neonatal death.[11-14]

❖ Presently, there is insufficient evidence to show that conservative management of idiopathic oligohydramnios at term is associated with a perinatal outcome comparable to that with induction of labour at 37–38 weeks.[9] Therefore, labour is commonly induced at 37–38 weeks of gestation in cases of idiopathic oligohydramnios.

POLYHYDRAMNIOS

INTRODUCTION

Polyhydramnios is defined as presence of AFV of 2,000 mL or greater at term (Fig. 32.2). The DVP in these cases is greater than or equal to 8 cm and AFI is above the 95th percentile for the particular gestational age. The value of AFI commonly used in the clinical practice for the diagnosis of polyhydramnios is greater than or equal to 24 cm. The varying degrees of polyhydramnios (Table 32.1) are based on the measurement of the largest vertical pocket of liquor.[15,16]

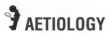

AETIOLOGY

In about two-thirds of cases, the causes of polyhydramnios are unknown and are therefore idopathic. Polyhydramnios could be related to increased urine production, and impaired swallowing and intestinal reabsorption of amniotic fluid. Polyhydramnios is more likely to occur due to the following causes:[17]

❖ *Foetal causes*:
   • Congenital abnormalities: The most common birth defects that cause polyhydramnios are those that hinder foetal swallowing, such as birth defects involving the GI tract (oesophageal or duodenal atresia), CNS (e.g. anencephaly, etc.) or muscular system (e.g. muscular dystrophy).
   • Twin-to-twin transfusion syndrome and Bartter's syndrome (both are likely to result in foetal polyuria)[18]
   • Parvovirus B19 infection (likely to result in foetal anaemia).
❖ *Maternal causes*:
   • Multiple pregnancies

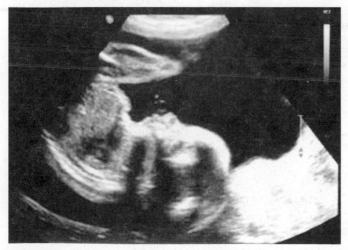

Fig. 32.2: Foetus with polyhydramnios

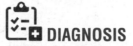

Table 32.1: Degrees of polyhydramnios

Grading	Criteria
Mild	Largest vertical pocket of liquor measures 8–11 cm
Moderate	Largest vertical pocket of liquor measures 12–15 cm
Severe	Largest vertical pocket of liquor measures >16 cm

   • Maternal diabetes mellitus (osmotic diuresis in the foetus)
   • Rh blood incompatibilities between mother and foetus (likely to result in foetal anaemia).

DIAGNOSIS

Clinical Presentation

Women with minor polyhydramnios experience few symptoms. Those who are more severely affected may experience the following symptoms:
❖ Difficulty in breathing
❖ Presence of large varicosities in the legs and/or vulva
❖ Presence of new haemorrhoids or worsening of those present previously.

Abdominal Examination

❖ Abdomen is markedly enlarged, along with fullness of flanks.
❖ The skin of the abdominal wall appears to be tense and shiny, and may show appearance of large striae.
❖ Clinically, the patients have a fundal height greater than the period of amenorrhoea.
❖ Foetal heart sounds may appear muffled as if coming from a distance.
❖ A fluid thrill may be commonly present.
❖ It may be difficult to palpate the uterus or the foetal presenting in parts due to presence of excessive fluid.

Investigations

Ultrasound examination: A comprehensive, high-resolution sonographic evaluation is recommended to establish the diagnosis of polyhydramnios, to identify multiple pregnancy and to determine if any foetal anomalies or foetal hydrops are present.[19,20] Detailed foetal assessment involves examination of foetal thorax, CNS, GI tract and renal system. The various grades of polyhydramnios based on the ultrasound findings have been previously described in Table 32.1.

Other investigations: Other laboratory evaluations, which may be required, depend upon the clinical circumstances and include tests such as:
❖ Screening for gestational diabetes
❖ Testing for foetomaternal haemorrhage if foetal anaemia is suspected. If polyhydramnios is associated with foetal anaemia, foetus is likely to be hydropic.
❖ Assessment of foetal middle cerebral artery peak systolic velocity helps in the identification of anaemic foetuses.

❖ Maternal serology to determine exposure to infectious agents (e.g. syphilis, parvovirus, cytomegalovirus, toxoplasmosis, rubella, etc.)[21]

❖ Appropriate tests for hereditary anaemias (e.g. α thalassemia) or metabolic abnormalities.

❖ Karyotype analysis may be offered in cases of severe polyhydramnios or in the presence of associated anatomic or structural anomalies.

❖ Biochemical analysis of amniotic fluid can help in the diagnosis of oesophageal atresia and Bartter's syndrome.

 ## MANAGEMENT

Mild degree of hydramnios usually resolves on its own without any treatment. No active management may be required in patients with asymptomatic hydramnios. For patients showing symptomatic hydramnios, the following treatment options are available:

❖ Treatment of the underlying cause

❖ *Decompression by amniocentesis*: Amniocentesis is a procedure involving the removal of a sample of amniotic fluid in order to provide relief against symptoms, such as respiratory embarrassment, excessive uterine activity or premature opening of cervical os, etc. Serial amnio-reduction in singleton pregnancies has been advocated but carries the risk of precipitating preterm labour and rapid reaccumulation of fluid following the procedure.[22,23] Treatment of polyhydramnios in relation to TTTS has been described in details in Chapter 23 (Multifoetal Gestation). Serial amnioreduction can be used for treatment of Stages I and II TTTS. Foetoscopic ablation of placental vascular anastomoses is the treatment of choice in more advanced cases (Stages III or IV).

❖ *Pharmacological management*: Pharmacological management can be initiated with the help of prostaglandin synthase inhibitors and cyclooxygenase-2 inhibitors (e.g. indomethacin and sulindac).[24-27] These drugs may help in reducing the AFV by reducing the foetal urinary output. However, drugs such as prostaglandin synthetase inhibitors may cause complications such as renal failure in neonates and premature closure of ductus arteriosus, thereby resulting in an increased perinatal mortality. Use of indomethacin in utero can also result in complications such as necrotising enterocolitis and intracranial haemorrhage.

Management in each case needs to be individualised based on the specific underlying aetiology. The specific therapeutic option is based on the gestational age, degree of maternal discomfort, and the likely indications or contraindications for using prostaglandin synthetase inhibitors. Treatment is usually indicated in cases of severe polyhydramnios (AFI > 40 cm; DVP > 12 cm), which causes a high intra-amniotic pressure resulting in maternal discomfort. If polyhydramnios persists despite therapy, delivery should be preferably conducted by 38 weeks of gestation in the view of increased risk of unexplained stillbirths. Management based on the period of gestation is as follows:

❖ *Less than 32 weeks of gestation*: In cases of severe symptomatic polyhydramnios at less than 32 weeks of gestation, amnioreduction (to normalise fluid volume) can be offered. Simultaneously, treatment with indomethacin can be commenced to maintain normal AFV. A course of corticosteroids is given prior to amnio-reduction because of the increased risk of preterm birth.

During indomethacin therapy, AFV must be monitored on at least weekly intervals and the indomethacin dosage must be adjusted based on the AFV changes. Blood flow through the ductus must be assessed through Doppler examination at every 2–7-day interval. Increased surveillance must be maintained after 28 weeks of gestation, to look for an early evidence of constriction. It may be possible to discontinue treatment with indomethacin, if polyhydramnios does not recur. In any case, indomethacin must be discontinued latest by 32 weeks because of the risk of premature ductal constriction.

❖ *Period of gestation between 32 weeks and 34 weeks*: For severe symptomatic polyhydramnios between 32 weeks and 34 weeks of gestation, amnioreduction is usually advised.

❖ *More than 34 weeks of gestation*: After 34 weeks, amniocentesis is offered to the woman for assessing foetal lung maturity. The baby is immediately delivered if the foetal maturity is confirmed. Administration of indomethacin is usually not recommended in these cases because of the high risk of premature closure of the ductus arteriosus at this gestational age.[28]

 ## COMPLICATIONS

Various complications which can occur due to polyhydramnios are as follows.[29-32]

Maternal

❖ Respiratory compromise and/or abdominal discomfort due to uterine distension

❖ Antepartum and postpartum haemorrhage (due to postpartum uterine atony)

❖ Abnormal foetal presentations or unstable lie

❖ Umbilical cord prolapse

❖ Uterine dysfunction, gestational diabetes

❖ Increased incidence of operative intervention

❖ Increased risk of premature delivery and PROM

❖ Increased risk of placental abruption and stillbirth

❖ Increased perinatal mortality (could be related to congenital malformations and preterm labour).

Foetal

❖ Congenital malformations

❖ Increased perinatal morbidity

❖ Stillbirths

❖ Preterm births.

CLINICAL PEARLS

❖ The outcome of pregnancies complicated by poly-hydramnios varies according to the severity and underlying aetiology of the excessive fluid accumulation.

❖ Vaginal delivery is possible in cases of hydramnios if the foetal head is reasonably fixed in the pelvis.

❖ Labour needs to be monitored in these cases due to an increased risk of cord prolapse and foetal distress.

EVIDENCE-BASED MEDICINE

❖ A careful search for the underlying cause is mandatory in the cases of polyhydramnios. In cases where no secondary cause can be identified, the gestational age for delivery may be prolonged by the use of cyclooxygenase inhibitors. However, this form of pharmacotherapy is not without risk.[24-27]

❖ Treatment for polyhydramnios in singleton pregnancy is recommended only if there is preterm labour or there is an evidence of significant maternal discomfort.[22,23]

REFERENCES

1. Rutherford SE, Phelan JP, Smith CV, Jacobs N. The four-quadrant assessment of amniotic fluid volume: an adjunct to antepartum fetal heart rate testing. Obstet Gynecol. 1987;70(3 Pt 1):353-6.

2. Sarno AP, Ahn MO, Brar HS, Phelan JP, Platt LD. Intrapartum Doppler velocimetry, amniotic fluid volume, and fetal heart rate as predictors of subsequent fetal distress. I. An initial report. Am J Obstet Gynecol. 1989;161(6 Pt 1):1508-14.

3. Yoshimura S, Masuzaki H, Gotoh H, Ishimaru T. Fetal redistri-bution of blood flow and amniotic fluid volume in growth-retarded fetuses. Early Hum Dev. 1997;47(3):297-304.

4. Peipert JF, Donnenfeld AE. Oligohydramnios: a review. Obstet Gynecol Surv. 1991;46(6):325-39.

5. Pryde PG, Hallak M, Lauria MR, Littman L, Bottoms SF, Johnson MP, et al. Severe oligohydramnios with intact membranes: an indication for diagnostic amnioinfusion. Fetal Diagn Ther. 2000;15(1):46-9.

6. Fisk NM, Ronderos-Dumit D, Soliani A, Nicolini U, Vaughan J, Rodeck CH. Diagnostic and therapeutic transabdominal amnioinfusion in oligohydramnios. Obstet Gynecol. 1991;78 (2):270-8.

7. Ashwal E, Hiersch L, Melamed N, Aviram A, Wiznitzer A, Yogev Y. The association between isolated oligohydramnios at term and pregnancy outcome. Arch Gynecol Obstet. 2014; 290(5):875-81.

8. Alchalabi HA, Obeidat BR, Jallad MF, Khader YS. Induction of labor and perinatal outcome: the impact of the amniotic fluid index. Eur J Obstet Gynecol Reprod Biol. 2006;129(2):124-7.

9. Ashwal E, Hiersch L, Melamed N, Aviram A, Wiznitzer A, Yogev Y. The association between isolated oligohydramnios at term and pregnancy outcome. Arch Gynecol Obstet. 2014;290(5): 875-81.

10. Ulkumen BA, Pala HG, Baytur YB, Koyuncu FM. Outcomes and management strategies in pregnancies with early onset oligohydramnios. Clin Exp Obstet Gynecol. 2015;42(3):355-7.

11. Dyer SN, Burton BK, Nelson LH. Elevated maternal serum alpha-fetoprotein levels and oligohydramnios: poor prognosis for pregnancy outcome. Am J Obstet Gynecol. 1987;157(2):336-9.

12. Richards DS, Seeds JW, Katz VL, Lingley LH, Albright SG, Cefalo RC. Elevated maternal serum alpha-fetoprotein with oligohydramnios: ultrasound evaluation and outcome. Obstet Gynecol. 1988;72(3 Pt 1):337-41.

13. Koontz WL, Seeds JW, Adams NJ, Johnson AM, Cefalo RC. Elevated maternal serum alpha-fetoprotein, second-trimester oligohydramnios, and pregnancy outcome. Obstet Gynecol. 1983;62(3):301-4.

14. Los FJ, Hagenaars AM, Cohen-Overbeek TE, Quartero HW. Maternal serum markers in second-trimester oligohydramnios. Prenat Diagn. 1994;14(7):565-8.

15. Pri-Paz S, Khalek N, Fuchs KM, Simpson LL. Maximal amniotic fluid index as a prognostic factor in pregnancies complicated by polyhydramnios. Ultrasound Obstet Gynecol. 2012;39(6): 648-53.

16. Hill LM, Breckle R, Thomas ML, Fries JK. Polyhydramnios: ultrasonically detected prevalence and neonatal outcome. Obstet Gynecol. 1987;69(1):21-5.

17. Pritchard JA. Fetal swallowing and amniotic fluid volume. Obstet Gynecol. 1966;28(5):606-10.

18. Rachid ML, Dreux S, Pean de Ponfilly G, Vargas-Poussou R, Czerkiewicz I, Chevenne D, et al. Prenatal diagnosis of Bartter syndrome: amniotic fluid aldosterone. Prenat Diagn. 2016;36(1):88-91.

19. Dashe JS, McIntire DD, Ramus RM, Santos-Ramos R, Twickler DM. Hydramnios: anomaly prevalence and sonographic detection. Obstet Gynecol. 2002;100(1):134-9.

20. Thompson O, Brown R, Gunnarson G, Harrington K. Prevalence of polyhydramnios in the third trimester in a population screened by first and second trimester ultrasonography. J Perinat Med. 1998;26(5):371-7.

21. Pasquini L, Seravalli V, Sisti G, Battaglini C, Nepi F, Pelagalli R, et al. Prevalence of a positive TORCH and parvovirus B19 screening in pregnancies complicated by polyhydramnios. Prenat Diagn. 2016;36(3):290-3.

22. Elliott JP, Sawyer AT, Radin TG, Strong RE. Large-volume therapeutic amniocentesis in the treatment of hydramnios. Obstet Gynecol. 1994;84(6):1025-7.

23. Dickinson JE, Tjioe YY, Jude E, Kirk D, Franke M, Nathan E. Amnioreduction in the management of polyhydramnios complicating singleton pregnancies. Am J Obstet Gynecol. 2014;211(4):434.e1-7.

24. Cabrol D, Landesman R, Muller J, Uzan M, Sureau C, Saxena BB. Treatment of polyhydramnios with prostaglandin synthe-tase inhibitor (indomethacin). Am J Obstet Gynecol. 1987; 157(2):422-6.

25. Hickok DE, Hollenbach KA, Reilley SF, Nyberg DA. The association between decreased amniotic fluid volume and treatment with nonsteroidal anti-inflammatory agents for preterm labor. Am J Obstet Gynecol. 1989;160(6):1525-30.

26. Kirshon B, Mari G, Moise KJ. Indomethacin therapy in the treatment of symptomatic polyhydramnios. Obstet Gynecol. 1990;75(2):202-5.

27. Rode L, Bundgaard A, Skibsted L, Odum L, Jørgensen C, Langhoff-Roos J. Acute recurrent polyhydramnios: a

CHAPTER 32

combination of amniocenteses and NSAID may be curative rather than palliative. Fetal Diagn Ther. 2007;22(3):186-9.

28. Aviram A, Salzer L, Hiersch L, Ashwal E, Golan G, Pardo J, et al. Association of isolated polyhydramnios at or beyond 34 weeks of gestation and pregnancy outcome. Obstet Gynecol. 2015;125(4):825-32.

29. Golan A, Wolman I, Sagi J, Yovel I, David MP. Persistence of polyhydramnios during pregnancy--its significance and correlation with maternal and fetal complications. Gynecol Obstet Invest. 1994;37(1):18-20.

30. Many A, Hill LM, Lazebnik N, Martin JG. The association between polyhydramnios and preterm delivery. Obstet Gynecol. 1995;86(3):389-91.

31. Smith CV, Plambeck RD, Rayburn WF, Albaugh KJ. Relation of mild idiopathic polyhydramnios to perinatal outcome. Obstet Gynecol. 1992;79(3):387-9.

32. Biggio JR, Wenstrom KD, Dubard MB, Cliver SP. Hydramnios prediction of adverse perinatal outcome. Obstet Gynecol. 1999;94(5 Pt 1):773-7.

Maternal Mortality

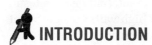 INTRODUCTION

Rate of maternal mortality in the world remains unacceptably high. Around the world about 830 women die every day. Women usually die as a result of complications during and following pregnancy and childbirth. Most of these obstetric complications develop during pregnancy and most are preventable or treatable. These complications can be prevented by provision of good maternal healthcare services. There are some medical complications, which may exist before pregnancy and may typically worsen during pregnancy. To prevent maternal mortality, these complications must be managed as part of the woman's ANC regimen. The major complications worldwide, accounting for nearly 75% of all maternal deaths include causes such as severe bleeding (e.g. postpartum haemorrhage), sepsis (usually after childbirth), high blood pressure during pregnancy (pre-eclampsia and eclampsia), complications during delivery and unsafe abortion.[1] Most maternal deaths are preventable, because healthcare solutions to prevent or manage complications are well known. All women require access to ANC during the antenatal period, skilled care during childbirth, and care and support during the postnatal period. Maternal health and newborn health are closely linked. Therefore, the rate of neonatal mortality is also high. Approximately 2.7 million newborn babies die every year worldwide.[2] Moreover, an additional 2.6 million babies are stillborn.[3] Therefore, it is predominantly important that all births are attended by skilled healthcare professionals, as timely obstetric management can help prevent both the maternal and neonatal mortality. While maternal mortality is discussed in this chapter, perinatal mortality is discussed in Chapter 55 (Care of a Newborn Child and Perinatal Mortality).

Definitions

Maternal Death

Maternal death is defined by the International Classification of Diseases, Injuries and Causes of Death (ICD9/10) as 'the death of a woman while pregnant or within 42 days of termination of pregnancy, from any cause related to or aggravated by pregnancy or its management, but not from accidental or incidental causes'. It does not matter if the pregnancy lasted only for a few weeks, as in miscarriage. The idea is to limit the definition of maternal death both in time and causation to produce agreed international definitions. Pregnancy should have contributed to the death, i.e. she would not have died if she had not been pregnant. In the UK, all maternal deaths are investigated by the confidential enquiries. Late deaths can be described as deaths occurring between 42 days and 1 year after pregnancy that are due to direct or indirect causes. Coincidental deaths are deaths from unrelated causes that happen to occur during pregnancy or the puerperium.

Maternity

A 'maternity' is any pregnancy going to 24 weeks or beyond or one resulting in a live birth before 24 weeks.

Maternal Mortality Rate

In the UK, the maternal mortality rate (MMR) can be defined as the number of 'direct' plus 'indirect' deaths (i.e. total number of maternal deaths) per 100,000 'maternities'. Direct deaths are deaths resulting from obstetric complications of the pregnant state (pregnancy, labour and puerperium), from interventions, omissions, incorrect treatment or from a chain of events resulting from any of the above, e.g. bleeding, eclampsia, etc. Indirect deaths are deaths resulting from a previously existing disease or disease that developed during pregnancy and which was not due to direct obstetric causes, but which was aggravated by the physiologic effects of pregnancy, e.g. cardiac disease. WHO, on the other hand, defines MMR as number of maternal deaths per 100,000 women of 'reproductive age group'. Maternal mortality ratio can be defined as number of maternal deaths per 100,000 live births.

WORLDWIDE TRENDS IN MATERNAL MORTALITY

According to WHO (2015), there was a worldwide drop in the MMRs by about 44% between the years 1990 and 2015. This was in form of decline in the worldwide MMRs from 385 deaths per 100,000 women of reproductive age group in 1990 to 216 deaths per 100,000 women of reproductive age group in 2015.[4] This mortality rate can be estimated as worldwide 287,000 maternal deaths per year. The MMRs remain high in developing countries and low-resource settings. Across the world MMR is presently 210 per 100,000 live births in 2015 (Fig. 33.1). The aim of WHO Sustainable Development Agenda is to reduce the global maternal mortality ratio to less than 70 per 100,000 women of reproductive age group between the years 2016 and 2030.[4]

Most of the load of maternal mortality and ill health is concentrated amongst the poorest populations in countries of sub-Saharan Africa and South Asia.[5] The highest rate of mortality is frequently observed among the marginalised and poor population, residing in remote and rural areas having limited access to healthcare services. This could be related to factors such as lack of access to quality health services, paucity of trained medical personnel, scarcity of transportation facilities, lack of knowledge about health services, poor sanitary conditions and poor environmental health due to factors such as overcrowding, poor air quality, poor sanitary conditions, etc. Improved maternal education is likely to bring about a reduction in the rate of maternal mortality. Various causes of maternal death in developing countries are listed in Table 33.1. The underlying factors for maternal mortality in developing countries include causes such as lack of access to contraception, unsafe abortion practices, lack of primary care or transport facilities, and inadequate staffing and equipment in the district hospitals.[6,7]

TRENDS IN MATERNAL MORTALITY IN THE UK

In developed countries such as the UK, the present MMR is around 10 per 100,000 maternities. In Britain between 1936 and 1985, the MMR fell due to the use of antibiotics, blood transfusion, ergometrine, better training of midwives and obstetricians, and the 1967 Abortion Act. There has been a statistically significant decrease in the maternal death rate between 2009–12 and 2011–13 in the UK. According to the Centre for Maternal and Child Enquiries (CMACE) report for the triennium 2006–2008, there were 261 maternal mortalities in the UK, which were directly or indirectly related to pregnancy. The overall MMR was 11.39 per 100,000 maternities.[8] There was a decline in the direct mortality rate, predominantly due to the reduction in deaths from thromboembolism and, to a lesser extent, haemorrhage. Despite a decline in the overall MMR in the UK, there has been an increase in deaths related to genital tract sepsis, particularly from community-acquired Group A streptococcal disease. The mortality rate related to sepsis increased from 0.85 deaths per 100,000 maternities in 2003–2005 to 1.13 deaths in 2006–2008, and sepsis has become the most common cause of direct maternal death. Cardiac disease is the most common cause of indirect death. However, indirect maternal death rates in the UK have continued to remain high with no significant change since 2003. Synchronised action across a wide range of healthcare services is required to deal with the problems mentioned in the Confidential Enquiries into Maternal Deaths (CEMD).

CONFIDENTIAL ENQUIRIES INTO MATERNAL DEATHS

All maternal deaths in the UK and Ireland are investigated by the national programme, the CEMD. These enquiries have been conducted in the UK since 1952. The committee directly responsible for the report was previously Confidential Enquiry into Maternal and Child Health (CEMACH). It was commissioned by the NICE. CEMACH had been incorporated into CMACE, which was the body primarily responsible for conducting these enquiries. Since June 2012, the CEMD has been carried out by the MBRRACE-UK (Mothers and Babies: Reducing Risk through Audits and Confidential Enquiries across the UK) collaboration.[9] The new MBRRACE-UK system applies to England, Wales and Scotland. Modified arrangements should be made in the north east of England and northern Ireland. The MBRRACE-UK is a secure web-based electronic data collection system. It operates through the NHS N3 gateway. While the CMACE produced a report

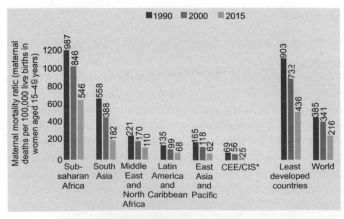

Fig. 33.1: Worldwide maternal mortality rates between the years 1990 and 2015[4]

*CEE/CIS: Central and Eastern Europe and the Commonwealth of Independent States

Table 33.1: Causes of maternal deaths in developing countries

Causes	Incidence (%)
Haemorrhage (both postpartum and antepartum)	22.9
Hypertensive diseases of pregnancy	18.5
Unsafe abortion	14.5
Hepatitis	12.5
Other infectious diseases	12.5
Sepsis	8.6
Syphilis	6.2
Obstructed labour	4.3

every triennium, analysing all maternal deaths from the previous 3 years divided into topic-specific chapters, the reports produced by the MBRRACE are now published on an annual basis, with each report focusing on a selection of chapters. Each MBRRACE-UK report now also contains 'Confidential Enquiry into Maternal Morbidity' (CEMM) elaborating details of women who survived the problems related to pregnancy. Besides this, MBRRACE-UK is also responsible for the surveillance of infant deaths up to age of 1 year and confidential enquiries on specific maternal and perinatal or infant morbidities (based on specific-topics). Reports from both maternal and infant programmes are issued on an annual basis from 2014. The topic for 2016 CEMM was pregnancy in women with artificial heart valves.

MBRRACE-UK is a collaboration led from the National Perinatal Epidemiology Unit, University of Oxford. It also includes collaborators from the Infant Mortality and Morbidity Studies group at the University of Leicester, the Universities of Liverpool and Birmingham, Imperial College, London, General Practice, and SANDS (the Stillbirth and Neonatal Death Charity). Participation in MBRRACE-UK is mandatory for all obstetric units in England. Deaths eligible for notification to the MBRRACE-UK are enlisted in Table 33.2.

The process of CEMD, also known as the 'audit loop', comprises of the five following steps, which eventually help in the formulation of recommendations to improve the quality of healthcare services:[10]

1. Identification of cases
2. Gathering information
3. Analysis of the results
4. Formulation of recommendations
5. Implementation of recommendations.

For the purpose of gathering information for CEMD, forms requesting the relevant information are sent to all clinicians involved in the case. The completed forms are then reviewed by national assessors in specialties such as obstetrics, pathology, midwifery, and if required, specialties such as anaesthesia, general medicine, intensive care and psychiatry may also be involved. The case studies are anonymised so that the assessors can comment freely and give their suggestions for improvement.

The latest CEMD was published in 2016. It focused on surveillance of all maternal deaths in the UK and Ireland from the period 2012–14 and includes Confidential Enquiries for women who died between 2009 and 2014. The figures for the MMR for the years 2010–12 and 2012–14 were 10 per 100,000 women and 8.5 per 100,000 women, respectively. There has been no statistically significant reduction in the rate of maternal deaths in the UK between 2009–11 and 2012–14. The report of the MBRRACE-UK Confidential Enquiry into Maternal Deaths and Morbidity (2016) is the third in the new annual series.[13] This thus, completes the full 3-year cycle (2014–2016) of chapters related to topic-based confidential enquiries, which has replaced the single previous triennial report. The features of these three series of MBRRACE reports are given in Table 33.3.

There has been no significant change in MMR from direct causes between the years 2009–11 to 2012–14. The deaths due to indirect causes remain high with no significant change since 2003, except for a decline in deaths due to influenza. This can be primarily attributed to a low level of influenza activity in 2012–14 in comparison to 2009–2010. Increasing immunisation rates in pregnancy against seasonal influenza should therefore be considered as a public health priority. Nevertheless, 14% cases of maternal deaths occurred due to pneumonia or influenza. Any one of the features, described

Table 33.2: Deaths eligible for notification to the MBRRACE-UK

Types of death	Definitions
Late foetal losses	The baby showing no signs of life is delivered between 22^{+0} and 23^{+6} weeks of gestation
Terminations of pregnancy	Pregnancy terminations from 22^{+0} weeks gestation onwards
Stillbirths	Delivery of the baby showing no signs of life after 24^{+0} weeks of pregnancy
Early neonatal deaths	Death of a neonate at 0–6 days following live birth of baby at any period of gestation of pregnancy
Late neonatal deaths	Death of a neonate at 7–27 days following live birth of a baby at any period of gestation
Postneonatal deaths	Death of an infant born at any period of gestation from 28 days after birth until the 1st year of life
Maternal deaths	All deaths of pregnant women and women up to 1 year following the end of the pregnancy (regardless of the circumstances and place of death)

Abbreviation: MBRRACE-UK, Mothers and Babies: Reducing Risk through Audits and Confidential Enquiries across the UK

Table 33.3: Features of three series of MBRRACE reports (2014–2016)[11-13]

Year of publication of MBRRACE report	Period of surveillance	Key areas targeted
2014	Surveillance data on maternal deaths from 2009–12	Confidential Enquiry reports on deaths and severe morbidity from sepsis, deaths from haemorrhage, amniotic fluid embolism, anaesthesia, neurological, respiratory, endocrine and other indirect causes
2015	Surveillance data on maternal deaths from 2011–13	Confidential Enquiry reports on deaths and morbidity from psychiatric causes, deaths due to thrombosis and thromboembolism, malignancy, homicides and late deaths
2016	Surveillance data on maternal deaths from 2012–14	Confidential Enquiry reports on deaths and severe morbidity from cardiac causes, deaths from pre-eclampsia and eclampsia and related causes, deaths in early pregnancy. Messages for management of pregnant patients in the critical care have also been provided

CHAPTER 33

PART II

Box 33.1: Red flag signs of maternal sepsis[14]

❑ Patient responses only to voice or pain/unresponsive
❑ Systolic BP ≤90 mmHg (or drop >40 from normal)
❑ Heart rate >130 beats/min
❑ Respiratory rate ≥25 breaths/min
❑ Oxygen supplementation is required to keep SpO_2 ≥92%
❑ Non-blanching rash, mottled/ashen/cyanotic
❑ Oliguria/anuria in last 18 hours
❑ Urine output <0.5 mL/kg/hr
❑ Lactate ≥2 mmol/L

Box 33.2: Key actions for diagnosis and management of sepsis[14]

❑ Timely recognition (imaging techniques are safe to use)
❑ Fast administration of intravenous antibiotics/antiviral agents
❑ Quick involvement of experts: Senior review is important

---

in Box 33.1, represents a 'red flag' in a sick pregnant or post-partum woman with suspected infection.[14] The key actions for diagnosis and management of maternal sepsis are described in Box 33.2.

Prevention of Mortality Related to Cardiovascular Diseases

The major focus of the MBRRACE (2016) report is maternal cardiovascular disease, which remains the largest single cause of maternal death during pregnancy and up to 6 weeks after pregnancy, responsible for nearly 23% cases. Thrombosis and thromboembolism, on the other hand, remains the leading cause of direct maternal death (responsible for 11% deaths).

Since deaths due to cardiovascular disease represent the leading cause of maternal death in the UK, it is important to take steps for prevention of these deaths (Box 33.3). The MBRRACE report (2016) highlighted many instances when death occurred due to failure of recognition of clear symptoms and signs of cardiac disease in a young pregnant woman.[13] Symptoms suggestive of cardiac disease should not be disregarded as exaggerated symptoms of normal pregnancy. Rather, these must always be fully investigated.

Prevention of Deaths due to Neurological Disorders

Neurological disorders were responsible for 11% deaths. In order to prevent deaths due to neurological causes, the steps given in Box 33.4 must be observed.

Prevention of Deaths due to Mental Health Problems

Mental health problems were identified as another important cause of maternal deaths, responsible for 9% cases. The major focus of the 2015 report was maternal mental health, and it is encouraging that there is an ongoing focus on improving maternal mental healthcare following the release of the report.[12] Due to identification of the importance of maternal suicide and its direct link with pregnancy, the WHO (2012) have recommended in their latest guidance on classification

---

Box 33.3: Key messages for the prevention of cardiac disease

❑ Complete investigation of important signs and symptoms such as increased respiratory rate, chest pain, persistent tachycardia, dyspnoea and orthopnoea, which could be indicative of underlying cardiac disease
❑ Repeated presentation of such symptoms should be considered as a 'red flag' sign by the staff caring for pregnant and postpartum women in any setting
❑ Presence of a normal ECG tracing and/or negative Troponin levels does not exclude the diagnosis of an acute coronary syndrome
❑ Prompt careful echocardiography and early review by a senior cardiologist is required in cases of new onset of cardiorespiratory symptoms and/or absence of valve clicks in women with prosthetic heart valves for exclusion of the possibility of valve thrombosis
❑ Urgent requirement for joint, co-ordinated, multidisciplinary, maternity and cardiac care of individuals
Autopsy where the clinical pathology points to cardiac disease
❑ Protocols in the Royal College of Pathologists' autopsy guidelines must be followed
❑ Molecular studies with the potential for family screening must be performed at the time of post-mortem examination in women having a morphologically normal heart, who have died from sudden cardiac arrest
❑ Family screening is required to rule out inherited aortopathy in cases of death due to aortic dissection in a young person

---

Box 33.4: Key messages for the prevention of neurological diseases

❑ Pregnant woman must be advised not to stop antiepileptic treatment on her own without taking an expert advise
❑ Worsening epilepsy or first seizure during pregnancy should be regarded as a red flag sign by the healthcare professional
❑ An urgent phone referral to neurology is essential

---

of maternal mortality, ICD-MM, that maternal suicides be classified as direct, rather than indirect, maternal deaths.[15] The same has been considered in the MBRRACE (2016) report. The 'red flag' signs indicative of severe maternal illness are listed in Box 33.5. Presence of these signs requires an urgent assessment by a senior psychiatrist.

Admission to a mother and baby unit should always be considered when a woman develops any of the signs mentioned in Box 33.6. Mental health assessments should always include an evaluation of woman's prior medical and obstetric history. Previous history of loss of a child, either by miscarriage, stillbirth, and intrauterine or neonatal death is likely to increase vulnerability of the mother to develop mental illness. Moreover previous history of psychiatric disorders or substance abuse further increases this risk. Such women must receive additional monitoring and support. Mental health assessment should also take into account the findings of recent presentations and increasing patterns of abnormal behaviour. Partners and other family members should be counselled and educated regarding maternal mental illness and its accompanying risks. Multiagency investigations into deaths from psychiatric causes at any stage during pregnancy and the first postnatal year should be conducted and must include the various services involved in caring for the woman.[12]

Box 33.5: The 'red flag' signs indicative of severe maternal illness

❏ Recent significant change in mental state or emergence of new symptoms
❏ Sudden onset or rapid worsening of mental symptoms
❏ New thoughts or acts of violent self-harm
❏ New and persistent expressions of incompetency as a mother
❏ Distancing from the infant

Box 33.6: Criteria for admission to a mother and baby unit

❏ Rapidly changing mental state
❏ Suicidal ideation (particularly of a violent nature)
❏ Pervasive guilt or hopelessness
❏ Significant estrangement from the infant
❏ New or persistent beliefs of inadequacy as a mother
❏ Evidence of psychotic behaviour

Prevention of Deaths due to Pre-eclampsia

Maternal deaths due to hypertensive disorders were found to be a lowest ever-recorded rate in the UK. There was less than one death due to hypertensive disorders for every million women giving birth. This can be considered as a major example of success and improvement in healthcare services as a result of research, audit and evidence-based guidelines. Contrary to the situation in the UK, pre-eclampsia remains one of the most common global causes of maternal death, which is likely to be responsible for a large number of deaths of women worldwide annually.

Though the mortality rates from pre-eclampsia have considerably reduced in the UK, steps must be taken for further improving certain aspects of care, which are mentioned in Box 33.7.

Reducing the Mortality Related to Early Pregnancy Complications

The following steps must be taken for reducing the mortality related to early pregnancy complications:

❖ Focused Assessment with Sonography for Trauma (FAST) scan must be performed in the women of reproductive age group, presenting to the emergency department in a collapsed state, with a suspicion of pulmonary embolism, especially if the woman is anaemic. FAST scan helps in excluding the diagnosis of intra-abdominal bleeding from a ruptured ectopic pregnancy before the administration of thrombolysis.
❖ Women of reproductive age group, who present in a state of shock and collapse in the community, with no obvious cause, should be immediately transferred to the hospital emergency department without delay for urgent assessment and management.
❖ The diagnosis of ectopic pregnancy should be considered in any woman of reproductive age presenting to the emergency department with collapse, acute abdominal/pelvic pain or gastrointestinal symptoms, including diarrhoea, vomiting and dizziness, regardless of whether or not she is pregnant. A bedside pregnancy test should be performed in these women.

Box 33.7: Key messages for the prevention of pre-eclampsia

❏ Maintenance of appropriate schedule of antenatal check-ups in women with risk factors for pre-eclampsia and those who develop hypertension or proteinuria during pregnancy
❏ Quick referral with clear communication between healthcare professionals in cases of new-onset hypertension or proteinuria
❏ Blood pressure monitoring and urinalysis for proteinuria must be performed during each antenatal visit in both primary and secondary care
❏ Blood pressure should be preferably maintained below 150/100 mmHg
❏ Urgent treatment of women with severe hypertension to bring down the blood pressure below 150/100 mmHg
❏ Transfer to a consultant-led unit in case the woman has a blood pressure over 140 mmHg systolic or 90 mmHg diastolic on two occasions in labour or immediately after birth
❏ Healthcare attendants must be made aware that agitation and restlessness may be a sign of an underlying problem in women with hypertension and must be considered as a red flag sign
❏ Neuroimaging should be performed urgently in any woman with hypertension or pre-eclampsia who has focal neurological signs or who has not recovered from a seizure

❖ Senior gynaecologist must urgently assess a woman with a suspected ectopic pregnancy showing deteriorating symptoms.

Messages Related to Critical Care Support

❖ A multidisciplinary team approach should be adopted for providing high quality care to the sick pregnant and postpartum women.
❖ Senior clinical staff must be promptly involved in the presence of reduced or altered consciousness level of a pregnant/postpartum woman, which must be considered as a red flag sign indicating established illness.
❖ Critical care support can be initiated in a variety of settings even prior to transfer to a critical care unit as a result of active collaboration between midwives and the critical care nurses.
❖ Important investigations in these cases must not be delayed due to pregnancy.
❖ Referral of a sick pregnant or postpartum woman within the hospital should be directed by the principle, 'one transfer to definitive care'.
❖ Pregnant and postpartum women with severe respiratory failure must be urgently referred to an ECMO (extra corporeal membrane oxygenation) centre.
❖ In critical care unit, both the obstetricians and obstetric anaesthetists must be closely involved in the clinical management of women with specific obstetric conditions such as pre-eclampsia. An appropriate balance must be maintained between clinical suspicion and a conclusive diagnosis.

CONCLUSION

In the UK maternal deaths are uncommon. Therefore, it is increasingly being recognised that the events surrounding

CHAPTER 33

individual maternal deaths may be unique. The CEMD, now run by MBRRACE-UK, is an integral component of the patient safety and risk management structure within UK maternity services, which is functioning since 1952. It has had an important positive influence on reducing the rate of maternal deaths from specific causes. Confidential enquiries aid detailed examination of the quality of care of individual cases against national guidelines or accepted best practice guidelines by multidisciplinary group of independent experts.

From the MBRRACE-UK (2015) report, it became evident that for many women who died due to mental health diseases in the years 2011–2013, the unique features of perinatal mental illness and their rapid deterioration had not been recognised by staff in general adult mental health services. The leading cause of maternal death in the UK has been identified as the maternal cardiovascular disease by the MBRRACE UK (2016) report. In these cases as well the healthcare professionals failed to recognise the symptoms related to underlying cardiac disorders. This emphasises the fact that the staff in maternity services and general practice must develop awareness regarding the 'red flag' symptoms of various likely causes of maternal deaths.

From the review of CEMD reports, it became clear that the postnatal care of women has been associated with evidence of fragmented care, gaps in postnatal care services, lack of co-ordination between various departments and lack of an individual taking overall responsibility. The CEMD report also highlights the urgent requirement for joint, multidisciplinary, maternity and medical care. It is the responsibility of every member of healthcare staff to ensure that women have appropriate care, even if it is outside their specialty area. They should take personal responsibility for ensuring that the woman has proper follow-up arrangements. Simply a letter to the general practitioner may not prove to be sufficient in many cases.

While there is still a scope for improvement in many of the healthcare services, the success of evidence-based quality care for women with hypertensive disorders and pre-eclampsia in the UK should be recognised. Presently, in the UK and Ireland, death of less than one woman in every million occurs as a result of pre-eclampsia or hypertensive disorder of pregnancy, a condition which is likely to result in a large number of deaths every day globally.

REFERENCES

1. Say L, Chou D, Gemmill A, Tunçalp Ö, Moller AB, Daniels JD, et al. Global causes of maternal death: a WHO systematic analysis. Lancet Glob Health. 2014;2(6):e323-33.
2. United Nations Children's Emergency Fund (UNICEF), World Health Organisation (WHO), World Bank, United Nations Population Division. The Inter-agency Group for Child Mortality Estimation (UN IGME). Levels and Trends in Child Mortality, Report 2015. New York: UNICEF; 2015.
3. Cousens S, Blencowe H, Stanton C, Chou D, Ahmed S, Steinhardt L, et al. National, regional, and worldwide estimates of stillbirth rates in 2009 with trends since 1995: a systematic analysis. Lancet. 2011;377(9774):1319-30.
4. World Health Organization (WHO), United Nations Children's Emergency Fund (UNICEF), United Nations Population Fund (UNFPA), World Bank Group and United Nations Population Division. Trends in maternal mortality: 1990 to 2015. Estimates by WHO, UNICEF, UNFPA, World Bank Group and the United Nations Population Division. Geneva: WHO; 2015.
5. Bhutta ZA, Black RE. Global maternal, newborn and child health--so near yet so far. N Engl J Med. 2013;369(23):2226-35.
6. Conde-Agudelo A, Belizan JM, Lammers C. Maternal-perinatal morbidity and mortality associated with adolescent pregnancy in Latin America: Cross-sectional study. Am J Obstet Gynecol. 2004;192(2):342-9.
7. Patton GC, Coffey C, Sawyer SM, Viner RM, Haller DM, Bose K, et al. Global patterns of mortality in young people: a systematic analysis of population health data. Lancet. 2009;374(9693): 881-92.
8. Cantwell R, Clutton-Brock T, Cooper G, Dawson A, Drife J, Garrod D, et al. Saving Mothers' Lives: Reviewing maternal deaths to make motherhood safer: 2006-08. The Eighth Report on Confidential Enquiries into Maternal Deaths in the United Kingdom. BJOG. 2011;118 (Suppl. 1):1–203.
9. Knight M. How will the new Confidential Enquiries into the Maternal and Infant Death in the UK operate? The work of MBRRACE-UK. Obstet Gynecol. 2013;15(1):65.
10. Lewis G. Saving Mothers' Lives: the continuing benefits for maternal health from the United Kingdom (UK) Confidential Enquires into Maternal Deaths. Semin Perinatol. 2012;36(1):19-26.
11. Mothers and Babies: Reducing Risk through Audits and Confidential Enquiries across the UK (MBRRACE-UK). Saving Lives, Improving Mothers' Care: Lessons learned to inform future maternity care from the UK and Ireland Confidential Enquiries into Maternal Deaths and Morbidity 2009-2012. Oxford: University of Oxford; 2014.
12. Mothers and Babies: Reducing Risk through Audits and Confidential Enquiries across the UK (MBRRACE-UK). Saving Lives, Improving Mothers' Care: Surveillance of maternal deaths in the UK 2011-13 and lessons learned to inform maternity care from the UK and Ireland Confidential Enquiries into Maternal Deaths and Morbidity 2009-13. Oxford: University of Oxford; 2015.
13. Knight M, Nair M, Tuffnell D, Kenyon S, Shakespeare J, Brocklehurst P, et al (Eds.) on behalf of MBRRACE-UK. Saving Lives, Improving Mothers' Care - Surveillance of maternal deaths in the UK 2012-14 and lessons learned to inform maternity care from the UK and Ireland Confidential Enquiries into Maternal Deaths and Morbidity 2009-14. Oxford: National Perinatal Epidemiology Unit, University of Oxford; 2016.
14. UK Sepsis Trust. (2016). Inpatient maternal sepsis tool. [Online] Available from http://sepsistrust.org/wp-content/uploads/2016/07/Inpatient-maternal-NICE-Final-1107-2.pdf. [Accessed December 2016].
15. World Health Organisation. (2012). The WHO Application of ICD-10 to deaths during pregnancy, childbirth and the puerperium: ICD-MM. [Online] Available from http://apps.who.int/iris/bitstream/10665/70929/1/9789241548458_eng.pdf?ua=1. [Accessed December 2016].

Medications during Pregnancy

INTRODUCTION

Over the past decade and a half, drugs, chemicals and other exogenous agents have been responsible for causing nearly 1% of the foetal congenital anomalies. Women are likely to ingest a variety of medications during pregnancy. Some medications may have taken before the pregnancy is recognised. On the other hand, some medicines are taken without the physician's advice, once the pregnancy is recognised. Overall, the prevalence of medicine use during pregnancy varies from less than 10% of pregnant women to more than 95%. In utero development of the baby can be divided into three phases: (1) preimplantation phase; (2) period of embryo; and (3) the foetal phase. Exposure to drugs during pregnancy must be separated into these time periods because the conceptus responds differently in each of the phases of development.[1]

1. *Preimplantation phase*: This phase begins from the formation of zygote and lasts until the blastocyst attaches to the uterine wall after the formation of chorionic villi. During this phase, the foetus is considered to be protected from the drugs or medications because there is no formal biological interface between the blastocyst and the mother. Errors occurring during this period can, however, result in prenatal death.

2. *Embryonic phase*: During the embryonic phase, various organs are being formed (Fig. 34.1).[2] In this phase, various undifferentiated cells form specialised cells which get converted into organs and tissues. The morphological architecture for a normal or abnormal human is laid down during the embryonic phase. Exposure to teratogenic agents during this phase may result in the development of congenital anomalies in the foetus. Also, during this phase, the drugs cannot be metabolised at adult or foetal rates, if at all.

3. *Foetal phase*: After embryogenesis (58–60 days post-conception) is completed, the embryo is converted into foetus. Most of the foetal period is occupied with the growth in the size of organs. The organs and structures, which had been formed during embryonic phase, simply grow in size and develop normal physiological functions during the foetal phase. Foetal enzyme systems involved in the drug metabolism are only beginning to function and some may not be active until after the neonatal period (e.g. cholinesterase). Organs, structures or functions formed normally during embryogenesis can be damaged due to teratogenic exposure in the foetal period.

Maternal Physiology during Pregnancy

The dynamic physiological changes occurring in the maternal-placental-foetal unit during pregnancy are likely to affect the pharmacokinetic processes of drug absorption, distribution and elimination. Some important physiological changes occurring during pregnancy are as follows:

❖ Pregnant women have the full enzyme complement for metabolising drugs, but most such systems (e.g. cholinesterase which metabolises cocaine) have lower activity during pregnancy.

❖ Maternal blood volume increases dramatically during pregnancy by approximately 40–50% to support the requirements of the developing foetus. Distribution of drugs in this increased blood volume may result in lower serum concentration of these drugs.

❖ Pregnancy is associated with a reduction in gastric motility and an increase in the gastric pH. However, these changes are unlikely to cause any measurable effect on the drug bioavailability due to this.

❖ Ventilatory changes may influence the pulmonary absorption of inhaled drugs.

❖ Absorption of the drug occurs with approximately the same kinetics as in the non-pregnant adult.

❖ As the GFR usually increases during pregnancy, renal drug elimination is generally enhanced. On the other hand, hepatic drug metabolism may increase, decrease or remain unchanged. Renal clearance of β-lactam

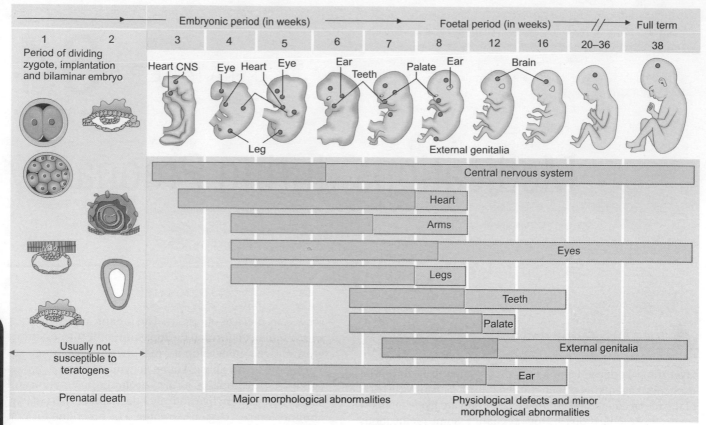

Fig. 34.1: Critical time for development of various foetal organs and structures

Source: Redrawn from Reference 2.

antibiotics (e.g. penicillin and cephalosporin) is increased during pregnancy. Although the level of these antibiotics may be lowered in plasma, their level is increased in the urine. This may be desirable for the treatment of urinary tract infection. Drugs such as LMWH may also be associated with an increased renal clearance during pregnancy, thereby requiring dose adjustments.[3]

❖ Renal clearance of the drug is increased and the enzyme activity is downregulated. Decreased enzyme activity is further exacerbated by increased blood volume, decreasing the overall effective serum concentration of a given dose.

❖ Pregnancy causes an increase in the volume of distribution as well as an increase in the fraction of unbound or active drug in the plasma. Volume of distribution can be defined as the volume in which an amount of drug would need to be distributed to produce a particular blood concentration. Volume of distribution is dependent on the plasma volume, tissue volume and the degree of binding of a drug to the tissues or the plasma proteins. For example, acidic drugs, such as warfarin, are bound to plasma proteins. The volume of distribution of such drugs is low but their plasma concentration is high. On the other hand, for basic drugs such as amphetamines, which are bound to the tissues, the volume of distribution is high, but the plasma concentration is low.

❖ Drugs that are tightly bound to the serum proteins have little chance to cross the placenta or enter the breast milk.

As a result, increased demands are placed on the maternal cardiovascular, hepatic and renal systems.

❖ Gravid uterus is vulnerable to a variety of effects not present in the non-pregnant state such as haemorrhage, rupture or preterm contractions.

❖ The concentration of two main drug-binding proteins, albumin and α1 glycoprotein, falls at term to around 70–80% of the prepregnancy levels. Pregnancy-related hypoalbuminaemia causes decreased protein binding, thereby resulting in increased free drug fraction. However, the overall effect is an unaltered free drug concentration because more amount of free drug is available for either hepatic biotransformation or renal excretion.

❖ Any drug administered to a pregnant woman must be considered as possibly harmful to the foetus, because all drugs administered to the mother are likely to cross the placental membrane, although at different rates.

❖ Most of the drugs cross placenta via passive diffusion. Therefore, small, non-ionised, lipid-soluble drugs are likely to cross the placenta at the highest rate. Recently, there has been a growing interest in the active transportation utilising energy-requiring drug transporters.[4] These may work against the concentration gradient and derive energy from adenosine triphosphate (ATP) or electrochemical gradients. These include P-glycoprotein which is able to transport drugs such as digoxin and dexamethasone. On the other hand, monocarboxylate and sodium or multivitamin transporters help in the transportation of drugs such as valproate and carbamazepine.

❖ Drugs such as steroids and alcohol may undergo metabolism in placenta because it expresses many enzymes capable of metabolising various drugs.

Medications during Lactation

❖ Most drugs are excreted into the breast milk by passive diffusion. Therefore, the drug concentration in milk is directly proportional to the corresponding concentration in maternal plasma. The milk to plasma (M:P) ratio, which compares milk with maternal plasma drug concentrations, serves as an index of the extent of drug excretion in the milk. For most drugs, the amount ingested by the infant rarely reaches the therapeutic levels. Therefore, drugs during pregnancy and breastfeeding should be preferably prescribed at the lowest effective dosage using the lowest number of drugs (monotherapy where possible).

❖ Transfer of the drug into breast milk is determined by the lipophilic drug properties, their molecular size and polarity. Highly plasma-bound drugs do not cross into the breast milk.

Drug Pharmacokinetics in Pregnancy

Presently, the data related to the pharmacokinetics of the various drugs during pregnancy is largely limited. Various studies related to pharmacokinetics of the same drug have presented with conflicting results. Therefore, no general statement about pharmacokinetic changes during pregnancy can be made. Each drug must be considered on an individual basis. Most of the pharmacokinetic changes are likely to cause a reduction in the drug plasma concentrations. When pharmacokinetic data are altered, increase in the drug dosage or schedules are required in order to maintain effective systemic drug levels.

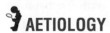

AETIOLOGY

Teratogenesis

Teratogenesis can be defined as structural or functional dysgenesis or malformation of the foetal organs. It can present in form of congenital malformations with varying severity, IUGR, carcinogenesis, foetal death, etc. A teratogen can be defined as any agent, physical force or other factor (e.g. maternal disease), which can induce a congenital anomaly through alteration of normal development during any stage of embryogenesis. Teratogenic agents include drugs and other chemicals; physical forces such as ionising radiation and physical restraint (e.g. amniotic banding); and maternal teratogenic diseases such as diabetes mellitus and phenylketonuria. Known human teratogenic drugs are listed in Box 34.1. Of these various teratogens, the most notorious human teratogen is thalidomide.

Teratogenic influence is likely to be strongest in the period of early organogenesis. The most important body

Box 34.1: Known human teratogenic drugs[5-7]

❑ ACE inhibitors	❑ Methotrexate
❑ Amiodarone	❑ Methylene blue
❑ Aminopterin	❑ Penicillamine
❑ Antiepileptic drugs	❑ Quinine
– Carbamazepine	❑ Radioiodine
– Clonazepam	❑ Retinoids (oral)
– Primidone	❑ Tetracycline derivatives
– Phenobarbital	❑ Thalidomide
– Phenytoin	❑ Fluconazole
– Valproic acid	❑ Methimazole
❑ Coumarin derivatives	❑ Misoprostol
❑ Cyclophosphamide	❑ Trimethadione,
❑ Danazol	paramethadione
❑ Diethylstilbestrol	❑ Trimethoprim
❑ Lithium	

structures of the foetus are formed in the first 12 weeks after conception, usually 20–55 days after conception. Interference in this process results in a teratogenic effect. Teratogenic influence is likely to be less strong if exposure to the drug is in the later period of foetal development. Though structural malformations are less likely to occur due to the exposure to the teratogen in later part of pregnancy, this can cause serious functional abnormalities, particularly of the neurobehavioural type.

Teratogenic Drugs in Pregnancy

❖ *Warfarin*: Warfarin is known to be teratogenic in the first trimester and can cause abnormalities such as intracerebral haemorrhage, nasal hypoplasia, stippling of the epiphyses, chondrodysplasia punctata and CNS abnormalities. Warfarin, unlike heparin has been shown to cause CNS damage in the foetus if given in the second and third trimesters. Warfarin is also not safe in the last 4 weeks of pregnancy because it crosses the placenta and causes haemorrhage.

❖ *Phenytoin*: Phenytoin can cause foetal hydantoin syndrome. Foetal hydantoin syndrome is a syndrome comprising of characteristic pattern of mental and physical birth defects, resulting from maternal use of the anticonvulsant drug, phenytoin during pregnancy. Some characteristic features of this syndrome may include distinctive skull and facial features, growth deficiencies (prenatal and postnatal growth restriction), hypoplastic nails of the fingers and toes, and/or mild developmental delays. Other findings occasionally associated with this syndrome include cleft lip and palate, short nose with a broad flattened nasal bridge, microcephaly, hypertelorism, strabismus, low set or abnormally formed ears, and skeletal malformations particularly of the fingers or hands. Various craniofacial and digital abnormalities, together with more major anomalies (cardiac defects, cleft lip and palate), and neural tube defects have also been associated with maternal phenytoin ingestion during pregnancy. Folic acid supplements reduce the incidence of neural tube defects and should be given to patients taking phenytoin.

- *Diethylstilbestrol*: Causes carcinoma of the vagina and vaginal adenosis in young women.
- *Quinine*: Causes blindness and deafness by causing hypoplasia of optic nerve.
- *Thalidomide*: Causes phocomelia, which involves absence of the long bones of the upper and/or lower limbs, amongst other defects.
- *Lithium*: Lithium may cause cardiac abnormalities.
- *Chlorpropamide*: Chlorpropamide may cause neonatal hypoglycaemia.
- *Pseudoephedrine*: Gastroschisis is a recognised effect of pseudoephedrine.
- *Irradiation*: Leukaemia, carcinoma of thyroid gland.
- *Valproate*: Valproate is associated with neural tube defects (extra folate should be prescribed in these cases).
- *Lisinopril*: This drug is teratogenic.
- *Losartan*: Losartan is contraindicated in pregnancy.
- *Statins*: Statins also are associated with teratogenicity.
- *Maternal hyperthermia*: This can result in CNS abnormalities in the foetus.
- *Glucocorticoids*: This can result in cleft lip.
- *Cyproterone acetate and possibly other '19-nor' steroids*: Androgenisation of the female foetus.
- *Rifampicin*: Rifampicin is an extremely powerful enzyme-inducer, so the combined OCP is contraindicated in those taking rifampicin. For such individuals, an alternative method of contraception is usually preferred. Even if rifampicin is taken only for a few days, its effect on the combined oral contraceptive should be assumed to last for at least a month. Besides being a powerful enzyme-inducer, rifampicin has been found to be associated with an increased incidence of neural tube defects and facial clefts in experimental animals. Despite the concerns, no teratogenic effect has been proved in the human. There also have been concerns regarding its potential to cause bleeding in terms of PPH and haemorrhagic disease of the newborn. Therefore, vitamin K should be prescribed in these cases.
- *Isotretinoin*: Treatment with isotretinoin is a recognised indication for termination of the pregnancy. Contraception is advised for 2 years after cessation of treatment. If consumed during pregnancy, it can result in anomalies such as hypoplastic ears, malformation of the facial bones, cardiac defects, hydrocephalus, thymic hypoplasia, etc.
- *Thiazide diuretics*: These have been shown to decrease placental perfusion.

Antibiotics to be Avoided during Pregnancy

Antibiotics are amongst the most common drugs used in pregnancy. None of the drugs prescribed in pregnancy can be guaranteed as 100% safe, but a few are significantly teratogenic. Some of the antibiotics which must be avoided during pregnancy include the following:

- *Aminoglycosides*: Aminoglycosides are known to be ototoxic. Aminoglycosides (streptomycin, gentamicin, tobramycin, etc.) may cause auditory or vestibular damage, especially when prescribed in the second or third trimester.
- *Co-trimoxazole*: It causes neonatal haemolysis and methaemoglobinaemia. It is also teratogenic in the first trimester.
- *Tetracycline*: Tetracycline causes dental discolouration (if taken in the second or third trimester) and maternal hepatotoxicity in large doses. Tetracycline is best avoided during pregnancy, but is not 'unsafe' if prescribed in limited doses during the first trimester.
- *Chloramphenicol*: Chloramphenicol may cause 'grey baby syndrome' usually in the third trimester. This syndrome occurs because the neonate cannot metabolise the drug, and therefore, suffers serious toxicity, which is often fatal. The term 'grey' refers to the description of the baby's appearance.
- *Ciprofloxacin*: This is a quinolone drug linked to arthropathy in animal experiments. Therefore, its use is restricted in pregnancy. However, the reports suggest that its use may be safe.
- *Nitrofurantoin*: This drug should be avoided in late pregnancy because of its links to neonatal haemolysis.
- *Trimethoprim*: Since this is a folate antagonist, there is concern that it may be teratogenic if taken in early pregnancy.
- *Metronidazole*: Metronidazole has not been shown to be teratogenic. In therapeutic doses, it is relatively safe during pregnancy. However, there is still reluctance to use it, particularly in the first trimester.

Safe Drugs during Pregnancy

Methyldopa is used for treatment of hypertension during pregnancy. It is the only hypotensive that is safe in all stages of pregnancy. Paracetamol is safe throughout a normal pregnancy. There is no evidence that ranitidine, metformin, aspirin or OCPs are teratogenic. Although it was once believed that aspirin and OCPs were teratogenic if consumed during pregnancy, studies indicate otherwise. Similarly, metformin is often used in cases of PCOS to induce fertility through reduction in insulin resistance. Antibiotics such as erythromycin and methylpenicillin are also largely safe during pregnancy.

Drugs Contraindicated during Lactation

Drugs contraindicated during lactation are listed in Box 34.2.[8] Some of these are described in details next:

- *Bromocriptine and cabergoline*: Both bromocriptine and cabergoline cause suppression of lactation. However, once lactation has been established, bromocriptine is not very effective in suppressing it. The British National Formulary states that although licensed, bromocriptine and cabergoline should not be routinely used for suppressing lactation during the puerperium. Pain and breast engorgement can be relieved with analgesics and good support. If a drug has to be used, cabergoline is preferred over bromocriptine. It has some very serious side effects;

Box 34.2: Drugs likely to have deleterious effects during lactation

- ❑ Amantadine
- ❑ Amiodarone
- ❑ Antineoplastic drugs
- ❑ Atropine
- ❑ Barbiturates
- ❑ Benzodiazepines
- ❑ Bromide
- ❑ Carbimazole
- ❑ Chloramphenicol
- ❑ Ephedrine
- ❑ Ergotamine
- ❑ Iodide
- ❑ Lithium
- ❑ Phenindione
- ❑ Primidone
- ❑ Radioactive agents
- ❑ Streptomycin
- ❑ Sulphonamides

fortunately these are rare. They include hypotension, hypertension, stroke, myocardial infarction and psychosis.

❖ *Sulphonamides*: Sulphonamides may worsen neonatal jaundice and cause haemolysis in the babies with glucose 6-phosphatase deficiency.

❖ *Labetalol*: Labetalol appears to cross to the baby in insufficient quantities to be able to cause problems of β-blockade. Nevertheless, the baby should be monitored if the mother is taking labetalol.

❖ *Tetracycline*: Tetracycline if taken in pregnancy may cause discolouration of the baby's teeth. It is thought that it is unlikely to do so via breast milk, but is best avoided to be safe.

❖ *Methyldopa*: Methyldopa is contraindicated during puerperium to avoid exacerbating postpartum depression (depression being a side effect of the drug). However, the amount secreted in breast milk is too small to affect the baby.

❖ *Androgens*: Androgens may cause masculinisation in the female infant or precocious development in the male infant. Therefore, they must not be used during puerperium.

❖ *Thiazide diuretics*: Thiazide diuretics in large doses may reduce or inhibit milk production.

Drugs Which can be Used During Breastfeeding

❖ *Propranolol*: Propranolol is secreted in breast milk and may be rarely associated to bradycardia but generally has little impact. Therefore, it can be administered to breastfeeding mothers.

❖ *Progesterone only contraceptive pill*: Progesterone only contraceptive pills are also not contraindicated in breastfeeding mothers.

❖ *Warfarin*: Warfarin is secreted in small amounts in breast milk and has little impact on foetal coagulation.

❖ *Ranitidine*: Significant amounts are present in breast milk but it is not known to be harmful during breastfeeding.

❖ *Antihypertensive agents*: ACE inhibitors may be used safely during the puerperium. They can be used if they were used preconceptually or they can be used for the first time. There is also no contraindication to the use of β-blockers during puerperium. Although antihypertensive agents, such as methyldopa, nifedipine or labetalol, are excreted into breast milk, no adverse effects on breast-fed infants exposed to these drugs have been reported. Therefore, these antihypertensive agents can be prescribed in puerperium.

❖ *Metronidazole*: Metronidazole is secreted in significant amounts in breast milk. Manufacturer advises avoiding single large doses. In clinical practice at normal doses, it appears to be safe and is widely used.

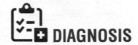

DIAGNOSIS

Prenatal Diagnosis

Exposure to certain medicines or substance abuse during pregnancy may not necessarily be an indication for termination of pregnancy. However, such exposure is definitely an indication for prenatal diagnosis. Prenatal diagnosis cannot rule out defects that are not related to gross structural anomalies. However, it can determine major congenital anomalies, such as spina bifida, structural heart defects, limb reduction, etc.

MANAGEMENT

Management of pregnant patients exposed to drugs or medication during pregnancy is described in Flow chart 34.1.[9]

Counselling and Evaluation of a Drug-exposed Pregnant Patient

All counselling regarding drug or medication exposure should be performed by a clinician, knowledgeable in both teratology and counselling. At the time of counselling, it is important for the clinician to maintain rapport with the patient, assuring confidentiality and establishing a basis for the patient's trust. The counsellor must convey the following to the patient:

❖ His or her understanding of the patient's concerns

❖ Explain to the patient that the purpose of the consultation is to deal directly with those concerns by ascertaining the magnitude of the risk for an adverse pregnancy outcome arising from the drug exposure.

Preconceptional Counselling

All counselling related to the use of drugs or medication during pregnancy should preferably occur prior to conception

Flow chart 34.1: Management of pregnant patients exposed to drugs or medication during pregnancy

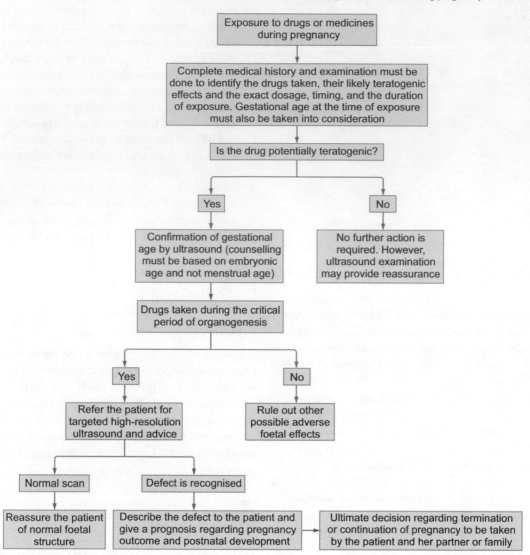

PART II

because during this time, the opportunity to prevent adverse events is optimal. Only medications which are known to be safe should be recommended for continued use while attempting to conceive.

Counselling the Exposed Gravida

Counselling the patient exposed to drugs or medication during pregnancy should be according to the protocol described in Flow chart 34.1. The concept of background risk for major congenital anomalies must be explained to the patient in a manner she can understand. This concept is particularly important because it conveys to the patient that even if the drug exposure is harmless, there is no guarantee that the foetus she carries will not have a congenital anomaly. Notwithstanding the exposure to various medicines, the background risk for development of major congenital anomalies varies between 3.5% and 5%.

At the time of taking history, it is important for the obstetrician to determine the exact medicines which were taken, their dosage, the timing, and the duration of exposure(s).

Besides this, the obstetrician must also enquire about the patient's medical, obstetric and genetic history in detail.[10]

Informed Consent and Postexposure Counselling

Before initiating informed consent regarding the exposure to medicines during pregnancy, factors such as the exact dosage administered, route and timing of administration must be ascertained as accurately as possible. Even if an agent is a potential teratogen (e.g. thalidomide) the actual risk to the foetus may be minimal if the timing of exposure occurred late during pregnancy or after the period of organogenesis. On the other hand, some teratogens such as radioactive iodine or the ACE inhibitors may be harmful only after early organogenesis.

After a detailed history is taken, the patient should be given full disclosure regarding the known or suspected risk of the agent, as well as the various therapeutic and diagnostic options available. This information should be accurate, yet easily understandable. All such information and counselling must be well-documented in the patient's notes.

Table 34.1: Adverse effects other than the birth defects on human foetus caused by various drugs

Maternal medications	Foetal or neonatal effects
Acetaminophen	Renal failure
Adrenocortical hormones	Adrenocortical suppression, electrolyte imbalance
Alcohol	Muscular hypotonia, hypoglycaemia, (?) withdrawal, IUGR, blood changes, effect on the mental ability
Alphaprodine	Platelet dysfunction
Amitriptyline	Withdrawal
Amphetamines	Withdrawal
Antihistamines	Infertility (?)
Antineoplastic agents	Transient pancytopenia, IUGR
Antithyroid drugs	Hypothyroidism
Barbiturates	Coagulation defects, withdrawal, IUGR
Chloral hydrate	Foetal death
Chloramphenicol	Death (Grey baby syndrome)
Chloroquine	Death (?)
Chlorpropamide	Prolonged hypoglycaemia, foetal death
Cocaine	Vascular disruption, withdrawal, IUGR
Coumarin anticoagulants	Haemorrhage, death , IUGR
Diazepam	Hypothermia, hypotonia, withdrawal
Ergot	Foetal death
Erythromycin	Liver damage (?)
Glutethimide	Withdrawal
Heroin/morphine/methadone	Withdrawal/neonatal death
Lithium	Cyanosis, flaccidity, polyhydramnios, toxicity

Contd...

Contd...

Maternal medications	Foetal or neonatal effects
Magnesium sulphate	Central depression and neuromuscular block
Meperidine	Neonatal depression
Mepivacaine	Foetal bradycardia and depression
Nitrofurantoin	Haemolysis
Novobiocin	Hyperbilirubinaemia (?)
Oral progestogens, androgens and oestrogens	Advanced bone age
Phenformin	Lactic acidosis
Phenothiazines	Hyperbilirubinaemia, depression, hypothermia (?), withdrawal
Prednisolone	Acute foetal distress, foetal death
Primidone	Withdrawal (?)
Quinine	Thrombocytopenia
Reserpine	Nasal congestion, lethargy, respiratory depression, bradycardia
Salicylates (excess)	Bleeding, foetal death
Sedatives	Behavioural changes
Smoking	Premature births, IUGR, perinatal loss (?)
Sulphonamides	Kernicterus (?), anaemia (?)
Tetracycline	Deposition in bones, inhibition of bone growth in premature infants, discolouration of teeth
Thiazide diuretics	Thrombocytopenia, salt and water depletion, neonatal death (?)
Tolbutamide	Thrombocytopenia, foetal deaths
Vitamin K analogues (excess)	Hyperbilirubinaemia

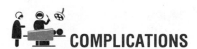

COMPLICATIONS

Potential Adverse Effects

Spontaneous Abortion

Nearly 50% of early pregnancies (0–58 days) may end in spontaneous miscarriages.

Congenital Anomalies

Congenital anomalies may be detected in nearly 3.5–5% cases. The frequency of congenital anomalies is several-folds higher amongst stillbirths and miscarriages than amongst live births, and is especially high amongst early (first-trimester) miscarriages.

Foetal Effects

Various foetal effects, which can occur, include:
❖ Damage to the organs or structures which are formed during organogenesis

❖ Damage to the systems undergoing histogenesis during the foetal period
❖ Foetal growth restriction
❖ Foetal deaths or stillbirths.

Neonatal and Postnatal Effects

Prenatal exposure to some drugs can cause adverse neonatal side effects such as difficulty in adaptation to life outside the uterus. Drugs causing such adverse neonatal side effects usually do not cause any teratogenic side effects. Some such effects include transient metabolic abnormalities, withdrawal and hypoglycaemia with the use of opiates, floppy infant syndrome with the use of benzodiazepines near term, patent ductus arteriosus with the use of prostaglandin synthase inhibitors (NSAIDs such as aspirin or indomethacin), grey baby syndrome with the use of high-dose chloramphenicol near delivery. Some such adverse effects other than the birth defects caused by drugs are listed in Table 34.1.[7]

CHAPTER 34

REFERENCES

1. Friedman JM, Little BB, Brent RL, Cordero JF, Hanson JW, Shepard TH. Potential human teratogenicity of frequently prescribed drugs. Obstet Gynecol. 1990;75(4):594-9.
2. Airëns ES, Simons AM. De Invlsed chemischestoffen op het angebaren kind. Natuuren Technieke. 1974;43.
3. Loebstein R, Lalkin A, Koren G. Pharmacokinetic changes during pregnancy and their clinical relevance. Clin Pharmacokinet. 1997;33(5):328-43.
4. Ito S. Transplacental treatment of fetal tachycardia: implications of drug transporting proteins in placenta. Semin Perinatol. 2001;25(3):196-201.
5. Polifka JE, Friedman JM. Medical genetics: 1. Clinical teratology in the age of genomics. CMAJ. 2002;167(3):265-73.
6. Shephard TH, Lemire RJ. Catalog of Teratogenic Agents, 11th edition. Baltimore: John Hopkins University Press; 2004.
7. Schardein JL. Chemically Induced Birth Defects, 3rd edition. New York: Marcel Dekker; 2000.
8. Buhimschi CS, Weiner CP. Medications in pregnancy and lactation: part 1. Teratology. Obstet Gynecol. 2009;113(1):166-88.
9. Lo WY, Friedman JM. Teratogenicity of recently induced medications in human pregnancy. Obstet Gynecol. 2002;100 (3):465-73.
10. Baird PA, Anderson TW, Newcombe HB, Lowry RB. Genetic disorders in children and young adults: a population study. Am J Hum Genet. 1988;42(5):677-93.

PART II

SECTION 5

Complications in the Early Pregnancy

OBSTETRICS

Ectopic Pregnancy

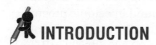 INTRODUCTION

The term 'ectopic' means 'out of place'. In an ectopic pregnancy, the fertilised ovum gets implanted outside the uterus, as a result of which the pregnancy occurs outside the uterine cavity. Most commonly, i.e. in nearly 95% of cases, the fertilised ovum gets implanted inside the fallopian tube. Other extrauterine locations where an ectopic pregnancy can get implanted include the ovary, abdomen or the cervix (Table 35.1 and Fig. 35.1). Since none of these locations have been equipped by nature to support a growing pregnancy, with continuing growth of foetus, the gestational sac and the organ containing it burst open. This can result in severe bleeding, sometimes even endangering the woman's life. The incidence of ectopic pregnancy has remained static in recent years (11.1/1,000 pregnancies). Nearly 32,000 cases of ectopic pregnancies were diagnosed in the UK within a 3-year period (2006–2008).[1]

AETIOLOGY

The major cause of ectopic pregnancy is acute salpingitis, accounting for 50% of cases. In nearly 40% of cases, the cause

Table 35.1: Average incidence for occurrence of ectopic pregnancy at various locations

Locations of extrauterine pregnancy	Incidence of occurrence (%)
Fallopian tube	97
Ampulla	80
Isthmus	11
Fimbria	4
Cornua	2
Interstitium	3
Abdominal cavity, ovary and cervix	3

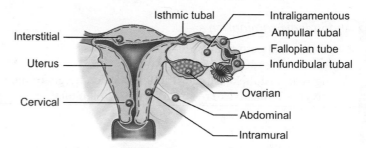

Fig. 35.1: Common sites for occurrence of ectopic pregnancy

remains unknown. The risk factors for ectopic pregnancy are as follows:[2,3]

❖ Prior history of an ectopic pregnancy
❖ *Pelvic infections*: History of pelvic infections, such as pelvic inflammatory disease (PID), STD, salpingitis and tuberculosis, is an important cause for ectopic pregnancy
❖ Prior surgeries of the fallopian tubes, including tubal reconstructive surgery, tubectomy, etc.
❖ Endometriosis and pelvic scar tissue (pelvic adhesions)
❖ Congenital abnormalities of tubes
❖ Smoking is a risk factor in about one-third of ectopic pregnancies
❖ Patients belonging to the age group of 35–44 years
❖ Infertility problems and use of ovulation induction drugs and other assisted reproductive techniques
❖ Use of progestin-only pills or progesterone-releasing intra-uterine device
❖ Salpingitis isthmica nodosa
❖ History of in utero exposure to diethylstilbestrol.

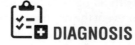 DIAGNOSIS

Clinical Presentation

❖ Initial symptoms are very much similar to those of a normal early pregnancy, e.g. missed periods, breast tenderness, nausea, vomiting or frequent urination.

❖ The typical triad on history for ectopic pregnancy includes bleeding, abdominal pain and a positive urine pregnancy test. These symptoms typically occur 6–8 weeks after the last normal menstrual period. Acute blood loss in some cases may result in the development of dizziness or fainting and hypotension.

❖ Many women with ectopic pregnancy may remain asymptomatic.

❖ Rarely there may be symptoms such as breast tenderness, gastrointestinal symptoms, dizziness, fainting or syncope, shoulder tip pain, urinary symptoms, passage of tissue, rectal pressure or pain on defecation, etc.

General Physical Examination

❖ Normal signs of early pregnancy (e.g. uterine softening)

❖ Sometimes there may be an evidence of haemodynamic instability [pallor, tachycardia (>100 beats/minute) or hypotension (less than 100/60 mmHg), shock or collapse and/or orthostatic hypotension].

Abdominal Examination

❖ Abdominal pain and tenderness

❖ Rebound tenderness

❖ Signs of peritoneal irritation (abdominal rigidity, guarding, etc.) are indicative of ruptured ectopic pregnancy.

Pelvic Examination

❖ Vaginal bleeding may be observed on per speculum examination

❖ Uterine or cervical motion tenderness on vaginal examination may suggest peritoneal inflammation.

❖ Uterus may be slightly enlarged and soft

❖ An adnexal mass may be palpated (with or without tenderness)

❖ There may be pelvic or adnexal tenderness

❖ Other reported signs of ectopic pregnancy include, cervical motion tenderness, abdominal distension and/or enlarged uterus.

Investigations

The following investigations must be done in the suspected cases of ectopic pregnancy:

Blood Group Typing (ABO and Rh Type)

Blood typing [ABO and rhesus (Rh)] and antibody screening should be done in all pregnant patients with bleeding to identify Rh-negative pregnant patients in whom bleeding would be associated with an increased risk of Rh isoimmunisation. Such patients require to be injected with 50 μg (280 IU) of anti-D immunoglobulins (Rhogam) to prevent the occurrence of haemolytic disease of the newborn. Blood must be typed and crossed in order to ensure availability of blood products in case of excessive blood loss.

Complete blood count and estimation of haemoglobin and/or haematocrit must be done in these patients for evaluation of maternal anaemia. In cases of tubal rupture with severe intra-abdominal bleeding, measurement of platelet count and/or coagulation tests is also indicated. If administration of methotrexate (MTX) is considered in cases of unruptured ectopic gestation, a CBC must be done as part of the pretreatment laboratory evaluation.

Urine or Serum β-hCG Levels

In the emergency department, pregnancy is diagnosed by determining the levels of β-hCG in the urine or serum. This hormone may be detected in the urine and blood as early as 1 week before an expected menstrual period. While urine testing may detect levels up to 20–50 IU/L, serum testing may detect levels as low as 5 IU/L. In most cases of suspected ectopic pregnancy, screening is initially done with urine pregnancy test. Determination of serum β-hCG levels is a time-consuming procedure and may not be a practical option at the time of emergency. However, if pregnancy is strongly suspected, even when the urine pregnancy test has a negative result, serum testing becomes necessary. The quantitative level of β-hCG found in ectopic pregnancy varies. In a normal pregnancy, the β-hCG levels double every 48–72 hours until it reaches 10,000–20,000 mIU/mL. Normal intrauterine pregnancies (IUPs) are associated with a doubling time of 1.4–2.1 days. According to the ACOG recommendations (2008),[4] an increase in serum hCG of less than 53% in 48 hours confirms an abnormal pregnancy. The increase in hCG concentration is at a much slower rate in most, but not all cases of ectopic and non-viable IUPs. A falling, slow-rising or plateauing hCG concentration is most consistent with a failed pregnancy (e.g. anembryonic pregnancy, tubal abortion, spontaneously resolving ectopic pregnancy, complete or incomplete abortion, etc.). A single serum measurement of the β-hCG concentration, however, cannot definitely identify the presence of an intrauterine gestational sac. Although women with an ectopic pregnancy tend to have lower β-hCG levels than those with an IUP, there is considerable overlap. Therefore, serial β-hCG measurement is often used for women with first-trimester bleeding or pain, or both. However, similar to a single measurement, serial measurement of β-hCG levels also cannot confirm the intrauterine location of the gestational sac. In a patient with a subnormal increase in β-hCG concentration, non-viability is assumed, and more invasive investigations must be used for differentiating between miscarriage and ectopic pregnancy. Though the falling β-hCG levels confirm non-viability, at the same time they do not rule out ectopic pregnancy. The lack of an IUP when the β-hCG level is above the discriminatory zone represents an ectopic pregnancy or a recent abortion.

Discriminatory zone of β-hCG: The discriminatory zone of β-hCG is the level above which a normal IUP is reliably visualised in nearly 100% cases. Ectopic pregnancy is suspected if transvaginal ultrasonography does not show an intrauterine gestational sac and the patient's β-hCG level is 1,000 mIU/mL (1,000 IU/L) or greater. A negative ultrasound examination at hCG levels below the discriminatory zone is suggestive of an early viable IUP or an ectopic pregnancy or non-viable IUP. Such cases where the location of gestational sac (whether intrauterine or extrauterine) cannot be identified on ultrasound examination are termed as 'pregnancy of unknown location'.[5]

The level of discriminatory zone may vary depending upon the patient's clinical scenario.[6-8] These levels are dependent upon the parameters such as quality of the ultrasound equipment, the experience of the sonographer, prior knowledge of the woman's risks, and symptoms and the presence of physical factors such as uterine fibroids and multiple pregnancy. A discriminatory zone of 1,000 IU/L can be used for specialised units performing high-resolution vaginal ultrasound, having prior knowledge about the woman's symptoms and serum β-hCG levels. Units where a diagnostic TVS is offered without a prior knowledge about the patient's clinical or biochemical parameters, a discriminatory zone of 1,500 IU/L or 2,000 IU/L is acceptable.

Serum hCG levels above the discriminatory zone: Visualisation of an intrauterine gestational sac at the serum hCG levels above the discriminatory zone almost always excludes the presence of an ectopic pregnancy. However, there may be some exceptions to this rule such as heterotopic pregnancy or the pregnancy in a rudimentary uterine horn or cornual pregnancy. Diagnosis of an extrauterine pregnancy is almost certain if there is absence of an intrauterine gestational sac and presence of a complex adnexal mass at hCG concentrations above the discriminatory zone. Presence of embryonic cardiac activity or a definite yolk sac in this adnexal mass is a certain evidence of an ectopic gestation. In these cases, treatment of ectopic pregnancy should be started. The diagnosis is less certain if there is absence of a complex adnexal mass or an intrauterine gestational sac on ultrasound examination with serum hCG levels greater than 1,500 IU/L. Absence of intrauterine gestational sac in presence of serum β-hCG levels above the discriminatory zone may sometimes be indicative of a multiple gestation, since there is no proven discriminatory level for multiple gestations. Therefore, in these cases, TVS examination and serum β-hCG concentration must be repeated again after 2 days. If an IUP is still not observed on TVS, then the pregnancy is abnormal. In these cases, serial follow-up with serum β-hCG levels is required:

❖ If the serum hCG concentration is observed to be increasing or has plateaued, treatment for ectopic pregnancy can be instituted.
❖ If the serum hCG concentration is observed to be decreasing, this is most consistent with a failed pregnancy (e.g. miscarriage, blighted ovum, tubal abortion, etc.).

The rate of fall is slower with an ectopic pregnancy than with a complete abortion. Weekly hCG concentrations should be monitored in these cases until the serum hCG levels become undetectable.

Serum hCG levels below the discriminatory zone: In case the serum β-hCG levels are below the discriminatory zone, evaluation of serum hCG levels must be repeated after 3 days in order to observe the trend. As previously mentioned, in normal viable intrauterine gestation, serum hCG concentration usually doubles every 1.4–2 days until

6–7 weeks of gestation. A normally rising hCG concentration should be evaluated with TVS examination when the serum hCG levels reach the discriminatory zone. At that time, an IUP or an ectopic pregnancy can be diagnosed. If the hCG concentration does not double over 72 hours, then the pregnancy is most likely abnormal (an ectopic gestation or IUP that is destined to abort).[9] The clinician can be reasonably certain that a normal IUP is not present in these cases. A falling hCG concentration is also most consistent with a failed pregnancy.

Imaging Studies

Ultrasonography, especially TVS or endovaginal ultrasonography should be the initial investigation of choice for symptomatic women in their first trimester. TVS can be performed either in the outpatient clinic or emergency department to diagnose IUP. Transvaginal ultrasonography has been reported to have sensitivity of 90%, specificity of 99.8%, with positive and negative predictive values of 93% and 99.8%, respectively.[10] Not only is this highly accurate in identifying ectopic pregnancy, but it also helps in determining the health and viability of the patient's IUP.

Signs of an intrauterine pregnancy on transvaginal sonography: Presence of a gestational sac with a sonolucent centre (>5 mm in diameter) is indicative of an IUP. Gestational sac is surrounded by a thick, concentric, echogenic ring located within the endometrium and contains a foetal pole, yolk sac, or both. A normal gestational sac, an ovoid collection of fluid adjacent to the endometrial stripe, can be visualised by means of the transvaginal probe at a gestational age of about 5 weeks. It can often be seen when it is 2 mm or 3 mm in diameter and should be consistently seen at 5 mm. Since a pseudogestational sac is often associated with an ectopic pregnancy, presence of a sac alone cannot confirm IUP. The earliest embryonic landmark, the yolk sac, appears when the sac is 8 mm or more in diameter, usually during the 5th week of gestation. Cardiac activity can be observed with endovaginal scanning when the embryo reaches 4–5 mm in diameter, at a gestational age of 6–6.5 weeks.

Probably abnormal intrauterine pregnancy: The IUP visualised on TVS is probably abnormal if the gestational sac is larger than 10 mm in diameter without a foetal pole or with a definite foetal pole but without cardiac activity. In these cases, the gestational sac frequently has an irregular or crenate border.

Definite ectopic pregnancy: Signs of a definite ectopic pregnancy on TVS examination are as follows:[11]

❖ *Presence of an extrauterine echogenic ring*: A thick, bright echogenic, ring-like structure, which is located outside the uterus, having a gestational sac containing an obvious foetal pole, yolk sac or both. This usually appears as an intact, well-defined tubal ring (Doughnut's or Bagel's sign, Fig. 35.2). Though this finding confirms the diagnosis of ectopic pregnancy, it may not always be present.
❖ *An empty uterus or presence of a pseudogestational sac*: Pseudogestational sac is typically formed due to endometrial changes and fluid collection in the endometrial

PART II

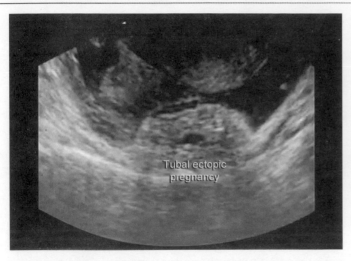

Fig. 35.2: Ultrasound examination showing the Bagel's sign, which can be defined as the thickened fallopian tube due to the presence of gestational sac inside it

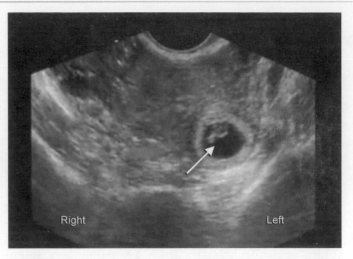

Fig. 35.3: Cornual ectopic pregnancy (indicated by arrow) shows presence of a gestational sac in the left horn of the bicornuate uterus. A gestational sac with a sonolucent centre can be identified

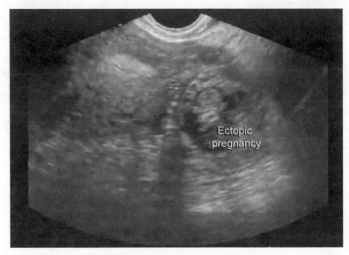

Fig. 35.4: Left-sided ectopic pregnancy

cavity occurring with implantation of extrauterine pregnancy. The gestational sac of a normal IUP is placed eccentrically, whereas a pseudogestational sac is centrally placed. An empty uterus on TVS images in patients with a serum β-hCG level greater than the discriminatory cutoff value is considered to be an ectopic pregnancy until proven otherwise. An empty uterus also may represent a recent abortion. However, in that case, serum β-hCG levels would not be greater than the discriminatory cutoff value.

❖ *Adnexal mass*: Cystic or solid adnexal or tubal masses (including the tubal-ring sign, representing a tubal gestational sac) (Figs 35.3 and 35.4) and severe adnexal tenderness with probe palpation are also suggestive of ectopic pregnancy.

❖ *Haematosalpinx*: There may be haematosalpinx (presence of free fluid or blood in the fallopian tubes) and echogenic or sonolucent cul-de-sac fluid.

❖ *Ruptured ectopic pregnancy*: In case of a ruptured ectopic pregnancy, the ultrasonographic findings include presence of free fluid or clotted blood in the cul-de-sac or in the intraperitoneal gutters (Morison's pouch).

The criteria for TVS diagnosis of ectopic pregnancy, given by Rottem et al. (1991), are described in Table 35.2.[12] If a low-risk patient's ultrasonography is negative for IUP, she is haemodynamically stable and has a β-hCG level less than 1,000 mIU/mL, the physician should take another β-hCG measurement after 48 hours. Patients with a non-diagnostic transvaginal ultrasonography results and a β-hCG level of 1,000 mIU/mL or greater are at an increased risk for ectopic pregnancy and may require a surgical consultation and must remain under vigilance. Serial measurement of β-hCG and progesterone concentrations may also be useful when the diagnosis remains unclear.[13,14]

Other Tests

Serum Progesterone Levels

Serum progesterone levels have been used by some in assessment of an ectopic pregnancy. While a value of 25 ng/mL

Table 35.2: The criteria for transvaginal ultrasonography diagnosis of ectopic pregnancy[12]

Stages	TVS finding
Type 1A	Well-defined tubal ring displaying foetal heart
Type 1B	Well-defined tubal ring displaying no foetal heart
Type 2	Ill-defined tubal mass
Type 3	Free pelvic fluid, empty uterus, displaying no adnexal mass

is associated with normal pregnancies in 98% of cases, a value of less than 5 ng/mL identifies a non-viable pregnancy without regards to the location of pregnancy. Most women with an ectopic pregnancy would show serum progesterone levels somewhere in between these two values, limiting the clinical usefulness of progesterone in diagnosing an ectopic pregnancy. Measurement of the serum concentration of progesterone has been investigated as a potentially useful adjunct to serum β-hCG measurement, since progesterone levels are stable and independent of gestational age in the first trimester. Rapid progesterone analysis can identify two important subgroups of patients in the emergency department with symptomatic first-trimester bleeding or pain, or both:

(1) stable patients with progesterone levels above 22 ng/mL, who have a high (but not certain) likelihood of viable IUP; and (2) patients with levels of 5 ng/mL or less, who almost certainly have a non-viable pregnancy. Invasive diagnostic testing (e.g. dilatation and curettage) could be offered to the latter, as could treatment with MTX, without fear of interrupting a potentially viable IUP. Serum progesterone levels can detect pregnancy failure and identify patients at risk for ectopic pregnancy, but they are not diagnostic of ectopic pregnancy. Sensitivity for diagnosis of ectopic pregnancy is very low (15%); therefore, 85% of patients with ectopic pregnancy will have normal serum progesterone levels. Therefore, serum progesterone levels are not routinely measured because the results of this test merely confirm the provisional diagnosis, which had already been established, by hCG measurements and TVS.

Colour Flow Doppler Examination

Blood flow in the arteries of the fallopian tube, which contains an ectopic pregnancy, is approximately 20–45% higher in comparison to the opposite tube. As a result, the Doppler waveforms in the tube containing an ectopic pregnancy show low impedance flow. Colour Doppler may also demonstrate a 'ring of fire' appearance due to an increased blood flow in the tubal mass (Figs 35.5A and B). However, investigations such as TVS and serum hCG measurements are usually sufficient for establishing the diagnosis in the usual clinical practice and routine Doppler ultrasound examination is not normally required.

Magnetic Resonance Imaging

Though MRI can be used for diagnosing ectopic pregnancy, it is not usually used due to high costs involved.

Diagnostic Procedures

Laparoscopic examination: Sometimes in case of doubt, laparoscopic examination may be performed to diagnose an ectopic pregnancy. In case, the diagnosis of ectopic pregnancy is confirmed on laparoscopic examination, definitive treatment (salpingectomy or salpingostomy) may be carried out.

DIFFERENTIAL DIAGNOSIS

Obstetric Causes

❖ Threatened or incomplete miscarriage or septic abortion
❖ Early pregnancy with pelvic tumours

Gynaecological Causes

❖ Pelvic inflammatory disease
❖ Ruptured or haemorrhagic corpus luteum
❖ Adnexal torsion
❖ Degenerating fibroids, dysfunctional uterine bleeding, endometriosis.

Non-gynaecological Diseases

❖ Appendicitis, urinary calculi, gastroenteritis
❖ Intraperitoneal haemorrhage, perforated peptic ulcer.

MANAGEMENT

Management plan of patients with bleeding during early pregnancy is summarised in Flow chart 35.1. The two most important differential diagnoses in these cases are threatened abortion and ectopic pregnancy. Management plan of patients with suspected diagnosis of ectopic pregnancy is described in Flow chart 35.2. Various treatment options for cases of ectopic pregnancy include expectant management, medical management and surgical treatment (Flow chart 35.3). The particular management option must be tailored according to the patient's clinical condition and her requirements for future fertility. Surgical treatment in form of open surgery (laparotomy) or minimal invasive surgery (laparoscopy) is the most commonly used treatment option. The procedures which can be performed at the time of both laparotomy and laparoscopy include salpingectomy or salpingotomy.

CHAPTER 35

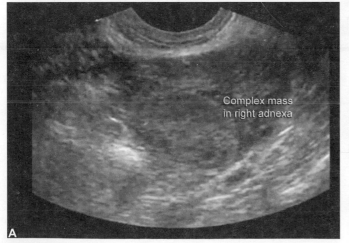

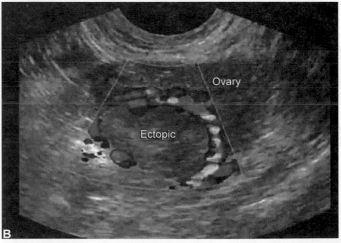

Figs 35.5A and B: (A) Complex right echogenic adnexal mass in this figure represents haematosalpinx (presence of free fluid or blood in the fallopian tubes); (B) Doppler ultrasound in the same case showing a 'ring of fire' appearance due to increased vascularity of the surrounding fallopian tube (*For colour version, see Plate 2*)

Flow chart 35.1: Management of early pregnancy bleeding

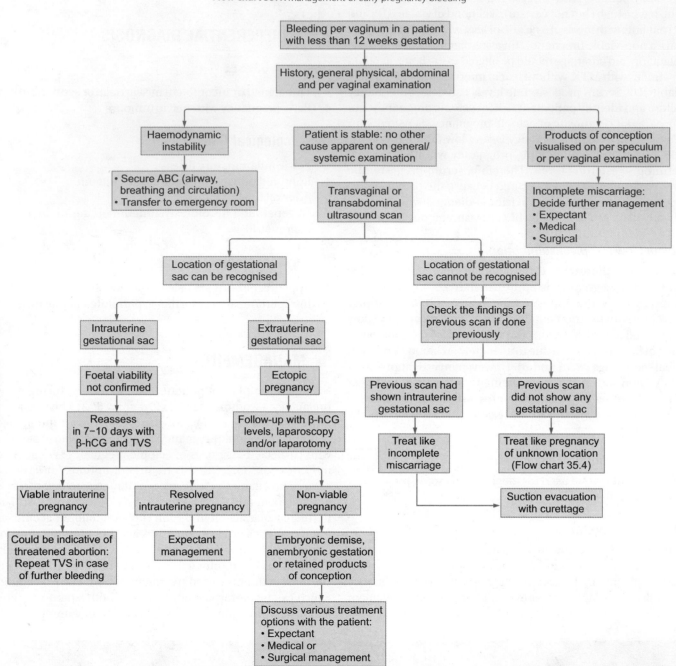

EXPECTANT MANAGEMENT

Expectant management is an option for women with minimal symptoms who are clinically stable with a pregnancy of unknown location or in cases of clinically stable asymptomatic women with an ultrasound diagnosis of ectopic pregnancy, showing declining serum hCG levels, initially less than 1,000 IU/L (Box 35.1). Contraindications for expectant management of ectopic pregnancy are enlisted in Box 35.2. Women who are being managed expectantly should be followed twice weekly with serial hCG measurements to ensure that the hCG levels are rapidly decreasing. Ideally, the hCG levels must become less than 50% of its initial level within 7 days. These women must also be followed weekly by transvaginal examinations to ensure that there is a reduction in the size of adnexal mass by 7 days. Measurement of weekly hCG levels and transvaginal ultrasound examinations are advised thereafter until serum hCG levels become less than 20 IU/L.

Pregnancy of Unknown Location

In the management of suspected ectopic pregnancy, the obstetrician must also keep in mind the probability of 'pregnancy of unknown location'. There is a serum hCG level at which it is assumed that all viable IUPs will be visualised by TVS. This is referred to as the discriminatory zone.[6]

Flow chart 35.2: Management of patients with suspected diagnosis of ectopic pregnancy

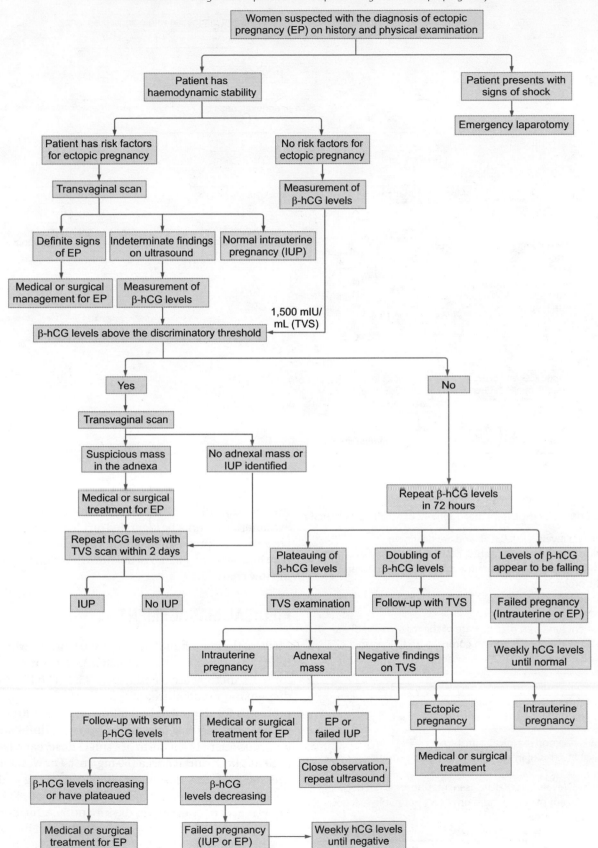

Flow chart 35.3: Treatment plan for patients with ectopic pregnancy

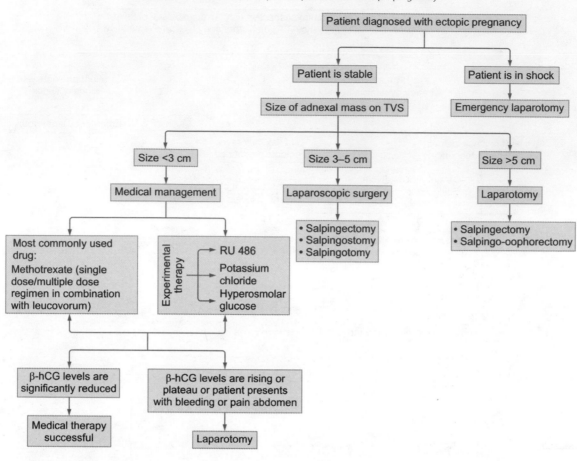

PART II

Box 35.1: Criteria for expectant management of ectopic pregnancy

❑ Serum hCG levels ≤1,000 IU/L and are declining
❑ Ectopic pregnancy is suspected, but TVS fails to reveal any gestational sac or an extrauterine mass suspicious for an ectopic pregnancy
❑ Size of ectopic pregnancy is <2 cm
❑ Haemoperitoneum is <50 mL
❑ The patient has been made aware of the risks involved; she accepts the risks and is able to comply with follow-up
❑ The patient should be within easy access to the hospital in question

Box 35.2: Contraindications for expectant management of ectopic pregnancy

❑ Patient is haemodynamically unstable
❑ Presence of signs of impending or on-going rupture of ectopic mass
❑ Serum hCG levels ≥1,000 IU/L, is increasing, or is not declining
❑ Non-compliant patient, who is unwilling or unable to follow-up with monitoring
❑ Patient does not have timely access to a medical institution

A negative ultrasound examination at hCG levels below the discriminatory zone is suggestive of an early viable IUP or an ectopic pregnancy or non-viable IUP. Such cases where the location of gestational sac (whether intrauterine or extrauterine) cannot be identified on ultrasound examination are termed as 'pregnancy of unknown location'.[7] Management plan in cases of pregnancy of unknown location is summarised in Flow chart 35.4.

MEDICAL MANAGEMENT

Medical therapy should be offered to suitable women, who fulfil the criteria mentioned in Box 35.3. Contraindications for MTX therapy are listed in Box 35.4. The hospital units dispensing medical treatment should have appropriate protocols for treatment and follow-up. Presently, the most widely used medical treatment option is administration of intramuscular MTX in form of a single dose, calculated from patient's body surface area (50 mg/m²). For women with an average BMI, this dose varies between 75 mg and 90 mg. Following the administration of this dose of MTX, serum hCG levels are checked on days 4 and 7. A further dose of MTX is given if hCG levels have failed to fall by more than 15% between days 4 and 7.[6-8] Box 35.5 describes the protocol for single-dose MTX. One of the most important advantages of outpatient medical therapy is that it is likely to result in considerable savings in the cost of treatment.

Flow chart 35.4: Management of pregnancy at unknown location

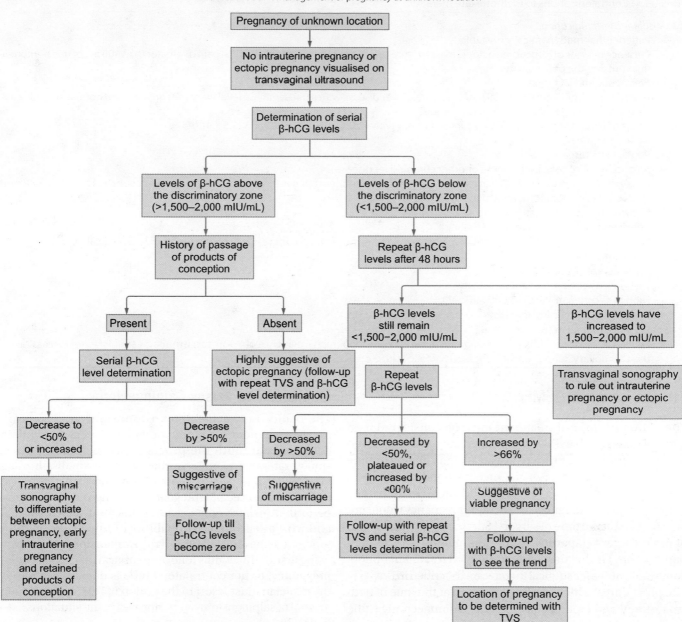

CHAPTER 35

Box 35.3: Prerequisites for starting medical treatment of ectopic pregnancy

❑ Patient is haemodynamically stable and does not have pelvic pain
❑ Patient desires future fertility
❑ Patient appears to be reliable and compliant who will return for post-treatment follow-up care
❑ Ectopic pregnancy smaller than 4 cm in diameter and no foetal heart activity on TVS or smaller than 3.5 cm with presence of cardiac activity and absence of any free fluid in the pouch of Douglas
❑ There is no evidence of tubal rupture
❑ Serum hCG is <3,000 IU/L, with minimal symptoms
❑ Availability of facilities for follow-up care following the use of methotrexate (MTX)
❑ Patient agrees to use reliable contraception for 3–4 months post-treatment
❑ Patient has no underlying severe medical condition or disorder
❑ There is no underlying abnormality of liver function test, kidney function test or CBC, suggestive of liver, renal or bone marrow impairment
❑ Patient does not have any known contraindications to MTX
❑ Patient is not currently taking non-steroidal anti-inflammatory drugs, diuretics, penicillin and tetracycline group of drugs
❑ Patient does not have a coexisting intrauterine pregnancy
❑ Patient is not breastfeeding

Box 35.4: Contraindications to methotrexate therapy

❑ *Absolute contraindications*
- Patient is haemodynamically unstable
- Presence of signs of impending ectopic mass rupture (i.e. severe or persistent abdominal pain or greater than 300 mL of free peritoneal fluid outside the pelvic cavity)
- Pregnancy and lactation
- Hepatic, renal, or haematological dysfunction, e.g. liver disease with a transaminase level two times greater than normal, renal disease with a creatinine level >1.5 mg/dL (133 µmol/L)
- Overt or laboratory evidence of immunodeficiency with a WBC count <1,500/mm^3 (1.5 × 10^9/L)
- Active pulmonary disease
- Peptic ulcer disease
- Alcoholism, alcoholic liver disease or other chronic liver disease
- Pre-existing blood dyscrasias, such as bone marrow hypoplasia, leucopenia, thrombocytopenia [platelet count less than 100,000/mm^3 (100 × 10^9/L) or significant anaemia
- Known sensitivity to methotrexate
- Coexistent viable intrauterine pregnancy
- Patient is unwilling to be compliant with post-therapeutic monitoring or there is lack of timely access to a medical institution

❑ *Relative contraindications*
- Large ectopic size (≥3.5 cm)
- Presence of embryonic cardiac activity
- High hCG concentration (>5,000 mIU/mL)
- Presence of foetal cardiac activity
- Presence of fluid in the peritoneal cavity
- *Other relative contraindications requiring further research*: Sonographic evidence of a yolk sac; isthmic location of ectopic mass rather than ampullary; high pretreatment levels of folic acid, etc.

SURGICAL MANAGEMENT

The option of surgical treatment must be considered if an adnexal mass suggestive of ectopic pregnancy can be observed on TVS examination or there are clear signs demonstrating presence of an ectopic pregnancy on ultrasound examination. If no abnormality is observed on the ultrasound examination, there is a high probability that an ectopic pregnancy would not be visualised at the time of surgery. Surgical treatment in form of open surgery (laparotomy) or minimal invasive surgery (laparoscopy) is the most commonly used treatment option. Some indications for surgical therapy are described in Box 35.6. The procedures, which can be performed at the time of both laparotomy and laparoscopy, include salpingectomy (tube removal) or the tube conserving procedures (salpingotomy or salpingostomy). Salpingotomy is the procedure involving surgical incision of the fallopian tube so that the contents of ectopic pregnancy can be removed or flushed out, following which the incision is closed. Salpingostomy is a similar tube conserving procedure where a surgical incision is given over the fallopian tube to remove the ectopic pregnancy. However, unlike salpingotomy where the incision is closed, in salpingostomy, the incision is not closed and is left to heal itself by secondary intent. Salpingectomy, on the other hand, is the surgical excision of the fallopian tube. In case of ruptured ectopic pregnancy, salpingectomy is invariably performed. Management of tubal pregnancy in the presence of haemodynamic instability should be by the most expedient and rapid method. In most cases this will be laparotomy. While in a haemodynamically stable patient, a laparoscopic approach is usually preferred over laparotomy, in cases of haemodynamic instability, laparotomy is the most preferred option.

Salpingostomy versus Salpingectomy

The choice between salpingostomy and salpingectomy for the treatment of ectopic pregnancy presently remains controversial. Both the procedures are associated with similar rates of operative morbidity. The main disadvantage of salpingostomy is the potential risk of persistent trophoblast and/or recurrent ectopic pregnancy. Salpingostomy is therefore performed in those women who are haemodynamically stable and with a reasonable probability of future normal tubal function in the affected tube. If the woman does not conceive in the first 12–18 months following surgical therapy for ectopic pregnancy, or her contralateral tube is damaged or absent, the clinician must resort to the option of IVF. Salpingectomy, instead of salpingostomy, is performed in the situations listed in Box 35.7.

According to two recent randomised trials, ESEP (European surgery in ectopic pregnancy) study[15] and DEMETER (Greek goddess of fertility) study,[16] presently there is no clear evidence regarding the use of salpingotomy in preference to salpingectomy in patients with a healthy contralateral tube. There are four cohort studies suggesting that salpingotomy may be associated with a higher rate of subsequent IUP.[17-20] However, the magnitude of this benefit is likely to be small. The use of conservative surgical technique is likely to expose the women to a small risk of tubal bleeding in the immediate postoperative period. There may be a potential requirement for further treatment of persistent trophoblast tissue. Therefore, if the option of salpingotomy is being considered, the surgeon must discuss both these risks and the possibility of further ectopic pregnancies in the conserved tube with the patient before undertaking such surgery.

Laparoscopic salpingotomy should be considered as the major treatment option for patient with ectopic pregnancy,

PART II

Box 35.5: Protocol for single-dose methotrexate (MTX)

- ❑ *Pretreatment investigations*
  - Complete blood count
  - Blood group typing (ABO and Rh) and antibody testing
  - Liver function and kidney function tests
  - Measurement of serum β-hCG levels
  - Transvaginal sonography
- ❑ *Pretreatment prerequisites*
  - Written informed consent must be obtained from the patient and her partner. They must be provided clear information (preferably written) about the possible requirement for further treatment and adverse effects following treatment
  - Woman's weight and height must be obtained and her body surface area (BSA) must be calculated
- ❑ *Day 0 (Day of treatment)*
  - Methotrexate needs to be injected in the dosage of 50 mg/m^2 of BSA by IM injection
  - Body surface area is calculated using the following formula:

$$BSA = \frac{\sqrt{(\text{Height in cm} \times \text{Weight in kg})}}{3,600}$$

  - RhoGAM® (300 µg) is administered intramuscularly if the patient is Rh negative
  - Advise patients not to take vitamins with folic acid until complete resolution of the ectopic pregnancy occurs
  - Folinic acid supplements to be discontinued
  - They should also refrain from strenuous exercises, alcohol consumption and intercourse for the same period
- ❑ *Day 4*
  - Measurement of the β-hCG levels must be performed and served as the baseline level against which subsequent levels are measured
- ❑ *Day 7*
  - Serum β hCG levels are measured on day 7
  - If serum hCG levels have failed to fall by more than 15% between days 4 and 7, a further dose of MTX is administered
  - If the β-hCG level has dropped by 15% or more since day 4, weekly hCG levels must be obtained until they have reached the negative level
  - If the weekly levels plateau or increase, a second course of MTX may be administered
  - Second dose of MTX may also be required if decline in β-hCG levels is <25% on day 7
  - If no drop has occurred by day 14, surgical therapy is indicated
  - If the patient develops increasing abdominal pain after MTX therapy, repeat a TVS to evaluate for possible rupture
  - Aspartate transaminase levels, CBC and TVS also need to be done
- ❑ *Weekly*
  - Measure serum β-hCG concentrations until levels become <15 IU/L
  - Perform TVS
- ❑ *Anytime*
  - Perform laparoscopy if the patient has severe abdominal pain, acute abdomen pain or if the ultrasound examination reveals blood in the abdomen

Box 35.6: Indications for surgical therapy

- ❑ Candidate not suitable for medical therapy (not willing to comply with post-treatment medical therapy follow-up or contra-indications to the use of methotrexate)
- ❑ Failed medical therapy
- ❑ Heterotopic pregnancy with a viable intrauterine pregnancy
- ❑ Patient is haemodynamically unstable and requires immediate treatment
- ❑ Impending or on-going rupture of the ectopic mass
- ❑ Absence of timely access to a medical institution for managing tubal rupture
- ❑ Patient desires permanent method of contraception

Box 35.7: Indications for performing salpingectomy instead of salpingostomy

- ❑ Uncontrolled bleeding from the implantation site
- ❑ Recurrent ectopic pregnancy in the same tube
- ❑ Severely damaged tube
- ❑ Large tubal pregnancy (i.e. >5 cm)
- ❑ Women who have completed their childbearing
- ❑ Women who may be treated with IVF in future

Moreover, in women with a damaged or absent contralateral tube, the procedure of IVF is likely to be required for future pregnancy if salpingectomy is performed. Due to the requirement for postoperative follow-up and the treatment of persistent trophoblast, the short-term costs of salpingotomy are greater than that of salpingectomy.[21] However, in the long term due to the requirement of assisted conception for future pregnancies with salpingectomy, salpingotomy is likely to be a more cost effective option in comparison to salpingectomy.[19] Therefore, in the presence of contralateral tubal disease, use of salpigotomy appears to be more appropriate.

Surgical treatment is associated with reduced requirement of time for resolution of the ectopic pregnancy and avoidance of the requirement for prolonged monitoring. Some prerequisites which must be taken into consideration before starting surgical therapy include the following:

❖ Treatment needs to be explained to the women and her partner and written informed consent must be obtained

❖ Patient's blood sample needs to be typed and cross-matched (ABO and Rh) and blood needs to be arranged. Anti-D immunoglobulins need to be administered to the women who are Rh negative. The following steps need to be taken in women who are haemodynamically unstable:

- Immediate resuscitation
- Securing immediate IV access by inserting large bore venous cannula
- Sending blood for CBC and cross matching and arranging at least 4 units of blood
- Informing the theatre staff, anaesthetist, and on-call gynaecology consultant
- Foley's catheter must be inserted prior to starting the procedure.

The urgency of the situation must be stressed to all concerned. The surgery must not be delayed and should be performed even before blood and fluid losses have been completely replaced.

who desires future fertility, in the presence of contralateral tubal disease. It is likely to be associated with a higher rate of subsequent IUP in comparison with laparoscopic salpingectomy in women with contralateral tubal disease.[17-20]

CHAPTER 35

Types of Surgical Approach

Surgical therapy may be either in form of open laparotomy or via the laparoscopic route. Nowadays, the trend is towards using a laparoscopic approach for surgery.[22] Numerous factors need to be considered before deciding the type of surgical approach to be used. Some of these factors include history of multiple prior surgeries, pelvic adhesions, skill of the surgeon and surgical staff, availability of the equipment, condition of the patient and size and location of ectopic pregnancy. As previously described, a laparoscopic approach to the surgical management of tubal pregnancy must be used in the haemodynamically stable patients. On the other hand, management of tubal pregnancy in the presence of haemodynamic instability should be by laparotomy. There is no role for medical management in the treatment of tubal pregnancy or suspected tubal pregnancy when a patient is showing signs of hypovolemic shock.

Laparoscopic Surgery

A laparoscopic approach to the surgical management of tubal pregnancy, in the haemodynamically stable patient is preferable to an open approach. Laparoscopic management is associated with considerably reduced postoperative morbidity, shorter operative times, reduced intraoperative blood loss, shorter duration of hospital stay, lower analgesic requirements, lower complication rate and time duration of return to normal activity level.[23-27] Most cases of ruptured as well as unruptured tubal pregnancy can be treated laparoscopically. The main advantages of laparoscopic surgery are enumerated in Box 35.8.

Complications due to laparoscopic management of ectopic pregnancy: In experienced hands there is no specific complication directly related to laparoscopic procedure, but if the surgeon is not trained enough in laparoscopy then there is the chance of the complications as described in Box 35.9. However, in experienced hands, the chances of these complications are extremely rare. Altogether, laparoscopic procedure

---

> **Box 35.8:** Advantages of laparoscopic surgery
>
> ❑ Reduced postoperative pain
> ❑ Faster recovery
> ❑ Short hospital stay
> ❑ Lower rate of postoperative complications like wound infection
> ❑ Cost-effectiveness
> ❑ Reduced postoperative analgesic requirement
> ❑ Reduced adhesion formation

> **Box 35.9:** Complications due to laparoscopic surgery
>
> ❑ Missed diagnosis
> ❑ Bleeding
> ❑ Incomplete removal of ectopic pregnancy
> ❑ Visceral injury
> ❑ Leakage of purulent exudates
> ❑ Intra-abdominal abscess
> ❑ Hernia

> **Box 35.10:** Indications for laparotomy
>
> ❑ Patient is haemodynamically unstable
> ❑ Cervical, interstitial or abdominal ectopic pregnancy
> ❑ Patients having large haematoma due to large ruptured ectopic pregnancy
> ❑ Presence of more than 1,500 cc haemoperitoneum
> ❑ Patients with underlying cardiac diseases and chronic obstructive pulmonary disease
> ❑ History of abdominal surgery in the past
> ❑ Patients at increased risk of complications with general anaesthesia

---

has a much lower complication rate in comparison to the conventional surgery.

Laparotomy

There are times when laparotomy is favoured over the laparoscopic approach. Some of these indications are described in Box 35.10. Laparotomy is usually preferred in cases of haemodynamic instability or when ectopic pregnancy is cervical, interstitial, abdominal, etc. Laparotomy is also preferred in patients having large haematoma due to large ruptured ectopic pregnancy or in case of presence of more than 1,500 cc haemoperitoneum. Patient with cardiac diseases and chronic obstructive pulmonary disease should not be considered a good candidate for laparoscopic management. Laparoscopic management of ectopic pregnancy may also be more difficult in patients who have had previous lower abdominal surgery or those who may also be at an increased risk for complications with general anaesthesia combined with pneumoperitoneum, e.g. the elderly patients.

Surgical Procedures at the Time of Laparotomy

Salpingectomy: The surgical procedure performed during laparotomy is usually salpingectomy. Salpingectomy involves removal of the ectopic pregnancy along with the fallopian tube of affected side. Milking of pregnancy through abdominal ostium (transfimbrial extraction) had been advocated in the past if the haemorrhage was easy to control and pregnancy was fimbrial. However, the risk of recurrent ectopic pregnancy in these cases is twice as high. Therefore, this procedure is no longer recommended. Regardless of the route of approach (whether laparotomy or laparoscopy), salpingectomy is indicated in the situations enumerated in Box 35.11. The clinician has the option for choosing between partial and total salpingectomy. The choice for partial versus total salpingectomy is based on the patient's age and her desire to conceive in future. Partial salpingectomy is usually done in cases where patient might opt for tubal anastomosis at a future date. Total salpingectomy is usually performed in those cases where IVF appears to be the likely treatment option.

Procedure of salpingectomy: The procedure of salpingectomy involves the following steps:

❖ The tube between the uterus and the ectopic pregnancy is clamped using a clamp. The pedicle is then cut and ligated.
❖ The tubo-ovarian artery is also clamped, cut and ligated, while preserving the utero-ovarian artery and ligament

CHAPTER 35

Box 35.11: Indications for salpingectomy

☐ The tube is severely damaged
☐ There is uncontrolled bleeding
☐ There is a recurrent ectopic pregnancy in the same tube
☐ There is a large tubal pregnancy of size >5 cm
☐ The ectopic pregnancy has ruptured
☐ The woman has completed her family and future fertility is not desired
☐ Ectopic pregnancy has resulted due to sterilisation failure
☐ Ectopic pregnancy has occurred in a previously reconstructed tube
☐ Patient requests sterilisation
☐ Haemorrhage continues to occur even after salpingotomy
☐ Cases of chronic tubal pregnancy

❖ The mesosalpinx must be continued to be clamped, cut and ligated until the tube is free and can be removed
❖ Following the excision and removal of the tube, the pedicles are ligated using a 2-0 or 3-0 synthetic absorbable suture.

Partial salpingectomy: Partial salpingectomy may be sometimes performed instead of complete salpingectomy if the pregnancy is in the midportion of the tube, none of the indications for salpingectomy are present and the patient appears to be a candidate for tubal reanastomosis in future. In these cases, a clamp is placed through an avascular area in the mesosalpinx under the ectopic pregnancy. This creates spaces through which two free ties are placed, which are tied around the tube on each side of the ectopic pregnancy. The isolated portion of the tube containing the ectopic pregnancy is then cut and removed.

Follow up: All patients who have not had the entire ectopic pregnancy removed by salpingectomy need to have their weekly hCG levels observed until these levels return to non-pregnant values. If, during this time span the hCG level either plateaus or rises, the patient must be treated with MTX. Patients should be advised to use some form of effective contraception until their hCG levels have returned to non-pregnant levels.

Salpingotomy: Tube-sparing salpingostomy or salpingotomy is a procedure in which the gestational sac is removed, without the removal of tube, through a 1 cm long incision on the tubal wall. This surgery is preferred over salpingectomy because not only is salpingotomy less invasive, but also associated with comparable rates of subsequent fertility and ectopic pregnancy. Laparoscopic salpingotomy should especially be considered as the primary modality of treatment if the woman has contralateral tube disease and desires future fertility. When salpingotomy is used for the management of tubal pregnancy, follow-up protocols (weekly serum β-hCG levels) are necessary for the identification and treatment of women with persistent trophoblastic disease. Persistent trophoblast is detected by the failure of serum hCG levels to fall as expected after initial treatment.

Procedure: After infiltrating the mesosalpinx with vasopressin (20 IU in 50 mL normal saline), 1–2 cm incision is made on the antimesenteric side of the tube. A syringe filled with saline is inserted deep into the incision and the fluid is injected forcefully in such a way so as to dislodge the ectopic pregnancy and clots. The contents of ectopic pregnancy and clots are then aspirated out. Following this, the bed of the ectopic pregnancy must be irrigated well. In case some trophoblastic tissue remains, prior injection of vasopressin may lead to anoxia and death of the trophoblasts, preventing postoperative growth. Bleeding may be controlled by applying pressure with blunt tissue forceps for 5 minutes.[28]

Postoperative follow-up: Regular follow-up must be done following surgery in order to ensure that the patient's hCG levels have returned to zero. This may take several weeks. Elevated hCG levels could mean that some ectopic trophoblastic tissue which was missed at the time of removal is still remaining inside. This tissue may have to be removed using MTX or additional surgery.

❖ The patient must be instructed to visit the clinician after 1 week for removal of sutures.
❖ The patient must be counselled that she may experience mild bleeding or pain during the 1st postoperative week. In case of mild pain, she can use simple analgesic drugs available over the counter. In case of pain or bleeding of severe intensity, she must be instructed to report to the clinician immediately.

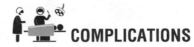

COMPLICATIONS

Ruptured ectopic pregnancy can result in life-threatening haemorrhage, hypovolaemic shock and/or DIC, which may even prove fatal. In the past few decades, ruptured ectopic pregnancy was amongst one of the leading causes of maternal mortality. Presently, with the improvement in imaging and minimal invasive procedures in cases of ectopic pregnancy, the mortality rate has considerably reduced. Nowadays, the trend is towards the use of minimal invasive surgery in cases of ectopic pregnancy. Although operative laparoscopy is associated with its own inherent complications, in experienced hands, there are usually minimal complications related to the laparoscopic procedure. However, if the surgeon is not trained enough in laparoscopy then there is a chance of complications as described in Box 35.9. In experienced hands, the chances of these complications are extremely rare. Altogether laparoscopic procedure has a much lower complication rate in comparison to the conventional surgery. Conventional surgery can also be associated with complications such as bleeding, infection and damage to the surrounding viscera such as bowel, bladder, ureters and other major vessels. Ectopic pregnancy can be associated with significant psychological distress to the parents because most mothers may perceive ectopic pregnancy as the loss of their pregnancy. Patient with a history of ectopic pregnancy is associated with an approximately 10% risk of developing ectopic pregnancy in the future. Conceiving a future intrauterine pregnancy is not a problem even if one of the tubes is removed. 65% of the women are likely to achieve a successful pregnancy in future within 18 months of having an ectopic pregnancy. Occasionally, fertility treatment such as IVF may be required.

CLINICAL PEARLS

❖ Ectopic pregnancy can be considered as the leading cause of pregnancy-related deaths during the first trimester.

❖ In a haemodynamically stable patient with ectopic pregnancy, laparoscopic approach is preferable to laparotomy.

❖ Non-sensitised women who are Rh negative with a confirmed or suspected ectopic pregnancy should receive anti-D immunoglobulins.

EVIDENCE-BASED MEDICINE

❖ If the patient has a healthy tube on the contralateral side, the available evidence does not clearly indicate whether or not salpingotomy should be used in preference to salpingectomy.[15-20]

❖ The available evidence indicates that laparoscopic salpingotomy is likely to be associated with a higher rate of subsequent IUP in future in comparison with laparoscopic salpingectomy in women with contralateral tubal disease.[17-20]

REFERENCES

1. Cantwell R, Clutton-Brock T, Cooper G, Dawson A, Drife J, Garrod D, et al. Saving Mother's Lives: Reviewing maternal deaths to make motherhood safer: 2006-2008. The Eight Report of the Confidential Enquiries into Maternal Deaths in the UK. BJOG. 2011;118 (Suppl 1):1-203.

2. Ankum WM, Mol BW, Van der Veen F, Bossuyt PM. Risk factors for ectopic pregnancy: a meta-analysis. Fertil Steril. 1996;65(6):1093-9.

3. Risk factor for ectopic pregnancy. Can Fam Physician. 1999;45:300, 309-10.

4. American College of Obstetricians and Gynecologists (ACOG). ACOG Practice Bulletin No. 94: Medical management of ectopic pregnancy. Obstet Gynecol. 2008;111(6):1479-85.

5. Mateer JR, Valley VT, Aiman EJ, Phelan MB, Thoma ME, Kefer MP. Outcome analysis of a protocol including bedside endovaginal sonography in patients at risk for ectopic pregnancy. Ann Emerg Med. 1996;27(3):283-9.

6. Sowter M, Frappell J. The role of laparoscopy in the management of ectopic pregnancy. Rev Gynaecol Practice. 2002;2: 73-82.

7. Saraj A, Wilcox J, Najmabadi S, Stein S, Johnson M, Paulson R. Resolution of hormonal markers of ectopic gestation. a randomized trial comparing single-dose intramuscular methotrexate with salpingostomy. Obstet Gynecol. 1998; 92 (6):989-94.

8. Sowter MC, Farquhar C, Petrie KJ, Gudex G. A randomized trial comparing single dose systemic methotrexate and laparoscopic surgery for the treatment of unruptured tubal pregnancy. BJOG. 2001;108(2):192-203.

9. Kadar N, DeVore G, Romero R. Discriminatory hCG zone: its use in the sonographic evaluation for ectopic pregnancy. Obstet Gynecol. 1981;58(2):156-61.

10. Cacciatore B, Stenman U, Ylöstolalo P. Diagnosis of ectopic pregnancy by vaginal ultrasonography in combination with a discriminatory serum hCG level of 1000 IU/L (IRP). BJOG. 1990;97(10):904-8.

11. Kirk E. Ultrasound in the diagnosis of ectopic pregnancy. Clin Obstet Gynecol. 2012;55(2):395-401.

12. Rottem S, Thaler I, Timor-Tritch E. Classification of tubal gestations by transvaginal sonography. Ultrasound Obstet Gynecol. 1991;1(3):197-201.

13. Casikar I, Reid S, Condous G. Ectopic pregnancy: Ultrasound diagnosis in modern management. Clin Obstet Gynecol. 2012;55(2):402-9.

14. Durston WE, Carl ML, Guerra W, Eaton A, Ackerson LM. Ultrasound availability in the evaluation of ectopic pregnancy in the ED: comparison of quality and cost-effectiveness with different approaches. Am J Emerg Med. 2000;18(4):408-17.

15. Mol F, van Mello NM, Strandell A, Strandell K, Jurkovic D, Ross J, et al. Salpingotomy versus salpingectomy in women with tubal pregnancy (ESEP study): an open-label, multicentre, randomised controlled trial. Lancet. 2014;383(9927):1483-9.

16. Fernandez H, Capmas P, Lucot JP, Resch B, Panel P, Bouyer J, et al. Fertility after ectopic pregnancy: the DEMETER randomized trial. Hum Reprod. 2013;28(5):1247-53.

17. Silva PD, Schaper AM, Rooney B. Reproductive outcome after 143 laparoscopic procedures for ectopic pregnancy. Obstet Gynecol. 1993;81(5 Pt 1):710-5.

18. Job-Spira N, Bouyer J, Pouly JL, Germain E, Coste J, Aublet-Cuvelier B, et al. Fertility after ectopic pregnancy: first results of a population-based cohort study in France. Hum Reprod. 1996;11(1):99-104.

19. Mol BW, Matthijsse HC, Tinga DJ, Huynh T, Hajenius PJ, Ankum WM, et al. Fertility after conservative and radical surgery for tubal pregnancy. Hum Reprod. 1998;13(7):1804-9.

20. Bangsgaard N, Lund C, Ottesen B, Nilas L. Improved fertility following conservative surgical treatment of ectopic pregnancy. BJOG. 2003;110(8):765-70.

21. Rulin MC. Is salpingostomy the surgical treatment of choice for unruptured tubal pregnancy? Obstet Gynecol. 1995;86(6):1010-3.

22. Royal College of Obstetricians and Gynaecologists (RCOG). The management of tubal ectopic pregnancy. Guideline No. 21. London: RCOG Press; 2010.

23. Murphy AA, Nager CW, Wujek JJ, Kettel LM, Torp VA, Chin HG. Operative laparoscopy versus laparotomy for the management of ectopic pregnancy. Fertil Steril. 1992;57(6):1180-5.

24. Vermesh M, Silva PD, Rosen GF, Stein AL, Fossum GT, Sauer MV. Management of unruptured ectopic gestation by linear salpingostomy: a prospective, randomized clinical trial of laparoscopy versus laparotomy. Obstet Gynecol. 1989;73(3 Pt 1):400-4.

25. Lundorff P, Thorburn J, Hahlin M, Kallfelt B, Lindblom B. Laparoscopic surgery in ectopic pregnancy: a randomized trial versus laparoscopy. Acta Obstet Gynecol Scand. 1991;70(4-5).343-0.

26. Lundorff P, Thorburn J, Lindblom B. Fertility outcome after conservative surgical treatment of ectopic pregnancy evaluated in a randomized trial. Fertil Steril. 1992;57(5):998-1002.

27. Gray DT, Thorburn J, Lundorff P, Strandell A, Lindblom B. A cost-effectiveness study of a randomised trial of laparoscopy versus laparotomy for ectopic pregnancy. Lancet. 1995; 345(8958):1139-43.

28. Kelley RW, Martin SA, Strickler RC. Delayed hemorrhage in conservative surgery for ectopic pregnancy. Am J Obstet Gynecol. 1979;133(2):225-6.

PART II

Spontaneous Miscarriage

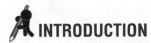

INTRODUCTION

Spontaneous abortion, also known as miscarriage refers to the spontaneous loss of pregnancy before attainment of the foetal viability. It can be considered as one of the most common complications of early pregnancy. According to the WHO and the CDC, spontaneous miscarriage can be defined as the termination of pregnancy prior to 20 weeks of gestation or birth of a foetus weighing less than 500 g in case the period of gestation is not known.[1] However, in the UK, miscarriage is defined as the loss of a pregnancy before 24 weeks of gestation. After 24 weeks, the pregnancy loss is defined as 'stillbirth'.

Miscarriage occurs in about 10–20% of all pregnancies.[2] Birth defects occur in about 3% of all pregnancies, some of which result in spontaneous miscarriage early in pregnancy. On the other hand, presence of chromosomal disorders, such as trisomy 21, 13, 18, monosomy XO, etc., may result in viable pregnancies and are associated with advanced maternal age. Approximately 75% of miscarriages occur before 16 weeks of gestation and of these nearly three-fourths occur within the first 2 months of pregnancy. Various types of spontaneous miscarriages (Table 36.1) are described herein.[3]

Threatened Abortion

Threatened abortion is a type of abortion where the process of abortion has begun, but has yet not progressed to a stage from where the recovery would be impossible. In case of threatened abortion, despite the occurrence of bleeding before 20 weeks of gestation, the cervical os is closed. The foetal heart rate is usually present and there may be normal intrauterine growth. The bleeding may sometimes stop on its own and pregnancy may continue normally. If the pregnancy continues, there may be increased chances of preterm labour, IUGR, placenta praevia, etc. Sonography can help differentiate between a viable or non-viable intrauterine pregnancy. Therapy should be directed towards treatment of the underlying cause. Treatment is mostly empirical. Bed rest along with sedation and painkillers is commonly prescribed.

Inevitable Abortion

Inevitable abortion is a type of abortion where the process of abortion has progressed to such an extent that the continuation of pregnancy is not possible. It is often associated with pain in abdomen and bleeding. The cervical os is open in these cases. This type of miscarriage may progress into either complete or incomplete miscarriage.

Incomplete Abortion

When the process of inevitable abortion has progressed to such an extent that part of foetal products has been expelled out and part of it is still within the uterine cavity, it is known as incomplete abortion. This type of abortion is associated with pain and bleeding. Cervical os is open and some of the foetal tissues may have been passed out.

Missed Abortion

Missed abortion is a condition in which the foetus becomes dead and is retained inside the uterine cavity. Beyond 12 weeks of gestation, the liquor amnii gets absorbed and the placenta becomes papery, pale and adherent. The patient is likely to present with features of threatened miscarriage. There may be presence of brownish vaginal discharge and subsidence of pregnancy symptoms such as retrogression of breast changes, cessation of uterine growth, etc. The foetal heart sounds may not be heard and the immunological tests for pregnancy may become negative. The uterus may be small for dates and ultrasound may reveal an empty gestational sac.

AETIOLOGY

Various causes of miscarriage (Flow chart 36.1) are as follows:
❖ Genetic causes
❖ Endocrinological causes
❖ Infections

Table 36.1: Various types of miscarriages[3]

Subcategory	Definitions	Clinical characteristics	Ultrasound criteria	Management
Threatened abortion	Bleeding before 20 weeks' gestation with closed cervix; pregnancy viable at time of presentation and may or may not result in a miscarriage	• Internal cervical os is closed	Findings appropriate according to the gestational age; subchorionic haemorrhage may be present	Mostly empirical treatment
Inevitable miscarriage	Miscarriage is imminent or is in the process of happening	• Leaking amniotic fluid • Cervical dilatation • Heavy bleeding • Severe pain • Miscarriage is unavoidable • Risk of incomplete abortion or sepsis	Products of conception are visible; foetal cardiac activity may or may not be present	Uterine evacuation
Incomplete abortion	A miscarriage where some parts of the foetus or placenta are unable to be naturally expelled by the mother	• Open internal cervical os • Bleeding • Ultrasound or pelvic examination shows products of conception • Complications such as haemorrhage and sepsis	Heterogeneous and/or echogenic material (suggestive of products of conception) along the endometrial stripe in endometrial cavity or in the cervical canal	Uterine evacuation
Complete abortion	All products of conception have been passed out through the cervical canal	• Closed internal cervical os	Empty uterine cavity; endometrial lining may be normal or thickened	No medical or surgical interventions are required because the uterine cavity is already empty
Missed abortion/ embryonic or foetal demise	A confirmed, non-viable pregnancy on ultrasound with no bleeding	• The foetus dies but the woman's cervical os stays closed • There is no bleeding • The foetus continues to stay inside the uterus • May be associated with coagulation defects	Embryonic pole ≥5 mm without foetal cardiac activity, or embryonic pole <5 mm and no interval growth over 1 week	Expectant, medical or surgical management
Anembryonic pregnancy/empty sac or blighted ovum	Pregnancy in which a gestational sac develops without development of any embryonic structures	• A fertilised egg implants into the uterine wall, but foetal development never begins • There is a gestational sac with or without a yolk sac, but there is an absence of foetal growth	Gestational sac >13 mm without yolk sac or >18 mm without embryonic pole, or empty sac beyond 38 days of gestation and no interval growth over 1 week	Expectant, medical or surgical management

PART II

Flow chart 36.1: Various causes of miscarriage

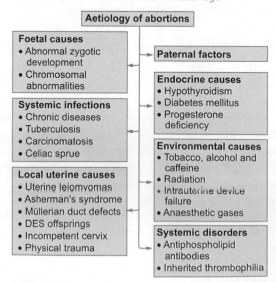

Abbreviation: DES, diethylstilbestrol

❖ Immunological causes
❖ Anatomical causes
❖ Antiphospholipid antibody syndrome
❖ Absence of blocking antibodies as a cause of miscarriage.

Genetic Causes

Genetic causes commonly include changes in the number of chromosomes, e.g. trisomy, polyploidy, etc. or structural abnormalities of chromosomes, e.g. translocations, deletions, etc. While nearly 33% of pregnancies that abort are anembryonic, 50% cases of spontaneous abortion occur due to chromosomal abnormalities (Table 36.2).

Endocrinological Causes

These include causes such as luteal phase defects, thyroid disorders including both hypothyroidism and hyperthyroidism, diabetes mellitus, etc.

Table 36.2: Various chromosomal abnormalities which can result in spontaneous miscarriage

Type of chromosomal abnormalities	Incidence (%)
Autosomal trisomies	52
Monosomy X	19
Polyploidies	22
Others	7

Infections

Infections include viral causes such as rubella, cytomegalovirus, HIV, etc.; parasitic causes such as Toxoplasma, malaria, etc.; and bacterial causes such as ureaplasma, Chlamydia, Brucella, etc.

Immunological Causes

Immunological causes include autoimmune diseases, alloimmune diseases, thrombophilias, etc.

Anatomical Causes

Anatomical causes can include reproductive tract abnormalities such as congenital uterine anomalies (bicornuate uterus, septate uterus, etc.), leiomyomas, shortened cervical canal (resulting in cervical incompetence), uterine adhesions, etc. Anatomic abnormalities of the uterus are associated with 10–15% cases of recurrent second-trimester miscarriages. Various müllerian abnormalities, such as septate uterus and bicornuate uterus, are commonly associated with recurrent miscarriage due to poor blood supply to the conceptus as a result of the implantation of the gestational sac over a relatively avascular septum. Müllerian anomaly, such as bicornuate uterus, could be responsible for producing an abnormal or irregularly shaped uterus, which could result in improper implantation and/or growth of the embryo, thereby resulting in recurrent miscarriages. Uterus didelphys is commonly associated with preterm labour, but can also sometimes cause recurrent miscarriage. Asherman's syndrome, characterised by presence of intrauterine adhesions and synechiae within the uterine cavity, is another cause of recurrent miscarriage. Diagnosis of Asherman's syndrome can be reached by doing tests like hysteroscopy, transvaginal ultrasound examination, hysterosalpingography, etc. Hysterosalpingogram revealing irregular filling defects in the endometrium is suggestive of endometrial adhesions. Hysteroscopic resection of the adhesions can be performed.

Antiphospholipid Antibody Syndrome

Antiphospholipid antibody syndrome is an autoimmune condition that has emerged as the most important treatable cause of recurrent miscarriage, early-onset pre-eclampsia, preterm labour, LBW babies and IUGR. This disease causes miscarriage by forming antibodies against the body's own tissues and placenta, resulting in thrombosis of vessels, placental infraction, foetal hypoxia and ultimately foetal death.

Absence of Blocking Antibodies as a Cause of Miscarriage

Allotypic antigens in the trophoblast may elicit the production of antibodies, which are cytotoxic to peripheral leucocytes in blood. These antigens are called trophoblast-lymphocyte cross-reactive (TLX) antigens. If the embryo contains paternal TLX antigens which do not exist in the mother, it may mount a protective reaction, resulting in abortion. If the mother produces antipaternal-blocking antibodies, these are able to produce a protective response, which helps in avoiding pregnancy rejection.

Box 36.1: Risk factors for spontaneous miscarriage

- ❑ Advancing maternal age
- ❑ Prior history of spontaneous miscarriage
- ❑ History of smoking (>10 cigarettes/day) or alcohol intake (moderate intake)
- ❑ Caffeine (high intake)
- ❑ History of cocaine use
- ❑ Maternal weight (BMI <18.5 or >25)
- ❑ Untreated celiac disease
- ❑ High gravidity
- ❑ Fever
- ❑ Low folate levels
- ❑ Chronic maternal diseases such as APS, PCOS, thyroid disorders, uncontrolled diabetes mellitus, etc.
- ❑ Use of medications such as itraconazole, methotrexate, NSAIDs, paroxetine, retinoids, etc.
- ❑ Exposure to toxins and occupational exposure (e.g. ionising radiation, pesticides, etc.)

Risk Factors

Various risk factors which could be associated with an increased risk of miscarriage and must be kept in mind while eliciting history are enumerated in Box 36.1.

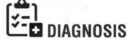

DIAGNOSIS

Clinical Presentation

Clinical presentation of a patient undergoing miscarriage is usually after first missed menses or after a period of amenorrhoea and may involve the following symptoms:

- ❖ First trimester bleeding or spotting
- ❖ There may be associated pain or cramping per abdomen. Pregnancy testing should be done in all women belonging to reproductive age group with abnormal vaginal bleeding. The β-hCG levels may be observed to be falling or abnormally rising.[4] Besides having vaginal bleeding and abdominal pain, patients with early pregnancy loss can have varied clinical presentation including:
  - Absent foetal heart tones on Doppler ultrasound
  - Size-dates discrepancy on bimanual examination
  - Routine ultrasonography indicating a non-viable pregnancy.

Abdominal Examination

Abdominal Palpation

- ❖ If an intrauterine pregnancy is more than 12 weeks gestation, it may be palpable per abdomen
- ❖ There may be extrauterine tenderness (suggestive of ectopic pregnancy). Rarely, there may be masses that may be palpated, indicative of ectopic pregnancy.

Vaginal Examination

❖ Products of conception can be visualised in the cervical os or vaginal vault upon per speculum examination. This is diagnostic of miscarriage (incomplete or inevitable). Any visible lesion on the cervix which may be responsible for producing bleeding (e.g. cervical erosions, polyps, malignancy, etc.) may also be visualised on per speculum examination.

❖ The cervix and uterus may appear to be soft upon vaginal examination.

❖ In cases of incomplete or inevitable miscarriage, the internal cervical os would felt to be open on per vaginal examination.

❖ In cases with early pregnancy bleeding where the internal cervical os is not open or products of conception cannot be visualised to be protruding from the cervical os, it is essential to rule out the diagnosis of ectopic pregnancy using TVS and determination of serial β-hCG levels, or both.

❖ A bimanual examination often helps in detecting size-dates discrepancy.

Investigations

Diagnosis of Miscarriage Using Ultrasound

Ultrasound examination forms an important investigation for arriving at a definitive diagnosis. Both TAS and TVS are complementary to one another in arriving at a diagnosis and the appropriate modality should be used depending upon the clinical situation. TVS has been shown to have a positive predictive value of 98% in confirming the diagnosis of complete miscarriage.[5] In a normal TVS, the yolk sac is normally visible by 5–5.5 weeks, foetal pole is visible by 5.5–6 weeks and foetal heart beat by 6 weeks. Gestational sac is the first to appear at 4.5–5 weeks. All these findings are likely to appear 1 week later on the TAS. Normally, when a gestational sac is observed on TVS, levels of β-hCG in the serum can vary between 1,500 IU/L and 2,000 IU/L. Features suggestive of non-viable pregnancy on ultrasound examination are described in Table 36.3. Other ultrasound features suggestive of non-viability on ultrasound examination are as follows:

❖ No embryonic growth on serial ultrasound scans

❖ Collapsed or distorted gestational sac

❖ Abnormalities of the yolk sac or its complete absence: Absence of yolk sac or presence of an abnormal yolk sac is associated with a positive predictive value of 95%.

Table 36.3: Predictors of non-viability on ultrasound examination

Ultrasound features which are present	Ultrasound features which are absent
• Gestational sac of 8 mm • Gestational sac of 16 mm • Gestational sac diameter >25 mm (TAS) or >18 mm (TVS) • Embryo with CRL of >5 mm • 7th week of gestation	• No yolk sac • No demonstrable embryo • Absent foetal poles • No cardiac activity (absent heart rate or heart rate <85 bpm)

Abbreviation: CRL, crown rump length

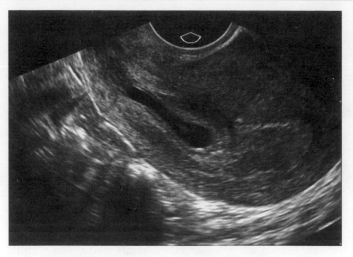

Fig. 36.1: Transvaginal ultrasound in case of inevitable abortion

❖ Absence of or an abnormality in foetal heart rate pattern

❖ Presence of subchorionic haematoma.

Figure 36.1 demonstrates the ultrasound findings in case of inevitable abortion. There is a loss of definition of gestational sac, resulting in a smaller diameter of gestational sac. There are no central echoes in the gestational sac which are normally indicative of a healthy pregnancy. Foetal cardiac activity is normally absent.

Role of Serial Human Chorionic Gonadotrophin Assessment in Predicting Pregnancy Outcome

Serial serum hCG assay is particularly useful in the diagnosis of cases of asymptomatic ectopic pregnancy. Modern monoclonal antibody based kits can detect hCG at concentrations of 25 IU/L, a level reached 9 days post conception (day 23 of a 28-day cycle).[6] Normally, a gestational sac would be visualised on TVS at β-hCG levels of 1,500–2,000 mIU/mL. This β-hCG level is known as the discriminatory zone and in a normal intrauterine gestation it is usually attained by 5 weeks of gestation.[7] This may, however, vary depending on the quality of the machine and the sonographer's skill. Discriminatory zones for serum hCG should be used to help exclude the diagnosis of possible ectopic pregnancy. At β-hCG levels above 1,500–2,000 IU/L, an ectopic pregnancy will usually be visualised with TVS. However, at the levels of β-hCG below the discriminatory zone, pregnancy of unknown location and miscarriage are both possible outcomes. Although a doubling of hCG titre is often expected to occur in cases of viable pregnancy within 48 hours, this can vary depending on the period of gestation. If the quantitative β-hCG level is greater than the 1,500–2,000 mIU/mL discriminatory zone, the pregnancy is likely to be viable. In these cases, an urgent TVS must be arranged to rule out an ectopic pregnancy and assess viability. If β-hCG levels are below the discriminatory zone, these levels must be followed at every 48 hours intervals until the discriminatory threshold is reached or until the diagnosis is clear from the trend of the β-hCG levels. Declining β-hCG levels are indicative of non-viable pregnancy or a miscarriage.

Role of Serum Progesterone Assay in Predicting Pregnancy Outcome

Measurement of serum progesterone level can be a useful adjunct in cases where ultrasound suggests pregnancy of unknown location. In these cases, TVS, measurement of serial serum hCG levels and progesterone levels may all be required in order to establish a definite diagnosis. When ultrasound findings suggest pregnancy of unknown location, serum progesterone levels below 25 nmol/L are usually associated with pregnancies subsequently confirmed to be non-viable.[7-11] However, viable pregnancies have been reported with initial serum progesterone levels of less than 15.9 nmol/L. In most cases, serum progesterone levels above 25 nmol/L are 'likely to indicate' and above 60 nmol/L are 'strongly associated with' pregnancies subsequently shown to be normal. Therefore, active intervention and uterine evacuation should not be undertaken based on low initial progesterone levels. Presently, it is not possible to define a specific discriminatory value for a single serum progesterone result that may allow absolute clinical confirmation of viability or non-viability. Therefore at present, pregnancy of unknown location is largely managed by TVS and serial β-hCG level determination.

Screening for infection: In women undergoing surgical evacuation, screening for infection, such as *Chlamydia trachomatis*, should be considered. If clinically indicated, the obstetrician can also consider vaginal swabs for excluding bacterial vaginosis. There is an increased risk of developing pelvic inflammatory disease in women, who have organisms such as *C. trachomatis, Neisseria gonorrhoea* or bacterial vaginosis in their lower genital tract at the time of suction evacuation.[12]

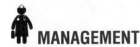

MANAGEMENT

In the past few years, the pattern of standard management in cases of miscarriage has changed with more emphasis being laid on the outpatient or clinic management rather than the inpatient management.

General Management

Treatment is usually directed towards the management of underlying cause. Beyond addressing modifiable risk factors and treating underlying maternal chronic conditions, no interventions have been shown to prevent miscarriage.

❖ Woman with loss of pregnancy should be treated with dignity and respect. Loss of pregnancy can cause significant distress to the woman and her partner. Taking into account the woman's individual circumstances and emotional response towards her loss, the obstetrician should provide information and support to the couple in a sensitive manner.[13] Healthcare professionals providing care for these women should be provided with appropriate training for

Table 36.4: Techniques for completion of abortion

Surgical techniques	Medical techniques

• Cervical dilatation followed by uterine evacuation
• Curettage
• Vacuum aspiration (suction curettage)
• Dilatation and evacuation
• Menstrual aspiration
• Laparotomy: hysterotomy
• Hysterectomy
	• Intravenous oxytocin
	• Intra-amniotic hyperosmotic fluid saline or urea
	• Prostaglandins:
	  – Intra-amniotic injection
	  – Vaginal insertion
	  – Parenteral injection
	  – Oral ingestion
	• Antiprogesterones—RU 486, mifepristone, etc.
	• Methotrexate—intramuscular and oral

communicating sensitively with the patient and her partner and breaking bad news to them.

❖ Tissue retained inside the uterine cavity as a result of miscarriage is associated with an increased risk of infection and haemorrhage and would not be passed spontaneously. The options for treatment include: expectant management, medical management and surgical uterine evacuation. A woman should be given the choice of various treatment options (Table 36.4) and should be counselled to choose the treatment option which she considers as the best.

❖ In cases with positive β-hCG results and absence of intrauterine gestational sac, ectopic pregnancy and pregnancy of unknown location must be ruled out [refer to Chapter 35 (Ectopic Pregnancy)]. The patient must be carefully observed for ectopic pregnancy if no products of conception are documented upon suction evacuation.

❖ Available evidence has shown that miscarriage is not prevented by strategies such as bed rest, vitamin supplementation, progestogen or hCG.[14]

❖ *Emotional support*: The woman undergoing miscarriage must be counselled that it has not occurred due to her fault. It was probably just bad luck, unless some obvious or recurrent cause can be detected, which warrants evaluation or intervention. She should be assured that there is nothing she has done that caused her pregnancy to fail. She must be encouraged to face her family and friends without any guilt. She must be encouraged to allow herself a normal grieving process by taking out time off from work and other commitments. The patient's partner must also be involved. The patient may require additional appointments to monitor the grief process and look for signs of depression.

Management in Specific Cases

Threatened Abortion

Administration of progestogens and hCG may prove to be useful in some cases. Anti-Rh immunoglobulins must be administered to Rh negative non-sensitised women with symptoms of threatened abortion, at or after 12 weeks of gestation. However, no treatment is available, which can stop the process of abortion.

Inevitable Abortion

In case of excessive bleeding, IV drip should be started with 5% dextrose in water or 5% dextrose in saline. Blood should be arranged and cross-matched, following which it may be transfused. In these cases, an IV injection of oxytocin 5–10 units or ergometrine 0.5 mg could be given. Arrangements should be made to evacuate the uterus as soon as possible. Suction evacuation can be used in case the period of gestation is less than 12 weeks. If the period of gestation is more than 12 weeks, the process of abortion can be accelerated using oxytocin infusion.

Incomplete Abortion

Treatment in cases of incomplete abortion is same as that discussed in cases of inevitable abortion. In case the size of uterus is more than 12 weeks, using a single dose of 600 μg misoprostol PO or 400 μg SL can facilitate the process of abortion to completion.

Missed Abortion

Before 12 weeks of pregnancy, the treatment comprises of suction evacuation. Oxytocin can be used for inducing uterine contractions after 12 weeks of gestation. Misoprostol (single oral dose of 600 μg) can be used for inducing uterine contractions both before and after 12 weeks of gestation. Passage of tissues should occur within a few days of receiving medical therapy. If it is not successful, surgical approach can be used to empty the uterine cavity.

Treatment of the Underlying Cause

When a specific cause of spontaneous miscarriage has been identified, treatment of that particular cause must be initiated.

Antiphospholipid antibody syndrome: Patients with recurrent pregnancy loss must be administered a prophylactic dose of subcutaneous heparin (preferably LMWH) and low-dose aspirin. In patients for whom the treatment with aspirin and heparin is not successful, use of IV immunoglobulins can be used. For details related to treatment of APS, kindly refer to Chapter 10 [Connective Tissue Disorders (Autoimmune Disorders)].

Absence of blocking antibodies as a cause of miscarriage: Immunotherapy with paternal pool leucocytes can be considered as an optimal solution for this problem. However, this therapy is presently in purely experimental stage and can be considered dangerous before further research is conducted.

Asherman's syndrome: The most accurate method of management of Asherman's syndrome is hysteroscopic resection via direct visualisation. These adhesions can also be removed on hysteroscopy. In order to prevent reformation of adhesions following surgery, prescription of oestrogen supplementation or placement of a splint, balloon or copper device may prove useful.

Uterine malformations: Surgical correction of the underlying uterine defect can be undertaken.

Expectant Management

Expectant management involves a 'wait and watch' policy to ensure that the process of miscarriage gets completed naturally without requiring any intervention. Various prerequisites before using expectant management have been described in Table 36.5. Patient counselling is particularly important for those women with an intact sac who wish to follow an expectant approach. They should be aware that complete resolution may take several weeks and that overall efficacy rates are low. If the patient so desires, she can quit expectant management at any stage and opt for a medical or surgical evacuation at a later date. In women undergoing expectant management, a follow-up visit may be required to assess if the process of expulsion is complete. Success can be defined as absence of gestational sac (or its remnants) and presence of an endometrial thickness less than or equal to 15 mm on TVS, 3 days to 6 weeks after diagnosis; absence of any vaginal bleeding; and 80% drop in the β-hCG levels 1 week following the passage of tissues. Since vaginal bleeding and positive urine pregnancy test can continue for 2–4 weeks, these cannot be considered as good measures of success. While using β-hCG levels to monitor resolution of pregnancy, for cases in which an intrauterine pregnancy has not been documented, it is important to follow β-hCG levels until they become zero because ectopic pregnancies can also present with declining β-hCG levels. Most expulsions occur in the first 2 weeks after diagnosis. Prolonged follow-up may be needed. It is acceptable and safe to wait up to 4 weeks postdiagnosis. It is associated with an overall success rate of 81%. Success rates can vary depending on the type of miscarriage. Expectant management is highly effective in cases of incomplete miscarriage (Table 36.6).

Table 36.5: Factors to be considered before undertaking expectant management

Prerequisites	Contraindications
• Less than 13 weeks of gestation • Stable vital signs • No evidence of infection or haemorrhage • Patient desires the use of expectant management	• Woman is at an increased risk of haemorrhage • She has a previous history of adverse and/or traumatic experience associated with pregnancy (e.g. stillbirth, miscarriage or antepartum haemorrhage) • She is at increased risk of adverse effects due to haemorrhage (e.g. coagulopathies or inability to have a blood transfusion) • Presence of infection

Table 36.6: Success rate with expectant management in case of various types of miscarriage

Types of miscarriage	Success rate with expectant management (%)
Incomplete/inevitable abortion	91
Missed abortion	76
Anembryonic pregnancies	66

PART II

Medical Management

Medical management can be offered as an effective alternative in the management of confirmed first-trimester miscarriage and is associated with several advantages (Box 36.2). To avoid unnecessary anxiety, women should be informed that bleeding may continue for up to 3 weeks after medical uterine evacuation. Medical evacuation is an alternative technique that complements, but does not replace, surgical evacuation. Various medical methods (Box 36.3) have been described using prostaglandin analogues (gemeprost or misoprostol) with or without antiprogesterone priming (mifepristone). Presently, there is no medical regimen for management of early pregnancy loss that is FDA approved. Misoprostol is a cheap, highly effective prostaglandin analogue that is active via PO, SL and PV routes. In case of missed miscarriages (closed cervix and intact sac), effective regimens involve use of a higher dose of prostaglandin for a longer duration of time or, alternatively, following priming with antiprogesterone. Prerequisites for medical management of spontaneous miscarriage are listed in Box 36.4. Though various regimens comprising of using different dosages (400–800 µg) through different routes (PO, SL and PV) have been tried, single dose of 800 µg misoprostol administered PV is associated with a high success rate and is normally used. This dose can be repeated if the process remains incomplete at 24 hours. Success rate depends on type of miscarriage—with incomplete abortion, this method can be 100% successful. SL route is associated with more side effects.

Mifepristone is progestin antagonist that binds to the progestin receptor. It may be used with misoprostol to 'destabilise' the implantation site. Current evidence-based regimen comprises of 200 mg mifepristone PO and 800 µg misoprostol PV. Other drug combinations which can be used are methotrexate and misoprostol. Methotrexate is a folic

Box 36.2: Advantages of using medical management

- May help in avoiding surgery
- Cost effective
- Few side effects (especially with vaginal application)
- Stable at room temperature
- Readily available

Box 36.3: Various options used for medical management of spontaneous abortion

- Misoprostol
- Mifepristone plus misoprostol
- Methotrexate plus misoprostol

Box 36.4: Prerequisites for medical management of spontaneous miscarriage

- Less than 13 weeks gestation
- Stable vital signs
- No evidence of infection
- No history of any allergies to medications used

Box 36.5: Indications for surgical management

- Patient is unstable
- Significant medical morbidity
- Excessive and persistent bleeding
- Patient desires immediate therapy
- Presence of retained infected tissue
- Suspected gestational trophoblastic disease
- Gestational sac continues to be present (as observed on ultrasound examination)
- Patient's preference

acid antagonist, which is cytotoxic to the trophoblast. It was initially used for medical management of ectopic pregnancy. It has also been used in combination with misoprostol to treat elective abortion medically. This combination has been found to be associated with success rates up to 98%. Misoprostol is administered 7 days after methotrexate injection.

With the use of medical method, the overall efficacy rates vary widely from 13% to 96%, with higher efficacy rates being associated with factors such as incomplete miscarriage,[15,16] use of higher dosage of misoprostol (1,200–1,400 µg),[14] vaginal administration of prostaglandins and clinical follow-up without routine ultrasound.[15-17]

Surgical Management

Despite the use of medical therapy, surgical management may still be used in presence of conditions described in Box 36.5.[18]

Surgical Uterine Evacuation

Surgical uterine evacuation has been the standard treatment offered to women who miscarry. It can be performed as manual vacuum aspiration under systemic analgesia or patient-controlled anaesthesia in an outpatient or clinic setting or as suction aspiration under general anaesthesia in an operation theatre. A surgical management option helps in providing immediate therapy and is associated with high success rates varying between 93% to 100%. Surgical uterine evacuation for miscarriage is commonly performed using suction curettage. Vacuum aspiration has been used as the method of choice for management of miscarriage where there is an intact intrauterine sac. A Cochrane review has established that vacuum aspiration is preferable to sharp curettage in cases of incomplete miscarriage because it is associated with a reduced risk of complications such as bleeding and pain as well as shortened duration of the procedure.[19] Prostaglandins are commonly administered prior to surgical evacuation. Their use is associated with several advantages such as significant reductions in dilatation force, haemorrhage and uterine or cervical trauma. Women, who are at an increased risk, must be administered antibiotics for treatment of infection. However, presently there is insufficient evidence to recommend routine antibiotic prophylaxis prior to surgical uterine evacuation. Antibiotic prophylaxis should therefore be administered based on individual clinical indications.

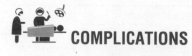

COMPLICATIONS

Complications Associated with Miscarriage Process

Septic Abortion or Miscarriage with Sepsis

In these cases, incomplete abortion is associated with ascending infection of the endometrium, parametrium, adnexa uteri or peritoneum. Ultrasound findings are consistent with those of incomplete abortion. Infection may also be associated with criminal abortion. Various organisms, which may be involved, include anaerobic bacteria, coliforms, *Haemophilus influenzae, Campylobacter jejuni,* group A streptococcus, etc. Infection, if not timely treated, may be associated with complications such as severe haemorrhage, bacterial shock, acute renal failure, uterine infection, parametritis, peritonitis, endocarditis, septicaemia, DIC, infertility, etc. Treatment involves supportive care, and use of antimicrobials and evacuation.

Complications Associated with Surgical Evacuation

Surgical evacuation could be associated with complications mentioned in Box 36.6.

Though small amount of cramping, pain and bleeding can commonly occur for 2–3 days after the procedure, severe degrees of persistent pain or amount of bleeding more than that associated with normal menstruation, especially in association with fever or fainting could be indicative of the underlying complications. Some of these are given hereafter.

Uterine Perforation

The most dreaded complication of the procedure is uterine perforation because the procedure of suction evacuation is essentially a blind one. The risk of uterine perforation becomes greater with the increasing gestational age of the foetus. Most uterine perforations are thought to occur during the process of uterine sounding or cervical dilation because the most common site of perforation is the junction of the cervix and the lower uterine segment. While the midline perforations in this region are usually benign, lateral perforations at this location may be particularly hazardous for the patient because they may extend to the branches of the uterine artery resulting in profuse haemorrhage.

A uterine perforation must be suspected, when no tissue is obtained; when the instruments appear to be inserted deeper than the depth expected, on the basis of the gestational age,

---

Box 36.6: Complications associated with surgical evacuation
❑ Uterine perforation
❑ Infection
❑ Incomplete evacuation
❑ Bleeding during and following the abortion
❑ Failure of the procedure
❑ Hypotension
❑ Asherman's syndrome
❑ Cervical lacerations or cervical incompetence

---

when haemorrhage occurs; or when obvious maternal tissues, such as omentum are obtained.

Sometimes, if the procedure is being performed under ultrasound guidance, uterine instrument (such as a uterine sound) may be visualised outside the uterine cavity. Sometimes when medical termination of pregnancy (MTP) is being performed during the procedure of laparoscopic sterilisation, the perforation may be visualised laparoscopically.

Treatment of perforation depends on the expected location, the woman's vital signs and condition, and whether the abortion is complete or not. In case of a suspected perforation, the patient must be observed for a few hours for the signs of hypovolaemia and shock. Intramuscular oxytocics (methergine) and antibiotics must be administered. If the patient's vitals are stable; the uterine perforation is midline; repeated pelvic examinations are negative; repeat haematocrit results are stable; the uterus is already empty and/or the amount of bleeding is minimal or none, then there is no need for patient hospitalisation. The patient may be discharged home in the company of a responsible adult and instructed to visit the hospital immediately, in case she experiences excessive pain or bleeding or some other complication at any time. She must be scheduled for a repeat general physical and pelvic examination, the next day. In case the patient continues to experience bleeding, pain or her vitals continue to remain unstable, she should be admitted to a hospital for observation and a possible laparoscopic examination. If the abortion is not complete at the time perforation is suspected, it should be completed with the aid of ultrasound or laparoscopy. Laparotomy may be required, in cases where intraperitoneal bleeding or bowel injury is suspected.

Infection

This can be easily avoided by the administration of broad-spectrum antibiotics. In case the infection is a result of incomplete evacuation, the surgeon first needs to completely evacuate the uterine cavity. Following this, the antibiotics must be given. In the cases of serious infection, IV antibiotics can be given. Laparotomy may be required in cases of peritonitis. If upon examination, the uterus appears to be tender and slightly enlarged, infection is a possibility. Infection in association with the retained products of conception is likely to result in the development of post-abortion endometritis, among women undergoing first trimester surgical abortion. Typically, the woman returns 3 or 4 days after the procedure with increased cramping and bleeding, sometimes accompanied by fever or nausea. The microorganism commonly involved in such cases is β-haemolytic streptococci. Endometritis should be treated immediately to avoid progression of infection. In most early cases, hospitalisation is not required and the outpatient treatment proves to be sufficient. Ampicillin usually works against microorganisms such as haemolytic streptococci. In case of infection with organisms, such as *Chlamydia* or bacterial vaginosis or other anaerobic organisms, combination of oral metronidazole and ofloxacin is commonly prescribed.

Incomplete Evacuation

The most common presentation in cases of incomplete evacuation is prolonged bleeding. In these cases the uterine contents have to be re-evacuated, under antibiotic coverage. Typical history suggestive of an incomplete evacuation is a woman returning several days after the procedure with the history of increased bleeding and cramping. On examination, she may have an enlarged uterus or tissue visible in the cervical os. Ultrasound examination is usually performed, but may not be always helpful because blood and debris are commonly present inside the uterus and the amount of retained tissue may be small.

Treatment of incomplete abortion may be pharmacological. Uterotonic drugs, such as methylergonovine (methergine) may help contract the uterus and expel the residual tissue. This method is appropriate when the amount of retained tissue is small and there are no signs of infection. If this method is chosen, the woman should be called for a follow-up visit within a few days, to make sure that her symptoms have resolved. If the amount of retained tissue inside the uterine cavity is large or if the woman cannot return for follow-up, then repeat suction should be done. Repeat suction is usually easy because the cervix is dilated and a cannula smaller than that used for the original procedure is adequate.

Bleeding During and Following Abortion

Most women have minimal bleeding during first trimester abortion. However, at times, there may be severe bleeding during and after the procedure. Uterine atony is the most likely cause of heavy and prolonged bleeding in these cases. Intravenous ergometrine (0.2 mg) or oxytocin (10–20 units) may be used to contract the uterus. Alternatively, misoprostol in the dosage of 400 µg may be prescribed either through oral or rectal route. Doses of misoprostol, as high as 1,000 µg, have been used per rectally in cases of atonic uterus. Prostaglandin F2α (carboprost) can be prescribed intramuscularly or into the uterus. In the absence of an obvious cervical or uterine injury, the surgeon should complete the abortion, evacuating the uterus rapidly, but gently. If the bleeding still continues to occur, the uterus is massaged between the two hands, e.g. bimanual compression.

The aspirated tissue is examined to assess the gestational age and to confirm that all foetal parts have been removed. If the bleeding still does not stop, the cervix should be explored for the presence of a likely laceration or for bleeding from the tenaculum site. Next, the uterus is gently explored with a sharp curette, preferably under ultrasound guidance, checking for uterine shape and size, retained tissue and uterine wall irregularities or defects. Repeat suction may remove clots and retained tissue and allow the uterus to contract. If bleeding persists even after the uterus has been emptied, the next manoeuvre is uterine tamponade. For details regarding control of bleeding from an atonic uterus, kindly refer to Chapter 50 (Postpartum Haemorrhage and Postpartum Collapse).

Failure of Procedure

The procedure, if not performed properly, may result in the continuation of the pregnancy. This may result in cases of very small sized uterus, where the suction cannula fails to suck out the products of conception. This may also occur in cases associated with a uterine anomaly (e.g. uterus didelphys or bicornuate uterus) or cases of ectopic pregnancy.

Hypotension

This could be related to excessive blood loss or due to a vaso-vagal response to pain. Management in these cases comprises of administration of IV fluids, oxygen, whole blood transfusion and corticosteroids.

Minor Complications

Minor complications like postoperative nausea and vomiting can be managed with antiemetics such as metoclopramide or ondansetron.

Asherman's Syndrome

This is a delayed complication, which can occur as a result of vigorous curettage. This complication is usually managed by hysteroscopic resection of intrauterine adhesions, followed by insertion of an intrauterine contraceptive device or a Foley's catheter, in order to keep the uterine wall apart.

Cervical Lacerations/Cervical Incompetence

Rarely, vigorous dilatation may result in the development of cervical lacerations and/or cervical incompetence in the subsequent pregnancies. This complication can be avoided by taking a good history and correct estimation of gestational age during the bimanual examination. Overzealous cervical dilation must be avoided. Dilatation is carried out using the smallest sized dilator. The Hegar's dilators are commonly used. These dilators must be held in a pen-holding fashion and must be gently inserted into the cervical canal. Undue force must not be used, while inserting the cannula. The dilatation must be started using the smallest size dilator. Gradually, larger sized dilators must be used. The cervix must be dilated about 0.5–1.0 mm more than the size of the suction cannula to be used. Cervical priming using prostaglandins, prior to the procedure, facilitates the process of dilatation without the use of undue force.

Complications Associated with Medical Method

Medical methods may be associated with complications such as increased duration of abdominal pain and bleeding, which may last between 14 days and 21 days. Also, the medical method is associated with a requirement for follow-up visit following the expulsion of the products of conception. This visit helps in confirming if the process of expulsion is complete or not. In case the process of expulsion is not complete, surgical evacuation is required.

PART II

CLINICAL PEARLS

❖ The obstetricians must always remain aware of the fact that women with a pregnancy of unknown location could have an ectopic pregnancy until the exact location of the gestational sac is determined.

❖ Efficacy rate associated with expectant management is comparatively reduced in presence of an intact gestational sac.

❖ Highest rates of efficacy with expectant management are observed in cases of inevitable miscarriage.

❖ Medical and expectant management should only be offered in units where women have an access to 24-hour telephone advice. Moreover, there should be facilities available for emergency admission if required.

EVIDENCE-BASED MEDICINE

❖ Current evidence indicates that miscarriage cannot be prevented by using strategies such as bed rest, vitamin supplementation, progestogen or β-hCG injections.[20-22]

❖ Present evidence is variable regarding the best route of misoprostol administration for pregnancy termination. Some RCTs indicate that the use of misoprostol as a medical method for pregnancy termination used through any of the following routes: oral, sublingual and vaginal may be equally effective.[23-25] On the other hand, one RCT has suggested that the vaginal route of administration may be associated with increased efficacy of misoprostol.[26]

REFERENCES

1. Centers of Disease Control and Prevention (CDC). (1997). State definitions and reporting requirements for live births, fetal deaths, and induced terminations of pregnancy (1997 revision). [online] Available at www.cdc.gov/nchs/products/other/miscpub/statereq.htm. [Accessed July, 2016].

2. Alberman E. Spontaneous abortion: epidemiology. In: Stabile I, Grudzinkas JG, Chard T (Eds). Spontaneous Abortion: Diagnosis and Treatment. London: Springer-Verlag; 1992. pp. 9-20.

3. Recommendations from the 33rd RCOG Study Group. In: Grudzinskas JG, O'Brien PM (Eds). Problems in Early Pregnancy: Advances in Diagnosis and Management. London: RCOG Press; 1997. pp. 327-31.

4. Royal College of Obstetricians and Gynaecologists (RCOG). The management of early pregnancy loss. Green-top Guideline No. 25. London: RCOG Press; 2006.

5. Jauniaux E, Johns J, Burton GJ. The role of ultrasound imaging in diagnosing and investigating early pregnancy failure. Ultrasound Obstet Gynecol. 2005;25(6):613-24.

6. Braunstein GD, Rasor J, Danzer H, Adler D, Wade ME. Serum human chorionic gonadotrophin levels throughout normal pregnancy. Am J Obstet Gynecol. 1976;126(6):678-81.

7. Condous G, Okaro E, Bourne T. The conservative management of early pregnancy complications: a review of the literature. Ultrasound Obstet Gynecol. 2003;22(4):420-30.

8. Hahlin M, Thorburn J, Bryman I. The expectant management of early pregnancy of uncertain site. Hum Reprod. 1995;10(5):1223-7.

9. Banerjee S, Aslam N, Woelfer B, Lawrence A. Elson J, Jurkovic D. Expectant management of pregnancies of unknown location: a prospective evaluation of methods to predict spontaneous resolution of pregnancy. BJOG. 2001;108(2):158-63.

10. McCord ML, Muram D, Buster JE, Arheart KL, Stovall TG, Carson SA. Single serum progesterone as a screen for ectopic pregnancy: exchanging specificity and sensitivity to obtain optimal test performance. Fertil Steril. 1996;66(4):513-16.

11. Mol BW, Lijmer JG, Ankum WM, van der Veen F, Bossuyt PM. The accuracy of a single serum progesterone measurement in the diagnosis of ectopic pregnancy: a meta-analysis. Hum Reprod. 1998;13(11):3220-7.

12. Royal College of Obstetricians and Gynaecologists (RCOG). The Care of Women Requesting Induced Abortion. Evidence-based Clinical Guideline No.7. London: RCOG Press; 2011.

13. National Institute of Clinical Excellence (NICE). (2012). Ectopic pregnancy and miscarriage: diagnosis and initial management. [online]. Available from www.nice.org.uk/guidance/cg154/chapter/1-recommendations. [Accessed July, 2016].

14. Jeve YB, Davies W. Evidence-based management of recurrent miscarriages. J Hum Reprod Sci. 2014;7(3):159-69.

15. Hinshaw K. Medical management of miscarriage. In: Grudzinskas JG, O'Brien PM (Eds). Problems in Early Pregnancy: Advances in Diagnosis and Management. London: RCOG Press; 1997. pp. 284-95.

16. Henshaw RC, Cooper K, El-Refaey H, Smith NC, Templeton AA. Medical management of miscarriage: nonsurgical uterine evacuation of incomplete and inevitable spontaneous abortion. BMJ. 1993;306(6882):894-5.

17. el-Refaey H, Hinshaw K, Henshaw R, Smith N, Templeton A. Medical management of missed abortion and anembryonic pregnancy. BMJ. 1992;305(6866):1399.

18. Ballagh SA, Harris HA, Demasio K. Is curettage needed for uncomplicated incomplete spontaneous abortion? Am J Obstet Gynecol. 1998;179(5):1279-82

19. Forna F, Gülmezoglu AM. Surgical procedures to evacuate incomplete abortion. Cochrane Database Syst Rev. 2001;(1):CD001993.

20. Haas DM, Ramsey PS. Progestogen for preventing miscarriage. Cochrane Database Syst Rev. 2013;(10):CD003511.

21. Aleman A, Althabe F, Belizán J, Bergel E. Bed rest during pregnancy for preventing miscarriage. Cochrane Database Syst Rev. 2005;(2):CD003576.

22. Morley LC, Simpson N, Tang T. Human chorionic gonadotrophin (hCG) for preventing miscarriage. Cochrane Database Syst Rev. 2013;(1):CD008611.

23. Tang OS, Lau WN, Ng EH, Lee SW, Ho PC. A prospective randomized study to compare the use of repeated doses of vaginal with sublingual misoprostol in the management of first trimester silent miscarriages. Hum Reprod. 2003;18(1):176-81.

24. Ngoc NT, Blum J, Westheimer E, Quan TT, Winikoff B. Medical treatment of missed abortion using misoprostol. Int J Gynecol Obstet. 2004;87(2):138-42.

25. Reynolds A, Ayres-de-Campos D, Costa MA, Montenegro N. How should success be defined when attempting medical resolution of first-trimester missed abortion? Eur J Obstet Gynecol Reprod Biol. 2005;118(1):71-6.

26. Creinin MD, Moyer R, Guido R. Misoprostol for medical evacuation of early pregnancy failure. Obstet Gynecol. 1997;89(5 Pt 1):768-72.

Gestational Trophoblastic Neoplasia

COMPLETE HYDATIDIFORM MOLE

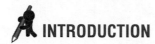 **INTRODUCTION**

Hydatidiform mole (H. mole) belongs to a spectrum of diseases known as gestational trophoblastic disease (GTD), resulting from overproduction of the chorionic tissue, which is normally supposed to develop into the placenta. H. mole can be considered as a neoplasm of trophoblastic tissue involving both syncytiotrophoblast and cytotrophoblast. H. moles are non-viable and genetically abnormal conceptions, showing excessive expression of paternal genes. It can be considered as an abnormal pregnancy in which placental villi become oedematous (hydropic) and start proliferating, resulting in the development of a cystic, grape-like structure filled with watery fluid. GTD forms a group of disorders covering a spectrum of conditions varying from benign disorders such as complete and partial molar pregnancies through to the malignant conditions, collectively known as gestational trophoblastic neoplasia (GTN) such as invasive mole, choriocarcinoma and the very rare placental site trophoblastic tumour (PSTT).

Comparison between a complete mole and partial mole has been illustrated in Table 37.1.

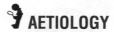 **AETIOLOGY**

Pathophysiology of molar gestation is described in Table 37.1 and Figures 37.1A to C.

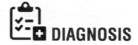 **DIAGNOSIS**

Clinical Presentation

❖ Initially, the symptoms may be suggestive of an early pregnancy; however, the uterus is often larger than the period of gestation
❖ The classic features of molar pregnancy include irregular vaginal bleeding, hyperemesis, excessive uterine enlargement and early failed pregnancy[1]
❖ The foetal movements and heart tones are usually absent. The uterus may appear doughy in consistency due to lack of foetal parts and amniotic fluid.

Table 37.1: Comparison between complete and partial mole

Parameters under consideration	Complete mole	Partial mole
Incidence	75–80%	15–25%
Cytogenetic studies	Diploid karyotype 46XX	Triploid karyotype 69XXY
Aetiology	Duplication of the haploid sperm following fertilisation of an 'empty' ovum or dispermic fertilisation of an 'empty' ovum	These contain two sets of paternal haploid genes and one set of maternal haploid genes. They usually occur following dispermic fertilisation of an ovum. Some cases of partial moles may represent tetraploid or mosaic conceptions
Histopathological analysis	There is no evidence of foetal tissue	There may be an evidence of foetal tissue or red blood vessels
Invasive potential and propensity for malignant transformation	Persistent trophoblastic disease following uterine evacuation may develop in about 15% cases with a complete mole	Persistent trophoblastic disease may develop in <5% of cases of partial mole

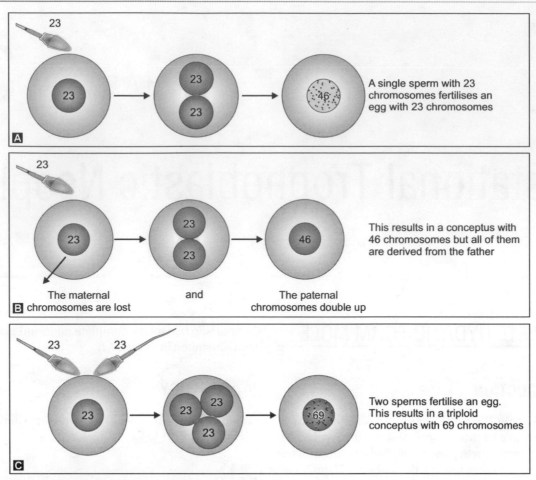

Figs 37.1A to C: Pathophysiology of molar gestation: (A) Normal process of fertilisation; (B) Complete hydatidiform mole; (C) Partial hydatidiform mole

❖ External ballottement is absent
❖ There may be history suggestive of vaginal bleeding or passage of grape-like tissue early in pregnancy
❖ There may be excessive nausea and vomiting. Hyperemesis may commonly occur
❖ There may be symptoms suggestive of hyperthyroidism
❖ Hydatidiform mole may be associated with early appearance of pre-eclampsia
❖ There may be abdominal distension due to theca lutein cysts
❖ Rarely, women may present with acute respiratory failure or neurological symptoms, such as seizures, which are likely to be due to metastatic disease.

General Physical Examination

❖ Signs suggestive of pre-eclampsia, hyperthyroidism and/or early pregnancy
❖ *Extreme pallor*: The patient's pallor may be disproportionate to the amount of blood loss due to concealed haemorrhage.

Vaginal Examination

There may be some vaginal bleeding or passage of grape-like vesicles. Internal ballottement cannot be elicited due to the lack of foetus. Unilateral or bilateral enlargement of the ovaries in the form of theca lutein cysts may be palpable.

Investigations

❖ Complete blood count, blood grouping and cross-matching
❖ *Serum β-hCG levels*: β-hCG levels in both serum and urine are raised. In cases of complete mole, β-hCG levels may be more than 100,000 mIU/mL.
❖ *Ultrasound of the pelvis*: Ultrasound examination is useful for establishing a pre-evacuation diagnosis of H. mole. However, the definitive diagnosis is made upon histological examination of the products of conception.[2] In case of a complete mole, the following features are observed on sonography:[3]
  • Features of missed miscarriage or anembryonic pregnancy (blighted ovum) may be observed
  • Characteristic vesicular pattern, also known as 'snow-storm appearance,' may be present due to generalised swelling of the chorionic villi and presence of multiple, small cystic spaces
  • There may be presence of an enlarged uterine endo-metrial cavity containing homogeneously hyperechoic endometrial mass with innumerable anechoic cysts (Fig. 37.2)
  • Ultrasound may also show the presence of theca lutein cysts in the ovaries.

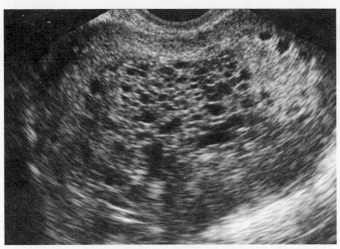

Fig. 37.2: Transvaginal sonogram of a second trimester complete hydatidiform mole (transverse section). There is presence of numerous anechoic cysts with intervening hyperechoic material

❖ *Histopathological examination*: As previously mentioned, histopathological examination helps in establishing the definitive diagnosis of H. mole. Pathologic evaluation may demonstrate swollen chorionic villi having a grape-like appearance, along with presence of hyperplastic trophoblastic tissue.

DIFFERENTIAL DIAGNOSIS

❖ *Anembryonic gestation*
❖ *Threatened abortion*: Both the conditions are associated with vaginal bleeding and similar sonographic findings
❖ *Presence of fibroid or an ovarian tumour with pregnancy*: They may cause the uterine size to be larger in relation to the period of gestation
❖ *Multiple pregnancies*: Both the conditions may be associated with early onset of pre-eclampsia before 20 weeks.

OBSTETRIC MANAGEMENT

Management in cases of molar gestation is described in Flow chart 37.1.
❖ The women with GTD (Box 37.1) must be registered at the trophoblastic screening centre and require follow-up as determined by the screening centre.
❖ All women diagnosed with GTD should be provided with written information about the condition and must be counselled regarding need for referral to trophoblastic screening centre for follow-up.
❖ The two main treatment options in case of H. mole are suction evacuation and hysterectomy.

Suction Evacuation

Suction curettage is the method of choice for evacuation of complete as well as partial molar pregnancies. In case of partial molar pregnancies, medical evacuation can be used when the size of the foetal parts prevents the use of suction curettage. Medical evacuation of complete molar pregnancies should be avoided as far as possible because of the theoretical potential of oxytocic agents to embolise and disseminate trophoblastic tissue through the venous system.[4,5]

❖ Cervix can be prepared immediately prior to the evacuation. Wherever possible prolonged cervical preparation, especially with prostaglandins, should be avoided. This is likely to reduce the risk of embolisation of trophoblastic cells.
❖ Due to the lack of foetal parts, a suction catheter, up to a maximum size of 12 mm, is usually sufficient to evacuate all complete molar pregnancies.
❖ In order to ensure that complete sustained remission has been achieved, serial assays of serum and urine β-hCG levels should be carried out on 2 weekly basis until three negative levels are obtained. Postevacuation, contraceptive measures should be instituted and the patient is advised to avoid pregnancy until hCG values have remained normal for 6 months.
❖ Excessive vaginal bleeding can be associated with molar pregnancy. Therefore, a senior surgeon must directly supervise surgical evacuation in cases of excessive bleeding.
❖ Anti-D prophylaxis is required following evacuation of a molar pregnancy
❖ The products of conception must be sent for histopathological examination.

Hysterectomy with Mole in Situ

Hysterectomy may serve as an option in the following cases of H. mole:
❖ Elderly multiparous women (age >40 years) who do not wish to become pregnant in the future
❖ Those women with H. mole desiring sterilisation
❖ Those with severe infection or uncontrolled bleeding
❖ Patients with non-metastatic persistent disease who have completed childbearing or are not concerned about preserving fertility.

If theca lutein cysts are present, they must be left as it is at the time of surgery or at the most, they can be aspirated in order to reduce their size. The ovaries must be conserved. At the time of surgery, it is important to inform the patient that since hysterectomy does not prevent metastatic disease, follow-up with β-hCG levels is essential even after surgery. Hysterectomy however does eliminate the complications related to local invasion.

Follow-up

Investigation for Persistent Gestational Trophoblastic Neoplasia after a Non-molar Pregnancy

Any woman who develops persistent vaginal bleeding after a pregnancy event is at risk of having GTN.[6-10] Therefore, a urine pregnancy test should be performed in all cases having persistent or irregular vaginal bleeding after a pregnancy event.

Flow chart 37.1: Management of molar pregnancy

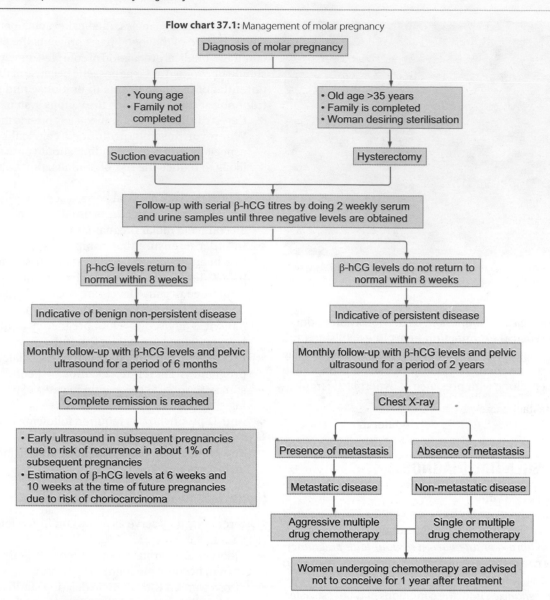

Box 37.1: Women with gestational trophoblastic disease who require registration at the trophoblastic screening centre

❑ Complete hydatidiform mole (H. mole)
❑ Partial H. mole
❑ Twin pregnancy with complete or partial H. mole
❑ Limited macroscopic or microscopic molar changes suggesting possibility of partial or early complete molar pregnancy
❑ Choriocarcinoma
❑ Placental-site trophoblastic tumour
❑ Atypical placental site nodules (characterised by nuclear atypia of trophoblast, areas of necrosis, calcification and increased proliferation within a placental site nodule)

Investigation for Persistent Gestational Trophoblastic Neoplasia after Gestational Trophoblastic Disease

❖ Follow-up after GTD should be individualised
❖ Measurement of hCG levels must be done 6–8 weeks following the end of the pregnancy to exclude recurrence of disease

❖ If hCG level has reverted to normal within 56 days (8 weeks) of the pregnancy event, then follow-up should be done after 6 months from the date of uterine evacuation
❖ If hCG has not reverted to normal within 56 days (8 weeks) of the pregnancy event, then follow-up should be done 6 months from the date of normalisation of the hCG level
❖ All women should be counselled to notify the screening centre at the end of any future pregnancy irrespective of its outcome
❖ Women should be advised not to conceive until their follow-up is complete.

Contraception Following Gestational Trophoblastic Disease

Women with GTD should be advised to use barrier methods of contraception until hCG levels have come back to normal. Once hCG level have normalised, the combined OCPs may be used. If the woman had started using oral contraception before the diagnosis of GTD was made, she can be advised to continue using oral contraception. There is no definite evidence regarding an increased risk of developing GTN due to the use of combined OCPs.[4,11] Also, there is little evidence regarding the adverse effects related to the use of single-agent progestogens in cases of GTD. Use of intrauterine contraceptive devices should be preferably avoided until hCG levels have normalised to reduce the risk of uterine perforation.

Hormone Replacement Therapy for Women after Gestational Trophoblastic Disease

Hormone replacement therapy may be used safely once hCG levels have returned to normal. Presently, there is no evidence regarding the adverse effects related to the use of hormone replacement therapy on the outcome of GTN. Women can be safely prescribed hormone replacement therapy, once hCG levels have returned to normal.

COMPLICATIONS

❖ The most important complication related to GTD is the development of GTN, which include conditions like invasive mole, choriocarcinoma and PSTT. All of these may metastasise and are potentially fatal if left untreated. GTN has been described in details later in the chapter.
❖ Benign forms of H. mole can result in complications like uterine infection, sepsis, haemorrhagic shock and pre-eclampsia, which may occur during early pregnancy.
❖ Recurrence of molar gestation may occur in 1–2% cases. This implies that nearly 98% of women who become pregnant following a molar pregnancy are unlikely to have a further molar pregnancy in future nor are they at an increased risk of obstetric complications.
❖ Excessive vaginal bleeding can be associated with molar pregnancy.
❖ Infection can commonly occur due to absence of the amniotic sac and due to the large surface area left after expulsion or evacuation of the mole.
❖ Gestational trophoblastic disease does not impair fertility or predispose to prenatal or perinatal complications (e.g. congenital malformations, spontaneous abortions, etc.).

CLINICAL PEARLS

❖ Royal College of Obstetrician and Gynaecologists recognises that the combined oral contraceptive and hormone replacement therapy are safe to use in women with H. mole once hCG levels have returned to normal.
❖ In case of twin gestation, where there is one viable foetus and the other pregnancy is molar, the pregnancy should be allowed to proceed if the mother wishes, following appropriate counselling regarding the increased risk of perinatal mortality and morbidity. Such women may be at an increased risk for developing complications such as pulmonary embolism, early foetal loss and premature delivery. There is no increased risk of developing GTN after a twin pregnancy.

EVIDENCE-BASED MEDICINE

❖ The use of oxytocic infusion prior to completion of the evacuation is not recommended.[4,5] If the woman is experiencing significant haemorrhage prior to evacuation, surgical evacuation should be expedited. In these cases, the obstetrician must weigh the use of oxytocin infusion to reduce the incidence of haemorrhage against the risk of tumour embolisation.[4,5]
❖ Presently, there is insufficient evidence regarding the use of mifepristone and misoprostol for management of molar pregnancies.[5]

PARTIAL MOLE

INTRODUCTION

Partial H. mole (PHM) is another form of benign disease belonging to the spectrum of GTDs. Difference between the complete and partial mole has already been described in Table 37.1.

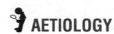

AETIOLOGY

Aetiology of partial mole is explained in Table 37.1 and is illustrated in Figure 37.1C.

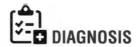

DIAGNOSIS

Clinical Presentation

The clinical features are same as that with complete H. mole (CHM), described previously in the text.

Investigations

Ultrasound examination: These include the following:
❖ Presence of a large placenta, cystic spaces within the placenta, an empty gestational sac or sac containing amorphous echoes or growth restricted foetus
❖ Increase in ratio of transverse to anterior-posterior dimension of the gestational sac to a value greater than 1.5
❖ Histopathological examination: Although complete mole does not contain any foetal tissue, non-viable foetal tissue may sometimes be present in PHM.

DIFFERENTIAL DIAGNOSIS

The conditions from which a PHM needs to be differentiated are same as that for CHM (as described previously).

MANAGEMENT

This is same as that described with CHM.

COMPLICATIONS

This is same as that described with CHM.

GESTATIONAL TROPHOBLASTIC NEOPLASIA

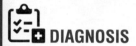

INTRODUCTION

Gestational trophoblastic neoplasia represents a variety of malignant diseases associated with the spectrum of GTDs. These include:

❖ Invasive mole
❖ Choriocarcinoma
❖ Placental site trophoblastic tumour
❖ Epithelioid trophoblastic tumour.

If the β-hCG level does not normalise within 10 weeks, the disease is classified as persistent. If metastasis is detected on various investigations (chest X-ray, CT, MRI, etc.), the disease is classified as metastatic. If no metastasis is detected, the disease is classified as non-metastatic.

DIAGNOSIS

Clinical Presentation

The metastatic disease can spread through the blood stream to lungs (80%), vagina (30%), pelvis (20%), brain (10%) and liver (10%). Metastasis to the lungs may result in symptoms like dyspnoea, cough, haemoptysis, chest pain, etc.

Investigations

❖ *Investigations to detect the metastatic disease*: Besides the investigations described with CHM previously, in the cases of GTN, investigations such as chest X-ray and CT scan of brain, chest, abdomen and pelvis need to be done in order to detect the metastatic disease. On chest X-ray the lungs may show presence of distinct nodules or cannon ball appearance.
❖ *β-hCG titres*: Women who have the malignant form of GTD may show β-hCG titres, which either plateau or rise and remain elevated beyond 8 weeks.

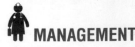

MANAGEMENT

The management plan for the treatment of persistent disease is shown in Flow chart 37.2. Any woman experiencing persistent or irregular vaginal bleeding following a pregnancy event (miscarriage, therapeutic termination of pregnancy or following the baby's delivery) is at risk of developing GTN. If the β-hCG level does not normalise within 8–10 weeks, the disease is classified as persistent.[12]

Persistent disease can be classified as metastatic or non-metastatic. In the cases of metastatic disease, chest X-ray and CT scan of brain, chest, abdomen and pelvis need to be done. If metastasis is detected on these investigations, the disease is classified as metastatic. If no metastasis is detected, the disease is classified as non-metastatic.

Non-metastatic Disease

In most of the cases, non-metastatic disease can be treated with a single chemotherapeutic drug, either methotrexate (more commonly used) or dactinomycin (used in cases of resistance to methotrexate). If single drug chemotherapy is ineffective, hysterectomy or multidrug chemotherapy can be tried.

Metastatic Disease

The system adopted by the WHO and FIGO for classifying gestational trophoblastic tumours (GTT) and treatment protocols is shown in Table 37.2.[13] Low-risk group has a score of 0–6; the moderate-risk group has a score between 5 and 7; and the high-risk group will have a score of 7 or higher.

Low-risk metastatic disease is treated with single or multiple drug chemotherapy (IM methotrexate or a combination of IV dactinomycin and etoposide). Moderate-risk metastatic disease is usually treated with multiagent chemotherapy. Women with high-risk GTT usually require combination chemotherapy along with selective use of surgery and radiotherapy. The standard multiagent chemotherapy regimen in high-risk group is EMA/CO (etoposide, methotrexate, actinomycin D, cyclophosphamide, vincristine) in which the drugs, like etoposide, dactinomycin and methotrexate, are alternated at weekly intervals with vincristine and cyclophosphamide.

Women who undergo chemotherapy are advised not to conceive for 1 year after completion of treatment. Women receiving chemotherapy for GTN, especially multiagent chemotherapy must be counselled that they may experience menopause at an earlier age in comparison to normal women in the same age-group.[14] They must also be advised about an increased risk of developing secondary cancers (e.g. acute myeloid leukaemia, breast cancer, melanoma, etc.) in future, especially with the use of multiagent chemotherapy which includes etoposide.

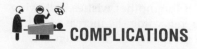

COMPLICATIONS

The development of GTT may result in conditions like invasive mole, choriocarcinoma and PSTT, all of which may metastasise and are potentially fatal if left untreated.

Flow chart 37.2: Management of persistent disease

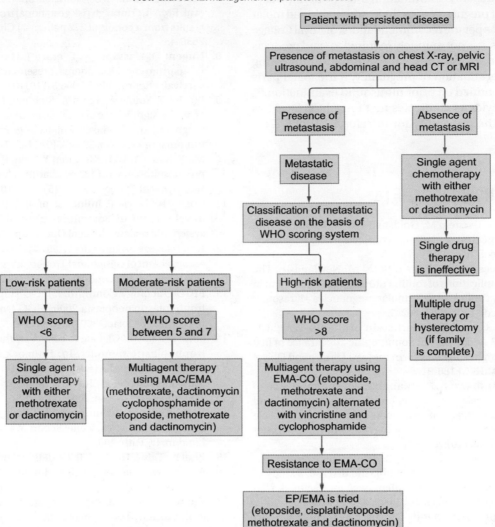

Table 37.2: The classification system by the WHO and FIGO for classifying gestational trophoblastic tumours and treatment protocols[13]

Risk factors	0	1	2	4
Age (years)	<40	≥40	—	—
Antecedent pregnancy	Mole	Abortion	Term	—
Interval (end of antecedent pregnancy to chemotherapy in months)	<4	4–6	7–13	>13
Human chorionic gonadotropin (IU/L)	$<10^3$	$10^3–10^4$	$10^4–10^5$	$>10^5$
Number of metastasis	0	1–4	5–8	>8
Site of metastasis	Lung	Spleen, kidney	Gastrointestinal tract	Brain, liver
Largest tumour mass	—	3–5 cm	>5 cm	—
Previous chemotherapy	—	—	Single drug	>2 drugs

CLINICAL PEARLS

❖ The lungs are the most common site for metastasis in case of malignant GTD
❖ Gestational trophoblastic neoplasia can occur after any GTD event, even when separated by a normal pregnancy.

EVIDENCE-BASED MEDICINE

❖ According to the recommendations by RCOG, products of conception obtained from the medical or surgical management of all failed pregnancies must be sent for histological assessment to exclude trophoblastic neoplasia.

PART II

In all cases, ultrasound examination must be done prior to termination of pregnancy to exclude non-viable and molar pregnancies. As per the recommendations of Royal College of Pathologists, it is not routinely required to send products of conception for histological examination following therapeutic termination of pregnancy, if the foetal parts have been identified on prior ultrasound examination.[15]

❖ The present evidence indicates that once hCG level has normalised, the possibility for development of GTN is very low.[16,17]

REFERENCES

1. Soto-Wright V, Berstein M, Goldstein DP, Berkowitz RS. The changing clinical presentation of complete molar pregnancy. Obstet Gynecol. 1995;86(5):775-9.

2. Sebire NJ, Rees H, Paradinas F, Seckl M, Newlands E. The diagnostic implications of routine ultrasound examination in histologically confirmed early molar pregnancies. Ultrasound Obstet Gynecol. 2001;18(6):662-5.

3. Benson CB, Genest DR, Bernstein MR, Soto-Wright V, Goldstein DP, Berkowitz RS. Sonographic appearance of first trimester complete hydatidiform moles. J Ultrasound Obstet Gynecol. 2000;16(2):188-91.

4. Stone M, Bagshawe KD. An analysis of the influence of maternal age, gestational age, contraceptive method and primary mode of treatment of patients with hydatidiform mole on the incidence of subsequent chemotherapy. Br J Obstet Gynaecol. 1979;86(10):782-92.

5. Tidy JA, Gillespie AM, Bright N, Radstone CR, Coleman RE, Hancock BW. Gestational trophoblastic disease: a study of mode of evacuation and subsequent need for treatment with chemotherapy. Gynecol Oncol. 2000;78(3 Pt 1):309-12.

6. Tidy JA, Rustin GJ, Newlands ES, Foskett M, Fuller S, Short D, et al. The presentation and management of women with choriocarcinoma after non molar pregnancy. Br J Obstet Gynaecol. 1995;102(9):715-19.

7. Bower M, Newlands ES, Holden L, Short D, Brock C, Rustin GJ, et al. EMA/CO for high risk gestational trophoblastic tumours: results from a cohort of 272 patients. J Clin Oncol. 1997;15(7):2636-43.

8. Nugent D, Hassadia A, Everard J, Hancock BW, Tidy JA. Postpartum choriocarcinoma: presentation, management and survival. J Reprod Med. 2006;51(10):819-24.

9. Powles T, Young A, Saniit A, Stebbing J, Short D, Bower M, et al. The significance of the time interval between antecedent pregnancy and diagnosis of high risk gestational trophoblastic tumours. Br J Cancer. 2006;95(9):1145-7.

10. Ma Y, Xiang Y, Wan XR, Chen Y, Feng FZ, Lei CZ, et al. The prognostic analysis of 123 postpartum choriocarcinoma cases. Int J Gynecol Cancer. 2008;18(5):1097-101.

11. Costa HL, Doyle P. Influence of oral contraceptives in the development of post molar trophoblastic neoplasia: a systematic review. Gynecol Oncol. 2006;100(3):579-85.

12. Royal College of Obstetrician and Gynaecologists (RCOG). The Management of Gestational Trophoblastic Disease. Green–top Guideline No. 38. London: RCOG Press; 2010.

13. FIGO Oncology Committee. FIGO staging for gestational trophoblastic neoplasia 2000. FIGO Oncology Committee. Int J Gynecol Obstet. 2002;77(3):285-7.

14. Seckl MJ, Rustin GJ. Late toxicity after therapy for gestational trophoblastic tumours. In: Hancock BW, Newlands ES, Berkowitz RS, Cole LA (Eds). Gestational Trophoblastic Disease, 3rd edition. London: International Society for the Study of Trophoblastic Disease; 2003. pp. 470-84.

15. Royal College of Pathologists (RCPath). Histopathology of Limited or no Clinical Value: Report of a Working Party Group. London: RCPath; 2002.

16. Pisal N, Tidy J, Hancock B. Gestational trophoblastic disease: is intensive follow up essential in all women? BJOG. 2004;111(12):1449-51.

17. Sebire NJ, Foskett M, Short D, Savage P, Stewart W, Thomson M, et al. Shortened duration of human chorionic gonadotrophin surveillance following complete or partial hydatidiform mole: evidence for revised protocol of a UK regional trophoblastic disease unit. BJOG. 2007;114(6):760-2.

SECTION 6

Foetal Complications (Diagnosis and Management)

OBSTETRICS

Foetal Growth Restriction

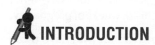 **INTRODUCTION**

Intrauterine growth restriction (IUGR) refers to low-birth-weight (LBW) infants whose birthweight is below the 10th percentile of the average for the particular gestational age, where the percentiles have been customised for maternal characteristics such as maternal height, weight, parity and ethnic group, gestational age at delivery, and infant sex.[1,2] IUGR infants are pathologically growth restricted due to some intrinsic or extrinsic pathological process. Therefore, they may manifest evidence of foetal compromise in form of abnormal results on Doppler studies, reduced liquor volume on ultrasound examination, etc. Intrinsic pathological process could be related to structural or chromosomal anomalies, inborn errors of metabolism and foetal infection, whereas extrinsic pathological process could be due to placenta-mediated growth restriction or maternal medical conditions such as pre-eclampsia, autoimmune disease, thrombophilias, renal disease, diabetes, essential hypertension, etc.

On the other hand, even if the infant's birthweight is less than 10th percentile, he or she may not be pathologically growth restricted. These infants have simply failed to achieve a specific weight or biometric size in accordance with the gestational age. These infants are termed as small for gestational age (SGA) infants and are defined as infants having an estimated foetal weight (EFW) or abdominal circumference (AC) less than the 10th percentile. Severe SGA infants have an EFW or AC less than the 3rd percentile.[3] LBW infant, on the other hand, refers to an infant with a birthweight of less than 2,500 g. Difference between the SGA infants and infants with pathological growth restriction is described in Table 38.1.

Pathologically growth-restricted infants can be of two types, i.e. symmetric intrauterine growth restricted and asymmetric intrauterine growth restricted, depending on the stage of foetal growth (Table 38.2) at which the pathological insult occurred. If the pathological insult occurs at Stage 1 of foetal growth, the process of cellular hyperplasia is mainly affected. This results in symmetrically growth restricted infants. If the pathological insult occurs at Stage 3 of foetal growth, cellular hypertrophy is

Table 38.1: Difference between the small for gestational age infants and infants with pathological growth restriction

Characteristics	Small for gestational age infants (normal)	Infants with pathological growth restriction
Birthweight	<10% of the average weight. Birth weight is usually <2.5 kg	<10% of the average weight, but may also be <25%. Birthweight is usually <2.5 kg, but may be larger
Ponderal index	Normal	Low
Amount of subcutaneous fat	Normal	Reduced
Neonatal course	Usually uneventful	May develop complications like hypoglycaemia, hypocalcaemia, hyperviscosity, hyperbilirubinaemia, necrotising enterocolitis, etc.
Perinatal mortality and morbidity	Occasionally, may be at an increased risk of perianal mortality and morbidity	Usually at an increased risk of perianal mortality and morbidity
RBC count	Normal RBC count	Elevated number of nucleated RBCs
Platelet count	Normal	Thrombocytopenia is usually present
Investigations	Foetal biometric tests, which help in measuring foetal size and gestational age are usually abnormal. Results of Doppler waveform analysis are within normal limits	Foetal biophysical tests, which help in assessing foetal well-being are usually abnormal. Doppler waveform analysis of umbilical and uterine arteries may be associated with reduced diastolic flow; absent or sometimes even reversed flow

Table 38.2: Stages of foetal growth

Stage of foetal growth	Growth characteristics	Weeks of gestation
Stage 1	Cell hyperplasia	4–20 weeks of gestation
Stage 2	Cellular hyperplasia	20–28 weeks of gestation
Stage 3	Cellular hypertrophy	28–40 weeks of gestation

mainly affected. This results in asymmetrically affected growth restricted infants. The other differences between symmetric and asymmetric IUGR infants are enumerated in Table 38.3.

🪡 AETIOLOGY

Maternal: Maternal causes are as follows:
- ❖ Constitutionally small mothers or low maternal weight
- ❖ Excessive alcohol intake
- ❖ Strenuous physical exercise
- ❖ Poor socioeconomic conditions
- ❖ Maternal anaemia, especially sickle cell anaemia
- ❖ Tobacco smoking, drug abuse during pregnancy
- ❖ Chronic placental insufficiency due to pre-eclampsia, chronic hypertension, renal disease, connective tissue disorders, gestational diabetes, etc.
- ❖ Maternal hypoxia (e.g. pulmonary diseases, cyanotic congenital heart disease, etc.)
- ❖ Endocrine disorders (e.g. diabetic nephropathy, hyperthyroidism, Addison's disease).

Foetal: Various foetal causes are as follows:
- ❖ Multiple pregnancy
- ❖ Congenital malformations (e.g. congenital heart disease, renal agenesis, etc.)
- ❖ Chromosomal abnormalities (e.g. trisomy 13, 16, 18, 21, etc.)
- ❖ Chronic intrauterine infection (e.g. congenital syphilis, TORCH, viral, bacterial, protozoan and spirochetal infections).

Placental: Placental abnormalities including chorioangioma, circumvallate placenta, marginal or velamentous cord insertion, placenta praevia, placental abruption, etc. may also be responsible.

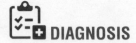

DIAGNOSIS

History

All pregnant women should be assessed at the time of their booking visit for identification of risk factors (Table 38.4) for an SGA foetus. This would help the clinicians in identifying neonates who require increased surveillance.

Identification of major risk factors: Women who have a major risk factor (OR > 2.0) as described in Table 38.4 should be referred for serial ultrasound examination involving the measurement of foetal size from 26–28 weeks of gestation. These patients should also be assessed for foetal well-being with umbilical artery Doppler from 26–28 weeks of pregnancy.

Identification of a minor risk factor: Women who have three or more minor risk factors (Table 38.4) should be referred for uterine artery Doppler at 20–24 weeks of gestation. Subsequent normalisation of flow velocity indices in women with an abnormal uterine artery Doppler at 20–24 weeks of pregnancy is still associated with an increased risk of an IUGR foetus. Therefore, repeating uterine artery Doppler is associated with limited value.

Serial ultrasound measurement of foetal size and assessment of well-being with umbilical artery Doppler starting at 26–28 weeks of pregnancy must be done in women who have an abnormal uterine artery Doppler at 20–24 weeks [defined as a pulsatility index (PI) > 95th percentile] and/or notching.

Table 38.3: Differences between symmetric and asymmetric IUGR

Symmetric IUGR	Asymmetric IUGR
Growth is affected before 16 weeks of gestation	Foetal growth is affected later in gestation
Foetus is proportionately small	Foetus is disproportionately small
Cell hyperplasia is affected	Cellular hypertrophy is mainly affected
Causes of symmetric IUGR mainly include congenital abnormalities, chromosomal aberrations, intrauterine infections, etc.	Causes of asymmetric IUGR include hypertension, anaemia, heart disease, accidental haemorrhage, etc.
Pathological process is intrinsic to the foetus	Pathological process is extrinsic to the foetus
Such neonates are small in all parameters	Head circumference is not as much affected as is AC
Catch-up growth occurs poorly after birth	Catch-up growth occurs reasonably well after birth
Neonatal prognosis is usually poor	Neonatal prognosis is usually good
Ponderal index is normal	Ponderal index is low
HC/AC and FL/AC ratios are normal. In normal pregnancies FL/AC is 22 for all gestational ages from 21 weeks onwards. Also, HC/AC at less than 32 weeks of normal gestation is more than 1; between 32–34 weeks of gestation is 1; at more than 34 weeks of gestation is less than 1	These ratios are elevated. HC and FL remain unaffected, whereas AC is reduced. As a result HC/AC and FL/AC are elevated
Also termed as type II (low profile IUGR)	Also termed as type I (late-flattening IUGR)
Less common: Usually responsible for 20% cases of IUGR	More common: Usually responsible for 80% cases of IUGR

Abbreviations: AC, abdominal circumference; FL, femur length; HC, head circumference; IUGR, intrauterine growth restriction

PART II

Table 38.4: Risk factors for SGA foetuses[4,5]

Major risk factors	Minor risk factors
• Maternal age >40 years	• Maternal age ≥35 years
• Smoking ≥11 cigarettes per day	• Nulliparity
• Cocaine	• BMI <20 kg/m²
• Daily vigorous exercise	• BMI ≥30 kg/m²
• Previous history of SGA/stillbirth baby	• Smoking 1–10 cigarettes per day
• Pre-eclampsia[6]	• IVF singleton pregnancy
• Chronic hypertension	• Low fruit intake prepregnancy
• Diabetes with vascular disease	• Pregnancy interval <6 months
• Renal impairment	• Pregnancy interval ≥60 months
• Antiphospholipid syndrome	• Mild pregnancy-induced hypertension
• Paternal or maternal history of SGA	• Placental abruption
• Heavy bleeding similar to menses at the time of threatened abortion	• Caffeine ≥300 mg/day in the third trimester
• Echogenic bowel on ultrasound	
• Unexplained APH	
• Low maternal weight gain	
• PAPP-A <0.4 MoM	

Abbreviations: SGA, small for gestational age; APH, antepartum haemorrhage; MoM, multiples of the median; PAPP-A, pregnancy-associated plasma protein-A

Abdominal Examination

❖ Serial measurement of symphysis-fundal height (SFH) is recommended during each antenatal visit from 24 weeks of pregnancy onwards. A lag of 4 cm or more on SFH measurement is suggestive of foetal growth restriction (FGR). To improve prediction of an SGA neonate, SFH should be preferably plotted on a customised chart.[7,8] Women in whom a single SFH measurement falls below the 10th percentile or in whom serial measurements demonstrate slow or static growth by crossing centiles should be referred for ultrasound measurement of foetal size.

❖ Reduced size of the foetus (in lieu of the gestational age) can be estimated on abdominal examination. This can be confirmed on ultrasound examination.

❖ Palpation of foetal head gives an estimation of foetal size and maturity.

❖ Abdominal palpation provides only a little accuracy regarding the prediction of an SGA neonate. Therefore, it is not routinely performed in this context.

Investigations

Biochemical Markers

The most important biochemical marker, which is used as screening tests for an IUGR foetus is measurement of serum pregnancy-associated plasma protein-A (PAPP-A) levels in the first trimester. Measurement of a low level [<0.415 multiples of the median (MoM)] of PAPP-A can be considered as a major risk factor for delivery of an SGA neonate.[9]

Ultrasound Biometry

This includes measurement of crown-rump length (Fig. 38.1); biparietal diameter (Fig. 38.2); AC (Fig. 38.3); femur length

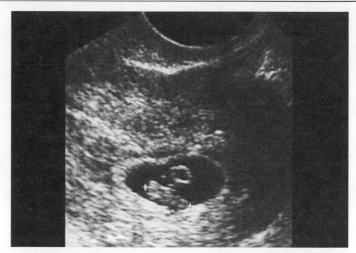

Fig. 38.1: Ultrasound measurement of crown-rump length

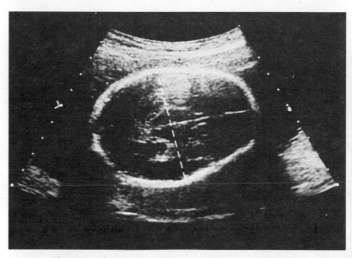

Fig. 38.2: Ultrasound measurement of biparietal diameter

CHAPTER 38

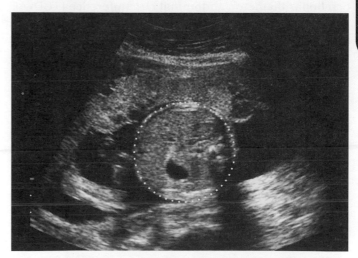

Fig. 38.3: Ultrasound measurement of abdominal circumference

(Fig. 38.4); transverse cerebellar diameter (TCD) (Fig. 38.5); and ultrasound EFW. In women undergoing serial assessment of foetal size, use of a customised foetal weight reference may help in improving the prediction of an SGA neonate and poor perinatal outcome.

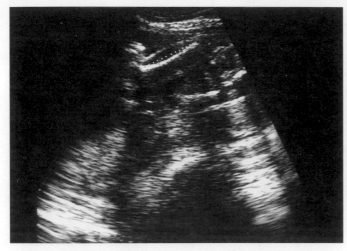

Fig. 38.4: Ultrasound measurement of femur length

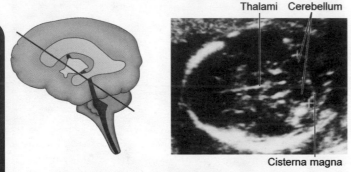

Fig. 38.5: Measurement of transverse cerebellar diameter

Ratio of various diameters, such as head circumference/ abdominal circumference (HC/AC ratio); transverse cerebellar diameter/abdominal circumference (TCD/AC ratio) and femoral length/abdominal circumference (FL/AC ratio), can also be used. Foetal ponderal index (FPI) is another ultrasound measured foetal index (FPI) for predicting IUGR, which is calculated with the help of the following formula:

$$FPI = \frac{\text{Estimated foetal weight}}{\text{Femur length}^3}$$

Measurement of foetal AC or EFW less than 10th percentile can be used for diagnosing an SGA foetus. However, routine measurement of foetal AC or EFW in the third trimester does not help in decreasing the incidence of an SGA neonate nor does it help in improving the perinatal outcome.[10] Use of routine foetal biometry in clinical practice is therefore not justified. If measurement of the foetal AC or EFW is less than 10th percentile or there is evidence of reduced growth velocity, the woman should be offered serial assessment of foetal size and umbilical artery Doppler. Measurement of AC or EFW, used for estimation of growth velocity, should be performed at least 3 weeks apart to help minimise the false-positive rates for diagnosing FGR.

Biophysical Tests

These tests help in assessing foetal well-being:
- ❖ Non-stress test
- ❖ Biophysical profile, amniotic fluid volume
- ❖ Foetal cardiotocography.

Changes Occurring in Various Doppler Velocity Waveforms in IUGR Foetuses (Flow chart 38.1)

Umbilical artery Doppler serves as the primary surveillance tool for management of IUGR foetuses.[11] The Doppler measurements from umbilical artery, uterine artery, middle cerebral artery (MCA) and ductus venosus (DV) are important for diagnosing placental insufficiency. The major Doppler detectable modifications in the foetal circulation associated with IUGR and foetal hypoxaemia include increased resistance in the umbilical artery, foetal peripheral vessels and maternal uterine vessels, in association with decreased resistance in the foetal cerebral vessels. The various types of indices which provide information regarding the amount of blood flow in various vessels are described in Table 38.5.

Uterine Artery Doppler

The uterine artery Doppler is indicative of uteroplacental circulation by showing presence or absence of resistance to

Flow chart 38.1: Changes occurring in various Doppler velocity waveforms in IUGR foetuses

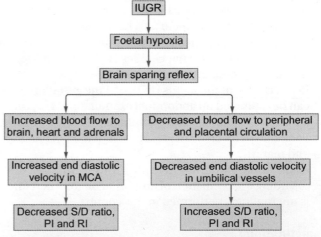

Abbreviations: IUGR, intrauterine growth restriction; S/D, systolic/diastolic; PI, pulsatility index; RI, resistance index; MCA, middle cerebral artery

Table 38.5: Types of Doppler indices

Doppler index	Calculation of Doppler index
Systolic/diastolic (S/D) ratio	$\dfrac{\text{Peak systolic blood flow}}{\text{End diastolic velocity}}$
Pulsatility index (PI)	$\dfrac{\text{Peak systolic velocity} - \text{end diastolic velocity}}{\text{Mean systolic velocity}}$
Resistance index (RI)	$\dfrac{\text{Peak systolic velocity} - \text{end diastolic velocity}}{\text{Peak systolic velocity}}$

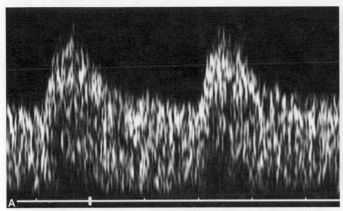
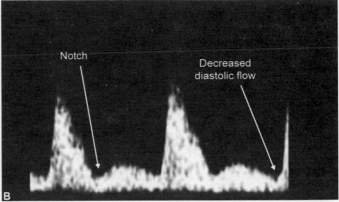

Figs 38.6A and B: Uterine artery blood flow patterns. (A) Normal uterine artery blood flow; (B) Abnormal uterine artery Doppler waveforms with decreased diastolic flow and early diastolic notching

the blood flow.[12,13] In normal pregnancy, both uterine artery in the placental bed and the foetal umbilical arteries circulations, exhibit high diastolic flow velocities caused by low resistance. With advancing gestational age, there occurs trophoblastic invasion of the uterine spiral arteries causing its dilatation and fall in the resistance to the blood flow. Uterine blood flow in a non-pregnant woman is about 50 mL/minute and increases to 700 mL/minute in the third trimester. Therefore, diastolic component in early pregnancy comprising of low peak flow velocity and early diastolic notch is transformed into one with high peak flow velocity and no diastolic notch by midgestation, and PI value is usually less than 1.2. Abnormal uterine artery Doppler studies characterised by reduced diastolic flow suggest a maternal cause for IUGR. Increased resistance to the blood flow in uterine vessels, resulting in reduced diastolic flow causes increased systolic-diastolic ratio of flow velocities in uterine vessels. PI greater than 1.45 with bilateral diastolic notches is suggestive of clinically significant uteroplacental vascular ischemia (Figs 38.6A and B).

Middle Cerebral Artery Doppler Studies

Middle cerebral artery can be easily demonstrated by colour Doppler in transverse foetal head position. In normal pregnancy, at 28–30 weeks, MCA is characterised by high systolic velocities and minimal diastolic velocities, resulting in high PI values greater than 1.45.[14] In IUGR, deficiency of oxygen causes the redistribution of blood flow resulting in increased blood flow to the brain causing a drop in the cerebral resistance. These changes can be attributed to the 'brain sparing effect', in which there is preferential perfusion of the brain, heart and adrenals at the expense of the integument and viscera, gut and kidneys in the hypoxic foetuses. This leads to a decrease in the systolic/diastolic (S/D) ratio as well as the PI and resistance index (RI) in the MCA. At the same time, there is reduced flow to the peripheral and placental circulations resulting in decreased end diastolic velocity in umbilical vessels and thereby increase in the S/D ratio, PI and RI. With the worsening of the foetal condition, as the blood flow to the brain also reduces, MCA blood flow velocity may return to normal. Changes in the cerebral flow parameters, however, have not been observed to correlate with the degree of asphyxic compromise. Therefore, these parameters are not helpful in choosing timing for delivery.

Umbilical Artery Doppler

In normal pregnancy, the placental vascular bed is a low-resistance bed, where impedance decreases with the advancing gestational age. The assessment of umbilical blood flow provides information regarding blood perfusion of the foetoplacental unit. In normal pregnancy, the foetal umbilical circulation is characterised by continuous forward flow. Characteristic umbilical blood flow has saw-tooth appearance of arterial flow in one direction and continuous umbilical venous blood flow in the other (Fig. 38.7A). The S/D ratio serves as an index of measurement which compares the systolic with the diastolic flow in the umbilical arteries and identifies the amount of resistance in the placental vasculature. The end diastolic blood flow in umbilical artery increases with advancing gestation in normal pregnancies. As a result there is a decline in both PI and S/D ratio with increasing gestation. As resistance decreases, RI values approach zero. On the other hand, when the resistance increases, end diastolic flow approaches zero, therefore, RI approaches one. If the end diastolic flow is absent, according to the equations mentioned in Table 38.5, S/D ratio would be equal to infinity and RI would be equal to one. Therefore, in these cases, the blood flow is assessed with the help of PI.

In cases of IUGR (especially due to placental insufficiency) if the resistance to blood flow does not decrease sufficiently, the umbilical circulation is characterised by presence of abnormal S/D ratio, PI or RI. The umbilical artery indices are considered as abnormal if they become greater than 95th percentile for the gestational age or there may be early diastolic notching (Fig. 38.7B) or the end diastolic flow may be either absent or reversed (Figs 38.7C and D). Generally, an S/D ratio of equal to or less than 3.0 is considered as normal. A rising S/D ratio indicates a worsening foetal prognosis and warrants closer more frequent monitoring. Absent end diastolic waveforms in umbilical arteries imply that nearly 75% of the vascular bed has been obliterated. There are 85% chances that the foetus would be hypoxaemic. Reverse end

CHAPTER 38

PART II

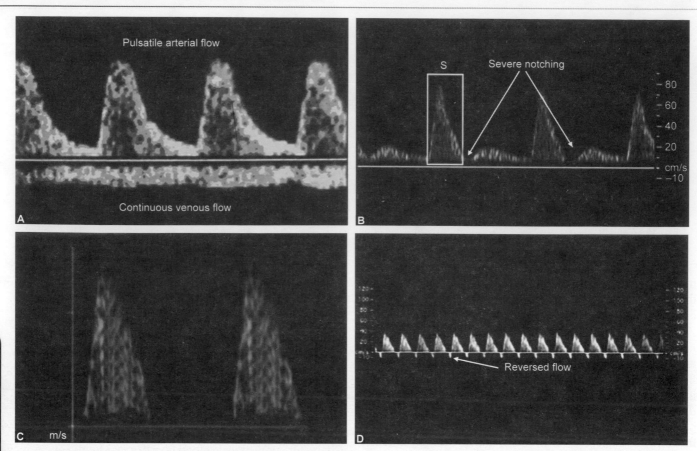

Figs 38.7A to D: Umbilical artery blood flow patterns: (A) Normal umbilical artery Doppler ultrasound waveforms; (B) Early diastolic notching; (C) Absent end diastolic flow; (D) Reversed end diastolic flow *(For colour version, see Plate 2)*

Box 38.1: Changes in umbilical blood flow with increasing vascular resistance

❖ Elevated pulsatility index and resistance index
❖ Early diastolic notch (Fig. 38.7B)
❖ Absent end diastolic blood flow (Fig. 38.7C)
❖ Reversed end diastolic blood flow (Fig. 38.7D)

diastolic frequencies, on the other hand, are associated with a 10-fold increase in perinatal mortality.[15] Abnormal waveforms on umbilical artery Doppler ultrasound should be followed-up with methods for enhanced foetal surveillance or delivery. Various changes in Doppler waveform analysis with increased resistance in umbilical vessels are summarised in Box 38.1.

Karyotyping

Karyotyping should be performed in severely SGA foetuses with structural anomalies. It should also be performed in women, in whom IUGR is diagnosed before 23 weeks of gestation, especially if uterine artery Doppler is normal.

Screening for infection: Serological screening for infections such as congenital cytomegalovirus and toxoplasmosis should be offered in severely IUGR foetuses. Testing for syphilis and malaria should be considered in high-risk populations.

 OBSTETRIC MANAGEMENT

Screening and management for cases of IUGR is described in Flow chart 38.2.[16]

ANTENATAL PERIOD

❖ Identifying the underlying cause for IUGR.
❖ Women must be advised to take rest in the left lateral position for a period of at least 10 hours everyday.
❖ *Daily foetal movement count*: In case the woman perceives less than 6 foetal movements within 2 hours, she should be advised to immediately consult her doctor.
❖ *Foetal surveillance in IUGR foetuses*: Umbilical artery Doppler should be considered as the primary tool for surveillance in case of IUGR foetuses. Use of umbilical artery Doppler in high-risk population has been shown to reduce perinatal morbidity and mortality associated with IUGR. Oligohydramnios may be often present in IUGR foetuses. Therefore, ultrasound assessment of liquor volume is often performed in cases of IUGR. However, ultrasound assessment of amniotic fluid volume should not be used as the only form of surveillance in SGA foetuses.[16] Interpretation of amniotic fluid volume should be based on single deepest vertical pocket.

Flow chart 38.2: Screening and management for cases of intrauterine growth restriction

Abbreviations: APH, antepartum haemorrhage; MoM, multiples of the median; PAPP-A, pregnancy-associated plasma protein-A; SFH, symphysis-fundal height; ANC, antenatal care

Management of the Diagnosed Cases of IUGR

If IUGR is identified during the ultrasound scan performed at 18–20 weeks; she must be offered a referral for a detailed foetal anatomical survey and uterine artery Doppler by a foetal medicine specialist. If the woman has abnormal uterine artery waveforms, she requires serial measurement of foetal size with the help of ultrasound and serial assessment of foetal well-being with the help of umbilical artery Doppler. On the other hand, women with normal uterine artery waveforms on Doppler analysis do not require serial measurement of foetal size and serial assessment of well-being with umbilical artery Doppler unless they develop specific pregnancy complications, such as antepartum haemorrhage (APH) or hypertension. Nevertheless, these women should be offered an ultrasound scan for foetal size and umbilical artery Doppler during the third trimester.

Normal Findings on Umbilical Artery Waveform Analysis

❖ If findings on umbilical artery waveform analysis are within normal limits, ultrasound examination must be repeated every fortnightly for estimation of AC and expected foetal weight. Umbilical artery and MCA Doppler must be performed in the third trimester after 32 weeks.

❖ *Timing of delivery*: In these cases, delivery must be offered after 37 weeks with the involvement of a senior clinician. The patient should be preferably delivered by 37 weeks if MCA Doppler PI is less than the fifth percentile. Delivery may be considered after 34 weeks if the growth appears to be static over 3 weeks.

Abnormal Findings on Umbilical Artery Waveform Analysis

❖ If the findings on umbilical artery Doppler analysis are abnormal, i.e. PI or RI greater than 2.5 S/D, but EDV is present, then ultrasound (AC and expected foetal weight) must be repeated at every weekly interval. Umbilical artery Doppler analysis must be performed twice weekly. Delivery is recommended by 37 weeks. Steroids must be considered if the patient is being delivered by caesarean section. Delivery after 34 weeks must be considered if growth appears to be static over 3 weeks.

❖ If Doppler waveform analysis shows absent or reversed end diastolic volume (AREDV), ultrasound examination (for assessment of AC and EFW) must be repeated on weekly basis. Investigations such as umbilical artery

CHAPTER 38

Doppler, ductus venosus (DV) Doppler and computerised cardiotocographic examination (cCTG) must be performed on daily basis.[17] Delivery may be considered before 32 weeks after a course of corticosteroids in case of abnormal DV Doppler or cCTG results, provided that the period of gestation is greater than or equal to 24 weeks and EFW is greater than or equal to 500 g. Even if the results of DV Doppler examination are within normal limits, delivery must be considered between 30 weeks and 32 weeks in these cases.

Intrapartum Period

- Early admission to the labour ward is recommended for women in spontaneous labour with an IUGR foetus in order to initiate continuous foetal heart rate monitoring in these patients.
- Presently, the RCOG (2013) recommends that the clinician needs to individualise each patient and decide the time for delivery by weighing the risk of foetal demise due to delayed intervention against the risk of long-term disabilities resulting from preterm delivery due to early intervention.[18]
- Since the growth-restricted foetus is especially prone to develop asphyxia, continuous foetal monitoring using external or internal CTG needs to be done in the intrapartum period. CTG tracing should preferably be interpreted based on short-term foetal heart rate variation from computerised analysis. If, at any time, the foetal heart rate appears to be non-reassuring, an emergency caesarean may be required. However, elective caesarean section is not justified for delivery of all IUGR foetuses.
- *Preterm IUGR foetus*: Administration of IM corticosteroids is required in case the delivery takes place between 24^{+0} weeks and 35^{+6} weeks of gestation.
- *Timing of delivery*: Preterm IUGR foetus with AREDV in the umbilical artery, prior to 32 weeks of gestation, must be delivered when DV Doppler becomes abnormal or umbilical vein pulsations appear, provided the foetus has attained viability. The course of corticosteroids must be administered prior to delivery in these cases. Even when DV Doppler waveforms are normal, delivery is recommended by 32 weeks of gestation in these cases and should be considered between 30 weeks and 32 weeks of gestation.

  A senior obstetrician should be preferably involved in determining the timing and mode of delivery for IUGR foetuses having normal umbilical artery Doppler waveforms after 32 weeks of gestation. Delivery should be offered at 37 weeks of gestation in these cases. IUGR foetus with abnormal umbilical artery Doppler waveforms detected after 32 weeks of gestation should be delivered no later than 37 weeks of gestation.

  In the term SGA foetus with normal umbilical artery Doppler, MCA Doppler waveforms should be used for deciding the timing for delivery. If MCA Doppler is abnormal (PI < 5th percentile), delivery should be recommended no later than 37 weeks of gestation.

In the preterm SGA foetus, MCA Doppler has limited accuracy to predict acidaemia and adverse outcome. Therefore, MCA Doppler should not be used to time delivery in case of preterm IUGR foetuses with abnormal umbilical artery Doppler waveform. In these cases DV Doppler should be used for surveillance and for timing the delivery.

- *Mode of delivery*: Delivery via caesarean section is recommended in the case of IUGR foetus with reversed or absent umbilical artery velocity. Induction of labour can be offered to the IUGR foetuses having normal umbilical artery Doppler waveforms or those where there is abnormal umbilical artery PI or RI but end-diastolic velocity is present. Induction of labour can be offered. However, in these cases, the rates of emergency caesarean section are increased. Therefore, continuous foetal heart rate monitoring is recommended from the onset of uterine contractions.

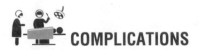

COMPLICATIONS

Foetal

Antepartum: This includes:
- Foetal hypoxia and acidosis
- Stillbirth
- Oligohydramnios.

Intrapartum: This includes:
- Neonatal asphyxia and acidosis
- Respiratory distress syndrome
- Meconium aspiration syndrome
- Persistent foetal circulation
- Intraventricular bleeding, neonatal encephalopathy.

Neonatal period: This includes:
- Hypoglycaemia (glucose levels of <30 mg/dL): It can be associated with symptoms like jitteriness, twitching, apnoea, etc.
- Hypoinsulinaemia, hypertriglyceridaemia
- Hypocalcaemia and hyperphosphataemia
- Meconium aspiration and/or birth asphyxia
- Hypothermia
- Hyperbilirubinaemia, polycythaemia, hyperviscosity syndrome
- Sepsis, necrotising enterocolitis
- Complications, such as cerebral palsy in long term.

CLINICAL PEARLS

- Second trimester markers for Down's syndrome (e.g. levels of α-foetoprotein, hCG levels, unconjugated oestriol levels, inhibin etc.) have a limited accuracy for predicting delivery of an IUGR neonate.[19]
- Crown-rump length of 15–60 mm (corresponding to gestational period varying from 8 weeks to 12.5 weeks) is found to have greatest accuracy in determining the period of gestation in the first trimester

❖ Biophysical profile should not be used for foetal surveillance in preterm SGA foetuses.[20]

EVIDENCE-BASED MEDICINE

❖ Serial ultrasound measurement of foetal size and assessment of well-being with umbilical artery Doppler should be offered in cases of foetal echogenic bowel.[4,5]
❖ The major Doppler detectable modifications in the foetal circulation associated with IUGR and foetal hypoxaemia include increased resistance in the umbilical artery, foetal peripheral vessels and maternal uterine vessels, in association with decreased resistance in the foetal cerebral vessels.[12-15]

REFERENCES

1. Clausson B, Gardosi J, Francis A, Cnattingius S. Perinatal outcome in SGA births defined by customised versus population-based birthweight standards. BJOG. 2001;108(8):830-4.
2. Figueras F, Figueras J, Meler E, Eixarch E, Coll O, Gratacos E, et al. Customised birthweight standards accurately predict perinatal morbidity. Arch Dis Child Fetal Neonat Ed. 2007;92(4):F277-80.
3. Chang TC, Robson SC, Boys RJ, Spencer JA. Prediction of the small for gestational age infant: which ultrasonic measurement is best? Obstet Gynecol. 1992;80(6):1030-8.
4. Kleijer ME, Dekker GA, Heard AR. Risk factors for intrauterine growth restriction in a socio-economically disadvantaged region. J Matern Fetal Neonatal Med. 2005;18(1):23-30.
5. McCowan L, Horgan RP. Risk factors for small for gestational age infants. Best Pract Res Clin Obstet Gynaecol. 2009;23(6):779-93.
6. Allen VM, Joseph K, Murphy KE, Magee LA, Ohlsson A. The effect of hypertensive disorders in pregnancy on small for gestational age and stillbirth: a population based study. BMC Pregnancy Childbirth. 2004;4(1):17.
7. Cnattingius S, Axelsson O, Lindmark G. Symphysis-fundus measurements and intrauterine growth retardation. Acta Obstet Gynecol Scand. 1984;63(4):335-40.
8. Neilson JP. Symphysis-fundal height measurement in pregnancy. Cochrane Database Syst Rev. 2000;(2):CD000944.
9. Fox NS, Shalom D, Chasen ST. Second-trimester fetal growth as a predictor of poor obstetric and neonatal outcome in patients with low first-trimester serum pregnancy-associated plasma protein-A and a euploid fetus. Ultrasound Obstet Gynecol. 2009;33(1):34-8.
10. Chitty LS, Altman DG, Henderson A, Campbell S. Charts of fetal size: 3. Abdominal measurements. Br J Obstet Gynaecol. 1994;101(2):125-31.
11. Morris RK, Malin G, Robson SC, Kleijnen J, Zamora J, Khan KS. Fetal umbilical artery Doppler to predict compromise of fetal/neonatal wellbeing in a high-risk population: systematic review and bivariate meta-analysis. Ultrasound Obstet Gynecol. 2011;37(2):135-42.
12. Lin S, Shimizu I, Suehara N, Nakayama M, Aono T. Uterine artery Doppler velocimetry in relation to trophoblast migration into the myometrium of the placental bed. Obstet Gynecol. 1995;85(5 Pt 1):760-5.
13. Prefumo F, Sebire NJ, Thilaganathan B. Decreased endovascular trophoblast invasion in first trimester pregnancies with high-resistance uterine artery Doppler indices. Hum Reprod. 2004;19(1):206-9.
14. Dubiel M, Gudmundsson S, Gunnarsson G, Marsal K. Middle cerebral artery velocimetry as a predictor of hypoxemia in fetuses with increased resistance to blood flow in the umbilical artery. Early Hum Dev. 1997;47(2):177-8.
15. Chang TC, Robson SC, Spencer JA, Gallivan S. Prediction of perinatal morbidity at term in small fetuses: comparison of fetal growth and Doppler ultrasound. Br J Obstet Gynaecol. 1994;101(5):422-7.
16. Alberry M, Soothill P. Management of fetal growth restriction. Arch Dis Child Fetal Neonatal Ed. 2007;92(1):F62-7.
17. Almström H, Axelsson O, Cnattingius S, Ekman G, Maesel A, Ulmsten U, et al. Comparison of umbilical-artery velocimetry and cardiotocography for surveillance of small-for-gestational-age fetuses. Lancet. 1992;340(8825):936-40.
18. Royal College of Obstetricians and Gynaecologists. The Investigation and Management of the Small-for-Gestational-Age Foetus. Green–top Guideline No. 31. London: RCOG; 2013.
19. Spencer K, Cowans NJ, Avgidou K, Molina F, Nicolaides KH. First-trimester biochemical markers of aneuploidy and the prediction of small-for-gestational age fetuses. Ultrasound Obstet Gynaecol. 2008;31(1):15-9.
20. Lalor JG, Fawole B, Alfirevic Z, Devane D. Biophysical profile for fetal assessment in high risk pregnancies. Cochrane Database Syst Rev. 2008;(1): CD000038.

CHAPTER 38

Foetal Infection

RUBELLA INFECTION IN PREGNANCY

INTRODUCTION

Rubella infection is caused by a single-stranded RNA virus. Rubella has an incubation period of 14–23 days and can be either acquired or congenital.

AETIOLOGY

Acquired infection usually occurs through inhalation. Congenital infection, on the other hand, occurs via transplacental spread. Nearly 80–90% of the individuals become immune by the age of 15 years.[1] About 10–20% of mothers are non-immune and therefore vulnerable to spread the virus to their foetus resulting in congenital infection.

In cases of congenital rubella, the virus spreads to the foetus through the bloodstream, causing death due to infection in early pregnancy; congenital malformations during the first trimester and more subtle damage in later infections. Congenital rubella infection is presumed to cause chromosomal breakages and inhibition of mitoses in infected embryonic cells.

DIAGNOSIS

Clinical Presentation

Acquired infection is usually associated with a mild illness called rubella or German measles. This illness is characterised by mild exanthematous fever, transient macular rash (lasting for ~3 days) and lymphadenopathy. In nearly 50% of the cases, the infection may be subclinical. The viraemia occurs nearly 1 week prior to the occurrence of rash and remains for nearly 12–14 days after its onset. Patients with acute rubella infection can transmit infection to others from around a week before to 4 days after the development of their rash.

Foetal damage caused by maternal rubella is related to the stage of pregnancy. Maternal rubella is associated with low birth weight and prematurity. Transplacental infection if occurring within the first 4 months of pregnancy can be associated with a high incidence of congenital anomalies, such as heart lesions (e.g. patent ductus arteriosus, ventricular septal defects, peripheral pulmonary artery stenosis, etc.), cataracts or congenital glaucoma, sensorineural deafness, pigmentary retinopathy, purpura, splenomegaly, jaundice, microcephaly, mental retardation, meningoencephalitis, radiolucent bone disease, etc. These anomalies constitute the classical congenital rubella syndrome.[2] In fact, rubella is the most common cause of congenital deafness in the developed countries. Foetal infection later in pregnancy may cause isolated deafness.

Pregnancy during which primary rubella infection is contracted has a higher incidence of miscarriage. Thereafter, rubella immunity is developed which protects subsequent pregnancies from this complication. Therefore, rubella infection in pregnancy is rarely associated with recurrent miscarriage.

Investigations

Fluorescent immunoassay techniques: Acute rubella specific immunoglobulin M (IgM) antibodies develop within 2–3 weeks of an acute infection.[3] These antibodies can be detected using fluorescent immunoassay techniques in the foetal blood sample.

Reverse transcriptase-polymerase chain reaction (RT-PCR): This test can be used for the detection of rubella virus RNA using primers.[4]

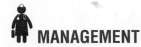
MANAGEMENT

Due to the absence of an antiviral drug for the treatment of rubella infection, the most important way of preventing this infection is prophylaxis against the rubella virus.

Prophylaxis

The disease being so mild, prophylaxis is directed only towards its teratogenic hazard and is therefore relevant only in women of childbearing age. An obvious method of protection is to acquire the infection before puberty. This was achieved by 'rubella parties', formerly practised in Australia, where adolescent girls voluntarily exposed themselves to known rubella cases.

Passive Prophylaxis

There is little evidence that administration of normal human immunoglobulins after contact reduces the risk of maternal rubella and foetal infection. However, this may help attenuate the severity of illness.

Active Prophylaxis

Several live-attenuated rubella vaccines have been developed by serial passage of the virus in tissue culture. The vaccine currently in use is the RA 27/3 strain grown in human diploid cell culture. It is administered by a single subcutaneous injection in the dose of 0.5 mL. The vaccine is available in combination with measles and mumps components as a part of measles, mumps and rubella (MMR) vaccine in the UK. Vaccine-induced immunity persists in most vaccines for at least 14 years and probably is lifelong.

The vaccine virus is apparently not teratogenic. The rubella vaccine contains a live virus with reduced ability to cause disease. Inadvertent administration of the vaccine to a pregnant woman may not therefore lead to congenital defects in the baby. Nevertheless, the vaccine must not be administered during pregnancy. Prophylaxis is relevant only in women of childbearing age and is best carried out by immunisation with a live-attenuated rubella vaccine. This vaccine is also administered to children at 15 months of age as such or in combination (MMR vaccine).

Foetal Management

* If the primary maternal infection has occurred in the first trimester, the woman must be counselled regarding the high risk of development of congenital malformations in the foetus. If the woman desires termination of pregnancy, the procedure can be carried out.
* In case of primary infection acquired between 12 weeks to 18 weeks, the risk of foetal congenital malformations is comparatively lower. This risk reduces to nil after 20 weeks. Therefore, in the second trimester the woman must be counselled for undergoing prenatal diagnostic procedures.[5]

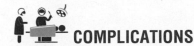
COMPLICATIONS

Complications due to congenital rubella syndrome have been described previously in the text.

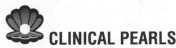
CLINICAL PEARLS

* Primary infection with rubella offers lifelong immunity and therefore congenital malformations are not due to secondary infections.
* Severe mental deficiency is uncommon in cases of congenital rubella infection.
* Multiple congenital defects are common if the transplacental passage of infection to the foetus occurred in the first 8 weeks of gestation.

TOXOPLASMOSIS

INTRODUCTION

Toxoplasmosis is caused by *Toxoplasma gondii,* an obligate intracellular parasite. The cat is the definitive host for this parasite and produces oocysts and sporozoites. The life cycle of *T. gondii* comprises three stages: (1) tachyzoite, (2) bradyzoite and (3) sporozoite. During the acute stage of infection, tachyzoites invade and replicate within cells of various organs such as heart, liver, spleen, lymph nodes, CNS and muscular tissues. Tachyzoites pass transplacentally to the foetus resulting in the congenital infection.[6] Bradyzoites are present in tissue cysts during the latent phase of infection. Sporozoite is the stage, in which the parasite resides within oocysts. When an oocyst is ingested by human or other hosts, sporozoites are released from it. Sporozoites usually infect the epithelial cells before converting to the proliferative tachyzoite stage.

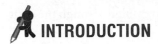
AETIOLOGY

The infection is usually transmitted through ingestion of water, soil, vegetables, or anything contaminated with oocysts shed in the faeces of an infected animal (most often cats) but can also be acquired through consumption of raw or undercooked meat containing *T. gondii* tissue cysts. Infection in the foetus occurs when the mother acquires a primary infection during or shortly before pregnancy. This is particularly the case in the immunocompromised host. Foetuses which acquire infection early in gestation (before 20 weeks of pregnancy) are likely to have more severe infection. Another factor which is likely to affect the disease severity is the parasitic load of the amniotic fluid, with a parasitic load of 1,100 parasites/mL or more in the amniotic fluid responsible for a more severe infection.

CHAPTER 39

PART II

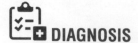

DIAGNOSIS

Clinical Presentation

In adults, it may cause a mild febrile illness resulting in lethargy, malaise and lymphadenopathy. Infection is a serious problem during pregnancy because foetal infection is associated with stillbirth, prematurity, IUGR, hepatitis, thrombocytopenia, neurological (hydrocephaly, microcephaly, etc.) and ophthalmological abnormalities (retinitis). Congenital toxoplasmosis is typically characterised by a triad comprising of chorioretinitis, intracranial calcifications and hydrocephalus.[7]

Investigations

Serological tests: Identification of IgM and immunoglobulin G (IgG) antitoxoplasma antibodies helps in confirming the diagnosis. Since false-positive serological tests may frequently occur, before initiating treatment, these tests must be confirmed at a Toxoplasma reference laboratory using enzyme-linked immunosorbent assay (ELISA) testing.

Infection in the foetus can be identified through the PCR of the amniotic fluid.[8]

MANAGEMENT

❖ Though the greatest risk of transmission to the baby is during the third trimester, disease is most severe when it is acquired during the first trimester.[9] Women in whom the foetus is infected before 20 weeks of gestation, parasite load of 1,100 parasites/mL or more is present in the amniotic fluid and/or there is a presence of foetal abnormalities on ultrasound examination, are more likely to be associated with a severe foetal infection having a poor prognosis. Termination of pregnancy can be considered in such woman, if the mother so desires.

❖ Women who acquire toxoplasmosis infection during pregnancy must be counselled regarding the risk of congenital infection and its clinical sequelae.[10] Pregnant women and other women of childbearing age must be educated about not ingesting raw or undercooked meat and using measures to avoid cross-contamination of other foods with raw or undercooked meat for prevention of congenital toxoplasmosis. They should also be counselled to protect themselves against exposure to cat litter or contaminated soil (e.g. use of gloves or other protective covering).[11]

❖ If the foetus is not infected, acute infection in pregnancy can be treated with spiramycin. However, there is limited evidence indicating the beneficial role of spiramycin in reducing the risk of foetal transmission.[12,13] Treatment with spiramycin should be preferably started within first 4 weeks of infection.[14]

❖ In case the foetus is infected, a combination of sulphadiazine and pyrimethamine may be used. Pyrimethamine is preferably avoided in the first trimester due to the risk of teratogenicity.

COMPLICATIONS

❖ Transmission of *T. gondii* infection to the foetus can result in serious foetal complications, such as mental retardation, seizures, blindness and death.

❖ Some health problems related to *T. gondii* may become apparent in the second or third decade of life.

CLINICAL PEARLS

❖ In the UK, there is no requirement for toxoplasmosis screening program because such a screening program is unlikely to be cost-effective.

❖ Women must be educated to take steps for preventing the spread of infection during pregnancy.

❖ The risk of transmission to the baby is highest during the third trimester. However, disease is most severe when the infection is acquired during the first trimester.

❖ Due to the potential ineffectiveness and risk related to treatment, educating the patient for prevention of infection is of prime importance for reducing the spread of infection.

EVIDENCE-BASED MEDICINE

❖ Though antibiotics (such as spiramycin and sulphonamides) are commonly prescribed to women with toxoplasmosis, the available evidence does not show that these medicines reduce the risk of mother-to-child transmission, or the severity of infection in the baby.[13,14] Moreover, these drugs are likely to have potential adverse toxic effects.

❖ Toxoplasmosis screening programs are not likely to be beneficial in reducing the risk of mother-to-child transmission.[8]

PARVOVIRUS INFECTION

INTRODUCTION

Parvoviruses are the smallest amongst the various DNA viruses (~20 nm). The only virus belonging to this group, which causes human infection, is parvovirus (B19).

AETIOLOGY

The main mode of spread of infection is via respiratory route, i.e. inhalation of the infected droplet. Infected individuals are contagious for about 5–10 days prior to the occurrence of the rash. Blood-borne transmission may also occur at times.

The life cycle of B19 includes binding of the virus to host cell receptors (particularly the P-receptor), internalisation of the virus particle, translocation of the genome to the host nucleus, DNA replication, RNA transcription, assembly of capsids and packaging of the genome and lastly cell lysis with release of the mature virions.

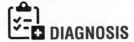

DIAGNOSIS

Clinical Presentation

Human parvovirus B19 may cause respiratory infection with an erythematous maculopapular rash (erythema infectiosum, slapped cheek disease or fifth disease), joint disease, aplastic crisis in children with chronic haemolytic anaemia (sickle cell disease), non-immune foetal hydrops following infection during pregnancy (second or third trimester of pregnancy) and persistent anaemia in immunodeficient individuals.[15] Symptomatic adults may often experience *polyarthropathy syndrome*. Parvovirus infection can cause severe foetal anaemia due to the infection of foetal erythroid progenitor cells, resulting in the shortened half-life of erythrocytes. There may be a transient, but severe pancytopenia. This may also eventually result in high output cardiac failure and non-immune hydrops foetalis (NIHF).[16-23] For details related to the management of NIHF, kindly refer to Chapter 40 (Non-immune Foetal Hydrops). Due to the expression of P antigen on foetal cardiac myocytes, the parvovirus B19 virus is able to infect myocardial cells causing myocarditis, which further aggravates cardiac failure.

Investigations

- *Serology*: This involves the measurement of parvovirus B19-specific IgG and IgM antibodies in the blood. Parvovirus B19 IgM antibodies usually appear within 2–3 days of acute infection and may persist for up to 6 months. On the other hand, parvovirus B19 IgG antibodies appear a few days after the appearance of IgM antibodies. Presence of IgG antibodies implies immunity to the parvovirus B19 infection.
- *Identification of viral DNA*: Viral DNA may also be identified by PCR of amniotic fluid or foetal blood by cordocentesis.
- *Measurement of middle cerebral artery peak systolic velocity*: Middle cerebral artery peak systolic velocity in high-risk pregnancies and in presence of some foetal pathology is an important indicator of foetal anaemia.[24]

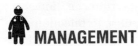

MANAGEMENT

- Pregnancy diagnosed with foetal hydrops should be referred to a tertiary care centre and be preferably managed by a maternal-foetal medicine specialist.
- No specific treatment or prophylaxis is available against B19 infection. Due to the self-limiting nature of parvovirus

infection, nearly 30% cases of hydrops are likely to resolve spontaneously.
- Non-immune mothers must be counselled regarding the risks of infection and methods for preventing them.
- Confirmed maternal infections must be actively monitored.
- Intervention such as correction of foetal anaemia helps in reducing the mortality rate. Cordocentesis must be performed for assessment of foetal haemoglobin levels and measuring the reticulocyte count. In presence of low blood counts, intrauterine transfusion may be performed. The upper limit of gestational age for transfusion varies from case to case and depends on the expertise available at a particular centre.
- Delivery should be considered if the foetus is at or near term. If delivery does not appear to be imminent, amniocentesis for the evaluation of foetal lung maturity may be considered. In case of lung immaturity, corticosteroids can be used for accelerating the lung maturity.

COMPLICATIONS

- Parvovirus B19 infection during the second and third trimesters of pregnancy can result in several harmful effects on the pregnant woman and her foetus.
- Effects may vary from an uncomplicated pregnancy to severe hydrops foetalis or intrauterine foetal death. In the foetus, this can then cause complications such as foetal anaemia, non-immune foetal hydrops and foetal death.
- The multisystem organ damage related to parvovirus B19 infection may result in spontaneous miscarriage, with the rate varying from 15% before 20 weeks of gestation to about 2% after 20 weeks.
- The neonatal complications of maternal parvovirus B19 infection include hepatic insufficiency, myocarditis, transfusion-dependent anaemia, and CNS abnormalities. However, most children born to mothers who develop parvovirus B19 infection in pregnancy do not appear to suffer long-term sequelae. The virus does not appear to cause long-term neurologic morbidity, but severe anaemia may be an independent risk factor for long-term neurologic sequelae. However, further future studies are required in this context.

CLINICAL PEARLS

- The parvovirus itself is not teratogenic agent.
- The risk of adverse foetal outcome due to parvovirus B19 infection is increased if maternal infection occurs during the first two trimesters of pregnancy. However, adverse outcomes can also occur due to infection in the third trimester.
- Risk of transplacental infection increases with the period of gestation, with the risk of transmission being almost 70% in the third trimester.

CHAPTER 39

❖ There occurs a time interval of 4–5 weeks between maternal infection and development of foetal consequences.

EVIDENCE-BASED MEDICINE

❖ Despite the various adverse effects caused by parvovirus, the virus does not appear to be a significant teratogen. Though there have been a few case reports[25,26] showing the association of parvovirus with some anomalies such as craniofacial and ophthalmic anomalies, and anomalies of the CNS, the available evidence does not demonstrate any significant association between parvovirus infection in pregnancy and an increased risk of congenital anomalies in human foetus.

❖ Presently, there are no randomised trials for the evaluation of the best management strategy for cases of foetal hydrops caused by parvovirus B19 infection.[24-26]

CYOTOMEGALOVIRUS INFECTION

INTRODUCTION

Cytomegalovirus (CMV) or HSV-5 is a double-stranded DNA virus belonging to the herpes virus family. CMV causes asymptomatic infection in immunocompetent hosts, with mononucleosis-like syndrome present in only a small percentage of cases. CMV causes latent infection; hence reactivation may result in a severe form of disease in patients who are immunocompromised. Mononucleosis-like syndrome commonly occurs in immunocompromised individuals.

AETIOLOGY

Cytomegalovirus is transmitted both orally and sexually, via blood transfusions, through tissue transplants, in utero, at birth, and by nursing. Infectious CMV may be shed in the bodily fluids of any previously infected person, and thus may be found in urine, saliva, blood, tears, semen and breast milk. CMV can cause congenital CMV infection, acquired CMV infection and infections in immunocompromised and immunocompetent adult hosts. CMV generally causes subclinical infection.

The principal reservoir of infection is small newborn children. The biggest risk is from the baby which is 'symptomatic' at birth following the intrauterine infection.[27] Such babies can excrete the virus for months from their urinary and respiratory tracts. The infected neonate can excrete the virus for 5 years or more. As a result, nurseries are a common source of infection. If the baby is infected in utero, and is born with the signs of infections, he or she is at a high risk of damage. However, if the baby is infected in utero and is born healthy or with no signs of infections, he or she is at a much lower risk of damage. Women seeking to avoid infection are advised to wash themselves carefully after dealing with infected children.

Sexual transmission of the virus can also occur, with infected men excreting the virus in semen for ages. Women should therefore avoid infected partners or ensure that they use condoms. Maternal infection is asymptomatic in 90% of the cases and the features are non-specific. It is not serious for the mother unless she is immunocompromised and usually produces a self-limiting illness with flu-like symptoms.

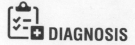

DIAGNOSIS

Clinical Presentation

In adults, the infection may be asymptomatic or result in symptoms such as fever, lymphadenopathy, muscular aches, loss of appetite, weakness, joint stiffness, etc.

Congenital CMV infection which occurs via transplacental passage is the most common congenital infection in the UK and developed part of the world. It may rarely cause lethal infection amongst the neonates. Nearly 5–10% of the congenitally infected babies may have symptoms apparent at birth. The cells of infected organs may show large intra-nuclear inclusions. CMV is a cause of non-immune hydrops due to haemolytic anaemia. Clinical features of congenital CMV infection include features such as microcephaly, sensorineural deafness, hepatosplenomegaly, chorioretinitis, evidence of IUGR, jaundice, skin rashes, echogenic bowel, intracranial calcification, hearing loss, anaemia, prolonged elevation of bilirubin and, rarely, inguinal hernia. Presence of intracranial calcification worsens the long-term prognosis of infected foetuses. Babies who are not symptomatic at birth may later show symptoms such as deafness (sensorineural), developmental delay, mental retardation and visual impairment. The severity of effect of CMV infection on the foetus is not dependent on the gestational age. However, the type of symptoms produced may vary with the gestational age. For example, foetal brain anomalies are more common if the infection occurs in the first trimester, whereas infection later in pregnancy is likely to be associated with symptoms such as hepatitis and thrombocytopenia.

Investigations

❖ *Serological tests*: The ELISA is the most commonly available serologic test for measuring antibodies to CMV. Assessment of the serum antibody levels help in knowing the stage of infection (recent or old) to some extent. Interpretation of IgG and IgM levels in maternal serum can, however, be difficult. IgM is the initial response to infection and is gradually replaced over a period of months by IgG. IgM is large antibody which is unable of crossing the placenta. Thus, in the early days of an infection, the baby gets no help from the maternal response as initially only IgM antibodies are formed which are unable to cross the placenta. Interpretation of anti-CMV antibodies in the serum is described in Table 39.1.[28]

PART II

Table 39.1: Interpretation of anti-cytomegalovirus antibodies in the serum

Antibody present	Interpretation
IgM only	Recent infection
IgG only	Old infection, presence of immunity
IgM + IgG	Recent infection with long-term immunity developing
Neither IgM nor IgG	No immunity

❖ *Identification of the virus*: Viral DNA can be identified in the amniotic fluid using PCR. The virus can also be sought in foetal blood obtained by cordocentesis. However, this is an invasive investigation and is associated with a high risk of foetal loss.

❖ *Histopathological examination*: Presence of 'Owl's-eye' inclusion body and basophilic intranuclear inclusion body on histopathology is the diagnostic feature of the cells infected by CMV.

❖ *Ultrasound examination*: Ultrasound is used for assessing for an evidence of foetal damage. Some of the classical features indicative of CMV infection on ultrasound examination include enlargement of the ventricles, and periventricular leucomalacia and calcification.

❖ *Magnetic resonance imaging*: MRI examination is sometimes performed. Its use, however, has not proved superior to ultrasound. Therefore, it is not recommended for routine use.

MANAGEMENT

❖ Primary maternal infection is immensely more dangerous than reinfection, which rarely occurs. Also, infection early in pregnancy is more likely to cause foetal damage than that occurring during the late pregnancy.

❖ *Vaccination*: Presently, no vaccination is available for CMV infection. CMV glycoprotein B vaccine is under research stages.[29]

❖ No effective foetal therapy is presently available. Antiviral drug such as ganciclovir, administered via IV route can help cause a temporary reduction in the shedding of virus and may also help in the reduction of audiological complications of CMV in some infants.[30] Valganciclovir syrup, prodrug of ganciclovir is associated with high oral bioavailability. It has also been administered orally in home settings.

❖ *Breast feeding*: Breast milk from mothers with primary infection in pregnancy usually contains the virus. However, the benefits of breastfeeding outweigh the risks to the baby. In addition, the mother is likely to transfer some protective IgG to the neonate, especially if she breast feeds. The virus can be transmitted vertically from the mother: across the placenta, directly from the genital tract during delivery and in breast milk.

CLINICAL PEARLS

❖ Screening for CMV infection during pregnancy is not recommended by the RCOG or the Department of Health.

❖ Laboratory diagnosis is used for confirming maternal CMV infection because the infection remains asymptomatic in most of the cases.

❖ Cytomegalovirus infection is one of the main causes of childhood deafness in the UK because MMR vaccination has helped in bringing down the incidence of infections such as measles, mumps and rubella. CMV also ranks second to Down's syndrome as a cause of mental retardation.

❖ Transmission through the breast milk is the most common source of infection of a neonate that was uninfected at birth.

SYPHILIS INFECTION

INTRODUCTION

Syphilis is an STD found worldwide, which only affects humans. Syphilis is a disease of blood vessels and of the perivascular areas. The incubation period is 9–90 days.

AETIOLOGY

Syphilis is an infection that is transmitted sexually. Congenital syphilis in the infant occurs as a result of transplacental transmission of infection. This may occur at any time during the period of gestation. However, the risk of transmission to the foetus depends on the stage of maternal infection. In general, the longer the time period for which the syphilis infection had occurred before pregnancy, the more benign would be disease outcome in the infant with respect to the rate and severity of infection. In the foetus, the skeletal system and the organs such as liver, pancreas, intestine, kidney and spleen are most frequently and severely involved.

DIAGNOSIS

Clinical Presentation

In case of maternal infection, the natural course of syphilis can be divided into primary, secondary and tertiary stages based on the clinical manifestations. The primary lesion in syphilis is the chancre. The chancre is a painless, relatively avascular, circumscribed, indurated, superficially ulcerated lesion. It is covered by a thick, glairy exudate very rich in bacteria. This is known as 'hard chancre' which most frequently occurs on the external genitalia, but it may also occur on the cervix, perianal area, in the mouth or anal canal. The regional lymph nodes become swollen, discrete, rubbery and non-tender. Secondary syphilis sets in 1–3 months after healing of the

PART II

primary lesion. In this stage, patients typically experience a 'flu-like' syndrome, lymphadenopathy, and a generalised mucocutaneous rash. Characteristic lesions of secondary syphilis are roseolar or papular skin rashes, *mucous* patches in the oropharynx and condylomata at the mucocutaneous junctions. For further details related to clinical presentation in cases of syphilis, kindly refer to Chapter 89 (Sexually Transmitted Infections).

Congenital syphilis could be either early or late. In early congenital syphilis, disease manifestations usually occur prior to 2 years of life. On the other hand, in cases of late syphilis, disease manifestations occur after 2 years of life. The severity of the manifestations is variable and can range from isolated abnormalities to fulminant involvement of multiple organ systems in cases of congenital syphilis. Amongst symptomatic infants, the most common clinical findings include the following: hepatomegaly, jaundice, rhinitis (nasal snuffles), rashes, generalised lymphadenopathy, skeletal abnormalities, etc.[31] Infected infants may suffer severe sequelae, including cerebral palsy, hydrocephalus, sensorineural hearing loss and musculoskeletal deformity. All these sequelae can be prevented with timely treatment during pregnancy.

Investigations

Diagnosis of the Mother

Two major types of serologic tests for syphilis exist: non-treponemal tests and treponemal tests. In non-treponemal tests or standard tests for syphilis (STS), cardiolipin or lipoidal antigen is used. Non-treponemal tests are flocculation tests and include VDRL test and rapid plasma reagin (RPR). On the other hand, treponemal tests are those in which treponemes are used as the antigen. These tests may use live *T. pallidum* strains (e.g. *T. pallidum* immobilisation test), killed *T. pallidum* (e.g. *T. pallidum* agglutination test, *T. pallidum* immune adherence test, and fluorescent treponema antibody test), or *T. pallidum* extracts as antigens (e.g. *T. pallidum* haemagglutination test and enzyme immunoassay).

Diagnosis of the Foetus

- *Serological tests*: It can be used for detecting the presence of the foetal syphilis-specific IgM antibodies in the foetal blood sample.
- *Identification of the treponemal DNA*: DNA of *T. pallidum* can also be detected by performing PCR in the amniotic fluid.
- *Ultrasound examination*: Features suggestive of congenital syphilis infection, which can be identified on ultrasound examination, include hepatomegaly, foetal hydrops, dilatation of the loops of small intestine, etc.[32]

MANAGEMENT

- Penicillin is the drug of choice for treating maternal infections with *T. pallidum*. So far, there have been no reports of penicillin-resistance. Serological tests must be performed at monthly intervals to evaluate the efficacy of treatment.

- Presently, no treatment is available for the infected foetus.[33] Foetal termination can be considered following discussion with the parents.

COMPLICATIONS

- Congenital syphilis remains the major cause of perinatal mortality and morbidity world-wide.
- It can result in the development of foetal complications such as cerebral palsy, hydrocephalus, sensorineural hearing loss, musculoskeletal deformity, etc.

CLINICAL PEARLS

- Women with untreated primary or secondary syphilis are more likely to transmit syphilis to their foetuses in comparison to the women with latent disease.
- Transplacental spread of syphilis infection can also occur when the disease is in its latent stage and there is absence of any clinical manifestations.
- Syphilis is the most important cause of foetal growth restriction and foetal hydrops, all across the world.[34]

REFERENCES

1. Freij BJ, South MA, Sever JL. Maternal rubella and the congenital rubella syndrome. Clin Perinatol. 1988;15(2):247-57.
2. Andrade JQ, Bunduki V, Curti SP, Figueiredo CA, de Oliveira MI, Zugaib M. Rubella in pregnancy: intrauterine transmission and perinatal outcome during a Brazilian epidemic. J Clin Virol. 2006;35(3):285-91.
3. Cradock-Watson JE. Laboratory diagnosis of rubella: past, present and future. Epidemiol Infect. 1991;107(1):1-15.
4. Bosma TJ, Corbett KM, O'Shea S, Banatvala JE, Best JM. PCR for detection of rubella virus RNA in clinical samples. J Clin Microbiol. 1995;33(5):1075-9.
5. Tang JW, Aarons E, Hesketh LM, Strobel S, Schalasta G, Jauniaux E, et al. Prenatal diagnosis of congenital rubella infection in the second trimester of pregnancy. Prenat Diagn. 2003;23(6):509-12.
6. Alford CA, Stagno S, Reynolds DW. Congenital toxoplasmosis: clinical, laboratory, and therapeutic considerations, with special reference to subclinical disease. Bull NY Acad Med. 1974;50(2):160-81.
7. Kimball AC, Kean BH, Fuchs F. Congenital toxoplasmosis: a prospective study of 4,048 obstetric patients. Am J Obstet Gynecol. 1971;111(2):211-8.
8. Guerina NG, Hsu HW, Meissner HC, Maguire JH, Lynfield R, Stechenberg B, et al. Neonatal serologic screening and early treatment for congenital Toxoplasma gondii infection. The New England Regional Toxoplasma Working Group. N Engl J Med. 1994;330(26):1858-63.
9. Wilson M, McAuley JM. Toxoplasma. In: Murray PR, Pfaller MA, Baron EJ (Eds). Manual of Clinical Microbiology, 7th edition. Washington, DC: American Society for Microbiology; 1999. pp. 1374-82.

10. Lynfield R, Guerina NG. Toxoplasmosis. Pediatr Rev. 1997; 18(3):75-83.

11. Dubey JP. Toxoplasmosis. J Am Vet Med Assoc. 1994;205(11): 1593-8.

12. Peyron F, Wallon M, Liou C, Garner P. Treatments for toxoplasmosis in pregnancy. Cochrane Database Syst Rev. 2000;(2): CD001684.

13. Dunn D, Wallon M, Peyron F, Petersen E, Peckham C, Gilbert R. Mother-to-child transmission of toxoplasmosis: risk estimates for clinical counselling. Lancet. 1999;353(9167):1829-33.

14. Budanov SV. [Spiramycin (Rovamycin) in the treatment of toxoplasmosis in pregnancy]. [Article in Russian]. Antibiot Khimioter. 2001;46(4):38-41.

15. Heegaard ED, Brown KE. Human Parvovirus B19. Clin Microbiol Rev. 2002;15(3):485-505.

16. Public Health Laboratory Service Working Party Fifth Disease. Prospective study of human parvovirus infection in pregnancy. Br Med J. 1990;300:1166-70.

17. Miller E, Fairley CK, Cohen BJ, Seng C. Immediate and long-term outcome of human parvovirus B19 infection in pregnancy. Br J Obstet Gynaecol. 1998;105(2):174-8.

18. Rodis JF, Quinn DL, Gary GW, Anderson LJ, Rosengren S, Cartter M, et al. Management and outcomes of pregnancies complicated by human B19 parvovirus infection: a prospective study. Am J Obstet Gynecol. 1990;163(4 Pt 1):1168-71.

19. Centers for Disease Control (CDC). Risks associated with human parvovirus B19 infection. MMWR Morb Mortal Wkly Rep. 1989;38(6):81-97.

20. Harger JH, Alder SP, Koch WC, Harger GF. Prospective evaluation of 618 pregnant women exposed to parvovirus B19: risks and symptoms. Obstet Gynecol. 1998;91(3):413-20.

21. Gratacos E, Torres PJ, Vidal J, Antolin E, Costa J, Jimenez de Anta MT, et al. The incidence of human parvovirus B19 infection during pregnancy and its impact on perinatal outcome. J Infect Dis. 1995;171(5):1360-3.

22. Guidozzi F, Ballot D, Rothberg A. Human B19 parvovirus infection in an obstetric population – a prospective study determining fetal outcome. J Reprod Med. 1994;39(1):36-8.

23. Rodis JF, Rodner C, Hansen AA, Borgida AF, Deoliveira I, Rosengren SS. Long-term outcome of children following maternal human parvovirus B19 infection. Obstet Gynecol. 1998;91(1):125-8.

24. de Jong EP, de Haan TR, Kroes AC, Beersma MF, Oepkes D, Walther FJ. Parvovirus B19 infection in pregnancy. J Clin Virol. 2006;36(1):1-7.

25. Levy R, Weissman A, Blomberg G, Hagay ZJ. Infection by parvovirus B19 during pregnancy: a review. Obstet Gynecol Surv. 1997;52(4):254-9.

26. Markenson GR, Yancey MK. Parvovirus B19 infection in pregnancy. Semin Perinatol. 1998;22(4):309-17.

27. Yinon Y, Farine D, Yudin MH, Gagnon R, Hudon L, Basso M, et al. Cytomegalovirus infection in pregnancy. J Obstet Gynaecol Can. 2010;32(4):348-54.

28. Lombardi G, Garofoli F, Stronati M. Congenital cytomegalovirus infection: treatment, sequelae and follow-up. J Matern Fetal Neonatal Med. 2010;23 Suppl 3:45-8.

29. Buonsenso D, Serranti D, Gargiullo L, Ceccarelli M, Ranno O, Valentini P. Congenital cytomegalovirus infection: current strategies and future perspectives. Eur Rev Med Pharmacol Sci. 2012;16(7):919-35.

30. Lackner A, Acham A, Alborno T, Moser M, Engele H, Raggam RB, et al. Effect on hearing of ganciclovir therapy for asymptomatic congenital cytomegalovirus infection: four to 10 year follow up. J Laryngol Otol. 2009;123(4):391-6.

31. Lago EG, Vaccari A, Fiori RM. Clinical features and follow-up of congenital syphilis. Sex Transm Dis. 2013;40(2):85-94.

32. Zenker PN, Berman SM. Congenital syphilis: trends and recommendations for evaluation and management. Pediatr Infect Dis J. 1991;10(7):516-22.

33. Rathbun KC. Congenital syphilis. Sex Transm Dis. 1983;10(2): 93-9.

34. Walker GJ, Walker DG. Congenital syphilis: A continuing but a neglected problem. Semin Fetal Neonatal Med. 2007;12(3): 198-206.

CHAPTER 39

Non-immune Foetal Hydrops

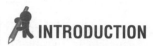 INTRODUCTION

Hydrops foetalis refers to abnormal collection of fluid in the foetal soft tissues and serous cavities. This condition is characterised by oedema in the skin and serous effusion in two or more body cavities. Hydrops foetalis is further classified as immune or non-immune hydrops foetalis (NIHF). While immune hydrops foetalis comprises of cases due to red cell alloimmunisation [e.g. Rh(D), Kell, etc.], NIHF comprises the subgroup of cases not caused by red cell alloimmunisation. For details related to immune hydrops, kindly refer to Chapter 26 (Rhesus Isoimmunisation). The widespread use of Rh(D) immune globulins in the UK has resulted in a drastic decline in the prevalence of Rh(D) alloimmunisation and associated hydrops. As a result, NIHF now accounts for almost 90% of hydrops cases.[1] The prevalence of NIHF ranges from 1/1,500 births to 1/3,800 births.[1-5]

AETIOLOGY

The pathogenesis of NIHF is not completely understood. Fluid homeostasis within the vascular and interstitial compartments is controlled by both hydrostatic and osmotic pressures as defined by the Starling equation. Several mechanisms at the macrovascular level are responsible for regulating the movement of fluid movement across the transmembraneous pathways. Various factors are responsible for dysregulation of the net fluid movement between the vascular and interstitial spaces and can include one of the following mechanisms caused by foetal disorders resulting in NIHF:[6]

❖ Obstructed or reduced lymphatic drainage in the thoracic and abdominal cavities
❖ Increased intravascular hydrostatic pressure
❖ Increased central venous pressure (CVP)
❖ Decreased intravascular oncotic pressure
❖ Increased interstitial oncotic pressure.

A disturbance in one of these factors may be responsible for development of foetal hydrops. Further research is required to understand the complex interplay between foetal cardiac dysfunction, maintenance of intravascular volume and increased CVP, role played by neural and circulating plasma proteins and hormones, and their respective contributions towards the development of foetal hydrops.

Disorders Associated with Non-immune Hydrops Foetalis

Foetal disorders associated with NIHF can be categorised into several groups (e.g. chromosomal, haematologic, cardiovascular, thoracic, infectious, etc.). Many of these disorders are listed in the Table 40.1. The probable aetiology behind NIHF may vary with the period of gestation. NIHF prior to 24 weeks of gestation is usually related to an aneuploidy, while majority of cases after 24 weeks of gestation may be related to cardiac (structural defects and rhythm disturbances), pulmonary and infectious aetiologies.[7,8] Homozygous α-thalassaemia is the most common cause of foetal hydrops in the Southeast Asia. However, this is an uncommon cause of this condition in the UK. In UK, causes such as aneuploidy, structural abnormalities and parvovirus infection are more commonly responsible for causing NIHF.

DIAGNOSIS

Clinical Presentation

Maternal Findings

Women carrying a hydropic foetus may have uterine size large for dates and may feel decreased foetal movements. Although hydrops is essentially a foetal condition, in many cases there may be associated maternal findings, such as theca lutein cysts, pre-eclampsia, anaemia, preterm labour and generalised oedema with or without pre-eclampsia (i.e. mirror syndrome). NIHF may also be associated with polyhydramnios and placental thickening.

Polyhydramnios: Polyhydramnios is generally defined as an AFI greater than 24 cm or a maximum vertical pocket greater than 8 cm.[9] It may be present in up to 75% of pregnancies complicated by NIHF. For details related to polyhydramnios, kindly refer to Chapter 32 (Liquor Abnormalities).

Table 40.1: Causes of non-immune foetal hydrops

Cardiovascular	Aneuploidy and structural abnormalities of chromosomes	Haematologic

Structural malformation
• Left heart hypoplasia
• Atrioventricular (AV) canal defect
• Right heart hypoplasia
• Closure of foramen ovale
• Single ventricle
• Transposition of the great arteries
• Ventricular septal defect
• Atrial septal defect
• Tetralogy of fallot
• Ebstein's anomaly
• Premature closure of ductus
• Truncus arteriosus
• Aortic or pulmonary stenosis
• Valvular insufficiency
Arrhythmia
• Tachyarrhythmia
  – Atrial flutter
  – Paroxysmal atrial tachycardia
  – Wolff-Parkinson-White syndrome
  – Supraventricular tachycardia
• Bradyarrhythmia including complete heart block
• Other arrhythmias (e.g. long QT)
High-output failure
• Neuroblastoma
• Sacrococcygeal teratoma
• Large foetal angioma
• Placental chorioangioma
• Umbilical cord haemangioma
Cardiac tumours
Other cardiac neoplasia
Cardiomyopathy
Cardiosplenic syndromes
	• 45, X
	• Trisomy 21
	• Trisomy 18
	• Trisomy 13
	• 18q$^+$
	• 13q$^-$
	• 45, X mosaic
	• Triploidy
	• 17q$^-$
	• Duplicated 11p
		• α-thalassaemia
		• Foetomaternal transfusion
		• Parvovirus B19 infection
		• In utero haemorrhage
		• Glucose-6-phosphate dehydrogenase (G6PD) deficiency
		• Red cell enzyme deficiencies
		• Thrombosis of major vessels
		• Leukaemia
		• Red cell aplasias
		• Pyruvate kinase deficiency

Thoracic	**Infections**	**Chondrodysplasias**
• Congenital cystic adenomatoid malformation of lung • Diaphragmatic hernia • Intrathoracic mass • Pulmonary sequestration • Chylothorax • Airway obstruction • Pulmonary lymphangiectasia • Pulmonary neoplasia • Bronchogenic cyst	• Parvovirus B19 (fifth disease) • Cytomegalovirus (CMV) • Toxoplasmosis • Syphilis • Herpes • Rubella • Coxsackievirus • Leptospirosis • *Trypanosoma cruzi*	• Thanatophoric dysplasia • Short rib polydactyly • Hypophosphatasia • Osteogenesis imperfecta • Achondrogenesis • Campomelic dysplasia • Lethal chondroplasia • Homozygous achondroplasia
Twin pregnancy	**Gastrointestinal**	**Urinary**
• Twin-twin transfusion syndrome (TTTS) • Acardiac twin	• Midgut volvulus • Malrotation of the intestines • Duplication of the intestinal tract • Meconium peritonitis • Hepatic fibrosis • Cholestasis • Biliary atresia • Hepatic vascular malformations • Hepatitis • Hepatic necrosis • Liver tumours or cysts	• Urethral stenosis or atresia • Posterior urethral valves • Congenital nephrosis (Finnish type) • Prune belly syndrome

Contd...

Contd...

Malformation sequences and genetic syndromes	Metabolic	Foetal/placental vascular tumours
• Congenital lymphoedema, e.g. Noonan's syndrome • Arthrogryposis • Multiple pterygium syndrome • Neu-Laxova syndrome • Pena-Shokeir syndrome • Myotonic dystrophy • Saldino-Noonan syndrome • Francois syndrome, type III • Familial Nuchal Bleb • Acrocephalopolydactylous dysplasia (Elejalde syndrome) • Thoracoabdominal syndrome • Lymphoedema distichiasis syndrome	• Gaucher's disease • GM$_1$ gangliosidosis • Sialidosis • Hurler syndrome • Mucopolysaccharidosis (MPS) IVa • Mucolipidosis type I+II • Galactosialidosis	*Foetal tumours* • Sacrococcygeal mediastinal or pharyngeal teratoma • Neuroblastoma • Large haemangiomas • Foetal tuberous sclerosis • Foetal tumours obstructing the vena cava, portal vein, or femoral vessels *Tumours of placenta/cord* • Chorioangiomas of the placenta (>4–5 cm in diameter) • Angiomyxoma, aneurysm, venous thrombosis • Umbilical vein torsion • True knots in the cord • Amniotic bands of the umbilical cord

Placental thickening: The placenta may appear thickened due to intravillous oedema. A placental thickness greater than or equal to 4 cm in the second trimester and greater than or equal to 6 cm in the third trimester is considered abnormal and should prompt further investigation.[10,11]

Mirror syndrome: Mirror syndrome (also called Ballantynes syndrome or triple oedema) refers to an unusual association of foetal and placental hydrops with maternal pre-eclampsia.[12] This condition is characterised by generalised maternal oedema, often in association with pulmonary involvement, which 'mirrors' the oedema of the hydropic foetus and placenta, thereby referring to the similarity between maternal oedema and foetal hydrops. Although usually associated with NIHF, this can also occur with immune-mediated hydrops. The pathogenesis of this syndrome remains unknown. Mirror syndrome can occur any time during the antepartum period and may persist during the postpartum period.[13] It may present with rapid onset of symptoms suggestive of pre-eclampsia such as weight gain, increasing peripheral oedema, progressive shortness of breath, etc. In mirror syndrome, the maternal haematocrit is often low in comparison to the high haematocrit or haemoconcentration in pre-eclampsia. Also, the amniotic fluid volume is often high (polyhydramnios) in comparison to oligohydramnios encountered in cases of pre-eclampsia. The foetus nearly always shows signs of hydrops.[14,15] Delivery is usually required to induce remission of maternal symptoms.

Investigations

Ultrasound Examination

The prenatal diagnosis of hydrops foetalis is based on ultrasound examination that shows two or more of the following foetal findings:

❖ *Ascites*: In its early stage, foetal ascites appears as a rim of echolucent fluid just interior to the abdominal wall or surrounding the bladder or liver.

❖ *Pleural effusion*: It may appear as a rim of echolucent fluid just interior to the chest wall, outlining the lungs. Persistent effusion that develops before 20 weeks of gestation may cause compression of the lung tissue, thereby retarding the growth and development of the lungs, resulting in the development of pulmonary hypoplasia. This may prove to be fatal in the neonatal period.

❖ *Pericardial effusions*: They appear as a rim of echolucent fluid surrounding the heart, which is usually visualised on the M-mode ultrasound.[2] Thickness of pericardial fluid greater than 2 mm, which increases on serial examinations, is suggestive of a pathologic aetiology.

❖ *Skin oedema (>5 mm)*: This is a late sign of foetal hydrops. Pathologic skin oedema has been defined as the thickness of subcutaneous tissues on the chest or scalp greater than 5 mm.[9]

Maternal Tests

Some tests must also be performed on the mother to identify the underlying cause of hydrops. These include indirect Coombs test (for identification of atypical antibodies), full blood counts, haemoglobin electrophoresis and TORCH titres. In selective cases, carrier status of glucose-6-phosphate dehydrogenase (G6PD) and pyruvate kinase can also be determined.

MANAGEMENT

Management in the Antenatal Period

❖ *Identification of underlying cause of hydrops*: An effort must be made by the clinician to determine the aetiology of hydrops at the time of diagnosis, since several aetiologies can be confirmed or omitted based upon the findings on ultrasound examination. The cause of hydrops can be determined prenatally or postnatally in 60–85% of cases. An attempt must be made to identify those cases caused by disorders which are treatable in utero by performing the following steps:

• Detailed family history: A genetic counsellor can be helpful in obtaining thorough history from the patient. The patient's ethnic background and personal and family history must be reviewed in order to identify any heritable disorders associated with hydrops, such as α-thalassaemia, inborn errors of metabolism and genetic syndromes. History of exposure to recent infection, particularly parvovirus infection must also be taken.[16]

- Sonography: Performing a thorough sonogram of the foetus, placenta, umbilical cord and amniotic fluid to look for causes of NIHF (e.g. foetal or placental structural abnormalities, arrhythmias, TTTS, etc.).
- Foetal echocardiogram: A foetal echocardiogram should be performed as it may detect previously unrecognised cardiac abnormalities. Atrial and ventricular rate and the heart rhythm must be evaluated on echocardiography.[17]
- Doppler assessment: Assessment of the peak systolic velocity (PSV) of foetal middle cerebral artery (MCA) on Doppler ultrasound helps in the evaluation of foetal anaemia. This has emerged as an accurate non-invasive tool for predicting foetal anaemia of any aetiology (whether immune or non-immune).[18,19] If MCA-PSV is elevated (>1.5 multiples of the median for the gestational age), the exact cause of the anaemia needs to be determined.
- Haemoglobin and haematocrit: Diagnosis of anaemia may be essential, because foetal anaemia is most likely to result in hydrops when the haemoglobin concentration becomes less than or equal to 5 g/dL. This usually corresponds to a haematocrit of less than 30%.[18]
- Complete blood count with red blood cell indices: A MCV less than 80 fL in the absence of iron deficiency is suggestive of thalassaemia. The father's MCV should also be determined. If MCV of both the parents is less than 80 fL, additional studies may be required. Haemoglobin electrophoresis helps in identifying the carriers of haemoglobin variants and β-thalassaemia. However, DNA-based genotyping is generally necessary to rule out α-thalassaemia in Asian couples. In these cases, haemoglobin electrophoresis is not recommended because it is non-diagnostic of α-thalassaemia.
- Blood type and antibody screen: A positive screen for antibodies directed against red cell antigens is suggestive of immune-mediated foetal anaemia.
- Kleihauer-Betke acid-elution smear or flow cytometry: This helps in detection of significant foetomaternal haemorrhage in case it had occurred.[10,20]
- Genetic testing: Foetuses with structural abnormalities should undergo genetic testing to identify an abnormal karyotype, if present. Karyotyping is mandatory in these cases. The samples can be obtained by amniocentesis, chorionic villus (placental) biopsy or foetal blood sampling.
- Serology: Maternal IgM and immunoglobulin G (IgG) serologies help in detecting the most common infectious causes of NIHF: parvovirus B19, cytomegalovirus (CMV), and toxoplasmosis. Foetal hydrops is also a characteristic finding of congenital syphilis. Therefore, a non-treponemal antibody test [e.g. VDRL test, Rapid Plasma Reagin (RPR) test should be obtained if not previously performed as part of routine prenatal care.

- Amniotic fluid analysis: At least 10 mL of amniotic fluid is required for PCR analysis for infections such as CMV, parvovirus B19 and toxoplasmosis.[1,21]

❖ *Multidisciplinary management*: Multidisciplinary team involving maternal-foetal medicine specialists and neonatologists should be involved in the management of these pregnancies.

❖ *Maternal surveillance*: Close monitoring of the maternal status is also important due to the increased risks of mirror syndrome.

❖ *Antepartum foetal surveillance*: In the absence of a lethal aetiology of NIHF, NST or foetal BPP must be done at least weekly. Delivery must be undertaken if there is evidence of foetal decompensation at a viable gestational age.
- Doppler assessment of the umbilical vein is performed because development of umbilical venous pulsations in hydropic foetuses is an ominous finding associated with foetal demise in over 70% of patients.
- Doppler velocimetry of the uterine artery is not useful in the absence of foetal growth restriction.
- Serial Doppler velocimetry of the MCA is also not useful in the absence of suspected foetal anaemia.

Management in the Intrapartum Period

❖ *Antenatal consultation*: Antenatal consultations with relevant subspecialty services (e.g. neonatology, foetal medicine) should be obtained. This may guide the clinician to make decisions regarding the appropriate extent of foetal monitoring and intervention.

❖ *Patient counselling*: Pregnancy counselling and management are dependent on the aetiology and severity of NIHF and whether it is possible to treat it successfully. Counselling should include a discussion of the potential risks and benefits of the available interventions versus expectant management. The patient should be counselled taking into account the severity of the underlying condition and the anticipated response to the intervention.

❖ *Antenatal surveillance*: In the absence of a lethal aetiology of NIHF, antenatal surveillance is generally performed because these pregnancies may be at a high risk of foetal death. In some cases early foetal delivery may be required. Methods for foetal surveillance in the antenatal period have previously been described.

❖ *Foetal therapy*: Urgent treatment must be instituted in case of conditions which are amenable to foetal therapy. Referral to a tertiary foetal medicine unit may be required. Termination of pregnancy can be considered as an option in cases where foetal prognosis appears poor. For cases in which the aetiology is not known and the prognosis appears uncertain, options which can be considered include antepartum monitoring with active intervention in case of foetal deterioration versus supportive therapy.

❖ *Corticosteroids*: Antepartum or intrapartum corticosteroid therapy is indicated if the gestational age is between 24 weeks to 34 weeks, the underlying aetiology of the hydrops is not believed to be lethal, and foetal delivery is planned in case there is deterioration of the foetal condition.[17]

CHAPTER 40

❖ *Timing of delivery*: Delivery of potentially viable neonates should occur at a tertiary care centre by a multidisciplinary team comprising of an obstetrician, maternal-foetal medicine specialist, neonatologist and paediatric sub-specialists. Elective preterm delivery prior to 34 weeks is associated with poor prognosis and should be avoided in the absence of deterioration in maternal or foetal status. However, delivery may be required if there is deterioration of maternal or foetal condition or there is worsening of NIHF in a pregnancy that has reached 34 weeks of gestation. However, in the absence of clinical deterioration or other indication for earlier intervention, the patient should be preferably delivered at 37–38 weeks.[17]

❖ *Mode of delivery*: Vaginal delivery is preferred if the foetal prognosis is poor and the clinician is unlikely to use any neonatal interventions. Caesarean birth is performed for routine obstetrical indications. However, caesarean delivery may be commonly required due to sudden deterioration in the foetal condition during the antenatal period or due to high frequency of occurrence of category II and III FHR patterns during the intrapartum period in the foetus which appears salvageable.

❖ *Stillborns and neonates*: Autopsy is recommended for all cases of foetal or neonatal deaths or pregnancy terminations associated with NIHF. Consultation with a medical geneticist is also advisable.

Treatment of the Underlying Condition

❖ *Foetal anaemia*: It can be treated by in utero IV transfusion.[22,23] This is the treatment of choice in case of immune hydrops where the foetuses are affected by red-cell alloimmunisation.

❖ *Treatment of foetal arrhythmias*: Arrhythmias of the foetal heart can be treated by either indirect administration or the direct administration of specific cardiotrophic drugs.

❖ *Treatment of pleural effusion*: This can be treated by pleuroamniotic shunting.[24,25]

❖ *Treatment of twin-twin transfusion*: Such cases can be treated by serial amnioreduction or direct foetoscopic laser ablation of the communicating placental vessels.

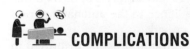

COMPLICATIONS

Some complications associated with NIHF are described in Table 40.2.

CLINICAL PEARLS

❖ The risk of recurrent NIHF can be high when hydrops has a genetic basis.

❖ Ultrasound-guided percutaneous in utero needle aspiration of a large collection of pleural fluid and/or ascites prior to delivery may reduce the risk of dystocia and facilitate neonatal resuscitation.

Table 40.2: Complications associated with non-immune hydrops

Antenatal period	Intrapartum period	Postpartum period
• Spontaneous or indicated preterm birth • Severe polyhydramnios • Maternal respiratory symptoms, which may require treatment or necessitate delivery • High foetal mortality rates	Shoulder dystocia	• Increased risk for retained placenta • Postpartum haemorrhage

❖ Non-immune hydrops foetalis is associated with an overall perinatal mortality rate of 50–98%.[2,3,20,26] Despite advances in foetal diagnosis and therapy, the mortality rate has not changed substantially over the past 15 years.

EVIDENCE-BASED MEDICINE

Anaemia caused by parvovirus infection is potentially the most treatable cause of NIHF. However, RCTs are required in future to be able to completely prove this.[23,27,28]

REFERENCES

1. Bellini C, Hennekam RC. Non-immune hydrops fetalis: a short review of etiology and pathophysiology. Am J Med Genet A. 2012;158A(3):597-605.
2. Pasman SA, Meerman RH, Vandenbussche FP, Oepkes D. Hypoalbuminemia: a cause of fetal hydrops? Am J Obstet Gynecol. 2006;194(4):972-5.
3. Takci S, Gharibzadeh M, Yurdakok M, Ozyuncu O, Korkmaz A, Akcoren Z, et al. Etiology and outcome of hydrops fetalis: report of 62 cases. Pediatr Neonatol. 2013;55(2):108-13.
4. Lin SM, Wang CH, Zhu XY, Li SL, Lin SM, Fang Q. Clinical study on 156 cases with hydrops fetalis. Zhonghua Fu Chan Ke Za Zhi. 2011;46(12):905-10.
5. Pfister KM, Schleiss MR, Reed RC, George TN. Non-immune hydrops fetalis caused by herpes simplex virus type 2 in the setting of recurrent maternal infection. J Perinatol. 2013; 33(10):817-20.
6. Essary LR, Vnencak-Jones CL, Manning SS, Olson SJ, Johnson JE. Frequency of parvovirus B19 infection in nonimmune hydrops fetalis and utility of three diagnostic methods. Hum Pathol. 1998;29(7):696-701.
7. Gest AL, Martin CG, Moise AA, Hansen TN. Reversal of venous blood flow with atrial tachycardia and hydrops in fetal sheep. Pediatr Res. 1990;28(3):223-6.
8. Giacoia GP. Severe fetomaternal hemorrhage: a review. Obstet Gynecol Surv. 1997;52(6):372-80.
9. Matsubara S, Ohmaru T, Ohkuchi A, Arai F, Kuwata T, Usui R, et al. Mirror syndrome associated with hydropic acardius in triplet pregnancy. Fetal Diagn Ther. 2008;24(4):429-33.
10. Liley AW. Liquor amnii analysis in the management of the pregnancy complicated by Rhesus sensitization. Am J Obstet Gynecol. 1961;82(6):1359-70.
11. Maternal-Fetal Medicine Committee, Clinical Practice Obstetrics Committee, Leduc L, Farine D, Armson BA, Brunner M,

PART II

et al. Stillbirth and bereavement: guidelines for stillbirth investigation. J Obstet Gynaecol Can. 2006;28(6):540-52.

12. Paternoster DM, Manganelli F, Minucci D, Nanhornguè KN, Memmo A, Bertoldini M, et al. Ballantyne Syndrome: a Case Report. Fetal Diagn Ther. 2006;21(1):92-5.

13. Nakamura K, Itoh H, Sagawa N, Kakui K, Nakayama T, Yamada S, et al. A case of peripartum cardiomyopathy with a transient increase of plasma interleukin-6 concentration occurred following mirror syndrome. J Perinat Med. 2002;30:426-8.

14. Andres RL, Brace RA. The development of hydrops fetalis in the ovine fetus after lymphatic ligation or lymphatic excision. Am J Obstet Gynecol. 1990;162(5):1331-4.

15. Aubard Y, Derouineau I, Aubard V, Chalifour V, Preux PM. Primary fetal hydrothorax: A literature review and proposed antenatal clinical strategy. Fetal Diagn Ther. 1998;13(6):325-33.

16. Daniel SJ, Cassady G. Non-immunologic hydrops fetalis associated with a large hemangioendothelioma. Pediatrics. 1968;42(5):828-33.

17. Brans YW, Milstead RR, Bailey PE, Cassady G. Blood-volume estimates in Coombs-test-positive infants. N Engl J Med. 1974;290(26):1450-2.

18. Carlson DE, Platt LD, Medearis AL, Horenstein J. Prognostic indicators of the resolution of nonimmune hydrops fetalis and survival of the fetus. Am J Obstet Gynecol. 1990;163(6 Pt 1): 1785-7.

19. Cowan RH, Waldo AL, Harris HB, Cassady G, Brans YW. Neonatal paroxysmal supraventricular tachycardia with hydrops. Pediatrics. 1975;55(3):428-30.

20. De Groot CJ, Oepkes D, Egberts J, Kanhai HH. Evidence of endothelium involvement in the pathophysiology of hydrops fetalis? Early Hum Dev. 2000;57(3):205-9.

21. Dumez Y, Mandelbrot L, Radunovic N, Révillon Y, Dommergues M, Aubry MC, et al. Prenatal management of congenital cystic adenomatoid malformation of the lung. J Pediatr Surg. 1993;28(1):36-41.

22. Montogomery LD, Belfort MA, Adam K. Massive foetal-maternal haemorrhage treated with serial combined intravenous and intraperitoneal fetal transfusions. Am J Obstet Gynecol. 1995;173(1):234-5.

23. Fairley CK, Smoleniec JS, Caul OE, Miller E. Observational study of the effect of intrauterine transfusions on the outcome of fetal hydrops after parvovirus B19 infection. Lancet. 1995;346(8986):1335-7.

24. Rodeck CH, Fisk NM, Fraser DI, Nicolini U. Long-term in utero drainage of foetal hydrothorax. N Engl J Med. 1988;319(17): 1135-8.

25. Chan V, Greenough A, Nicolaides KN. Antenatal and postnatal treatment of pleural effusion and extralobar pulmonary sequesteration. J Perinat Med. 1996;24(4):335-8.

26. Graves GR, Baskett TF. Nonimmune hydrops fetalis: antenatal diagnosis and management. Am J Obstet Gynecol. 1984;148(5): 563-5.

27. Simms RA, Liebling RE, Patel RR, Denbow ML, Abdel-Fattah SA, Soothill PW, et al. Management and outcome of pregnancies with parvovirus B19 infection over seven years in a tertiary fetal medicine unit. Fetal Diagn Ther. 2009;25(4): 373-8.

28. Odibo AO, Campbell WA, Feldman D, Ling PY, Leo MV, Borgida AF, et al. Resolution of human parvovirus B19-induced nonimmune hydrops after intrauterine transfusion. J Ultrasound Med. 1998;17(9):547-50.

Foetal Anomalies and Their Management

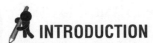 INTRODUCTION

Congenital defects can be considered as the most important cause of foetal anomalies. These anomalies are responsible for the death of nearly 303,000 newborn children worldwide, within 4 weeks of birth.[1] They also can be an important cause of long-term disability which can have a significant impact on the individuals, families, healthcare system as well as the society as a whole. During the last few decades, the use of ultrasonography for the detection of foetal abnormalities has become widespread in many parts of the world. This has enabled an early diagnosis of the congenital abnormalities in infants during the prenatal period. This has resulted in major repercussions for both clinicians and the involved parents. Several options for the obstetric management are possible in these cases, ranging from standard care and continuation of pregnancy to the termination of pregnancy. The statistics by Department of Health related to the number of abortions performed in the year 2008, shows that nearly 200,000 abortions were performed amongst the women aged 15–44 years in England and Wales.[2] Nearly 66% of these terminations were performed prior to 20 weeks of gestation. The overall percentage of terminations, which were performed specifically for foetal abnormality, presently remains unknown because there may be many indications for termination before 24 weeks of gestation [refer to Chapter 93 (Medical Termination of Pregnancy)].

The couple is often ill-prepared for bad news related to the health of their unborn child in the case of abnormal findings. Therefore, the couple should be provided complete psychological support in decision-making when a foetal abnormality is diagnosed. When parents consider end-of-life decisions, they experience both ambivalent and emotional feelings. On the one hand, they may want to save their pregnancy. On the other hand, they want to protect their child, themselves and the family from the burden of severe disability.

These complex parental reactions need to be delicately and sensitively handled by the healthcare professionals.

With the technological developments in field of imaging (especially, sonography and MRI), many advances have been made in the field of foetal surgery. However, there still remains a wide potential for further development and many obstacles still need to be overcome. Currently, foetal endoscopic surgery is being performed for limited but ever-increasing indications in select centres throughout the world. While performing these procedures, the surgeon has a moral and ethical responsibility of weighing maternal risks against foetal benefits. It may be reasonable to withhold a particular surgical procedure, especially that having questionable foetal outcome, so as not to endanger the mother's life.

AETIOLOGY

Most common causes of foetal anomalies are tabulated in Box 41.1. Please note that the list is exhaustive and the box enumerates only the most commonly identified foetal anomalies.

DIAGNOSIS

Clinical Presentation

'Serious handicap' implies that a child has serious physical or mental disability which may result in significant suffering or long-term impairment of his/her ability to function in society. Assessment of foetal disability is an extremely difficult area. Presently, it is still not clear regarding what constitutes a serious handicap because an accurate prognosis and description of many prenatally detected abnormalities is yet not possible. Therefore, assessment of the seriousness of a foetal abnormality should be preferably individualised, taking into account all available clinical information.

Box 41.1: Most common causes of foetal anomalies

Chromosomal abnormalities
❑ Down's syndrome
Genetic defects
❑ Cystic fibrosis
Structural defects
❑ Congenital heart defects
❑ Cleft lip or palate
❑ *Neural tube defects:* Spina bifida (spina bifida occulta, meningocele, and myelomeningocele); anencephaly, enecephalocele, etc.
❑ Clubfoot
Functional/developmental defects
Disorders of nervous system
❑ Learning disabilities, mental retardation
❑ Behavioural disorders
❑ Speech or language difficulties
❑ Convulsions, autism
❑ Prader-Willi syndrome
❑ Fragile X syndrome
Disorders of sensory system
❑ Blindness, cataracts
❑ Hearing loss including deafness
Metabolic disorders
❑ Phenylketonuria (PKU)
❑ Hypothyroidism
Degenerative disorders
❑ Muscular dystrophies, lysosomal disorders, etc.
Environmental defects
❑ Maternal exposure to various drugs, infections (e.g. rubella), toxins, etc.

Investigations

❖ *Foetal anomaly ultrasound screening:* According to the current national guidelines, routine screening for trisomy 21 should be performed before 14 completed weeks of gestation to allow early decisions to be made, including the options for performing invasive diagnostic tests or to have the pregnancy terminated if the diagnosis is confirmed.[3] For details, kindly refer to Chapter 4 (Biochemical and Ultrasound Screening for Foetal Anomalies).

Foetal anomaly screening using ultrasound scanning is usually performed in all women from 18^{+0} days to 20^{+6} weeks of gestation.[4] If the scan reveals either a suspected or confirmed abnormality, the woman should be informed by the sonographer in a sensitive manner at the time of the scan because such information may have significant emotional impact over the patient. Healthcare professional must be present to provide immediate psychological support for women who are being provided with distressing news about their baby during the scan. The sonographer may take a second opinion from the senior sonographer colleague for confirming the findings. If an abnormality is confirmed or suspected, referral to an expert in foetal ultrasound, such as a foetal medicine specialist is usually required. An appointment should be arranged as soon as possible and preferably within 3 working days. Referral may not be required in the presence of some obvious major foetal abnormalities, such as anencephaly because

in these cases decision is guided by local guidelines. If the specialist cannot confirm the abnormality and is confident that the foetus is developing normally, the woman should still be referred back to her obstetrician for further discussion. Once an abnormality has been confirmed, arrangements should be made for the woman to take advice of an expert who has knowledge about the prognosis of the abnormality and the management options available. With technical improvements in ultrasound equipment, 3-D ultrasound technology has been introduced for diagnostic purposes. However, its exact role remains unclear.

❖ *MRI scan*: MRI scan serves as an effective adjunct to ultrasound for diagnosis and evaluation of foetal structural abnormalities, particularly those involving the foetal CNS.

❖ *Prenatal diagnostic techniques*: Prenatal diagnostic techniques such as amniocentesis, chorionic villus sampling and foetal blood sampling remain standard methods for the diagnosis of foetal chromosomal or genetic abnormalities such as aneuploidy. For details related to these procedures, kindly refer to Chapter 5 (Invasive Prenatal Diagnosis).

However, non-invasive techniques which are likely to reduce the requirement for invasive procedures in the future are being developed. One such non-invasive technique involves the detection of cell free, foetal-specific segments of DNA (free foetal DNA or ffDNA) in the maternal circulation.[5] With technological advancements, techniques such as polymerase chain reaction or fluorescence in situ hybridisation are able to diagnose chromosomal anomalies such as trisomy 21, within 24–48 hours.

MANAGEMENT

❖ *Multidisciplinary team approach*: Management of pregnancy in which an abnormal foetus is identified requires a multidisciplinary team approach comprising a sonologist, obstetrician, foetal medicine specialist, paediatricians, paediatric surgeons, geneticists and neonatologists, nurse specialist, etc.

❖ *Breaking bad news*: Once the diagnosis of foetal abnormality has been made, parents must be informed in a sensitive manner about the baby's condition, the prognosis, whether the baby would be born alive or not, and the level of disability if the baby would be born alive.

❖ *Psychological support*: Telling the parents about an abnormal foetus may elicit much grief and shock for the parents. It may be difficult for them to make decisions related to the management of abnormal foetus, especially when they have to make decisions related to the foetal termination. Therefore, they must be handled in a very sensitive manner. Written information must be preferably provided. Psychological support must be provided to the parents as well as the family. They must also be provided contact information for communicating with the various

Flow chart 41.1: Management of cases of foetal anomalies

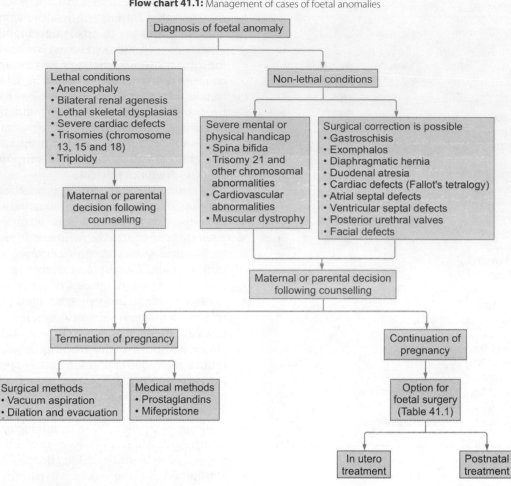

PART II

relevant support groups. Women and their partners must be provided with as much information as possible regarding the implications of the diagnosis, especially if the prognosis remains uncertain. This information should not only be provided by the obstetricians, but also other medical specialists, such as paediatricians, paediatric surgeons, geneticists, neonatologists, foetal medicine specialists or subspecialists.

❖ *Counselling and support*: Following the diagnosis of foetal abnormality, the process of decision-making may prove to be a difficult one for women and their partners. Such kind of diagnosis can cause considerable emotional shock and distress. In such sensitive circumstances, appropriate counselling and support must be provided to the woman and her partner by the healthcare practitioners involved. A non-directive, non-judgemental and supportive approach must be preferably adopted by all the staff involved in the care of a woman or couple facing a possible termination of pregnancy. At no point must the woman be pressurised to make a quick decision. However, once the decision has been made, the procedure should be organised with minimal delay.

❖ *Deciding the further course of management*: Once the foetal anomaly has been diagnosed, the algorithm for deciding further course of management available is described in Flow chart 41.1 and includes options such as termination

of pregnancy, or continuation of pregnancy, supported with or without in utero or postnatal treatment. The various treatment options are discussed in details next.

Termination of Pregnancy

The most important decisions which the parents need to take regarding the further course of management is deciding whether to continue or terminate the pregnancy. Termination of pregnancy may be an option in conditions which are likely to be fatal or those conditions which are likely to result in significant physical or mental harm. However, whether or not a woman undergoes termination for a particular foetal anomaly solely depends upon her consent to do so. Even in the presence of an obviously fatal foetal condition such as anencephaly, a woman may not choose to undergo a termination. A woman's decision to decline the offer of termination must be fully supported by the clinician.

Termination of Pregnancy before 21⁺⁶ Weeks of Gestation

Live birth following termination of pregnancy before 21^{+6} weeks of gestation is very uncommon. Still, the women and their partners should be counselled regarding this unlikely possibility. Staff should also be trained to deal with this rare possibility. A foetus which is born alive following termination of pregnancy is considered to be a live birth, irrespective of the gestational age at birth. Such a child should be registered as a live birth. According to law, a child is born alive when it is capable of maintaining an existence independent of its mother. A foetus which is born alive with abnormalities incompatible with life should be managed so as to maintain its comfort and dignity during its terminal care. Thus, before deciding the termination of pregnancy, it is important to define whether the foetus would be born alive or not.

Termination of Pregnancy after 21⁺⁶ Weeks of Gestation

Termination of pregnancy with option for foeticide: After 22 weeks of gestation, live birth becomes increasingly common. Therefore, when termination of pregnancy for a foetal abnormality is decided after 21⁺⁶ weeks, RCOG recommends that intrauterine foeticide should also be routinely offered.[6] This is usually attained by intracardiac administration of potassium chloride under ultrasound control into the foetal circulation.[7] Prior to the procedure, foetal sedation can be achieved by administering diazepam or pethidine into the foetal circulation. Following 1 hour after the procedure, an ultrasound examination must be performed to ensure the cessation of foetal pulsations.

Termination of pregnancy without the option for foeticide: In cases of pregnancy termination after 22 weeks of gestation where the foetal abnormality is not compatible with survival, termination of pregnancy without prior foeticide may be preferred by some women.

Where the foetal abnormality is not lethal and termination of pregnancy is being undertaken after 21⁺⁶ weeks of gestation, failure to perform foeticide could result in the live birth and survival of the baby. In such situations, the child should receive appropriate support in the neonatal ICU.

Method for Termination of Pregnancy

Once the decision to terminate the pregnancy has been reached, the method and place for termination of pregnancy along with the decision for foeticide must be discussed with the patient and her partner. Prior to pregnancy termination, there must be discussions regarding various options for pain relief and whether the woman might want to see the dead baby and have mementos such as photographs, locks of hair, and prints of the baby's hands and feet. She must also be provided information related to the effect of termination on her physical health in the postnatal period and the possibility of a postmortem examination being performed. She will need to be made aware of the fact that information obtained from a postmortem examination may be relevant for her subsequent pregnancies.

Pregnancy can be terminated using medical or surgical methods. Surgical methods of pregnancy termination include vacuum aspiration or suction curettage and dilatation and evacuation. Vacuum aspiration is a process involving aspiration or suction of contents in the uterine cavity using plastic tube attached to the vacuum machine following cervical dilation. Cervix can either be dilated using graduated plastic or metallic dilators or vaginal prostaglandin preparations. Vacuum aspiration can be used until the end of first trimester. The procedure of dilatation and evacuation, on the other hand, is performed in some units up to 20 weeks of gestation. This procedure involves extraction of foetal parts using appropriate instruments following mechanical dilatation of cervix up to the diameter of 14 mm. Cervical priming agents such as mifepristone, misoprostol and gemeprost can be used for achieving cervical dilation in a safe and effective manner. Dilatation and evacuation is a distressing procedure, which is not widely available. The main disadvantage of this procedure is that it does not allow the full postmortem examination of the foetus if required. Medical method of termination of pregnancy involves the use of prostaglandins and antiprogesterone (e.g. mifepristone). The standard regimen for medical termination involves the administration of 200 mg of mifepristone orally followed 36–48 hours later by misoprostol 800 µg vaginally then 400 µg of misoprostol orally (for a maximum of 4 doses). The patient should be made aware about the fact that within the NHS, medical abortion induced by drugs is usually offered after 14 weeks of gestation. Medical method of termination is associated with an additional advantage of providing the opportunity for postmortem examination. Details related to the methods of pregnancy termination are described in Chapter 93 (Medical Termination of Pregnancy).

Post-termination Follow-up

After a termination for foetal abnormality, well-organised follow-up care is essential. Appropriate time for grieving must be allowed for the parents. It is essential to maintain good communication with primary care to ensure that the woman's general practitioner remains well-informed. Following discharge, she must be offered a home visit by the community midwife.[8] During the post-termination follow-up appointment with the obstetrician, the autopsy findings must be discussed with the patient and the risk of recurrence explained. It may also be necessary to obtain genetic advice. Follow-up with the paediatric or the neonatal team is also an important part of bereavement counselling. Lastly, a discharge letter summarising the details related to the diagnosis and the procedure performed must be sent to the patient.

Postmortem Examination

Postmortem examination of the dead foetus is a vital part of management. However, this may at times be very distressing for the parents or family. Though it is possible to accurately identify most major foetal anomalies using high-resolution ultrasound examination, postmortem examination is still required because it provides further details. This information may prove useful in subsequent pregnancies and enable a more specific genetic counselling for future. Referral to a genetic specialist may be required in order to assess the risk of recurrence of the diagnosed pathology and the possibility to investigate other family members. Before performing postmortem examination for foetuses of any gestational age, consent is required. If the parents do not give their consent for postmortem examination, the clinician can request for photographs, X-rays, tissue samples (e.g. skin, placental specimen, etc.) for cytogenetic analysis.

Decision for Continuation with Pregnancy

If the woman wants to continue her pregnancy, her decision must be fully supported by the healthcare professional even if the woman does not give her consent for termination in the presence of an obviously fatal foetal condition. If the woman wishes to continue with the pregnancy, she should be managed either at the foetal medicine unit (depending on the abnormality) or in combination with her referring obstetrician. If the woman chooses the option of palliative care after delivery, this decision must be respected, supported and an individualised care plan must be agreed to. According to the Royal College of Paediatrics and Child Health document, 'Withholding or Withdrawing Life Sustaining Treatment in Children: A Framework for Practice', palliative neonatal care may be offered to the child in following three situations:[9]

1. *The 'no chance' situation*: The child has such severe disease that life-sustaining treatment is likely to simply delay death without causing any significant improvement of suffering. Treatment for sustaining life appears to be inappropriate in these cases.

2. *The 'no purpose' situation*: Although the child in these cases may be able to survive with treatment, the degree of physical or mental impairment may be so great in these cases that the treatment appears to serve no purpose.

3. *The 'unbearable' situation*: The child has progressive and irreversible illness. The family wishes to have a particular treatment withdrawn or to refuse further treatment, because they feel it would be difficult to tolerate further treatment.

Women who decline termination for non-lethal conditions must be referred to the specialists such as paediatricians, paediatric surgeons or neonatologists. They may be offered in utero or postnatal foetal surgery.

Foetal Surgery

❖ A number of interventions (Table 41.1) are currently being performed in specialist centres to improve foetal outcome following in utero diagnosis of foetal pathology.

❖ Parents who are willing to continue their pregnancies must be provided with complete information regarding the underlying condition, its treatment and the possible long-term outcomes of the procedure. This information should be preferably provided by the paediatric surgeon who shall be performing the surgery.

❖ Continued foetal surveillance in the form of regular ultrasound examinations may be required for some foetal conditions (e.g. gastroschisis) in the antenatal period due to the risk of development of potential complications during the intrapartum period.

❖ Continuous psychological counselling of the parents may also be required during the antepartum period. Serial ultrasound examinations may be performed to provide the reassurance to the parents that their baby is growing normally. Parents must be provided information regarding the time, place and mode of delivery for their baby, the baby's appearance following birth, any postnatal procedure which may be performed on the baby, etc.

Table 41.1: Indications for foetal surgery and their recommended treatment options

Foetal structural defect	Recommended treatment

• Urinary tract obstructive defects
  – Pelviureteric junction obstruction
  – Ureterovescical junction obstruction
  – Urethral obstruction
  – Ureterocele
	• Vesicocentesis
	• Vesicoamniotic shunt
	• Foetoscopic vesicostomy
	• Laser ablation

• Lung defects
  – Cystic adenomatoid malformations
  – Pleural effusion
  – Pulmonary sequestration
	• Pleuroamniotic shunt
	• Thoracoamniotic shunt
	• Open pulmonary lobectomy

• Diaphragmatic hernia	• Open complete repair • Temporary tracheal occlusion

• Multiple pregnancy
  – Twin-to-twin transfusion syndrome
  – Acardiac twins
	• Laser ablation
	• Cord occlusion

• Foetal anaemia	• Intrauterine foetal transfusion of red blood cells
• Sacrococcygeal teratoma	• Resection of tumour • Radiofrequency ablation • Foetoscopic vascular occlusion
• Ovarian cysts	• Cyst aspiration

• Placenta or amnion
  – Chorioangioma of placenta
  – Amniotic band syndrome
	• Vascular occlusion

• Central nervous system defects
  – Aqueductal stenosis
  – Dandy-Walker syndrome
  – Myelomeningocele
	• Ventriculoamniotic shunt
	• Open ventriculoperitoneal shunt
	• Foetoscopic coverage
	• Open repair

• Facial defects – Cleft lip and palate	• Foetoscopic coverage • Open repair

❖ An alternative approach to foetal therapy is the administration of drugs to the mother. These drugs are likely to produce an affect in the foetus after passing through the placenta. The most common examples include the use of steroids to induce maturation of the foetal lungs before preterm delivery, maternal steroids and immunoglobulin to treat foetal alloimmune thrombocytopenia and maternal administration of antiarrhythmic drugs (e.g. digoxin, flecainide, amiodarone, etc.) for the treatment of foetal arrhythmias.

❖ There are some foetal surgery-related procedures performed in utero, which are likely to improve the foetal or neonatal outcomes in presence of major foetal abnormalities. Three such procedures, which are presently being evaluated as part of research protocols include the following:

1. *In Utero Closure of Spina Bifida*

In utero closure of spina bifida during the second trimester of pregnancy is done by performing a maternal hysterotomy.[10]

PART II

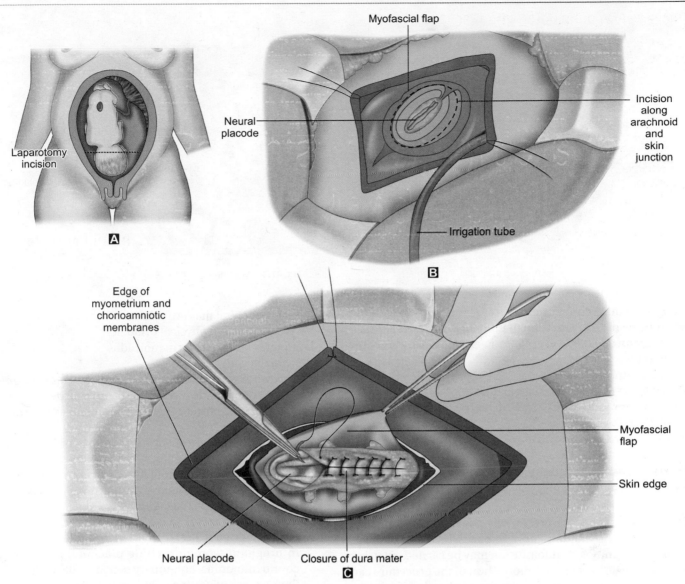

Figs 41.1A to C: Steps of foetal surgery involving repair of a meningomyelocele

Though spina bifida is not a fatal condition, it has been found that repairing the defect in utero helps in minimising the damage caused by spina bifida including paralysis, hydrocephalus, etc. According to the recently published results of the first part of 'MOMS trial' (Management of Myelomeningocele Study), an ongoing RCT since 2003, prenatal surgery for myelomeningocele at 26 weeks of gestation has been found to be associated with reduced requirement for postnatal shunting (at 12 months of age) and improved motor outcomes at 30 months.[11] However, the procedure has been found to be associated with significant maternal and foetal risks (prematurity, default hysterotomy scar, etc.). Therefore, potential benefits of prenatal surgery need to be balanced against the risks of prematurity and maternal morbidity. The prenatal surgery for myelomeningocele repair involves a laparotomy, hysterotomy and amniotomy to expose the foetal back in the defect. The closure of the defect is performed in a similar way as that performed in the postnatal stage (Figs 41.1A to C).

2. Clip or Balloon Foetal Endoscopic Tracheal Occlusion (FETO)

Endoscopic placement of an inflated balloon in the foetal trachea helps in improving growth of the lungs in cases with congenital diaphragmatic hernia.[12] This procedure is performed at about 23–27 weeks of gestation. Preoperatively, the patient is given betamethasone for attaining foetal lung maturity. In this surgery, a 5-mm trocar is inserted inside the uterine cavity. Through this, a 4-mm perfusion hysteroscope is guided through the foetal vocal cords under the guidance of a foetoscope and ultrasound examination. A detachable silicone balloon is placed in the foetal trachea midway between the carina and vocal cords (Fig. 41.2). It is then inflated with iso-osmotic contrast material so as to fill the foetal trachea to a diameter of about 0.5 mm and a length of at least 2 cm following which it is detached, so that it remains in place.[13,14] At the time of delivery of foetal head during caesarean section, ex utero intrapartum therapy (EXIT) procedure is done. The

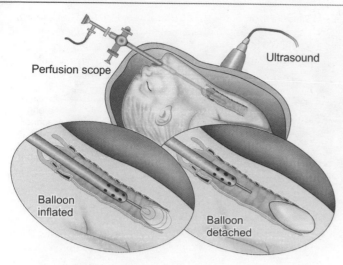

Fig. 41.2: Foetal endoscopic tracheal occlusion

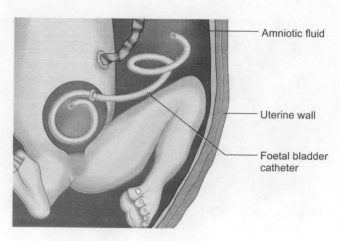

Fig. 41.3: Diagrammatic representation of vesicoamniotic shunt

EXIT procedure comprises the following steps, which are executed prior to the division of umbilical cord:

❖ Deflation and removal of the balloon under bronchoscopic guidance
❖ Suctioning of the airway
❖ Insertion of the endotracheal tube
❖ Administration of an exogenous surfactant (in the dosage of 3 mg/kg body weight)
❖ Starting assisted ventilation.

3. Percutaneous Vesicoamniotic Shunting

This procedure may be useful in male foetuses with presumed posterior urethral valves.[11] This shunt procedure is performed if the kidney is functioning normally, the karyotype is normal and there are no major malformations in the foetus. In case of oligohydramnios, amnioinfusion may be carried out using warmed Ringer's lactate solution. Though the procedure can be performed under local, regional or general anaesthesia, local anaesthesia is usually preferred. Foetal analgesia is administered in the form of 0.2 mg/kg pancuronium and 10 mg/kg fentanyl. A small 3–5 mm stab incision is made below the umbilicus, avoiding entry into vessels as observed by colour Doppler. The shunt trocar is then carefully introduced into the amniotic space near the lower part of the foetal abdomen into a foetal amniotic pocket. It is then quickly inserted into the foetal bladder using sharp, shift movements of the hand and placed in a central position. Urine sample is aspirated and sent for culture and analysis of renal function. A double pigtail 'Rodeck' or 'Harrison' shunt catheter is then gently straightened and threaded into the trocar sheath before removing the internal stylet wire. The proximal segment of the catheter is pushed into the foetal bladder and the distal end of the catheter is positioned in the amniotic space (Fig. 41.3).

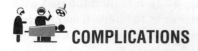

COMPLICATIONS

Complications associated with abnormal foetus are described next.

❖ Lethal congenital malformations
❖ Severe mental and physical disability
❖ Long-term and short-term morbidity
❖ Psychological trauma
❖ *Complications related to the procedure of pregnancy termination:* These include haemorrhage, uterine perforation, cervical trauma, postabortion infections, failed abortion, etc.
❖ *Complications related to foetal surgery:* Some of the complications related to foetal surgery are as follows:[15]
  • *Maternal complications:* In foetal surgery, mother is an innocent bystander, who is at risk of various complications related to anaesthesia and surgery, e.g. blood loss, infection, injury to the surrounding organs, bowel obstruction, etc. Other complications related to surgery in pregnant women include placental abruption, chorioamnionitis, pulmonary oedema due to tocolytic therapy, risk of uterine dehiscence and rupture.
  • *Preterm labour:* Though the laparoscopic procedures are associated with much lower risk in comparison to the endoscopic procedures, all the procedures are associated with a substantial risk of preterm prelabour rupture of the membranes, preterm labour and birth of a premature baby.
  • *Injury to the foetus during surgery:* The foetus may get injured at the time of foetoscopic surgery.
  • *Requirement of caesarean delivery for future pregnancies:* In cases of open foetal surgery, caesarean delivery is required for all future pregnancies for the mother because of the hysterotomy.
  • *Foetal demise:* This could occur as a result of cord compression and/or placental abruption.

CLINICAL PEARLS

❖ Under the Abortion Act, 1967 (amended 1990), termination of pregnancy after 24 weeks of gestation has become legal in presence of a lethal abnormality or if there is sufficient evidence to show that the infant would be born with serious mental or physical disability.

❖ It is the duty of the healthcare professional to fully support a woman's decision even if she declines termination in the presence of an obviously fatal foetal condition such as anencephaly.

❖ Risks associated with termination procedures are lower if they are performed earlier during the gestation.

❖ In accordance with the RCOG guidance, foeticide should be routinely offered for terminations over 21[+6] weeks of gestation.[6]

❖ Termination of pregnancy may be associated with high parental psychological stress, with nearly 40% women showing signs of psychiatric morbidity.

❖ A well-organised follow-up care plan is essential for following termination in case of foetal abnormality.

EVIDENCE-BASED MEDICINE

❖ The available evidence shows that once a serious foetal anomaly has been diagnosed, majority of patients (80–90%) are likely to opt for the termination of their pregnancy. Termination of pregnancy is most likely to be associated with lethal defects in the CNS. Patients who have foetuses with abnormalities associated with uncertain prognoses (particularly neural defects which could be correctable in utero or neonatal period) are more likely to opt for continuation of pregnancy.[16-18]

❖ Though in utero treatment of some structural abnormalities has been practised for a number of years, presently there is no good evidence regarding their efficacy. There is requirement for well-designed prospective randomised studies in future to establish the efficacy of such interventions.[9]

REFERENCES

1. World Health Organization (WHO). (2016). Congenital anomalies. [online]. Available from www.who.int/mediacentre/factsheets/fs370/en. [Accessed October, 2016].

2. Department of Health. Statistical Bulletin: Abortion Statistics, England and Wales: 2009. London: Department of Health; 2009.

3. National Institute for Clinical Excellence (NICE). Antenatal care: Routine care for the Healthy Pregnant Woman. Clinical Guideline CG62. London: NICE; 2008.

4. UK National Screening Committee. (2016). UK Screening Panel. Foetal Anomalies: The UK NSC policy on foetal anomaly screening in pregnancy. [online]. Available from www.legacy.screening.nhs.uk/fetalanomalies. [Accessed November, 2016].

5. Hahn S, Chitty LS. Noninvasive prenatal diagnosis: current practice and future perspectives. Curr Opin Obstet Gynecol. 2008;20(2):146-51.

6. Royal College of Obstetricians and Gynaecologists (RCOG). Termination of Pregnancy for Foetal Abnormality in England, Scotland and Wales: Report of a Working Party. London: RCOG; 2010.

7. Pasquini L, Pontello V, Kumar S. Intracardiac injection of potassium chloride as a method for feticide: experience from a single UK tertiary centre. BJOG. 2008;115(4):528-31.

8. Statham H, Solomou W, Green JM. When the Baby has an Abnormality: A Study of Parents' Experiences. Cambridge: Centre for Family Research, University of Cambridge; 2001.

9. Royal College of Paediatrics and Child Health. Withholding or Withdrawing Life Sustaining Treatment in Children: A Framework for Practice, 2nd edition. London: RCPCH; 2004.

10. Walsh DS, Adzick NS. Foetal surgery for spina bifida. Semin Neonatol. 2003;8:197-205.

11. Adzick NS, Thom EA, Spong CY, Brock JW, Burrows PK, Johnson MP, et al. A randomized trial of prenatal versus postnatal repair of myelomeningocele. N Engl J Med. 2011;364(11):993-1004.

12. Doné E, Gucciardo L, Van Mieghem T, Jani J, Cannie M, Van Schoubroeck D, et al. Prenatal diagnosis, prediction of outcome and in utero therapy of isolated congenital diaphragmatic hernia. Prenat Diagn. 2008;28:581-91.

13. VanderWall KJ, Skarsgard ED, Filly RA, Eckert J, Harrison MR. Fetendo-clip: a foetal endoscopic tracheal clip procedure in a human fetus. J Pediatr Surg. 1997;32(7):970-2.

14. Harrison MR, Albanese CT, Hawgood SB, Farmer DL, Farrell JA, Sandberg PL, et al. Fetoscopic temporary tracheal occlusion by means of detachable balloon for congenital diaphragmatic hernia. Am J Obstet Gynecol. 2001;185(3):730-3.

15. Golombeck K, Ball RH, Lee H, Farrell JA, Farmer DL, Jacobs VR, et al. Maternal morbidity after maternal-foetal surgery. Am J Obstet Gynecol. 2006;194(3):834-9.

16. Schechtman KB, Gray DL, Baty JD, Rothman SM. Decision-making for termination of pregnancies with foetal anomalies: analysis of 53,000 pregnancies. Obstet Gynecol. 2002;99(2):216-22.

17. Pryde PG, Isada NB, Hallak M, Johnson MP, Odgers AE, Evans MI. Determinants of parental decision to abort or continue after non-aneuploid ultrasound-detected foetal abnormalities. Obstet Gynecol. 1992;80(1):52-6.

18. Bijma HH, van der Heide A, Wildschut HI. Decision-making after ultrasound diagnosis of foetal abnormality. Reprod Health Matters. 2008;16(31 Suppl):82-9.

SECTION 7

Intrapartum Period

OBSTETRICS

Normal and Abnormal Progress of Labour

NORMAL LABOUR AND DELIVERY

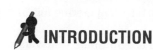 INTRODUCTION

Labour comprises of a series of events taking place in the woman's genital organs, which help to expel the foetus and other products of conception outside the uterine cavity into the outer world. It can be defined as the onset of painful uterine contractions accompanied by any one of the following: ROM; bloody show; cervical dilatation and/or effacement. It normally comprises of four stages which are described in Table 42.1. Graphical representation of normal labour for both nulliparous and multiparous women as described by Friedman (1955) is shown in Figure 42.1.[1,2]

The first stage of labour begins with the onset of regular uterine contractions and ends with complete dilatation and effacement of cervix. It is divided into two phases given next.

1. Latent phase (preparatory phase)
2. Active phase.

Latent Phase (Preparatory Phase)

Latent phase begins with onset of regular contractions, with contractions occurring after every 15–20 minutes, lasting 20–30 seconds. Gradually, the frequency of contractions increases and they can occur after every 5–7 minutes, lasting for 30–40 seconds. This phase ends when cervix becomes about 3–5 cm dilated. The latent phase lasts for approximately 8–9 hours in the primi, and less than 6 hours in multigravida. Prolonged latent phase can be defined as greater than 20 hours in primigravida and greater than 14 hours in the multigravida. During the latent phase, there may be subtle cervical changes and it may be difficult to assess them accurately. The cervix shortens from 3 cm in length to less than 0.5 cm and dilates up to 3 cm.

Table 42.1: Various stages of labour

Stages of labour	Description	Characteristics	Duration in primigravida (in mins)	Duration in multigravida (in mins)

Stage I	Starts from the onset of true labour pains and ends with complete dilatation of cervix	Can be divided into:
		• *Latent phase:* Slow and gradual cervical effacement and dilatation (up to 3 cm)
		• *Active phase:* Active cervical dilatation (3–10 cm) and foetal descent. It comprises of:
		  – Acceleration phase
		  – Phase of maximum slope
		  – Deceleration phase
			—	—

Stage II	Starts from full dilatation of cervix and ends with expulsion of the foetus from birth canal	—	50	20
Stage III	Begins after expulsion of the foetus and is associated with expulsion of placenta and membranes	—	15	15
Stage IV	Stage of observation which lasts for at least 1 h after the expulsion of afterbirths	—	60	60

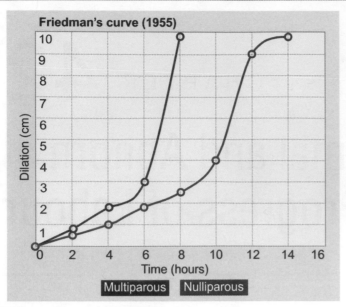

Fig. 42.1: Graphical representation of normal labour depicted by Friedman's curve[1,2]

Active Phase

Active phase begins when the cervix is about 4 cm dilated and ends when it becomes fully dilated. It comprises of the three following phases:

1. *Phase of acceleration*: This phase lies between the latent phase and the phase of maximum slope.
2. *Phase of maximum slope*: During this phase there is linear dilatation with time. According to Friedman, during this phase the minimum rate of progression is at least 1 cm/h.
3. *Phase of deceleration*: This phase occurs at the end of active phase prior to complete dilatation.

AETIOLOGY

The exact mechanism for the initiation of labour is still unclear. However, the most likely mechanisms are as follows:

❖ *Mechanical factors*: Uterine distension
❖ *Endocrine factors*: There is increased cortisol secretion by foetal adrenals and increased production of oestrogens and prostaglandins from the placenta. Together, these cause an increased release of oxytocin from the maternal pituitary and increased synthesis of contraction-associated proteins.

DIAGNOSIS

Clinical Presentation

Symptoms indicating the onset of labour are as follows:

❖ *Lightening*: At the onset of labour, engagement of foetal head in the pelvis causes the baby to move lower down into the pelvis. This relieves pressure over the mother's diaphragm and lungs, causing her lungs to expand, thereby helping her to breathe easily. However, there is increased pressure in the pelvis, which may put pressure over her bladder and rectum.

❖ *Bloody show*: Cervical dilatation and effacement occur at the onset of labour. Cervical discharge mixed with blood from ruptured capillaries presents as a pinkish-brown discharge called 'show'.

❖ *Increased frequency and strength of Braxton Hicks contractions*: The uterine contractions are likely to become more frequent, intense and painful.

❖ *Rupture of membranes*: There may be rupture of the amniotic sac resulting in the leakage of amniotic fluid through the vaginal opening.

General Physical Examination

❖ Assessment of patient's vital signs
❖ Assessment of FHR
❖ Character of uterine contractions.

Abdominal Examination

❖ The abdominal examination must comprise of the following:
❖ *Uterine height*: Estimation of the height of uterine fundus (Fig. 42.2)
❖ *Foetal lie*: The foetal lie may be longitudinal, transverse or oblique (Fig. 42.3)
❖ *Foetal presentation*: Foetal presentation can be described as the foetal body part which occupies the lower pole of the uterus and thereby first enters the pelvic passage. Foetal presentation is determined by foetal lie and may be of three types: (1) cephalic, (2) podalic (breech) or (3) shoulder (Fig. 42.3). Foetal malpresentation can be described as any presentation other than the vertex presentation. Presentations which can be delivered vaginally at term include vertex, face (mentoanterior) and breech presentation. On the other hand, presentations which cannot be delivered vaginally at term include face (mentoposterior), brow and shoulder presentation. Cord presentation is another foetal malpresentation where the umbilical cord presents either through the cervix alongside

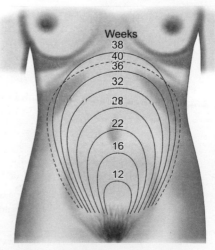

Fig. 42.2: Estimation of the height of uterine fundus

the presenting part (occult presentation) or past it (overt presentation) in the presence of ruptured membranes. Babies with cord presentation may be delivered vaginally when diagnosed late in the second stage of labour and in cases where a quick vaginal delivery can be safely anticipated. The obstetrician must remember that all malpresentations may deliver vaginally in form of an extremely preterm foetus.

❖ Obstetric grips [Leopold's manoeuvres (Fig. 42.4)]
❖ *Uterine contractions*: The frequency and duration of uterine contractions must be measured either through internal or external cardiotocography.
❖ Assessing the engagement of foetal presenting part by feeling how many fifths of the head are palpable above the brim of the pelvis (Figs 42.5A and B)
❖ Auscultation of foetal heart.

Per Speculum Examination

Per speculum examination enables inspection the cervix and vaginal walls. It is especially useful in cases of preterm labour or PROM and antepartum haemorrhage (APH) for assessment of the leaking fluid or blood, respectively. Per speculum examination also helps in accessing the cervix and fornices for the purpose of taking bacteriological swabs and cervical smears.

Indicators of ruptured membranes on per speculum examination are as follows:
❖ Gross vaginal pooling of fluid
❖ Positive results on nitrazine and fern testing of vaginal secretions
❖ Evidence of meconium.

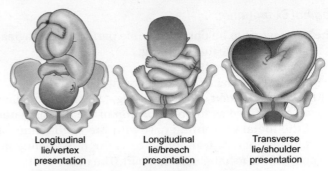

Fig. 42.3: Different types of foetal lies and presentation

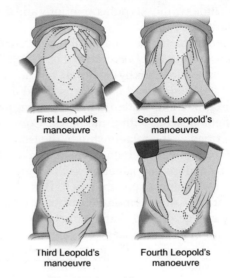

Fig. 42.4: Leopold's manoeuvres

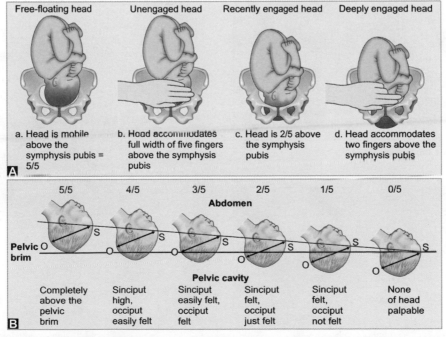

Figs 42.5A and B: Estimation of foetal descent through abdominal examination

Vaginal Examination

The parameters to be observed while performing a vaginal examination include the following:

❖ Cervical dilatation (Fig. 42.6)
❖ Cervical consistency and effacement (Fig. 42.7)
❖ *Foetal presentation and position* (Fig. 42.8): Foetal position can be defined as the relationship of the denominator of the foetal presenting part with the fixed points of maternal pelvis. Denominator is the most definable point of the foetal presenting part. The denominator for vertex presentation is occiput; for breech presentation is sacrum; acromion for shoulder presentation and mentum for face presentation. The fixed points of the maternal pelvis include symphysis pubis anteriorly and the sacrum posteriorly.
❖ Assessment of foetal membranes and amount of liquor
❖ *Foetal descent* [*station of foetal head* (Fig. 42.9)]: According to the recommendations by the Royal College of Midwives, the decent of foetal head must be assessed during each vaginal examination.[3] Station of the presenting part relates to the foetal descent within the pelvis. Conventionally, it is described as the relationship to the ischial spine in centimetres above and below this landmark. It can be defined by abdominal palpation as the number of fifths of foetal head palpable per abdomen. This is particularly important when there is moulding of foetal head because this may exaggerate the shape of foetal head, giving an impression of better descent on vaginal examination. Therefore, the station of the foetal presenting part must be defined vaginally only after an abdominal examination has been done.

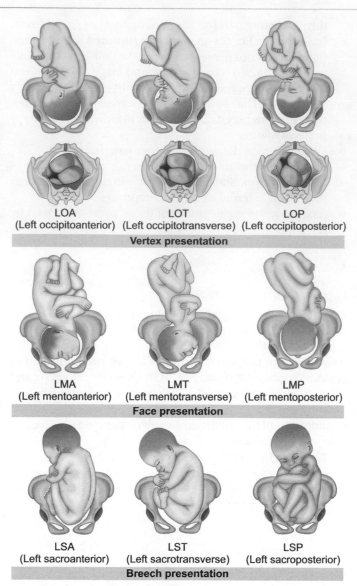

LOA
(Left occipitoanterior) LOT
(Left occipitotransverse) LOP
(Left occipitoposterior)

Vertex presentation

LMA
(Left mentoanterior) LMT
(Left mentotransverse) LMP
(Left mentoposterior)

Face presentation

LSA
(Left sacroanterior) LST
(Left sacrotransverse) LSP
(Left sacroposterior)

Breech presentation

Fig. 42.8: Various positions possible with different presentations

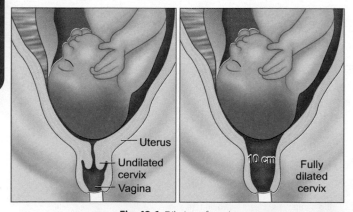

— Uterus
— Undilated cervix
— Vagina

10 cm Fully dilated cervix

Fig. 42.6: Dilation of cervix

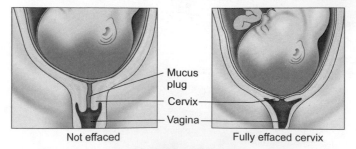

Mucus plug
Cervix
Vagina

Not effaced Fully effaced cervix

Fig. 42.7: Effacement of cervix

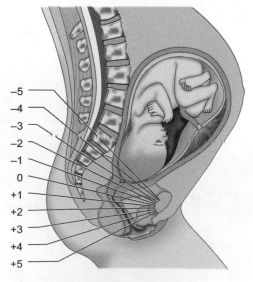

−5
−4
−3
−2
−1
0
+1
+2
+3
+4
+5

Fig. 42.9: Station of foetal head

PART II

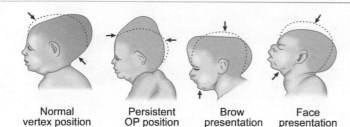

| Normal vertex position | Persistent OP position | Brow presentation | Face presentation |

Fig. 42.10: Moulding of the foetal skull
Abbreviation: OP, occipito-posterior

Table 42.2: Degree of moulding of foetal skull

Degree of moulding	Description
0 (normal)	Normal separation of the bones with open sutures
1+ (mild moulding)	Bones touching each other
2+ (moderate moulding)	Bones overlapping, but can be separated with gentle digital pressure
3+ (severe moulding)	Bones overlapping, but cannot be separated with gentle digital pressure

❖ *Moulding of foetal skull* (Fig. 42.10): Determination of the degree of moulding of foetal head forms an important part of the vaginal examination as it relates to the fit of foetal head through the pelvis. Degree of moulding of foetal skull is described in Table 42.2. Caput succedaneum, another type of foetal head swelling is a reflection of scalp oedema.

The presence of caput succedaneum (soft tissue oedema of foetal scalp) can also be felt as a soft, boggy swelling, which may make it difficult to identify the presenting part of the foetal head clearly. With severe caput, the sutures may be impossible to feel. Although, presence of caput is usually indicative of prolonged labour, it may sometimes be even present in normal cases and therefore may not be useful in planning the management.

❖ *Pelvic assessment*: Preparations for delivery are made as the cervical dilatation and effacement approaches completion and/or crowning of the foetal presenting part becomes evident at the vaginal introitus.

Investigations

❖ Haematocrit with CBC
❖ Urine for proteins (dipstick examination)
❖ Blood typing (ABO and Rh)
❖ Blood typing and screening (in case caesarean section is anticipated)
❖ Venereal disease research laboratory, TORCH, HIV, hepatitis B surface antigen (HBsAg) (in case they have not been done in the antenatal period).

MANAGEMENT OF NORMAL LABOUR AND DELIVERY

Predelivery Preparation

❖ *Patient position*: The patient is commonly placed in the dorsal lithotomy position with left lateral tilt

❖ Vulvar and perineal cleaning and draping with antiseptic solution must be done
❖ The sterile drapes must be placed in such a way that only the area immediately around the vulva and perineum is exposed
❖ If at any time during the abdominal examination, the bladder is palpable, the patient must be encouraged to void. If, despite of distended bladder, the patient is unable to void, catheterisation is indicated
❖ *Patient monitoring*: Maternal BP and pulse should be recorded every hour during the first stage of labour and every 10 minutes during the second stage of labour. The FHR should be recorded immediately after a contraction at least every 30 minutes during the active phase of the first stage of labour and at least every 15 minutes during the second stage
❖ *Induction of labour*: This has been described in detail in Chapter 43 (Induction of Labour).
❖ *Foetal monitoring*: Antepartum and intrapartum foetal monitoring has been discussed in Chapter 49 (Antepartum and Intrapartum Foetal Asphyxia)
❖ *Partogram*: Normal labour should be plotted graphically on a partograph (Fig. 42.11). Various parameters observed at the time of vaginal examination must be graphically plotted on the partogram and carefully documented during each vaginal examination. The partograph is divided into a latent phase and an active phase. The latent phase ends while the active phase begins when the cervix is 3 cm dilated. Cervical dilation and descent of the presenting part are plotted in relation to an alert line and an action line. Alert line starts at the end of latent phase and ends with the full dilation of the cervix (10 cm) within 7 hours (at the rate of 1 cm/h). The action line is drawn 4 hours to the right of the alert line. Labour is considered to be abnormal when the cervicograph crosses the alert line and falls on zone II, and intervention is required when it crosses the action line and falls in the zone III.

Despite the widespread use of partograms in almost all labour wards, there is much debate regarding the benefits of partograms in improving neonatal outcomes. A Cochrane review has determined that routine use of partogram as part of standard management and care is not recommended.[4] However, presently its use has been established as a part of clinical practice and should be continued to be done unless there is strong evidence to indicate otherwise. Future evidence is required to establish the efficacy of partogram use.

Delivery

Mechanism of normal labour has been described in Figure 42.12 and comprises of the following steps as described next.

Delivery of Foetal Head

❖ With the increasing descent of the head, the perineum bulges and thins out considerably. As the largest diameter of the foetal head distends the vaginal introitus, crowning is said to occur.

CHAPTER 42

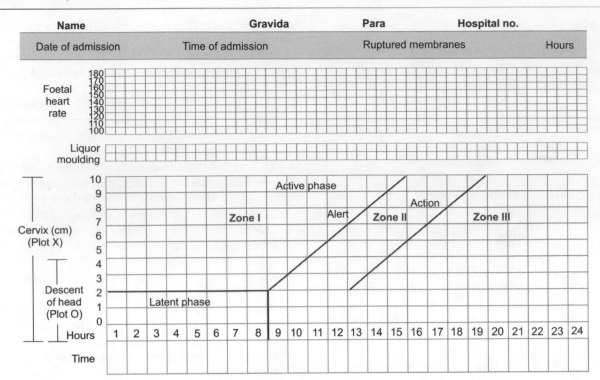

Fig. 42.11: Partograph

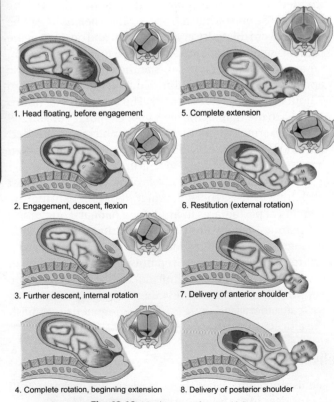

Fig. 42.12: Mechanism of normal labour

1. Head floating, before engagement
2. Engagement, descent, flexion
3. Further descent, internal rotation
4. Complete rotation, beginning extension
5. Complete extension
6. Restitution (external rotation)
7. Delivery of anterior shoulder
8. Delivery of posterior shoulder

* As the head distends the perineum and it appears that tears may occur in the area of vaginal introitus, mediolateral surgical incision called episiotomy may be given.
* As the foetal head progressively distends the vaginal introitus, the healthcare professional, in order to facilitate the controlled birth of the head, must place the fingers of one hand against the baby's head to keep it flexed and apply perineal support with the other hand. Delivery of the foetal head can be achieved with the help of Ritgen manoeuvre. This helps in providing controlled delivery of the head and favours extension at the time of actual delivery so that the head is delivered with its smallest diameter passing through the introitus and minimal injury occurs to the pelvic musculature.

* Once the baby's head is delivered, the woman must be encouraged not to push. The baby's mouth and nose must be suctioned.
* The obstetrician must then feel around the baby's neck in order to rule out the presence of cord around the foetal neck.

Delivery of Shoulders

* Following the delivery of foetal head, the foetal head falls posteriorly, while the face comes in contact with the maternal anus. As the restitution or external rotation of the foetal head occurs, the occiput turns towards one of the maternal thighs, and the head assumes a transverse position. This movement implies that bisacromial diameter has rotated and has occupied the A-P diameter of the pelvis. Soon the anterior shoulder appears at the vaginal introitus.
* Following the delivery of the anterior shoulder, the posterior shoulder is born.

Delivery of Rest of the Body

This is followed by delivery of the rest of the body by lateral flexion.

Clamping the Cord

The umbilical cord must be clamped and cut if not done earlier.

Postdelivery Care

❖ The baby must be placed over the mother's abdomen and then handed over to the assisting nurse or the paediatrician

❖ The baby's body must be thoroughly dried, the eyes be wiped and breathing must be assessed

❖ In order to minimise the chances of aspiration of amniotic fluid, soon after the delivery of the thorax, the face must be wiped and the mouth and the nostrils must be aspirated

❖ The baby must be covered with a soft, dry cloth and then with a blanket to ensure that the baby remains warm and no heat loss occurs

❖ Following the delivery of baby, the placenta needs to be delivered

❖ The obstetrician must look for signs of placental separation following the delivery of the baby

❖ The third stage of labour must actively be managed.

 CLINICAL PEARLS

❖ The most common causes for abnormal hardness and tenderness of the uterus include abruptio placentae or a ruptured uterus.

❖ Intermittent auscultation of the foetal heart has been found to be equivalent to continuous electronic monitoring for the assessment of foetal well-being, provided that the nurse-to-patient ratio is 1:1.

PROLONGED LABOUR

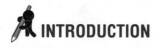 **INTRODUCTION**

If a woman's cervix fails to dilate as per the standards of Friedman's curve, she is traditionally assigned to the diagnosis of failure to progress and is usually delivered by caesarean section. 'Failure to progress' is one of the most important causes for unplanned caesarean deliveries in the United States.

Though the Friedman's curve was published nearly 60 years ago, it still continues to serve as the basis of how most physicians describe normal labour (Gabbe et al. 2014).[5] According to the Friedman's curve, abnormal progress of labour can be defined as the lack of changes or minimal change in cervical dilatation or effacement during a 2-hour period (for each of the phase: latent and active phase) in a woman having regular uterine contractions before the beginning of second stage of labour or as a descent of less than or equal to 1 cm/h in nullipara and less than or equal to 2 cm/h in multipara during the second stage of labour (from complete cervical dilatation to delivery). Indicators for abnormal labour have been described in Table 42.3.

Table 42.3: Diagnostic criteria for abnormal labour

Indicator	Nullipara	Multipara
Prolonged latent phase	>20 h	>14 h
Average second stage	50 min	20 min
Prolonged second stage without (with) epidural	>2 h (>3 h)	>1 h (>2 h)
Protraction disorders		
Protracted active-phase dilation	<1.2 cm/h	<1.5 cm/h
Protracted descent	≤1 cm/h	≤2 cm/h
Arrest disorders		
Prolonged deceleration	>3 h	>1 h
Secondary arrest of dilation*	>2 h	>2 h
Arrest of descent*	>1 h	>1 h
Failure of descent	No descent in the deceleration phase or the second stage of labour	
Third-stage disorders		
Prolonged third stage	>30 min	>30 min

*Adequate contractions >200 Montevideo units per 10 minutes for 2 hours

Modern researchers, however, feel that the Friedman's curve can no longer be applied to the modern day women because there have been many changes in the medical practice since 1955. Women are no longer sedated during labour. However, epidurals are commonly used. Use of epidural analgesia is likely to lengthen both the first and second stages of labour.[6,7] Also, oxytocin is much more frequently used for both labour induction and augmentation. Women in labour tend to belong to older age groups in comparison to the average age of 20 years included in the Friedman's study.

A study by Zhang et al. (2010) has shown that in the modern times, mothers do not rapidly start dilating at 3 cm as was observed by Dr Friedman in 1955.[8] Instead most modern women (both nullipara and multipara) begin active labour when they are 6 cm dilated. Before the cervical dilatation of 6 cm was reached, the progress in both nulliparas and multiparas appeared at a similar pace. However, after 6 cm, labour accelerated at a much faster pace in multiparas in comparison to the nulliparas. Majority of women took less than 2 hours to dilate by 1 cm during the active phase of labour. Interestingly, no dilatation occurred in many women for long periods, nevertheless they had a normal vaginal delivery.

The average rate of dilatation for the modern women was 1.2 cm/h during the active stage of labour. These results were different from those described by Friedman, according to whom 1.2 cm/h was the lowest acceptable rate of cervical dilation. In other words, what Friedman considered as slow labour is actually the normal rate of dilatation in the present time. Due to this discrepancy in Friedman's data and that in the modern times, many women may be incorrectly diagnosed as having failure to progress, when in fact they may be having normal labour.

The average duration of second stage of labour for nulliparous women was 1.1 hours with an epidural and 0.6 hours without an epidural. On the other hand, the average duration of second stage of labour for multiparous women was less than

Table 42.4: New definitions for normal labour and arrested labour[9,10]

Condition describing abnormal labour	Old definition (based on the ACOG Practice Bulletin, 2003)[10]	New evidence-based definition (Joint Workshop, 2014)[9]
Labour dystocia	Slow, abnormal progression of labour	This terminology is no longer used
Failure to progress	A vague term implying lack of progressive cervical dilatation, lack of descent of the baby's head or both	The workshop authors recommend that adequate time must be allowed for the normal latent and active phases of the first stage and for the second stage as long as the maternal and foetal conditions remain within normal limits.
Active labour	A woman is said to be in active labour after she attains a dilatation of about 3–4 cm. This is the time after which there should be a rapid increase in cervical dilatation	A woman is said to be in active labour after she attains a dilatation of about 6 cm. Multiparous women are likely to progress faster in comparison to the nulliparous women after this point.
Arrest of first stage of labour	Labour in the first stage is diagnosed as arrested when the woman in active labour has no change in cervical dilatation even after 2 h despite of having adequate contractions	Labour in the first stage is diagnosed as arrested when the woman with cervical dilatation of 6 cm and with ruptured membranes has no cervical changes for 4 h or more despite of having adequate contractions or for 6 h or more of inadequate contractions. In case the woman's cervix has dilated less than 6 cm, she requires additional time and interventions before arrest of labour can be diagnosed.
Arrest of second stage of labour	This can be diagnosed in the presence of following conditions: • >3 h in a nulliparous woman with an epidural • >2 h in a nulliparous woman without an epidural • >2 h in a multiparous woman with an epidural • >1 h in a multiparous woman without an epidural	This can be diagnosed in the presence of following conditions provided there is no descent or rotation of the baby: • After ≥4 h in nulliparous women with an epidural • After ≥3 h in nulliparous women without an epidural • After ≥3 h in multiparous women with an epidural • After ≥2 h in multiparous women without an epidural.
Failed induction of labour	Progression of labour differs significantly for women with an elective induction of labour in comparison with women who have had a spontaneous onset of labour. At least 12–18 h of latent labour must be allowed before arriving at the diagnosis of failed induction. This practice may help in reducing the rate of caesarean deliveries	Failure to have regular contractions (every 3 min) and failure of the cervix to change after at least 24 h of oxytocin (and ruptured membranes, if possible). This time should be measured following the completion of cervical ripening

0.5 hours with an epidural and about 0.25 hours without an epidural.

In the year 2012, ACOG, the Society for Maternal Foetal Medicine, and the National Institute for Maternal and Child Health came together in a joint workshop and proposed new definitions for normal labour and arrested labour (Table 42.4).[9]

AETIOLOGY

Various causes for abnormal progress of labour include abnormalities in the passage (bony pelvis and the soft tissues within the semirigid structure), passenger (baby) and the power (expulsive uterine contractions). These comprise of the following abnormalities:

Abnormalities in expulsive forces: These include:
❖ Hypotonic uterine dysfunction (uterine inertia)
❖ Hypertonic uterine dysfunction
❖ Poor maternal expulsive efforts (related to maternal fatigue or epidural analgesic use).

Foetal abnormalities: These include:
❖ Abnormalities in foetal size (e.g. foetal macrosomia, with foetal weight ≥4,000 g)
❖ Abnormalities in foetal presentation (e.g. brow, shoulder, face)
❖ Abnormalities in foetal position (e.g. occiput posterior, occiput transverse, etc.): Foetal malpresentations and malpositions may cause larger diameter of the foetal presenting part to present at the pelvic inlet. This may interfere with the rotation of foetal head, thereby impeding progress.
❖ Abnormalities in foetal attitude (extension, asynclitism, etc.)
❖ Foetal congenital abnormalities (anencephaly, foetal ascites, foetal tumours, etc.).

Pelvic abnormalities: These include:
❖ Cephalopelvic disproportion (CPD)
❖ Cervical dystocia.
Deformities of bony pelvis are rare in developed countries where the nutritional status during childhood is adequate. However, soft tissue abnormalities can also influence the

outcome of labour, e.g. abnormalities in the remodelling of cervix and space occupying lesions in the pelvis such as cervical fibroids, ovarian cysts, etc.

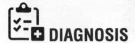

DIAGNOSIS

Clinical Presentation

These include the following:

❖ Lack of change or minimal change in cervical dilatation or effacement during a 2-hour period (for each of the phase: latent and active phase) in a woman having regular uterine contractions before the beginning of the second stage of labour

❖ Descent of less than or equal to 1.0 cm/h in nullipara and less than or equal to 2.0 cm/h in multipara during the second stage of labour.

Abdominal Examination

❖ Establishing and documenting an estimated foetal weight

❖ Monitoring the FHR and uterine contraction patterns.

Vaginal Examination

Vaginal examination should be regularly performed to monitor the progress of cervical dilation and descent of the foetal presenting part as described in the clinical presentation. Vaginal examination should also involve the following:

❖ *Clinical pelvimetry*: This is important for assessing the pelvic type (android, gynaecoid, platypelloid, anthropoid) and the presence of CPD, if any.

❖ *Evaluation of the position of foetal head*: This should be preferably done early in labour, because as labour progresses, caput and moulding may interfere with the correct assessment.

Investigations

❖ *Imaging studies*: X-ray pelvimetry and CT pelvimetry may be helpful for assessment of the maternal bony pelvis. These studies will help reassure the clinician regarding pelvic adequacy and for ruling out cephalopelvic disproportion as the probable cause of abnormal labour.

❖ *Partogram*: The simplest test used for evaluating abnormal progress of labour is to plot the patient's progress (cervical dilation and the decent of foetal presenting part) on a partogram.

❖ *Cardiotocography*: Intermittent auscultation and cardio-tography can be used for monitoring the FHR, especially when the labour is progressing abnormally. The clinician should make sure that the foetal heart tracing remains reassuring throughout the course of labour. Cardiotcography also helps in the evaluation of uterine contractions (especially their strength and frequency).

❖ *Ultrasound*: Examination by ultrasound helps in confirming an abnormal position, e.g. occiput posterior position as a cause of abnormal progress of labour. This may be sometimes useful when the diagnosis by clinical examination appears questionable.

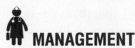

MANAGEMENT

Patients with prolonged latent phase can be managed in the following ways:

❖ *Optimisation of maternal well-being*: This can be ensured by provision of maternal hydration, pain relief and provision of one-to-one care or professional maternal companion, if not already provided. The carer need not necessarily be the midwife and should not be the husband or partner. Meta-analysis of RCTs has shown that the continuous presence of a caregiver is likely to reduce the likelihood of medication for pain relief, instrumental vaginal delivery, caesarean section and a 5-min APGAR score of less than 7.[11] Continuous support is also associated with a slight reduction in the overall length of labour.

❖ *Amniotomy*: Though amniotomy is traditionally practiced to shorten the duration of labour, meta-analysis has shown that amniotomy is not associated with a statistically significant reduction in the duration of first stage in nulliparous or multiparous women.[12] Amniotomy is therefore not recommended to be used routinely as part of standard labour management and care.

❖ *Mobilisation during labour*: According to the present recommendations, women in low-risk labour should be informed about the benefits of upright positions, and encouraged and assisted to assume whatever positions they choose.[13]

❖ *Stimulation with oxytocin*: It is possible to manipulate the component of 'power' or abnormalities in expulsive function to some extent. The frequency, intensity and duration of uterine contractions can be augmented through the use of oxytocin. However, use of oxytocin may not be practical in all situations. Also, it has the potential for inducing iatrogenic foetal compromise. Women with dysfunctional labour are likely to gain some benefit.

Use of oxytocin is encouraged by NICE (2007) for nulliparous women and has been shown to shorten the duration of labour.[14] However, it is not likely to bring down the rate of first-stage caesarean sections. However, in case of multiparous women, if there are chances of obstructed labour, forcing uterine contractions with oxytocin can result in uterine rupture. Therefore, NICE has recommended that oxytocin should only be started in multiparous women once the obstetrician has made full assessment. Current guidelines do not recommend the use of syntocinon in the second stage whether or not the regional anaesthesia is in place. The only exception to this would be cases where there are poor contractions at the beginning of second stage in nulliparous women with regional anaesthesia.

In cases of uterine hypocontractility, oxytocin (30 units diluted in 500 mL of saline) must be started at a rate of 0.5–1.0 mU/min and gradually increased by 1–2 mU/min at every 20–30 minutes, until an adequate pattern of contractions is achieved. Oxytocin should be titrated to provide a contraction frequency of 4–5 per 10 minutes with each contraction lasting for approximately 40 seconds. Oxytocin takes 30–45 minutes to reach the steady state levels following intravenous administration. Increment of oxytocin dosage should not be performed more frequently than half-hourly intervals. Such regimen has been found to be compatible with normal progress of labour with minimal adverse sequela. Appropriate steps must be taken if signs of maternal or foetal distress appear at any time. Amniotomy and oxygen infusion can also be tried in cases with reduced uterine activity. If there is no response even after 3 hours of augmentation with oxytocin, caesarean section may be required in most of the cases due to the possibility of an underlying CPD.

Continuous foetal monitoring is required with the use of oxytocin irrespective of the patient's parity. Once oxytocin has been commenced, vaginal examination must be done at every 4-hourly intervals. If there has been less than 2 cm progress, decision should be made regarding the requirement for caesarean section. Presently, there is paucity of evidence demonstrating that the use of oxytocin for augmenting labour is likely to improve either maternal or foetal outcome.

❖ *Assisted vaginal delivery*: Assisted vaginal delivery in the form of vacuum or forceps application can serve as a good option in cases of delayed second stage.
❖ *Caesarean section*: This may appear to be treatment of choice when vaginal delivery appears to be unsafe.

COMPLICATIONS

Maternal: There is an increased incidence of the following:
❖ Traumatic injuries (cervical tears, uterine rupture, etc.)
❖ Increased incidence of operative deliveries
❖ Chorioamnionitis
❖ Postpartum haemorrhage
❖ Puerperal sepsis, subinvolution.

Foetal: These include:
❖ Foetal hypoxia, thick meconium stained liquor
❖ Intracranial stress or haemorrhage
❖ Variable or delayed decelerations
❖ Foetal acidosis
❖ Five-minute APGAR score of less than 7
❖ Increased rate of admission to the NICU
❖ Increased perinatal morbidity and mortality.

CLINICAL PEARLS

❖ The evaluation of the descent of foetal head may be complicated due to development of moulding and caput formation.
❖ In nulliparous patients, inadequate uterine activity is a common cause of primary dysfunctional labour, while in multiparous patients CPD is the common cause.

❖ Women should be given an adequate time for both the first and second stages of labour. Also, an 'adequate' time is much longer than what has traditionally been allowed by Friedman in the past.

EVIDENCE-BASED MEDICINE

❖ The Friedman's criteria for normal labour, which is currently being used by most of the healthcare providers has now largely become obsolete. The new, evidence-based definitions of normal labour, labour arrest and failed induction, which have been proposed by ACOG, the Society for Maternal Foetal Medicine, and the National Institute for Maternal and Child Health in a joint workshop, should now be adopted by the obstetricians.[9] As long as mother and baby are both healthy, and as long as the length of labour does not qualify for being labelled as 'arrested labour', labouring women should be treated as if they are having normal progression of labour. More time must be allowed to women, who are being medically induced, for completion of the early phase of labour. Essentially, 6 cm and not 3–4 cm should be considered as the beginning of the active phase. Caregivers should always remember that during the normal latent phase of labour (before the dilatation of 6 cm), sometimes there may be no change in the cervical dilation for several hours.

❖ Immobilisation in the first stage has been associated with longer duration of labour and NICE discourages women from staying supine.[14] Not lying down in supine position and not being in lithotomy position has been associated with shorter duration of second stage and lower rates of caesarean section. The present evidence indicates that walking and upright positions in the first stage of labour is likely to reduce the duration of labour, the risk of caesarean birth and the requirement for epidural analgesia.[13] Moreover, this does not seem to be associated with increased requirement for intervention or cause any adverse effect on maternal and neonatal well-being. Better quality trials are still required in future to confirm the true risks and benefits of upright and mobile positions in comparison with recumbent positions for all women during labour.[15]

REFERENCES

1. Friedman EA. Primigravid labor; a graphicostatistical analysis. Obstet Gynecol. 1955;6(6):567-89.
2. Friedman EA. Labor in multiparas; a graphicostatistical analysis. Obstet Gynecol. 1956;8(6):691-703.
3. Royal College of Midwives (RCM). Evidence Based Guidelines for Midwifery-Led Care in Labour. London: Royal College of Midwives; 2012.
4. Lavender T, Hart A, Smyth RM. Effect of partogram use on outcomes for women in spontaneous labour at term. Cochrane Database Syst Rev. 2013;(7):CD005461.

PART II

5. Gabbe SG, Niebyl JR, Galan HL, Jauniaux ERM, Landon MB, Simpson JL, et al. Obstetrics: Normal and Problem Pregnancies, 6th edition. Philadelphia: Elsevier; 2014.

6. Alexander JM, Sharma SK, McIntire DD, Leveno KJ. Epidural analgesia lengthens the Friedman active phase of labor. Obstet Gynecol. 2002;100(1):46-50.

7. Frigo MG, Larciprete G, Rossi F, Fusco P, Todde C, Jarvis S, et al. Rebuilding the labor curve during neuraxial analgesia. J Obstet Gynaecol Res. 2011;37(11): 1532-9.

8. Zhang J, Landy HJ, Branch DW, Burkman R, Haberman S, Gregory KD, et al. Contemporary patterns of spontaneous labor with normal neonatal outcomes. Obstet Gynecol. 2010; 116(6):1281-7.

9. Spong CY, Berghella V, Wenstrom KD, Mercer BM, Saade GR. Preventing the first cesarean delivery: summary of a joint Eunice Kennedy Shriver National Institute of Child Health and Human Development, Society for Maternal-Fetal Medicine, and American College of Obstetricians and Gynecologists Workshop. Obstet Gynecol. 2012;120(5):1181-93.

10. American College of Obstetrics and Gynecology (ACOG) Committee on Practice Bulletins-Obstetrics. ACOG Practice Bulletin Number 49, December 2003: Dystocia and augmentation of labor. Obstet Gynecol. 2003;102(6):1445-54.

11. Hodnett ED, Gates S, Hofmeyr GJ, Sakala C. Continuous support for women during childbirth. Cochrane Database Syst Rev. 2013;7:CD003766.

12. Smyth RM, Markham C, Dowswell T. Amniotomy for shortening spontaneous labour. Cochrane Database Syst Rev. 2013;(6):CD006167.

13. Lawrence A, Lewis L, Hofmeyr GJ, Styles C. Maternal positions and mobility during first stage labour. Cochrane Database Syst Rev. 2013;(8):CD003934.

14. National Institute of Clinical Excellence (NICE). Intrapartum care: Care of healthy women and their babies during childbirth. NICE clinical guideline 55. London: NICE; 2007.

15. Royal College of Obstetricians and Gynaecologist (RCOG); Royal College of Midwives (RCM); Royal College of Anaesthetists (RCoA); and Royal College of Paediatrics and Child Health (RCPCH). Safer Childbirth: Minimum Standards for the Organisation and Delivery of Care in Labour. London: RCOG Press; 2007.

CHAPTER 42

Induction of Labour

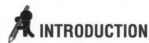

INTRODUCTION

Induction of labour (IOL) can be defined as commencement of uterine contractions before the spontaneous onset of labour with or without ruptured membranes. It is indicated when the benefits of delivery outweigh the benefits of continuing the pregnancy to either mother or the foetus. IOL comprises of cervical ripening (in case of an unfavourable cervix) and labour augmentation. While cervical ripening aims at making the cervix soft and pliable, augmentation refers to stimulation of spontaneous contractions which may be considered inadequate due to failed cervical dilation or foetal descent.[1] Dilatation and effacement of cervix associated with cervical ripening and labour augmentation ultimately results in delivery of the baby.

Cervical ripening is a complex process, primarily occurring under the influence of prostaglandins whereby prostaglandins cause the breakdown of the cervical proteoglycan ground substance, scattering of the collagen fibres, an increase in the content of substances such as elastase, glycosaminoglycans, dermatan sulphate and hyaluronic acid in the cervix.[2]

Induction of labour must be considered only when vaginal delivery appears to be an appropriate route of delivery and no contraindications for the vaginal route are present. IOL helps in expediting the process of vaginal delivery. It is a commonly used procedure in the UK, with labour in nearly every one out of five pregnancies being induced. IOL using pharmacological methods is likely to result in spontaneous labour without further intervention in about two-thirds of women, 10–15% are likely are likely to have instrumental births and 22% may require emergency caesarean sections. IOL can be done by using both medical and surgical methods.

Induction of labour needs to be clinically justified because this may has a huge impact on the maternal and neonatal mortality and morbidity. Increased gestational age beyond 40 weeks is associated with an increased risk of perinatal mortality. Birth after 42 weeks of gestation is likely to result in an increased rate of intrapartum and neonatal deaths. Therefore, women with uncomplicated pregnancies should be given every opportunity to go into spontaneous labour. IOL must be offered to women with uncomplicated pregnancies between 41+0 to 42+0 weeks of gestation to avoid the risks related to prolonged pregnancy. Women who do not wish to have IOL should be offered additional antenatal monitoring which should include as a minimum, an electronic foetal monitoring and measurement of liquor volume twice weekly. IOL can be carried out in the outpatient setting, with safety and support procedures in place. IOL when carried out in the inpatient setting, it should be preferably during the morning hours due to higher maternal satisfaction rates. The exact timing for induction must be based on the woman's preferences and clinical circumstances.

INDICATIONS

Induction of labour is indicated only in those situations where it becomes apparent that both the mother and the foetus would be associated with a higher likelihood of better outcome, if the foetal birth is expedited.[3] Before taking the decision for IOL, the obstetrician must weigh the benefits of labour induction against the potential maternal and foetal risks. Though there are no absolute indications for IOL, some common clinical indications and contraindications for IOL are discussed in Tables 43.1 and 43.2 respectively.

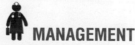

MANAGEMENT

Preprocedure Preparation

Prior to the IOL, following steps must be performed:
❖ *Patient counselling:* Before IOL is undertaken, the patient must be carefully counselled. She should be explained about the reason for induction, end points of the process, requirement for LSCS in case the induction

Table 43.1: Indications for induction of labour

Maternal indications	
Indications specific to pregnancy	*Maternal disease*
• Prolonged pregnancy • Prelabour rupture of membranes at term • Premature prelabour rupture of membranes • Polyhydramnios/oligohydramnios • Ruptured membranes with pre-eclampsia or eclampsia or non-reassuring foetal heart status • Abruptio placentae • Chorioamnionitis • Rh isoimmunisation • Maternal request • Advanced maternal age • Multifoetal pregnancy	• Diabetes mellitus • Renal disease • Chronic pulmonary disease • Obstetric cholestasis • Chronic hypertension
Foetal indications	
• Postmaturity • Intrauterine growth restriction • Premature rupture of membranes • Foetus with congenital anomalies • Intrauterine foetal death • Suspected foetal macrosomia	

Table 43.2: Contraindications for induction of labour

Absolute	Relative
• Transverse lie • Vasa praevia, placenta praevia • Previous caesarean delivery/scarred uterus (especially with the involvement of uterine cavity)	• Previous lower segment caesarean section • Breech presentation • Multiple pregnancy • Maternal heart disease

fails, options for mode of delivery, neonatal outcomes and complications, when, where and how induction would be carried out, the alternative options if the woman chooses not to have IOL, the risks and benefits of IOL in specific circumstances, the proposed methods for induction, the arrangements for providing support and pain relief, etc. Provision of pain relief may be particularly important because women are likely to find induced labour more painful than spontaneous labour. All relevant information should be made available to the woman and she should be helped to be able to make an informed choice regarding her care or treatment plan.

❖ *Evaluation of the state of cervix:* This is done by calculation of the Bishop's score (Table 43.3). A maximum score of 13 is possible with this scoring system. Labour is most likely to commence spontaneously with a score of 9 or more, whereas lower scores (especially those <5) may require cervical ripening and/or augmentation with oxytocin.[4] Bishop score should be again reassessed 6 hours after vaginal instillation of PGE$_2$ tablet or gel and 24 hours following the vaginal insertion of PGE$_2$ controlled-release pessary.

Table 43.3: Bishop's score (modified)

Score	Dilation (cm)	Effacement (%)	Station of the presenting part	Cervical consistency	Position of cervix
0	Closed	0–30	−3	Firm	Posterior
1	1–2	40–50	−2	Medium	Mid position
2	3–4	60–70	−1, 0	Soft	Anterior
3	>5	>80	+1, +2	–	–

❖ *Ultrasound assessment of gestational age:* This would help to prevent induction in premature babies.

❖ *Assessment of foetal lung maturity:* This may not be required in case where induction is medically indicated and the risk of continuing the pregnancy is greater than the risk of delivering a baby before lung maturity has been attained.

❖ *Maternal and foetal monitoring:* Before the initiation of IOL, healthcare professional should make sure that the facilities are available for continuous electronic FHR and uterine contraction monitoring. Once the cardiotocographic trace comes out as normal while the patient is being induced, intermittent auscultation can be used.

❖ *Pain relief:* Women being offered IOL should be informed that induced labour is likely to be more painful in comparison to the spontaneous labour. Women should therefore be informed regarding the availability of various pain relief options ranging from simple analgesics to epidural analgesia. For the purpose of pain relief, the opportunity to labour in water is also sometimes recommended.

METHODS FOR INDUCTION

Methods of cervical ripening include pharmacological methods, non-pharmacological methods and use of mechanical cervical dilators.[5]

Pharmacological Methods

Medical methods for labour induction commonly comprise of prostaglandins [dinoprostone (PGE$_2$) or misoprostol (PGE$_1$)] and/or oxytocin.

Dinoprostone

Vaginal instillation of dinoprostone (PGE2) gel is the preferred method for IOL. Advantages of using prostaglandins over oxytocin for IOL are listed in Box 43.1. Dinoprostone helps in cervical ripening and is available in the form of gel (Prepidil or Cerviprime) or vaginal tablet or controlled-release vaginal insert (Cervidil®). Prepidil comprises of 0.5 mg of dinoprostone in a 2.5 mL syringe.[6] The gel is injected intracervically every 6 hours for up to the maximum of two doses in a 24-hour period. Cervidil, on the other hand, is a vaginal insert containing 10 mg of dinoprostone. One cycle of vaginal PGE$_2$ controlled-release pessary is administered over 24 hours. The main advantage of

Box 43.1: Advantages of using prostaglandins over oxytocin for induction of labour

❑ Use of prostaglandins over oxytocin for induction of labour facilitates ambulation
❑ The labour contractions are less painful
❑ The risk of postpartum haemorrhage is lower in comparison with oxytocin
❑ No danger of fluid overload and neonatal jaundice as observed with oxytocin

Cervidil is that it can be immediately removed in case it causes hyperstimulation.

On the other hand, the main advantage of using oxytocin is that it is possible to control the augmented labour while using oxytocin infusion with the help of continuous monitoring of the uterine activity and FHR. The rate of infusion is controlled by the healthcare provider and can be stopped, reduced or increased at any moment whenever the need arises. On the contrary, the IOL cannot be controlled while using prostaglandins. Once a prostaglandin tablet has been consumed orally or the prostaglandin gel has been instilled, the effect of the drug cannot be as reversed unlike in case of oxytocin. Use of prostaglandins is favoured over oxytocin in cases where labour is induced in either nulliparous or multiparous women with intact membranes, regardless of the fact whether the cervix is favourable or not. However, if the membranes have ruptured, both prostaglandins and oxytocin may be used, as both of them are equally effective in such cases.

Misoprostol

Misoprostol (Cytotec) is a synthetic PGE_1 analogue. This drug has not been currently approved by the United States Food and Drug Administration (US FDA) for cervical ripening or IOL. Misoprostol, however, has been approved for the prevention of peptic ulcers. Use of misoprostol for cervical ripening is an off-label use, which is still considered controversial by some clinicians. However, its use is recommended by the ACOG. A dose of 25 mg is placed transvaginally at every 3 hourly interval for a maximum of 4 doses or it may be prescribed in the oral dosage of 50 mg orally at every 4 hourly interval.[7] Also, presently, the available evidence supports the intravaginal or oral use of 25–50 µg of PGE_1 for cervical ripening or IOL. The same dosage can be repeated after 4–6 hours, if required.

100 µg of oral or 25 µg of vaginal misoprostol has been found to be similar in efficacy to IV oxytocin for labour induction. In comparison to the PGE_2 analogues, PGE_1 analogues are cheaper, can be stored at room temperature and are easy to administer. PGE_1 is a more effective method of cervical ripening than either intravaginal or intracervical PGE_2 or oxytocin. PGE_1 in comparison to PGE_2 has been found to be associated with an increased incidence of hyperstimulation.[8] The safety issues concerning the use of vaginal misoprostol are presently unclear and it has yet not got FDA approval for its use as an inducing agent. Misoprostol overdosage, however, can be associated with complications such as tachysystole, uterine hyperstimulation, which may be associated with

birth asphyxia and/or rupture uterus. Another complication, which may occur, is meconium-stained liquor (resulting in meconium aspiration). Presently, as recommended by NICE (2008), use of misoprostol for the purpose of IOL is limited to the cases of intrauterine foetal death or in the context of a clinical trial.[9]

Oxytocin

Oxytocin is a uterotonic agent which stimulates uterine contractions and is used for both induction and augmentation of labour. It can be started in low dosage regimens of 0.5–1.5 mU/min or the high dosage regimen of 4.5–6.0 mU/min, with incremental increases of 1.0–2.0 mU/min at every 15–40 minutes.[10] If an intrauterine pressure catheter is in place, measurement of intrauterine pressure ranging between 180 Montevideo units/10 minutes to 200 Montevideo units/10 minutes is an indicator of adequate oxytocin dosing.

Other Pharmacological Methods for Induction of Labour

Mifepristone (Mifeprex) is an antiprogesterone agent, which is able to stimulate the uterine contractions.[11] It may be offered as a method of IOL to women who have intrauterine foetal death.

Isosorbide mononitrate is another agent, which can be used for cervical ripening without stimulating uterine activity. Breast massage and nipple stimulation is a non-pharmacologic method, which is thought to stimulate uterine contractions by facilitating the release of oxytocin from the posterior pituitary gland. The most commonly used technique involves gentle massage of the breasts or application of warm compresses to the breasts for 1 hour, three times a day.

Non-pharmacological or Surgical Management

Various non-pharmacological methods for labour induction comprise of the following:
❖ Low ROM
❖ Stripping of membranes.

Low Rupture of Membranes

Artificial rupture of membranes (ARM) is used as a method of induction only in the patients where the cervix is favourable. ARM induces labour by causing the release of prostaglandins.[12]

Procedure for Rupture of Membranes

❖ Before proceeding with ARM, the FHR must be checked.
❖ After placing the woman in lithotomy position, under all aseptic precautions, two fingers smeared with antiseptic ointment are introduced inside the vagina.
❖ The index finger is passed through the cervical canal beyond the internal cervical os.
❖ Using the index and the middle fingers, the foetal membranes are swept free from the lower uterine segment as far as can be reached with fingers.
❖ While the fingers are still in the cervical canal, with the palmar surface upward, a long Kocher's forceps with closed blades is introduced along the palmar aspect of the fingers up to the membranes.

* The blades of the Kocher's forceps are opened to grasp the membranes and tear it using twisting movements.
* When the membranes rupture, there is a visible gush of amniotic fluid.
* The colour of the escaping liquor must be noted. Meconium-stained liquor is suggestive of foetal distress.
* If the head is not engaged, an assistant must push the head to fix it to the brim in order to prevent cord prolapse.

Advantages: Advantages of amniotomy or ROM are as follows:

* The process of ARM, by providing extensive contact between the foetal presenting part and the cervix, encourages release of endogenous prostaglandins, thereby augmenting labour and shortening its duration.
* The escape of liquor at the time of ARM provides the opportunity for early detection of meconium-stained liquor amnii and the possibility of foetal distress, thereby instigating closer observation of foetal well-being.

Stripping of Membranes

As the name implies, the process involves stripping of membranes by inserting the examining finger through the internal cervical os and moving it in a circular direction to detach the inferior pole of the membranes from the lower uterine segment. The process is thought to augment labour by causing the release of prostaglandins ($PGF_{2\alpha}$) and phospholipase A_2.

Mechanical Methods

This may include natural osmotic dilators (e.g. laminaria tents) and synthetic osmotic dilators. The natural dilators are hygroscopic in nature and are capable of absorbing endocervical and local tissue fluids, which cause the device to enlarge within the endocervical canal, thereby exerting controlled mechanical pressure. Balloon devices such as 24/26-French Foley's balloon can also be used to provide mechanical pressure directly in the cervix as the balloon is inflated.

POSTPROCEDURAL CARE

Artificial Rupture of Membranes

Following the process of ARM, the following steps must be observed:

* Colour of liquor and cervical status following ROM is observed.
* The clinician must detect cord prolapse, if present.
* Quality of FHR must be assessed following ROM. In case the FHR is less than 100 beats/min or more than 180 beats/min, foetal distress must be suspected.
* Foetal electrode may be applied in high-risk cases in order to assess the foetal heart status.
* A sterile vulvar pad is applied.
* Prophylactic antibiotics may be administered in case delivery is not anticipated within 18 hours.

* If good labour is not established 1 hour after ARM, oxytocin infusion must be started. In case of the presence of severe maternal disease (e.g. sepsis, eclampsia, etc.), oxytocin infusion must begin at the same time as ARM.

INDUCTION OF LABOUR IN SPECIFIC CIRCUMSTANCES

Preterm prelabour rupture of membranes: Induction of labour should not be carried out before 34 weeks unless there is presence of an additional obstetric indications such as infection, foetal compromise, etc. In case of preterm prelabour ROM after 34 weeks, the decision regarding whether or not to induce labour, using vaginal PGE_2 must be taken after taking into consideration several factors such as risks to the woman (e.g. sepsis, possible requirement for caesarean section), risks to the baby (e.g. sepsis, problems relating to preterm birth) and local availability of neonatal intensive care facilities. Women with prelabour ROM at term (at or over 37 weeks) can be offered a choice between IOL with vaginal PGE_2 or expectant management.[9]

Previous caesarean section: Women with a previous history of caesarean delivery undergoing VBAC may be offered IOL with vaginal PGE_2 based on the woman's individual circumstances and wishes.[9] Women undergoing VBAC, in whom labour is induced, must be counselled regarding the increased requirement for emergency caesarean section during induced labour as well as an increased risk of uterine rupture.

Maternal request: Induction of labour should not be routinely offered on maternal request alone except under exceptional circumstances when induction may be considered at or after 40 weeks.

Breech presentation: Induction of labour is not generally recommended in the cases of breech presentation. IOL can be offered in certain circumstances such as external cephalic version is unsuccessful, declined or contraindicated, and the woman does not give consent for an elective caesarean section. In such cases, IOL can be offered after discussing the associated risks with the woman.

Foetal growth restriction: Induction of labour is not recommended in cases of severe foetal growth restriction with confirmed foetal compromise.

Suspected foetal macrosomia: Labour should not be routinely induced in cases of suspected foetal macrosomia.

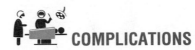 COMPLICATIONS

Induction of labour, in general, can be associated with the following complications:

* Uterine hyperstimulation (with oxytocin and misoprostol) may result in uteroplacental hypoperfusion and FHR deceleration. Use of tocolysis can be considered if uterine hyperstimulation occurs during IOL.

❖ Prostaglandins may produce tachysystole, which may be controlled with terbutaline.

❖ Maternal systemic effects, such as fever, vomiting and diarrhoea, may be infrequently observed.

❖ *Failure of induction*: Induction can be considered as failed if labour does not start after one cycle of treatment. If induction fails, decisions about further management should be made in accordance with the woman's wishes, and her clinical circumstances. If IOL fails, the subsequent management options include a further attempt to induce labour or caesarean delivery.

❖ *Uterine rupture*: Increased incidence of uterine rupture is likely to occur in women with previous caesarean delivery undergoing VBAC in whom labour is induced. If uterine rupture is suspected during induced labour, the baby should be delivered by emergency caesarean section.

❖ Uterine atony and postpartum haemorrhage

❖ Increased rate of caesarean delivery

❖ Chorioamnionitis

❖ The obstetrician is compelled to accomplish delivery within a reasonable period of time.

❖ Oxytocin may be responsible for producing water intoxication.

Complications associated with ARM are as follows:

❖ Reduction in amniotic fluid may result in cord compression and/or head compression.

❖ The intensity of pains may increase to undesirable levels, adversely affecting the foetus.

❖ There may be a danger of cord prolapse and/or limb prolapse.

❖ Predisposition to a premature separation of the placenta

❖ The risk of ascending infection, which further increases with the passage of time.

To reduce the incidence of cord prolapse, one of the most important complications of ARM, the obstetricians and midwives should observe the following precautions:

❖ Before induction, engagement of the presenting part should be assessed.

❖ The healthcare professional should try palpating for umbilical cord presentation at the time of preliminary vaginal examination. If umbilical cord is felt at the time of vaginal examination, obstetrician must avoid dislodging the baby's head.

❖ Amniotomy should be avoided if the baby's head is high.

Complications associated with sweeping and stretching of membranes include risk of infection, bleeding, accidental rupture of the membranes and discomfort to the patient.

CLINICAL PEARLS

❖ Most women are likely to go into labour spontaneously by 42 weeks of gestation.

❖ Intracervical application of dinoprostone (PGE$_2$, 0.5 mg gel) has been the gold standard for cervical ripening. On the other hand, oxytocin is the most commonly used drug all over the world to augment labour.

Table 43.4: Methods for induction of labour not supported by the available evidence[9]

Pharmacological methods	Non-pharmacological methods
• Oral PGE$_2$	• Herbal supplements
• Intravenous PGE$_2$	• Acupuncture
• Extra-amniotic PGE$_2$	• Homeopathy
• Intracervical PGE$_2$	• Castor oil
• Intravenous oxytocin alone	• Hot baths
• Hyaluronidase	• Enemas
• Corticosteroids	• Sexual intercourse
• Oestrogen	
• Vaginal nitric oxide donors	

❖ Amniotomy, alone or with oxytocin, should not be used as a primary method of IOL unless there are specific clinical reasons for not using vaginal PGE$_2$ (e.g. risk of uterine hyperstimulation).

❖ Mechanical procedures (balloon catheters and laminaria tents) should not be routinely used for IOL.

❖ Vaginal PGE$_2$ has been used in UK practice for many years in women with ruptured membranes. However, as per recommendations by NICE (2008), vaginal PGE$_2$ should be either not used or should be used with caution in women with ruptured membranes.[12] Before prescribing vaginal PGE$_2$ for women with ruptured membranes, the healthcare professionals must obtain informed consent and document it in the patient's notes.

EVIDENCE-BASED MEDICINE

❖ The present evidence has shown that the labour induced by prostaglandins is likely to have a longer interval between ROM and delivery in comparison to that induced with oxytocin and ROM, especially in cases where the cervix is ripe.[13] However, in cases where the cervix is unripe, prostaglandins are likely to be more successful than oxytocin in inducing labour.[14]

❖ The available evidence does not support use of various methods enlisted in Table 43.4 for IOL.[9]

REFERENCES

1. ACOG Committee on Practice Bulletins—Obstetrics. ACOG Practice Bulletin No. 107: Induction of labor. Obstet Gynecol. 2009;114(2 Pt 1):386-97.
2. Friedman E. Labor: Clinical Evaluation and Management, 2nd edition. New York: Appleton-Century-Crofts; 1978.
3. Royal College of Obstetricians and Gynaecologists. (2001). Induction of labour. Evidence-based Clinical Guideline Number 9. [online] Available from www.perinatal.sld.cu/docs/guiasclinicas/inductionoflabour.pdf. [Accessed August, 2016].
4. Hadi H. Cervical ripening and labor induction: clinical guidelines. Clin Obstet Gynecol. 2000;43(3):524-36.
5. Adair CD. Nonpharmacologic approaches to cervical priming and labor induction. Clin Obstet Gynecol. 2000;43(3):447-54.

6. Arias F. Pharmacology of oxytocin and prostaglandins. Clin Obstet Gynecol. 2000;43(3):455-68.

7. Hofmeyr GJ, Gülmezoglu AM, Pileggi C. Vaginal misoprostol for cervical ripening and induction of labour. Cochrane Database Syst Rev. 2010;(10):CD000941.

8. Buser D, Mora G, Arias F. A randomized comparison between misoprostol and dinoprostone for cervical ripening and labor induction in patients with unfavorable cervices. Obstet Gynecol. 1997;89(4):581-5.

9. National Institute of Clinical Excellence. (2008). Induction of labour. Clinical Guideline 70. [online] Available from www.nice.org.uk/guidance/cg70/resources/inducing-labour-975621704389. [Accessed June, 2016].

10. Keirse MC. Augmentation of labor. In: Chalmers I, Enkin M, Keirse MC (Eds). Effective Care in Pregnancy and Childbirth. Oxford: Oxford University Press; 1989. pp. 951-66.

11. Neilson JP. Mifepristone for induction of labour. Cochrane Database Syst Rev. 2000;(4):CD002865.

12. Bricker L, Luckas M. Amniotomy alone for induction of labour. Cochrane Database Syst Rev. 2000;(4):CD002862.

13. Bhasin A. Comparison of maternal complications in patients induced with oral PGE2 and oxytocin. J Obstet Gynaecol India. 1993;43:553.

14. Witter FR. Prostaglandin E2 preparations for preinduction cervical ripening. Clin Obstet Gynecol. 2000;43(3):469-74.

CHAPTER 43

Anaesthesia and Analgesia in Labour

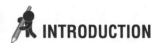 INTRODUCTION

Provision of effective and safe analgesia during labour has remained an ongoing challenge for the healthcare professionals. In the middle of 20th century, neuraxial techniques were introduced for providing pain relief during labour. Since the past two decades,[1] there have been numerous developments that have led to comprehensive and evidence-based management of labour pain. The availability of regional analgesia for labour reflects the standard obstetric care. The National Health Services Maternity Statistics of 2005–2006 in the UK reported that one-third of the pregnant patients chose epidural analgesia during labour. Currently, the rate of regional analgesia in the UK is approximately 22.7%. Epidural analgesia has presently become a commonly employed technique for providing pain relief during labour. Epidural analgesia should be administered only once the diagnosis of labour has been established and the patient requests for pain relief. Use of early neuraxial labour analgesia does not negatively affect the mode of delivery. Moreover, it results in an improved level of maternal satisfaction.

METHODS OF PAIN RELIEF IN LABOUR

Non-pharmacological Methods

Various non-pharmacological methods such as use of trans-cutaneous electrical nerve stimulation (TENS), continuous support in labour, touch and massage, water bath, intradermal sterile water injections, acupuncture and hypnosis may be beneficial for the management of pain during labour.[2] TENS involves application of electrical impulses to the skin via flexible electrodes that are placed over T10 to L1 dermatomes on either side of the spinous process to provide analgesia for the first stage of labour. However, the trials evaluating such methods have small number of women and

they do not provide sufficient evidence regarding the quality of pain relief provided by these techniques. While there is some evidence suggesting that water immersion during the first stage of labour helps in reducing the requirement for epidural analgesia, there is no evidence to show that the use of TENS provides better analgesia in comparison to placebo. Nevertheless, TENS can reduce the requirement for other analgesic interventions and is free from side effects.

Parenteral Narcotics

Systemic opioids are the most widely used medications for labour analgesia. Though their efficacy during labour is limited, they invariably provide sedation. However, all opioids can cause reduced APGAR and neurobehavioural scores, and neonatal respiratory distress even when administered few hours before birth. It may also inhibit maternal gastric emptying, thereby increasing the occurrence of nausea and vomiting.

Neonatal respiratory depression caused by opioids can be reversed through direct IV/IM injection of 0.1 mL/kg body weight of naloxone, a specific opioid antagonist, to the newborn. There is no benefit of administering naloxone to the mother during labour or just before delivery. Naloxone use may sometimes precipitate a withdrawal in the newborn of the opioid-dependent mother.[3]

Opioid drugs can be prescribed and administered by the midwives in accordance with the rules of Nursing and Midwifery Council and locally agreed upon policies and procedures.

Pethidine: Pethidine (meperidine), an opioid agonist, is the most frequently used opioid in the UK as well as across the globe. Its effect on progress of labour presently remains puzzling. Pethidine should not be preferably administered in patients with cervical dystocia as there is no evidence of beneficial action, rather there is an increased risk of neonatal adverse outcome.[4]

Ketamine: Ketamine, categorised as a 'dissociative anaesthetic agent' also acts on the opioid receptors. Besides its use for initiation and maintenance of anaesthesia, it is also commonly used for providing pain relief. Use of IV ketamine as a sole anaesthetic agent for labour pains is not considered safe because the labouring mother may often require anaesthetic dosages which may compromise the baby's airways. Furthermore, the benzodiazepines administered for counteracting delirium, resulting from ketamine use, can cause neonatal respiratory depression. Its usage during labour should preferably be discouraged.

Fentanyl: Fentanyl is a highly lipid-soluble synthetic opioid with a high analgesic potency.[5] It can be considered as a useful drug for labour analgesia due to its rapid onset of action within 2–3 min after IV route, with short duration of action and with no major metabolites. It can be administered in boluses of 25–50 µg every hour or as a continuous infusion of 0.25 µg/kg/h. Due to the rapid onset of action and delayed clearance, fentanyl is perhaps the drug of choice administered by patient-controlled intravenous analgesia (PCA). It is administered as the bolus dosage of 20–30 µg and 5-minutes lockout period.

Tramadol: Tramadol is a pethidine-like synthetic opioid having only 10% potency in comparison to that of morphine. When administered in the dosage of 1–2 mg/kg body weight, it does not cause clinically significant respiratory depression. The onset of action of tramadol occurs within 10 minutes of IM administration and the duration lasts for approximately 2–3 h. Though tramadol is capable of easily crossing the placenta, the neonates are able to completely metabolise tramadol via hepatic route.[6]

Butorphanol: Butorphanol is an opioid having agonist-antagonist properties similar to that of pentazocine. It offers analgesia with sedation. It is five times as potent as morphine and 40 times as potent as pethidine. Butorphanol is administered in the dosage of 2–4 mg intramuscularly. Butorphanol is not commonly used for labour analgesia because it is associated with high rates of sedation.

Remifentanil: Remifentanil is an ultrashort-acting synthetic opioid with a high potency. It has a rapid onset of action and is readily metabolised by plasma and tissue esterases into an inactive metabolite. The effective analgesic half-life is approximately 6 minutes. It thus allows effective analgesic action for consecutive uterine contractions. It readily crosses the placenta. However, it is largely metabolised by the foetus. Due to its pharmacokinetic profile, this drug is preferred over other opioids for labour PCA.[7] The recommended dose of remifentanil is an IV bolus of 20 µg, with a lockout interval of 3 minutes on the PCA pump. However, there appear to be wide variations in the dosage required for effective labour analgesia. During IV PCA with remifentanil, the mother should be monitored on a one-to-one basis because maternal hypoventilation may be commonly present. IV administration of remifentanil by PCA system is useful for women with thrombocytopenia or other haematological abnormalities because it helps in avoiding the requirement for regional analgesia or IM injection. This appears to be a promising technique for women whom requesting labour analgesia, in neuraxial techniques are contraindicated.

Inhalation Methods

The most commonly used anaesthetic agent which helps in provision of analgesia through inhalation is nitrous oxide (Entonox®). It is administered as a 50:50 mixture of oxygen and nitrous oxide. Other inhalational agents which have been tried in the recent times include the volatile anaesthetic agents, such as sevoflurane (Sevox), isoflurane and enflurane. Sevoflurane has a short onset and offset of action. It, therefore, appears to be the best-suited inhalational agent for labour analgesia and can be administered as patient-controlled inhalation analgesia.[8] These agents are, however, not widely accepted in the clinical practice.

Entonox

Entonox® is usually self-administered by inspiration through a facemask or mouthpiece. Inhalation of the gas should preferably begin as soon as the contraction begins to allow maximum drug effect during the peak of contraction. Hyperventilation with Entonox® can be followed by a period of apnoea. Therefore, the woman should always hold the mouthpiece by herself. In case, she becomes unconscious and experiences apnoea, she would let go of the mask. A few breaths of air would eliminate nitrous oxide and her consciousness would be invariably regained soon.

The drug is non-cumulative and does not affect the foetus. Prolonged inhalation of Entonox® can, however, inactivate vitamin B12 and inhibit DNA synthesis. A systemic review of literature regarding the use of Entonox® in labour has not shown Entonox® to be a potent analgesic agent.[9] Pain is still perceived under the influence of this drug. In fact, it is rendered more bearable due to the intoxicated state. Nearly 30–40% of women in labour derive no benefit. This review demonstrates the beneficial action of Entonox® only in cases where the method of inhalation is properly followed. Entonox® inhalation can serve as a useful method in places where neuraxial techniques are not practiced, and in patients with a short duration of labour. It can cause highly variable maternal sedative effect. According to the guidelines by the Obstetric Anaesthetists Association, UK (2013), Entonox® is being rapidly discontinued from the UK due to its poor analgesic efficacy and potential to cause environmental pollution.[10]

Regional Analgesia in Labour

Central neuraxial analgesia is currently the gold standard technique for pain control in obstetrics.[11] It helps in providing pain relief through the blockade of sensory nerves as they enter the spinal cord. Local anaesthetic agents and/or opioids can be introduced into the epidural and/or the subarachnoid (intrathecal) space. The use of neuraxial techniques has increased dramatically in the last 20 years, especially in the western world. There are few dedicated centres in India as well. The satisfaction of birth experience is greater with the use of neuraxial techniques. Nearly 90% of the consultant obstetric units in the UK provide a 24-hour regional analgesia service.

INDICATIONS

Indications for the use of obstetric analgesia are as follows:

❖ Provision of pain relief during first and second stages of labour

❖ Facilitation of patient cooperation during labour and delivery

❖ Provision of anaesthesia for episiotomy or forceps delivery, or extension for caesarean delivery.

CONTRAINDICATIONS

Contraindications for administration of epidural analgesia are as follows:

❖ Epidural analgesia must not be administered in presence of active maternal haemorrhage, coagulation disorders, maternal septicaemia and/or infection at the insertion site.

❖ *Administration of low-molecular-weight heparin:* Administration of LMWH in previous 10–12 hours is a relative contraindication.

❖ *Previous spinal surgery:* Previous history of spinal surgery is a contraindication for epidural analgesia because scar tissue from previous spinal surgery can make the identification of epidural space difficult and impede the spread of local anaesthetic solution.

❖ *Untreated pyrexia:* In these cases, there is a risk of bacteraemia and possibility for the development of vertebral canal abscess in case bleeding occurs from the epidural veins.

❖ *Hypovolaemia or active haemorrhage:* There is a risk of cardiovascular collapse secondary to the sympathetic blockade.

❖ Patient refusal

❖ *Lack of sufficient resources:* Epidural analgesia is also contraindicated in situations where there is a lack of sufficiently trained midwives for the continuous maternal and foetal care and monitoring for the entire duration of the epidural block.

SURGICAL MANAGEMENT (EPIDURAL ANALGESIA)

Preoperative Preparation

❖ Informed consent must be obtained from the patient.

❖ Prehydration with 500–1,000 mL of crystalloid solution in order to prevent the development of postprocedural hypotension

❖ Patient is placed in lateral decubitus or sitting position.

Steps of Surgery

❖ Under all aseptic precautions, the epidural Tuohy's needle is inserted in the epidural space between the vertebra L3 and L4. Epidural space lies between the dura mater and the ligamentum flavum in the space between the vertebra L3

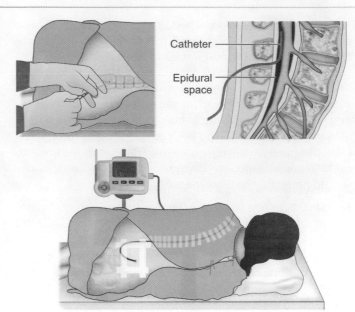

Fig. 44.1: Administration of epidural analgesia

and L4 (Fig. 44.1). It can be identified by loss of resistance at the time of needle insertion.

❖ An epidural catheter is threaded by 3–5 cm into the epidural space. An indwelling catheter is usually kept in place for repeated bolus top-up injections or continuous infusion.

❖ A test dose of 3 mL of 1.5% lidocaine with 1:200,000 epinephrine or 3 mL of 0.25% bupivacaine with 1:200,000 epinephrine is injected.

❖ If the test dose is negative, approximately 10 mL of 0.25% bupivacaine (Marcaine) or 0.25% of ropivacaine, with or without a small dose of a lipid-soluble opioid (e.g. fentanyl or sufentanil) is injected. Synergistic mixture of local anaesthetic agent and opioids has enabled significant reductions in the amount of local anaesthetic agent used. While the local anaesthetic prevents the conduction of nerve impulses, opioids act on specific receptors in the spinal cord.

❖ Following this, epidural analgesia may be maintained either with intermittent bolus injections or continuous epidural infusion. Patient-controlled epidural analgesia (PCEA) may also be used.

❖ In case of spinal analgesia, the needles used for spinal injection are much finer than the Tuohy's needle. Also, the subarachnoid space, which contains the cerebrospinal fluid is a few millimeters deep inside the meninges.

Postoperative Care

❖ Following the administration of epidural analgesia, the woman is placed in lateral or semilateral position in order to avoid aortocaval compression.

❖ Blood pressure must be recorded at every 5–15 minutes interval for an hour following the procedure.

❖ Continuous FHR monitoring at least for an hour following the procedure is required to detect any abnormalities in the FHR.

❖ Hourly monitoring of the level of analgesia and intensity of motor blockade is required.

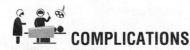

COMPLICATIONS

Immediate

These include:

- *Maternal hypotension:* Intracranial hypotension due to low pressure of cerebrospinal fluid can be rarely complicated by the cranial subdural haematoma secondary to the tearing of dural bridging veins.
- *Toxicity of local anaesthetics:* In case of an inadvertent injection of a local anaesthetic agent in the epidural vein, signs and symptoms of local anaesthetic toxicity can arise due to the high concentration of local anaesthetic agent in the CNS. Rarely convulsions and/or cardiac arrest may be induced by local anaesthetics. A new and effective treatment, IV Intralipid® 20% has been introduced for local anaesthetic-induced cardiac arrest.[12] The dose for a 70-kg adult is 100 mL. In the most recent report by the CEMD, one of the deaths was due to IV administration of bupivacaine from an infusion bag intended for epidural use. This death might have been avoided if Intralipid® therapy had been available.
- *Side effects specific to opioids:* In the most likely event of the cephalad spread of opioids to the brainstem, maternal respiratory depression can occur. Another side effect related to the use of opioids is pruritus.
- *Total spinal:* Any inadvertent communication between the epidural and subarachnoid space may be associated with the risk of introduction of large dose of local anaesthetic agent, which was ideally intended for the epidural space, to reach the subarachnoid space. 'Total spinal' can be described as a block high enough to impair the diaphragmatic innervation, thereby causing respiratory arrest. Emergency tracheal intubation and treatment of hypotension may be required for the mother. An emergency caesarean delivery may be required based on abnormal FHR pattern. Once the high block has regressed, tracheal extubation may be carried out.
- Increase in the duration of labour (controversial, discussed later)
- Increased requirement for instrumental vaginal delivery and caesarean section (controversial, discussed later)
- *Epidural and breastfeeding*: Presently, there is conflicting evidence regarding the effect of epidural analgesia on lactation failure. The available evidence has failed to demonstrate a significant association between epidural and lactation failure.[13] Further studies are required to assess the impact, if any, of epidural analgesia on breastfeeding.
- Backache
- *Maternal pyrexia*: Epidural analgesia during labour is likely to be associated with maternal pyrexia, the exact cause of which remains unknown. Epidural analgesia rarely causes temperature rise above 1°C. In case the temperature rise is more than 1°C, any underlying cause must be ruled out and appropriately treated. Irrespective of the cause, any pyrexia during the intrapartum period needs to be aggressively treated with hydration, antipyretics (e.g. acetaminophen) and other appropriate measures. Intrapartum pyrexia due to epidural does not require evaluation for neonatal sepsis.[14]

Delayed

The delayed complications include the following:

- *Postdural puncture headache*: Accidental meningeal puncture with a Tuohy's needle is known as the dural tap. This may be associated with the leakage of cerebrospinal fluid, which may result in the development of severe postural headache in nearly 85% of women. Presence of only headache due to dural tap is an indication for elective forceps or vacuum application at the time of full dilatation. The definitive treatment for this is epidural blood patch that involves epidural injection of up to 20 mL of autologous blood preferably within 24–48 hours postdelivery.
- *Transient backache:* Presently, there is no study demonstrating any significant association between the epidural pain relief and the incidence of long-term back pain.[15]
- Rarely, there may be epidural abscess, meningitis, or permanent neurologic deficit.

CLINICAL PEARLS

- Use of epidural analgesia helps in avoiding opioid-induced maternal and neonatal respiratory depression.
- During the second stage of labour, it is important to ensure that the segmental extent of epidural analgesia has spread to include the S2-S4 nerve roots in order to maintain analgesia in the perineal region.
- For placement of neuraxial analgesia or anaesthesia in difficult cases, the use of ultrasound guidance and continuous intrathecal analgesia via microcatheters may help in overcoming difficulties.
- Administration of naloxone is not recommended during the primary steps of neonatal resuscitation.

EVIDENCE-BASED MEDICINE

Technical Advances

There have been several exciting advances in the field of neuraxial analgesia.[15,16] This includes the refinement of techniques [sequential combined spinal epidural analgesia (CSEA)]; availability of newer drugs and adjuvants and the introduction of various novel modalities of drug delivery systems, like patient-controlled infusion regimes.

Combined Spinal Epidural Analgesia Technique

The CSEA technique can be safely used to provide labour analgesia. It combines the rapid, reliable onset of profound analgesia resulting from spinal injection with the flexibility and longer duration of epidural techniques.[16] This technique, in the UK, involves an initial subarachnoid injection of fentanyl mixed with a small amount of local anaesthetic. The CSEA kit spinal needle comprises of a fine pencil-point needle and a locking device. Use of the spinal opioids provides immediate analgesia, usually within 5 minutes as opposed to at least 20 minutes with the epidural. Since no motor block is produced, the patient retains her capacity for ambulation. However, depending on the drug regimen, proprioception may be impaired resulting in an inability to maintain joint balance. This technique is also associated with a minimal risk of postdural puncture headache and failed spinals.

Low-dose Epidural Regimes

Traditionally, a high concentration (0.2–0.25%) of local anaesthetic has been used to maintain epidural analgesia during labour. Since the past decade, the concentration of local anaesthetic agent used for maintaining labour epidural analgesia has been reduced to about 0.0625–0.125%. With the emergence of the concept of low-dose and minimal local anaesthetic dose and volumes (MLAD and MLAV), all present-day labour epidurals can be considered as being low-dose epidurals. The technique of using low concentration of local anaesthetic agent has helped in reducing the total dose of local anaesthetic used as well as the occurrence of side effects.[17,18]

Results of the COMET (Comparative Obstetric Mobile Epidural Trial Group) Study Group, UK have shown that the use of low-dose epidural techniques for labour analgesia is associated with beneficial delivery outcome.[19] Therefore, continued routine use of traditional epidurals might not be justified. These techniques, CSEA and low-dose infusion epidurals are associated with a lower incidence of instrumental vaginal deliveries in comparison with the traditionally administered intermittent bolus epidurals by the midwives. This is probably due to the preservation of motor tone and bearing down reflex.

A Cochrane review has failed to find differences in the overall rates of maternal satisfaction, mode of delivery and ability to ambulate with CSEA in comparison with epidural analgesia.[20,21] Side effects and complications which can occur with CSEA include pruritus, nausea and vomiting, hypotension, uterine hyperstimulation, foetal bradycardia and maternal respiratory depression.[22,23] The use of small-bore 'atraumatic' spinal needles is likely to reduce the incidence of postdural puncture headache in patients receiving CSEA to approximately 1% or less. Also, several recent reports have failed to find an increase in these complications or an increased rate of caesarean section.

The guidelines issued by the Obstetric Anaesthetists Association, UK in 2005[24] limit the routine use of CSEA. This technique is presently indicated only in certain specific situations, such as very early stage of labour where local anaesthetic agents need to be avoided, advanced stages of labour where rapid analgesia is desirable and difficult epidurals because CSEA is likely to reduce the failure rate of epidurals.

Patient-controlled Epidural Analgesia

Patient-controlled epidural analgesia is a novel method of the drug delivery system, which favours self-administration of epidural opioids and local anaesthetics. This method is being advocated in several units in the UK because it provides several advantages, such as ability to lower the drug dosage, reduced degree of motor blockade, decrease in the requirement for anaesthetic interventions, etc. This technique is associated with a feeling of self-control and self-esteem, which may be important for a positive experience during childbirth. Some studies suggest that analgesia may be improved by a continuous background infusion.

Presently, the ideal PCEA regimen to be used remains controversial. Lim et al.[25] have demonstrated that demand-only PCEA (5 mL bolus, 15-minute lockout interval) was associated with reduced consumption of local anaesthetic agents, but an increased incidence of complications such as breakthrough pain, higher pain scores, shorter duration of effective analgesia and lower maternal satisfaction in comparison with PCEA with background infusion (5 mL bolus, 10–12-minute lockout interval and 5–10 mL/h infusion).

Computer-integrated Patient-controlled Epidural Analgesia

Another adaptation of the epidural delivery pump technology is computer-integrated PCEA (CI-PCEA). This technique controls background infusion rates depending on the previous hour's demand boluses. This technique appears to have a potential for improving the administration of epidural medication, especially for women with prolonged labours.[26]

Continuous Spinal Analgesia with Microcatheters

The FDA has restricted the use of spinal microcatheters due to the possible risk of cauda equina syndrome.[27]

Newer Local Anaesthetics and Adjuvants

The availability of newer local anaesthetics like ropivacaine and levo bupivacaine are associated with increased maternal safety due to their potential of being less cardiotoxic after an inadvertent IV injection.

Alpha-2 agonist, clonidine and cholinesterase inhibitor, neostigmine have also been used as adjuvants for labour analgesia.[28,29] Both these drugs can be administered either epidurally or via the intrathecal route. Spinal clonidine, in doses of 100–200 µg, produces excellent labour analgesia of short duration. However, it may be associated with side effects such as excessive sedation and hypotension. Clonidine is not approved for use in obstetric patients in the United States.

Use of Ultrasound to Study Neuraxial Anatomy and Localise Epidural Space

Ultrasound imaging of the spine has recently been projected to help identify the epidural space and predict difficult spine score, especially in women with abnormal lumbosacral anatomy (scoliosis) and those who are obese. Arzola et al.[30] have found a good agreement between ultrasound depth and the needle depth.

Myths and Controversies

Epidural Analgesia: Increased Rate of Operative and Instrumental Delivery

A Cochrane review after analysing 38 RCTs involving 9,658 women has shown that epidural analgesia does not appear to have any statistically significant influence on the risk of caesarean delivery, rate of maternal satisfaction in relation with pain relief and long-term backache.[31] It also did not appear to have an immediate effect on neonatal status as determined by the APGAR score. A systematic review comparing two different meta-analyses of randomised trials, has also not shown any direct relationship between epidural analgesia and increased rate of caesarean section.[13] Future studies are required to evaluate rare, but potentially severe adverse effects of epidural analgesia on women in labour and long-term neonatal outcomes.

Use of neuraxial analgesia, however, has been shown to prolong the duration of labour on an average by an hour. Moreover, the patients receiving epidural analgesia are associated with relatively higher rates of occipitoposterior position, augmentation with oxytocin and instrumental delivery. However, the use of low-dose epidural regimens has helped in decreasing the overall incidence of these undesirable adverse effects. A large randomised trial, COMET study involving 1,054 patients has shown the low dose of epidural infusion to be associated with nearly 25% reduction in the rate of the instrumental vaginal delivery in comparison with conventional epidural regimen.[19]

Timing of Epidural Analgesia during Labour

When epidural is initiated early in labour, it is associated with a higher rate of caesarean delivery. A randomised, controlled, prospective trial has suggested that epidural analgesia may be delayed until a cervical dilation of 4–5 cm has been reached.[32] On the other hand, RCT by Wong et al.[33] has shown that there was no difference in the rate of caesarean delivery when neuraxial analgesia was administered early in labour (2 cm) versus administration of epidural analgesia was administered late in labour (4–5 cm). Based on the results of this study, the ACOG and the American Society of Anesthesiologists (ASA) have jointly emphasised that there is no need to wait subjectively till the cervical dilation has reached 4–5 cm, and have recommended that 'maternal request is a sufficient indication for pain relief in labour.'[34]

Early versus Delayed Pushing

Delayed pushing has been advocated in patients with epidural analgesia to effectively increase spontaneous vaginal births, decrease instrument-assisted deliveries and shorten the pushing time. 'The Pushing Early or Pushing Late with Epidural' (PEOPLE) study also recommends the policy of delayed pushing for nulliparous women who have full dilatation while they are under epidural anaesthesia because of better outcomes associated with delayed pushing.[35]

Vaginal Birth after Caesarean and Epidural

Taskforce guidelines jointly issued by the ASA and the Society of Obstetric Anaesthesiologists and Perinatologists (SOAP) in 2007 recommend that neuraxial techniques may be offered to patients attempting VBAC.[36] In these patients, it is appropriate to consider early placement of a neuraxial catheter which can be used later for labour analgesia or for anaesthesia in case the patient eventually has an operative delivery.

REFERENCES

1. Lieberman E, O'Donohue C. Unintended effects of epidural analgesia during labor: A systematic review. Am J Obstet Gynecol. 2002;186:S31-68.
2. Simkin PP, O'hara M. Nonpharmacologic relief of pain during labor: systemic reviews of five methods. Am J Obstet Gynecol. 2002;186:S131-59.
3. Chestnut DH, Polley LS, Tsen LC, Wong CA (Eds). Chestnut's Obstetric Anesthesia: Principles and Practice. Philadelphia, PA: Mosby Elsevier; 2009. pp. 405-501.
4. Sosa CG, Balaguer E, Alonso JG, Panizza R, Laborde A, Berrondo C. Meperidine for dystocia during the first of labor: a randomized controlled trial. Am J Obstet Gynaecol. 2004; 191(4):1212-8.
5. Rayburn W, Rathke A, Leuschen MP, Chleborad J, Weidner W. Fentanyl citrate analgesia during labor. Am J Obstet Gynecol. 1989;161(1):202-6.
6. Claahsen-van der Grinten HL, Verbruggen I, van den Berg PP, Sporken JM, Kollée LA. Different pharmacokinetics of tramadol in mothers treated for labour pain and in their neonates. Eur J Clin Pharmacol. 2005;61(7):523-9.
7. D'Onofrio P, Novelli AM, Mecacci F, Scarselli G. The efficacy and safety of continuous intravenous administration of remifentanil for birth pain relief: an open study of 205 Parturients. Anesth Analog. 2009;109(6):1922-4.
8. Yeo ST, Holdcroft A, Yentis SM, Stewart A, Bassett P. Analgesia with sevoflurane in labour. II. Sevoflurane compared with entonox for labour analgesia. Br J Anaesth. 2007;98(1):110-5.
9. Rosen MA. Nitrous oxide for relief of labor pain: a systematic review. Am J Obstet Gynecol. 2002;186:S110-26.
10. Association of Anaesthetists of Great Britain & Ireland (AAGBI), Obstetric Anaesthetists Association (OAA). (2013). OAA/AAGBI Guidelines for Obstetric Anaesthetic Services 2013. [online] Available from www.aagbi.org/sites/default/files/obstetric_anaesthetic_services_2013.pdf. [Accessed August, 2016].
11. Hawkins JL. Epidural analgesia for labour and delivery. N Engl J Med. 2010;362(16):1503-10.
12. Corman SL, Skledar SJ. Use of lipid emulsion to reverse local anesthetic-induced toxicity. Ann Pharmacother. 2007;41(11): 1873-7.
13. Leighton BL, Halpern SH. The effects of epidural analgesia on labor, maternal, and neonatal outcomes: a systematic review. Am J Obstet Gynecol. 2002;186:S69-77.
14. Birnbach DJ. Advances in labour analgesia. Can J Anesth. 2004;51:R1-3.
15. Lim Y, Sia AT. Dispelling the myths of epidural pain relief in childbirth. Singapore Med J. 2006;47(12):1096-100.

16. Macarthur AJ, Gerard W. Ostheimer "What's New in Obstetric Anesthesia" Lecture. Anesthesiology. 2008;108(5):777-85.

17. Lacassie HJ, Habib AS, Lacassie HP, Columb MO. Motor blocking minimum local anesthetic concentrations of bupivacaine, levobupivacaine, and ropivacaine in labor. Reg Anesth Pain Med. 2007;32(4):323-9.

18. Boulier V, Gomis P, Lautner C, Visseaux H, Palot M, Malinovsky JM. Minimal concentration of ropivacaine and levobupivacaine with sufentanil for epidural analgesia in labour. Internl J Obstet Anaesth. 2009;18(3):226-30.

19. Comparative Obstetric Mobile Epidural Trial (COMET) Study Group UK. Effect of low-dose mobile versus traditional epidural techniques on mode of delivery: a randomised controlled trial. Lancet. 2001;358(9275):19-23.

20. Norris MC, Fogel ST, Conway-Long C. Combined spinal-epidural versus epidural labor analgesia. Anesthesiology. 2001;95(4):913-20.

21. Simmons SW, Cyna AM, Dennis AT, Hughes D. Combined spinal-epidural versus epidural analgesia in labour. Cochrane Database Syst Rev. 2007;(3):CD003401.

22. Clarke VT, Smiley RM, Finster M. Uterine hyperactivity after intrathecal injection of fentanyl for analgesia during labor: a cause of fetal bradycardia? Anesthesiology. 1994;81(4):1083.

23. Nielsen PE, Erickson JR, Abouleish EI, Perriatt S, Sheppard C. Fetal heart rate changes after intrathecal sufentanil or epidural bupivacaine for labor analgesia: incidence and clinical significance. Anesth Analg. 1996;83:742-6.

24. Obstetric Anaesthesia Association (OAA). (2005). OAA/AAGBI Guidelines for Obstetric Anaesthetic Service. [online] Available from www.aagbi.org/sites/default/files/obstetric05.pdf. [Accessed August, 2016].

25. Lim Y, Ocampo CE, Supandji M, Teoh WH, Sia AT. Randomized controlled trial of three patient-controlled epidural analgesia regimens for labor. Anesth Analg. 2008;107(6):1968-72.

26. Sng BL, Sia AT, Lim Y, Woo D, Ocampo D. Comparison of computer integrated patient controlled analgesia and patient controlled epidural analgesia with a basal infusion for labour and delivery. Anaesth Intensive Care. 2009;37(1):46-53.

27. Arkoosh VA, Palmer CM, Yun EM, Sharma SK, Bates JN, Wissler RN, et al. A randomized, double-masked, multicenter comparison of the safety of continuous intrathecal labor analgesia using a 28-gauge catheter versus continuous epidural labor analgesia. Anesthesiology. 2008;108(2):286-98.

28. Van de Velde M, Berends N, Kumar A, Devroe S, Devlieger R, Vandermeersch E, et al. Effects of epidural clonidine and neostigmine following intrathecal labour analgesia: a randomised, double-blind, placebo-controlled trial. Int J Obstet Anaesth. 2009;18(3):207-14.

29. Wallet F, Clement HJ, Bouret C, Lopez F, Broisin F, Pignal C, et al. Effects of a continuous low-dose clonidine epidural regimen on pain, satisfaction and adverse events during labour: a randomized, double-blind, placebo-controlled trial. Eur J Anaesthesiol. 2010;27(5):441-7.

30. Arzola C, Davies S, Rofaeel A, Carvalho JC. Ultrasound using the transverse approach to the lumbar spine provides reliable landmarks for labour epidurals. Anesth Analg. 2007; 104(5):1188-92.

31. Anim-Somuah M, Smyth RMD, Jones L. Epidural versus non-epidural or no analgesia in labour. Cochrane Database Syst Rev. 2011;(12):CD000331.

32. Thorp JA, Hu DH, Albin RM, McNitt J, Meyer BA, Cohen GR, et al. The effect of intrapartum epidural analgesia on nulliparous labor: a randomized, controlled, prospective trial. Am J Obstet Gynecol. 1993;169(4): 851-8.

33. Wong CA, Scavone BM, Peaceman AM, McCarthy RJ, Sullivan JT, Diaz NT, et al. The risk of caesarean delivery in neuraxial analgesia given early vs late in labour. N Engl J Med. 2005;352(7):655-65.

34. American College of Obstetricians and Gynecologists Committee on Obstetric Practice. ACOG committee opinion. No. 339: Analgesia and aesarean delivery rates. Obstet Gynecol. 2006;107(6):1487-8.

35. Petrou S, Coyle D, Fraser WD. Cost-effectiveness of a delayed pushing policy for patients with epidural anesthesia. The PEOPLE (Pushing Early or Pushing Late with Epidural) Study Group. Am J Obstet Gynecol. 2000;182(5):1158-64.

36. American Society of Anesthesiologists Task Force on Obstetric Anesthesia. Practice guidelines for obstetric anesthesia: an updated report by the American Society of Anesthesiologists Task Force on Obstetric Anesthesia. Anesthesiology. 2007;106(4):843-63.

PART II

SECTION 8

Delivery and Its Complications

OBSTETRICS

Caesarean Delivery

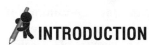

INTRODUCTION

Caesarean section (CS) is a surgical procedure commonly used in the obstetric practice. In this procedure, the foetal delivery is attained through an incision made over the abdomen and uterus, after 28 weeks of pregnancy.[1] If the removal of foetus is done before 28 weeks of pregnancy, the procedure is known as hysterotomy. Presently, there has been a considerable rise in the rate of caesarean deliveries. Caesarean delivery has become a commonly performed surgery in the clinical obstetric practice. Though the procedure is associated with its own inherent complications, its use does help in avoiding difficult vaginal deliveries, which could have led to considerable maternal morbidity and mortality. On the other hand, caesarean delivery on its own, being a major surgery is associated with some inherent complications of laparotomy, such as haemorrhage, infections, damage to the bladder and other pelvic organs, etc. With the advancement in medical technology, an increasing rate of caesarean delivery has led to an important question, 'should the women with previous caesarean delivery (for a non-recurrent cause), be posted for an elective repeat CS or be considered for trial of vaginal delivery?' The answers to this problem largely remain controversial and are discussed in Chapter 30 (Pregnancy after Previous Caesarean Delivery). Though a large number of patients with previous caesarean delivery are being considered for VBAC, the risk of scar rupture, although small, still remains.

INDICATIONS

Abdominal delivery through a CS is usually performed when a vaginal delivery is likely to put the baby's or mother's life or health at risk. Women requiring caesarean delivery can be categorised into three groups: (1) those who have clinical indications for caesarean delivery; (2) women with previous caesarean delivery who may opt for VBAC or ERCS; (3) women requesting for caesarean delivery without any clinical

---

Box 45.1: Indications for primary caesarean delivery

Common indications
- ❑ Failure to progress during labour or dystocia (18%)
- ❑ Non-reassuring foetal status (32%)
- ❑ Foetal malpresentation (19%)
- ❑ Suspected macrosomia (5,000 g in women without diabetes; 4,500 g in women with diabetes) (10%)
- ❑ Pre-eclampsia (10%)
- ❑ Maternal request (8%)

Less common indications
- ❑ Abnormal placentation (e.g. placenta praevia, vasa praevia, placenta accreta) (3%)
- ❑ Multiple pregnancy (with first foetus in non-cephalic presentation)
- ❑ Foetal bleeding diathesis
- ❑ Cord presentation or cord prolapse
- ❑ Maternal infection (e.g. herpes simplex or HIV)

---

indication (maternal request for caesarean delivery, MRCS). Clinical indications for CS are listed in Box 45.1.[2] Majority of caesarean deliveries are performed for causes such as failure to progress in labour, presumed foetal compromise, breech presentation and ERCS. Some such indications are described next:

- ❖ *Breech presentation*: Caesarean section should be offered to pregnant women with a singleton breech presentation at term, where external cephalic version is contraindicated or has been unsuccessful, because it helps in reducing perinatal mortality and neonatal morbidity.
- ❖ *Twin presentation*: Routine CS in uncomplicated twin pregnancies at term where the first twin is in cephalic presentation is likely to result in an increased perinatal mortality and morbidity in the second twin. In twin pregnancies where the first twin is in non-cephalic presentation, the effect of CS in improving perinatal outcomes is uncertain. However, the current practice is to offer a planned CS in these cases.
- ❖ *Placenta praevia*: Caesarean section should be offered to the women where the placenta partly or completely covers the internal cervical os (minor or major placenta praevia).

Colour Doppler ultrasound is highly accurate in making a diagnosis of placenta praevia and morbidly adherent placenta (MAP). Grey scale ultrasound should generally not be used for making a decision about placenta praevia or MAP. Though MRI scan is better for a more complete diagnosis and is associated with higher accuracy, it is not routinely used because many women may not wish to undergo MRI scan due to numerous reasons such as discomfort of being enclosed in a small space, the risk of supine hypotension, the noise of the machine, the length of the procedure, etc. The risks and benefits of using MRI scan must be discussed with the mother. If a colour-flow Doppler ultrasound scan result suggests the diagnosis of MAP, the woman can be counselled regarding the improved accuracy of MRI for diagnosing MAP and verifying the degree of invasion.

❖ *Morbidly adherent placenta*: Nearly 0.6–1.3% women with a previous caesarean delivery are at the risk of developing placenta praevia. Approximately, 11–14% of these women are likely to develop MAP.[3] As the number of previous caesarean deliveries increase, risk of developing placenta praevia and MAP increases in subsequent pregnancies (Table 45.1). At the time of CS, if the placenta fails to separate following the administration of oxytocin, diagnosis of MAP can be established. In these cases, the following options can be used:

• Manual or piecemeal placental removal: This method may be associated with blood loss and may not be effective in removing all the placental bits.

• Hysterectomy with placenta in situ: This may appear to be a suitable option if the patient does not require preservation of fertility.

• Conservative management with placenta in situ: This option can be considered if the woman wants to preserve her fertility, there has been no antenatal bleeding and the placenta has not been breached at the time of caesarean delivery.

When performing a CS for women suspected to have MAP, presence of the following healthcare professionals should be ensured in the multidisciplinary team: consultant obstetrician, consultant anaesthetist, an experienced paediatrician and a senior haematologist. Besides this, a critical care bed and sufficient cross-matched blood and blood products must be readily available. All hospitals should have locally agreed protocols for the management of MAP.

❖ *Cephalopelvic disproportion*: Pelvimetry is not useful for predicting patients with cephalopelvic disproportion who are likely to experience 'failure to progress' in labour.

Therefore, there is no requirement of pelvimetry for decision-making regarding mode of birth.

❖ *Foetal distress*: Abnormal cardiotocographic tracing is often considered as an indication for caesarean delivery. Use of electronic foetal monitoring is likely to be associated with an increased likelihood of caesarean delivery. When CS is contemplated because of an abnormal FHR pattern, in cases where foetal acidosis is suspected, foetal blood sampling should be offered, provided that it is technically possible and no contraindications are present (e.g. maternal infection such as HIV, hepatitis viruses or herpes simplex virus); foetal bleeding disorders such as haemophilia and prematurity, etc. In cases where there is clear evidence of acute foetal compromise, e.g. prolonged decelerations (>3 minutes), the baby should be delivered urgently. There is no need to do foetal blood sampling in these cases.

Maternal Request for Caesarean Delivery

There has been a worldwide increase in the number of caesarean deliveries performed in response to maternal request. The main reason of maternal preference of CS is that the mother perceives it to be the safest option for the baby. A consistent relation has been found between MRCS and the history of previous CS, previous negative birth experience, a complication in the current pregnancy or a fear of giving vaginal birth.[4] If a mother requests for CS, the obstetrician needs to counsel the patient and search, examine and note down the specific reasons for the request.[5] If a woman requests a CS when there is no other obstetric indication for CS, the obstetrician must counsel her regarding the overall risks and benefits of CS in comparison with the vaginal birth.[6] When a woman requests a CS because she has anxiety about the vaginal route of childbirth, she should be offered referral to a healthcare professional with expertise in providing perinatal mental health support.[7] If despite of these, the woman is unable to consider the vaginal birth as an acceptable option and still requests a CS, she should be offered a planned CS. An obstetrician unwilling to perform a CS in such cases should refer the woman to an obstetrician who agrees to perform the surgery.

 SURGICAL MANAGEMENT

Preoperative Preparation

The steps discussed below should be observed for preoperative preparation.

Empty stomach: In order to prevent the risk of aspiration of gastric contents and/or aspiration pneumonitis at the time of administration of anaesthesia, the patient should be nil per mouth for at least 12 hours before undertaking a CS. In case the patient is full stomach, she should be administered H_2 receptor blocker or proton pump inhibitors) to reduce gastric volumes and acidity before CS. Women undergoing a CS should also be offered antiemetics (either pharmacological agents or acupressure) to reduce the risk of nausea and

Table 45.1: Risk of development of placenta praevia and morbidly adherent placenta (MAP) in patients with a previous caesarean delivery[3]

No. of previous caesarean deliveries	Risk of developing placenta praevia (%)	Risk of developing MAP (%)
One previous CS	0.6–1.3	11–14
Two previous CS	1.1–2.3	23–40
Three or more previous CS	1.8–3.7	35–67

PART II

vomiting during CS. Each maternity unit should have a drill for failed intubation during obstetric anaesthesia.

Patient position: The patient is placed with 15° lateral tilt on the operating table, in order to reduce the chances of hypotension.

Preoperative blood test: A haemoglobin assessment must be offered prior to CS to identify women having anaemia. Although blood loss of more than 1,000 mL is an infrequent complication after CS, it may, nevertheless, occur in 4–8% of cases of CS. CS in pregnant women at risk of having blood loss greater than 1,000 mL (e.g. women having CS for antepartum haemorrhage, abruption, placenta praevia, uterine rupture, etc.) should be preferably carried out at a maternity unit with onsite blood transfusion services. Such women must be offered the following tests before CS: grouping and saving of serum; cross-matching of blood; a clotting screen and preoperative ultrasound for localisation of the placenta.

Safe surgical practice: Double gloves should be worn by the healthcare professionals while performing surgery on women, who have tested positive for HIV. Other general recommendations for safe surgical practice should also be followed at the time of CS to reduce the risk of transmission of HIV infection to the healthcare professionals at the time of surgery.

Anaesthesia: While CS can be performed under general or regional anaesthesia, nowadays regional anaesthesia is favoured.[8] Spinal and epidural anaesthesia have become the most commonly used forms of regional anaesthesia in the recent years. Regional anaesthesia is safer and is associated with significantly lower maternal and neonatal morbidity, in comparison to general anaesthesia. General anaesthesia, if used for unplanned CS, should include preoxygenation, cricoid pressure and rapid sequence induction to reduce the risk of aspiration. Women who are having a CS under regional anaesthesia should be offered IV ephedrine or phenylephrine and volume preloading with crystalloids or colloids, in order to reduce the risk of hypotension occurring at the time of surgery. Before cleaning and draping the patient, it is a good practice to check the foetal lie, presentation, position and foetal heart sounds once again. Foley's or plain rubber catheter must be inserted, following which the cleaning and draping of the abdomen is done.

Urinary catheter: Women having CS with regional anaesthesia require an indwelling urinary catheter to prevent overdistension of the bladder because the anaesthetic block is likely to restrict the normal bladder function.

Antibiotic prophylaxis: Preoperative antibiotic prophylaxis is recommended 0–60 minutes prior to giving the incision. Single dose of a narrow spectrum antibiotic (cefazolin) 2 g (for a patient <120 kg) is usually preferred. Co-amoxiclav is usually not prescribed because it may be associated with an increased risk of necrotising enterocolitis in babies. This strategy helps in reducing the risk of postoperative infections. There is no evidence regarding the beneficial effect of multiple doses or broad-spectrum antibiotics.

Thromboprophylaxis: Mechanical thromboprophylaxis is recommended for all women undergoing caesarean delivery.

For women who are at a high risk of thromboembolism, a combination of mechanical and pharmacological thromboprophylaxis is suggested until the woman starts ambulating after the surgery. Pharmacological treatment (where required) is begun 6–12 hours following the surgery.

Preparation of the skin: The area around the proposed incision site must be washed with antiseptic solution (e.g. povidone iodine solution). Antiseptic skin cleansing before surgery is thought to reduce the risk of postoperative wound infections. The antiseptic solution must be applied at least three times over the incision site, using a high-level disinfected sponge-holding forceps and cotton or gauze swab. The surgeon must begin at the proposed incision site and move outwards in a circular motion away from the incision site. After reaching the edge of the sterile field, the previous swab must be discarded and new swab must be used. At the end, the inner aspects of thighs and umbilicus must be swabbed. Some surgeons prefer preparing the umbilicus in the beginning using a sterile cotton-tipped applicator, dipped in antiseptic solution, which is discarded after application. Inner aspect of the thighs are then prepared in the end. The surgeon must keep his or her arms and elbows high and surgical gown away from the surgical field. The woman must be draped using sterile drapes immediately after the area of surgery has been adequately prepared, in order to avoid contamination. If the drape has a window, it should be placed directly over the incision site.

The woman's pubic hair must not be shaved prior to surgery, as this may increase the risk of wound infection. The hair may be trimmed, if necessary.

Timing of caesarean delivery: A planned CS should not routinely be carried out before 39 weeks because of an increased risk of respiratory morbidity in babies born by CS before labour. This risk, however, decreases significantly after 39 weeks.

Classification of caesarean delivery: Previously, CS had been classified as either elective or emergency procedures. Since the year 2000, a new system of categorisation has been adopted throughout the UK, which groups the caesarean deliveries as 'planned' and 'unplanned' (Table 45.2). Unplanned groups of caesarean deliveries belong to categories 1 and 2, where there is an immediate threat to the life of mother or the foetus (e.g. cord prolapse, prolonged bradycardia, pH <7.20, uterine rupture, etc.) or in cases where there is maternal or foetal compromise, which is not immediately life-threatening (e.g. failure to progress in labour; a patient booked as category 4 CS admitted

Table 45.2: NCEPOD (National Confidential Enquiry into Patient Outcome and Death) classification system for caesarean delivery on the basis of urgency[9]

Type	Category	Description
Unplanned CS	1	Immediate threat to the life of the woman or foetus
	2	Maternal or foetal compromise which is not immediately life-threatening
Planned CS	3	No maternal or foetal compromise, but nevertheless early delivery is required
	4	Delivery timed to suit woman or staff

in labour). In cases where there is an immediate threat to the life of either mother or foetus, a CS should be done as soon as possible, preferably within 30 minutes. In cases where there is no immediate threat to the mother or foetus, a CS should be performed as soon as possible, preferably with 75 minutes. Planned groups of caesarean deliveries belong to categories 3 and 4. These include cases where there is no maternal or foetal compromise, yet early delivery is required (e.g. failed induction with no maternal or foetal compromise, patient booked as category 4 CS presented with ruptured membranes, not in labour) or in cases where CS can be performed at a time to suit the woman and her maternity service (e.g. elective CS).

Surgical Steps

The essential steps in a caesarean delivery are summarised in Figures 45.1A to H and are described next in details.

Giving an Abdominal Skin Incision

A vertical or transverse incision can be given over the skin. The vertical skin incision can be either given in the midline or at paramedian location, extending just above the pubic symphysis to just below the umbilicus. Previously, vertical skin incision at the time of CS was favoured, as it was supposed to provide far more superior access to the surgical field in

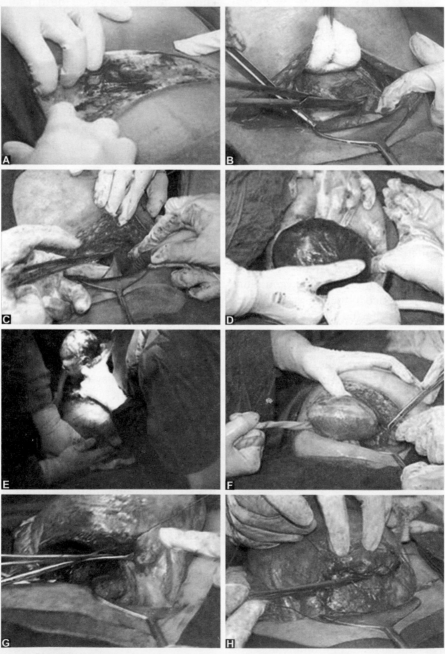

Figs 45.1A to H: Steps of caesarean delivery: (A) Giving an incision over the abdomen and dissecting out different layers of skin; (B) Application of Doyen's retractor after dissection of parietal peritoneum followed by incision of visceral peritoneum; (C) Giving a uterine incision; (D) Delivery of foetal head; (E) Delivery of the entire baby out of the uterine cavity; (F) Delivery of the placenta; (G) Clamping the uterine angles with Green Armytage clamps; (H) Stitching the uterine cavity *(For colour version, see Plate 3)*

comparison to the transverse incision. Also, the vertical incision showed potential for extension at the time of surgery. However, it was associated with poor cosmetic results and an increased risk of wound dehiscence and hernia formation. Therefore, nowadays, transverse incision is mainly favoured due to better cosmetic effect, reduced postoperative pain and improved patient recovery. Two types of transverse incisions are mainly used, while performing CS: (1) the sharp (Pfannenstiel) type and (2) the blunt (Joel-Cohen) type.[10,11]

1. *Sharp Pfannenstiel transverse incision*: In this type, a slightly curved, transverse skin incision is made at the level of pubic hairline, about an inch above the pubic symphysis and is extended somewhat beyond the lateral borders of rectus abdominis muscle. The rectus sheath is incised in the middle and the incision is extended on both sides with the help of scissors. The rectus sheath is held on both sides by Allis forceps and dissected upwards. In case the superior epigastric vessels are injured and start bleeding, they can either be suture ligated or coagulated with the help of diathermy. Following the separation of the muscles, pyramidalis and rectus abdominis, the parietal peritoneum is identified and grasped with the help of two artery forceps. An incision is placed between the two artery forceps after ensuring that no other structure has been grasped. The incision is then carefully extended upwards and downwards, to ensure that the bladder is not injured.

   Pfannenstiel incision is associated with better cosmetic results, reduced rate of postoperative pain, fascial wound dehiscence and incisional hernia. The use of Pfannenstiel incision is discouraged in situations, where a large operating space is required or in cases, where access to the upper abdomen may be required. Also, in cases of repeat CS, re-entry through a Pfannenstiel incision may be difficult and time-consuming, due to the formation of adhesions and scars. In cases, where more room is required at the time of surgery, but a transverse incision is preferred, a Maylard incision may be used instead of a Pfannenstiel incision. In these cases, the rectus muscles are sharply divided. This incision may be typically useful in cases of repeat CS with previous transverse incision.

2. *Joel-Cohen blunt incision*: In this type, a straight skin incision about 3 cm in size is given above the pubic symphysis and 3 cm below the line, which joins anterior superior iliac spines. Subsequent tissue layers are opened bluntly, without using a sharp scalpel. The initial cut is given only through the cutis. In the midline, which is free from large blood vessels, the cut is deepened to meet the fascia. If necessary, the incision can be extended with scissors and not with a knife.

   A small transverse opening is made in the fascia with the scissors. The rest of the fascia is then opened transversely, by pushing the slightly open tip of a pair of straight scissors, first in one direction and then in the other. The fascia is stretched caudally and cranially, using the index fingers to make room for the next step.[12] The muscle and fat tissue is separated by applying manual bilateral skin traction, using the index and middle fingers of both the surgeon and his assistant. The use of surgical knife must be avoided as far as possible and, if required, the scissors can be used instead. Parietal peritoneum is identified and finger dissection is done. A hole is made in the parietal peritoneum, which is then extended by the pull of surgeon and his/her assistant. Haemostasis is achieved with the help of diathermy.

Comparison between sharp (Pfannenstiel) versus blunt (Joel-Cohen) skin incisions: Presently, the transverse incision of choice is Joel-Cohen incision because it is associated with shorter operating times, and reduced postoperative febrile morbidity, blood loss, postoperative pain, and time from skin incision up to the baby's birth.[13,14]

Excision of Previous Scar

Excision of the existing previous scar must always be performed at the beginning of surgery, by either giving an elliptical incision incorporating the scar or giving an incision over the previous scar with trimming of the fibrosed edges of the wound. Excision of the previous scar is usually difficult at the end of the surgery, but must be done, if it has not been done previously.

Dissecting the Rectus Sheath

After dissecting through the skin, subcutaneous fat and fascia, as the anterior rectus sheath is reached, sharp dissection may be required. A scalpel can be used to incise the rectus sheath throughout the length of the incision. The cut edges of the incised rectus sheath are held with the help of Allis forceps and then carefully separated out from the underlying rectus muscle and pyramidalis. These muscles are then separated with the help of blunt and sharp dissection, to expose transversalis fascia and peritoneum.

Opening the Peritoneum

The transversalis fascia and peritoneal fat are dissected carefully to reach the underlying peritoneum. After placing two haemostats about 2 cm apart to hold the peritoneum, it is carefully opened. The layers of peritoneum are carefully examined to be sure that omentum, bowel or bladder is not lying adjacent to it. This may be especially important in cases of obstructed labour, where the bladder has been pushed cephalad almost to the level of umbilicus. The peritoneum is superiorly incised up to the level of incision and inferiorly to a point just above the peritoneal reflection over the bladder.

Insertion of the Doyen's Retractor

Following the dissection of parietal peritoneum and the identification of the lower uterine segment, the surgeon must then check, if the uterus is dextrorotated, by identifying the round ligaments. In the dextrorotated uterus, the left round ligament in comparison to the right round ligament may be anterior and closer to the midline. Following the identification of lower uterine segment, some surgeons prefer to put a moistened laparotomy pack in each of the paracolic gutters. The loose fold of the uterovesical peritoneum over the lower

PART II

uterine segment is then grasped with the help of forceps and incised transversely with the help of scissors. The lower flap of the peritoneum is held with artery forceps and the loose areolar tissue pushed down. The underlying bladder is then separated by blunt dissection. Finally, the lower flap of peritoneum and the areolar tissue is retracted by the Doyen's retractor to clear the lower uterine segment. The upper flap of the peritoneum is pushed up to leave about 2 cm wide strip on the uterine surface, which is not covered with peritoneum.

Giving a Uterine Incision

An incision is made in the lower uterine segment about 1 cm below the upper margin of peritoneal reflection and about 2–3 cm above the bladder base. While making an incision in the uterus, a curvilinear mark of about 10 cm length is made by the scalpel, cutting partially through the myometrium. The uterine incision must be gently given, taking care to avoid any injury to the underlying foetus. Following this, a small cut (~ 3 cm in size) is made, using the scalpel in the middle of this incision mark, reaching up to, but not through the membranes. The rest of the incision can be completed either by stretching the incision, using the tips of two index fingers along both the sides of the incision mark or using bandage scissors, to extend the incision on two sides. The bandage scissors are introduced into the uterus over the two fingers, in order to protect the foetus. The use of bandage scissors may be especially required in cases, where the lower uterine segment is thickened and the uterine incision cannot be extended using the fingers. There has been much controversy regarding, whether a blunt or sharp uterine incision must be used. The National Collaborating Centre for Women's and Children's Health (NCCWCH, 2011)[15] recommends that blunt rather than sharp extension of the uterine incision should be used when the uterine segment is well formed because it is supposed to reduce amount of blood loss, incidence of postpartum haemorrhage and the requirement for transfusion at the time of CS. If the lower uterine segment is very thin, injury to the foetus can be avoided by using the handle of the scalpel or a haemostat (an artery forceps) to open the uterus. The uterine incision must be large enough to allow the delivery of the head and trunk without the risk of extension of the incision laterally into the uterine vessels. One must remember that in patients with advanced second stage of labour, the lower uterine segment may be excessively stretched. In these cases, it may be required to place the incision relatively higher, in order to avoid the extension towards the vagina. In case the surgeon feels that lateral extension of the uterine incision is a possibility, he/she can use several alternatives, such as making a J-shaped, U-shaped or a T-shaped incision. As the foetal membranes bulge out through the uterine incision, they are ruptured. The amniotic fluid, which is released following the ROMs, is sucked with the help of a suction machine.

Location of the Uterine Incision

Lower segment uterine scar or the upper segment uterine scar: While in the past, a vertical incision (classical) was commonly used, this was associated with a high risk of scar rupture during future pregnancies. There are two types of vertical incisions: (1) low vertical (limited to the lower uterine segment) and (2) the classical vertical (extending up to the uterine fundus). The low vertical incision appears to be as safe and strong as the low transverse incision.[16] The classical incision is rarely performed at or near term because it is associated with a high rate of scar rupture in future pregnancies. As a result, lower segment transverse incisions are nowadays preferred. Indications for considering a vertical uterine incision are as follows:

❖ Poorly developed lower uterine segment in settings where marked degree of intrauterine manipulation is anticipated (e.g. extremely preterm breech presentations, foetus in transverse lie where the back faces downwards).
❖ Presence of pathology in the lower uterine segment due to which it may not be possible to give a transverse incision (e.g. large myoma, anterior placenta praevia or accreta).
❖ Densely adherent bladder
❖ Postmortem delivery.

The lower segment uterine scar is considered sounder than the upper segment scar due to the following reasons:

❖ The lower uterine segment is thinned out during labour. As a result, the thin margins of the lower segment can be easily apposed at the time of uterine repair without leaving behind any dead space pocket. In case of the classical scar, it may be difficult to appose the thick muscle layer of the upper segment. Blood filled pockets may be formed. This may be later replaced by fibrous tissues, resulting in the weakening of the scar.
❖ The lower segment usually remains inert in the post-partum period. On the other hand, the upper segment undergoes rapid contractions and retractions, resulting in the loosening of the uterine sutures. This can result in imperfect healing and further weakening of the uterine scar.
❖ When the uterus stretches in the future pregnancy, the stretch is along the line of the scar in the case of the lower segment scar, whereas in cases of vertical scar, the uterus stretches in the direction perpendicular to the scar, thereby resulting in the scar weakness.
❖ Chances of the placental implantation in the area of the scar at the time of the future pregnancy are highly unlikely in the case of the lower segment scar. However, in case of the classical scar, the placental tissue is quite likely to implant in the area of the scar at the time of future pregnancy. Penetration and the invasion of the scar by the placental trophoblasts is likely to produce further weakening of the scar.

As a result of the previously mentioned reasons, the lower-segment scar is much stronger as compared to the upper-segment scar and is unlikely to give way during subsequent pregnancies. Lower-segment scar may rupture occasionally at the time of labour. On the other hand, upper-segment scar is weak and may rupture, both during the antenatal period and at the time of labour.

Delivery of the Infant

In case of cephalic presentation, once the foetal presenting part (head) becomes visible through the uterine incision, the surgeon places his/her right hand below the foetal presenting part and grasps it. In case of cephalic presentation, the foetal head is then elevated gently, using the palms and fingers of the hand. Delivery of the foetal head should be in the same way as during the normal vaginal delivery.

There is no need for routine use of forceps, in order to deliver foetal head. Forceps should be used for the delivery of foetal head at the time of caesarean delivery, only if there is difficulty, while delivering the baby's head. At times, the foetal head may be wedged in the birth canal. In these cases, the assistant by placing his or her hand in the vagina may be required to exert pressure in the upwards direction. The Doyen's retractor is inserted again, once the foetal presenting part has been grasped. In order to facilitate delivery, fundal pressure is applied by the assistant. Delivery is completed in the manner similar to normal vaginal delivery. Once the baby shoulders have delivered, an IV infusion containing 20 U of oxytocin per litre of crystalloids is infused at a rate of 10 mL/min, until effective uterine contractions are obtained. Bolus doses of oxytocin must be avoided due to risk of hypotension. Fundal massage, following the delivery of the baby, helps in reducing bleeding and hastens the delivery of placenta. Following the delivery of the baby, the cord is clamped and cut, and the baby handed over to the paediatrician. A single dose of prophylactic antibiotics in the dose of ampicillin 2 g or cefazolin 1 g is administered intravenously after the cord is clamped and cut (if not previously administered at the time of giving the incision). It helps in providing adequate prophylaxis. No additional benefit has been demonstrated with the use of multiple dose antibiotic regimens. If the woman shows signs of infection, e.g. fever, urinary tract infections, sepsis, etc., antibiotics must be continued until the woman becomes free of fever for at least 48 hours.

Some obstetricians tend to delay the clamping of cord because it is likely to be associated with numerous benefits such as reduced incidence of neonatal anaemia; enhanced systemic and pulmonary perfusion; and improved breast-feeding outcomes. However, this practice can also be associated with adverse effects such as polycythaemia, hyper-viscosity, hyperbilirubinaemia, transient tachypnoea of the newborn and risk of maternal foetal transfusion in rhesus negative women. Since the present studies provide conflicting results, future RCTs are required to determine the effect of delayed cord clamping on the various neonatal outcomes.

Placental Removal

At the time of CS, the placenta should be removed, using controlled cord traction or awaiting spontaneous expulsion and not manually removed as this reduces the risk of endometritis.[17] Following the delivery of the placenta, the remnant bits of membranes and decidua are removed using a sponge-holding forceps. The cut edges of the uterine incision are then identified and grasped with the help of Green-Armytage clamps. The uterine angles are usually grasped with Allis forceps. Additionally, some surgeons practice routine dilatation of internal os, in order to allow better drainage of lochia postdelivery.[18] This strategy has not been shown to reduce the risk of postoperative maternal fever,

wound infection, or bring about a change in haemoglobin concentration. Prior to the closure of uterine incision, it is a good practice to inspect the adnexa (both the tubes and ovaries).

Closing the Uterine Incision

The main controversies related to the closure of the uterine incision are whether the closure should be in the form of a single-layered or a double-layered closure and whether the uterus should be exteriorised or not at the time of closure. Before repair of the uterine incision, some surgeons prefer to exteriorise the uterus in order to improve exposure and facilitate closure of uterine incision. Moreover, uterine exteriorisation has some inherent advantages. A relaxed atonic uterus can be easily recognised and massage can therefore be applied. The uterine incision, its extension and bleeding points can be visualised more easily and repaired. Adnexal exposure is superior and it may be easier to carry out tubal sterilisation.

According to the results of a large randomised trial (CORONIS), there were no statistically significant differences in maternal outcome based on the method of entry into the uterine cavity (blunt versus sharp entry), method of repair of the uterine incision (exterior versus intra-abdominal repair), method of closure (single-layer versus double-layer closure) and choice of suture material (chromic catgut versus polyglactin-910).[19] Therefore, until there is emergence of better quality evidence proving otherwise, any of these surgical techniques is acceptable. Choice of using a particular method depends on personal preference and the specific clinical settings.[19-21]

However, exteriorisation of the uterus while repairing the uterine incision is not recommended because it is likely to be more painful and is not likely to improve operative outcomes such as haemorrhage and infection. Also, uterine exteriorisation has been found to be associated with a higher rate of intraoperative nausea and vomiting. Therefore, intraperitoneal repair of the uterus at the time of CS should be preferably undertaken. Rarely, exteriorisation of the uterus may help in better visualisation of the uterine incision in case of extensions, thereby making repair easier. In such cases, it is the obstetrician's duty to ensure that both the patient and the anaesthetist have been warned that the uterus would be exteriorised.

Single-layered or double-layered closure of uterine incision: Both single-layered and double-layered closure of uterine incision is being currently practiced. Though single-layered closure is associated with reduced operative time and reduced blood loss in the short term, the risk of the uterine rupture during subsequent pregnancies is increased.[22,23]

The CAESAR (CAESARean section surgical techniques) trial, the largest RCT of CS surgical techniques undertaken till date, has not shown any significant differences in the various short-term outcomes such as length of hospital stay, preterm delivery, amnionitis, postpartum endometritis, placental abruption, postpartum haemorrhage, blood transfusion, uterine dehiscence, etc. with the single- versus double-layered closure of the uterine incision.[24] However, there are concerns related to the risk of uterine rupture in the future with the use of single-layered technique of closure. Therefore, two-layered technique of closure is presently recommended until the results from the CAESAR follow-up trial become available. Currently, single layer closure of the uterine incision is best performed in the research settings. The current recommendation by NCCWCH, 2011 is also to close the uterus in two layers, as the safety and efficacy of closing uterus in a single layer presently remains uncertain.[15]

Peritoneal Closure

The current recommendation by the RCOG is that neither the visceral nor the parietal peritoneum should be sutured at the time of CS as this reduces the operative time and the requirement for the postoperative analgesia.[25]

Closure of the Rectus Sheath

Rectus sheath closure is performed after identifying the angles and holding them with Allis forceps. The angles must be secured using 1-0 Vicryl sutures. The rectus layer is closed with the help of continuous locked sutures placed no more than 1 cm apart. Haemostasis must be checked at all levels.

Closure of Subcutaneous Space

There is no need for the routine closure of the subcutaneous tissue space, unless there is more than 2 cm of subcutaneous fat, because this practice has not been shown to reduce the incidence of wound infection.

Skin Closure

Obstetricians should be aware that presently the differences between the use of different suture materials and methods of skin closure at the time of CS are not certain. Skin closure can be either performed using subcutaneous, continuous repair absorbable or non-absorbable stitches or using interrupted stitches with non-absorbable sutures or staples.[26] In women who are at an increased risk of haematoma formation or infection, an interrupted method of closure can be adopted because with this method, there is an advantage of removal of one or two sutures to allow drainage when required. Closure of the anterior abdominal wall depends on the type of incision. In the rare situations where a vertical midline abdominal incision is used at the time of CS, mass closure of the rectus sheath and subcutaneous tissues with slowly absorbable continuous sutures should be used because this is likely to be associated with fewer complications such as incisional hernias, dehiscence, sinus formation, pain, etc. in comparison to the layered closure. In case of transverse incision, each tissue layer is closed separately in a layer-by-layer manner.

Following the skin closure, the vagina is swabbed dried and dressing applied to the wound.

Postoperative Care

Immediate Postoperative Care

❖ After surgery is completed, the woman needs to be monitored in the recovery area.

❖ Monitoring of routine vital signs (blood pressure, temperature, breathing), urine output, vaginal bleeding, bleeding from the incision site and uterine tonicity (to check, if the uterus remains adequately contracted), needs to be done at hourly intervals for the first 4 hours. Thereafter, the monitoring needs to be done at every four hourly intervals for the first postoperative day at least. Adequate analgesia needs to be provided, initially through the IV line and later with oral medications.

❖ When the effects of anaesthesia have worn off, about 4–8 hours after surgery, the woman may be transferred to the postpartum room.

❖ Following the baby's birth, umbilical artery pH should be measured in all cases of CS performed for suspected foetal compromise to help ensure the foetal well-being and care of the baby.

Pain Management after Caesarean Section

Adequate postoperative pain control is important. A woman, who is in severe pain, may not recover well. However, excessive use of sedative drugs must be avoided, as this may limit the patient's mobility, which is important to prevent thromboembolism. Patient-controlled analgesia, using opioid analgesics should be offered after CS because it is associated with higher rate of patient satisfaction. Women could be offered diamorphine (0.3–0.4 mg intrathecally) for intra- and postoperative analgesia. NSAIDs may be used postoperatively, as an adjunct to other analgesics because they help in reducing the requirement for opioids. Adding acetaminophen also increases the effects of the other medications with very little additional adverse risk. Analgesic rectal suppositories can also be used for providing relief from pain in women following CS.

Fluids and Oral Food after Caesarean Section

As a general rule, about 3L of fluids must be replaced by IV infusion during the first postoperative day, provided that the woman's urine output remains greater than 30 mL/h. If the urine output falls below 30 mL/h, the woman needs to be reassessed to evaluate the cause of oliguria. In uncomplicated cases, the urinary catheter can be removed by 12 hours postoperatively. IV fluids may need to be continued, until she starts taking liquids orally. The clinician needs to remember that prolonged infusion of IV fluids can alter electrolyte balance. If the woman receives IV fluids for more than 48 hours, her electrolyte levels need to be monitored every 48 hours. Balanced electrolyte solution (e.g. potassium chloride 1.5 g in 1L IV fluids) may be administered.

In case of uneventful surgery, early oral intake (preferably within 6 hours of surgery) is encouraged. If the surgery was uncomplicated, the woman may be given a light liquid diet in the evening after the surgery. If there were signs of infection or if the CS was for obstructed labour or uterine rupture, bowel sounds must be heard before prescribing oral liquids to the patient. In these cases, the woman can be given solid food, when she starts passing gas. Women who are recovering well and who do not have complications after the surgery can be advised to eat and drink, whenever they feel hungry or thirsty. The clinician must ensure that the woman is eating a regular diet before she is discharged from the hospital.

Ambulation after Caesarean Section

The woman must be encouraged to ambulate as soon as 6–8 hours following surgery. In case, she finds it difficult to get up from the bed and walk, she can be asked to remain in bed and do simple limb exercises (e.g. leg elevation, foot dorsiflexion, plantar flexion, etc.) and breathing exercises on the bed itself. Early ambulation enhances circulation, encourages early return of normal gastrointestinal function and facilitates general well-being. Even in cases, where complications were encountered at the time of surgery, mobilisation must be preferably begun within 24 hours after the surgery.

Dressing and Wound Care

The dressing must be kept on the wound for the first 2–3 days after surgery, to provide a protective barrier against infection. Thereafter, dressing is usually not required. If blood or fluid is observed to be leaking through the initial dressing, the dressing must not be changed. The amount of blood or fluid lost must be monitored. If bleeding increases or the bloodstain covers half the dressing or more, the dressing must be removed and replaced with another sterile dressing. The dressing must be changed while using a sterile technique. The surgical wound also needs to be carefully inspected. Staples or non-absorbable sutures (whichever were applied) can be removed by 3–4 days in case of transverse incision and minimal traction on the skin edges. In case of presence of risk factors for wound complications (e.g. diabetes, obese patients, etc.) or in case of vertical incision, the staples or sutures can be left in place for at least 5–7 days or longer depending upon the clinical situation.

Length of Hospital Stay

Length of hospital stay is likely to be longer after a CS (an average of 3–4 days) in comparison to that after a vaginal birth (average 1–2 days). However, women who are recovering well and have not developed complications following CS may be offered early discharge. Some operative and postoperative interventions, which can be used for reducing CS-related morbidity, include use of regional anaesthesia rather than general anaesthesia, antibiotic prophylaxis to prevent infection and use of thromboprophylaxis, to prevent thromboembolism.

ALTERNATIVE TECHNIQUES FOR CAESAREAN DELIVERY

In order to further reduce the operation time and reduce the complications associated with Joel-Cohen technique of caesarean delivery, several modifications of caesarean delivery have been introduced, some of which have been discussed next.

Misgav-Ladach Technique

This technique is a modified Joel-Cohen technique and is also known as Joel-Cohen-Stark technique. In this technique, the Joel-Cohen abdominal incision is used and the uterus is also opened in a manner similar to the Joel-Cohen method.[27] Following the manual removal of the placenta, the uterus is exteriorised. The myometrial incision is closed with one layer of locked continuous sutures. A second layer of sutures is placed only if required. The peritoneal layers (both the visceral and peritoneal) are not sutured. The fascia is re-approximated with a continuous running stitch. The skin is closed with two or three mattress sutures. The skin edges between these sutures are approximated with the help of Allis forceps. Similar to the Joel-Cohen technique, the Misgav-Ladach technique also favours minimisation of sharp dissection. It has been shown that the use of Misgav-Ladach technique is associated with fewer intraperitoneal adhesions at the time of repeat caesarean delivery.[28]

Pelosi's Technique

Pelosi's technique can be described as a simple, least traumatic approach towards caesarean delivery. It is associated with short operating time, minimal instrumentation, reduced surgical dissection and reduced rate of postoperative complications such as pain, blood loss, infection and wound complications.[29,30] In this technique, a Pfannenstiel abdominal incision is given. Electrocautery is used for transversely cutting the subcutaneous tissues and the fascia. The rectus muscles are separated with the help of blunt dissection, using both the index fingers. The peritoneum is opened with blunt finger dissection, following which all the layers of the abdominal wall are stretched manually to the extent of the skin incision. The bladder is not reflected inferiorly. A small transverse incision is made over the lower uterine segment. It is extended laterally, curving upwards with blunt finger dissection or scissors. The baby is delivered with external fundal pressure. Following the delivery of the baby, oxytocin is administered and the placenta removed after spontaneous separation. The uterus is massaged. The myometrial incision is closed with single layer chromic catgut continuous locking sutures. Neither visceral nor parietal peritoneal layer is sutured. The fascia is closed with a continuous synthetic absorbable suture. If the subcutaneous layer is thick, interrupted 3-0 absorbable sutures are used for obliterating the dead space. The skin is closed with staples. Presently, there are no randomised trials comparing Pelosi's technique to other techniques.

Haemostatic Caesarean Section

This is a new surgical technique used for managing pregnant women infected with HIV-1. The surgeon must adorn double gloves while performing CS in women who are HIV-positive. Haemostatic CS is a type of elective CS with technical modifications, which is used in all patients receiving antiretroviral treatment and in whom breastfeeding has been prohibited. The patient is scheduled for surgery at 38 weeks of gestation, while the patient is not in labour and membranes are intact. The technique involves management of lower uterine segment while maintaining the integrity of membranes. This helps in avoiding massive contact between maternal blood and the foetus. Thus, this technique helps in reducing the rate of vertical transmission to less than 2%.

Classical Caesarean Section

Classical CS involves giving a vertical uterine incision. Indications of the classical CS have been previously described in the text.

Procedure

In case of a classical CS, the uterine incision is given vertically. The lower limit of the uterine incision is initiated as low as possible, usually above the level of bladder. The uterine incision is extended in the cephalad direction using bandage scissors, until the incision becomes large enough to facilitate delivery. Following the delivery of the baby and the placenta, the uterine incision is closed in layers. A three-layered closure is usually used in case of classical incision due to an increased vascularity of the upper segment. The deeper layers are approximated using a layer of continuous 0 or no. 1 chromic catgut sutures. The outer layer is closed using figure-of-eight continuous sutures. The edges of the uterine serosa are approximated using continuous 2-0 chromic catgut sutures.

Avoiding a Classical Uterine Incision

A classical caesarean delivery is associated with a weaker scar in comparison to a transverse incision due to the reasons previously described in the text. Therefore, rather than performing a classical CS, the clinicians prefer to use some kind of variations in the lower-segment uterine incision. Mostly, the surgeon is able to decide the exact incision only at the time of surgery. Variations of the lower-segment incision are commonly used, in cases where there is a requirement for an extended surgical field, in order to avoid scar extension, e.g. transverse lie with hand prolapse and large baby, etc. Some of the variations include the following:

- *An inverted T-shaped incision*: This incision involves cutting upwards from the middle of the transverse incision
- *J-shaped or hockey-stick incision*: This incision involves extension of one end of the transverse incision upwards
- *U-shaped or trap-door incision*: This incision involves extension of both ends of the transverse scar upwards. Of all these various choices, the T-shaped scar is the worst choice due to its difficult repair, poor healing and chances of scar rupture during subsequent pregnancies.

COMPLICATIONS

Various complications associated with caesarean delivery are tabulated in Box 45.2 and are described next in details.

Uterine Rupture

Uterine rupture has been discussed in details in Chapter 30 (Pregnancy after Previous Caesarean Delivery). Causes of a

---

> **Box 45.2:** Complications associated with caesarean delivery
>
> - ❑ Abdominal pain
> - ❑ Injury to bladder, ureters, etc.
> - ❑ Increased risk of rupture uterus and maternal death
> - ❑ Neonatal respiratory morbidity
> - ❑ Hysterectomy
> - ❑ Thromboembolic disease
> - ❑ Increased duration of hospital stay
> - ❑ Antepartum or intrapartum intrauterine deaths in future pregnancies
> - ❑ Patients with a previous history of caesarean delivery are more prone to develop complications, like placenta praevia and adherent placenta during future pregnancies

> **Box 45.3:** Causes of a weak scar
>
> - ❑ Improper haemostasis at the time of surgery
> - ❑ Imperfect coaptation of uterine margins at the time of surgery
> - ❑ Extension of the angles of uterine incision
> - ❑ Infection during healing
> - ❑ Placental implantation at the site of incision

weak scar due to the various techniques adopted at the time of caesarean delivery are described in Box 45.3.

Infection

Infection is a complication, which can commonly develop after CS. Endometritis or infection of the endometrial cavity must be suspected, if there is excessive vaginal bleeding or discharge following the surgery. Infection of the urinary tract can result in symptoms like dysuria, increased urinary frequency, pyuria, etc.

Trauma to the Urinary Tract

This complication can occur during the caesarean surgery and, if not appropriately handled, can result in development of urinary tract fistulas.

Thromboembolism

Thromboembolism must be suspected if the patient develops cough, swollen calf muscles or positive Homan's sign. A positive Homan's sign is associated with DVT and is said to be present when passive dorsiflexion of the ankle by the examiner elicits sharp pain in the patient's calf

Obstetric or Caesarean Hysterectomy

Caesarean or obstetric hysterectomy may be required in cases of uncontrollable maternal haemorrhage, a situation frequently encountered with a MAP. Obstetric hysterectomy refers to the removal of the uterus at the time of a planned or unplanned CS. It involves either the removal of pregnant uterus with pregnancy in situ (in cases of cervical cancer) or a recently pregnant uterus due to some complications of delivery. Sometimes, hysterectomy may be required following delivery, either vaginal or caesarean in order to save mother's life. Emergency obstetric hysterectomy has become an indispensable life-saving procedure in the obstetric practice. Obstetric hysterectomy can also be performed in the peripartum or the postpartum period. If performed within the short time after vaginal delivery, it is termed as postpartum hysterectomy. In most cases of hysterectomy following vaginal birth, the indication for the procedure is uterine atony with uncontrolled haemorrhage that has failed to respond to conservative measures. The most common indication for hysterectomy at the time of CS is rupture uterus. In contrast, placenta accreta with or without an associated placenta praevia is the most common indication for emergency post-caesarean hysterectomy. History of a previous CS increases the likelihood of placenta praevia, placenta accreta, scar dehiscence and overt uterine rupture. Each of these diagnosis increases the risk for emergency hysterectomy.

Some important causes for emergency obstetric hysterectomy are enumerated in Box 45.4.[3]

Obstetric hysterectomy could be performed as an emergency or an elective procedure depending upon the indications and circumstances under which it is performed. It could be of subtotal or supracervical type (involving the removal of the uterus above the cervix), total (involving the removal of both uterus and cervix) or the radical type (with foetus in utero). In cases of severe haemorrhage or DIC, supracervical

hysterectomy should preferably be used in place of a total hysterectomy, as it is likely to reduce the operative time as well as minimise the extent of surgical dissection and blood loss. In all other cases, total hysterectomy is usually preferred.

Presently, there is no clinical standard at which hysterectomy is recommended. Local protocols must be formulated to address this issue and guide the clinicians in case of uncontrollable blood loss (e.g. that exceeding 2.5 L). From an early stage, these cases must be managed by an experienced obstetrician. The obstetrician should not delay the procedure for too long due to an increased risk of maternal mortality and morbidity with increasing haemorrhage. Previous confidential enquiries into maternal deaths have shown a delay in performing obstetric hysterectomy as an avoidable cause of maternal mortality.[31] Prior to the surgery, the patient must be adequately counselled and appropriate consent must be taken from the patient.

Hysterectomy is sometimes used for the pregnant woman with gynaecological disorders, such as leiomyomas or the high-grade cervical intraepithelial neoplasia, but this surgery usually can be safely delayed until the pelvic structures return to their prepregnant state. Elective hysterectomy at the time of delivery is a controversial procedure due to the increased morbidity related to the surgery being performed on highly vascular pelvic organs.

Box 45.4: Indications for obstetric hysterectomy

Obstetric emergencies
- ❑ Postpartum haemorrhage (PPH):
  - Intractable uterine atony
  - Inverted uterus
  - Coagulopathy
  - Laceration of a pelvic vessel
- ❑ Sepsis:
  - Chorioamnionitis with sepsis
  - Myometrial abscesses

Caesarean delivery
- ❑ Ruptured uterus:
  - Traumatic
  - Spontaneous
  - Extending pelvic haematoma
  - Lateral extension of the uterine incision with the involvement of uterine vessels
- ❑ Placental implantation in the lower segment (placenta accreta, increta or percreta)
- ❑ Presence of large or symptomatic leiomyomas, which may prevent effective uterine repair
- ❑ Uncontrollable PPH
- ❑ Couvelaire uterus
- ❑ Severe uterine infection particularly that caused by *Clostridium welchii*

Non-emergency situations (peripartum hysterectomy)
- ❑ Coexisting gynaecological disorders:
  - Multiple uterine myomas
  - Stage I cervical carcinoma
  - Cervical intraepithelial neoplasia
  - Ovarian malignancy
- ❑ Previous gynaecological disorders:
  - Endometritis
  - Pelvic inflammatory disease
  - Heavy and irregular menstrual bleeding
  - Pelvic adhesions

CLINICAL PEARLS

❖ The use of caesarean delivery helps in avoiding difficult cases of vaginal delivery, which may be associated with considerable maternal and foetal mortality and morbidity.

❖ Caesarean delivery may be associated with certain advantages in comparison to the vaginal delivery. Some such advantages of caesarean delivery include reduced incidence of perineal pain, urinary incontinence and uterovaginal prolapse.

❖ At the time of CS, the obstetrician must try to accommodate as far as possible the woman's preferences for the birth, such as playing music playing in theatre, lowering the screen to see the baby being born, or observing silence in the operation theatre so that the mother's voice is the first voice which the baby hears.

EVIDENCE-BASED MEDICINE

❖ Presently, there is no evidence to support the routine use of drains at the time of caesarean delivery. In case the obstetrician feels that there is a risk of ongoing bleeding at the time of caesarean delivery, intraperitoneal drains can be used. Preferably, these drains should be wide-bored and of non-suction variety. CAESAR study has showed no benefit regarding the routine use of subcutaneous drains. They should be used only if clinically indicated. If the drains are used, the abdominal peritoneum must be closed. Use of superficial drains is not likely to reduce the incidence of infection or haematoma and is therefore best avoided.[24] Better-designed RCTs in future are required to determine the effect of wound drainage on postoperative morbidity, especially in women more at risk of such adverse outcomes (e.g. obese women).

❖ Presently, there is inadequate evidence to determine the effectiveness of adhesive drapes at the time of caesarean delivery for reducing the chances of blood spillage and cross infection, thereby improving safety for the staff in the operating room.[32,33] Also, the practice of using separate surgical knives for incising the skin and the deeper tissues at the time of CS is not recommended because it is not likely to reduce the occurrence of wound infection.[34,35]

REFERENCES

1. National Institutes of Health. Caesarean childbirth. NIH Publication No. 82–2067. Bethesda MD: US Department of Health and Human Services; 1981.

2. Barber EL, Lundsberg LS, Belanger K, Pettker CM, Funai EF, Illuzzi JL. Indications contributing to the increasing Caesarean delivery rate. Obstet Gynecol. 2011;118(1):29-38.

3. Guise JM, Eden K, Emeis C, Jonas DE, Morgan LC, Reuland D, et al. Vaginal birth after cesarean: new insights. Evid Rep Technol Assess (Full Rep). 2010;191:1-397.

4. Gamble JA, Creedy DK. Women's request for a cesarean section: a critique of the literature. Birth. 2000;27(4):256-63.

5. Grant A, Glazener CMA. Elective caesarean section versus expectant management for delivery of the small baby. Cochrane Database Syst Rev. 2001;(2):CD000078.

6. Hofmeyr GJ, Hannah ME. Planned caesarean section for term breech delivery. Cochrane Database Syst Rev. 2000;(2): CD000166.

7. Crowther CA. Caesarean delivery for the second twin. Cochrane Database Syst Rev. 2000;(2):CD000047.

8. Afolabi BB, Lesi FE, Merah NA. Regional versus general anaesthesia for Caesarean section. Cochrane Database Syst Rev. 2006;(4):CD004350.

9. National Confidential Enquiry into Perioperative Deaths (NCEPOD). (1995). Report of the National Confidential Enquiry into Perioperative Deaths 1992/3. [online]. Available from www.ncepod.org.uk/1992report/Full%20Report%201991-1992.pdf. [Accessed August, 2016].

10. Franchi M, Ghezzi F, Raio L, Di Naro E, Miglierina M, Agosti M, et al. Joel-Cohen or Pfannenstiel incision at Caesarean delivery: does it make a difference? Acta Obstet Gynecol Scand. 2002;81(11):1040-6.

11. Mathai M, Hofmeyr GJ. Abdominal surgical incisions for CS. Cochrane Database Syst Rev. 2007;(1):CD004453.

12. Song SH, Oh MJ, Kim T, Hur JY, Saw HS, Park YK. Finger-assisted stretching technique for Caesarean section. Int J Gynaecol Obstet. 2006;92(3):212-6.

13. Hofmeyr JG, Novikova N, Mathai M, Shah A. Techniques for Caesarean section. Am J Obstet Gynecol. 2009;201(5):431-44.

14. Rietberg CC, Elferink-Stinkens PM, Brand R, van Loon AJ, Van Hemel OJ, Visser GH. Term breech presentation in The Netherlands from 1995 to 1999: mortality and morbidity in relation to the mode of delivery of 33824 infants. Int J Obstet Gynaecol. 2003;110(6):604-9.

15. National Collaborating Centre for Women's and Children's Health. Caesarean section. NICE Clinical Guideline. London: RCOG Press; 2011.

16. Shipp TD, Zelop CM, Repke JT, Cohen A, Caughey AB, Lieberman E. Intrapartum uterine rupture and dehiscence in patients with prior lower uterine segment vertical and transverse incisions. Obstet Gynecol. 1999;94(5 Pt 1):735-40.

17. Wilkinson C, Enkin MW. Manual removal of placenta at CS. Cochrane Database Syst Rev. 2000;(2):CD000130.

18. Ahmed B, Abu Nahia F, Abushama M. Routine cervical dilatation during elective cesarean section and its influence on maternal morbidity: a randomized controlled study. J Perinat Med. 2005;33(6):510-3.

19. CORONIS Collaborative Group, Abalos E, Addo V, Brocklehurst P, El Sheikh M, Farrell B, et al. CS surgical techniques (CORONIS): a fractional, factorial, unmasked, randomised controlled trial. Lancet. 2013;382(9888):234-48.

20. Siddiqui M, Goldszmidt E, Fallah S, Kingdom J, Windrim R, Carvalho JC. Complications of exteriorized compared with in situ uterine repair at Caesarean delivery under spinal anesthesia: a randomized controlled trial. Obstet Gynecol. 2007;110(3):570-5.

21. Coutinho IC, Ramos de Amorim MM, Katz L, Bandeira de Ferraz AA. Uterine exteriorization compared with in situ repair at caesarean delivery: a randomized controlled trial. Obstet Gynecol. 2008;111(3):639-47.

22. Enkin MW, Wilkinson C. Single versus two layer suturing for closing the uterine incision at CS. Cochrane Database Syst Rev. 2000;(2):CD000192.

23. Gyamfi C, Juhasz G, Gyamfi P, Blumenfeld Y, Stone JL. Single-versus double-layer uterine incision closure and uterine rupture. J Matern Fetal Neonatal Med. 2006;19(10):639-43.

24. CAESAR study collaborative group. Caesarean section surgical techniques: a randomised factorial trial (CAESAR). BJOG. 2010;117(11):1366-76.

25. Lyell DJ, Caughey AB, Hu E, Daniels K, et al. Peritoneal closure at primary caesarean delivery and adhesions. Obstet Gynecol. 2005;106(2):275-80.

26. Alderdice F, McKenna D, Dornan J. Techniques and materials for skin closure in caesarean section. Cochrane Database Syst Rev. 2003;(2):CD003577.

27. Fatušié Z, Hudié I, Musié A. Misgav-Ladach Caesarean section: general consideration. Acta Clin Croat. 2011;50(1):95-9.

28. Holmgren G, Sjöholm L, Stark M. The Misgav Ladach method for cesarean section: method description. Acta Obstet Gynecol Scand. 1999;78(7):615-21.

29. Pelosi MA, Pelosi MA. Pelosi minimally invasive technique of cesarean section. Surg Technol Int. 2004;13:137-46.

30. Nabhan AF. Long-term outcomes of two different surgical techniques for Caesarean. Int J Gynaecol Obstet. 2008;100(1):69-75.

31. Confidential enquiries into maternal deaths in the United Kingdom. Why mother's die 1997-1999. London: RCOG Press; 2001.

32. Ward HR, Jennings OG, Potgieter P, Lombard CJ. Do plastic adhesive drapes prevent post caesarean wound infection? J Hosp Infect. 2001;47(3):230-4.

33. Cordtz T, Schouenborg L, Laursen K, Daugaard HO, Buur K, Munk Christensen B, et al. The effect of incisional plastic drapes and redisinfection of operation site on wound infection following caesarean section. J Hosp Infect. 1989;13(3):267-72.

34. Johnson CD, Serpell JW. Wound infection after abdominal incision with scalpel or diathermy. Br J Surg. 1990;77(6):626-7.

35. Pearlman NW, Stiegmann GV, Vance V, Norton LW, Bell RC, Staerkel R, et al. A prospective study of incisional time, blood loss, pain, and healing with carbon dioxide laser, scalpel, and electrosurgery. Arch Surg. 1991;126(8):1018-20.

PART II

Instrumental Vaginal Delivery

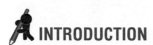 INTRODUCTION

Operative delivery can be of two types: (1) abdominal method (caesarean section) and (2) vaginal-assisted delivery (forceps delivery or vacuum extraction). Over the past 10–15 years, the rate of caesarean delivery has increased, while that of instrumental vaginal delivery has fallen. The present trend is towards increasing use of vacuum delivery and this method is rapidly replacing forceps as the predominant method for instrumental vaginal delivery.

Vaginal instrumental delivery involves the use of either forceps or vacuum to facilitate the delivery of foetal head. Both the types of assisted vaginal deliveries aid the delivery of foetal head either through application of manual traction (forceps) or suction force (vacuum cup). Although the most important function of forceps is application of traction, they also prove useful for rotating the foetal head, particularly those lying in the occiput transverse or occipitoposterior positions. The force produced by the forceps on foetal skull is a complex function of the strength of pull and compression exerted by the forceps and friction produced by maternal tissues.

While forceps are usually used for speeding up the delivery, occasionally they can also be used for slowing down delivery, e.g. while delivering the after-coming head of the breech. Therefore, it is of utmost importance that the clinicians involved in maternal care are well acquainted with the technique of performing an operative vaginal delivery either using forceps or vacuum. However, none of these methods, neither vacuum nor forceps, is 100% perfect, because each method is associated with its own advantages and disadvantages. While the use of forceps is associated with an increased risk of injuries to the woman's genital tract, vacuum usage is associated with an increased risk of foetal scalp injuries, such as neonatal cephalohaematoma or subgaleal haematoma.

The term 'ventouse' is derived from a French word meaning a soft cup. This device is known as vacuum extractor in the USA, while it is referred to as ventouse in Europe.[1] In the recent times, increasing interest in the use of vacuum extractor can be largely considered due to the fact that it is relatively safer for both the mother and infant in comparison to forceps delivery. Suction force by the vacuum creates an artificial caput or chignon within the cup. This helps in the firm hold of vacuum cup and allows adequate traction. The original vacuum extractor was designed by Sir John Young in Edinburgh in 1849.[2]

Soon after, Malmström developed the prototype of the modern vacuum extractor in Sweden.[3] The Malmström extractor consisted of a metal cup with a flat plate inside it and a chain attached to the plate. The chain was placed inside a rubber tube, which was necessary to develop the vacuum, and was attached to a traction bar. Traction is applied to the vacuum cup by the chain and plate.[4] The metal cup comes in four sizes and it is recommended that the largest cup possible should be used for delivery. It was not until 1973, when Kobayashi developed the soft silastic cup in the USA.[5,6] The silastic cup has many advantages over the metal cup. Compared with metal-cup vacuum extractors, soft-cup devices are easier to use and cause fewer neonatal scalp injuries.[7-10] The chance of injury to the foetal scalp is relatively less because the vacuum can be developed quickly and, therefore, can be released between contractions.[8] However, the major disadvantage associated with the use of vacuum extractors is that they are likely to detach more frequently in comparison to the metallic cups, which detach less frequently.[9,10] Today, more and more healthcare attendants are showing preference towards the use of silastic vacuum extractor as an alternative to delivery, when the foetal head is stuck up in the midpelvis rather than proceeding directly with caesarean section.[11] While forceps is an instrument which helps in the delivery of foetal head through transmission of the mechanical force to the base of skull, ventouse is an instrument, which assists in delivery by creating a vacuum between it and the foetal scalp. The pulling force in case of vacuum extraction helps in dragging the cranium.[12]

SURGICAL EQUIPMENT USED

Forceps

Forceps are instruments that help in the delivery of the foetus, by applying traction to the foetal head. The credit for the invention of the precursor of the modern forceps, which is presently used for the delivery of live infants, goes to Peter Chamberlen of England (1600 c).[13] Modifications in the forceps design have led to the development of more than 700 different types and shapes of forceps. Presently, the use of forceps has decreased to a great extent in the clinical practice due to an improvement in the foetal monitoring and surveillance techniques. Many different types of forceps are being used at different centres. Wrigley's forceps are most commonly used for forceps delivery, whereas Keilland's forceps are commonly used for the rotation of foetal head. Another type of forceps commonly used are the Piper's forceps, which are used for the delivery of the after-coming head in cases of breech vaginal deliveries. Use of Piper's forceps helps in reducing traction on the foetal neck during breech vaginal delivery.

Forceps are composed of two branches, each of which has four major components: blades, shank, lock and handle. The forceps blades have two curves, i.e. the cephalic curve and the pelvic curve. The cephalic curve is adapted to provide a good application to the foetal head. In cephalic application, the forceps blades are applied along the sides of the head, grasping the biparietal diameter in between the widest part of the blades. The long axis of the blades corresponds more or less to the occipitomental plane of the foetal head. Since this method of application results in negligible compression effect on the cranium, this method of application is favoured over pelvic method of application. On the other hand, the pelvic curve conforms to the axis of birth canal and allows the blades to fit in with the curve of the birth canal. Pelvic application consists of application of forceps blades along the sides of lateral pelvic wall, ignoring the position of foetal head. Therefore, this type of application can result in serious compression on the cranium, especially in case of unrotated head.

The ACOG criteria for classification of instrumental delivery (both forceps and vacuum) according to the station and rotation of foetal head are described in Table 46.1.[14,15] The revised classification uses the level of the leading bony point of the foetal head in centimetres, measured from the level of the maternal ischial spines to define station (±5 cm). High forceps deliveries, used in previous classification systems, defined them as procedures performed when the head was not engaged. High forceps application is not included in the present classification system. According to ACOG (1994) and the SOGC (2005), 'high forceps deliveries are not recommended in modern obstetric practice'.[11,15,16]

Types of Vacuum Devices

Originally, vacuum devices as invented by Malmström had a rigid metal cup with a separate suction catheter attached laterally and connected to a foot- or hand-operated pedal. Nowadays, besides the rigid cups (made of metal), flexible

Table 46.1: The ACOG criteria for classification of instrumental delivery[14,15]

Procedure	Criteria
Outlet forceps	• The foetal scalp is visible at the introitus, without separating the labia • The foetal skull has reached the pelvic floor • The sagittal suture is in anteroposterior diameter or right or left occiput anterior or posterior position • The foetal head is at or on the perineum • The rotation does not exceed 45°

Low forceps	• Leading point of foetal skull is at station ≥+2 and not on the pelvic floor
	• The degree of rotation does not matter. It could be either:
	  – Rotation is 45° or less (left or right occiput anterior to occiput anterior or left or right occiput posterior to occiput posterior)
	  – Rotation is 45° or more

Mid pelvic	Station is above +2 cm, but the head is engaged
High pelvic application	Not included in the classification system

Table 46.2: Types of vacuum delivery suction-cup devices

Names	Size (in mm)	Material
Soft cups (silicone or plastic)		
Gentle Vac	60	Soft rubber
Kiwi ProCup	65	Soft plastic
Mityvac Bel	60	Soft silicone
Secure Cup	63	Rubber
Silc Cup	50–60	Silicone rubber
Soft Cup	60	Soft polyethylene
Tender Touch	60	Soft silicone
Vac-U-Nate 65 Soft Silicone	65	Soft silicone
Rigid 'anterior' cups (plastic or metal)		
Flex Cup	60	Polyurethane
Kiwi OmniCup	50	Rigid plastic
Malmström	40–60	Metal
Mityvac 'M' Style	50	Rigid polyethylene
Rigid 'posterior' cups (plastic or metal)		
Bird Posterior Cup	40–60	Metal
Kiwi OmniCup	50	Rigid plastic
Mityvac 'M' Select	50	Rigid polyethylene

or soft cup (made of plastic, silicone or silastic material) and semi-rigid cups are also available (Table 46.2). Metallic cups are preferred over flexible cups in case of occipitoposterior positions and difficult occipitoanterior positions. Soft or semi-rigid vacuum cups may be available in different shapes: mushroom-shaped and bell-funnel shaped. Mushroom-shaped devices are associated with a lower failure rate in comparison to the bell-shaped devices. Examples of different types of cups include soft or rigid anterior cups and rigid posterior cups. Posterior cups are flatter, which allow for better placement at the flexion point on the foetal head, which is usually much further back in the sacral hollow during occipitoposterior presentation. Most of the newer devices use hand-pump suction, which requires an assistant or can be used by the healthcare attendant (herself or himself).[17] In the United States, these handheld devices are intended for single use and are disposable.

Presently, the use of silastic vacuum extractor is gaining popularity in various parts of the world. However, the procedure must be performed by an experienced healthcare attendant and it must be immediately abandoned, if it does not proceed smoothly or the cup dislodges more than three times. The healthcare attendant must consider vacuum extraction as a trial. There should be a progressive descent of foetal head with each traction attempt. If there is no clear evidence regarding the descent of foetal head, an alternative delivery approach must be considered. Delivery by vacuum extractor is being considered less traumatic for the mother, in comparison to the forceps delivery. Moreover, complications to the foetus may be minimised, if the physician recognises contraindications to the use of vacuum extraction and follows the procedure correctly. Although a simple procedure, it still demands proper knowledge of the indications, careful use of technique, meticulous care and most importantly operator experience.

INDICATIONS

Indications for instrumental vaginal deliveries are identical for forceps and vacuum extractors. No indication for operative vaginal delivery is absolute and largely depends upon the skill and preference of the operator. Many times, the clinician may prefer a caesarean section rather than a difficult forceps delivery. The use of mid-forceps delivery in modern obstetric practice still remains controversial.[18,19] Many clinicians favour the use of caesarean delivery over difficult mid-forceps application. The various maternal and foetal indications for operative vaginal delivery are described below.[20,21]

Maternal Indications

❖ *Termination of second stage of labour*: This may be required in case of conditions which are threatening to the mother (maternal exhaustion, severe pre-eclampsia, severe bleeding, cardiac or pulmonary disease, history of spontaneous pneumothorax, chorioamnionitis, acute pulmonary oedema, etc.).[22]
❖ *Prolonged second stage*: If the second stage of labour is too prolonged, it requires to be terminated. Prolonged second stage of labour has been described by Friedman,[23] as nulliparous women, who fail to deliver after 3 hours with the use of regional anaesthesia and 2 hours without its use or a lack of continuing progress for 1 hour without regional anaesthetics, or 2 hours with regional anaesthetics in multiparous women. Prolonged second stage of labour may be related to inadequate uterine contractions, ineffective maternal efforts, malrotation of foetal head

(e.g. occipitoposterior position), perineal rigidity, epidural analgesia, etc.

Foetal Indications

❖ Suspicion of immediate or potential foetal compromise in the second stage of labour, in the form of non-reassuring foetal heart sounds on continuous cardiotocographic machine trace (particularly foetal heart decelerations with reduced or absent variability). This may be related to conditions, such as foetal umbilical cord prolapse, premature separation of placenta, etc.
❖ In the hands of an experienced healthcare attendant, foetal malpositions, such as the after-coming head in breech vaginal delivery and occipitoposterior positions can be considered as indications for forceps delivery.[24] Presently, there is no evidence regarding the beneficial use of prophylactic forceps application in an otherwise normal term labour and delivery.

The classification, indications and contraindications for vacuum delivery are almost the same as that utilised for forceps delivery. However, unlike the forceps, vacuum extractors cannot be used in cases of face presentation or after-coming head of breech.[25] The vacuum must never be applied to an unengaged head, i.e. above zero station.[26]

Other indications for vacuum application include the following:[11,27]

❖ As an alternative to forceps operation (e.g. occipitotransverse or occipitoposterior position)
❖ Shortening of the second stage of labour for maternal benefit (e.g. maternal exhaustion)
❖ Delay in descent of the head in the second stage of labour (e.g. case of the second baby of twins)
❖ Prolonged second stage of labour.

Contraindications

Use of Vacuum for Operative Vaginal Delivery

Absolute contraindications: Some absolute contraindications for the use of vacuum for operative vaginal delivery are as follows:[28]
❖ Cephalopelvic disproportion
❖ Non-engagement of foetal head or presence of the head at a high station
❖ Operator inexperience.

Relative contraindications: Some relative contraindications to vacuum delivery are as follows:
❖ *Foetal prematurity*: Gestational age less than 34 weeks has been considered as a relative contraindication to foetal delivery, due to an increased risk for intracranial haemorrhage.[29]
❖ Known foetal conditions that affect the bones or disorders of foetal bone mineralization
❖ Foetal coagulation defects or active bleeding disorders
❖ Non-cephalic or facial presentation
❖ Foetal macrosomia.

Contraindications for Forceps Application

The following are the contraindications for forceps-assisted vaginal deliveries:

- ❖ Any contraindication for normal vaginal delivery (a total placenta praevia, cephalopelvic disproportion, etc.)
- ❖ Refusal of the patient to give verbal consent for the procedure
- ❖ Cervix is not fully dilated or effaced.
- ❖ Inability to determine the foetal presentation or position of foetal head
- ❖ Inadequate pelvic size or cephalopelvic disproportion
- ❖ Previous unsuccessful attempts of vacuum extraction (relative contraindication)
- ❖ Absence of adequate anaesthesia or analgesia
- ❖ Setup with inadequate facilities and support staff
- ❖ Inexperienced operator.

MANAGEMENT

Forceps Delivery

Prerequisites for Forceps Delivery

Before the application of forceps, it is important for the healthcare attendant to review the indications for operative vaginal delivery and confirm the presence of all the following prerequisites for forceps application:[30]

- ❖ *Maternal verbal consent*: Maternal verbal consent should be obtained prior to the application of forceps. However, in some circumstances, it may not be possible to take the maternal consent, especially if the procedure needs to be performed as an emergency or if the mother is sedated. In these cases, consent may be taken from the patient's partner or relatives. If a forceps delivery has been planned in advance (i.e. for maternal medical indications), it is possible to counsel the patient and take her consent prior to the onset of active labour.
- ❖ *Assessment of the maternal pelvis*: The maternal pelvis must be adequately assessed before proceeding with a forceps delivery. The type of pelvis (i.e. gynaecoid, android, anthropoid or platypelloid) and adequacy of the pelvis for delivery of the baby must be clinically assessed prior to undertaking delivery. It should be emphasised that adequate pelvic size depends not just on the pelvic assessment, but also on the size and presentation of the foetus.
- ❖ *Engagement of the foetal head*: The foetal head must be engaged before application of forceps. Engagement of the foetal head implies that the largest diameter of the foetal presenting part (biparietal diameter in case of cephalic presentation) has passed through the pelvic inlet. Engagement of the foetal presenting part is of great importance, as it helps in ruling out foetopelvic disproportion.
- ❖ *Presentation, position and station of the presenting part*: The presentation, position and station of the foetal presenting part must be reconfirmed just before the procedure. The foetus must present as vertex or face with

the chin anterior. The station of the foetal head must be at or below the zero station. If the leading part of the foetal head is at the zero station or below, the foetal head is said to be engaged. This implies that the biparietal plane of the foetal head has passed through the pelvic inlet. However, in the presence of excessive moulding or caput formation, engagement may not have taken place, even if the head appears to be at zero station. In these cases, the healthcare attendants can improve their clinical estimate of engagement by using the abdominal palpation, to estimate how much of the foetal head is above the upper level of the pubic symphysis. A recently engaged foetal head may be two-fifths palpable per abdominally. The presence of the sagittal sutures in the anteroposterior diameter of the pelvic outlet must be also confirmed before application of forceps. Determination of foetal position by examination of sagittal sutures and fontanels is possible when the head is low in the pelvis. However, when the head is at a higher station, an absolute determination of the position of foetal head may not be possible. In these cases, foetal position can be determined by locating the foetal ear. Forceps are applied across the ears to the mandibular region.

- ❖ *Cervical dilatation and effacement*: The cervix must be fully dilated and effaced. If the forceps are applied before complete cervical dilatation and effacement has been attained, the procedure may produce severe maternal lacerations and haemorrhage.
- ❖ *Status of the membranes*: The foetal membranes must have ruptured prior to the application of forceps.
- ❖ *Bladder to be emptied*: The bladder should be emptied in preparation for forceps operative deliveries, regardless of the type of anaesthesia used. Except for the cases where the foetal head is on the perineum, the bladder should be emptied with the help of a catheter.
- ❖ *The woman's position*: The labouring woman, in whom forceps have to be applied, should be preferably placed in the 'lithotomy position'. However, some practitioners prefer to use the left lateral position instead. After placement in the proper position, the woman must be adequately cleaned and draped, while observing aseptic precautions in order to minimise the chances of maternal infection.
- ❖ *Adequate analgesia*: The patient must be administered adequate analgesia prior to the application of forceps. The decision regarding the type of anaesthesia to be used should be made before initiating the delivery. An adequate level of anaesthesia is an important prerequisite before forceps application. Attempts to undertake the instrumental delivery without adequate anaesthesia may be extremely painful for the mother and may end up in failure. While some healthcare attendants use only local infiltration of anaesthesia to the perineal body prior to forceps application, others may prefer to use pudendal block anaesthesia augmented with IV sedation. In some cases, adequate anaesthesia may also be obtained using regional or general anaesthesia. Regional anaesthesia using epidural or spinal block is more commonly used, while general anaesthesia is usually reserved for very complicated situations.

PART II

❖ *Operator's competence and facilities for operative delivery*: Adequate facilities for caesarean section should be available in case the delivery by forceps fails. Operator's skill, training and competence in the use of forceps, play an important role in the eventual success of the procedure. The operator should not only be competent in the use of the forceps, but he or she should be promptly able to recognize and manage potential complications. It is very important for the operator to know when he or she must abandon the attempts at forceps delivery and resort to caesarean section.

Steps for Application of the Forceps[13,14]

Steps for application of forceps are described in Figures 46.1A to F and comprise of the following.

Identification of the Forceps Blades

In order to identify the blade of the forceps, whether left or right, the blades must be articulated and then placed in front of the pelvis with the tip of the blades pointing upwards and the concave side of the pelvic curve forwards. In this position, the forceps blade which corresponds to the left side of the maternal pelvis is the left blade and the one which corresponds to the right side of the maternal pelvis is the right blade.

The success of instrumental vaginal delivery using forceps largely depends upon the technique of forceps application. Knowledge regarding the exact position of the foetal head is of utmost importance before the application of forceps. The term 'pelvic application' is used when the left blade is applied on the left side of the pelvis and the right blade is applied on the right side of the pelvis, regardless of the foetal position. The 'cephalic application', on the other hand, involves application of blades of forceps on the two sides of foetal head. Since pelvic application is more dangerous due to the risk of significant maternal injury involved, this type of forceps application is not commonly used in clinical practice. The cephalic application of forceps is largely preferred over the pelvic application. Once the blades of the forceps have been identified, other steps involved in simple outlet forceps delivery for an occipitoanterior position are as follows:

❖ *Checking the prerequisites for forceps application*: After ensuring proper anaesthesia, an empty bladder and other prerequisites for forceps application (as described previously), the foetal position and FHR are checked again.

❖ *Application of the left blade of the forceps*: Before the application of forceps blades, the operator places his or her back towards the maternal right thigh and holds the left handle of the left branch of forceps between the fingers of left hand, as if holding a pencil. The shank is held perpendicular to the floor, and under the guidance

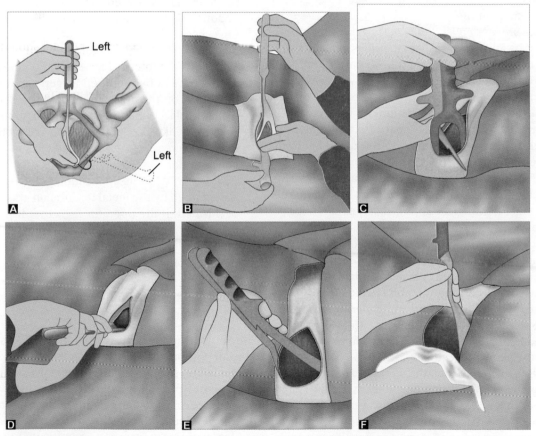

Figs 46.1A to F: (A) The left blade is introduced into the left side of the maternal pelvis; (B) The left blade is in place and the right blade is introduced by the right hand; a median or mediolateral episiotomy may be performed at this point; (C) The forceps have been locked; (D) Application of horizontal traction with the operator seated; (E) As the foetal occiput bulges out, the traction is applied in the upward direction; (F) Following the distension of vulval outlet by the foetal head, the branches of forceps are disarticulated and delivery of rest of the head is completed by modified Ritgen's manoeuvre

CHAPTER 46

of the fingers of the right hand, the left blade is inserted into the posterior half of the left side of the pelvis along the left vaginal wall. The force necessary to insert the blade is exerted by the pressure of the thumb, which is placed over the heel of the forceps blade. The left hand guides the handle in a wide arc until the blade is in place. As the blade is introduced into the vagina, it is brought to a horizontal position. This blade may be either left in place to stand freely on its own or is held in place without pressure by an assistant. The blades of the forceps are usually applied when the uterus is relaxed and not when the woman is experiencing uterine contraction. However, once properly applied the blades may be left in place, if a contraction occurs at the time of placement.

❖ *Application of the right blade of the forceps*: The right blade of the forceps is held in the right hand and introduced into the right side of the pelvis in the similar manner, with the operator's back towards the patient's left thigh.

❖ *Locking the blades of the forceps*: After proper placement of the left blade, it should lie almost parallel to the floor. With insertion of the right blade, the forceps should be locked without pressure. In case there is trouble in locking the blades of the forceps, it implies that they have not been properly applied. Even if the blades do get locked up, they might just slip off when the traction is applied. Therefore, before locking the forceps blades and application of traction, it is important to check if the blades have been properly applied or not.

❖ *Checking the proper application of the forceps*: The forceps blades must be applied directly to the sides of foetal head along the occipitomental diameter. In case of occiput anterior position, appropriately applied blades are equidistant from the sagittal sutures. The shanks of the blades must be perpendicular to the sagittal suture and there must be only a fingertip or less space between the heel of the blade and sagittal suture. On the other hand, in case of occipitoposterior position, the blades would be equidistant from the midline of the face and brow. The biparietal diameter of the foetal head corresponds to the greatest distance between the appropriately applied blades. Consequently, in a proper cephalic application, the long axis of the blades corresponds to the occipitomental diameter, with the ends of the blades lying over the posterior cheeks. When the forceps have been correctly applied, the blades lie over the parietal eminence, the shank should be in contact with the perineum and the superior surface of the handle should be directed upwards. In this position, the forceps should lock easily without any force and stand parallel to the plane of the floor.

❖ *Application of traction*: When the operator is sure that the blades have been placed appropriately, traction can be applied. At all times, the operator should be careful towards avoiding the use of undue force. The traction is usually applied in the direction of pelvic axis and at all times must be gentle and intermittent. The operator should be seated in front of the patient, with elbows kept pressed against the sides of the body. To avoid excessive force during traction,

the force should be exerted only through the wrist and forearms. Initially, the traction is applied in a horizontal direction until the perineum begins to bulge. With the application of traction, as the vulva starts getting distended by the foetal occiput, an episiotomy may be performed if the operator feels that it would facilitate the delivery process. As the foetal occiput emerges out, the handles of forceps are gradually elevated, eventually pointing almost directly upwards as the parietal bones emerge. As the handles are raised, the head delivers by extension. While applying traction in the upwards direction, the operator's four fingers should grasp the upper surface of the shanks and handles, while the thumbs must exert the necessary force on their lower surface. Traction should be applied intermittently, synchronous with the uterine contractions and the foetal head should be allowed to recede inside during the periods of uterine relaxation. This helps in simulating normal delivery as much as possible and helps in preventing undue compression over the foetal head. In an emergency situation, applying continuous traction may be necessary until the foetal head delivers. The safe limit for the amount of traction to be applied, in order to accomplish safe foetal head descent has been considered to be about 45 pounds in primiparas and 30 pounds in multiparas.[13]

Though there is no fixed limit for the number of traction attempts to be applied before abandoning the procedure, in case there is no descent of the foetal head, abdominal delivery should be considered following three unsuccessful attempts at the forceps. Once the vulva has been distended by the foetal head, some operators prefer to remove the forceps blades and complete the delivery of foetal head by modified Ritgen's manoeuvre. Some operators, on the other hand, prefer to keep the forceps blades in place, while the foetal head is emerging out. This practice is likely to increase the total foetal dimension, thereby increasing the likelihood of causing injury to the vulvar outlet.

❖ *Episiotomy*: With the application of traction, as the vulva is distended by the foetal occiput, an episiotomy may be performed, if the operator feels that it would facilitate the delivery of foetal head. The utility of episiotomy in preventing short- and long-term maternal injury presently remains controversial.

Steps of Vacuum Extraction in Occipitoanterior Position

The actual steps of vacuum extraction in case of occipito-anterior position are shown in Figures 46.2A to D. These steps are described here in details. Under all aseptic precautions, the patient's perineum and external genitalia are cleaned and draped. The patient's labia are separated, following which the vacuum (soft) cup, which has been compressed and folded, prior to insertion, is applied. The cup is inserted gently by pressing it in inwards and downwards direction, so that the inferior edge of the cup lies close to the posterior fourchette.

PART II

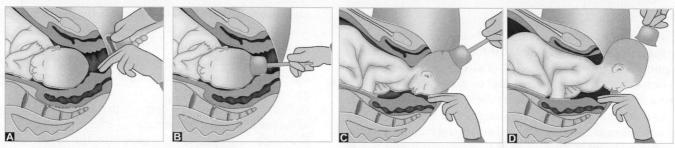

Figs 46.2A to D: (A) Insertion of the vacuum cup into the vagina following the separation of patient's labia; (B) Application of the vacuum cup over the foetal head in such a way that the cup is placed as far posteriorly as possible; (C) Application of traction at right angles to facilitate the delivery of foetal head; (D) As the head clears the pubic symphysis, the delivery of head is completed by modified Ritgen's manoeuvre

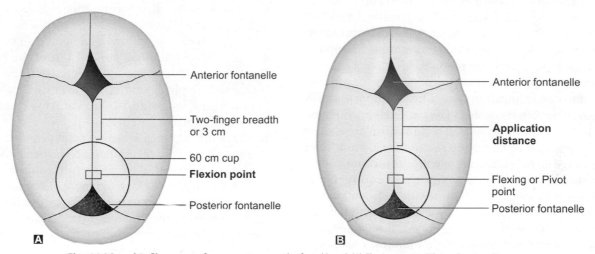

Figs 46.3A and B: Placement of vacuum cup over the foetal head: (A) Flexion point; (B) Application distance

Placement of Vacuum Cup over the Foetal Head

The vacuum cup should be so positioned as to prevent the deflexion and asyncylitism of foetal head. The cup should be placed in such a way that the centre of the cup lies directly over the flexion point or the pivot point which can be defined as a point over the sagittal suture, about 6 cm behind the anterior fontanelle or 3 cm in front of the posterior fontanelle (Figs 46.3A and B). As a general rule, the cup must be placed as far posteriorly as possible. This implies that the edge of the cup having a diameter of 5–7 cm would be approximately 3 cm from the anterior fontanelle and would lie over the posterior fontanel. This is known as the application distance. Four different types of cup applications are possible: (1) flexing median, (2) flexing paramedian, (3) deflexing median and (4) deflexing paramedian. In the flexing median type of cup application, the centre of cup lies over the flexion point. This positioning helps in maintaining flexion of the foetal head and avoids traction over the anterior fontanel. If the cup is placed anteriorly on the foetal cranium near the anterior fontanelle rather than over the occiput, this may result in undue extension of the cervical spine. Similarly, if the cup is asymmetrically placed in relation to the sagittal suture, it is likely to worsen asyncylitism. While positioning the cup, the healthcare attendant must be careful that no maternal soft tissues get trapped between the vacuum cup and foetal head. Moreover, the cup should not be twisted because this is likely to result in lacerations or injury to the foetal head. In order to prevent the entrapment of maternal tissues within the vacuum cup, the full circumference of the vacuum cup must be palpated, both before and after the vacuum has been created, as well as prior to the application of traction. While applying the vacuum cup, the knob on the metal cup or the ridge on the silastic cup should be in line with the posterior fontanel.

Creation of Vacuum Suction

Once the cup has been properly placed, vacuum must be created. The healthcare attendant must place the fingers of one hand against the suction cup and grasp the handle of the instrument with the other hand, following which the vacuum is applied. In order to achieve effective traction, a pressure of at least 0.6–0.8 kg/cm^2 must be created. The pressure must be gradually created, by increasing suction at the rate of 0.2 kg/cm^2 every 2 minutes. With the use of soft cups, it is possible to create negative pressure of 0.8 kg/cm^2 over as little as 1 minute. Prior to the application of traction, an episiotomy may be performed. With the vacuum extractor, a midline or mediolateral episiotomy is adequate and a pudendal nerve block serves as an optimal form of anaesthesia.

Force of Traction

When using a metal cup or a Kiwi Omnicup for vacuum extraction, a chignon needs to form before traction is applied and this would take 1–2 minutes. '*Chignon*' is a French word meaning a large coil or lump of hair (bun) at the back. In obstetrics, *chignon* refers to a swelling over the scalp (artificial caput succedaneum) that develops inside the cup when vacuum is induced and is the means by which the cup adheres to the scalp. It is observed immediately after the removal of cup from the scalp. However, it rapidly decreases in size 1 hour after birth to become a diffuse swelling. It usually disappears over a period of 1–2 days. As soon as the vacuum has been built up and the operator has checked that no vaginal tissue is trapped inside the silastic cup, traction should be applied with each uterine contraction in line of pelvic axis. Initially, the traction must be applied in the direction perpendicular to the base of cup, i.e. in the downward direction. Once crowning of the head occurs, the direction must be changed to downwards and forwards in relation to the maternal position. The patient is encouraged to push at the same time, so that a minimum amount of traction is required to complete the delivery. More than three good attempts of pulling are usually not recommended. Delivery should be achieved within three contractions. Descent should, however, be achieved with each contraction. The procedure should be discontinued if unintended cup detachments or 'popups' of the cup occur three times or if extraction is not achieved within 15–20 minutes of initiation. In case the cup gets dislodged, it should be reapplied only after careful inspection of foetal scalp for any injury. In order to prevent 'pop-offs' during traction, the healthcare attendant must keep a thumb on the anterior part of the cup and index finger on the scalp to detect any detachment of the cup. Early detachment of the silastic cup can be detected if the edges of the cup begin to roll over. Traction should be repeated with each contraction, until crowning of the foetal head occurs. As the head clears the pubic symphysis, the delivery of head is completed by modified Ritgen's manoeuvre. Once the foetal head has delivered, suction is released and the cup is removed. Delivery can then proceed as usual. The procedure should be abandoned, if delivery is not achieved or the labour does not progress. Under ordinary circumstances, the procedure must be abandoned after three successive cup detachments. In these cases, forceps delivery or abdominal delivery must be considered. The procedure should also be stopped, if there appears any evidence of maternal or foetal trauma.

Using the 'ABCDEFGHIJ' Mnemonic

The steps performed in vacuum extraction can be described using the mnemonic 'ABCDEFGHIJ'.[31] This acronym has been reviewed as follows:

❖ **A:** Prior to delivery, the healthcare attendant should **a**ddress the patient and discuss the risks and benefits of operative vaginal delivery. At the time of delivery, extra **a**ssistance is required. This includes nursing care professionals, midwives, anaesthetists, paediatricians and neonatal resuscitation team. Adequate **a**nalgesics should be administered before carrying out vacuum delivery. Though pudendal anaesthesia suffices in most of the cases, regional anaesthesia may be sometimes required for vacuum delivery.

❖ **B:** The **b**ladder should be emptied prior to the application of vacuum in order to avoid risk of injury.

❖ **C:** Prior to the application of vacuum, the **c**ervix should be completely dilated.

❖ **D:** The position of the foetal head should be **d**etermined prior to vacuum application.

❖ **E:** The vacuum **e**quipment should be checked by the healthcare attendant, to ensure adequate suction.

❖ **F:** The centre of the cup should be placed at the **f**lexion point, which can be defined as a point over the sagittal suture, approximately 3 cm in front of the posterior fontanelle and approximately 6 cm from the anterior fontanel. The placement of cup over the flexion point is important, as it helps in maximising traction and minimising detachment of the cup.

❖ **G:** The healthcare attendant must apply **g**entle traction and increase the force of vacuum suction with the manometer at the recommended range. While some healthcare attendants prefer to lower the force of suction between contractions to decrease rates of scalp injury, others prefer to maintain continuous suction, especially in cases where rapid foetal delivery is required, e.g. in cases of non-reassuring foetal heart tones.

❖ **H:** It is important for the healthcare attendant to know when to **h**alt the procedure for instrumental delivery. Use of vacuum should be **h**alted, when there are three disengagements of the vacuum (or 'pop-offs'), more than 20 minutes have elapsed or three consecutive pulls result in no progress or delivery.

❖ **I:** The healthcare attendant must evaluate each individual patient, regarding whether or not to give an **i**ncision for a possible episiotomy, when the perineum gets distended by the foetal head.

❖ **J:** The vacuum cup must be removed as soon as the foetal **j**aw is reachable.

Postdelivery Examination

The postoperative steps for vacuum delivery are same as that of forceps delivery. Following instrumental vaginal delivery, thorough examination of both the mother and the newborn is advisable.

Maternal Examination

The mother's external genitalia must be carefully examined, in order to rule out the presence of any cervical, vaginal, perineal and paraurethral lacerations or tears. In case of the presence of significant maternal vulvar oedema, measures such as perineal ice application and painkillers may prove to be useful. A postoperative haemogram should be obtained in patients who experience excessive bleeding. Before discharging patients who had undergone forceps delivery, pelvic and rectal examinations must be performed in order to exclude any bleeding and presence of entities, such as pelvic haematoma, rectal tears, misplaced sutures, unrecognised lacerations, etc.

Neonatal Examination

The newborn must be examined for lacerations, bruising and other injuries over the scalp and face.

Follow-up

In case no forceps-related complications are found at the time of discharge, the mother should be asked to come for a follow-up postpartum examination within 4–6 weeks, where the usual protocol for postpartum care, including a thorough pelvic examination must be performed.

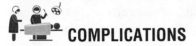

COMPLICATIONS

Forceps

The use of forceps has been found to be associated with long-term maternal and foetal morbidity. Mid-forceps application is associated with higher rates of maternal and neonatal morbidity in comparison to outlet-forceps or low-forceps application.

Maternal Complications

❖ *Injury to the maternal tissues*: Even with use by an experienced operator, forceps deliveries may be associated with an increased risk of perineal tears and lacerations (both vaginal and cervical).[30] This could be related to the more rapid and extensive stretching of the maternal tissues with delivery of the foetal head. Perineal tears are likely to especially occur in the cases, where the episiotomy is not given at the right time.[32-34]

❖ *Haemorrhage*: Severe maternal tissue injury and lacerations due to forceps application can sometimes result in extensive bleeding and maternal haemorrhage.

❖ *Febrile morbidity*: This could be the manifestation of postpartum uterine infection and pelvic cellulitis, resulting from the infection caused by trauma to the tissues.

❖ *Urinary retention and bladder dysfunction*: Damage to the urethral sphincters may result in urinary retention and bladder dysfunction.

❖ *Late maternal complications*: Late maternal complications could be related to damage caused to the pelvic support tissues. This damage could manifest in the form of genitourinary fistulae or pelvic organ prolapse. Injury caused by forceps may in the long-term result in the development of faecal incontinence due to damage to the rectal sphincter function or urinary incontinence due to damage to the urethral sphincters.[35,36]

Injuries to Baby

Foetal injury: Various foetal injuries which can be caused by the application of forceps, include cephalohaematoma, facial nerve injury, depressed skull fractures, intracranial bleeding, shoulder dystocia, etc.[37,38] Additionally, cerebral palsy and subtly lower IQ (2.5 points) levels have also been described in infants delivered by forceps.

Vacuum

Some of the major complications for vacuum application include neonatal injuries. Use of vacuum can result in development of injuries, such as scalp lacerations, bruising, subgaleal haematomas, cephalohaematomas, intracranial haemorrhage, neonatal jaundice, subconjunctival haemorrhage, clavicular fracture, shoulder dystocia, injury of sixth and seventh cranial nerves, Erb's palsy, retinal haemorrhage and foetal death.[39,40] Signs and symptoms of serious intracranial injury in a neonate include apnoea, bradycardia, bulging fontanels, convulsions, irritability, lethargy and poor feeding. Various neonatal injuries, which can occur as a result of vacuum application, are described below.

Cephalohaematomas

Vacuum deliveries are associated with higher chances of development of neonatal cephalohaematoma, in comparison with forceps delivery. The resolution of cephalohaematomas can result in the development of hyperbilirubinaemia over long term. In case of cephalohaematoma (Fig. 46.4A), bleeding occurs beneath the periosteum, between the skull and the periosteum. As a result, the boggy swelling associated with cephalohaematoma is limited by the suture lines in contrast to the subgaleal haematomas, which are not limited by the suture lines.

Subgaleal or Subaponeurotic Haematomas

Subgaleal haematoma occurs as a result of bleeding in the potential space between the skull periosteum and epicranial aponeurosis (Fig. 46.4B). Since the collection occurs above the periosteum, it can cross the suture lines. Subgaleal haematoma must be suspected in case of boggy scalp swelling, swelling crossing the suture lines and an expanding head circumference.[41,42] The diffuse head swelling shifts with repositioning and indents on palpation. Swelling is not limited by suture lines (unlike in the cases of cephalohaematoma). The infants may also have signs of hypovolaemia (hypotension, pallor, tachycardia, tachypnoea and a falling haematocrit).

Intracranial Haemorrhage

These can be of various types, depending upon the location of the blood collection. Epidural haematoma occurs in the potential space between the dura mater and the skull. Subdural haematoma occurs in the potential space between the dura mater and arachnoid mater. Subarachnoid haemorrhage occurs in the subarachnoid space between the arachnoid mater and pia mater.

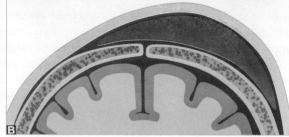

Figs 46.4A and B: (A) Cephalohaematoma and (B) Subgaleal haematoma

Shoulder Dystocia

Operative vaginal delivery is a risk factor for shoulder dystocia and it occurs more commonly with vacuum delivery, in comparison to the forceps delivery. The incidence of shoulder dystocia increases in cases of foetal macrosomia.

Retinal Haemorrhage

These usually resolve within several weeks and are unlikely to be associated with long-term morbidity.

Transient Neonatal Lateral Rectus Palsy

Since this usually resolves spontaneously, it is unlikely to have much clinical importance.

CLINICAL PEARLS

Vacuum versus Forceps

❖ *Failed forceps*: This is a term implying that an attempt to deliver with forceps had been unsuccessful. If the operator is not sure regarding whether the attempt at forceps delivery would be successful or not, the attempt is considered to be a trial of forceps delivery. The patient undergoing trial of forceps must be delivered in a setup, well equipped with facilities for an emergency caesarean delivery, in case the need arises. In case the satisfactory application of the forceps cannot be achieved or there is no descent of foetal head even after three attempts of traction application through forceps, the procedure must be abandoned and delivery accomplished with the help of vacuum extraction or caesarean section. Some of the causes of failed forceps are as follows:
  • Unsuspected cephalopelvic disproportion
  • Misdiagnosis of the position of the head
  • Incomplete dilation of the cervix
  • Outlet contraction (very rare in an otherwise normal pelvis).
❖ *Administration of an episiotomy*: It is not necessary to routinely perform an episiotomy with instrumental vaginal delivery.[43] If the tissues feel rigid and there is a probability for occurrence of tears, a mediolateral episiotomy can be considered.

EVIDENCE-BASED MEDICINE

Forceps versus Vacuum[44-49]

Vacuum extractors have replaced forceps in many situations, where instrumental vaginal delivery is required, in order to avoid abdominal caesarean delivery. Vacuum extraction is associated with a higher rate of neonatal injury, in comparison to the forceps delivery. In comparison with metal-cup vacuum extractors, soft-cup vacuum devices are easier to use and are associated with fewer neonatal scalp injuries. However, the soft cups are likely to detach more frequently.

The 'ventouse' delivery is considered to be more physiological and similar to normal vaginal delivery, in comparison to the forceps delivery. The comparison between vacuum and forceps delivery has been tabulated in Table 46.3. Theoretically, the use of vacuum extractor has several advantages over obstetric forceps. The use of vacuum helps in avoiding the insertion of space-occupying steel blades within the vagina. On the other hand, with a forceps delivery the foetal biparietal diameter is increased by the thickness of each forceps blade. Unlike forceps, the vacuum cup takes up minimal space in a mother's birth canal and, therefore, it is less likely to result in accidental maternal injuries. Additionally, with the use of vacuum extractor, there is no requirement for precise rotation of foetal head prior to the application of the vacuum cup. Thus, the vacuum can be used, even if the healthcare attendant is unsure about the exact foetal position. Since the vacuum extractor helps in the application of traction only, therefore, even if the occiput is not directly anterior or the head is in an unrotated position, it is most likely to rotate, when it reaches the perineum, similar to the case of spontaneous vaginal delivery. Moreover, even if the foetal head is deflexed, vacuum extraction often helps in flexing it. Vacuum application is associated with a much reduced maternal trauma. The amount of traction applied to the foetal head remains uncontrollable with forceps delivery, but it can be controlled with the use of a vacuum extractor. As a result, a high incidence of third- and fourth-degree maternal lacerations is associated with the use of forceps. However, use of vacuum is likely to result in serious foetal complications, including significant craniofacial injuries, retinal haemorrhages and transient lateral rectus palsy. An increased incidence of cephalohaematomas has also been noted after vacuum deliveries. The incidence of foetal injuries is likely to be higher with the use of Malmström vacuum cup, in comparison to the use of soft silastic cups.

Table 46.3: Comparison between forceps and vacuum delivery

Parameters	Delivery by forceps	Vacuum extraction
Effect on biparietal diameter (BPD) of foetal head	Space-occupying steel blades within the vagina cause an increase in the foetal BPD	Vacuum cup is not a space occupying device, therefore no change in foetal BPD
Amount of traction required	More traction force is required	Lesser traction force is needed
Maternal injuries	More chances of perineal injuries and lacerations	Lower chances of perineal injuries and lacerations
Foetal injuries	Lesser chances of injury to the foetal scalp and brain	More chances of injury to the foetal scalp and brain
Technical skill required	More technical skill is required on the part of the operator	Less technical skill is required on the part of the operator
Application in case of unrotated foetal head or occipitoposterior position	Must not be applied in cases of unrotated foetal head or occipitoposterior position	Can be applied in cases of unrotated foetal head or occipitoposterior position
Cervical dilation	Must be applied only in cases of fully dilated cervix	Can be applied even through incompletely dilated cervix
Safety feature	Not present	Present (when the traction is high, cup dislodges or pops off on its own)
Autorotation of foetal head	Cannot occur	Can occur along with traction
Use in other foetal presentations	Can be used in cases of mentoanterior position and after-coming head of the breech	Cannot be used in cases of mentoanterior position and after-coming head of the breech
Failure rate	Lower	Higher
Maternal morbidity	Higher	Lower

Moreover, the technique of vacuum application is easier to learn and quicker to apply in comparison to forceps application. Overall, vacuum application is associated with higher rate of successful vaginal delivery. Another major advantage of vacuum extractor is that when traction is too great, the cup dislodges or pops off. This acts as a safety feature of the vacuum device. The vacuum cup has a traction limit of 23 lbs, which is much less than that with forceps delivery and therefore can be considered as an additional safety factor. However, during vacuum extraction, patient's active participation is essential. Therefore, ventouse delivery can be considered more physiological than the forceps delivery.

Vacuum delivery, however, is associated with some complications as follows:

❖ Vacuum cannot be used in cases of preterm delivery, face presentation, after-coming head of the breech or in cases of maternal exhaustion where she is unable to bear down.
❖ Vacuum delivery is likely to cause more trauma to the baby in comparison to the delivery by forceps.

❖ Requirement of complex equipment (especially in cases of older instruments), which is subject to failure if not well maintained.

REFERENCES

1. Meniru GI. An analysis of recent trends in vacuum extraction and forceps delivery in the United Kingdom. Br J Obstet Gynaecol. 1996;103(2):168-70.
2. McQuivey RW. Vacuum-assisted delivery: a review. J Matern Fetal Neonatal Med. 2004;16(3):171-80.
3. Lucas MJ. The role of vacuum extraction in modern obstetrics. Clin Obstet Gynecol. 1994;37(4):794-805.
4. Donald I (Ed). Practical Obstetric Problems. London: Lloyd-Luke; 1969. p. 608.
5. Dell DL, Sightler SE, PlauchéAL WC. Soft cup vacuum extraction: a comparison of outlet delivery. Obstet Gynecol. 1985;66(5):624-8.
6. Ross MG. Vacuum delivery by soft cup extraction. Contemp Ob Gyn. 1994;39:48-53.
7. Berkus MD, Ramamurthy RS, O'Connor PS, Brown K, Hayashi RH. Cohort study of silastic obstetric vacuum cup deliveries: I. Safety of the instrument. Obstet Gynecol. 1985;66(4):503-9.
8. Johanson R, Menon V. Soft versus rigid vacuum extractor cups for assisted vaginal delivery. Cochrane Database Syst Rev. 2000;(2):CD000446.
9. Kuit JA, Eppinga HG, Wallenburg HC, Huikeshoven FJ. A randomized comparison of vacuum extraction delivery with a rigid and a pliable cup. Obstet Gynecol. 1993;82(2):280-4.
10. Groom KM, Jones BA, Miller N, Paterson-Brown S. A prospective randomised controlled trial of the Kiwi Omnicup versus conventional ventouse cups for vacuum-assisted vaginal delivery. BJOG. 2006;113(2):183-9.
11. American College of Obstetricians and Gynecologists (ACOG): Operative Vaginal Delivery. Technical Bulletin No. 196. Washington, DC: ACOG; 1994.
12. O'Grady JP. Modern Instrumental Delivery. Baltimore: Williams & Wilkins; 1988. pp. 155-85.
13. Hale R. Dennen's Forceps Deliveries, 4th edition. Philadelphia: FA Davis; 2001.
14. American Academy of Pediatrics and American College of Obstetricians and Gynecologists. Guidelines for Perinatal Care, 6th edition. Washington, DC; 2007. p. 158.
15. American College of Obstetricians and Gynecologists. Operative vaginal delivery. Clinical management guidelines for obstetricians-gynecologists. Int J Gynaecol Obstet. 2001;74(1):69-76.
16. Society of Obstetricians and Gynaecologists of Canada. Guidelines for operative vaginal birth. Number 148, May 2004. Int J Gynaecol Obstet. 2005;88(2):229-36.
17. Attilakos G, Sibanda T, Winter C, Johnson N, Draycott T. A randomised controlled trial of a new handheld vacuum extraction device. BJOG. 2005;112(11):1510-5.
18. Friedman EA. Midforceps delivery: no? Clin Obstet Gynecol. 1987;30(1):93-105.
19. Hayashi RH. Midforceps delivery: yes? Clin Obstet Gynecol. 1987;30(1):90-2.
20. Dauphin-McKenzie N, Celestin MJ, Brown D, González-Quintero VH. The advanced life support in obstetrics course as an orientation tool for obstetrics and gynecology residents. Am J Obstet Gynecol. 2007;196(5):e27-8.

CHAPTER 46

21. Healy DL, Laufe LE. Survey of obstetric forceps training in North America in 1981. Am J Obstet Gynecol. 1985;151(1):54-8.

22. Cheng YW, Hopkins LM, Caughey AB. How long is too long: Does a prolonged second stage of labor in nulliparous women affect maternal and neonatal outcomes? Am J Obstet Gynecol. 2004;191(3):933-8.

23. Friedman EA. Patterns of labor as indicators of risk. Clin Obstet Gynecol. 1973;16(1):172-83.

24. Schifrin BS. Polemics in perinatology: disengaging forceps. J Perinatol. 1988;8(3):242-5.

25. Vacca A. Handbook of Vacuum Extraction in Obstetric Practice, 1st edition. London, UK: E. Arnold; 1992. p. 32.

26. Johanson R. Choice of instrument for vaginal delivery. Curr Opin Obstet Gynecol. 1997;9(6):361-5.

27. ACOG committee opinion. Delivery by vacuum extraction. Number 208, September 1998. Committee on Obstetric Practice. American College of Obstetricians and Gynecologists. Int J Gynaecol Obstet. 1999;64(1):96.

28. Williams MC. Vacuum-assisted delivery. Clin Perinatol. 1995;22(4):933-52.

29. Morales R, Adair CD, Sanchez-Ramos L, Gaudier FL. Vacuum extraction of preterm infants with birth weights of 1,500- 2,499 grams. J Reprod Med. 1995;40(2):127-30.

30. Bofill JA, Rust OA, Perry KG, Roberts WE, Martin RW, Morrison JC. Operative vaginal delivery: a survey of fellows of ACOG. Obstet Gynecol. 1996;88(6):1007-10.

31. Damos JR, Bassett R. Chapter H. Assisted vaginal delivery. In: Advanced Life Support in Obstetrics (ALSO) Provider Syllabus, 4th edition. Leawood, Kan: American Academy of Family Physicians; 2003. pp. 3-8.

32. Angioli R, Gómez-Marín O, Cantuaria G, O'sullivan MJ. Severe perineal lacerations during vaginal delivery: the University of Miami experience. Am J Obstet Gynecol. 2000;182(5):1083-5.

33. Youssef R, Ramalingam U, Macleod M, Murphy DJ. Cohort study of maternal and neonatal morbidity in relation to use of episiotomy at instrumental vaginal delivery. BJOG. 2005;112(7):941-5.

34. Hirsch E, Haney EI, Gordon TE, Silver RK. Reducing high-order perineal laceration during operative vaginal delivery. Am J Obstet Gynecol. 2008;198(6):668.e1-5.

35. Andrews V, Sultan AH, Thakar R, Jones PW. Occult anal sphincter injuries–myth or reality? BJOG. 2006;113(2):195-200.

36. Donnelly V, Fynes M, Campbell D, Johnson H, O'Connell PR, O'Herlihy C. Obstetric events leading to anal sphincter damage. Obstet Gynecol. 1998;92(6):955-61.

37. Demissie K, Rhoads GG, Smulian JC, Balasubramanian BA, Gandhi K, Joseph KS, et al. Operative vaginal delivery and neonatal and infant adverse outcomes: population based retrospective analysis. BMJ. 2004;329(7456):24-9.

38. Towner DR, Ciotti MC. Operative vaginal delivery: a cause of birth injury or is it? Clin Obstet Gynecol. 2007;50(3):563-81.

39. PlaucheÅL WC. Fetal cranial injuries related to delivery with the MalmstroÅNm vacuum extractor (review). Obstet Gynecol. 1979;53(6):750-7.

40. Aguero O, Alvarez H. Fetal injury due to the vacuum extractor. Obstet Gynecol. 1962;19:212-7.

41. Boo NY, Foong KW, Mahdy ZA, Yong SC, Jaafar R. Risk factors associated with subaponeurotic haemorrhage in full-term infants exposed to vacuum extraction. BJOG. 2005;112(11):1516-21.

42. Chadwick LM, Pemberton PJ, Kurinczuk JJ. Neonatal subgaleal haematoma: associated risk factors, complications and outcome. J Paediatr Child Health. 1996;32(3):228-32.

43. Hudelist G, Mastoroudes H, Gorti M. The role of episiotomy in instrumental delivery: is it preventative for severe perineal injury? J Obstet Gynaecol. 2008;28(5):469-73.

44. Damron DP, Capeless EL. Operative vaginal delivery: a comparison of forceps and vacuum for success rate and risk of rectal sphincter injury. Am J Obstet Gynecol. 2004;191(3):907-10.

45. Johanson RB, Menon BK. Vacuum extraction versus forceps for assisted vaginal delivery. Cochrane Database Syst Rev. 2000;(2):CD000224.

46. Caughey AB, Sandberg PL, Zlatnik MG, Thiet MP, Parer JT, Laros RK Jr. Forceps compared with vacuum: rates of neonatal and maternal morbidity. Obstet Gynecol. 2005;106(5 Pt 1):908-12.

47. Gardella C, Taylor M, Benedetti T, Hitti J, Critchlow C. The effect of sequential use of vacuum and forceps for assisted vaginal delivery on neonatal and maternal outcomes. Am J Obstet Gynecol. 2001;185(4):896-902.

48. Bhide A, Guven M, Prefumo F, Vankalayapati P, Thilaganathan B. Maternal and neonatal outcome after failed ventouse delivery: comparison of forceps versus cesarean section. J Matern Fetal Neonatal Med. 2007;20(7):541-5.

49. Wen SW, Liu S, Kramer MS, Marcoux S, Ohlsson A, Sauvé R, et al. Comparison of maternal and infant outcomes between vacuum extraction and forceps deliveries. Am J Epidemiol. 2001;153(2):103-7.

PART II

Shoulder Dystocia

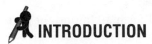 **INTRODUCTION**

Shoulder dystocia can be defined as the inability to deliver the foetal shoulders after the delivery of the foetal head without the aid of specific manoeuvres (other than the gentle downward traction on the head).[1] The chances for the occurrence of shoulder dystocia are high when the diameter of the foetal shoulders (bisacromial diameter) is relatively larger than the biparietal diameter of foetal head. Shoulder dystocia occurs as a result of disproportion between the bisacromial diameter of the foetus and the anteroposterior diameter of the pelvic inlet, which causes impaction of the anterior shoulder behind the symphysis pubis. Shoulder dystocia can occur during a normal vaginal delivery or an assisted instrumental (ventouse or forceps) delivery. Shoulder dystocia occurs in about 0.5% births and can be of two types: (1) high shoulder dystocia and (2) the low shoulder dystocia.[2] Low shoulder dystocia results due to the failure of engagement of the anterior shoulder and impaction of anterior shoulder over the maternal symphysis pubis. This type of the shoulder dystocia is also known as unilateral shoulder dystocia. This is the more common type and is easily dealt with using standard techniques. There can be a high perinatal mortality and morbidity associated with this complication and therefore it needs to be managed appropriately. Since it is difficult to predict shoulder dystocia or prevent its occurrence, all the obstetrician must be well-versed with its management. Shoulder dystocia is an important obstetric emergency, which must be managed within minutes in order to avoid any significant maternal and foetal complications.

Presently, there is no way for the obstetrician to determine with any degree of accuracy, which babies are likely to be macrosomic or to experience shoulder dystocia at the time of delivery. Since both the prediction and the prevention of shoulder dystocia are difficult, it is important for the obstetrician to be well versed with this technique for immediately managing this condition in case it occurs.

Following the delivery of foetal head, as the baby's anterior shoulder passes under the mother's pubic bone, an effort must be made to deflect the baby's head in the downwards direction and applying traction to release the anterior shoulder. An important thing for the healthcare attendants is not to apply undue traction over the foetal head at the time of delivery as it is likely to result in foetal injuries such as injury to the brachial plexus. Another important thing for the healthcare attendant to remember is not to panic when faced with such a situation. Most cases of shoulder dystocia can be resolved by practicing the above-described manoeuvres with a cool mind.

AETIOLOGY

Shoulder dystocia is a largely unpredictable and unpreventable event as a large majority of cases occur in the women with no risk factors. Moreover, ultrasound prediction of foetal weight may be grossly inaccurate. However, the clinicians must be aware of existing risk factors (Box 47.1) and remain alert regarding the possibility of shoulder dystocia with any delivery.[3-5] Maternal history of diabetes mellitus is considered as an important risk factor for the development

---

Box 47.1: Risk factors for shoulder dystocia[4,5]

❏ *Prelabour factors*
  – Previous history of shoulder dystocia
  – Macrosomia
  – Diabetes mellitus
  – Maternal BMI >30 kg/m²
  – Multiparity
❏ *Intrapartum factors*
  – Induction of labour
  – Prolonged first stage of labour
  – Secondary arrest
  – Oxytocin augmentation
  – Prolonged second stage of labour
  – Failure of descent of the head
  – Increased rate of assisted vaginal delivery

of shoulder dystocia.[6] The ACOG has recommended that an estimated foetal weight of over 4.5 kg should be considered as an indication for delivery by caesarean section in order to reduce the potential morbidity and mortality in pregnancies complicated with maternal diabetes mellitus.[7] Shoulder dystocia has been observed to recur in about 1–16% cases.

DIAGNOSIS

Diagnosis of shoulder dystocia is made on the basis of clinical presentation at the time of vaginal delivery.

Clinical Presentation

There are two main signs that indicate the presence of shoulder dystocia and must be routinely looked for by the birth attendants to make a timely diagnosis of shoulder dystocia:[8,9]

1. *Non-emergence of the baby's body:* The baby's body does not emerge out even after the application of routine traction, and maternal pushing following the delivery of baby's head. Routine traction is defined as 'the traction required for delivery of the shoulders in a normal vaginal delivery where there is no difficulty with the shoulders'. Routine traction in an axial direction can be used for establishing the diagnosis of shoulder dystocia. However, any other traction should be avoided. There is also difficulty with the delivery of foetal face and chin.

2. *The 'Turtle sign':* The foetal head suddenly retracts back against the mother's perineum after it emerges from the vaginal introitus. The baby's anterior shoulder is caught on the back of the maternal pubic bone, causing retraction of the foetal head and preventing delivery of the remainder of the baby. The baby's cheeks bulge out, resembling a turtle pulling its head back into its shell. There is failure of restitution of the foetal head and the descent of shoulders.

MANAGEMENT

Management of shoulder dystocia has been summarised in Flow chart 47.1.[4] While different birth attendants may follow different combination of manoeuvres, it is important for them to have a well thought-out, clear cut sequence of manoeuvres as recommended by some authentic source in his or her mind. Management of shoulder dystocia comprises of the following steps:

❖ Shoulder dystocia drill should form an important part of training for the junior doctor and the nurses. Drill is a practice run-through of the labour and delivery team for a simulated case of shoulder dystocia. The initial management in the cases of shoulder dystocia has also been summarised by the mnemonic HELPERR, which is described in Table 47.1.[9] The immediate steps which need to be taken in case of an anticipated or a recognised case of shoulder dystocia are described next.

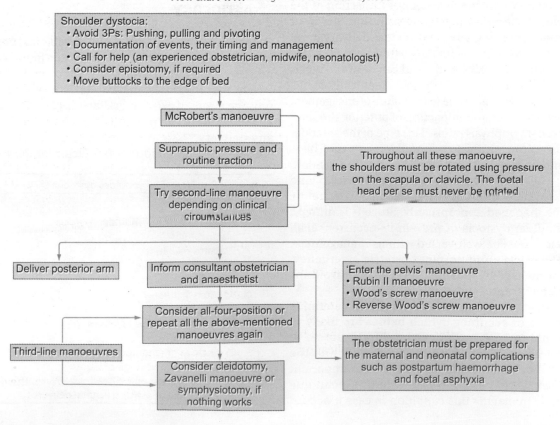

Flow chart 47.1: Management of shoulder dystocia

Shoulder dystocia:
- Avoid 3Ps: Pushing, pulling and pivoting
- Documentation of events, their timing and management
- Call for help (an experienced obstetrician, midwife, neonatologist)
- Consider episiotomy, if required
- Move buttocks to the edge of bed

↓

McRobert's manoeuvre

↓

Suprapubic pressure and routine traction

↓

Try second-line manoeuvre depending on clinical circumstances

→ Throughout all these manoeuvre, the shoulders must be rotated using pressure on the scapula or clavicle. The foetal head per se must never be rotated

Deliver posterior arm

Inform consultant obstetrician and anaesthetist

'Enter the pelvis' manoeuvre
- Rubin II manoeuvre
- Wood's screw manoeuvre
- Reverse Wood's screw manoeuvre

Third-line manoeuvres

Consider all-four-position or repeat all the above-mentioned manoeuvres again

↓

Consider cleidotomy, Zavanelli manoeuvre or symphysiotomy, if nothing works

The obstetrician must be prepared for the maternal and neonatal complications such as postpartum haemorrhage and foetal asphyxia

PART II

Table 47.1: Mnemonic for describing initial management in the cases of shoulder dystocia

H	Call for **h**elp
E	**E**valuate for episiotomy
L	**L**egs (the McRoberts' manoeuvre)
P	Suprapubic **p**ressure
E	**E**nter the pelvis manoeuvres (internal rotation), such as Rubin II manoeuvre, Wood's screw manoeuvre and reverse Wood's screw manoeuvre
R	**R**emove the posterior arm
R	**R**oll the patient

❖ After recognition of shoulder dystocia, extra help should be summoned immediately. This should include further midwifery assistance, an experienced obstetrician, a paediatric resuscitation team and an anaesthetist. One person should be assigned the task of recording the time since the time of onset of dystocia and saying it loud after every 30 seconds. The team arriving for help should be immediately notified about the diagnosis of shoulder dystocia.

❖ As soon as the shoulder dystocia has been identified, maternal pushing, and foetal pulling and pivoting should be discouraged, as this may lead to further impaction of the shoulders.

❖ The woman should be manoeuvred to bring her buttocks to the edge of the bed. She should be laid flat and if any pillows are present under her back, they should be removed. If the woman is in the lithotomy position, her legs must be removed from the supports. One assistant should be on the either side of the mother to provide support. The woman's legs should be hyperflexed following which routine traction in an axial direction should then be applied to the foetal head to evaluate if the shoulders have been released. The same degree of strength should be applied at the time of traction as applied during a normal delivery.

❖ Pushing by the mother should be discouraged, because this may worsen the impaction of shoulders.

❖ Fundal pressure should not be employed. It is associated with a high rate of neonatal complications and may sometimes even result in uterine rupture.

❖ Enlarging the episiotomy may facilitate the delivery of shoulders in some cases. However, the routine use of episiotomy is not necessary in all cases. The clinicians should apply their own discretion regarding whether an episiotomy needs to be given or not; or if already given, does it need to be enlarged or not.

❖ Management of shoulder dystocia needs to be done within 5–7 minutes of the delivery of the foetal head in order to prevent irreversible foetal injury due to foetal hypoxic acidosis.[10-12]

❖ Following the delivery of baby, the clinicians should be alert regarding the possibility of maternal complications such as postpartum haemorrhage, and third- and fourth-degree perineal tears. If the above-mentioned steps do not prove to be useful, the various manoeuvres described next can be undertaken.

❖ Of the various manoeuvres mentioned next, McRobert's manoeuvre is a simple, rapid, non-invasive and effective intervention, which is associated with a minimal rate of complications and should be performed first. Application of suprapubic pressure can be used to improve the efficacy of the McRobert's manoeuvre.

McRobert's Manoeuvre

McRobert's manoeuvre is the single most effective intervention, which is associated with success rate as high as 90% and should be the first manoeuvre to be performed.[13] Prophylactic McRobert's position may also be recommended in cases where shoulder dystocia is anticipated. The McRobert's manoeuvre (Figs 47.1A and B) involves sharp flexion and abduction of the maternal hips and positioning the maternal thighs on her abdomen. This manoeuvre helps in cephalad rotation of the symphysis pubis and the straightening of lumbosacral angle. This manoeuvre, by straightening the sacrum tends to free the impacted anterior shoulder.[14] It also helps in rotating the maternal pelvis towards the maternal head, thereby increasing the relative anterior-posterior diameter of the pelvis.

Suprapubic Pressure

Suprapubic pressure (also known as Rubin I manoeuvre) in conjunction with McRobert's manoeuvre is often all that is required to resolve 50–60% cases of shoulder dystocia. By application of suprapubic pressure, the obstetrician makes an attempt to manually dislodge the anterior shoulder from behind the pubic symphysis. In this manoeuvre, the attendant makes a fist and places it just above the maternal pubic bone and pushes in downwards and lateral direction to push the posterior aspect of the anterior shoulder towards the foetal chest for a period of at least 30 seconds (Fig. 47.2). Application of suprapubic pressure helps in reducing the foetal bisacromial diameter and rotating the anterior foetal shoulder into the wider oblique diameter of the pelvis. With the help of routine axial traction, the shoulder is then freed to slip underneath the symphysis pubis. Since shoulder dystocia is caused by an infant's shoulders entering the pelvis in a direct anterior-posterior orientation instead of the more physiologic oblique diameter, pushing the baby's anterior shoulder to one side or the other from above often helps in changing its position to the oblique, which would facilitate its delivery.

If these simple measures (the McRobert's manoeuvre and suprapubic pressure) fail then a choice needs to be made between the all-four-position and internal manipulation. Some of the manoeuvres for internal manipulation include Wood's screw manoeuvre, Rubin II manoeuvre and reverse Wood's screw manoeuvre. These manoeuvres are more commonly used in comparison to the all-four-position.

Enter the Pelvis Manoeuvres[15]

❖ *Rubin II manoeuvre*: In this manoeuvre, the obstetrician inserts the fingers of his or her right hand into the vagina and applies digital pressure onto the posterior aspect

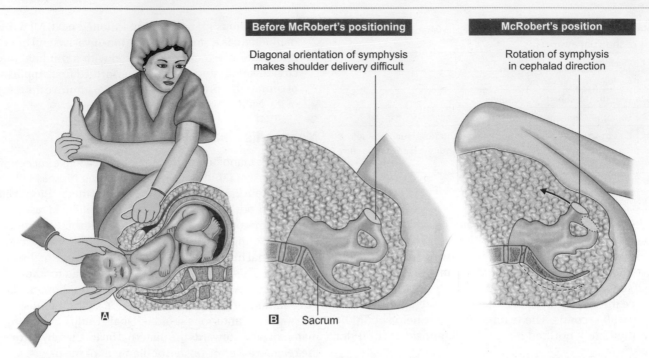

Figs 47.1A and B: (A) McRobert's manoeuvre (exaggerated hyperflexion of the thighs upon the maternal abdomen) and application of suprapubic pressure; (B) McRobert's manoeuvre causes the pubic symphysis to rotate in cephalad direction and straightening of lumbosacral angle

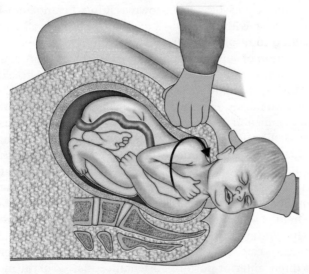

Fig. 47.2: Application of suprapubic pressure in the direction of foetal face

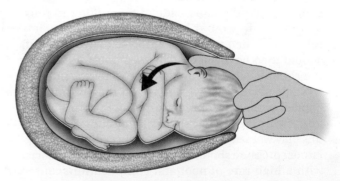

Fig. 47.3: Rubin II manoeuvre

of the anterior shoulder (or the most accessible foetal shoulder) making an attempt to push it towards the foetal chest (Fig. 47.3). This rotates the shoulders forward into the more favourable oblique diameter. The delivery is likely to be successful if attempted after the application of this manoeuvre.

❖ *Wood's screw manoeuvre*: In this manoeuvre, the obstetrician's hand is placed behind the posterior shoulder of the foetus (Fig. 47.4). The shoulder is rotated progressively by 180° in a corkscrew manner so that the impacted anterior shoulder is released. A variation of this is the Rubin II manoeuvre, which involves pushing on the posterior surface of the posterior shoulder. In addition to the corkscrew effect, pressure on the posterior shoulder has

the advantage of flexing the foetal shoulders across the chest. This decreases the distance between the shoulders, thereby reducing the dimension that must come out through the pelvis.

The force with which the infant's shoulder is compressed against the maternal pubic bone and the pressure applied by the clinician's hands on the foetus while performing various manoeuvres to facilitate delivery may often result in bruises over the baby's body.

❖ *Reverse Wood's screw manoeuvre*: In this manoeuvre, the obstetrician applies pressure to the posterior aspect of the posterior shoulder and attempts to rotate it through 180° in the direction opposite to that described in the Wood's screw manoeuvre (Fig. 47.5).

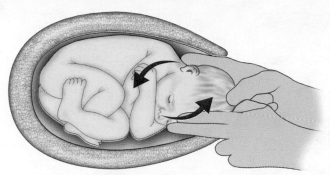

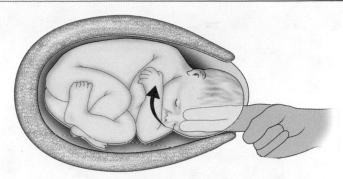

Fig. 47.4: Wood's screw manoeuvre: The hand is placed behind the posterior shoulder of the foetus. The shoulder is rotated progressively by 180° in a corkscrew manner so that the impacted anterior shoulder is released

Fig. 47.5: Reverse Wood's screw manoeuvre: The shoulder is rotated progressively by 180° in a direction opposite to that described in the Wood' screw manoeuvre

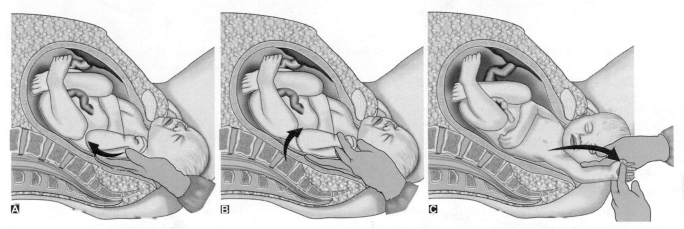

Figs 47.6A to C: Delivery of posterior arm. (A) The clinician's hand is introduced into the vagina along the posterior shoulder. Keeping the arm flexed at the elbow, it is swept across the foetal chest; (B) The foetal hand is grasped and the arm is extended out along the side of the face; (C) The posterior arm and shoulder are delivered from the vagina

CHAPTER 47

Delivery of the Posterior Arm

Another effective manoeuvre for resolving shoulder dystocia is the delivery of the posterior arm. In this manoeuvre, the obstetrician places his or her hand behind the posterior shoulder of the foetus and locates the arm. This arm is then swept across the foetal chest and delivered (Figs 47.6A to C). With the posterior arm and shoulder now delivered, it is relatively easy to rotate the baby, dislodge the anterior shoulder and allow delivery of the remainder of the baby.

All-Four Manoeuvre[16]

In this manoeuvre, the patient is instructed to roll over from her existing position and to take a knee chest position on all her four limbs. This allows rotational movement of the sacroiliac joints, resulting in a 1–2 cm increase in the sagittal diameter of the pelvic outlet. This disimpacts the shoulders, allowing them to slide over the sacral promontory.

Third-Line Manoeuvres

Several third-line methods have been described for cases, which are resistant to all simple measures. Some of these manoeuvres include cleidotomy, symphysiotomy and the Zavanelli manoeuvre. These manoeuvres are rarely employed in today's modern obstetric practice.

❖ Cleidotomy: This involves bending the clavicle with a finger or its surgical division.
❖ *Symphysiotomy*: This involves surgical division of the symphyseal ligament.[17]
❖ *Zavanelli manoeuvre*: The Zavanelli manoeuvre involves cephalic replacement of the head followed by caesarean section. In this manoeuvre, firstly, the foetal head is rotated back into its prerestitution position, i.e. occiput anterior (Fig. 47.7A). Following this, the head is flexed and pushed back up into the vagina (Fig. 47.7B). Once the foetal head gets back into the pelvis, an emergency caesarean section is performed to deliver a live baby.[18]

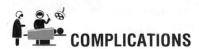

COMPLICATIONS

Foetal and Neonatal Complications

Following shoulder dystocia deliveries, 20% of babies may suffer some sort of injury, either temporary or permanent. The most common of these injuries are damage to the brachial

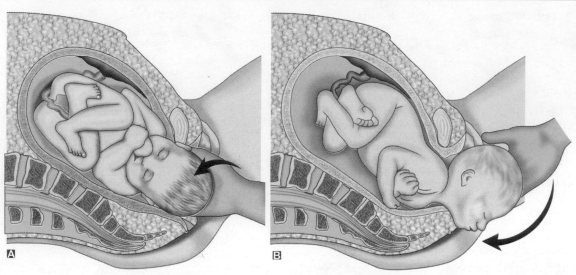

Figs 47.7A and B: Zavanelli manoeuvre: (A) The head is manually rotated to occipitoanterior position; (B) Flexion of the foetal head and returning it into the vagina while applying constant pressure. This is followed by an immediate caesarean section

plexus nerves, fracture of clavicles, fracture of humerus, contusions, lacerations and birth asphyxia.[19] Some of the foetal complications resulting due to shoulder dystocia are described next.

Brachial Plexus Injuries[20]

Brachial plexus injury (BPI) is one of the most important foetal complications of shoulder dystocia. Most cases of BPI resolve without leaving any permanent disability. However, permanent neurological dysfunction can develop in fewer than 10% cases. In the UK and Ireland, the incidence of BPI was 0.43 per 1,000 live births. Neonatal BPI is the most common cause for litigation related to shoulder dystocia and the third most litigated obstetric-related complication in the UK.

The brachial plexus consists of the nerve roots of spinal cord segments C5, C6, C7, C8 and T1. These nerve roots form three trunks, upper, middle and lower, which further divide into anterior and posterior divisions. The upper trunk is made up of nerves from C5 and C6, the middle trunk from undivided fibres of C7 and the lowermost trunk is made up of nerves from C8 to T1. Injury to the upper part of the brachial plexus is called Erb's palsy (C5 to C7) while injury to the lower nerves of the plexus is called Klumpke's palsy (C8 to T1). Both types of injuries can cause significant, lifelong disability. Erb's palsy affects the muscles of the upper arm and shoulders causing 'winging' of scapula.[21,22] Due to impaction of shoulder as a result of shoulder dystocia, application of upwards lateral traction on the foetal head results in the stretching of brachial plexus (Fig. 47.8). This type of injury also causes adduction and internal rotation of humerus with the forearm extended. This has also been described as the 'waiters tip' position. Klumpke's palsy involves lower trunk lesions from nerve roots C7, C8 and T1. In this injury, the elbow becomes flexed and the forearm supinated (opened up, palm upwards) with a characteristic claw-like deformity of the hand.

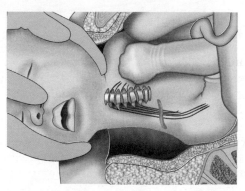

Fig. 47.8: Mechanism of injury to brachial plexus as a result of shoulder dystocia

Fractured Clavicle

The second most common type of injury suffered by infants following shoulder dystocia deliveries is fracture of clavicle, which has an incidence rate of nearly 10%.

Neurological Injury

If the head-shoulder delivery interval is greater than 7 minutes, chances of the brain injury are high as a result of neonatal asphyxia and acidosis.[23]

Maternal

Besides the foetal complications, shoulder dystocia can also cause some complications in the mother. The most common maternal complications include postpartum haemorrhage, third- and fourth-degree perineal tears, cervical lacerations and vaginal and vulvar lacerations.

CLINICAL PEARLS

❖ Throughout the various manoeuvres described previously, the shoulders must be rotated using pressure on the

PART II

scapula or clavicle. The foetal head per se must never be rotated.

❖ Mild cases of shoulder dystocia can be managed through the application of suprapubic pressure, and McRobert's manoeuvre. Moderate cases of shoulder dystocia require management with manoeuvres such as Wood's screw manoeuvre, Rubin II manoeuvre and delivery of the posterior arm. Zanvelli manoeuvre may be rarely required in undeliverable or severe cases of shoulder dystocia.

❖ Infants of diabetic mothers have a two- to four-fold increased risk of shoulder dystocia compared with infants of the same birthweight born to non-diabetic mothers.

❖ Decision regarding the mode of delivery (either caesarean section or vaginal delivery) in the women with previous history of shoulder dystocia should be made jointly by the woman and her carers following discussion regarding severity of any previous neonatal or maternal injury, predicted foetal size and maternal choice.

EVIDENCE-BASED MEDICINE

❖ The present evidence indicates that induction of labour does not prevent shoulder dystocia in non-diabetic women with a suspected macrosomic foetus.[3] Incidence of dystocia is, however, reduced in women with gestational diabetes where the labour is induced at term.

❖ As per the recommendations of the NICE guidelines for pregnant women with diabetes, elective birth through induction of labour, or by elective caesarean section (in presence of indications) after 38 completed weeks of gestation must be offered to pregnant women with diabetes who have a normally grown foetus.[3] On the other hand, elective caesarean delivery should be preferably considered in pregnant women with gestational or pre-existing diabetes having an estimated foetal weight of greater than 4.5 kg due to an increased risk of shoulder dystocia in such women. This is likely to reduce the potential neonatal morbidity especially that associated with BPI.

REFERENCES

1. Royal College of Obstetricians and Gynecologists (RCOG). (2012). Shoulder dystocia. [online] Available from www.rcog.org.uk/globalassets/documents/guidelines/gtg_42.pdf. [Accessed August, 2016].

2. Dystocia and abnormal labor. In: Cunnigham FG, Leveno KJ, Bloom SL, Hauth JC, Gilstrap LC, Wenstrom KD (Eds). William's Obstetrics, 23rd edition. US: McGraw Hill; 2010. pp. 513-7.

3. National Institute for Health and Clinical Excellence. Diabetes in Pregnancy: Management of Diabetes and Its Complications from Preconception to the Postnatal Period. London: RCOG Press; 2008.

4. Sokol RJ, Blackwell SC. American College of Obstetricians and Gynecologists. Committee on Practice Bulletins—Gynecology. ACOG practice bulletin no. 40: shoulder dystocia. Int J Gynaecol Obstet. 2003;80(1):87-92.

5. Acker DB, Sachs BP, Friedman EA. Risk factors for shoulder dystocia. Obstet Gynecol. 1985;66(6):762-8.

6. Geary M, McParland P, Johnson H, Stronge J. Shoulder dystocia—is it predictable? Eur J Obstet Gynecol Reprod Biol. 1995;62(1):15-8.

7. Gross SJ, Shime J, Farine D. Shoulder dystocia: predictors and outcome. A five-year review. Am J Obstet Gynecol. 1987;156(2):334-6.

8. Gurewitsch ED, Johnson TL, Allen RH. After shoulder dystocia: managing the subsequent pregnancy and delivery. Semin Perinatol. 2007;31(3):185-95.

9. Baxley EG, Gobbo RW. Shoulder dystocia. Am Fam Physician. 2004;69(7):1707-14.

10. Wood C, Ng KH, Hounslow D, Benning H. The influence of differences of birth times upon foetal condition in normal deliveries. J Obstet Gynaecol Br Commonw. 1973;80(4):289-94.

11. Wood C, Ng KH, Hounslow D, Benning H. Time—an important variable in normal delivery. J Obstet Gynaecol Br Commonw. 1973;80(4):295-300.

12. Beer E, Folghera MG. Time for resolving shoulder dystocia. Am J Obstet Gynecol. 1998;179(5):1376-7.

13. Gherman RB, Goodwin TM, Souter I, Neumann K, Ouzounian JG, Paul RH. The McRobert's maneuver for the alleviation of shoulder dystocia: how successful is it? Am J Obstet Gynecol. 1997;176(3):656-61.

14. Gherman RB, Tramont J, Muffley P, Goodwin TM. Analysis of McRobert's maneuver by x-ray pelvimetry. Obstet Gynecol. 2000;95(1):43-7.

15. Gherman RB, Ouzounian JG, Goodwin TM. Obstetric maneuvers for shoulder dystocia and associated foetal morbidity. Am J Obstet Gynecol. 1998;178(6):1126-30.

16. Bruner JP, Drummond SB, Meenan AL, Gaskin IM. All-four maneuver for reducing shoulder dystocia during labor. J Reprod Med. 1998;43(5):439-43.

17. Crichton D, Seedat EK. The technique of symphysiotomy. S Afr Med J. 1963;37:227-31.

18. Sandberg EC. The Zavanelli maneuver: 12 years of recorded experience. Obstet Gynecol. 1999;93(2):312-7.

19. Baskett TF, Allen AC. Perinatal implications of shoulder dystocia. Obstet Gynecol. 1995;86(1):14-7.

20. Hankins GD, Clark SL. Brachial plexus palsy involving the posterior shoulder at spontaneous vaginal delivery. Am J Perinatol. 1995;12(1):44-5.

21. Gherman RB, Ouzounian JG, Miller DA, Kwok L, Goodwin TM. Spontaneous vaginal delivery: a risk factor for Erb's palsy? Am J Obstet Gynecol. 1998;178(3):423-7.

22. Sandmire HF, DeMott RK. Erb's palsy: concepts of causation. Obstet Gynecol. 2000;95(6 Pt 1):941-2.

23. Stallings SP, Edwards RK, Johnson JW. Correlation of head-to-body delivery intervals in shoulder dystocia and umbilical artery acidosis. Am J Obstet Gynecol. 2001;185(2):268-74.

CHAPTER **48**

Perineal Injuries

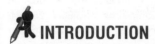 INTRODUCTION

Perineal injury can be defined as the injury which occurs to the perineum during the process of childbirth. Perineal and vaginal tears can commonly occur at the time of vaginal deliveries. The perineal injury can be classified into the following degrees as described in Box 48.1 and Figures 48.1A to D.[1-3]

There is occurrence of the injuries to the perineum at the time of vaginal delivery, especially in cases of instrumental delivery and/or the use of midline episiotomy. The third- and fourth-degree tears occur at the rate ranging from 0% to 8% in the UK, with the incidence in the primipara being about 6.1% and that in multipara about 1.7%.[4] Repair of the perineal injuries, especially those related to the injuries to the anal sphincter can help in considerably reducing morbidity related to the development of faecal incontinence or haemorrhage. Employing proper technique for surgical repair is also important. The aims of surgery in these cases are to help in the restoration of pelvic and perineal anatomy as far as possible and prevention of immediate as well as long-term morbidity.

Box 48.1: Sultan's classification of perineal injuries[2,3]

- ❑ *First degree*: Injury to the perineal skin and/or vaginal mucosa not involving the perineal muscles
- ❑ *Second degree*: Injury to the perineum involving the perineal muscles, but not the anal sphincters
- ❑ *Third degree*: Injury to the perineum involving the anal sphincter complex (external and internal anal sphincters):
  - *3a*: Less than 50% of external anal sphincter is torn
  - *3b*: More than 50% of external anal sphincter is torn
  - *3c*: Internal anal sphincter also gets involved
- ❑ *Fourth degree*: Injury to the perineum involving the anal sphincter complex (external and internal anal sphincters) and rectal mucosa

---

AETIOLOGY

Anatomical Considerations

Perineum is a diamond-shaped aperture corresponding to the pelvic outlet. It is bounded on the anterior side by pubic symphysis, coccyx on the posterior side and ischial tuberosities on the lateral sides. It is divided into a urogenital triangle anteriorly and an anal triangle posteriorly. The pelvic diaphragm is a muscular partition, which separates the pelvic cavity above from the perineal region below. It mainly comprises the muscles, levator ani and coccygei, along with the associated fascia on their upper and lower aspects.[5,6] Together these muscles provide resistance to the continuous downward force of intra-abdominal pressure. Acting together with the muscles of the abdomen, these muscles deflect the direction of this pressure away from the genital hiatus, through which the pelvic organs may otherwise descent, resulting in prolapse. These muscles are closely associated with pelvic viscera and are most likely to be damaged during the process of childbirth and delivery. Levator ani muscle, one each situated on the either side of the pelvis, supports the viscera in pelvic cavity, and surrounds the various structures (cervix, vaginal canal, anal canal and neck of urethra), which pass through the genital hiatus. The levator ani is the main muscle of the pelvic floor that is composed of three parts: (1) pubococcygeus, (2) ischiococcygeus and (3) iliococcygeus. The pubo-coccygeus, the main part of the levator, takes its origin from the posterior surface of pubis and anterior half of fascial line over obturator internus and it runs backward from the body of the pubis towards the coccyx to get inserted into the anococcygeal body. It may be damaged during parturition. Damage to all the nerves supplying levator ani, either due to delivery or other reasons, is likely to affect the function of pelvic floor. Injury and/or the weakening of the muscles of pelvic floor may result in urinary incontinence, faecal incontinence and vaginal prolapse.

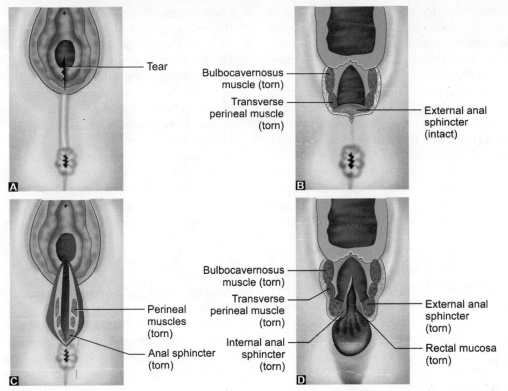

Figs 48.1A to D: (A) First-degree perineal tear involving only the vaginal mucosa and not the perineal muscles; (B) Second-degree perineal tear involving the perineal muscles as well; (C) Third-degree perineal tear involving the anal sphincter complex; (D) Fourth-degree perineal tear involving the rectal mucosa as well

The central tendon of perineum or the perineal body plays an important role in anchoring the musculofascial support of the pelvic floor.

Central tendon of the perineum is formed by the convergence of tendinous attachments of the following: bulbocavernosus, external anal sphincter and, levator ani muscles, deep and the superficial transverse perineal muscles of both the sides. Tearing or stretching of the central tendon during delivery is likely to cause damage to the support of posterior vaginal wall, resulting in anal incontinence or anal prolapse.

Both internal and external anal sphincters help in maintaining anal continence. External anal sphincter has three parts that have no distinct separation from each other. These parts are:
1. *Subcutaneous part* having no bony attachment
2. *Superficial oval part*: Fibres arise from the coccyx and anococcygeal ligament and pass anteriorly around the anus to get inserted into the perineal body.
3. *Deep part*: The muscle fibres arise from the perineal body and after encircling the lower half of anal canal, they get fused with the puborectalis.

Internal anal sphincter, which is involuntary, is formed by the smooth muscles of the rectum. It is innervated by the sympathetic fibres from the presacral ganglia (L5) and parasympathetic fibres from sacral segments (S2 to S4).

At the time of vaginal delivery, the vaginal introitus either stretches beyond its elastic capacity or expands too quickly. The tissues thus tend to tear resulting in perineal trauma. Anal incontinence, on the other hand, can occur due to the disruption of sphincter muscles, traction neuropathy of the pudendal nerve or a combination of both.

Risk Factors

Various obstetric risk factors responsible for the occurrence of vaginal tears are enlisted in Box 48.2 and are described below:[7-12]
- *Vaginal delivery*: Vaginal deliveries, specifically instrumental vaginal deliveries (irrespective of the fact whether an episiotomy was given or not) may be associated with the occurrence of vaginal tears.
- *Epidural analgesia*: Due to prolongation of the second stage of labour, there is an increased requirement for episiotomy and instrumental delivery in women who have received epidural analgesia. This may result in an increased risk of perineal trauma.
- *Parity*: Primiparas are more at risk of perineal trauma in comparison to multigravidas.

Box 48.2: Risk factors for occurrence of perineal injury[13,14]

- ❑ Asian ethnicity
- ❑ Nulliparity
- ❑ Birthweight >4 kg
- ❑ Shoulder dystocia
- ❑ Occipitoposterior position
- ❑ Prolonged second stage of labour
- ❑ Instrumental delivery

CHAPTER 48

❖ *Episiotomy*: Initially, episiotomies were introduced to prevent damage to the pelvic floor. However, evidence till date shows that a midline episiotomy is likely to place the sphincter at an increased risk for injury. Presently, there is no scientific justification for the use of episiotomy. An appropriately placed mediolateral episiotomy may, however, cause fewer tears. Its use is recommended by the RCOG in situations where deems necessary, ensuring that it is directed approximately 45–60° away from the midline when the perineum is distended. An episiotomy performed at an angle of 60° from the centre of the introitus at the time of crowning of foetal head, is likely to result in a postdelivery angle of 45°.[15] It is also preferable to consider mediolateral episiotomy at the time of instrumental deliveries.

❖ *Other intrapartum risk factors*: They include macrosomia (weight >4 kg), shoulder dystocia, occipitoposterior positions, history of third-degree tears in previous deliveries and prolonged second stage of labour.

MANAGEMENT

Repair of Perineal Tears

The repair of perineal tears is essentially done in the manner similar to that of an episiotomy and is discussed next.

Preoperative Preparation

❖ Repair of third- or fourth-degree perineal tears should be performed by appropriately trained practitioners, who have received formal training in techniques for repairing anal sphincter injury at the time of their obstetric training. Before undertaking the repair of perineal tears, the healthcare professionals should explain to the woman what they plan to do and how they would go about the procedure.

❖ Before proceeding with the repair, thorough exploration of the vulva, vagina and perineal area following delivery of the baby and the placenta is required. Amount of trauma and injury over the vaginal mucosa, vulva, cervix and perineal areas must be carefully assessed. Per speculum examination helps in the visualisation of cervix and lower genital tract to exclude lacerations. Any injury, if found, must adequately be sutured and repaired. Before performing the repair, the perineum along with the site of incision must be well swabbed with an antiseptic solution.

❖ Endoanal ultrasound using high frequency (10 MHz) can be considered as the best imaging modality for the diagnosis of perineal trauma.[16]

❖ In case of deep tears, involvement of anal sphincters must also be assessed by placing a gloved finger in the anus and gently lifting it. The tightness or tone of the sphincter must also be assessed. If there is no tear in the sphincters, one must proceed with the suturing of vaginal tears. Small first-degree tears that are not actively bleeding may be left without being sutured.

❖ Under all aseptic precautions after cleaning and draping the perineum, the proposed site of repair is infiltrated with 10 mL of 1% lignocaine. Anaesthesia in the form of nerve blocks or local injections of anaesthetic drug is given if the patient has not received regional anaesthesia (e.g. epidural anaesthesia) for the delivery. If proper visualisation of lower genital tract does not appear to be possible, it may be necessary to take the woman to theatre for examination under anaesthesia.

❖ While performing the repair of the vaginal or cervical tears, the patient must be placed in lithotomy position, with a good source of light from behind.

❖ The obstetrician must ensure that adequate assistance and instruments are also available in order to provide adequate exposure of the genital tract.

Surgical Steps

Repair of vaginal tears: The steps for repair of vaginal tears are as follows:

❖ Any tear in the vaginal mucosa is sutured with 2-0 Vicryl Rapide™ or chromic catgut sutures with the help of continuous stitches. The first stitch must be taken 1 cm above the apex of tear in the vaginal mucosal tissue. This stitch is particularly important because if apex is not securely closed it can be associated with continuing bleeding or a vulvar haematoma.

❖ Perineal muscles are approximated with 2-0 chromic catgut sutures with the help of interrupted stitches.

❖ Skin is closed with the help of interrupted mattress sutures using silk or subcuticular stitches.

❖ At the end of vaginal tear repair, a per rectal examination may be performed to ensure that no stitches have been taken through the rectal mucosa.

Repair of a fourth-degree laceration: The steps for repair of a fourth-degree laceration are as follows:

❖ In case of injury to the anal sphincters and rectal mucosa, the area is well irrigated with saline and antiseptic solution. The most experienced obstetrician available must be called.

❖ In case of fourth-degree laceration, it is important to approximate the torn edges of the anorectal mucosa with fine absorbable sutures.

❖ Approximation of the anorectal mucosa and submucosa is done using 3-0 polyglactin sutures in a running or an interrupted manner (Fig. 48.2A). Sutures are preferably placed in the muscularis avoiding the mucosa. 3-0 polyglactin sutures are preferred over polydioxanone sutures (PDS) because they are likely to cause less irritation and discomfort in comparison to the PDS sutures.

❖ The superior extent of the anterior anal laceration is identified and sutures are placed through the submucosa of the anorectum starting above the apex of the tear and extending down until the anal verge.

❖ A second layer of sutures is placed through rectal muscularis using 3-0 polyglactin sutures in a running or interrupted fashion (Fig. 48.2B). This layer of sutures acts as a reinforcing layer and incorporates the anal sphincter at the distal end.

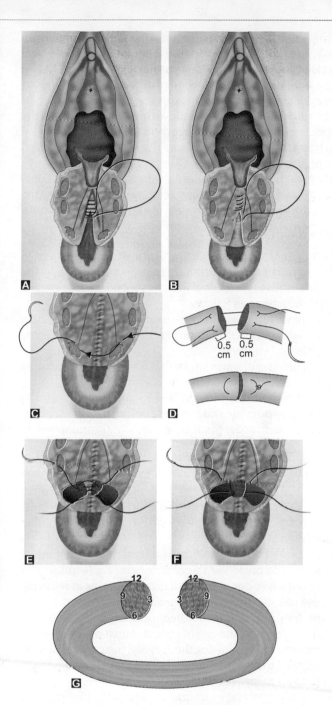

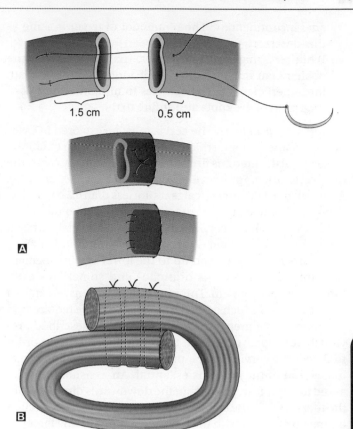

Figs 48.3A and B: (A) Overlap method of suturing the anal sphincters; (B) Appearance of the anal sphincter following repair through overlap method

Figs 48.2A to G: Repair of a fourth-degree laceration: (A) Approximation of anorectal mucosa and submucosa using continuous sutures; (B) Second layer of sutures placed through the rectal muscularis; (C) End-to-end approximation of the external anal sphincter. Sutures being placed through the posterior wall of external anal sphincters (these would be tied in the end); (D) Close-up view of the external anal sphincters showing end-to-end approximation; (E) End-to-end sutures taken through the interior of external anal sphincter (shown in deep purple); (F) Approximation of the anterior wall of external anal sphincter; (G) Appearance of the anal sphincter following repair through end-to-end method

❖ Finally, the torn edges of the anal sphincter are isolated, approximated and sutured together with three or four interrupted stitches using either monofilament sutures such as 3-0 PDS or modern braided sutures such as 2-0 polyglactin. The anal sphincters need to be repaired in case of fourth-degree tears as well as some third-degree tears. The internal anal sphincter is identified as the thickening of the circular smooth muscle layer at the distal 2–3 cm of the anal canal. It appears as the glistening white fibrous structure lying between the anal canal submucosa and the fibres of external anal sphincter. In case the internal anal sphincters have retracted laterally, they need to be sought and brought together after holding them with Allis forceps.

❖ Following the repair of internal anal sphincters, the torn edges of external anal sphincters are identified and grasped with Allis clamp. The repair of these sphincters can be performed either using end-to-end repair (Figs 48.2C to G) or the overlap method (Figs 48.3A and B).[17,18] For end-to-end approximation of the external anal sphincters,[17-19] simple interrupted sutures using 3-0 PDS or 2-0 polyglactin are placed through the edges of external anal sphincter and its connective tissue capsule at 3, 6, 9 and 12 O'clock positions. The sutures are first placed through the inferior and posterior portions of the sphincter; these stitches are tied last in order to facilitate the repair.

❖ The overlap method involves taking two sets of sutures: the first row of sutures is taken 1.5 cm from the edge on one side and 0.5 cm on the other side in such a way that when the sutures are tied, the free ends overlap one another. The free end is then sutured to the rest of the sphincter. The overlap method was considered superior to the end-to-end method as it was thought to be associated with fewer postoperative complications such as faecal urgency and

CHAPTER 48

anal incontinence.[20] The remainder of repair is same as that described for an episiotomy.

❖ While repairing the internal or external anal sphincter, the obstetrician must try burying of surgical knots beneath the superficial perineal muscles to minimise the risk of migration of the knots and suture to the skin.

Repair of cervical tears: The cervix must be explored in cases of unexplained haemorrhage after the third stage of labour, especially if the uterus is firmly contracted. In many cases, the deep cervical tears present as the likely cause for haemorrhage. Although most of the cervical tears are less than 0.5 cm in size, deep cervical tears may at times even extend into the upper third of vagina. If the cervix is partially or completely avulsed from the vagina, the condition is known as colporrhexis. Rarely, such tears may also extend up to the lower uterine segment and uterine artery or its branches and sometimes even through the peritoneum. This may result in extensive external haemorrhage. In such cases, laparotomy may be required.

Preoperative preparation is same as that described previously for repair of vaginal tears and laceration. In order to detect the cervical tears, proper visualisation and visual inspection of the cervix is essential. An assistant must be asked to apply firm pressure in the downwards direction over the uterus, while the surgeon must exert downwards traction on the lip of cervix with the help of sponge-holding forceps.

The procedure of repair comprises the following steps (Fig. 48.4):

❖ Direct visualisation and inspection of the cervix is done using three sponge-holding forceps. The anterior lip of cervix is grasped with one forceps at 12 O'clock position, the second forceps is placed at 2 O'clock position and the third one is placed at 4 O'clock position. The position of these three forceps is progressively changed, i.e. the first forceps is placed at 2 O'clock position, second one is placed at 4 O'clock position and third one at 6 O'clock position.

❖ The changes in the position of forceps are done until the entire cervical circumference has been inspected.

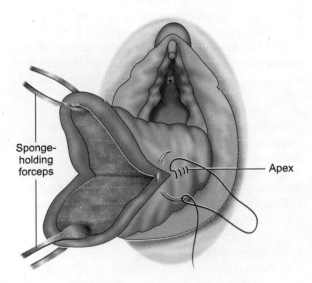

Fig. 48.4: Repair of a cervical tear

Small, non-bleeding lacerations of the cervix can be left unsutured. Lesions larger than 2 cm in size or those with a bleeding vessel need to be sutured.

❖ The lacerations can be stitched with the help of continuous interlocking chromic catgut sutures.

❖ The stitch must begin 1 cm above the apex of the tear. If the apex cannot be visualised, gentle traction must be applied to bring the apex into the view. The stitch must be placed as high as possible.

❖ After stitching the laceration, the healthcare professional must look for any continuing bleeding. Pressure or packing over the area of repair may help in achieving haemostasis.

Postoperative Care

❖ *Care of anal sphincter injuries*: The postoperative steps in case of repair of anal sphincter injuries are essentially the same as those for repair of first- or second-degree vaginal tears, which are as follows:

• Application of an ice pack over the stitches may help in reducing inflammation in the area, thereby reducing pain and swelling.

• Regular use of warm sitz bath is also helpful in reducing pain and inflammation over the site of incision.

• The patient must be advised to ambulate around as much as possible and regularly perform the pelvic floor exercises in order to stimulate circulation and speed up the process of healing.

• Use of painkillers, such as paracetamol, may help in providing pain relief.

❖ Due to the involvement of anal sphincters and rectal mucosa in cases of third- and fourth-degree perineal injuries, additional steps may be required, which are described as follows:

• In case of third- and fourth-degree tears, the patient should be prescribed stool softeners (e.g. lactulose) for about a week or two. Use of laxatives helps in reducing the risk of wound dehiscence. Bulking agents should preferably not be prescribed routinely with laxatives.[21] In these cases, the use of enemas must be avoided.

• Immediately following the surgery, the patient must be advised to take liquid diet for a day and then gradually convert to low-residue diet over a few days.

• Vaginal or rectal examination and sexual intercourse must be avoided for at least 2 weeks following the repair.

• Broad-spectrum antibiotics must be prescribed following the repair of anal sphincters in order to reduce the risk of postoperative infections and wound dehiscence.[22]

• Women should be advised that physiotherapy following repair of anal sphincters could prove to be beneficial.

❖ Daily follow-up is required to look for any evidence of wound infection. The patient should be called at around 6–12 weeks postpartum for review. Women should be advised that approximately 60–80% of women who underwent repair of anal sphincters are likely to become asymptomatic 12 months following delivery. If the woman complains of incontinence or pain during this follow-up visit, she must be preferably referred to a specialist gynaecologist or a colorectal surgeon.

❖ *Future deliveries*: All women who sustained injury to the anal sphincters in the previous pregnancy should be counselled regarding the mode of delivery during her future pregnancy and this should be clearly documented in her notes.

All women who had sustained injury to the anal sphincters in their previous pregnancies and are symptomatic or have abnormal endoanal ultrasonography and/or manometry should be counselled regarding the option of elective caesarean birth during their future pregnancies.

COMPLICATIONS

Perineal injury can be associated with extensions or tears into the muscle of the rectum or even the rectum itself. Some of the complications, which are likely to occur as a result of perineal injuries, are as follows:

❖ *Bleeding*: There may be continuing bleeding which may or may not be accompanied by a haematoma formation. In case a haematoma is observed, the repair has to be opened and haematoma drained.
❖ Wound breakdown
❖ Infection
❖ *Perineal pain*: While a slight amount of pain which gets relieved on taking painkillers is a common occurrence with an episiotomy, persistent severe pain at the episiotomy site could be an indicator of presence of a large vulvar, paravaginal or ischiorectal haematoma, thereby necessitating a thorough exploration in these cases. There may be an accompanying superficial dyspareunia.
❖ Extension of the episiotomy into third- and fourth-degree vaginal lacerations
❖ Longer healing times
❖ Increased discomfort when intercourse is resumed
❖ Swelling
❖ *Persistence of incontinence*: Continuing faecal incontinence for 6 or more months calls for a repeat surgery. In order to restore sphincteric function and muscle bulk, augmented biofeedback physiotherapy can be done.
❖ *Abnormal signs of tissue healing*: Abnormal signs of tissue healing in the form of perineal granulation tissue, skin bridges, atrophy, localised scarring, etc. may be visible. In these cases, localised injection of corticosteroids or hyaluronidase may prove to be helpful.

CLINICAL PEARLS

❖ The integrity of internal anal sphincter is likely to play a role in the maintenance of continence. Injury to internal anal sphincter may result in incontinence, which can be defined as the involuntary passes of flatus or faeces affecting the quality of life.
❖ Perineal support or protection at the time of crowning can be protective against obstetric anal sphincter injuries. The

risk of such injuries can also be reduced by the application of warm compression during the second stage of labour.[23]

❖ In case of lacerations or tears involving the anal sphincter complex, special attention must be paid towards the maintenance of anatomical integrity.
❖ Application of figure-of-eight sutures should be avoided during the repair because they are haemostatic in nature and may cause ischaemic injury.

EVIDENCE-BASED MEDICINE

❖ The present evidence related to the protective effect of episiotomy in preventing obstetric anal sphincter injuries has presented with conflicting results. While the NHS Hospital Episode Statistics data (April 2000 to March 2012) has shown that episiotomy is associated with the lowest risk of third- and fourth-degree perineal tears, some other studies have also shown a protective effect while others have not.[13,24-27]
❖ Rectal buttonhole tears can be defined as tears involving the rectal mucosa while the anal sphincter complex remains intact. This type of injury cannot be classified as a fourth-degree tear. This type of injury is documented as a rectal buttonhole tear in the patient's notes and if not recognised and repaired on time, there is evidence to suggest that this type of tear may lead to the development of a rectovaginal fistula.[28]
❖ Presently, there is uncertain evidence regarding the use of best suture material for repairing the injury to anal sphincters.[29]

REFERENCES

1. Rock JA, Jones HW. Te Linde's Operative Gynecology, 10th edition. Philadelphia: Lippincott Williams & Wilkins; 2011.
2. Andrews V, Shelmeridine S, Sultan AH, Thakar R. Anal and urinary incontinence 4 years after a vaginal delivery. Int Urogynecol J. 2013;24(1):55-60.
3. Sultan AH. Obstetric perineal injury and anal incontinence. Clin Risk. 1999;5:193-6.
4. Thiagamoorthy G, Johnson A, Thakar R, Sultan AH. National survey of perineal trauma and its subsequent management in the United Kingdom. Int Urogynecol J. 2014;25(12):1621-7.
5. Snell RS. Clinical Anatomy by Regions, 8th edition. Philadelphia: Lippincott Williams & Wilkins; 2008.
6. Wester C, Brubaker L. Normal pelvic floor physiology. Obstet Gynecol Clin North Am. 1998;25(4):707-22.
7. Snooks SJ, Swash M, Henry MM, Setchell M. Risk factors in childbirth causing damage to the pelvic floor innervation. Int J Colorectal Dis. 1986;1(1):20-4.
8. Andrews V, Sultan AH, Thakar R, Jones PW. Risk factors for obstetric anal sphincter injury: a prospective study. Birth. 2006;33(2):117-22.
9. Faltin DL, Sangalli MR, Roche B, Floris L, Boulvain M, Weil A. Does a second delivery increase the risk of anal incontinence? BJOG. 2001;108(7):684-8.
10. Jones KD. Incidence and risk factors for third degree perineal tears. Int J Gynaecol Obstet. 2000;71(3):227-9.

11. O'Herlihy C. Obstetric perineal injury: risk factors and strategies for prevention. Semin Perinatol. 2003;27(1):13-9.

12. Rizk DE, Thomas L. Relationship between the length of the perineum and position of the anus and vaginal delivery in primigravidae. Int Urogynecol J Pelvic Floor Dysfunct. 2000;11(2):79-83.

13. Gurol-Urganci I, Cromwell DA, Edozien LC, Mahmood TA, Adams EJ, Richmond DH, et al. Third- and fourth-degree perineal tears among primiparous women in England between 2000 and 2012: time trends and risk factors. BJOG. 2013;120(12):1516-25.

14. McLeod NL, Gilmour DT, Joseph KS, Farrell SA, Luther ER. Trends in major risk factors for anal sphincter lacerations: a 10-year study. J Obstet Gynaecol Can. 2003;25(7):586-93.

15. Kalis V, Landsmanova J, Bednarova B, Karbanova J, Laine K, Rokyta Z. Evaluation of the incision angle of medio-lateral episiotomy at 60 degrees. Int J Gynaecol Obstet. 2011;112(3):220-4.

16. Cornelia L, Stephan B, Michel B, Antoine W, Felix K. Trans-perineal versus endo-anal ultrasound in the detection of anal sphincter tears. Eur J Obstet Gynecol Reprod Biol. 2002;103(1):79-82.

17. Royal College of Obstetricians and Gynaecologists (RCOG). (2015). The Management of Third- and Fourth-Degree Perineal Tears. Green-top Guideline No. 29. [online] Available from www.rcog.org.uk/globalassets/documents/guidelines/gtg-29.pdf. [Accessed June, 2016].

18. Fernando RJ, Sultan AH, Kettle C, Radley S, Jones P, O'Brien PM. Repair techniques for obstetric anal sphincter injuries: a randomized controlled trial. Obstet Gynecol. 2006;107(6):1261-8.

19. Sze EH, Ciarleglio M, Hobbs G. Risk factors associated with anal sphincter tear difference among midwife, private obstetrician, and resident deliveries. Int Urogynecol J Pelvic Floor Dysfunct. 2008;19(8):1141-4.

20. Thakar R, Fenner DE. Perineal and anal sphincter trauma. In: Sultan AH, Thakar R, Fenner DE (Eds). Anatomy of the Perineum and the Anal Sphincter. London: Springer; 2007. pp. 1-12.

21. Eogan M, Daly L, Behan M, O'Connell PR, O'Herlihy C. Randomised clinical trial of a laxative alone versus a laxative and a bulking agent after primary repair of obstetric anal sphincter injury. BJOG. 2007;114(6):736-40.

22. Buppasiri P, Lumbiganon P, Thinkhamrop J, Thinkhamrop B. Antibiotic prophylaxis for third- and fourth-degree perineal tear during vaginal birth. Cochrane Database Syst Rev. 2010;(11):CD005125.

23. Aasheim V, Nilsen AB, Lukasse M, Reinar LM. Perineal techniques during the second stage of labour for reducing perineal trauma. Cochrane Database Syst Rev. 2011;(12) CD006672.

24. De Leeuw JW, Vierhout ME, Struijk PC, Hop WC, Wallenburg HC. Anal sphincter damage after vaginal delivery: functional outcome and risk factors for fecal incontinence. Acta Obstet Gynecol Scand. 2001;80(9):830-4.

25. Fritel X, Schaal JP, Fauconnier A, Bertrand V, Levet C, Pigné A. Pelvic floor disorders 4 years after first delivery: a comparative study of restrictive versus systematic episiotomy. BJOG. 2008;115(2):247-52.

26. de Vogel J, van der Leeuw-van Beek A, Gietelink D, Vujkovic M, de Leeuw JW, van Bavel J, et al. The effect of a mediolateral episiotomy during operative vaginal delivery on the risk of developing obstetrical anal sphincter injuries. Am J Obstet Gynecol. 2012;206(5):404.e1-5.

27. Räisänen S, Vehviläinen-Julkunen K, Heinonen S. Need for and consequences of episiotomy in vaginal birth: a critical approach. Midwifery. 2010;26(3):348-56.

28. Sultan AH, Kettle C. Diagnosis of perineal trauma. In: Sultan AH, Thakar R, Fenner DE (Eds). Perineal and Anal Sphincter Trauma: Diagnosis and Clinical Management, 1st edition. London: Springer; 2007. pp. 13-9.

29. Williams A, Adams EJ, Tincello DG, Alfirevic Z, Walkinshaw SA, Richmond DH. How to repair an anal sphincter injury after vaginal delivery: results of a randomised controlled trial. BJOG. 2006;113(2):201-7.

Antepartum and Intrapartum Foetal Asphyxia

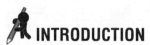

INTRODUCTION

Foetal hypoxia is associated with a prolonged drop in oxygen level (hypoxaemia) and an increase in carbon dioxide level (hypercapnia) in the foetal blood. Foetal asphyxia or intrauterine asphyxia is a common cause of long-term neurologic dysfunction and can cause damage to the brain, CNS and other organs, and sometimes can even result in death. Combinations of patient education, clinical examination, sonographic assessment, Doppler ultrasound and electronic foetal monitoring (EFM) are used for diagnosis of foetal hypoxia in the antepartum period. Various tests for antepartum foetal assessment late in pregnancy include daily foetal movement count (DFMC), NST, contraction stress test (CST), BPP, modified BPP, etc. With technological advancements, the foetal surveillance can also extend into the intrapartum period. Internal cardiotocographic monitoring and foetal scalp blood sampling are the most commonly used diagnostic tests for foetal well-being during labour. A significant rise in the rates of caesarean section over the past few years has been largely attributed to increasing use of EFM for ensuring foetal well-being at the time of labour. In view of the ongoing debate regarding the use of EFM, the obstetrician must also use other methods of intrapartum monitoring such as foetal scalp sampling for appropriate evaluation of the cases of intrapartum asphyxia and hypoxia.

AETIOLOGY

Foetal hypoxia can be described as reduced oxygen supply to the foetus. This is usually associated with a prolonged drop in oxygen level (hypoxaemia) and an increase in carbon dioxide level (hypercapnia) in the foetal blood. Various causes of foetal hypoxia are listed in Box 49.1. Foetal hypoxia is the result of impairment in the placental gas exchange that results in significant changes in the foetal pH. Prolonged foetal hypoxia creates a hostile environment in various vital organs. When

---

Box 49.1: Causes of foetal hypoxia

❑ Uterine hyperstimulation
❑ Maternal disease (placental disease, placental abruption, etc.)
❑ Cord compression
❑ Intrinsic foetal disease
❑ Maternal supine hypotension syndrome
❑ Compression of the umbilical cord
❑ Drugs administered for analgesia and anaesthesia

---

the foetal heart is affected, cardiac output decreases, thereby leading to foetal hypotension and causes further decrease in foetal circulation and blood flow to the heart and the brain. Prolonged and sustained hypoxaemia result in decreased oxygen levels in the tissues (hypoxia) that lead to foetal asphyxia.[1] Prolonged and uncorrected foetal asphyxia can produce potential damage to the brain, CNS and other organs, and sometimes even cause death.[1] Hence, it is mandatory to carry out routine foetal surveillance for detection of asphyxia in the antepartum and intrapartum period.

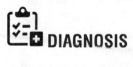

DIAGNOSIS

FOETAL HYPOXIA IN THE ANTEPARTUM PERIOD

Electronic foetal monitoring with the help of cardiotocography (CTG) is the most commonly used method for foetal monitoring during the antenatal period. This method is also used during the intrapartum period and is described next. Various other methods for diagnosis of foetal hypoxia in the antepartum period such as DFMC, NST, CST, BPP, modified BPP, etc. have been discussed in Chapter 6 (Tests for Foetal Well-being).

Electronic Foetal Monitoring

Electronic foetal monitoring has been defined by both the ACOG and the RCOG as monitoring the baby's heart rate for indicators of stress, usually during labour and birth using electronic foetal heart-rate monitoring device.[2,3] EFM can be of two types: (1) external and (2) internal cardiac monitoring. External foetal heart monitoring is performed by attaching the cardiotocograph machine through external transducers to the mother's abdomen with elastic straps. Though routine use of continuous EFM in every pregnancy is not recommended, it is widely used in the assessment of foetal health particularly in high-risk pregnancies [refer to Chapter 6 (Test for Foetal Well-being)] where there is an increased risk of perinatal death, cerebral palsy or neonatal encephalopathy. Current evidence does not support the use of the admission CTG in normal, healthy low-risk pregnancy and it is therefore not recommended. In such cases, intermittent auscultation with a handheld Doppler must be preferably done.

Continuous EFM should also be used in cases where oxytocin is being used for induction or augmentation of labour or in the presence of other intrapartum risk factors (e.g. epidural analgesia, vaginal bleeding in labour, maternal pyrexia, fresh meconium-stained liquor, etc.).

Features of the Heart Rate Observed on the Cardiotocograph

A foetal heart tracing should be interpreted using a systematic approach. Four main features of the heart rate must be observed on the cardiotocograph. These include: (1) baseline heart rate; (2) baseline variability; (3) decelerations; and (4) acceleration. Most FHR features in isolation, except the presence of late decelerations, are below par at predicting poor neonatal outcome. Each of these features is described next.

Baseline heart rate: The normal average baseline FHR in the third trimester is between 120 bpm to 160 bpm. Foetal hypoxaemia and metabolic acidosis are often associated with baseline bradycardia (Fig. 49.1), reduced baseline variability (Fig. 49.2) and late FHR decelerations (Figs 49.3A and B). Though bradycardia is indicative of foetal distress, it is important to remember that bradycardia is a late sign of foetal hypoxia (a continued lack of oxygen supply to the foetus). Baseline tachycardia (FHR exceeds 160 bpm) may also be an early clinical sign of foetal hypoxia (Fig. 49.4). In order to compensate for early hypoxic changes, the baseline FHR may rise to increase the cardiac output, which would help in maintaining the oxygenation of foetal vital centres in the brain. However, complicated baseline tachycardia, i.e. that associated with loss of baseline variability or deceleration of any type and/or heart rate of more than or equal to 200 bpm is extremely ominous and may be associated with foetal acidosis and high risk of foetal decompensation.[4] Such a heart rate pattern requires urgent foetal blood sampling (FBS) and pH estimation, followed by immediate delivery. However, in the presence of good variability, tachycardia is usually not a sign of foetal distress.

Baseline variability: Baseline variability can be defined as the minor fluctuations which occur in baseline FHR at 3–5 cycles per minute. It is measured by approximating the difference in bpm between the highest peak and lowest trough of fluctuation in a 1-minute segment of the FHR trace. Normal baseline variability can be considered to be greater than or equal to 5 bpm between contractions. Reduced baseline

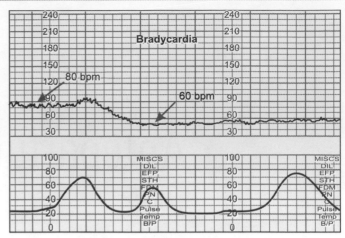

Fig. 49.1: A heart rate tracing showing foetal bradycardia

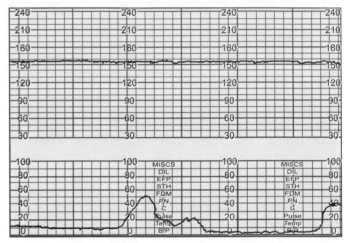

Fig. 49.2: Reduced baseline variability of <5–10 bpm over a period of time

variability commonly occurs during foetal sleep cycles. Also, it may commonly occur for up to 40 minutes during labour. The predictive value of reduced baseline variability as an isolated feature remains unclear. However, reduced baseline variability, in association with late or variable decelerations, is associated with an increased risk of cerebral palsy.

Deceleration: A sudden decrease in FHR by more than 15 bpm lasting for more than 15 seconds but less than 2 minutes from the baseline is considered as a deceleration.[3,5] There are three types of decelerations: (1) early, (2) late and (3) variable decelerations (Table 49.1). The obstetrician should always remember that the presence of decelerations during labour is not always ominous because during labour it is possible for some non-pathological type of decelerations to occur as well. However, their occurrence during the antenatal period should always be considered pathological. Different types of decelerations have been described next.

Early decelerations: Early decelerations begin at about the same time as the onset of the uterine contraction. The nadir of early decelerations coincides with the peak of contraction (Figs 49.5A and B). Presence of these decelerations is usually not indicative of foetal compromise. They may occur due to head compression during uterine contractions.

Late decelerations: Late decelerations are the most ominous FHR pattern.[6] The onset of these decelerations occurs after the beginning of the contraction, and the nadir of the deceleration occurs after the peak of the contraction. They are usually caused by reduced blood flow or lack of blood flow to the uterus and placenta during a contraction. They are associated with reduced placental perfusion resulting in uteroplacental insufficiency. Uteroplacental insufficiency can result in hypoxia and metabolic abnormalities. Presence of repeated late decelerations are associated with an increased risk of cerebral palsy, umbilical artery acidosis and an APGAR score of less than 7 at 5 minutes.

Variable decelerations: Uncomplicated variable decelerations are not consistently found to be associated with poor neonatal outcome (reduced 5-minute APGAR scores or metabolic acidosis). Variable decelerations are commonly present in association with other FHR abnormalities, e.g. baseline changes and reduced variability. Such variable decelerations are likely to be associated with poor adverse neonatal outcomes (such as an increased risk of umbilical artery acidosis and an APGAR score of less than 7 at 5 minutes) in comparison with 'uncomplicated' variable decelerations.

Acceleration: Acceleration can be defined as transient increases in FHR of 15 bpm or more, which lasts for 15 seconds or more. Presence of FHR accelerations is associated with good outcome. The significance of absent accelerations on an otherwise normal CTG presently remains unclear.

Sinusoidal Pattern

A sinusoidal pattern is one in which the amplitude of oscillations and period of short-term (beat-to-beat variability) remains more or less constant. This gives the trace a smooth,

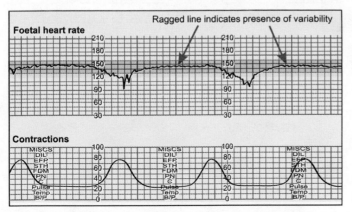

Fig. 49.3A: Late deceleration with preserved baseline variability

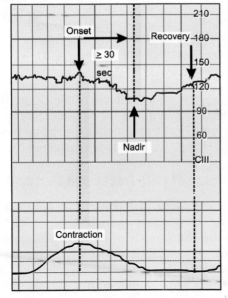

Fig. 49.3B: Late deceleration (magnified view)

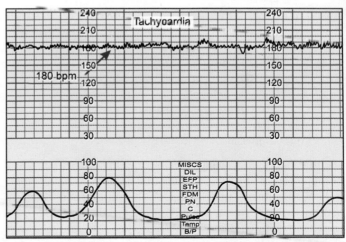

Fig. 49.4: A tracing showing foetal tachycardia

Table 49.1: Different types of decelerations

Parameters	Early deceleration	Late deceleration	Variable deceleration
Onset	Decrease in the FHR, starts at about the same time as the onset of the contraction (Figs 49.5A and B)	Onset of the deceleration occurs after the beginning of the contraction (Figs 49.3A and B)	Can occur any time during the contraction
Nadir of deceleration	The nadir of deceleration coincides with the peak of contraction	The nadir of the deceleration occurs after the peak of contraction	Characterised by the presence of short acceleration followed by rapid deceleration which is not related to the timing of uterine contraction
Significance	Normal and common	Most ominous FHR	Severe, atypical types may be ominous
Examples	May occur due to foetal head compression during uterine contractions	Usually occurs due to uteroplacental insufficiency	Usually occurs due to cord compression

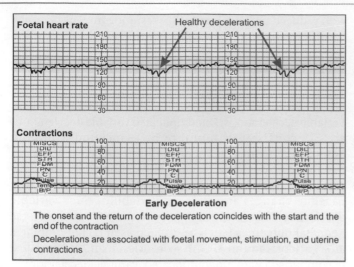

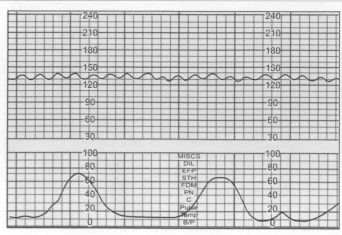

Fig. 49.5A: Early deceleration with preserved baseline variability

Fig. 49.6: Foetal heart tracing showing sinusoidal pattern

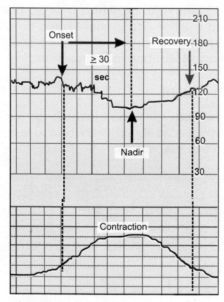

Fig. 49.5B: Early deceleration (magnified view)

Box 49.2: Criticisms for the widespread use of cardiotocography

- ❏ Indirect signal of the foetal condition
- ❏ Substantial intra- and interobserver variation regarding the interpretation
- ❏ Increase in medicolegal vulnerability
- ❏ Low validity, high incidence of false-positive findings
- ❏ Lack of uniform classification systems
- ❏ Increase in the number of operative deliveries
- ❏ Confusion due to many influences on foetal heart rhythm
- ❏ Differences in recording techniques

undulating, regular wavy appearance (Fig. 49.6). The foetal heart pattern is labelled as sinusoidal if this pattern lasts for at least 10 minutes. In this pattern, the amplitude of oscillations usually varies between 5 to 15 bpm with a fixed period of 3–5 cycles per minute.[7] Foetal activity may be minimal or absent, and FHR accelerations are usually lacking. A true sinusoidal pattern is rare but ominous and is associated with high rates of foetal morbidity and mortality.[8] Some of the causes for sinusoidal pattern include the following: foetal anaemia, massive foetal haemorrhage due to causes such as maternal anticoagulation therapy (aspirin, warfarin, etc.), bleeding vasa praevia, cordocentesis, Rh isoimmunisation, etc. Maternal administration of some sedative and analgesic drugs like meperidine, pethidine, butorphanol, alphaprodine (but not other narcotics) can also cause sinusoidal pattern. Sinusoidal pattern due to pethidine can be treated by administration of naloxone.

The incidence of perinatal death associated with sinusoidal FHR patterns appears to be low in uncomplicated labours. In uncompromised babies, these patterns do not appear to be associated with poor outcome. In clinical practice, if this pattern appears in labour, a foetomaternal haemorrhage must be clinically excluded and, hence, presence of sinusoidal waves on CTG must be viewed with suspicion.

Categorisation of FHR Traces and Outcome

The impact of various FHR features on perinatal outcome remains unclear. Recently, there has been a lot of criticism related to the routine use of EFM for antepartum foetal surveillance (Box 49.2), because it is thought to result in an increased rate of operative delivery. In clinical practice, CTG traces are not evaluated on the basis of individual features. Instead, an overall assessment is made on the basis of a number of features. This is used for making clinical decisions in the light of clinical factors and the stage of labour. Categorisation of FHR traces is described in Table 49.2. This is based on NICE classification of FHR features (Table 49.3), which classifies the cardiotocographic traces as normal, non-reassuring and abnormal based on the four important characteristics of foetal heart trace, i.e. (1) baseline heart rate, (2) variability, (3) decelerations and (4) accelerations. Traces classified as 'abnormal' are likely to be associated with an increase in the incidence of neonatal encephalopathy, cerebral palsy, neonatal acidosis and APGAR score of less than 7 at 5 minutes.

While taking a CTG trace, the CTG machines should be standardised in such a way that the paper speed is set to 1 cm/min, sensitivity displays are set to 20 bpm, and FHR range displays of 50–210 bpm are used.

Table 49.2: Categorisation of foetal heart rate traces

Category	Definition
Normal	A cardiotocograph where all four features fall into the reassuring category
Suspicious	A cardiotocograph whose features fall into one of the non-reassuring categories and the remainder of the features are reassuring
Pathological	A cardiotocograph whose features fall into two or more non-reassuring categories or one or more abnormal categories

Table 49.3: NICE classification of foetal heart rate features

	Baseline rate (bpm)	Variability	Decelerations	Acceleration
Normal	110–160	≥5	None	Present
Non-reassuring	100–109 161–180	<5 for ≥ 40, but <90 minutes	• *Early decelerations* • *Variable decelerations*: Dropping from baseline by 60 bpm or less and taking 60 seconds or less to recover; present for >90 minutes, with >50% of contractions Or • *Variable decelerations*: Dropping from baseline by >60 bpm or taking >60 seconds to recover; present for up to 30 minutes, occurring with >50% of contractions • Single prolonged deceleration up to 3 minutes	Absence of accelerations in an otherwise normal CTG is of uncertain significance
Abnormal	<100 >180 Sinusoidal pattern ≥10 minutes	<5 ≥90 minutes	• *Atypical variable decelerations*: Non-reassuring >30 minutes after conservative measures, >50% contractions • *Late decelerations*: >30 minutes with >50% contraction • *Bradycardia/prolonged deceleration*: Single prolonged deceleration present for >3 minutes	

FOETAL HYPOXIA IN THE INTRAPARTUM PERIOD

With technological advancements, the foetal surveillance can also extend into the intrapartum period. Some of these tests used for intrapartum monitoring have been mentioned in Box 49.3. In clinical practice, the diagnostic tests for foetal well-being during labour commonly include internal cardiotocographic monitoring and FBS. The results on intrapartum foetal monitoring tests help in assuring the obstetrician that the foetus is able to obtain enough oxygen inside the intrauterine cavity. Thus, these techniques act as principal procedures for screening foetal distress and hypoxia during labour.

Intermittent Auscultation

For the purpose of foetal monitoring during the intrapartum period in an otherwise healthy woman with uncomplicated pregnancy, intermittent auscultation should be offered. During the active stages of labour, intermittent auscultation should be preferably done after each contraction, for a minimum period of 60 seconds. The frequency of intermittent auscultation should be at least after every 15 minutes during the first stage and after every 5 minutes during the second stage of labour. In the pregnancies previously monitored with intermittent auscultation, continuous EFM is recommended in the following situations:

❖ Evidence of a foetal heart baseline less than 110 bpm or greater than 160 bpm on auscultation
❖ Evidence of any decelerations on auscultation
❖ Development of any risk factors during labour.

Box 49.3: Intrapartum tests

❏ Internal electronic foetal monitoring
❏ Foetal blood sampling
❏ Pulse oximetry
❏ ST analysis on foetal electrocardiography
❏ Foetal scalp lactate measurement
❏ Near-infrared spectroscopy

Adjuvant Tests of Foetal Well-being

Foetal Scalp Blood Sampling

Foetal scalp blood sampling is a widely used method for assessing foetal condition in the event of ominous FHR patterns on EFM (Fig. 49.7). This method was introduced by Saling in 1960 as a diagnostic tool in cases with non-reassuring or ominous FHR tracings.[9] Foetal scalp blood sampling has been considered as a gold standard in order to identify foetal hypoxia. Concurrent use of foetal scalp sampling with EFM may not only help in improving the foetal outcome but also reducing the rate of operative delivery.[10] However, the study by Goodwin et al. has shown that the process of foetal scalp sampling does not offer significant benefits in intrapartum foetal monitoring.[11] The results of foetal scalp blood sampling, their interpretation and the most appropriate clinical intervention are shown in Table 49.4.

Principle: Under normal conditions, when the foetus receives sufficient supply of oxygenated blood from the mother via the placenta, aerobic metabolism occurs. Glucose is broken down through the aerobic pathway, which uses oxygen to produce energy in the form of adenosine triphosphate (ATP), along with

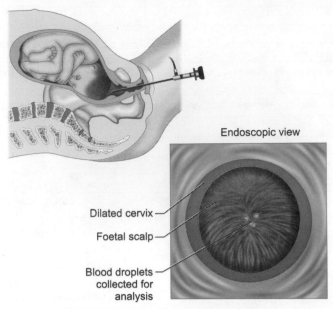

Endoscopic view

Dilated cervix

Foetal scalp

Blood droplets
collected for
analysis

Fig. 49.7: Procedure of foetal scalp pH sampling

Table 49.4: Interpretation of foetal blood sampling

Scalp blood pH*	Pathology	Intervention
<7.20	Foetal acidosis	Urgent intervention
7.21–7.24	Borderline (preacidaemia)	Sampling to be repeated within 30 minutes
>7.25	Reassuring (normal)	Normal monitoring to be performed, repeat if cardiotocograph continues to deteriorate

* All scalp pH estimations should be interpreted taking into account the initial pH measurement, the rate of progress in labour and the clinical condition of the mother and baby.

carbon dioxide (CO_2) and water. Under normal circumstances, the CO_2 is removed from the foetus via the placenta. However, in cases of foetal hypoxia or in case of conditions, such as cord compression causing obstruction to blood flow, there is accumulation of CO_2 and deficiency of oxygen resulting in the development of respiratory acidosis. In case of reduced oxygen supply to the foetus, it has to engage in anaerobic metabolism. The end product of anaerobic metabolism is lactic acid. Lactic acid is a strong monocarboxylic acid, which disassociates easily at the physiological pH into hydrogen ions (H^+) and lactate. The accumulation of these substances can result in the development of metabolic acidosis and lactoacidosis. Metabolic acidosis results in multiorgan dysfunction in the newborn and poor long-term neonatal outcome.

Cases where delivery is anticipated due to the presence of an abnormal FHR pattern or in the cases of suspected foetal acidosis, FBS should be undertaken in the absence of technical difficulties or any contraindications. Contraindications to FBS are enlisted in Box 49.4. However, in cases where there is clear evidence of acute foetal compromise, e.g. presence of a prolonged deceleration (>3 minutes), FBS need not be undertaken. In these cases, the baby should be delivered urgently.

Box 49.4: Contraindications to foetal blood sampling

❑ Maternal infection such as HIV, hepatitis viruses or herpes simplex virus
❑ Foetal bleeding disorders such as haemophilia
❑ Prematurity (<34 weeks)
❑ Acute foetal compromise

Foetal Scalp Lactate Measurement

Lactate analysis on foetal scalp blood during labour might serve as an alternative method in the management of intrapartum foetal distress. Since a past few years, reliable lactate meters (Lactate Pro™) have become available for bedside obstetric practice. It is a simple technique requiring only 5 µL of blood. Report is usually obtained digitally at the end of 1 minute.

Principle: Lactate is the main fixed organic acid in the metabolic acidosis, and the major contributor to base deficit. Recently, a bedside-held lactate meter (Lactate Pro™) has been developed. It has greatly simplified the process of FBS, as it requires much less amount of blood in comparison to that required for FBS (5 µL vs 35–50 µL). Since the concentration of lactate is highest in plasma, lower in haemolysed blood and lowest in whole blood (with intact erythrocytes), different types of lactate meters are used for measurement in different blood compartments.

The use of foetal scalp lactate estimation is not likely to result in reduction in the incidence of adverse neonatal or maternal outcomes. However, its use is associated with a significant reduction in sampling failure in comparison to EFM with foetal scalp pH estimation.

Foetal Pulse Oximetry

Presently, there is no evidence regarding the benefit of foetal pulse oximetry. The largest RCT till date has failed to show any benefit in terms of reduction in the rate of caesarean delivery or improvement of neonatal condition.[12] Foetal pulse oximetry is therefore not used in the UK.

Foetal Electrocardiogram Analysis

In response to foetal hypoxaemia, there occur changes in the foetal PR interval and ST segment of electrocardiogram (ECG). Due to this, foetal ECG analysis is commonly used in combination with conventional CTG monitoring during labour. ST waveform analysis of foetal ECG for intrapartum surveillance (STAN®) is a newly introduced method for foetal surveillance.[13] Cochrane review by Neilson (2015) has shown that the combination of ST analysis and CTG monitoring was associated with a lower risk of neonatal encephalopathy.[14] It was also associated with a reduction in the requirement for FBS and fewer operative vaginal deliveries. Foetal monitoring with the analysis of PR interval is not likely to be associated with any clinical benefit. According to this review, the use of ST analysis in labour appears to be promising. However, it is likely to be associated with several disadvantages such as the use of spiral foetal scalp electrode, requirement for FBS if there are abnormalities on the CTG trace. Foetal ECG can now be acquired through abdominally sited electrodes. This technique is likely to avoid the use of foetal scalp electrodes and allows earlier foetal ECG monitoring in labour.

Other Tests

Near-infrared spectroscopy (NIRS) is a new technique for foetal monitoring, which is still in the developmental phase. This technique helps in directly measuring the cerebral oxygen concentration. The principle of this modality is based on the differing absorption characteristics of oxygenated and reduced haemoglobin molecules. The mean oxygen saturation of cerebral haemoglobin can be calculated by measuring the changes in oxygenated and deoxygenated haemoglobin at the time of uterine contractions.

MANAGEMENT

General Management

❖ If a woman appears to be in foetal distress, the obstetrician should immediately implement the general steps mentioned in Box 49.5.

❖ The use of tocolytic therapy during episodes of foetal distress helps in reducing abnormal FHR patterns but is not likely to reduce the rate of caesarean section.

Box 49.5: General steps for management of foetal distress

❑ *Strategies for improvement of placental blood supply*
  - Patient to be placed in propped up position or in the left lateral position to avoid aortocaval compression
  - Administration of oxygen via a face mask[15]
  - Reduction of uterine activity, especially if excessive
  - Correction of maternal hypovolaemia and/or hypotension
  - Maintenance of maternal hydration (use of IV fluids)[16]
  - Use of ephedrine for lower limb vasodilatation secondary to epidural analgesia

❑ *Strategies for reduction of uterine activity especially if excessive*
  - Stop oxytocin, if it is being administered
  - Remove vaginal prostaglandins if it had been recently administered
  - Vaginal lavage may be useful if prostaglandin gel had been administered
  - Consider administration of tocolytic agents (0.25 mg subcutaneous terbutaline)

❑ *Evidence of foetal distress not secondary to oxytocin infusion*
  - Administration of tocolytic agents for foetal distress IV or subcutaneous terbutaline (250 μg), sublingual trinitroglycerine (GTN) spray (400 μg) or IV salbutamol (100 μg)][17]
  - Avoiding use of medications that could depress FHR

❑ *Reduction of umbilical cord compression*
  - Transcervical amnioinfusion

❑ *Maternal tachycardia/pyrexia*
  - If maternal temperature ≥37.8°C, consider screening for infection and treatment
  - If pulse ≥140 bpm, reduce tocolytic infusion
  - Check BP; administer 500 mL crystalloids if appropriate

❖ *Transcervical amnioinfusion*: The process of transcervical amnioinfusion is likely to bring about an increase in the amniotic fluid volume (AFV), thereby reducing the occurrence of umbilical cord compression. The commonly used protocol involves the infusion of 500 mL of Hartmann's solution over 20–30 minutes followed by an infusion at the rate up to 250 mL/h. A Cochrane review by Hofmeyr (2012) has shown that amnioinfusion causes an improvement in the FHR by reducing the rate of variable decelerations.[18] Though there are methodological limitations to the trials reviewed in this Cochrane review, amnioinfusion is also likely to improve the short-term measures of neonatal well-being, thereby lowering the rate of caesarean delivery. More research in the future is required to assess the impact of amnioinfusion on the rates of caesarean section rates in cases with a stringent diagnosis of foetal distress.

Definite Management

Management protocol for foetal surveillance in cases of foetal asphyxia is described in Flow chart 49.1. Management algorithm in high-risk pregnancy (e.g. pre-eclampsia, gestation diabetes, IUGR, etc.) where there is an evidence of antepartum asphyxia is described in Flow chart 49.2.

❖ If the exact cause for foetal distress can be identified, definite treatment should be instituted as shown in Table 49.5.

❖ In cases of abnormal/pathological CTG trace or cases with confirmed acute foetal compromise, delivery should be accomplished as soon as possible. The accepted standard has been that, ideally, this should be accomplished within 30 minutes. There is no need to perform FBS in such cases. Urgency of delivery should take into account the severity of the FHR abnormality and relevant maternal factors. The anaesthetist and paediatrician should be urgently called for help.

❖ On the other hand, conservative management (Box 49.5) must be used in cases where the CTG falls into the suspicious/non-reassuring category.

❖ In cases where the CTG is abnormal, but foetal compromise cannot be confirmed, FBS should be done in cases where appropriate/feasible. If the results of FBS are within normal limits, conservative management approach can be adopted. In situations where FBS is not possible or appropriate, or FBS shows a pH ≤7.2, delivery should be expedited.

❖ Where delivery is contemplated because of an abnormal FHR pattern, in cases of suspected foetal acidosis, FBS should be undertaken in the absence of technical difficulties or any contraindications.

Planning Delivery

Decision for delivery is based on the results of the clinical tests such as CTG and secondary tests of foetal well-being, particularly FBS and the patient's overall clinical picture. This should include the evaluation of obstetric risk factors, progress in labour and presence of untreatable foetal/maternal complications such as abruption, cord prolapse, chorioamnionitis and scar dehiscence.

Flow chart 49.1: Management protocol for foetal surveillance in case of foetal asphyxia during pregnancy

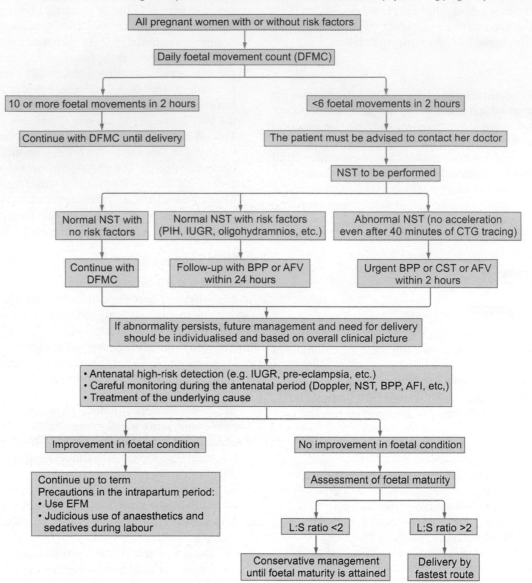

PART II

If FHR abnormalities persist or there are additional signs of distress (thick meconium-stained fluid), an emergency delivery must be planned by the obstetrician in cases where foetal maturity has been attained. When the baby's heart rate pattern demonstrates a lack of oxygen, it is necessary for the baby to be born immediately. According to the present guidelines of RCOG, delivery must be achieved within 30 minutes following the diagnosis of foetal distress. However, this is rarely achieved in clinical practice and its clinical significance has been called to question.[19] The healthcare attendant/clinician must make it a norm to keep the women and her relatives apprised of the situation regarding the labour at all times and involve them in the clinical decision-making. This small step goes a long way in preventing the future medicolegal complications. The delivery must be planned by the fastest route. If the woman is not in active labour, caesarean section appears to be the only option for the obstetrician. If the woman is in active labour, there are two options, that are described next.

1. If the cervix is fully dilated and the foetal head is not more than one-fifth above the symphysis pubis or the leading bony edge of the head is at zero station (head is engaged), the obstetrician can deliver the baby by vacuum extraction or forceps application.
2. If the cervix is not fully dilated or the leading bony edge of the head is above zero station (head is not yet engaged), the obstetrician needs to deliver the baby by caesarean section.

Following delivery, umbilical cord samples should be taken, 1- and 5-minute APGAR scores calculated and all results recorded in the mother's and newborn's notes. There has been a significant rise in the rates of caesarean section over the past few years.[20] This can be largely attributed to increasing use of EFM for ensuring foetal well-being at the time of labour. The EFM has not been found to be associated with any long-term benefits in either low- or high-risk pregnancies, in comparison to the use of intermittent auscultation for foetal monitoring.[3]

Flow chart 49.2: Management algorithm in high-risk pregnancy

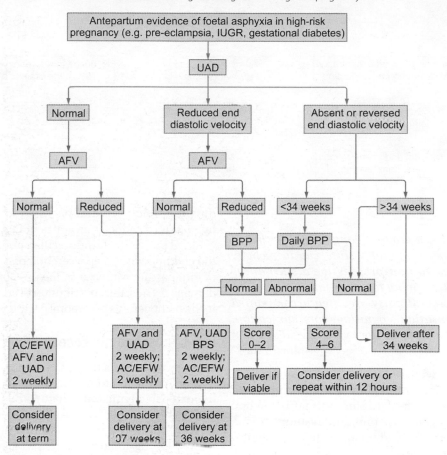

Abbreviations: AC, abdominal circumference; AFV, amniotic fluid volume; BPS, biophysical profile score; EFW, estimated foetal weight; UAD, umbilical artery Doppler

Table 49.5: Definite treatment for foetal distress

Cause of foetal distress	Treatment
Abruptio placentae	Delivery by fastest route
Chorioamnionitis (fever, foul-smelling vaginal discharge, etc.)	Immediate administration of antibiotics
Cord prolapse	Emergency caesarean section

Also, the use of EFM has been found to bring about increase in the rates of caesarean and vaginal instrumental delivery, infection, cerebral palsy in premature babies, etc.[21] The use of foetal distress as an indication for caesarean delivery has been largely in debate. It has been shown that the baby's heart rate during labour correlates poorly with measures of the baby's condition at birth. Also, measures of the baby's condition at birth correlate poorly with long-term outcomes.[22-24] In view of this ongoing debate and the high false-positive rate associated with the use of EFM, the obstetricians must use other methods of intrapartum monitoring such as foetal scalp sampling and internal CTG to adequately evaluate the cases with intrapartum asphyxia and hypoxia. If none of these intrapartum techniques are available, the obstetricians must observe their own clinical discretions and judgement and resort to operative delivery only when it appears fully justifiable in view of optimal maternal and neonatal outcome.

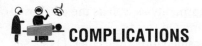

COMPLICATIONS

Careful antepartum and intrapartum foetal surveillance helps in preventing asphyxia and thereby avoiding the development of foetal distress. A cascade of events exists from hypoxic acidaemia through metabolic acidosis, neonatal encephalopathy, cerebral palsy and long-term sequelae. The likelihood of development of long-term sequelae is dependent upon the nature and duration of the insult, and the vulnerability of the foetus. Most term infants subject to hypoxia of short duration will completely recover. Umbilical cord blood gas analysis at birth can provide a measure of the severity of the metabolic acidosis but not the duration of the hypoxic insult. Some of these negative consequences related to foetal distress are described in Flow chart 49.3 and are discussed next.

Meconium Aspiration Syndrome

The babies in distress are more likely to release meconium in the amniotic fluid due to increased peristaltic activity of the GI tract. Thus, they are also more likely to aspirate meconium and develop meconium aspiration syndrome.

CHAPTER 49

Flow chart 49.3: Consequences of foetal hypoxia

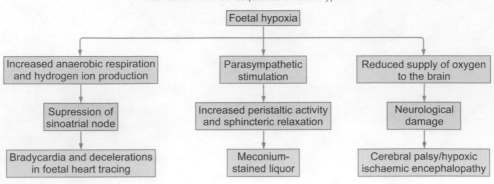

Cerebral Palsy

'Cerebral palsy describes a group of long-term disorders of the development of movement and posture, causing activity limitation, attributed to non-progressive disturbances that occurred in the developing foetal or infant brain. The motor disorders of cerebral palsy are often accompanied by disturbances of sensation, cognition, communication, perception, and/or behaviour, and/or by a seizure disorder.'
—**Martin Bax**[25]

Cerebral palsy is a well-recognised, non-progressive neurodevelopmental condition beginning in early childhood and persisting through the lifespan. Since this term 'cerebral palsy' refers to a heterogeneous condition, resulting from a multitude of different causes and includes different clinical presentations, the term, 'cerebral palsies'[25] is sometimes preferred instead. Cerebral palsy most commonly results from the distortion of normal brain development that occurs over a short period of time. They are most commonly classified on the basis of the motor abnormality as well as the diagnosed movement disorders present. On this basis, cerebral palsies can be most commonly classified into three types: (1) spastic type; (2) ataxic type and (3) athetoid type.

Relationship between intrapartum foetal asphyxia and cerebral palsy: There appears to be an association between intrapartum foetal asphyxia and development of cerebral palsy in the child. Traditionally, it has been believed that cerebral palsy is related to intrapartum asphyxia and difficult labour. Poor obstetrical care is often blamed for cerebral palsy, thus resulting in much legal litigation against obstetricians for not observing proper medical care during labour and delivery. The relation between the quality of care, which is provided to a mother during labour and delivery, and the death of her baby or cerebral palsy in her surviving child is a continuing source of debate involving obstetricians, paediatricians, parents, and lawyers. Over the past 10 years, there has been a considerable change in the views held by obstetricians, paediatricians, and lawyers regarding the origin of cerebral palsy. The present evidence base does not suggest a strong link between intrapartum asphyxia and cerebral palsy. It has been observed that most children who develop cerebral palsy often do not show any intrapartum clinical signs which could be attributed to the hypoxic injury.[26] Also most babies with clinical markers of hypoxia at the time of labour and delivery

do not develop cerebral palsy.[27] Additionally, intrapartum hypoxia is only one of several aetiological factors resulting in cerebral palsy.[28] In a study by Blair and Stanley, only 8% of all the children with spastic cerebral palsy had previous history of intrapartum asphyxia as the possible cause of their brain damage.[29] Thus, the contribution of adverse antenatal factors in the pathogenesis of cerebral palsy requires further research.

Hypoxic-ischaemic Encephalopathy

Damage to the cells in the CNS due to inadequate supply of oxygen may result in development of a condition known as hypoxic-ischaemic encephalopathy (HIE). This condition may be responsible for causing death in the newborn period or result in future developmental abnormalities, mental retardation, disabilities or cerebral palsy. Development of HIE due to intrapartum asphyxia is an issue related to considerable medical and medicolegal debate. HIE is characterised by clinical and laboratory evidence of acute or subacute brain injury due to asphyxia. Most often, the underlying cause remains unknown. Inspite of major advancements in foetal monitoring technology, HIE remains a serious condition, causing significant mortality and long-term morbidity. The incidence of HIE is particularly high in developing countries which may not have adequate resources.[30,31]

Neonatal encephalopathy is *'a clinically defined syndrome of disturbed neurological function in the earliest days of life in the term infant, manifested by difficulty with initiating and maintaining respiration, depression of tone and reflexes, subnormal level of consciousness, and often by seizures.'*
—**Nelson and Leviton**[32]

Diagnosis

The criteria described by the American Academy of Pediatrics (AAP)[33] and ACOG to assist in the diagnosis of severe HIE is described in Box 49.6.

Pathophysiology:[33-37]

The primary event in the development of HIE is brain hypoxia and ischaemia due to systemic hypoxaemia and/or reduced cerebral blood flow (CBF). The cellular events at neuronal level, which are responsible for producing the neuronal damage related to HIE, are summarised in Flow chart 49.4. In the foetuses and newborn suffering from acute asphyxia,

Box 49.6: Criteria for the diagnosis of severe hypoxic-ischaemic encephalopathy

❑ Profound metabolic or mixed acidaemia (pH <7.00)
❑ Persistence of an APGAR score of 0–3 for longer than 5 minutes after birth
❑ Neonatal neurologic sequelae (e.g. seizures, coma, hypotonia)
❑ Multiple organ involvement (e.g. kidney, lungs, liver, heart, intestines, etc.)

the CBF falls below critical levels, and the brain continues to suffer from diminished blood supply and a lack of sufficient oxygen to meet its needs. Initial reduction in CBF causes hypoxia, hypoglycaemia and severe anaemia. This leads to intracellular energy failure or energy crisis. The energy crisis triggers off a large cascade of events at the biochemical level, following HIE injury.

Classification of the Degree of Encephalopathy

The staging system proposed by Sarnat and Sarnat in 1976[38] is often useful for classifying the degree of encephalopathy. This system classifies HIE into three stages: stages 1, 2 and 3 (Table 49.6).

Treatment[39]

There is no treatment for HIE per se. Symptomatic therapies (physiotherapy, muscle relaxants, etc.) can help with muscle tone and control. Traditional therapies include physical therapy for gross motor control, occupational therapy for small muscle control and for assistance with activities of daily living, and speech and language therapy for dysarthria and other speech abnormalities.

Medical Treatment

The patient must be provided standard intensive care support involving the correction of metabolic acidosis, limiting fluid intake to two–thirds the maintenance volume for the first 3–4 days, and keeping the infant nil per os (NPO) during the first 3 days of life or until the general level of alertness and consciousness improves.

Medical treatment involving the use of anticonvulsants forms the main element of treatment. Seizures can be treated with medicines like phenobarbital, lorazepam, phenytoin, etc.[40] Supportive care in form of maintenance of adequate ventilation, perfusion and metabolic status may be required. The blood gases and acid-base status must be maintained in the physiological ranges including partial pressure of arterial oxygen (PaO_2): 80–100 mmHg; partial pressure of arterial carbon dioxide ($PaCO_2$): 35–40 mmHg; and pH: 7.35–7.45. The mean BP must be maintained above 35 mmHg (for term infants). Inotropic agents including dopamine and dobutamine, which help in increasing BP and combating shock, can also be used. However, presently no clear information is available on the effects of these drugs on CBF in neonates. Since both hypoglycaemia and hyperglycaemia are known to cause brain injury, efforts must be made to avoid both of them. In the first 2 days of life, IV fluids must be

Flow chart 49.4: Pathophysiology of hypoxic-ischaemic encephalopathy

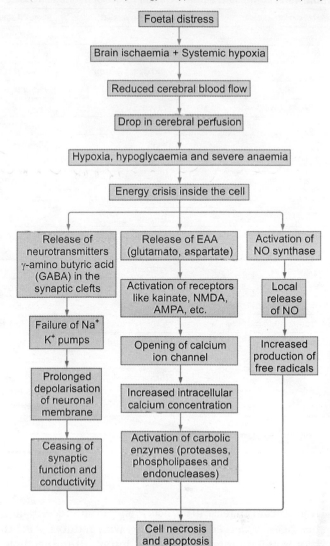

Abbreviations: EAA, excitatory amino acids; NMDA, N-methyl-D-aspartate; AMPA, amino-3-hydroxy-5-methyl-4 isoxazole propionate; NO, nitric oxide

restricted to about two-thirds of the normal daily requirement for that particular gestational age. Fluid and electrolyte therapy must be individualised for each patient depending upon the clinical course of the disease, changes in weight, urine output, and the results of serum electrolyte and renal function studies. Hypothermia is emerging as a new and evolving therapy for mild-to-moderate cases of HIE. Brain cooling to about 3–4°C below the baseline temperature (i.e. to 33–34°C) may help in protecting the neurons from injury.[41] The method could involve either the provision of whole body cooling[42] or selective cooling over the head.[43]

CLINICAL PEARLS

❖ Interpretation of FHR traces is significantly affected by intra- and interobserver errors. The use of computerised systems for FHR analysis helps in improving the consistency of interpretation.

CHAPTER 49

Table 49.6: Sarnat and Sarnat's clinical stages of perinatal hypoxic-ischaemic brain injury[38]

Level of consciousness	Stage 1 (Hyperalert)	Stage 2 (Lethargic or obtunded)	Stage 3 (Stuporous)
Neuromuscular control			
Muscle tone	Normal	Mild hypotonia	Flaccid
Posture	Mild distal flexion	Strong distal flexion	Intermittent decerebration
Stretch reflexes	Overactive	Overactive	Decreased or absent
Segmental myoclonus	Present	Present	Absent
Complex reflexes			
Suck	Weak	Weak or absent	Absent
Moro	Strong, low threshold	Weak, incomplete; high threshold	Absent
Oculovestibular	Normal	Overactive	Weak or absent
Tonic neck	Slight	Strong	Absent
Autonomic function			
Autonomic function	Generalised sympathetic depression	Generalised parasympathetic depression	Both systems depressed
Pupils	Mydriasis	Miosis	Variable, often unequal, poor light reflex
Heart rate	Tachycardia	Bradycardia	Variable
Bronchial and salivary secretions	Sparse	Profuse	Variable
Gastrointestinal motility	Normal or decreased	Increased; diarrhoea	Variable
Seizures	None/uncommon	Common; focal or multifocal	Uncommon (excluding decerebration)
Electroencephalogram findings			
	Normal (awake)	*Early*: Low voltage continuous delta and theta *Later*: Periodic pattern (awake) *Seizures*: Focal 1–1.5-Hz spike-and-wave	*Early*: Periodic pattern with isopotential phases *Later*: Totally isopotential
Duration			
	<24 hours	2–14 hours	Hours to weeks

❖ A significant increase in the occurrence of late decelerations has been observed in the babies with reduced APGAR scores at 5 minutes of birth and intrapartum metabolic acidosis.

❖ Presently, the gold standard for decision to delivery interval in cases of confirmed foetal compromise has been accepted as 30 minutes. However, the evidence supporting this standard is presently weak and inconclusive. Therefore, achievability of safe delivery within 30 minutes time period presently remains uncertain.

EVIDENCE-BASED MEDICINE

Presently, there is insufficient evidence to support the efficacy of administration of maternal oxygen for the treatment of foetal distress. The present evidence also does not support the use of prophylactic oxygen therapy in the second stage of labour. If maternal oxygen therapy is required, in no case should it be used for a long period unless there is documented low oxygen saturation. There is no evidence of benefit of such practice. In fact, there is a possibility of occurrence of detrimental effect when it is applied for more than a few minutes.[16,44,45]

REFERENCES

1. Grovitz S, Borten M. (2015). Our focus is medical malpractice. [online] Available from www.gbmedlaw.com/Fetal_Asphyxia.html. [Accessed August, 2016].
2. Foetal heart-rate patterns: monitoring, interpretation, and management. ACOG technical bulletin no. 207. Washington, DC: ACOG; 1995.
3. Royal College of Obstetrics and Gynaecologists (RCOG). (2001). The use of electronic foetal monitoring. [online]. Available from www.ctgutbildning.se/Course/referenser/index.php. [Accessed August, 2016].
4. Nielsen PV, Stigsby B, Nickelsen C, Nim J. Intra-and Interobserver variability in the assessment of intrapartum cardiotocograms. Acta Obstet Gynecol Scand. 1987;66(5):421-4.
5. Ingemarsson I, Herbest A. The role of electronic foetal monitoring in labour. J Perinat Med. 1991;19(1):134-8.
6. MacDonald D, Grant A, Sheridan-Pereira M, Boylan P, Chalmers I. The Dublin randomised controlled trial of intrapartum foetal heart-rate monitoring. Am J Obstet Gynecol. 1985;152(5):524-39.
7. Tomoaki I, Yuji M, Quilligan EJ, Cifuentes, P, DoiS, Soung-Day P. Two sinusoidal heart-rate patterns in fetal lambs undergoing extracorporeal membrane oxygenation. Am J Obstet Gynecol. 1999;180(2):462-8.

8. Nielsen TF. Cesarean section. In: Sachs BP, Beard R, Papiernik E, Russell C (Eds). Reproductive Health Care for Women and Babies. New York: Oxford University Press; 1995. pp. 279-90.

9. Saling HE. The first blood gas analysis and pH measurements on the fetus during labor and the clinical significance of this new technique. Arch Gynakol. 1963;198:82-6.

10. Gardosi J. Monitoring technology and the clinical perspective. Bailliere's Clin Obstet Gynaecol. 1996;10(2):325-40.

11. Goodwin TM, Milner ML, Paul RH. Elimination of foetal scalp blood sampling on a large clinical service. Obstet Gynecol. 1994;83(6):971-5.

12. Bloom SL, Spong CY, Thom E, Varner MW, Rouse DJ, Weininger S, et al. Fetal pulse oximetry and cesarean delivery. N Engl J Med. 2006;355(21):2195-202.

13. Taylor MJ, Thomas MJ, Smith MJ, Oseku-Afful S, Fisk NM, Green AR, et al. Non-invasive intrapartum foetal ECG: preliminary report. BJOG. 2005;112(8):1016-21.

14. Neilson J. Foetal electrocardiogram (ECG) for foetal monitoring during labour. Cochrane Database Syst Rev. 2015;(12): CD000116.

15. Hofmeyr GJ. Maternal oxygen administration for foetal distress. Cochrane Database Syst Rev. 2000;(2):CD000136.

16. Hofmeyr GJ, Gülmezoglu AM. Maternal hydration for increasing amniotic fluid volume in oligohydramnios and normal amniotic fluid volume. Cochrane Database Syst Rev. 2002;(2):1-20.

17. Kulier R, Hofmeyr GJ. Tocolytics for suspected intrapartum foetal distress. Cochrane Database Syst Rev. 2000;(2):1-19.

18. Hofmeyr GJ, Lawrie TA. Amnioinfusion for potential or suspected umbilical cord compression in labour. Cochrane Database Syst Rev. 2012;(1):CD000013.

19. Mackenzie IZ, Cooke I. Prospective 12 month study of 30 minutes decision to delivery intervals for "emergency" caesarean section. BMJ. 2001;322(7298):1334-5.

20. Taffel SM. Cesarean delivery in the United States, 1990. National Center for Health Statistics. Vital Health Statistics, Series 21, no. 51. Washington DC: Government Printing Office; 1994.

21. NICE. (2014). Intrapartum care—care of healthy women and their babies during childbirth. NICE clinical guidelines 55. [online] Available from www.nice.org.uk/guidance/cg190/resources/intrapartum-care-for-healthy-women-and-babies-35109066447557. [Accessed August, 2016].

22. Chauhan SP, Magann EF, Scott JR, Scardo JA, Hendrix NW, Martin JN. Cesarean delivery for foetal distress: rate and risk factors. Obstet Gynecol Surv. 2003;58(5):337-50.

23. Hendrix NW, Chauhan SP. Cesarean delivery for nonreassuring foetal heart rate tracing. Obstet Gynecol Clin North Am. 2005;32(2):273-86.

24. James D. Caesarean section for foetal distress. BMJ. 2001;322 (7298):1316-7.

25. Bax M, Goldstein M, Rosenbaum P, Leviton A, Paneth N. Proposed definition and classification of cerebral palsy, April 2005. Dev Med Child Neurol. 2005;47(8):571-6.

26. Hall DM. Birth asphyxia and cerebral palsy. BMJ. 1989;299 (6694):279-82.

27. Levene MI, Sands C, Grindulis H, Moore JR. Comparison of 2 methods of predicting outcome in perinatal asphyxia. Lancet. 1986;1(8472):67-9.

28. Himmelmann K, Hagberg G, Beckung E, Hagberg B, Uvebrant P. The changing panorama of cerebral palsy in Sweden. IX. Prevalence and origin in the birth-year period 1995-1998. Acta Paediatr. 2005;94(3):287-94.

29. Blair E, Stanley FJ. Intrapartum asphyxia: a rare cause of cerebral palsy. J Pediatr. 1988;112(4):515-9.

30. Badawi N, Kurinczuk JJ, Keogh JM, Alessandri LM, O'Sullivan F, Burton PR, et al. Intrapartum risk factors for newborn encephalopathy: The Western Australian case-control study. BMJ. 1998;317(7172):1554-8.

31. Adamson SJ, Alessandri LM, Badawi N, Burton PR, Pemberton PJ, Stanley F. Predictors of neonatal encephalopathy in full term infants. BMJ. 1995;311(7005):598-602.

32. Nelson KB, Leviton A. How much of neonatal encephalopathy is due to birth asphyxia? Am J Dis Child. 1991;145(11):1325-31.

33. Berger R, Garnier Y. Pathophysiology of perinatal brain damage. Brain Res Brain Res Rev. 1999;30(2):107-34.

34. De Haan HH, Hasaart TH. Neuronal death after perinatal asphyxia. Eur J Obstet Gynecol Reprod Biol. 1995;61(2):123-7.

35. Depp R. Perinatal asphyxia: assessing its causal role and timing. Semin Pediatr Neurol. 1995;2(1):3-36.

36. Papile LA, Rudolph AM, Heymann MA. Autoregulation of cerebral blood flow in the preterm foetal lamb. Pediatr Res. 1985;19(2):159-61.

37. Patel J, Edwards AD. Prediction of outcome after perinatal asphyxia. Curr Opin Pediatr. 1997;9(2):128-32.

38. Sarnat HB, Sarnat MS. Neonatal encephalopathy following foetal distress: a clinical and electroencephalographic study. Arch Neurol. 1976;33(10):696-705.

39. Vannucci RC, Perlman JM. Interventions for perinatal hypoxic-ischemic encephalopathy. Pediatrics. 1997;100(6):1004-14.

40. Hall RT, Hall FK, Daily DK. High-dose phenobarbital therapy in term newborn infants with severe perinatal asphyxia: a randomized, prospective study with three-year follow-up. J Pediatr. 1998;132(2):345-8.

41. Thorngren-Jerneck K, Alling C, Herbst A, Amer-Wahlin I, Marsal K. S100 protein in serum as a prognostic marker for cerebral injury in term newborn infants with hypoxic ischemic encephalopathy. Pediatr Res. 2004;55(3):406-12.

42. Shankaran S, Laptook AR, Ehrenkranz RA, Tyson JE, McDonald SA, Donovan EF, et al. Wholebody hypothermia for neonates with hypoxic-ischemic encephalopathy. N Engl J Med. 2005;353(15):1574-84.

43. Gluckman PD, Wyatt JS, Azzopardi D, Ballard R, Edwards AD, Ferriero DM, et al. Selective head cooling with mild systemic hypothermia after neonatal encephalopathy: multicenter randomised trial. Lancet. 2005;365(9460):663-70.

44. Young DC, Popat R, Luther ER, Scott KE, Writer WD. Influence of maternal oxygen administration on the term fetus before labor. Am J Obstet Gynecol. 1980;136(3):321-4.

45. Ramanathan S, Gandhi S, Arismendy J, Chalon J, Turndorf H. Oxygen transfer from mother to fetus during cesarean section under epidural anesthesia. Anesth Analg. 1982;61(7):576-81.

CHAPTER 49

SECTION 9

Postpartum Period

OBSTETRICS

Postpartum Haemorrhage and Postpartum Collapse

POSTPARTUM HAEMORRHAGE

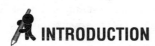 **INTRODUCTION**

According to the World Health Organization, postpartum haemorrhage (PPH) can be defined as excessive blood loss per vaginum (>500 mL in case of normal vaginal delivery or >1,000 mL following a caesarean section) from the time period extending within 24 hours of delivery and lasting until the end of the puerperium.[1] PPH is described as minor when there is blood loss between 500 mL to 1,000 mL or as major when there is blood loss of more than 1,000 mL. Major PPH can be further divided as moderate where the blood loss is between 1,000 mL to 2,000 mL or severe where blood loss is more than 2,000 mL. The ACOG has defined PPH as a decrease in haematocrit by 10% or requirement of blood transfusion 24 hours after the delivery. The WHO has classified PPH into two categories: (1) primary PPH and (2) secondary PPH. Primary PPH can be defined as blood loss, estimated to be greater than 500 mL, occurring from the genital tract, within 24 hours of delivery. Secondary PPH, on the other hand, can be defined as abnormal bleeding from the genital tract, occurring 24 hours after delivery until 6 weeks postpartum.[2]

According to the UK CEMD 2003-2005 report, obstetric haemorrhage was identified as the third highest direct cause of maternal death. It was responsible for 6.6 deaths per million maternities. This rate was almost similar to that in the previous triennium.[3,4] Majority of maternal deaths due to haemorrhage in the UK were due to substandard care and therefore were largely considered as preventable. The CEMD 2009-2012 report showed that in nearly 61% cases of maternal death due to PPH, the severity of PPH was not identified. This has highlighted the importance of correlating clinical signs and symptoms with the severity of PPH.

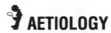 **AETIOLOGY**

The mnemonic '4 Ts' (tone, trauma, tissue and thrombin) helps in describing the four important causes of PPH, which are enumerated in Table 50.1.

Table 50.1: Causes of postpartum haemorrhage

Causes	Description
Tone: Atonic uterus (most common cause)	Overdistension of uterus, induction of labour, prolonged/precipitate labour, anaesthesia (use of halogenated drugs like halothane), analgesia, grand multiparity, placenta praevia, use of uterine relaxants, previous history of PPH, etc.
Trauma	Large episiotomy and extensions, tears and lacerations of perineum, vagina or cervix, pelvic haematomas, uterine inversion, ruptured uterus, etc.
Tissue	Retained placental fragments, retained products of conception, invasive placenta
Thrombin	Drugs (e.g. aspirin, heparin, warfarin, alcohol, chemotherapy), liver diseases, severe vitamin K deficiency, Von Willebrand's disease, haemophilia, pre-eclampsia, placental abruption, coagulopathies, DIC, etc.

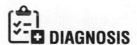 **DIAGNOSIS**

Clinical Presentation

General Physical Examination

❖ Features of shock, such as hypotension and tachycardia, may be present. Clinicians should be aware that the visual estimation of peripartum blood loss may be inaccurate and assessment of severity of PPH should take into consideration the patient's signs and symptoms, especially the symptoms of hypovolaemia.

Abdominal Examination

On abdominal palpation, the uterus may appear to be atonic.

Per Speculum Examination

- ❖ Bleeding through the cervical os may be observed.
- ❖ Tears or lacerations of the genital tract (particularly vagina and cervix), which may be responsible for bleeding, may be visualised.

Investigations

- ❖ Complete blood count with peripheral smear
- ❖ *Coagulation profile*: Platelet count, PT, APTT, thrombin time, etc.
- ❖ Urine analysis (for haematuria)
- ❖ *High vaginal swab*: To rule out infection (especially gonorrhoea, chlamydia, etc.)
- ❖ *Transabdominal or transvaginal ultrasound*: Ultrasound examination may especially, be required if retained products of conception are suspected.

MANAGEMENT

Antenatal Period

- ❖ Women having low haemoglobin levels (<11 g/dL) in the antenatal period should be investigated and aptly treated to optimise haemoglobin levels prior to delivery.
- ❖ Iron-deficiency anaemia should be corrected prior to delivery because depleted uterine myoglobin levels can contribute to atony because myoglobin is essential for muscle action.
- ❖ Women with a history of previous caesarean section must have their placental site determined by ultrasound examination. MRI can be used, where facilities are available, in women at risk of placenta accreta, increta or percreta. Such women are at very high risk of major PPH.[5] In such cases, delivery must be managed by consultant-led multidisciplinary team. Before undertaking delivery, the obstetrician should confirm the availability of blood, fresh frozen plasma (FFP) and platelets.

Intrapartum Period

- ❖ Most mothers in the UK are able to cope up with a blood loss between 500 mL to 1,000 mL.[6,7] In these cases, basic measures such as close monitoring, IV access, full blood count and blood grouping and screening must be initiated. Protocol of emergency measures to achieve resuscitation and haemostasis should be started if the estimated loss becomes more than 1,000 mL.[8]
- ❖ Active management of the third stage of labour involving the use of interventions (such as the use of uterotonics, early clamping of the umbilical cord and controlled cord traction to expedite delivery of the placenta) are likely to help reduce the blood loss.[9,10] Delayed clamping of cord for

at least 2 minutes is likely to be beneficial for the newborn baby. This benefit is also likely to extend into the infancy. Therefore, NICE guidelines recommend that the umbilical cord should not be clamped earlier than 1 minute from delivery of the baby, provided that there are no concerns over cord integrity or the baby's well-being.[11]

- ❖ Prophylactic oxytocics should be offered routinely in the management of the third stage of labour in all women. Intramuscular oxytocin (5 IU or 10 IU) is the agent of choice for prophylaxis in the third stage of labour for women delivering vaginally.[12] For women delivering by caesarean section, NICE has recommended that oxytocin in the dose of 5 IU be administered by slow IV injection following the delivery of placenta to help reduce the amount of blood loss.[11] Use of IV tranexamic acid (0.5–1.0 g) can be considered in addition to oxytocin, at the time of caesarean section in women at increased risk of PPH to reduce the amount of blood loss.
- ❖ Syntometrine® (Alliance), combination of ergometrine-oxytocin in the dose of 500 mL, helps in reducing the risk of minor PPH. However, there may be an increased risk of vomiting or increased blood pressure. Therefore, before using Syntometrine, the advantage of a reduction in the risk of PPH must be weighed against the risk of adverse effects associated with its use.[13]
- ❖ Misoprostol (600 µg orally) can be used in cases where oxytocin is not available, e.g. home-birth settings. However, it is not as effective as oxytocin.[14]
- ❖ Carbetocin, an 8 amino acid long analogue of oxytocin, is licensed in the UK specifically for the prevention of PPH in the cases of caesarean delivery. Cochrane review has shown high efficacy of carbetocin in the prevention of PPH.[15]
- ❖ According to the guidelines by the Scottish Executive Committee of the RCOG, the immediate management in case with PPH comprises of steps that are enumerated in Box 50.1,[16] all of which may be required to be undertaken simultaneously. These steps mainly comprise of the following components: communication with all significant professionals; patient's resuscitation; monitoring and investigation; and measures to stop the bleeding. In case of major PPH with continuing bleeding, a consultant obstetrician should be alerted and should normally attend the delivery unit to provide hands-on care to the patient. Communication with the patient and her birthing partner is also important and clear information of the events must be provided to them. According to the guidelines from the British Committee for Standards in Haematology (2006), the main therapeutic goals for resuscitation in case of massive blood loss are summarised in Box 50.2.[17]
- ❖ While awaiting the results of coagulation studies, up to 1 L of FFP and 10 units of cryoprecipitate may be administered empirically.[18]
- ❖ Once the patient has been stabilised, next step of management depends on whether the placenta has delivered or not (Flow chart 50.1).

PART II

Box 50.1: Steps involved in the immediate management of patients with postpartum haemorrhage

- ❑ Communicate (call for additional staff to manage the obstetric emergency)
- ❑ Resuscitation of the patient (evaluation of ABC: Airway, Breathing and Circulation)
- ❑ Blood to be sent for typing and cross-matching. Blood transfusion can be considered in these cases
- ❑ Administration of oxygen via a face mask
- ❑ The woman should be kept in a flat position and should be kept warm using appropriate available measures
- ❑ Establishment of IV access (via a 14-gauge cannula) and infusion of crystalloids. Until blood is available, up to 3.5 L of clear fluid (up to 2 L of warmed crystalloid Hartmann's solution) and/or colloid (1.5 L) must be infused as rapidly as required
- ❑ Special blood filters should not be used because they are likely to slow down the infusions
- ❑ Blood must be transfused as soon as possible (cross-matched blood is preferably used; if it is unavailable, uncross-matched group-specific blood or 'O RhD negative' blood can be transfused
- ❑ Monitoring the patient
- ❑ Identifying and treating the underlying cause of bleeding
- ❑ *Blood coagulation studies*: Recombinant factor VIIa therapy can be used based on the results of coagulation (dosage of 90 μg/kg, which may be repeated within 15–30 minutes)[16]
- ❑ Use of uterotonics to control the bleeding

Box 50.2: Therapeutic goals for resuscitation in case of massive blood loss[16]

- ❑ Haemoglobin >8 g/dL
- ❑ Platelet count >75 × 10⁹/L (platelets concentrates must be administered if platelet count <50 × 10⁹)
- ❑ Prothrombin <1.5 × mean control
- ❑ Activated prothrombin time <1.5 × mean control
- ❑ Fibrinogen >1.0 g/L (cryoprecipitate must be administered if fibrinogen level <1 g/L)
- ❑ Four units of fresh frozen plasma must be administered for every six units of red cells transfused or prothrombin time/activated partial thromboplastin time >1.5 × normal (12–15 mL/kg or total 1 L)

Management of Atonic Uterus

❖ If the placenta has delivered, but the uterus is not hard and contracted, instead appears to be atonic and flabby, the PPH is of atonic type. In this case, the following steps need to be carried out:
  - The urinary bladder must be emptied
  - The uterine cavity must be explored for any retained placental bits
  - The vagina and cervix must be still inspected for presence of lacerations and tears (traumatic PPH is commonly present in association with atonic PPH)
  - Repeat administration of uterotonics
  - *Bimanual uterine massage*: If the clinician finds the uterus to be soft upon bimanual examination, a bimanual uterine massage must be performed to contract the myometrial muscles. The manoeuvre involves the massage of the posterior aspect of the uterus with the abdominal hand and that of the anterior aspect of the uterus with the vaginal hand (Fig. 50.1). Though bimanual uterine massage is commonly being performed for the management of atonic uterus, the recent-most green-top guidelines by the RCOG (December, 2016) for prevention and management of PPH, have shown limited scope of uterine massage for further reduction in postpartum blood loss, once an oxytocic agent has been administered.[19]

- If the above-mentioned steps are unable to control the PPH, medical methods must be used. Medical management of PPH includes use of uterotonic agents such as oxytocin (Syntocinon), ergot alkaloids (methyl ergometrine), prostaglandin analogues (misoprostol), recombinant factor VIIa (rFVIIa), etc. (Table 50.2).

❖ In UK settings where women with PPH require transfer from midwife-led to consultant-led units, use of a non-pneumatic antishock garment may be helpful.

❖ Surgical management becomes necessary if the uterus remains atonic and flabby despite of conservative or medical management. First-line 'surgical' intervention for most women where uterine atony is the only or main cause of haemorrhage is intrauterine balloon tamponade. Balloon tamponade can be attempted using a Foley catheter,[20] Bakri balloon,[21] Sengstaken-Blakemore oesophageal catheter,[22,23] condom catheter[24] or the urological Rusch balloon.[25] Prior to the initiation of uterine tamponade, tamponade test can be performed to assess the effectiveness of tamponade. In this test, a catheter is inserted into the uterine cavity via the cervix, using ultrasound guidance when possible, and filled with warm saline until the distended balloon is palpable per abdomen. The balloon is to be surrounded by the well-contracted uterus and must be visible at the lower portion of the cervical canal. Test is considered as positive if there is no or only minimal bleeding via the cervical canal. Cases where tamponade test is positive, uterine tamponade is likely to be successful and no further surgical intervention or hysterectomy is usually required. On the other hand, if significant bleeding continues via the cervix, the tamponade test can be considered as a failure and other surgical interventions must be performed. There is no clear evidence regarding the time duration for which the balloon tamponade should be left in place. In most cases, 4–6 hours of tamponade is usually sufficient in achieving haemostasis. Preferably, it should be removed during daytime hours, in the presence of appropriate senior staff, because further intervention may be required in case bleeding still occurs.[21,22]

❖ If uterine tamponade fails to stop the bleeding, the following conservative surgical interventions may be attempted, depending on clinical circumstances and available expertise:
  - Application of aortal compression at the time of surgery
  - *Haemostatic brace sutures*: Brace sutures of uterus (B-lynch compression sutures) may be particularly suitable when the uterus has already been opened

Flow chart 50.1: Management of postpartum haemorrhage

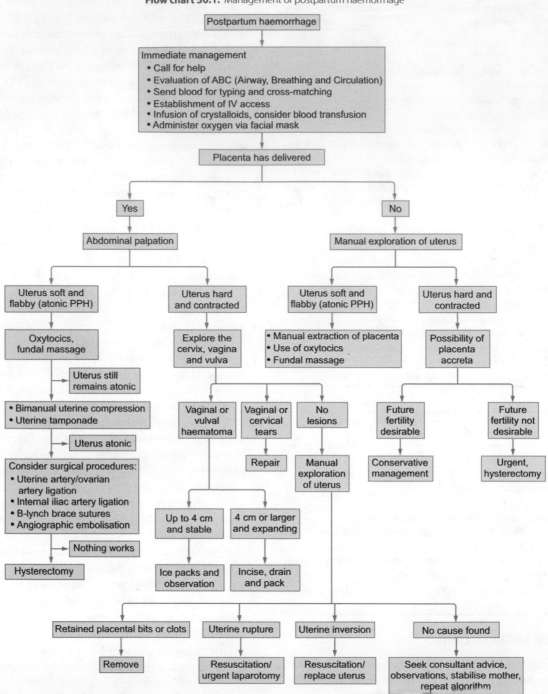

at caesarean section (Fig. 50.2). Besides the B-lynch compression sutures, several other techniques have also been described by various researchers. In a technique of modified compression sutures described by Hayman et al. (2002), there is no requirement for hysterotomy as required by the B-lynch technique (Fig. 50.3).[26] Some observational studies[27-29] suggest that haemostatic suture techniques are effective in controlling severe PPH and in reducing the requirement for hysterectomy. However, presently, there is no study to indicate the superiority of one technique over the other. Obstetricians are encouraged to familiarise themselves with one technique,

under the guidance of an experienced colleague. It is recommended that a laminated diagram of the brace technique must be kept in operation theatre. Presently, there is limited experience with the technique and few complications have been by far reported.

- Uterine artery or utero-ovarian artery ligation (Fig. 50.4)
- Bilateral ligation of internal iliac (hypogastric arteries) (Figs 50.5A to C)
- Angiographic embolisation
- *Hysterectomy (as a last option if nothing seems to work)*: A second consultant clinician should be preferably involved while taking the decision for hysterectomy.

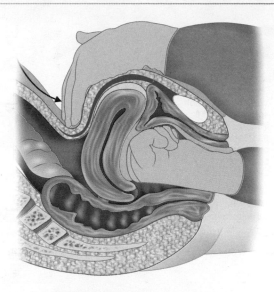

Fig. 50.1: Bimanual uterine compression

Table 50.2: Various oxytocics used for controlling postpartum haemorrhage

Drug	Dosage	Side effects	Contraindications
Oxytocin	5 units of oxytocin may be administered by slow IV injection (dosage may be repeated if required) or it can be given as Syntocinon infusion (40 units in 500 mL Hartmann's solution at 125 mL/h). When administered as an IV bolus, oxytocin should be given slowly in a dose of not more than 5 units	Water intoxication and nausea at high dosage	Nil
Methylergometrine (methergine)	0.5 mg by slow intramuscular or IV injection	Nausea, vomiting, hypertension, retained placenta, if given before placental separation occurs	Hypertension, heart disease
Carboprost (15-methyl PGF2α)	250 µg given as intramuscular injection, not less than every 15 minutes for a maximum of 8 doses. Carboprost can be given via direct intramyometrial injection in the dosage of 0.5 mg	Diarrhoea, vomiting, flushing, pyrexia, hypertension, bronchoconstriction, etc.	Significant pulmonary disease (asthma), cardiac, hepatic or renal disease
Misoprostol	600–1,000 µg per rectally or orally Dose and frequency have yet not been standardised	Diarrhoea, pyrexia (>40°C)	Significant pulmonary, cardiac, hepatic or renal disease

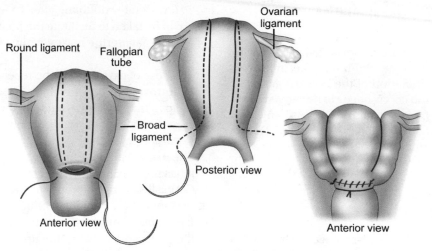

Fig. 50.2: B-lynch suture

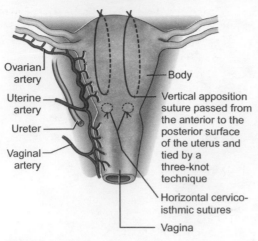

Fig. 50.3: Application of the Hayman compression suture

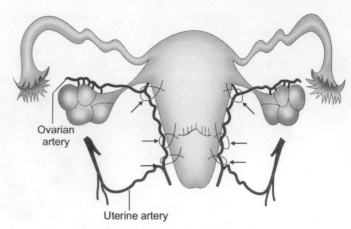

Fig. 50.4: Various sites of uterine artery ligation

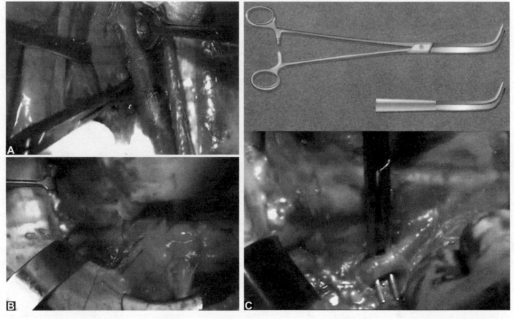

Figs 50.5A to C: Process of internal iliac artery ligation: (A) Dissection of the retroperitoneal tissues to identify the internal iliac artery; (B) Mixter's forceps and placement of Mixter's forceps around the internal iliac artery; (C) The ligation of internal iliac artery *(For colour version, see Plate 3)*

Repair of Vaginal and Perineal Injuries

The perineal and vaginal injuries commonly occur during the process of childbirth and are important causes of PPH. Since traumatic injury to the genital tract is an important cause of PPH, careful examination of the external genitalia, vulva, perineum, vagina and cervix needs to be carried out in good light to rule out any tears or injuries. In case any tears or lacerations are present, these need to be repaired. Details related to the repair of perineal injuries have been described in Chapter 48 (Perineal Injuries).

The Placenta has yet not Delivered or Non-adherent Placenta

The mean time from delivery until placental expulsion is 8–9 minutes. Longer intervals are associated with an increased risk

of PPH, with rates doubling after 10 minutes. The following steps can be taken to facilitate the placental delivery:

1. A maternal uterine massage must be performed to expel any clot.
2. The dose of oxytocics can be repeated, e.g. syntocinon 10 IU intravenous or 10 IU intramuscular. Ergometrine or syntometrine must be avoided for retained placenta because they may cause tonic uterine contraction, which may delay expulsion.
3. The urinary bladder must be emptied by catheterising if it has previously not been done.
4. Controlled cord traction must be repeated to deliver the placenta.
5. If possible a portable ultrasound scan must be done to see if the placenta is still in the upper segment or whether it has separated and is in the lower segment of the uterus.

6. If the placenta appears to be trapped in the lower uterine segment, a vaginal examination must be performed to remove the placenta and other clots.

7. Injection to the umbilical vein with 20 mL solution of 0.9% saline and 20 units of oxytocin significantly helps in reducing the need for manual removal of the placenta in comparison with injection of saline alone.

8. If the placenta does not deliver even within 30 minutes of the delivery of the baby, the patient must be taken to the operation theatre for manual exploration of placenta under general anaesthesia. Further clinical management depends on whether or not a distinct cleavage plane between the placenta and the uterine wall can be located or not. If a distinct cleavage plane between the placenta and the uterine wall can be located, management options include manual removal of the placenta, using appropriate analgesia.

Adherent Placenta

If a distinct cleavage plane between the placenta and the uterine wall cannot be located and if the tissue plane between the uterine wall and placenta cannot be developed through blunt dissection with the edge of the gloved hand, diagnosis of invasive or adherent placenta should be considered.

Invasive placenta can be a life-threatening condition. The incidence has increased from 0.003% to 0.04% of deliveries since 1950s; this increase is likely as a result of an increase in caesarean section rates. Adherent placenta can be classified into three categories: (1) placenta accreta; (2) placenta increta; and (3) placenta percreta. In placenta accreta, the abnormally firm attachment of the placenta to the uterine wall prevents the placenta from separating normally after delivery. The retained placenta interferes with uterine contraction that is necessary to control bleeding after delivery, thereby resulting in PPH. Several risk factors for placenta accreta have been identified. Among these, the most important one appears to be placenta praevia. For details related to placenta praevia, kindly refer to Chapter 25 (Antepartum Haemorrhage).

In patients with placenta praevia the incidence of placenta accreta appears to correlate with the number of previous caesarean sections. Maternal age greater than 35 years and placental location overlying the previous uterine scar also increases the risk of accreta. Other reported risk factors include multiple previous pregnancies, previous uterine surgery and previous dilatation and curettage (D&C). In a patient with a previous caesarean section and a placenta praevia, the risk of placenta accreta is dependent upon the number of previous caesarean sections as follows:

❖ Woman with previous one caesarean section has 14% risk of placenta accreta.
❖ Woman with previous two caesarean sections has a 24% risk of placenta accreta.
❖ Woman with previous three caesarean sections has 44% risk of placenta accreta.

Management of an Adherent Placenta

Conservative management: The conservative management comprises of the following steps that are described next.

1. In case of densely adherent placenta, the clinician must not try to remove any non-adherent portions of the placenta.
2. The cord can be trimmed.
3. The patient's vital signs and amount of bleeding should be closely observed.
4. Antibiotics should be administered.
5. In the woman who is stable, hysterectomy may be avoided by the use of methotrexate.

Surgical management: If the bleeding remains uncontrolled despite of using conservative management, the following surgical options can be used:

❖ Uterine artery embolisation
❖ Low and high bilateral uterine vessel ligation
❖ Ligation of internal iliac arteries.

If the above-mentioned surgical options are unable to control the haemorrhage, hysterectomy is the only choice left to save the woman's life.

Management of Secondary Postpartum Haemorrhage

The most common cause for secondary PPH is presence of retained tissue fragments inside the uterine cavity. Treatment of secondary PPH involves the following:

❖ Stabilisation of the patient; blood may be transfused if required.
❖ *Administration of antibiotics*: Secondary PPH is often associated with endometritis. When antibiotics are clinically indicated, a combination of ampicillin and metronidazole is usually appropriate.[30] In cases where the patient is allergic to penicillin, clindamycin can be administered in place of ampicillin. This antibiotic therapy combination also does not contraindicate breastfeeding. The addition of gentamicin is recommended where there is endomyometritis (tender uterus) or overt sepsis.
❖ In women presenting with secondary PPH, high vaginal and endocervical swabs for the assessment of vaginal microbiology may be required. A pelvic ultrasound is commonly performed which may help in excluding the presence of retained products of conception. However, this may not always be reliable.
❖ *Surgical evacuation of the retained products of conception*: Surgical measures may nevertheless be required if there is excessive or continuing bleeding, irrespective of ultrasound findings. A senior obstetrician should be involved in the decision-making process. Evacuation of retained products of conception must also be done by the senior obstetrician because these women are associated with a high risk for uterine perforation.

COMPLICATIONS

Postpartum haemorrhage is one of the important causes of maternal morbidity and mortality. Some of the complications are as follows:

❖ Blood loss resulting in shock, DIC
❖ Septicaemia and death
❖ Renal failure

- Puerperal sepsis; failure of lactation
- Blood transfusion reaction, thromboembolism, Sheehan's syndrome, hypovolemic shock, puerperal shock and multiple organ failure associated with circulatory collapse and decreased organ perfusion.

CLINICAL PEARLS

- Visual estimation of peripartum blood loss may be inaccurate. Therefore, the healthcare professionals must make use of the patient's clinical signs and symptoms for assessing the cases of PPH.
- Presently, there are no firm criteria for initiating red cell transfusion in cases of PPH. Blood transfusion is usually initiated based on both clinical and haematological assessment.
- The routine use of rFVIIa is not recommended for the management of major PPH, except in research settings.
- For control of major PPH, clinicians may have to resort to hysterectomy sooner rather than later, especially in cases of placenta accreta or uterine rupture.
- Every maternity unit should have a multidisciplinary protocol for the management of PPH. All staff involved in maternity care should receive training in the management of various obstetric emergencies, including management of PPH. Regular drills and team rehearsals must be conducted to train the healthcare professionals in the management of PPH. A formal clinical incident review must be done in all cases of PPH involving a blood loss of greater than 1,500 mL.
- Both active management and the use of prophylactic uterotonics in the third stage of labour help in reducing the risk of PPH.

EVIDENCE-BASED MEDICINE

- Present evidence has shown that the active management of third stage of labour (including the use of a uterotonic agents, usually 0.25 mg of methergine or ergometrine 0.2 mg) soon after the delivery of the anterior shoulder and/or oxytocin 10 IU within 1 minute of birth of the baby; clamping of the umbilical cord within the first minute of life; uterine massage after birth and before or after delivery of the placenta, or both and controlled cord traction or Brandt-Andrews manoeuvre to deliver the placenta (Fig. 50.6) has been associated with reduced maternal blood loss and lower risk of PPH. However, active management is also associated with an increased risk of side effects such as nausea, vomiting and raised blood pressure. Therefore, the most important step, which must routinely be used in the third stage for prevention of PPH, is the active management of third stage of labour.[9,10]
- Presently, there is limited evidence regarding the efficacy of prophylactic arterial catheterisation with the view

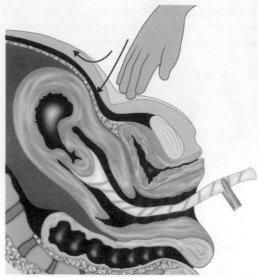

Fig. 50.6: Method of controlled cord traction. This involves applying firm traction on the umbilical cord with one hand and suprapubic counter-pressure with the other hand

of balloon occlusion or embolisation of pelvic arteries (e.g. internal iliac arteries, anterior division of internal iliac or uterine arteries) for control of PPH in cases of antenatally diagnosed placenta accreta.[31-37] Use of arterial embolisation has been found to be beneficial in controlling primary as well as secondary PPH. Till there is availability of further evidence, these techniques can be considered in units where appropriate facilities are available.

- Cell salvage can be described as the process in which the blood shed during an operation is collected, filtered and washed to produce autologous RBCs, which are then transfused to the patient. The presently available evidence supports the use of cell salvage in cases of obstetric haemorrhage. This therapy is likely to become increasingly common in future. However, further studies are required concerning its clinical use.[38] Intraoperative cell salvage may be a useful technique in women who refuse blood or blood products (Jehovah's Witnesses) or in patients where massive blood loss is anticipated (e.g. placenta percreta or accreta).

POSTPARTUM COLLAPSE

Maternal collapse is defined by RCOG as an acute event involving the cardiorespiratory systems and/or brain, which leads to a reduced or an absent level of consciousness (and potentially death) in the immediate postpartum period or up to 6 weeks postdelivery.[39] The UK Obstetric Surveillance System (UKOSS), run by the National Perinatal Epidemiology Unit (NPEU), plays a vital role in the study of rare events and maternal morbidity during pregnancy. Severe maternal morbidity event has been defined as an event associated with a high risk for maternal death without timely intervention.[40] Some cases of maternal morbidity may involve maternal collapse during the postpartum period. Though it is a rare event (rate varying between 0.14 to 6 per 1,000 births), it can

PART II

Table 50.3: Differential diagnosis of postpartum collapse

Obstetric causes	Non-obstetric causes	Anaesthetic causes
• Acute obstetric haemorrhage (antepartum haemorrhage, PPH) • Placental abruption • Atonicity of the uterus • Rupture of the uterus • Pre-eclampsia or eclampsia • Peripartum cardiomyopathy	• Vasovagal attacks • Postictal state (following an epileptic seizure) • Pulmonary embolism • Air embolism • Anaphylaxis • Aspiration • Aortic dissection • Sepsis/septic shock • Cardiac arrhythmias • Cerebrovascular accident	• High spinal anaesthesia • Aspiration • Local anaesthetic toxicity • Drug toxicity ($MgSO_4$, eclampsia, etc.)

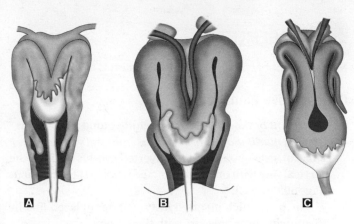

Figs 50.7A to C: Degrees of uterine inversion (A) first degree; (B) second degree and (C) third degree

have potentially devastating consequences and may at times precede death. Therefore, the healthcare providers must be skilled in the initial effective resuscitation techniques. They must also be able to investigate and diagnose the cause of the collapse, thereby enabling appropriate management. Various causes of postpartum collapse are described in Table 50.3. The most common non-obstetric causes of maternal collapse include vasovagal attacks and the postictal state following an epileptic seizure. The potentially preventable life-threatening obstetric causes of postpartum collapse, such as uterine inversion, amniotic fluid embolism and pulmonary embolism are discussed next.

UTERINE INVERSION

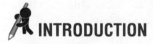 **INTRODUCTION**

Uterine inversion during the acute postpartum period is a relatively rare complication in which the uterus is turned inside out either partially or completely.[41] The uterine endometrium with or without attached placenta may be visible. Uterine inversion can be classified as follows (Figs 50.7A to C):
- *First degree*: Dimpling of the uterine fundus which remains well above the level of internal os.
- *Second degree*: Uterine fundus passes through the cervix, but lies inside the vagina.
- *Third degree (complete)*: The uterus protrudes completely out of the vaginal introitus. The uterine endometrium with or without the attached placenta may be visible.

In terms of onset of the inversion, it can be classified as acute, subacute and chronic.

AETIOLOGY

The exact aetiology behind uterus inversion remains unclear. The most likely factors include the following:
- Spontaneous prolapse is commonly associated with a sharp rise in intra-abdominal pressure accompanied with uterine atony

- Strong traction on the umbilical cord, particularly when the placenta is in a fundal location, during the third stage of labour
- Placenta accreta, particularly involving the uterine fundus
- Short umbilical cord
- Antepartum use of magnesium sulphate or oxytocin
- *Iatrogenic causes*: Mismanaged third stage of labour, pulling the cord, Crede's method of placental delivery, application of fundal pressure in an atonic uterus.

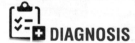 **DIAGNOSIS**

Clinical Presentation

- Severe hypotension with shock
- Acute pain in the lower abdomen with bearing down sensation.

Abdominal Examination

Absence of uterine fundus or presence of an obvious defect of the fundus upon abdominal palpation.

Bimanual Examination

Bimanual examination helps in conforming the diagnosis and degree of prolapse and reveals the features described next:
- Profuse bleeding through the cervical os
- Palpation of the inverted fundus at the cervical os or vaginal introitus
- In cases of incomplete inversion, the fundal wall may be palpated in the lower uterine segment and cervix.

Investigations

- *Ultrasound*: On transverse scans, a hyperechoic mass in the vagina with a central hypoechoic H-shaped cavity may be visualised. A depressed longitudinal groove, extending from the uterine fundus to the centre of the inverted part may be observed on longitudinal scans.
- *Magnetic resonance imaging*: Appearance of the uterus is similar to that found in sonographic imaging; however, MRI findings are much more accurate.

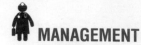

MANAGEMENT

Management of cases of uterine inversion is as follows:[42,43]

Conservative Management

❖ *Treatment of shock*: This may include blood transfusion.
❖ *Manual manipulation of the uterus (Johnson's manoeuvre)*: This consists of pushing the inverted fundus through the cervical ring with pressure directed towards the umbilicus (Figs 50.8A to C):
  • The part which inverted last must be replaced first by applying firm pressure with the fingers.
  • Counter-pressure must be applied by the hand placed over the abdomen.
  • Following the replacement, hand must remain inside the vagina until the uterus is contracted.
  • Following uterine replacement, the vagina must be packed with antiseptic roller gauze and the foot end of the bed must be elevated.
❖ *Use of pharmacological agents*: Most commonly used uterine relaxants comprise of magnesium sulphate or terbutaline. In extreme cases, IV nitroglycerine or general anaesthetic agent, such as halothane, can also be used.
❖ Use of oxytocic agents must be withheld if the diagnosis of uterine inversion is made.
❖ *O'Sullivan's method*: Use of hydrostatic pressure to correct the inversion.

Surgical Management

Surgical intervention may be required if conservative management is unsuccessful.

❖ *Huntington procedure*: A laparotomy is performed to locate the cup of the uterus. Gentle traction is applied in an upward direction after placing the clamps in the cup of the inversion below the cervical ring. Repeated clamping and traction must be continued until the inversion is corrected.

❖ *Haultain procedure*: An incision is made in the posterior portion of the inversion ring through the abdomen, to increase the size of the ring and allow repositioning of the uterus.

COMPLICATIONS

❖ Postpartum haemorrhage and shock[44]
❖ Maternal death
❖ Pulmonary embolism
❖ Untreated cases may develop infection and/or sloughing.

CLINICAL PEARLS

❖ Uterine inversion can be a life-threatening obstetric complication, which must be treated like an obstetric emergency.
❖ The best prognosis is achieved by prompt recognition of the condition and immediate attempts to correct the inversion.

AMNIOTIC FLUID EMBOLISM

INTRODUCTION

Amniotic fluid embolism is a catastrophic syndrome occurring during labour and delivery or in the immediate postpartum period. This condition occurs when amniotic fluid, foetal cells, hair or other debris enter the maternal circulation via the placental bed of the uterus and trigger an allergic reaction. This reaction then results in cardiorespiratory collapse and DIC.

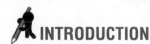

AETIOLOGY

The pathophysiology of amniotic fluid embolism is presented in Flow chart 50.2.[45]

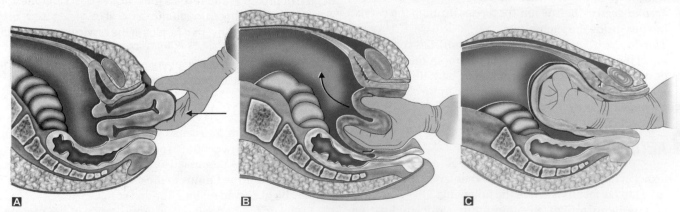

Figs 50.8A to C: Reduction of uterine inversion using Johnson's method. (A) The protruding fundus is grasped with fingers directed towards the posterior fornix; (B and C) The uterus is returned to position by pushing it through by steady application of pressure towards the fundus

PART II

Flow chart 50.2: Pathophysiology of amniotic fluid embolism

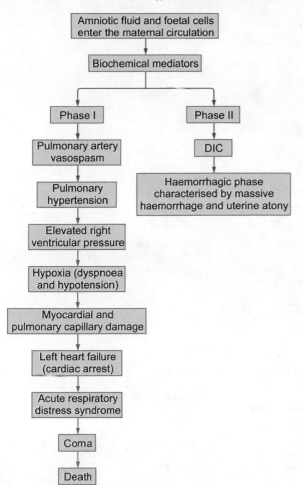

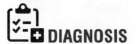 **DIAGNOSIS**

The diagnosis of amniotic fluid embolism is one of exclusions and is based on the assessment of symptoms and clinical course, and not on the basis of laboratory or pathology findings.[46]

Clinical Presentation

- ❖ Dyspnoea
- ❖ Non-reassuring foetal status (in case of pregnant women)
- ❖ Altered mental status followed by sudden cardiovascular collapse
- ❖ Profound respiratory failure with deep cyanosis
- ❖ Cardiovascular shock
- ❖ Convulsions and profound coma
- ❖ Disseminated intravascular coagulation and maternal death.

Investigations

- ❖ *Echocardiography*: This helps in evaluating cardiac function and intravascular volume status.
- ❖ *Electrocardiography*: This may show a right strain pattern with changes in ST segment and T-waves, and tachycardia.

- ❖ *Complete blood count*: Complete blood count including the coagulation parameters such as PT, APTT, FDP and fibrinogen levels may be required.
- ❖ Arterial blood gases
- ❖ Chest X-ray
- ❖ Ventilation-perfusion scanning.

 MANAGEMENT

Management in cases of amniotic fluid embolism is as follows:[46,47]

- ❖ The goals of management are to restore cardiovascular and pulmonary equilibrium by maintaining the systolic blood pressure greater than 90 mmHg; urine output greater than 25 mL/h and arterial pO_2 greater than 60 mmHg.
- ❖ In case of uterine atony, efforts must be made to re-establish uterine tone.
- ❖ Efforts must be made to correct coagulation abnormalities.
- ❖ Control of the airway is done with tracheal intubation and administration of 100% O_2 with positive-pressure ventilation.
- ❖ Venous access must be maintained with large bore IV catheters.
- ❖ Infusion of crystalloids must be started to treat hypotension, increase the circulating volume and cardiac output. Dopamine infusion may be started if patient still remains hypotensive.
- ❖ An immediate caesarean delivery is required in patients who have yet not delivered.
- ❖ *Blood and blood products*: This may include use of FFP, platelets, cryoprecipitate, rFVIIa, etc. Cryoprecipitate must be administered for a fibrinogen level less than 100 mg/dL, and platelet transfusion given for platelet count less than 20,000/mm³.

 COMPLICATIONS

- ❖ *High maternal and foetal morbidity and mortality*: Various causes of maternal death include sudden cardiac arrest, DIC, acute respiratory distress syndrome, multiple organ failure, etc. European guidelines for resuscitation following cardiac arrest are described in Flow chart 50.3.[48]
- ❖ There may be neurological impairment amongst the mothers and foetuses that survive.

 CLINICAL PEARLS

- ❖ The main clinical symptom, which should lead the clinician to suspect amniotic fluid embolism, is sudden onset of dyspnoea in the face of cardiovascular collapse and DIC.
- ❖ A multidisciplinary team approach comprising of an obstetrician, anaesthesiologist and intensivist is necessary for a successful outcome.

CHAPTER 50

Flow chart 50.3: Guidelines for advanced life support in adults[48]

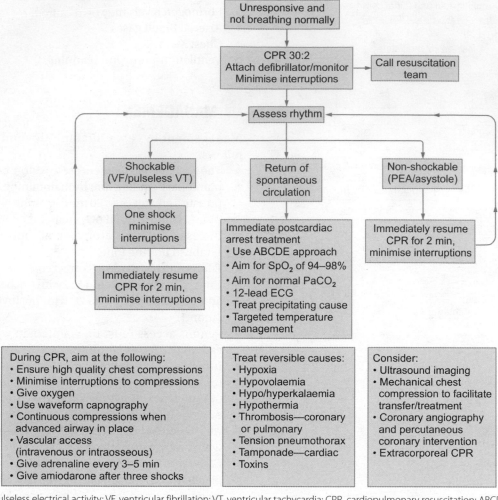

Abbreviations: PEA, pulseless electrical activity; VF, ventricular fibrillation; VT, ventricular tachycardia; CPR, cardiopulmonary resuscitation; ABCDE, Airway, Breathing, Circulation, Disability and Exposure

PULMONARY EMBOLISM

Pulmonary embolism can be considered as another important cause of postpartum collapse and has been described in details in Chapter 14 (Anaemia and Other Haematological Abnormalities).

REFERENCES

1. Mousa HA, Alfirevic Z. Treatment for primary postpartum haemorrhage. Cochrane Database Syst Rev. 2007;(1):CD003249.
2. Alexander J, Thomas PW, Sanghera J. Treatments for secondary postpartum haemorrhage. Cochrane Database Syst Rev. 2002;(1):CD002867.
3. Confidential Enquiry into Maternal and Child Health. Why Mothers Die 2000–2002. The Sixth Report of the Confidential Enquiries into Maternal Deaths in the United Kingdom. London: RCOG Press; 2004.
4. Confidential Enquiry into Maternal and Child Health. Saving Mothers Lives: Reviewing maternal deaths to make motherhood safer. 2003–2005. Seventh Report of the Confidential Enquiries into Maternal Deaths in the United Kingdom. London: CEMACH; 2007.
5. You WB, Zahn CM. Postpartum haemorrhage: abnormally adherent placenta, uterine inversion, and puerperal haematomas. Clin Obstet Gynecol. 2006;49:184-97.
6. The management of postpartum haemorrhage. Drug Ther Bull. 1992;30:89-92.
7. de Groot AN. Prevention of postpartum haemorrhage. Baillieres Clin Obstet Gynaecol. 1995;9:619-31.
8. Drife J. Management of primary postpartum haemorrhage. Br J Obstet Gynaecol. 1997;104.275-7.
9. Prendiville WJP, Elbourne D, McDonald SJ. Active versus expected management in the third stage of labour. Cochrane Database Syst Rev. 2000;(3):CD000007.
10. Westhoff G, Cotter AM, Tolosa JE. Prophylactic oxytocin for the third stage of labour to prevent postpartum haemorrhage. Cochrane Database Syst Rev. 2013;(10):CD001808.
11. National Institute for Health and Care Excellence. Intrapartum Care: Care of Healthy Women and their Babies during Childbirth. NICE Clinical Guideline 190. Manchester: NICE; 2014.
12. Gulmezoglu AM, Forna F, Villar J, Hofmeyr GJ. Prostaglandins for prevention of postpartum haemorrhage. Cochrane Database Syst Rev. 2007;(3):CD000494.
13. McDonald SJ, Abbott JM, Higgins SP. Prophylactic ergometrine oxytocin versus oxytocin for the third stage of labour. Cochrane Database Syst Rev. 2004;(1):CD000201.

14. Alfirevic Z, Blum J, Walraven G, Weeks A, Winikoff B. Prevention of postpartum hemorrhage with misoprostol. Int J Gynaecol Obstet. 2007;99(Suppl 2):S198-201.

15. Su LL, Chong YS, Samuel M. Carbetocin for preventing postpartum haemorrhage. Cochrane Database Syst Rev. 2012; (4):CD005457.

16. Stainsby D, MacLennan S, Thomas D, Isaac J, Hamilton PJ. Guidelines on the management of massive blood loss. Br J Haematol. 2006;135:634-41.

17. Franchini M, Lippi G, Franchi M. The use of recombinant activated factor VII in obstetric and gynaecological haemorrhage. BJOG. 2007;114:8-15.

18. Walker ID, Walker JJ, Colvin BT, Letsky EA, Rivers R, Stevens R. Investigation and management of haemorrhagic disorders in pregnancy. J Clin Pathol. 1994;47:100-8.

19. Mavrides E, Allard S, Chandraharan E, Collins P, Green L, Hunt BJ, et al. Prevention and management of postpartum haemorrhage: Green-top Guideline No. 52. BJOG. 2016. [Epub ahead of print].

20. Ikechebelu JI, Obi RA, Joe-Ikechebelu NN. The control of postpartum haemorrhage with intrauterine Foley catheter. J Obstet Gynecol. 2005;25:70-2.

21. Bakri YN, Amri A, Abdul Jabbar F. Tamponade-balloon for obstetrical bleeding. Int J Gynaecol Obstet. 2001;74:139-42.

22. Chan C, Razvi K, Tham KF, Arulkumaran S. The use of a Sengstaken-Blakemore tube to control postpartum haemorrhage. Int J Obstet Gynecol. 1997;58:251-2.

23. Condous GS, Arulkumaran S, Symonds I, Chapman R, Sinha A, Razvi K. The 'tamponade test' in the management of massive postpartum haemorrhage. Obstet Gynecol. 2003;101:767-72.

24. Akhter S, Begum MR, Kabir Z, Rashid M, Laila TR, Zabeen F. Use of a condom to control massive postpartum haemorrhage. MedGenMed. 2003;5(3):38.

25. Keriakos R, Mukhopadhyay A. The use of the Rusch balloon for management of severe postpartum haemorrhage. J Obstet Gynecol. 2006;26:335-8.

26. Hayman RG, Arulkumaran S, Steer PJ. Uterine compression sutures: surgical management of postpartum hemorrhage. Obstet Gynecol. 2002;99:502-6.

27. Ghezzi F, Cromi A, Uccella S, Raio L, Bolis P, Surbek D. The Hayman technique: a simple method to treat postpartum haemorrhage. BJOG. 2007;114:362-5.

28. Hwu YM, Chen CP, Chen HS, Su TH. Parallel vertical compression sutures: a technique to control bleeding from placenta praevia or accreta during caesarean section. BJOG. 2005;112:1420-3.

29. Kafali H, Demir N, Soylemez F, Yurtseven S. Hemostatic cervical suturing technique for management of uncontrollable postpartum haemorrhage originating from the cervical canal. Eur J Obstet Gynecol Reprod Biol. 2003;110:35-8.

30. Mackeen A, Packard RE, Ota E, Speer L. Antibiotic regimens for postpartum endometritis. Cochrane Database Syst Rev. 2015;(2):CD001067.

31. Levine AB, Kuhlman K, Bonn J. Placenta accreta: comparison of cases managed with and without pelvic artery balloon catheters. J Matern Fetal Med. 1999;8:173-6.

32. Alvarez M, Lockwood CJ, Ghidini A, Dottino P, Mitty HA, Berkowitz RL. Prophylactic and emergent arterial catheterization for selective embolization in obstetric hemorrhage. Am J Perinatol. 1992;9:441-4.

33. Mitty HA, Sterling KM, Alvarez M, Gendler R. Obstetric haemorrhage: prophylactic and emergency arterial catheterization and embolotherapy. Radiology. 1993;188:183-7.

34. Dubois J, Garel L, Grignon A, Lemay M, Leduc L. Placenta percreta: balloon occlusion and embolization of the internal iliac arteries to reduce intraoperative blood losses. Am J Obstet Gynecol. 1997;176:723-6.

35. Hansch E, Chitkara U, McAlpine J, El-Sayed Y, Dake MD, Razavi MK. Pelvic arterial embolization for control of obstetric haemorrhage: a five-year experience. Am J Obstet Gynecol. 1999;180:1454-60.

36. Ojala K, Perala J, Kariniemi J, Ranta P, Raudaskoski T, Tekay A. Arterial embolization and prophylactic catheterization for the treatment for severe obstetric hemorrhage. Acta Obstet Gynecol Scand. 2005;84:1075-80.

37. Bodner LJ, Nosher JL, Gribbin C, Siegel RL, Beale S, Scorza W. Balloon-assisted occlusion of the internal iliac arteries in patients with placenta accreta/percreta. Cardiovasc Intervent Radiol. 2006;29:354-61.

38. Allam J, Cox M, Yentis SM. Cell salvage in obstetrics. Int J Obstet Anesth. 2008;17:37-45.

39. Royal College of Obstetricians and Gynaecologists. Maternal Collapse in Pregnancy and the Puerperium. Green-top Guideline No. 56. London: RCOG Press; 2011.

40. Knight M, Kurinczuk JJ, Tufnell D, Brocklehurst P. The UK Obstetric Surveillance System for rare disorders of pregnancy. BJOG. 2005;112:263 5.

41. Ripley DL. Uterine emergencies: atony, inversion, and rupture. Obstet Gynecol Clin North Am. 1999;26:419-34.

42. Wendel PJ, Cox SM. Emergent obstetric management of uterine inversion. Obstet Gynecol Clin North Am. 1995;22:261-74.

43. Hostetler DR, Bosworth MF. Uterine inversion: a life-threatening obstetric emergency. Journal of the American Board of Family Practice. 2000;13:120-3.

44. Furukawa S, Sameshima H. The importance of the monitoring of resuscitation with blood transfusion for uterine inversion in obstetrical hemorrhage. Obstet Gynecol Int. 2015;2015: 269156.

45. Knight M, Tuffnell D, Brocklehurst P, Spark P, Kurinczuk JJ; UK Obstetric Surveillance System. Incidence and risk factors for amniotic-fluid embolism. Obstet Gynecol. 2010;115:910-7.

46. Morgan M. Amniotic fluid embolism. Anaesthesia. 1979;4:20-32.

47. Conde-Agudelo A, Romero R. Amniotic fluid embolism: an evidence-based review. Am J Obstet Gynecol. 2009;201:445. e1-13.

48. European Resuscitation Council. (2015). Guidelines for advanced life support in adults. [online] Available from www.resus.org.uk. [Accessed December, 2016].

CHAPTER 50

Puerperal Pyrexia

INTRODUCTION

Puerperal pyrexia is characterised by a rise in temperature of 38°C (100.4°F) or higher in the puerperium (i.e. within 6 weeks of giving birth). This temperature rise must be observed on two separate occasions, 24 hours apart, usually within the first 10 days following delivery, excluding the first 24 hours after delivery. In the past, before the advent of antimicrobial therapy, group A β-haemolytic streptococci (GAS) was the most common cause of postpartum sepsis. Though the prognosis has been considerably improved with the advent of antibiotic therapy, recently, again there has been a dramatic rise in the cases of maternal deaths attributable to GAS. Three cases of maternal deaths due to puerperal sepsis were described by the Seventh Report on CEMD in the UK for the years 2003–2005[1] and 26 cases of maternal deaths due to puerperal sepsis were reported by the Eight Report on CEMD in 2006–2008, out of which 13 cases were due to GAS.[2] Therefore, postpartum sepsis remains an important cause of maternal deaths in the UK. The most common site of sepsis during puerperium is the genital tract, especially the uterus, resulting in endometritis.

AETIOLOGY

Puerperal pyrexia is usually related to one of the following factors:

❖ *Benign fever*: Though most cases of puerperal pyrexia are related to infection, some cases may be non-infectious in nature. Features that are more typical of benign fever are the presence of early low-grade fever in absence of any other symptomatology.
❖ *Breast engorgement*
❖ *Infection of the urogenital tract*: This may include infections such as endometritis, urinary tract infection, infections due to perineal repair, etc. Uterine infection known as endometritis, which is the most common of all genital tract infections, especially occurs following caesarean delivery. Endometritis is a polymicrobial infection associated with mixed aerobic and anaerobic flora. The microorganisms, which are most commonly involved, include GAS (also known as *Streptococcus pyogenes*), *Escherichia coli, Staphylococcus aureus, Streptococcus pneumoniae,* methicillin-resistant *S. aureus* (MRSA), *Clostridium septicum, Morganella morganii,* etc. The CEMD report (2006–2008) identified one case of maternal death due to Panton-Valentine leukocidin (PVL)-producing MRSA following caesarean section.[1] Gram-negative bacteria that produce extended-spectrum β-lactamases (ESBL) are becoming an increasingly common cause of urinary tract infections resistant to antibiotics such as coamoxiclav and cephalosporins in the UK. Infection with ESBL was responsible for one case of maternal death in the CEMD report (2006–2008).[1] In the cases of infection with ESBL, antibiotics such as carbapenems or novel IV antimicrobials such as colistin may be used. *Clostridium* spp. remain an uncommon cause of death due to sepsis in the puerperium, with one case of maternal death being reported due to *C. septicum* post-termination of pregnancy.[1]
❖ *Distant infection*: Besides infection of the urogenital tract, other causes of puerperal pyrexia, which may be due to distant infections, include causes such as mastitis, infection of the caesarean wound, pulmonary infection or pneumonia, thrombophlebitis, skin and soft-tissue infection, gastroenteritis, pharyngitis and rarely meningitis, etc. The most important causative organism of mastitis is *S. aureus*, most commonly CA-MRSA. It is important for the healthcare professional to examine the woman's breasts because mastitis is often clinically overlooked. However, it may result in complications such as breast abscesses,[3-6] necrotising fasciitis and toxic shock syndrome.[1,6] During the CEMD report (2005-2008), two women were reported to have died due to mastitis-related sepsis, one with

Box 51.1: Risk factors for maternal sepsis as identified by the Confidential Enquiries into Maternal Deaths[1,2]

❑ Obesity
❑ Impaired glucose tolerance or diabetes mellitus
❑ Impaired immune status or woman is on immunosuppressant medication
❑ Anaemia
❑ Vaginal discharge
❑ History of pelvic infection in the past
❑ Amniocentesis and other invasive procedures
❑ Cervical cerclage
❑ Prolonged spontaneous rupture of membranes
❑ Perineal trauma at the time of vaginal birth
❑ Caesarean section, wound haematoma
❑ Retained products of conception
❑ GAS infection in close contacts/family members
❑ Ethnicity: Black or minority group origin

Abbreviation: GAS, group A β-haemolytic streptococci

necrotising mastitis resulting from GAS and the other with *S. aureus*.

Multiple risk factors for maternal sepsis as identified by the CEMD reports are tabulated in Box 51.1.[1,2]

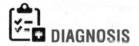

DIAGNOSIS

A general history and examination should be carried out in order to identify the source of sepsis. Women should be evaluated clinically for any symptoms of shock. If they appear to be unusually unwell or present with symptoms of dehydration or vomiting, hospital admission should be considered.

Clinical Presentation

All health professionals should be familiar with the signs and symptoms of maternal sepsis and critical illness. They should also be aware of the rapid, potentially lethal course of severe sepsis and septic shock. In case the physician at primary care suspects sepsis, the patient should be urgently referred to the secondary care. While taking history related to past infectious diseases, it is important to ask if she recently had any illness or was exposed to any illness, particularly streptococcal infections (pharyngitis, impetigo, cellulitis, etc.), in close contacts or family members.

Clinical signs suggestive of sepsis include one or more of the following:

❖ *Fever and malaise*: Degree of fever is proportional to the extent of infection and sepsis. Chills and rigors may accompany fever. Rigors may be associated with persistent spiking temperature, which is suggestive of an abscess. The obstetrician needs to be aware of the fact that sometimes the patients may have a normal temperature, which may be due to antipyretics or NSAIDs. In fact, sometimes hypothermia is present which is indicative of shock. Malaise may be associated with reduced appetite, lethargy, etc.

❖ *Maculopapular rash*: A generalised maculopapular rash could be indicative of staphylococcal or streptococcal sepsis. Any widespread rash could be suggestive of early toxic shock syndrome, especially if conjunctival hyperaemia is also present.

❖ *Diarrhoea or vomiting*: They may be due to exotoxin production and may be indicative of an early toxic shock.

❖ *Features suggestive of shock*: Along with pyrexia or occasionally hypothermia, there could be clinical features suggestive of shock such as tachycardia, tachypnoea, hypoxia, hypotension, oliguria, impaired consciousness, failure to respond to treatment, etc.

❖ *Abdominal palpation*: Uterus may be subinvoluted and tender. Genital tract sepsis may present with constant severe abdominal or pelvic pain and tenderness, which may not be relieved by the usual analgesic medications. Agonising pain out of proportion to the clinical signs is suggestive of a deep infection. In these cases, diagnosis of necrotising fasciitis or myositis must be considered.[5,7-9] A pain scoring system is also useful for charting the patient's progress.

❖ *Breast examination*: Examination of both the breasts is important because mastitis could be the underlying cause of puerperal sepsis. In cases of mastitis, the breast would appear tender, red and inflamed on examination. Breast engorgement may be also sometimes present.

❖ *Caesarean wound inspection*: In the presence of infection, the wound may become red and inflamed. There may be spreading cellulitis or discharge. This may result in a collection of pus, which may eventually cause wound disruption.

❖ *Vaginal examination*: Infected episiotomy may be present. Parametrial tenderness can be elicited. There may be presence of foul smelling lochia or offensive vaginal discharge, suggestive of infection. Smelly vaginal discharge is suggestive of anaerobic infection, whereas serosanguinous discharge is suggestive of streptococcal infection.

Investigations

Investigations should be directed at identifying the cause of infection:

❖ *Urinary tract infection*: If the patient presents with the clinical symptoms of urinary tract infection, a midstream specimen of urine must be sent for routine and microscopy examination. Presence of leucocytes, protein and blood in a midstream specimen of urine may be suggestive of current infection and a specimen should be sent for culture.

❖ *Pneumonia*: In presence of pulmonary infection, sputum specimen may be required for culture and sensitivity.

❖ *Throat swabs*: A throat swab should be sent for culture in any woman with symptoms of tonsillitis or pharyngitis.

❖ *Skin and soft-tissue infection*: A woman with suspected bacterial sepsis should be carefully examined for skin and soft-tissue infection, particularly at the insertion sites of IV cannulae, drains, vascular access devices, any indwelling devices or injection sites and caesarean or episiotomy wounds. In case of any discharge, swabs should be taken and sent for culture and sensitivity. If any indwelling device has been identified as the source of infection, it should be removed as soon as is practicable. This is particularly important because skin and soft-tissue infections may be typically associated with toxic shock syndromes.[5-11] Moreover, recurrent abscess formation in the soft tissues, especially labial abscesses, is a feature of PVL-producing staphylococci.[12]

❖ *Culture and sensitivity*: High vaginal, endocervical swabs and urine analysis for culture and sensitivity may be required in suspected urogenital infections.

   Other samples for culture are guided by the clinical suspicion of focus of infection and may include throat swabs, midstream urine, placental swabs, sputum samples, cerebrospinal fluid, epidural site swab, caesarean section or episiotomy site wound swabs and expressed breast milk. Samples should ideally be obtained prior to starting antibiotic therapy as the results may become uninformative within a few hours of starting antibiotics.

   In case of diarrhoea, routine culture (e.g. *Salmonella*, *Campylobacter*) of the stool sample must be done. If diarrhoea particularly occurs following antimicrobial therapy, a stool sample should be submitted for *C. difficile* toxin testing.[13]

   If there is a clinical indication of investigations for unusual pathogens, the laboratory should be informed in advance, e.g. *Listeria monocytogenes* due to the consumption of soft cheese or cured meats, or if there is a history of foreign travel (parasites, typhoid or cholera).

❖ *Blood cultures*: This is one of the most important investigations and should be obtained prior to the administration of antibiotics. However, antibiotic treatment in these cases should be started without waiting for microbiology results.

❖ *Serum lactate measurement*: Serum lactate levels should be measured within 6 hours of the suspicion of severe sepsis to aid the management plan. Serum lactate levels greater than or equal to 4 mmol/L is indicative of tissue hypoperfusion.

❖ *Imaging*: Appropriate imaging studies should be performed in order to confirm the source of infection based on the clinical suspicion of the focus of infection. This could include a chest X-ray, pelvic ultrasound scan or CT scan. Pelvic ultrasound helps in detection of any retained placental bits. Persistent puerperal infection can be evaluated on CT or MRI. CT scan is also indicated if a pelvic abscess is suspected.

❖ *Blood investigations*: These consist of performing the tests such as full blood count, including haematocrit (especially haemoglobin estimation), TLC, DLC and platelet count, serum urea, serum electrolytes, and C-reactive protein (CRP) levels. Leucocytosis to the extent of 15,000–30,000 cells/μL may be present in the cases of sepsis. Thrombocytosis (high-platelet count) with a rising CRP and 'rising and falling' pyrexia usually indicates a collection of pus or an infected haematoma in the woman.

❖ *MRSA status*: If the MRSA status of the woman is not known, a premoistened nose swab may be sent for rapid MRSA screening at a place where such test is available.

MANAGEMENT

General Management

❖ *Multidisciplinary team approach*: Monitoring of the woman with suspected severe sepsis should be done by a multidisciplinary team including a senior obstetrician, an intensivist, microbiologist or infectious disease clinician. However, a single consultant must lead this team.

❖ *Monitoring of the vitals*: Regular observations of all vital signs (including temperature, pulse rate, BP and respiratory rate) should be recorded on a modified early obstetric warning score (MEOWS) chart. While MEOWS charts are commonly being used, there is no standardisation and various units are using different charts.

❖ *Antibiotic prophylaxis*: Antibiotic prophylaxis against infection is especially important in cases of caesarean delivery for prevention of puerperal sepsis. However, there is no good evidence supporting the use of antibiotics at the time of instrumental delivery. Recent recommendations by NICE suggest that antibiotic prophylaxis against infective endocarditis is not required in women with congenital heart disease.[14] However, if the woman with congenital heart disease develops fever, puerperal pyrexia must be ruled out in close consultation with the cardiologist.

• *Sepsis care bundle*: Box 51.2 enumerates the steps, which should be performed within the first 6 hours of the identification of cases of severe sepsis. These steps together are known as the 'sepsis care bundle'.[15] In case the woman has hypotension and/or a serum lactate levels greater than 4 mmol/L, she must be administered crystalloid or an equivalent in an initial minimum dose of 20 mL/kg body weight. If hypotension does not respond to initial fluid resuscitation and the mean arterial pressure remains below 65 mmHg, use of vasopressors may be required.

   If the patient is in septic shock and continues to have severe persistent hypotension despite fluid resuscitation and/or serum lactate levels greater than 4 mmol/L, the physician must at least try to achieve the following: central venous pressure of greater than or

---

Box 51.2: Tasks to be performed within the first 6 hours of the identification of severe sepsis (sepsis care bundle)[15]

❏ Administration of high-flow oxygen (to maintain saturation >94%)
❏ Blood cultures to be obtained prior to antibiotic administration
❏ Broad-spectrum antibiotic must be administered within 1 hour of recognition of severe sepsis
❏ Serum lactate levels and full blood count must be measured
❏ Intravenous fluid resuscitation to be started
❏ Accurate measurement of urine output

PART II

equal to 8 mmHg and central venous oxygen saturation greater than or equal to 70% or mixed venous oxygen saturation greater than or equal to 65%.

❖ *Referral to the hospital*: Community carers should be aware of the signs and symptoms of puerperal sepsis (as previously described) and should refer these women to hospital as early as possible.

❖ *Antibiotics*: Early treatment with antibiotics, whether oral or parenteral, may be crucial in determining the outcome. In case of clinical features such as abdominal pain, fever (>38°C) and tachycardia (>90 bpm), the patient should be admitted to the hospital for administration of IV antibiotics. A clinical review by the senior obstetrician is also required in these cases.

❖ Nonsteroidal anti-inflammatory drugs should be avoided for providing pain relief in cases of sepsis as they inhibit the polymorphs to fight against GAS infection. Paracetamol can be administered in the cases of pyrexia. Not only does it act as an antipyretic, it also helps in improving patient's comfort while at the same time not altering the disease course.

❖ Management of severe pneumonia (if present) should be in consultation with a respiratory physician and a medical microbiologist. Most commonly used antibiotic combination in these cases is a β-lactam antibiotic together with a macrolide antibiotic.

❖ Presence of any intercurrent illness necessitating antimicrobial therapy should be noted at the time of admission. Ingestion of unpasteurised milk products raises the possibility of infection with *Salmonella*, *Campylobacter* or *Listeria*. History of recent travel to foreign lands or tropical countries may be associated with a high rate of carriage of multiresistant organisms. In these cases, appropriate consultation with a microbiologist is required to ensure that appropriate isolation procedures and diagnostic tests have been implemented. Q fever is caused by *Coxiella burnetii* after inhalation of infectious particles from cattle, sheep and other domesticated animals.

❖ *Involvement of other specialists in care*: All cases of sepsis in the puerperium should be managed by the obstetrician in consultation with a clinical microbiologist or infectious diseases physician. Women with earlier history of carrier status or infection with multiresistant organisms (e.g. ESBL producing organisms, MRSA, etc.) should be notified to the infection control team as early as possible. If the diagnosis of necrotising fasciitis is suspected, intensive care physicians must be involved as quickly as possible. Referral for surgical opinion, ideally from plastic and reconstructive surgeons may also be required.[13]

❖ In case of severe septicaemia, transfer to the critical care unit may be required so that isotropic support can be initiated.

Specific Management

❖ In case the woman shows signs suggestive of influenza or GAS or either of these conditions is suspected, immediate consultation with a consultant microbiologist is required.

❖ Appropriate cultures including throat swabs must be taken and the health protection units must be informed.

❖ Antibiotics or antivirals must be commenced without waiting for the results of these cultures.

❖ Contacts of the patient who show signs and symptoms of non-invasive GAS infection must be traced and treated with penicillin V. If the patient is allergic to penicillin, azithromycin can be used.

❖ Patients thought to have H1N1 infection should be treated with oseltamivir.

❖ In case wound infection or endometritis are both complicated by abscess formation, antibiotics alone may be insufficient. In these cases, surgical drainage is also required.

COMPLICATIONS

❖ Wound infection or dehiscence
❖ Necrotising fasciitis, peritonitis, adnexal infections
❖ *Parametrial phlegmon*: This is characterised by parametrial cellulitis and areas of induration or phlegmon within the leaves of broad ligament.
❖ Pelvic thrombophlebitis
❖ Infection of perineum, vagina and cervix.

CLINICAL PEARLS

❖ Early presentation of sepsis (<12 hours postbirth) is more likely to be caused by streptococcal infection, particularly GAS. Severe continuous pain is usually suggestive of necrotising fasciitis.

❖ When a woman who has recently delivered presents with persistent vaginal bleeding and abdominal pain, infection must also be suspected and actively ruled out. In cases of even a slight suspicion of puerperal infection, the woman must be referred back to the maternity unit as soon as possible.

❖ Intravenous drug abusers are associated with a high risk of staphylococcal and streptococcal sepsis as well as generalised immunosuppression, endocarditis and harbouring blood-borne viruses. Appropriate precautions for infection control should be instituted in such women.

❖ Implementation of the sepsis bundles has helped in reducing mortality from sepsis in the general population.

EVIDENCE-BASED MEDICINE

❖ In the women suspected to be suffering from puerperal sepsis, high-dose IV broad-spectrum antibiotics should be immediately commenced in the hospital without waiting for the results of investigations because if the infection becomes systemic, the woman's condition can deteriorate extremely rapidly if left untreated, with death resulting within a few hours. It is essential to note the speed of onset or worsening of symptoms and signs. Early treatment with antibiotics, whether oral or parenteral, may be fundamental in determining the outcome.

The obstetrician needs to check and regularly record the laboratory tests in consultation with the medical microbiologist to ensure that the specimens are processed appropriately and to enable the communication of the results at the earliest opportunity. Antimicrobial therapy must be tailored according to the results of Gram stain, and culture and sensitivities. No single antibiotic regimen has yet been shown to be superior over the others. Therapy should, therefore, be determined by local hospital policies based on the antibiotic sensitivities of bacteria isolated locally in line with the standards of quality assurance. These policies need to be reviewed, easily accessible and well promoted throughout the hospital.[1,2,13]

❖ Use of prophylactic antibiotics is likely to reduce the occurrence of endometritis following caesarean delivery. Antibiotics covering *Bacillus fragilis* and other penicillin-resistant anaerobic bacteria must be preferably used. In cases of uncomplicated endometritis, there is no need of oral therapy following IV therapy because IV therapy alone is sufficient.[16]

REFERENCES

1. Centre for Maternal and Child Enquiries (CMACE). Saving Mothers' Lives: reviewing maternal deaths to make motherhood safer: 2006–08. The Eighth Report on Confidential Enquiries into Maternal Deaths in the United Kingdom. BJOG. 2011;118 (Suppl 1):1-203.
2. Lewis G (Ed). The Confidential Enquiry into Maternal and Child Health (CEMACH). Saving Mothers' Lives: Reviewing Maternal Deaths to Make Motherhood Safer 2003–2005. The Seventh Report on Confidential Enquiries into Maternal Deaths in the United Kingdom. London: CEMACH; 2007.
3. Lee IW, Kang L, Kuo PL, Chang CM. Puerperal mastitis requiring hospitalization during a nine-year period. Am J Obstet Gynecol. 2010;203(4):332.e1-6.
4. McAdoo GL, Monif GR. Expanding disease spectrum associated with puerperal mastitis. Infect Dis Obstet Gynaecol. 1997;5:376-9.
5. Stafford I, Hernandez J, Laibl V, Sheffield J, Roberts S, Wendl G. Community-associated methicillin-resistant Staphylococcus aureus among patients with puerperal mastitis requiring hospitalization. Obstet Gynecol. 2008;112(3):533-7.
6. Tillett RL, Saxby PJ, Stone CA, Morgan MS. Group A streptococcal necrotising fasciitis masquerading as mastitis. Lancet. 2006;368(9530):174.
7. Lappin E, Ferguson AJ. Gram-positive toxic shock syndromes. Lancet Infect Dis. 2009;9(5):281-90.
8. Stevens DL. Streptococcal toxic shock syndrome. Clin Microbiol Infect. 2002;8(3):133-6.
9. Morgan MS. Diagnosis and management of necrotising fasciitis: a multiparametric approach. J Hosp Infect. 2010;75(4):249-57.
10. Barnham MR, Weightman NC. Bacteraemic Streptococcus pyogenes in the peri-partum period: now a rare disease and prior carriage by the patient may be important. J Infect. 2001;43(3):173-6.
11. Yamada T, Yamada T, Yamamura MK, Karabami K, Hayakawa M, Tomaru U, et al. Invasive group A streptococcal infection in pregnancy. J Infect. 2010;60(6):417-24.
12. Jung N, Lehmann C, Hellmann M, Seifert H, Valter MM, Hallek M, et al. Necrotizing pneumonia caused by Panton-Valentine leucocidin-producing Staphylococcus aureus originating from a Bartholin's abscess. Infect Dis Obstet Gynaecol. 2008;2008:491401.
13. Rouphael NG, O'Donnell JA, Bhatnagar J, Lewis F, Polgreen PM, Beekmann S, et al. Clostridium difficile-associated diarrhea: an emerging threat to pregnant women. Am J Obstet Gynecol. 2008;198:625.e1-6.
14. National Institute of Clinical Excellence (NICE). (2008). Prophylaxis against infective endocarditis: antimicrobial prophylaxis against infective endocarditis in adults and children undergoing interventional procedures. [online]. Available from www.nice.org.uk/guidance/cg64. [Accessed August, 2016].
15. Dellinger RP, Levy MM, Carlet JM, Bion J, Parker MM, Jaeschke R, et al. Surviving Sepsis Campaign: International guidelines for management of severe sepsis and septic shock. Crit Care Med. 2008;36(1):296-327.
16. Royal College of Obstetricians and Gynaecologists. Bacterial sepsis following pregnancy. Green-top Guideline No. 64b. London: RCOG Press; 2012.

Psychiatric Disorders in the Puerperium (Mood Disturbances)

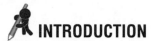 INTRODUCTION

The postpartum period is a vulnerable time for women. Besides being associated with joy at the arrival of the new baby, this period is also associated with increased responsibilities for the new mother and her partner. Woman with a past medical history of psychiatric illness or a family history of psychiatric illness are particularly vulnerable. If psychiatric disorders in the postpartum period are not treated, it can have several short- and long-term consequences for both the infant and the mother. Psychiatric disorders during pregnancy can be a cause of significant mortality and morbidity. In the last CEMD reports, 12 cases of indirect death were due to suicide. Moreover, psychiatric causes were also responsible for another 22 cases of late maternal deaths. Of the 12 cases of indirect deaths, 5 had a previous history of psychosis, whereas 7 had a previous history of severe depressive illness. 10 out of these 12 patients died in the immediate postpartum period.[1,2] Also majority of these patients who died had a previous history of depressive illness or puerperal psychosis.

Management of mood-related disorders during the antenatal period must involve the management of pre-existing psychiatric diseases. Disorders of mood in the postnatal period can be divided into three categories: (1) baby blues, (2) postpartum depression (PPD) and (3) puerperal psychosis.

Baby Blues and Postpartum Depression

Postpartum blues is a relatively common condition. Nearly 50% of the women suffer from postpartum blues, whereas postnatal depression may occur in approximately 10–15% cases. Postpartum blues frequently occurs in the first few days following delivery, whereas PPD occurs within 4 weeks of childbirth, with a peak of incidence within the first 4 months postpartum.[3,4] In both of these conditions, the mother experiences symptoms such as transient experience of tearfulness, anxiety and irritability in the first few days following delivery. Symptoms of baby blues usually taper off by second postpartum week, while symptoms of PPD may last longer. Also, the symptoms of PPD are more intense (e.g. suicidal thoughts or inability to care for the infant). Administering a screening test, such as the Edinburgh Postnatal Depression Scale, can help identify women who require treatment.

Puorperal Psychosis

Puerperal psychosis is even rarer entity occurring in approximately 0.1% cases.

It can be defined as a severe mental disorder, usually occurring in the first 4 weeks of delivery. It is characterised by irrational ideas and unusual reactions to the baby. Additionally, the patient may suffer from symptoms such as restlessness, irritability and mood liability.

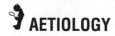 AETIOLOGY

Antenatal Psychiatric Disorders

The pre-existing mood disorders (e.g. anxiety, depression schizophrenia, maniac-depressive illness, etc.) can be precipitated for the first time during the antenatal period because pregnancy itself can be considered as a significant life-changing event. The stress related to pregnancy may be secondary to the social limitations of pregnancy rather than pregnancy itself. Pregnancy can place an additional strain on the relationship with the partner and may also be associated with worries about financial constraints. These stress factors may be sufficient to destabilise a susceptible individual.

Postpartum Blues

The immediate postpartum period is the time of significant social and psychological changes. This can cause mood disorders in a significant proportion of postpartum women, commonly termed as postpartum blues. The likely pathogenesis of this condition could be related to factors such as lack of sleep, hospitalisation and pain. Postpartum baby blues is a self-limiting condition, which is not associated with any specific metabolic or endocrinological disturbance. This condition is likely to be more common following the first delivery. The sufferers of this disorder are not more likely to have a past psychiatric history in comparison to the non-sufferers.

Postpartum Depression

Social and physiological changes occurring during the postpartum period could be related to the pathogenesis of PPD. No specific endocrinological change has been found to be associated with the pathogenesis of PPD. Previously, it was believed that the reduction in serum concentration of progesterone and oestrogen after birth was responsible for this condition because both of these hormones are believed to have psychoactive properties. Unlike postpartum blues, postnatal depression is associated with a history of psychiatric illness. Many experts do not even recognise this condition as a separate disease entity. Several factors, which may increase the risk for the development of PPD, include:

- A previous history of PPD[5]
- A history of depression prior to conception
- A family history of depression, particularly PPD[6,7]
- Poor social support
- Experience of adverse life events during the postpartum period
- Marital instability
- Young maternal age
- Infants with health problems or perceived 'difficult' temperaments.

Puerperal Psychosis

It is not clear if puerperal psychosis is a separate disease entity or a rapidly evolving affective psychosis. The aetiology of puerperal psychosis is poorly understood. It, however, does appear to be more common following first delivery, in patients with previous history of bipolar disorders or psychosis and in patients with family history of psychotic illness (e.g. schizophrenia or bipolar disorder). This disease is associated with nearly 25% risk of recurrence in the subsequent pregnancies. Many patients also suffer from recurrent relapsing affective disorders for the rest of their lives.

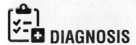

DIAGNOSIS

Clinical Presentation

Postpartum Blues

Postpartum blues is a transient condition characterised by symptoms such as irritability, anxiety, reduced concentration, insomnia, tearfulness, and mild, often rapid, mood swings from joy to sadness. Symptoms usually reach their peak on the fifth postpartum day and usually resolve within 2 weeks.

Box 52.1: Criteria for a major depressive episode[3]

- ❑ Five or more of the following symptoms* must be present daily or almost daily for at least 2 consecutive weeks:
  1. Depressed mood
  2. Loss of interest or pleasure
  3. Significant increase or decrease in appetite
  4. Insomnia or hypersomnia
  5. Psychomotor agitation or retardation
  6. Fatigue or loss of energy
  7. Feelings of worthlessness or guilt
  8. Diminished concentration
  9. Recurrent thoughts of suicide or death
- ❑ The symptoms do not meet the criteria for other psychiatric conditions
- ❑ The symptoms cause significant impairment in usual functioning at work, school, and in social activities
- ❑ The symptoms are not caused by the direct effects of a substance or a general medical condition
- ❑ The symptoms are not better accounted for by the loss of a loved one

*At least one of which must be 1 or 2.

Postpartum Depression

Symptoms of PPD are similar to that of a major depressive episode experienced at any time in the non-gravid women (Box 52.1). There may be slight differences, as described next:

- Difficulty in sleeping when the baby sleeps
- Lack of enjoyment in the maternal role
- Feelings of guilt related to parenting ability
- Concomitant symptoms of anxiety, including panic attacks and obsessional fears
- Frightening experiences for mother (e.g. visualisation of images of harm occurring to their babies).

Puerperal Psychosis

This condition has a rapid onset, usually manifesting itself within the first 2 weeks after childbirth or, at most, within 3 months postpartum. Patients may present with symptoms resembling an acute manic episode or a psychotic depression. They may have delusions or hallucinations, which may be a frightening experience for them. Many patients also have additional symptoms resembling delirium, labile mood, transient confusion, etc. Such patients may lose touch with reality and are at risk of harming themselves or their babies.

Investigations

A very useful and easily administered, self-reporting screening tool for PPD is the validated Edinburgh Postnatal Depression Scale (Fig. 52.1).[8-10] This tool comprises of a series of 10 questions, which the patient can complete at her physician's office prior to her first postpartum follow-up appointment or when she brings her baby for immunisation. For each question, there are four possible replies. She has to choose one reply which best reflects her feelings over the past 7 days. Responses are scored as 0, 1, 2 or 3. A maximum score that a woman can get is 30. A minimum score of 12 has been associated with the diagnosis of PPD. The detection rates of

Name:_____ Date: _____ Number of months postpartum: _____

As you have recently had a baby, we would like to know how you are feeling. Please mark the answer which comes closest to how you have felt in the past 7 days, not just how you feel today.

Here is an example, already completed:

I have felt happy:

☐ Yes, all the time

☒ Yes, most of the time

☐ No, not very often

☐ No, not at all

This would mean "I have felt happy most of the time during the past week", Please complete the following questions in the same way.

In the past 7 days:

1. I have been able to laugh and see the funny side of things

☐ As much as I always could   0

☐ Not quite so much now   1

☐ Definitely not so much now   2

☐ Not at all   3

2. I have looked forward with enjoyment to things

☐ As much as I ever did   0

☐ Rather less than I used to   1

☐ Definitely less than I used to   2

☐ Hardly at all   3

3. I have blamed myself unnecessarily when things went wrong

☐ Yes, most of the time   3

☐ Yes, some of the time   2

☐ Not very often   1

☐ No, never   0

4. I have been anxious or worried for no good reason

☐ No, not at all   0

☐ Hardly ever   1

☐ Yes, sometimes   2

☐ Yes, very often   3

5. I have felt scared or panicky for no very good reason

☐ Yes, quite a lot   3

☐ Yes, sometimes   2

☐ No, not much   1

☐ No, not at all   0

6. Things have been getting on top of me

☐ Yes, most of the time I haven't been able to cope   3

☐ Yes, sometimes I haven't been coping as well as usual 2

☐ No, most of the time I have coped quite well   1

☐ No, I have been coping as well as ever   0

7. I have been so unhappy that I have had difficulty in sleeping

☐ Yes, most of the time   3

☐ Yes, sometimes   2

☐ Not very often   1

☐ No, not at all   0

8. I have felt sad or miserable

☐ Yes, most of the time   3

☐ Yes, quite often   2

☐ Not very often   1

☐ No, not at all   0

9. I have been so unhappy that I have been crying

☐ Yes, most of the time   3

☐ Yes, quite often   2

☐ Only occasionally   1

☐ No, never   0

10. The thought of harming myself has occurred to me

☐ Yes, quite often   3

☐ Sometimes   2

☐ Hardly ever   1

☐ Never   0

Fig. 52.1: Edinburg postnatal depression score[8-10]

CHAPTER 52

postnatal depression in the community can be improved by the implementation of Edinburgh Postnatal Depression Scale at 6 weeks postnatal check.

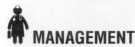

MANAGEMENT

Preconceptional Period

❖ Before establishing a psychiatric diagnosis in the post-partum period, it is important to rule out any underlying medical condition. Women suffering from anaemia in the early postpartum period may be at increased risk of developing PPD.[11] Abnormalities in thyroid function could also be responsible for producing psychiatric symptoms.[12] Testing for CBC and thyroid function tests should therefore be done.

❖ The women with their consent, their partners and families should be actively involved in the decision-making process.

❖ As per the recommendations by the NICE guidelines, women identified as having serious mental disorders in the prepregnancy period should be referred for advice to specialised perinatal mental health services (Box 52.2).[13] In the event of unavailability of such services, women can be referred to general psychiatric services. However, presently, NICE does not recommend the requirement of antenatal screening programmes for identification of these women because such programmes have largely proved to be unsuccessful.[13]

❖ Women suffering from or having a high risk of developing major mental illness should be recognised by ensuring that they are examined during their antenatal booking visit before 12 completed weeks of gestation.

Antenatal Period

❖ Management of psychiatric illness during pregnancy is similar to that in the non-pregnant woman.

Box 52.2: Indications for referral to specialised perinatal mental health services[13]

❑ Woman with current illness showing severe psychiatric symptoms, (e.g. psychosis, severe anxiety, severe depression, suicidal tendency, self-neglect, harm to others, significant interference with day-to-day functioning, etc.)

❑ Women with present or previous history of severe mental illness, e.g. psychotic disorders, severe anxiety or depression, obsessive compulsive disorders, eating disorders, bipolar disorders, schizophrenia, etc.

❑ Previous history of serious postpartum mental illness (e.g. puerperal psychosis)

❑ Women who have been prescribed complex psychotropic medication regimens prior to pregnancy

❑ Psychiatric illness of moderate severity developing in late pregnancy or the early postpartum period

❑ Family history of psychiatric disorders (e.g. first-degree relative with bipolar disorder or puerperal psychosis)

❖ The main concern during the antenatal period is the effect of psychotropic drugs on the foetus due to the high rates of transplacental transfer of these drugs. Though these drugs are not licensed for use during pregnancy, it is a well-established fact that there is likely to be a high risk of complications such as relapse of psychiatric conditions, anxiety disorders, schizophrenia, etc., if the medications for mood disorders are withdrawn during the antenatal period.

❖ Use of antidepressant group of drugs during pregnancy is usually not associated with an increased risk of major malformations. The United States FDA has issued a warning regarding cardiac malformations following the use of paroxetine in the first trimester. Moreover, use of drugs such as lithium, benzodiazepines and antipsychotic medications in the first trimester of pregnancy is likely to be associated with small but significantly increased risk of teratogenicity in the offspring.

❖ Women should be counselled regarding the possible adverse effects of psychotropic drugs and the risks from an untreated mental disorder on their pregnancy. They should also be counselled about the risks of abruptly stopping these medications without prior discussion with their doctor.

❖ To reduce the risk of harm to the foetus or child, psychotropic drugs should be prescribed cautiously during pregnancy. Before prescribing these drugs, the healthcare professional must maintain a balance between the risks of taking psychotropic drugs and the risks due to an untreated mental disorder or due to abruptly stopping the medication.[14]

❖ During the postpartum period, infants of mothers who have taken psychotropic medication in pregnancy should be observed for signs of neonatal adaptation syndrome. Neonatal assessment is required even if these symptoms are mild and self-limiting.

Postpartum Blues

❖ Provision of a supportive environment for the new mother, with both the healthcare professionals and family working together usually proves to be sufficient. Since this condition is largely self-limiting, drug therapy is usually not required.

❖ Minor tranquilisers at low doses (e.g. lorazepam 0.5 mg) may be prescribed on a short-term basis for the management of insomnia.

❖ Careful maternal monitoring is essential during this period because a small percentage of women with postpartum blues may eventually develop PPD. Women who are facing marital difficulties or those in whom the condition persists beyond 10–14 days are at an increased risk of developing PPD.

❖ According to the recommendations by the NICE, if the resolution of the above-mentioned symptoms does not occur between 10–14 days postdelivery, the patient must be assessed for PPD.[13] She may be referred to psychiatric services where deemed appropriate.

Postpartum Depression

❖ Early treatment is essential in these cases because post-natal depression is likely to have a significant effect on the maternal-infant relationship and the infant's development.

❖ In the past, treatment of PPD comprised of social support, supportive therapy, administration of hormones (oestrogen and progestogens) and prescription of antidepressants. However, the present Cochrane review has demonstrated discouraging results with the use of hormonal therapy for treatment of PPD.[15] Hormonal therapy is presently not recommended for treatment of women with PPD. Modern therapy for PPD, therefore, revolves around the use of supportive and pharmacological therapy.

❖ A combination of cognitive behavioural therapy and antidepressants appears to be the best treatment option for PPD.[16,17] NICE has recommended that interventions such as self-help strategies, non-directive counselling and short courses of cognitive behavioural therapy and/or interpersonal psychotherapy act as the first-line therapy and must be offered first to the patients with mild-to-moderate postnatal depression.[13] In case the woman is resistant to this therapy, those with severe depression or those who decline psychological treatment must be offered treatment with antidepressants. If either of these treatment strategies fails, the woman can be offered a combination of these two therapies.

❖ Psychiatrist having experience in postpartum mental health disorders must be involved at an early stage.

❖ In case the patient is hospitalised, her separation from the baby should be avoided and she should be preferably admitted in the specialised mother and baby unit.

Puerperal Psychosis

❖ This is a psychiatric emergency and the women with this condition must be hospitalised. Failure to treat this condition may be associated with high infanticide rates.

❖ The mother together with her infant must be preferably admitted in a specialised mother-child unit to prevent separation from her child.

❖ Antidepressant and neuroleptic medications must be initiated under psychiatric supervision.

❖ Aggressive treatment in unresponsive cases may include electroconvulsive therapy.

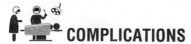

COMPLICATIONS

Maternal

Untreated depression can result in the development of a chronic depressive illness and increased risk for suicide.

Neonatal

Untreated PPD can have the following negative consequences for the infant:

❖ The negative interactive patterns formed between the mother and child during the critical early period of bonding may affect the child's development in future.

❖ Children exposed to maternal psychiatric illnesses may develop the following disorders in the future: Conduct disorders, inappropriate aggression, cognitive and attention deficits, etc.

CLINICAL PEARLS

❖ Assessment of the woman's risk for developing psychiatric illness should begin prepregnancy and preferably continue throughout the pregnancy and the early postpartum period.

❖ Most women who commit suicide following or during pregnancy are likely to have a significant history of mental health disorders.

❖ Despite the presence of safety concerns, most drugs used for treating psychiatric conditions during pregnancy can be considered relatively safe.

❖ The presence of a psychotic disorder may prevent a woman from obtaining adequate prenatal and postpartum care.

EVIDENCE-BASED MEDICINE

❖ The present evidence shows that oestrogen therapy may be of uncertain value for the treatment of severe PPD. Its role in the prevention of recurrent PPD has also not been meticulously assessed. Moreover, use of oestrogen therapy may be associated with potential side effects such as thromboembolic disorders, endometrial hyperplasia, inhibition of lactation, etc.

❖ Synthetic progestogens should preferably not be used in the postpartum period because therapy with synthetic progestogens is likely to be associated with higher incidence of PPD in comparison to the placebo. The natural progestogens are likely to be associated with mood-elevating properties. However, their role in the prevention and treatment of PPD has yet to be evaluated in a randomised, placebo-controlled trial.[15]

❖ Randomised control trial has shown that fluoxetine is as effective as cognitive behavioural therapy for treatment of PPD.[18] Therefore, the decision regarding choice of treatment (antidepressants vs. cognitive behavioural therapy) must be left to the women themselves.

REFERENCES

1. Lewis G (Ed). The Confidential Enquiry into Maternal and Child Health (CEMACH). Why Mothers Die 2000–2002. The Sixth Report on Confidential Enquiries into Maternal Deaths in the United Kingdom. London: RCOG Press; 2004.

2. Lewis G (Ed). The Confidential Enquiry into Maternal and Child Health (CEMACH). Saving Mothers' Lives 2003–2005. The Seventh Report on Confidential Enquiries into Maternal Deaths in the United Kingdom. London: CEMACH; 2007.

3. American Psychiatric Association. Diagnostic and Statistical Manual of Mental Disorders, 4th edition, Text Revision. Washington, DC: American Psychiatric Association; 2000.

4. Steiner M. Postpartum psychiatric disorders. Can J Psychiatry. 1990;35:89-95.

5. Lewellyn AM, Stowe ZN, Nemeroff CB. Depression during pregnancy and the puerperium. J Clin Psychiatry. 1997;58 (Suppl 15):26-32.

6. O'Hara MW. Social support, life events, and depression during pregnancy and the puerperium. Arch Gen Psychiatry. 1986;43(6):569-73.

7. Kumar R, Robson MK. A prospective study of emotional disorders in childbearing women. Br J Psychiatry. 1984;144:35-47.

8. Cox JL, Holdon JM, Sagovsky R. Detection of postnatal depression: development of the 10-item Edinburgh Postnatal Depression Scale. Br J Psychiatry. 1987;150:782-6.

9. Murray L, Carothers AD. The validity of the Edinburgh Post-natal Depression Scale on a community sample. Br J Psychiatry. 1990;157:288-90.

10. Beck CT, Gable RK. Further validation of the postpartum depression screening scale. Nurs Res. 2001;50(3):155-64.

11. Corwin EJ, Murray-Kolb LE, Beard JL. Low haemoglobin level is a risk factor for postpartum depression. J Nutr. 2003;133(12):4139-42.

12. Lucas A, Pizarro E, Granada ML, Salinas I, Sanmartí A. Postpartum thyroid dysfunction and postpartum depression: Are they two linked disorders? Clin Endocrinol (Oxf). 2001; 55(6):809-14.

13. National Collaborating Centre for Mental Health, National Institute for Health and Clinical Excellence. Antenatal and postnatal mental health. The NICE Guideline on Clinical Management and Service Guidance. London: The British Psychological Society and the Royal College of Physicians; 2007.

14. Ryan D, Kostaras X. Psychiatric disorders in the postpartum period. BC Med J. 2005;47(2):100-3.

15. Dennis CL, Ross LE, Herxheimer A. Oestrogens and progestins for preventing and treating postpartum depression. Cochrane Database Syst Rev. 2008;(4):CD001690.

16. Altshuler LL, Cohen L, Szuba MP, Burt VK, Gitlin M, Mintz J. Pharmacologic management of psychiatric illness during pregnancy: Dilemmas and guidelines. Am J Psychiatry. 1996;153(5):592-606.

17. Molyneaux E, Howard LM, McGeown HR, Karia AM, Trevillion K. Antidepressant treatment for postnatal depression. Cochrane Database Syst Rev. 2014;(9):CD002018.

18. Appleby L, Warner R, Whitton A, Faragher B. A controlled study of fluoxetine and cognitive-behavioural counselling in the treatment of postnatal depression. BMJ. 1997;314(7085): 932-6.

Problems with Breastfeeding

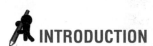 INTRODUCTION

There is extensive data in the literature supporting the concept that breast milk is the optimum food for the babies. It may be associated with several benefits such as reduced morbidity from respiratory, gastrointestinal, urinary tract and the middle ear infection as well as reduced tendency towards atopy, obesity, type 1 and type 2 diabetes, leukaemia, sudden infant death syndrome, etc. Breastfeeding is also likely to be beneficial for the mothers, resulting in a reduced incidence of epithelial ovarian cancers, premenopausal breast cancers, myocardial infraction, type 2 diabetes, metabolic syndrome, etc.[1] Conditions, which interfere with breastfeeding, are likely to result in important epidemiological health issues. Internal audit in the UK (2010) showed that nearly 76% of the women in the UK commence breastfeeding.[2] Breastfeeding is more common amongst the women from social class I than in the socioeconomic class V. Also, it is more common in England than in the other parts of the UK. In the UK, these rates fall to approximately 48% at 6 weeks and 25% at 6 months. At 6 months postpartum less than 1% of the women are exclusively breastfeeding. The proportion of women who breastfeed has been identified as a high priority by the government in their white paper, 'Our Healthier Nation'.[3] The WHO recommends exclusive breastfeeding until the age of 6 months. For these targets to be reached, interventions of proven benefit need to be employed throughout the health services. UNICEF and WHO have jointly developed a programme, Baby-Friendly Hospital Initiative (BFHI), where the maternity services that employ their 10 steps to successful breastfeeding can apply for the baby-friendly status. These 10 steps are evidence-based standards designed to protect, promote and support breastfeeding. These steps include management of issues such as establishment of local policies, training of staff, antenatal and postnatal education of women and establishment of support groups. As an incentive to maternity services, many primary care trusts in England are working towards the

Table 53.1: Global criteria for the baby-friendly hospital initiative[4]

Steps	Criteria
Step 1	The hospital should have a written breastfeeding policy, which is routinely communicated to all healthcare staff
Step 2	All the healthcare staff must be trained in skills necessary to implement the policy
Step 3	Informing all pregnant women about the benefits and management of breastfeeding
Step 4	Helping mothers to initiate breastfeeding within half an hour of the baby's birth
Step 5	Teaching mothers the method of breastfeeding and maintenance of lactation, even if they should be separated from their infants
Step 6	No food or drink other than breast milk to be given to the infant, unless medically indicated
Step 7	Rooming-in must be practiced and the mothers and infants must be allowed to remain together, 24 hours a day
Step 8	Breastfeeding on demand must be encouraged
Step 9	No artificial teats or pacifiers (also known as dummies or soothers) must be provided to breastfeeding infants
Step 10	Establishment of breastfeeding support groups must be encouraged and mothers must be referred to them at the time of discharge from the hospital

achievement of baby-friendly status. The global criteria for the BFHI is described in Table 53.1[4] and serves as the standard for measuring adherence to each of the 10 steps for successful breastfeeding.[4]

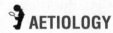 AETIOLOGY

Normal Lactation

Lactation is the process of milk production, which occurs from the mammary glands. Establishment of lactation is dependent on a variety of factors including production of prolactin from the anterior pituitary gland and production of oxytocin from the posterior pituitary gland. The endocrine control of lactation can be divided into the following stages:

❖ *Mammogenesis*: This stage is associated with preparation of the breast tissues. During pregnancy, there is growth of both ductal and lobuloalveolar systems.

❖ *Lactogenesis*: There is synthesis and secretion of milk by breast alveoli during this phase. Although some amount of secretions are produced from the breasts throughout the pregnancy, actual milk secretion starts by 3rd or 4th postpartum days. With the decline in the levels of oestrogen and progesterone following delivery, prolactin is able to initiate its milk secretory activity in the previously fully developed mammary glands. Other hormones, which may enhance the secretory activity of mammary glands, include growth hormone, thyroxine, glucocorticoids and insulin.

❖ *Galactokinesis*: During this phase, there is ejection of milk. Due to this, the milk is forced down the ampulla of lactiferous ducts from where it can be sucked by the infant.

❖ *Galactopoiesis*: This phase is associated with maintenance of lactation. Prolactin is the most important hormone, which is responsible for galactopoiesis. Sucking is essential for maintenance of effective lactation. It helps in removal of milk produced by the glands as well as causes release of prolactin.

Abnormalities in Lactation

Problems with lactation are rarely due to dysfunction at the pituitary-hypothalamic axis. The main reasons why the women are neither able to initiate or continue breastfeeding is usually due to social and cultural causes. Other reasons for abnormalities in breastfeeding could be due to medical causes such as breast engorgement, mastitis, breast abscess, enforced separation of the mother and the baby, poor infant feeding, etc.[5]

Breast Engorgement

This condition is related to imbalance between production of milk and its intake by the infant. Some predisposing factors for breast engorgement include delayed initiation of feeds, infrequent feeds, time limited feeds, a late shift from colostrum to milk production and administration of supplementary feeds. When the production of milk exceeds its consumption, the alveolar spaces within the breasts get distended. As a result, the breasts become swollen, tender and hot. This causes compression of the capillaries, which increases arterial pressure in the breast tissues. This eventually results in the compression of connective tissues and reduced lymphatic drainage, causing obstructive mastitis (breast engorgement and oedema).

Infective Mastitis

Infection in cases of obstructive mastitis results in development of infective mastitis. Mastitis can be defined as the parenchymatous infection of the mammary glands. The most important causative organism is *Staphylococcus aureus*,

most commonly CA-MRSA. Other organisms, which can be involved, include *S. epidermidis* A, B and F, β-*haemolytic streptococcus*, *Haemophilus influenzae* and *Escherichia coli*.

Enforced Separation of the Mother and the Baby

Enforced separation of the mother and baby could be related to the ill health of the mother or baby or both. This separation may have a significant impact on the establishment of breastfeeding because frequent feeding is essential for the successful long-term breastfeeding.[6] This is obviously not possible if the mother and baby are physically separated or they are too ill to feed. One of the important steps of the '10 steps to successful breastfeeding' promoted by UNICEF is ensuring that the mother and baby remain together. Systematic reviews of RCTs have shown that prolonged breastfeeding is not more prevalent in women who perform their first breastfeed within 30 minutes of birth.[7] Early contact is likely to be associated with greater communication between mothers and infants.

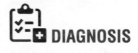

DIAGNOSIS

MASTITIS

Clinical Presentation

❖ Clinical symptoms usually appear by 3rd to 4th weeks of puerperium
❖ The infection is usually unilateral and is associated with marked breast engorgement and inflammation
❖ Fever may be associated with chills or rigors
❖ Hardening and reddening of the breast tissue and intense pain
❖ Development of abscesses and presence of fluctuation.

Investigations

❖ *Ultrasound examination*: This is done to detect the presence of breast abscess.
❖ *Culture and sensitivity*: Culture and sensitivity of the breast milk help in identifying the causative organism.

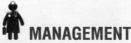

MANAGEMENT

Breast Engorgement

❖ Prevention of breast engorgement can be achieved by avoiding stasis of milk. This can be prevented by using the technique of 'feeding on demand' and attaching the baby to the nipple in the correct position from the first feed onwards.[8]
❖ Supportive counselling and warm or cold compresses
❖ Anti-inflammatory agents are useful in cases of breast engorgement.
❖ Antibiotics are usually not required in the early stages of obstructive mastitis, when signs and symptoms of mastitis

Box 53.1: Indications for administration of antibiotics in cases of breast engorgement

- ❑ Acute pain
- ❑ Severe symptoms
- ❑ Symptoms present for more than 12–24 h
- ❑ Fever
- ❑ Systemic infection
- ❑ Positive microbiology studies

are not severe or have not been present for more than 12–24 hours. Antibiotics, however, may be required in presence of conditions tabulated in Box 53.1.

❖ Although some interventions such as hot or cold packs, Gua-Sha (scraping therapy), acupuncture, ultrasound therapy, cabbage leaves and proteolytic enzymes may appear to be a beneficial treatment option for the patients with breast engorgement, presently, there is insufficient evidence from published trials regarding significant efficacy of any intervention.[9] Therefore, routine implementation of any of these techniques cannot be presently justified.

Mastitis

❖ Treatment of infective mastitis mainly comprises of antibiotic treatment after bacterial identification and sensitivity. Infection usually resolves within 48 hours with treatment. Treatment with antibiotics will also be required in case of breast abscess.

❖ Women with both obstructive and infective mastitis must continue to breastfeed. In case the mother is not breastfeeding, she should be encouraged to manually express the milk.[10] However, breastfeeding should be discontinued in women with breast abscess. Abscesses either require surgical drainage under general anaesthesia or needle aspiration (with or without ultrasound control).

Breast Abscesses

❖ In case of an abscess in early stages, presenting as an indurated mass, a course of antibiotics usually proves to be sufficient. The most common cause of infection in these cases is CA-MRSA. If clinician is sure about the absence of MRSA, a breast abscess can be treated with an antibiotic which is active against methicillin-sensitive staphylococci. This can be administered orally or intravenously depending upon the severity of infection. In cases of suspected or confirmed CA-MRSA, or in patients who are allergic to penicillin, antibiotics such as trimethoprim or sulfamethoxazole, doxycycline, or clindamycin can be used.[11] Vancomycin may be used in more severe cases and in hospitalised patients where hospital-acquired MRSA is suspected.

❖ In case of a mature abscess (e.g. fluctuant mass), surgical intervention along with antibiotics is indicated. In most cases of small abscesses (<5 cm in size), needle aspiration with or without ultrasound guidance can be used to drain an abscess.[12] Sometimes, multiple aspirations over

time (daily aspiration for 5–7 days) may be required for complete drainage. Ultrasound examination can be used to check the completion of drainage. In presence of large abscesses (>5 cm in diameter), incision and drainage may be required. The drained out or aspirated purulent material should be submitted for microbiology studies and cytological examination. Antibiotics should be continued for up to 10 days postdrainage in abscesses greater than 5 cm in size.

Enforced Separation of the Mother and the Baby

If breastfeeding is established in these cases, the mother should be advised to express her breast milk either by hands or mechanically and collect it in a container to feed the infant later. This is especially important in case of babies admitted to the neonatal units because of many previously mentioned advantages of breastfeeding. Many neonatal units have established milk banks to store this milk. In mothers where breastfeeding is contraindicated (e.g. maternal HIV infection or severe maternal ill health), a dopamine agonist such as cabergoline may be prescribed to stop milk production.

CLINICAL PEARLS

❖ Pain in the breasts due to mastitis (both obstructive and infective) can be considered as the third most common cause for discontinuation of breastfeeding. Nearly one-fourth of the women discontinue due to this reason.

❖ Poor technique of breastfeeding is an important cause for discontinuation of breastfeeding.

❖ Treatment of choice in cases of breast engorgement is anti-inflammatory agent (ibuprofen, paracetamol, etc.)

❖ Early skin-to-skin contact between the mother and the child is likely to be associated with several benefits such as improved breastfeeding outcomes, cardiorespiratory stability and reduced infant crying.[6]

EVIDENCE-BASED MEDICINE

❖ When surgical drainage is performed for breast abscesses, the choice of incision for drainage, whether radial or circumferential, presently remains controversial. While the best cosmetic results are associated with circumferential incisions, they may be associated with damage to the surrounding ducts. Radial incisions, on the other hand, may be associated with poor cosmetic results. However, they carry a minimal risk of damage to the surrounding lactiferous ducts. Therefore, circumferential incisions are preferred for draining superficial abscesses, while the radial incisions are used for draining deep abscesses.[10-12]

❖ It has been speculated that the timing of a baby's first breastfeed may affect the total duration of breastfeeding as well as emotional attachment between the mother and child. Systematic reviews have, however, failed to show improved prevalence of long-term breastfeeding in the groups of women who commence feeding early in comparison to those who commence feeding their infants between 4 hours and 8 hours postdelivery. No differences were found between early and delayed contact with regards to the duration of breastfeeding.[7] Early contact, however, does result in an improved communication between the mother and the child.

❖ Support from a professional person (especially UNICEF trained) is associated with a significant reduction in the rate of discontinuation of breastfeeding.[13,14]

REFERENCES

1. Stuebe A. The risks of not breastfeeding for mothers and infants. Rev Obstet Gynecol. 2009;2(4):222-31.
2. The Health and Social Care Information Centre. (2012). The infant feeding survey: 2010. [online]. Available from www.hscic.gov.uk/catalogue/PUB08694/Infant-Feeding-Survey-2010-Consolidated-Report.pdf. [Accessed July, 2016].
3. Department of Health. Our Healthier Nation: A Contract for Health. London: HSMO; 1998.
4. World Health Organization. Baby Friendly Hospital Initiative: Revised, Updated and Expanded for Integrated Care. Geneva: World Health Organization; 2009.
5. Bharat A, Gao F, Aft RL, Gillanders WE, Eberlein TJ, Margenthaler JA. Predictors of primary breast abscesses and recurrence. World J Surg. 2009;33(12):2582-6.
6. Moore ER, Anderson GC, Bergman N, Dowswell T. Early skin-to-skin contact for mothers and their healthy newborn infants. Cochrane Database Syst Rev. 2012;(5):CD003519.
7. Renfrew MJ, Lang S, Woolridge MW. Early versus delayed initiation of breastfeeding. Cochrane Database Syst Rev. 2000;(2):CD000043.
8. Wight NE. Management of common breastfeeding issues. Pediatr Clin North Am. 2001;48(2):321-44.
9. Mangesi L, Zakarija-Grkovic I. Treatments for breast engorgement during lactation. Cochrane Database Syst Rev. 2016;(6):CD006946.
10. British Medical Journal (BMJ) Best Practice. Mastitis and Breast Abscess. London: BMJ; 2016.
11. Lam E, Chan T, Wiseman SM. Breast abscess: evidence based management recommendations. Expert Rev Anti Infect Ther. 2014;12(7):753-62.
12. Dener C, Inan A. Breast abscesses in lactating women. World J Surg. 2003;27(2):130-3.
13. Berens PD. Prenatal, intrapartum and postpartum support of the lactating mother. Pediatr Clin North Am. 2001;48(2):365-75.
14. Renfrew MJ, McCormick FM, Wade A, Quinn B, Dowswell T. Support for healthy breastfeeding mothers with healthy term babies. Cochrane Database Syst Rev. 2012;(5):CD001141.

SECTION 10

The Newborn Infant

OBSTETRICS

Asphyxia Neonatorum

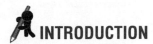

INTRODUCTION

Asphyxia neonatorum occurs due to non-establishment of satisfactory pulmonary respiration at birth. If allowed to progress, this condition can result in hypoxia, hypercarbia and metabolic acidosis.

AETIOLOGY

Continuation of intrauterine hypoxia: The main cause for asphyxia neonatorum includes perinatal asphyxia and foetal distress linked to many causes before birth (Table 54.1).[1]

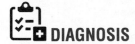

DIAGNOSIS

Clinical Presentation

❖ *Evaluation of APGAR score*: **A**ppearance, **p**ulse, **g**rimace, **a**ctivity and **r**espiration (APGAR) score (Table 54.2) helps in the assessment of foetal condition and is usually calculated at 1, 5 and 15 minutes of birth. Persistence of APGAR score of 0–3 for greater than 5 minutes after birth may be associated with neonatal asphyxia.[2]
❖ Neurological manifestations such as hypotonia, coma, seizures, etc.
❖ Multiorgan dysfunction.

Investigations

❖ *Antepartum/intrapartum tests of foetal surveillance*: These tests, such as NST, contraction stress test, BPP, electronic foetal monitoring (both external and internal) may be abnormal.
❖ *Foetal blood pH sampling*: Metabolic acidosis (<7.2).
❖ *Foetal blood lactate sampling*: Presence of lactic acidosis (>4.8 mmol/L).

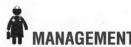

MANAGEMENT

Steps for Neonatal Resuscitation

Most babies, even those born apnoeic, will resuscitate themselves if a clear airway is provided. The algorithm for neonatal resuscitation is described in Flow chart 54.1.[3] However, the basic approach to resuscitation is Airway, Breathing and Circulation, with the following initial actions:[4]

Step 1: The clock is started as soon as the baby is born. Extra help should be called for. Initial step of resuscitation involves providing warmth by placing the baby under a radiant warmer. The baby is placed with his or her head in a 'sniffing' position, with the eyes looking directly upwards. This position helps in opening the airway. The airway is then cleared with a bulb syringe or suction catheter, which helps in clearing the secretions from the oropharynx. Routine oropharyngeal suction is not required because most of the normally vigorous babies are able to clear these secretions on their own. Suctioning is only required in cases of infants with excessive secretions or those with blood or meconium in their secretions. The suction catheter must be gently inserted inside the oropharynx, not further than 5 cm. A suction pressure of 100 mmHg is usually sufficient. The term and larger preterm baby should be dried with a warm towel by rubbing it vigorously so as to stimulate the baby.

Very-low-birthweight (<1,500 g) preterm babies are particularly at the risk of hypothermia despite the use of traditional techniques for reducing heat loss.[5] Currently, it is recommended that such babies must be covered by food-grade, heat-resistant plastic wrapping without drying them and placed under radiant heat. This technique is likely to provide additional warming to the child. Temperature must be monitored closely because of the slight risk of hyperthermia possible with this technique.[6] Other techniques to maintain

Table 54.1: Causes of foetal distress[1]

Foetal	Antepartum	Intrapartum	Postpartum
• Multiple pregnancy • Prematurity • Post-term birth • Intrauterine growth restriction • Congenital abnormalities • Liquor disturbances (oligohydramnios and polyhydramnios) • Hydrops • Immunisation • Intrauterine infection	• Abruptio placentae • Oxytocin induction • Strong hypertonic uterine contractions • Placental insufficiency (pre-eclampsia, IUGR, etc.) • Hypertensive disorders of pregnancy • Maternal hypotension (supine position, epidural anaesthesia) • Chorioamnionitis • Postmaturity • Chronic ill health • Drug digestion (legal or illegal) • Anatomical abnormalities	• Foetal distress • Abnormal presentations • Antepartum haemorrhage • Uterine rupture/scar dehiscence • *Oxytocin induction*: Strong uterine contractions • Operative vaginal delivery due to vacuum or forceps application • Cord around the neck and cord compression • Cord prolapse • Prolonged second stage of labour/rupture of membranes • Thick meconium • Instrumental delivery • Abnormal uterine contractions (dystocia)	• Pulmonary, cardiovascular and neurological abnormalities in the neonate

Table 54.2: APGAR score

Signs	0	1	2	Component of acronym
Colour	Blue, pale	*Acrocyanosis*: Body pink, extremities blue	Complete pink	**A**ppearance
Heart rate	Absent	Slow (<100 bpm)	>100 bpm	**P**ulse
Reflex irritability	No response	Grimace/ feeble cry	Strong cry, cough or sneeze	**G**rimace
Muscle tone	Flaccid	Flexion of extremities	Active body movements	**A**ctivity
Breathing	Apnoea	Slow, irregular	Good, crying	**R**espiratory effort

Note: Total score: 10; No depression/normal: 7–10; Mild depression: 4–6; Severe depression: 0–3

Flow chart 54.1: Algorithm for neonatal resuscitation[3]

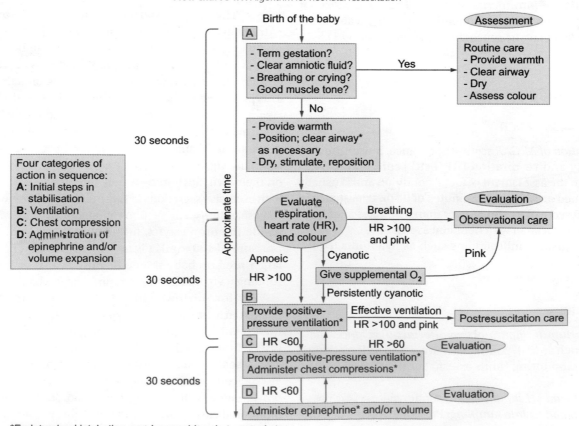

*Endotracheal intubation may be considered at several steps

temperature during stabilisation of the baby in the delivery room (e.g. drying and swaddling, warming pads, increased environmental temperature, placing the baby skin-to-skin with the mother and covering both with a blanket) have been used. However, none of them have been evaluated in controlled trials nor compared with the plastic wrap technique for premature babies.

These initial techniques should not take more than 20–30 seconds.

Clearing the Airway of Meconium

Aspiration of meconium before delivery, during birth, or during resuscitation can cause severe aspiration pneumonia. One technique of reducing aspiration is suctioning the meconium from the infant's airway following the delivery of the head but before delivery of the shoulders (intrapartum suctioning). However, routine intrapartum oropharyngeal and nasopharyngeal suctioning for infants born to mothers with meconium staining of amniotic fluid is no longer recommended. According to the traditional recommendations,[7-9] endotracheal intubation must be performed in meconium-stained infants (who are not vigorous) immediately following birth, and suction must be applied to the endotracheal tube as it is withdrawn. RCTs[10,11] have indicated that this practice is unlikely to be beneficial in case of vigorous infants. A vigorous infant can be considered as the one having strong respiratory efforts, good muscle tone, and a heart rate (HR) greater than 100 bpm.

Further Management

Step 2: Following the immediate postbirth assessment and administration of initial steps, further resuscitative efforts should be guided by simultaneous assessment of respirations, HR, and baby's colour, i.e. calculation of the APGAR score. This score should be evaluated by 30 seconds of life. Further management depends on the APGAR score (Table 54.3). Repeat scores should be performed at an interval of every 30 seconds depending on the baby's condition. Gasping and apnoea indicate the requirement for assisted ventilation.[12] Increasing or decreasing HR can also provide evidence of improvement or deterioration.

Step 3: *Administration of oxygen*: Use of supplemental oxygen should be considered in cases where the baby continues to have central cyanosis despite the use of initial steps. In these cases, free-flow oxygen is administered. Supplementary oxygen is also recommended in cases where positive-pressure ventilation is indicated for resuscitation. Mode of delivery and concentration of oxygen administered depends on the state of respiratory efforts.

There are concerns regarding the potential adverse effects of 100% oxygen on respiratory physiology and cerebral circulation. 100% oxygen is also likely to cause potential damage to the tissues resulting in the formation of oxygen-free radicals. There are concerns regarding the risk of potential injury due to oxygen-free radicals, especially in the premature infant. The clinician needs to remain cautious regarding the use of excessive oxygen. On the contrary, there are also concerns about the damage to the tissues due to oxygen deprivation during and after asphyxia.

The standard approach to resuscitation is to use 100% oxygen. Some clinicians may begin resuscitation with an oxygen concentration of less than 100%, while some may start with room air, i.e. using no supplementary oxygen. If the clinician begins resuscitation with room air, it is recommended that supplementary oxygen must be available for use, in case there is no appreciable improvement within 90 seconds after birth. If supplementary oxygen is not easily available, positive-pressure ventilation should be administered with room air.

Step 4: *Positive-pressure ventilation*: If the infant is still apnoeic, is gasping or shows no response, or if the HR remains below 100 bpm, or if an infant remains cyanosed even after 30 seconds of administration of step 3, step 4 should be considered. At this stage of resuscitation, the infant is usually no more than 1 minute of age. Positive-pressure ventilation

Table 54.3: Further management based on APGAR score[4]

APGAR score	Baby's characteristics	Management
APGAR score between 7 and 10	These are healthy babies. The child is pink in colour centrally, has a heart rate (HR) >100 bpm and shows a good respiratory effort	They should be kept warm and given to their mothers
APGAR score between 4 and 6	Babies may be cyanosed, with normal or reduced tone, having a poor respiratory effort, with or without a slow HR (<100 bpm)	If the baby responds to tactile stimulation and suctioning of the oropharynx, then no further resuscitation is needed. If there is no response, the clinician must progress to assisted ventilation. Oxygen by bag and mask ventilation (Fig. 54.1) at a pressure of 30–40 cm of H_2O must be given. Once the lungs have inflated and the HR has increased or if the chest has been seen to move in response to passive inflation, then ventilation should be continued at a rate of 30–40 breaths/min. Ventilatory support must be continued until regular breathing is established
APGAR score of <4	The baby may be blue or white and/or floppy. There may be absent breathing, or gasping with absent HR or profound bradycardia (<100 bpm)	Full intensive resuscitation would be required in such infants. Tracheal intubation (Figs 54.2A and B) remains the gold standard for airway management

CHAPTER 54

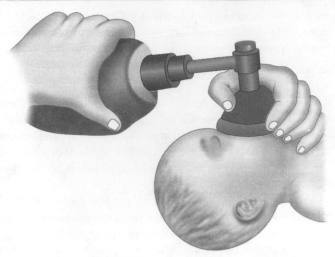

Fig. 54.1: Bag and mask ventilation

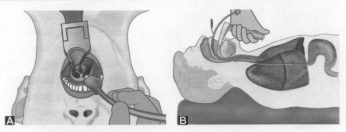

Figs 54.2A and B: (A) Tracheal intubation; (B) Magnified view of endotracheal intubation

can be performed with a bag-valve-mask apparatus or a facemask along with a T-piece connector. Assisted ventilation should be delivered at a rate of 40–60 breaths per minute to promptly achieve or maintain a HR of greater than 100 bpm. While starting positive-pressure ventilation, initially five rescue breaths are administered. These are the more sustained breaths, which help in overcoming the high airway resistance present in the lungs of the infant who has yet not breathed. The infant's response following these rescue breaths must be assessed. If there is still concern regarding respiration, regular ventilation must be commenced. This is administered at the rate of 30–40 breaths per minute, with each breath lasting for 0.5 seconds. Clinically, the physician can evaluate the adequacy of these breaths by noting the chest movement, hearing the breath sounds and observing the infant's colour and HR. Once good spontaneous respiratory rate has been established, ventilation should be stopped.

Step 5: Placement of endotracheal tube: If there is no response or poor respiratory effort despite positive-pressure ventilation even after 30–60 seconds, endotracheal intubation may be considered. Endotracheal intubation may also be indicated at several points during neonatal resuscitation:

❖ Requirement of tracheal suctioning for meconium-stained liquor
❖ Anticipated requirement for long-term ventilatory support
❖ Ineffective or prolonged bag-mask ventilation
❖ Performance of chest compressions
❖ Requirement for endotracheal administration of medications
❖ Resuscitation in special circumstances, e.g. presence of congenital diaphragmatic hernia or extremely low-birthweight babies (<1,000 g).

Increase in HR following endotracheal intubation and administration of intermittent positive pressure can be considered as the best indicator for correct placement of endotracheal tube and effective ventilation.[13] Detection of levels of exhaled CO_2 serves as an effective method for confirmation of endotracheal tube placement in infants, including very low-birthweight infants.[14-17] Once the vocal cords are visualised following insertion of the laryngoscope

with blade of an appropriate size (size 1 blade for a term infant and size 0 blade for preterm infant), an endotracheal tube is inserted inside. Once the endotracheal tube has been positioned in place, ventilatory circuit is attached, following which the ventilatory breaths are delivered at the rate of 30–40 breaths per minute. The act of intubation, starting right from the time of insertion of laryngoscope blade in the mouth until the time of attachment of the endotracheal tube to the ventilator circuit should not take longer than 20–30 seconds.

Step 6: Chest compression: Once the airway and breathing have been assessed, circulation must then be evaluated. The best sites to check for the HR and pulse include the base of umbilical cord and brachial pulse. Chest compressions may be required if the HR is less than 60 bpm despite adequate ventilation with supplementary oxygen for 30 seconds. Before starting chest compressions, rescuers should ensure that assisted ventilation is being delivered optimally. Compressions should be delivered on the lower third of the sternum to a depth of approximately one-third of the anterior-posterior diameter of the chest.[18,19] Two techniques have been described:[20-22]

1. *Compression with two thumbs with fingers encircling the chest and supporting the back*: The two-thumb encircling hands technique is most effective technique of giving chest compressions and comprises of encircling the chest with both hands, so that the fingers lie behind the baby and the thumbs are opposed on the sternum just below the inter-nipple line (Figs 54.3A and B). The two thumb-encircling hands technique is recommended for performing chest compressions in newly born infants because this technique is likely to generate higher peak systolic and coronary perfusion pressure in comparison to the two-finger technique.

2. *Compression with two fingers (index and middle fingers) with a second hand supporting the back*: The two-finger technique may be preferable when access to the umbilicus is required during insertion of an umbilical catheter.

Current recommendation is to perform three compressions for each ventilation breath (3:1 ratio), with 90 compressions and 30 breaths to achieve approximately 120 events per minute. Thus, each event will be allotted approximately half a second. During the phase of relaxation, the chest should be permitted to fully re-expand. However, the rescuer's thumbs should not leave the chest. Respirations, HR, and colour should be reassessed about every 30 seconds, and coordinated chest compressions and ventilations should continue. Once the

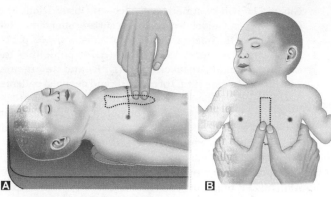

Figs 54.3A and B: Infant chest compression: (A) Two-finger compression; (B) Chest-encircling technique

HR increases above 60 bpm and the chest is seen rising, chest compressions can be discontinued.

Step 7: *Use of medications*: If after adequate lung inflation and chest compressions, the HR has not responded, vascular access, medications and volume expansion as described in Table 54.4 should be considered. Umbilical vein is the quickest and most effective means for achieving vascular access. Drugs are rarely indicated in resuscitation of the newly born infant.[23] Bradycardia in the newborn infant is usually the result of inadequate lung inflation or profound hypoxaemia. Therefore, the most important step for its correction is establishment of adequate ventilation. However, if the HR remains below 60 bpm despite adequate ventilation with 100% oxygen and chest compressions, administration of epinephrine or volume expansion, or both, may be considered.

COMPLICATIONS

❖ *Neurological damage*: Neurological deprivation of the oxygen supply to the brain can result in neurological damage, cerebral oedema, seizures, cerebral palsy, hypoxic ischaemic encephalopathy, etc.
❖ *Cardiovascular complications*: Hypotension, cardiac failure
❖ *Renal complications*: Acute cortical necrosis, renal failure
❖ *Impaired LFTs*
❖ *Gastrointestinal complications*: Ulcers and necrotising enterocolitis
❖ *Lungs*: Persistent pulmonary hypertension.

Table 54.4: Drugs to be used for neonatal resuscitation

Drugs	Indication	Dosage
Adrenaline (epinephrine): Most important medicine available	Profound unresponsive bradycardia or circulatory standstill	10–30 µg/kg (0.1–0.3 mL/kg of 1:10,000 solution) adrenaline may be given intravenously or via endotracheal tube. Higher IV doses are not recommended. Following administration, 1–2 minutes of ventilation and chest compressions are performed. Further doses of 10–30 µg/kg may be tried at 3–5-min intervals if there is no response.
Sodium bicarbonate: Its use remains controversial	*Metabolic acidosis*: It can be used in cases where sustained cellular acidosis affects myocardial contractility. Its use is likely to improve the myocardial contractility as well as facilitate the beneficial action of adrenaline	1–2 mmol/kg (2 mL/kg of 4.2% solution) may be used to raise the pH
Dextrose	Hypoglycaemia	A slow bolus of 5 mL/kg of 10% dextrose is administered intravenously, followed by secure IV dextrose infusion at a rate of 100 mL/kg/day
Fluid (volume expansion): This is considered when blood loss is suspected or the infant appears to be in shock (pale skin, poor perfusion, weak pulse) and has not responded adequately to other resuscitative measures	Hypovolaemia due to circulatory disturbances	Volume expansion, initially with 10 mL/kg of normal saline
Blood	Hypovolaemia due to haemorrhage	10–20 mL/kg of O-negative blood as a bolus dose
Naloxone: Use of naloxone should be avoided in babies whose mothers are suspected of having had long-term exposure to opioids because it can result in a severe withdrawal state in these infants	Alleviation of effects of maternal opiates	It is administered in the dose of 0.1 mg/kg preferably by IM or IV routes. Neonate should be monitored closely for recurrent apnoea or hypoventilation, and subsequent doses of naloxone may be required. Naloxone has a shorter half-life than most opiates. Therefore, repetition of the dosage may be required. Endotracheal administration of naloxone is not recommended

CLINICAL PEARLS

❖ Careful antepartum and intrapartum foetal surveillance helps in preventing asphyxia and thereby avoiding the development of foetal distress.

❖ Usually, the first indication of success of neonatal resuscitation is an increase in the baby's HR.

EVIDENCE-BASED MEDICINE

Neuroprotective Nature of Hypothermia

❖ There is insufficient evidence regarding the maintenance of hypothermia in the delivery room because recent multicentric trials have shown that hypothermia may be neuroprotective in term infants with moderate or severe perinatal asphyxial hypoxia. These studies managed infants with core temperatures of about 33.5°C for up to 72 hours. The current recommendation is that for acute resuscitation, normothermia should be maintained and hyperthermia should certainly be prevented.[24,25]

❖ There is increasing evidence regarding the detrimental effects of hyperoxia on the lungs and eyes in the preterm infants. Therefore, initial approach to resuscitation should be only with air. In the event of poor response to air, introduction of oxygen can be considered. A better approach could be to use an oxygen or air blender for managing the concentration of oxygen used.[26,27]

❖ Some clinicians tend to perform intrapartum suction of oropharyngeal tube in infants born to mothers with meconium-stained liquor. Though there is some evidence to illustrate that intrapartum suctioning might be effective for reducing the risk of aspiration syndrome,[28,29] subsequent evidence from large multicentre randomised trials[30,31] did not show such an effect. A Cochrane review of the topic published in 2001 further affirmed these findings.[32] Therefore, current recommendations no longer advise routine intrapartum oropharyngeal and nasopharyngeal suctioning for vigorous infants born to mothers with meconium staining of amniotic fluid for prevention of meconium aspiration syndrome.[33] It still remains debatable if it would be ethically possible to carry out the study of non-vigorous babies. However, based on the previous discussion, it appears reasonable that intrapartum oropharyngeal suctioning must be performed in non-vigorous or depressed infants with meconium-stained liquor.

REFERENCES

1. Overview and principles of resuscitation. In: American Academy of Pediatrics, American Heart Association, Kattwinkel J, Short J (Eds). Textbook of Neonatal Resuscitation, 5th edition. Dallas, Tx: American Academy of Pediatrics; 2006.

2. Gilstrap LC, Oh W. American College of Obstetricians and Gynecologists. Guidelines for Perinatal Care, 5th edition. Elk Grove Village, IL: American Academy of Pediatrics; 2002. p. 187.

3. 2005 American Heart Association (AHA) guidelines for cardiopulmonary resuscitation (CPR) and emergency cardiovascular care (ECC) of pediatric and neonatal patients: neonatal resuscitation guidelines. Pediatrics. 2006;117:e1029.

4. International consensus on cardiopulmonary resuscitation and emergency cardiovascular care science with treatment recommendations. Part 7: Neonatal resuscitation. Resuscitation. 2005;67:293-303.

5. Costeloe K, Hennessy E, Gibson AT, Marlow N, Wilkinson AR. The EPICure study: outcomes to discharge from hospital for infants born at the threshold of viability. Pediatrics. 2000;106(4):659-71.

6. Vohra S, Roberts RS, Zhang B, Janes M, Schmidt B. Heat Loss Prevention (HeLP) in the delivery room: a randomized controlled trial of polyethylene occlusive skin wrapping in very preterm infants. J Pediatr. 2004;145(6):750-3.

7. Gregory GA, Gooding CA, Phibbs RH, Tooley WH. Meconium aspiration in infants: a prospective study. J Pediatr. 1974;85(6): 848-52.

8. Rossi EM, Philipson EH, Williams TG, Kalhan SC. Meconium aspiration syndrome: intrapartum and neonatal attributes. Am J Obstet Gynecol. 1989;161(5):1106-10.

9. Davis RO, Philips JB, Harris BA, Wilson ER, Huddleston JF. Fatal meconium aspiration syndrome occurring despite airway management considered appropriate. Am J Obstet Gynecol. 1985;151(6):731-6.

10. Wiswell TE, Gannon CM, Jacob J, Goldsmith L, Szyld E, Weiss K, et al. Delivery room management of the apparently vigorous meconium-stained neonate: results of the multicenter, international collaborative trial. Pediatrics. 2000;105(1 Pt 1):1-7.

11. Halliday HL. Endotracheal intubation at birth for preventing morbidity and mortality in vigorous, meconium-stained infants born at term. Cochrane Database Syst Rev. 2001;(1):CD000500.

12. Dawes GS. Foetal and Neonatal Physiology. A Comparative Study of the Changes at Birth. Chicago, IL: Year Book Medical Publishers Inc; 1968.

13. Palme-Kilander C, Tunell R. Pulmonary gas exchange during facemask ventilation immediately after birth. Arch Dis Child. 1993;68(1 Spec No):11-6.

14. Aziz HF, Martin JB, Moore JJ. The pediatric disposable end-tidal carbon dioxide detector role in endotracheal intubation in newborns. J Perinatol. 1999;19(2):110-3.

15. Bhende MS, Thompson AE. Evaluation of an end-tidal CO_2 detector during pediatric cardiopulmonary resuscitation. Pediatrics. 1995;95(3):395-9.

16. Repetto JE, Donohue P-CP, Baker SF, Kelly L, Nogee LM. Use of capnography in the delivery room for assessment of endotracheal tube placement. J Perinatol. 2001;21(5):284-7.

17. Roberts WA, Maniscalco WM, Cohen AR, Litman RS, Chhibber A. The use of capnography for recognition of esophageal intubation in the neonatal intensive care unit. Pediatr Pulmonol. 1995;19(5):262-8.

18. Orlowski JP. Optimum position for external cardiac compression in infants and young children. Ann Emerg Med. 1986;15(6):667-73.

19. Phillips GW, Zideman DA. Relation of infant heart to sternum: its significance in cardiopulmonary resuscitation. Lancet. 1986;1(8488):1024-5.

20. Thaler MM, Stobie GH. An improved technique of external cardiac compression in infants and young children. N Engl J Med. 1963;269:606-10.

21. David R. Closed chest cardiac massage in the newborn infant. Pediatrics. 1988;81(4):552-4.

22. Todres ID, Rogers MC. Methods of external cardiac massage in the newborn infant. J Pediatr. 1975;86(5):781-2.

23. Perlman JM, Risser R. Cardiopulmonary resuscitation in the delivery room: associated clinical events. Arch Pediatr Adolesc Med. 1995;149(1):20-5.

24. Gunn AJ, Bennet L. Is temperature important in the delivery room resuscitation? Semin Neonatol. 2001;6(3):241-9.

25. Jacobs SE, Berg M, Hunt R, Tarnow-Mordi WO, Inder TE, Davis PG. Cooling for newborns with hypoxic ischaemic encephalopathy. Cochrane Database Syst Rev. 2013;(1): CD003311.

26. Rabi Y, Rabi D, Yee W. Room air resuscitation of the depressed newborn: a systemic review and metaanalysis. Resuscitation. 2007;72(3):353-63.

27. Saugstad OD, Rootwelt T, Aalen OO. Resuscitation of the newborn infant with room air or oxygen. Tidsskr Nor Laegeforen. 2000;120(1):25-8.

28. Falciglia HS, Henderschott C, Potter P, Helmchen R. Does DeLee suction at the perineum prevent meconium aspiration syndrome? Am J Obstet Gynecol. 1992;167(5):1243-9.

29. Carson BS, Losey RW, Bowes WA Jr, Simmons MA. Combined obstetric and pediatric approach to prevent meconium aspiration syndrome. Am J Obstet Gynecol. 1976;126(6):712-5.

30. Vain NE, Szyld EG, Prudent LM, Wiswell TE, Aguilar AM, Vivas NI. Oropharyngeal and nasopharyngeal suctioning of meconium-stained neonates before delivery of their shoulders: multicentre, randomised controlled trial. Lancet. 2004;364(9434):597-602.

31. Wiswell TE, Gannon CM, Jacob J, Goldsmith L, Szyld E, Weiss K, et al. Delivery room management of the apparently vigorous meconium-stained neonate: results of the multicenter, international collaborative trial. Pediatrics. 2000;105(1 Pt 1):1-7.

32. Halliday HL. Endotracheal intubation at birth for preventing morbidity and mortality in vigorous, meconium-stained infants born at term. Cochrane Database Syst Rev. 2001;(1):CD000500.

33. Kattwinkel J, Zaichkin J, Denson S, Niermeyer S (Eds). Textbook of Neonatal Resuscitation, 4th edition. Texas: American Academy of Pediatrics and American Heart Association; 2000.

CHAPTER 54

Care of a Newborn Child and Perinatal Mortality

Care of a Newborn Child and Its Associated Common Problems

 INTRODUCTION

Examination of a newborn baby allows the midwife, paediatrician or the obstetrician to assess and monitor the baby's condition and promptly provide appropriate care and treatment as soon as possible. Every newborn must be examined thoroughly within the first 72 hours of birth.[1]

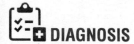 **DIAGNOSIS**

Clinical Presentation

General Physical Examination

Both parents should be encouraged to be present during the time of the physical examination of their baby to enable them to understand their baby's requirements.

❖ *Vital signs*: Normal respiratory rate in a newborn child varies between 30 breaths per minute to 60 breaths per minute, whereas the pulse rate varies between 100 bpm to 160 bpm. Normal range of blood pressure in a newborn child is 45–60 mmHg systolic and 25–40 mmHg diastolic. Normal body temperature in a newborn baby varies between 36.4°C to 37.5°C. Baby's temperature is recorded through rectal, oral or axillary route.

❖ *Skin colour*: A normal baby is usually pink in colour. Pallor may be due to anaemia, birth asphyxia or shock. Cyanosis or bluish discolouration of the skin may be indicative of cardiorespiratory dysfunction. Yellowish discolouration of the baby's skin, nail beds or the sclera could be indicative of jaundice (bilirubin levels >5 mg/dL).

❖ *Congenital anomalies*: There should be no major visible **abnormality** such as cleft lip and palate, congenital heart **disease**, etc.

❖ *Infant's weight*: There is 7–10% weight loss during the first week of life. Weight gain begins from 2nd week onwards.

❖ *Infant's length*: Crown-foot length varies between 48 cm and 53 cm. Normal weekly gain in length is 0.8–1 cm for the first 8–12 weeks of life.

❖ *Dermatological changes*: Various types of non-pathological skin rashes which may be present in the newborn child, include milia, Mongolian spots, erythema toxicum, capillary haemangiomas or stork bites, etc. They are usually of no significance and generally disappear with time. Some pathological skin changes include port wine stain, strawberry naevus, etc.

❖ *Examination of the head*: The head circumference is measured with a paper tape. Head circumference on an average is 33–38 cm and increases by 0.5–0.8 cm per week. The head fontanelles and sutures are palpated. Bulging fontanelles may be due to the increased intracranial pressure, meningitis or hydrocephalus. Depressed fontanelles are seen with dehydration. The baby's head must also be examined for the presence of any abnormal swellings such as caput succedaneum, cephalohaematoma, chignon, moulding, etc.

❖ *Neck*: It is checked for movements and presence of abnormal swellings such as goitre, thyroglossal cysts, sternomastoid haematoma, etc. and abnormal shortening (indicative of Turner's syndrome).

❖ *Eyes*: They are checked with an ophthalmoscope for abnormalities such as cataracts, retinoblastoma and corneal opacities. They must also be checked for any abnormal or sticky discharge that could be indicative of infection.

❖ *Face and mouth*: Face of the newborn is evaluated for various dysmorphic features such as hypertelorism (eyes widely separated) or low set ears (trisomy 9, 18, triploidy) or the facial nerve injury. Mouth is checked for cleft palate or lip, deciduous teeth, lingual frenulum (tongue-tie), macroglossia or oral thrush (candidal infection). Excessive drooling from the mouth could be indicative of condition such as oesophageal atresia.

❖ *Chest*: Breathing and chest wall movements are observed for the signs of respiratory distress. Presence of wheeze or crepitations must be noted. While examining the chest, the breasts of the newborn are also evaluated. They may sometimes be enlarged under the effect of maternal oestrogen.

❖ *Heart*: It is examined for rate, rhythm, and the quality of heart sounds and presence of any murmurs. Presence of murmurs in the newborn child could be indicative of congenital heart disease.

❖ *Abdomen*: On palpating the abdomen, the liver normally extends 1–2 cm below the costal margin; the spleen tip may be palpable, as may be the kidney on the left side. Any intra-abdominal masses may require further investigations. Umbilicus is examined for any discharge, redness or infection and presence of hernia. The cut end of the cord must also be inspected for the number of umbilical arteries and veins.

❖ *Genitalia*: It should be examined carefully before gender assignment. Anus and rectum are checked to rule out imperforation and their position. A normal baby must pass meconium within 48 hours of the birth.

❖ *Limbs*: Extremities, spine and joints must be examined for abnormalities such as syndactyly (fusion of the digits), polydactyly (multiple digits), simian crease (Down's syndrome), talipes equinovarus and hip dislocation (Ortolani and Barlow manoeuvres).

❖ *Nervous system*: The baby must be examined for any irritability, abnormal muscle tone, reflexes, cranial and peripheral nerves.

❖ *General foetal characteristics*: These may vary based on the gestational age (Table 55.1).

Investigations

Haematological findings: Normal haematological parameters in a newborn child are RBC count: 6–8 million; Hb: 18–20 g%; WBC: 10,000–17,000/mm³; Platelets: 35,000/mm³; sedimentation rate—markedly elevated.

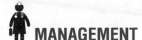

MANAGEMENT

❖ Immediately following birth, the baby must be placed on a cot where neutral thermal condition is being maintained. Hypothermia must be avoided. The baby must be dried immediately after birth and must be covered from head to toe with a prewarmed towel. Early breastfeeding must be encouraged.

❖ Routine baby bath must be delayed until the baby is able to maintain the body temperature and breastfeeding has been started. The excessive blood, vernix, blood or meconium must be wiped off from the baby's skin using sterile moist swabs, following which the skin is dried using a soft towel.

❖ Daily cleansing of the umbilical cord stump with spirit and antibiotic powder must be done.

❖ Single dose of vitamin K (0.5–1 mg) is given to all newborn babies within 6 hours of birth. This helps in preventing bleeding due to the deficiency of vitamin K.

❖ Hepatitis B vaccine is administered at birth.

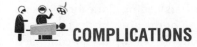

COMPLICATIONS

The important danger signs, which require medical attention, include the following terms.

Transient Tachypnoea of the Newborn

Also known as the wet lung syndrome, transient tachypnoea of the newborn (TTN) is characterised by a temporary difficulty in breathing and low oxygen levels. The affected neonates breathe rapidly, may grunt while breathing out and may show drawing in of the chest wall while breathing in.[2] TTN is probably related to the delayed clearance of the lung fluid by the neonatal lungs. This may be a sign of disease in the alveoli, which are unable to absorb the lung fluid. If the infants' alveoli are not opening up adequately, they may try to open them up by increasing their intrathoracic pressure. This may result in tachypnoea with variable grunting, and flaring and retractions of the chest wall. This sign may be present within a few hours after birth and may disappear within 24–48 hours after birth. Infants born by caesarean delivery (especially elective delivery) are likely to be an increased risk of developing TTN.[3,4] The diagnosis is based on clinical presentation, chest X-ray and after exclusion of other common respiratory conditions such as pneumothorax, respiratory distress syndrome (RDS), etc. Most newborns completely recover within 2–3 days. Affected newborns usually require treatment with oxygen and need some assistance with breathing. Signs and symptoms of acute respiratory embarrassment in such babies may be indicative of severe underlying disease. If the signs do not appear to settle down within a few hours, they appear to be worsening, or there is a presence of other risk factors; infant should be admitted to neonatal unit for further investigations and management.

Hypoglycaemia

Neonatal hypoglycaemia can be defined as blood glucose levels of less than 30 mg/dL (2.6 mmol/L).[5] It can be associated with symptoms like jitteriness, twitching, apnoea, etc. The infants at high risk of developing hypoglycaemia include preterm infants, growth-restricted infants, infants of diabetic mothers, infants

Table 55.1: Foetal characteristics based on the period of gestation

	Preterm	Term	Post-term
Breast nodule	≤2 mm	2–4 mm	4–7 mm
Scalp hair	Fine hair	Fuzzy, fine hair	Coarse hair
Ear lobe	No cartilage	Moderate amount of cartilage	Thick cartilage, resulting in a stiff ear lobe
Testes and scrotum	Partially descended testis; small scrotum with few rugae	Testes have usually descended and rugae are present	Fully descended testes with normal sized scrotum having prominent rugae

PART II

with prenatal asphyxia, septic infants, infants with inborn errors of metabolism, etc. It can occur due to reduced glycogen stores or glycogenolysis or gluconeogenesis, increased metabolic rate and deficient release of catecholamines in these babies.[6] Hypoglycaemia can be associated with symptoms such as hypotonia, lethargy, apathy, poor feeding, jitteriness, seizures, cyanosis, apnoea, hypothermia, tachycardia, pallor, etc. Early feeding of the newborn baby with breast milk can help prevent hypoglycaemia. The mainstay of therapy for babies who are alert and have an intact airway include administration of orange juice (20 mL/kg). 10% dextrose via IV, nasogastric or intraosseous routes may be employed in babies who are unable to feed, drink or cannot protect their airways. Boluses of 10% dextrose (2–3 mL/kg) may be followed by continuous infusion.

Rubbing of 40% dextrose gel over the infant's buccal membrane is more effective than feeding alone for reversing hypoglycaemia in the first 48 hours after birth. The Sugar Babies Study: a randomised, double-blind, placebo-controlled trial has shown that dextrose gel should be considered as first-line treatment to reverse hypoglycaemia in individuals at risk of hypoglycaemia.[7]

Hypothermia

Hypothermia may be defined as the rectal temperature of less than 36°C. Factors responsible for producing hypothermia include reduced amount of subcutaneous fat, increased surface-volume ratio, decreased heat production, etc. Hypothermia could be related to environmental factors or an underlying illness (neonatal sepsis, intracranial haemorrhage, etc.). This commonly occurs in preterm and growth-restricted babies.

Hypothermia can be associated with considerable neonatal morbidity in the form of lethargy, poor feeding, hypoglycaemia, metabolic acidosis, respiratory distress, neonatal sepsis, etc.[8] Treatment of hypothermia involves rewarming the infants by immediately drying the newborn after birth, wrapping them in a warm towel or blanket and placing them in an incubator or a radiant warmer. If hypothermia is related to an underlying cause, steps must be taken for its rectification.

Prematurity

The preterm baby is usually deficient in subcutaneous fat. As a result, the baby's skin appears pink in colour, feels very thin and can easily wrinkle. The preterm baby's head circumference may exceed the waist circumference. Birthweight of a normal term infant varies from 2,500 g to 3,999 g. Most preterm babies may be of low weight. Low birthweight can be defined as weight less than 2,500 g. Length of a preterm baby may be less than 47 cm. A premature baby is likely to suffer from complications such as patent ductus arteriosus, poor sucking and swallowing reflexes, episodes of apnoea, intraventricular haemorrhage, developmental and/or cognitive delays, retinopathy of prematurity, necrotising enterocolitis (NEC), feeding intolerance, growth failure, RDS, bronchopulmonary dysplasia, hypothermia, hypoglycaemia, hyperbilirubinaemia, etc.[9] In a premature infant, Dubowitz (Ballard) examination is used for assessing foetal maturity based on the physical characteristics as well as the maturity of neuromuscular system (Fig. 55.1).

Dubowitz (Ballard) examination for newborn: Points are given for each parameter, which is assessed. Low scores (–1 or 0) are given in case of extreme prematurity. High scores (4, 5) are

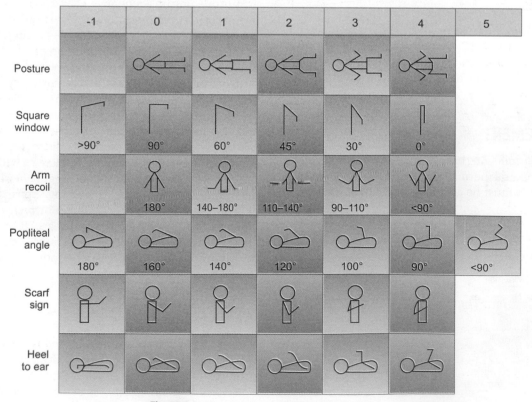

Fig. 55.1: Dubowitz (Ballard) examination for newborn

given in case of postmaturity. Physical characteristics, which are assessed, include parameters such as skin texture, lanugo hair, plantar creases, breasts, eyes, ear and appearance of the genitalia. Assessment of neuromuscular maturity includes evaluation of parameters such as posture, square window (flexion of baby's hand towards the wrist); arm recoil (angle of recoil following very brief extension of the upper extremity); heel to ear movement (passive resistance to extension of posterior hip flexor muscles); popliteal angle (resistance of baby's knee to extension) and scarf sign (how far the elbow can be moved across the baby's chest).

Jaundice

Most common cause of jaundice in the newborns is physiological jaundice. Physiological jaundice occurs during the first few days of life because RBCs in the neonate breakdown at a slightly increased rate, resulting in the accumulation of unconjugated bilirubin in the blood. This occurs because the liver and the digestive tract are relatively immature during the first few days of life. The physiological jaundice typically appears between day 2 and 4 days after birth and is usually asymptomatic. It usually resolves by 1–2 weeks of life. Low levels of unconjugated bilirubin are not harmful and can be treated with simple therapy such as phototherapy.

However, high levels of unconjugated bilirubin may be associated with severe haemolysis occurring due to rhesus or ABO incompatibility.[10] Jaundice due to acute haemolytic disease presents during the first 24–48 hours of life. Therefore, jaundice occurring in a baby during the first 1–2 days of life is likely to be pathological and requires investigations. Such babies may develop high levels of unconjugated bilirubin, which may cause damage to the specific areas of the neonatal brain, causing permanent brain damage (kernicterus). This can lead to a range of neurodevelopmental problems such as cerebral palsy, deafness, motor and speech delay, and sometimes even death. Most infants with postnatal jaundice can be treated with phototherapy.[11] Exchange transfusion may be required in serious cases.

Prolonged jaundice (with duration >2 weeks in term baby and >3 weeks in a preterm baby) is a cause of concern. One of the most common causes for this is breast milk jaundice. This condition is likely to occur due to the presence of a high level of a substance in the breast milk, which slows bilirubin excretion, thereby causing an increase in the bilirubin levels. However, breast milk jaundice is a diagnosis of exclusion and must be reached after excluding other common causes of jaundice (e.g. obstruction due to biliary atresia, hereditary liver disorders, e.g. Dubin-Johnson syndrome, Crigler-Najjar syndrome, etc.).[12]

Respiratory Distress Syndrome

The neonatal RDS or infant RDS, previously also known as hyaline membrane disease, occurs in infants that lack adequate amounts of pulmonary surfactant at birth.[13] RDS affects about 1% of newborn infants and is the leading cause of death among the preterm infants, with its incidence decreasing with advancing gestational age.[14]

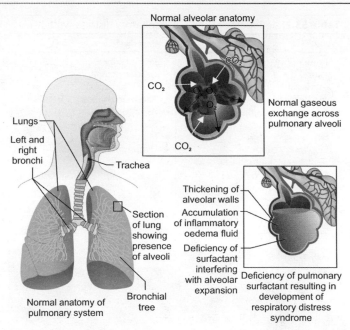

Fig. 55.2: Pathophysiology of respiratory distress syndrome

Normally, when the lungs initially inflate with the baby's first breath, the alveolar sacs expand, fill with air, and remain open. As the alveolar sacs remain open, the surface area within the lungs becomes quite large. The larger the surface area of lungs exposed to the air, the more opportunity oxygen has to pass from the alveoli into the blood. A foamy, fatty liquid-like substance called surfactant is an essential part of this process and helps the alveoli to remain open even at the time of expiration. Without the surfactant, the alveolar sacs may have difficulty in remaining open because they tend to stick together. Surfactant usually appears in the foetal lungs at about 24th week of pregnancy and gradually increases in amount by about the 35th week. Additionally, at the time of labour, there is production of natural steroids in the mother's body, which pass on to the baby through the placenta. These steroids or those that have been artificially administered to the mother, speed up production of surfactant in the lungs in preparation for a baby's first breath. Babies born prematurely may develop a pathological condition called RDS due to the presence of immature lungs or inadequate pulmonary surfactant production (Fig. 55.2). Aetiology of the RDS is described in Table 55.2.

The clinical presentation of RDS is usually in the form of a premature infant of 28–32 weeks gestation, who breathes initially, but soon develops breathing problems. If there are no major complications, recovery is usually quite satisfactory. Whether treated or not, the clinical course for the acute disease lasts about 2–3 days. Despite huge advances in care, RDS remains the most common single cause of death in the first month of life.

The exact diagnosis of the condition is made based on the clinical picture and the chest X-ray.

The X-ray of a premature baby with RDS would show the following features (Fig. 55.3):
❖ Small lung volume (bell-shaped chest)
❖ *Air bronchograms*: Presence of air in the airways of the lung gives a black appearance in comparison to the

Table 55.2: Aetiopathogenesis of respiratory distress syndrome

Causes	Predisposing factors
• Prematurity (most important cause) • Maternal oversedation during the delivery • Traumatic brain injury of the foetus at birth • Ischaemic necrosis of the respiratory centres • Birth trauma or umbilical cord strangulation • Blockage of the air passages due to particulate matter, blood clots or aspirated meconium from the amniotic fluid	• Prematurity • *Gender:* Boys more than girls • *Race:* Caucasian • Caesarean delivery • Asphyxia • Maternal diabetes • Multiple birth • Hypothermia • Infection

Box 55.1: Complications of respiratory distress syndrome

❑ Retinopathy of prematurity
❑ Retrolental fibroplasia
❑ *Bronchopulmonary dysplasia:* Exudative inflammation in the alveoli resulting in the formation of granulation tissue, which later progresses to fibrosis. In final stages, the lungs show focal fibrosis and bullous emphysema. Bronchopulmonary dysplasia may eventually result in the development of pulmonary hypertension, cor pulmonale, focal emphysema, atelectasis, etc.
❑ *Patent ductus arteriosus:* Incomplete conversion of the foetal circulation into an adult one
❑ Intraventricular haemorrhage
❑ *Necrotising enterocolitis:* Anoxic necrosis of intestinal mucosal cells, leading to ulceration, perforation, and finally peritonitis
❑ Chronic pulmonary disease leading to peripheral vasodilatation and pulmonary vasoconstriction

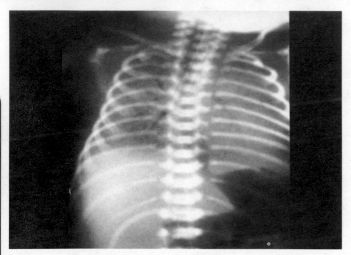

Fig. 55.3: X-ray appearance of respiratory distress syndrome

surrounding white areas that do not contain air, resulting in the formation of air bronchograms.

❖ *Ground glass granularity:* Granular-looking areas, which resemble white salt and black pepper being sprinkled over it, appear on the film. The more the presence of pepper (black areas), the more the aeration; the more salt (white areas), more the collapse or presence of fluid. In terminal stages, the fluid-filled alveoli contribute to the complete 'white-out' of the chest. In severe cases, this becomes exaggerated until even the cardiac borders become inapparent (a complete 'white-out' appearance). Complications of RDS are listed in Box 55.1

Treatment of RDS comprises the following:

❖ *Antenatal corticosteroid administration:* Nowadays, premature birth may be sometimes iatrogenically produced. In these cases, the patient is usually administered steroids in order to speed up production of surfactant in the foetal lung and reduce the chances of the baby developing RDS.

❖ *Supplemental oxygen:* With the occurrence of RDS, the baby's breathing needs to be stabilised with either supplemental oxygen or some form of ventilation that assists the baby with his or her breathing.

❖ Surfactant replacement therapy.

❖ *Intravenous fluids:* Administration of IV fluids is required for stabilising the blood sugar, blood salts and blood pressure.

Meconium Aspiration Syndrome

The passage of meconium into the amniotic fluid is especially important because of the potential risk of development of meconium aspiration syndrome (MAS) and its sequelae. Though freshly passed meconium is sterile and does not contain any bacterial contamination, the infants are likely to aspirate this meconium into the lungs resulting in the development of respiratory failure and hypoxaemia. Infants delivered through meconium-stained amniotic fluid are more likely to be depressed at birth and to require resuscitation and neonatal intensive care.

Meconium aspiration syndrome is a disease of term and post-term infants and its severity is linked to coexisting foetal asphyxia. Aspiration of meconium into the distal airways can occur either antenatally or postnatally. Sometimes, when foetal gasping is initiated before delivery, meconium aspiration can occur in utero, before the baby is born. Normally, there is little peristaltic activity in foetal bowel. Also, the anal sphincters remain in the contracted state. It is believed that hypoxia and acidaemia stimulate the parasympathetic system. This causes the anal sphincter to relax, whilst at the same time increasing the production of motilin, which promotes intestinal peristalsis resulting in passage of meconium into the amniotic cavity.[15-17]

Postnatal inhalation can occur late in the second stage or immediately after delivery if the infant gasps or makes breathing movements while the oropharynx, nasopharynx or trachea contains meconium-stained liquor. Meconium has a number of adverse effects on the neonatal lung, which may ultimately result in the development of MAS that can lead to respiratory failure and hypoxaemia. The series of events involved in production of foetal asphyxia and acidosis due to aspiration of meconium by the foetus has been illustrated in Flow chart 55.1.

Meconium aspiration syndrome is diagnosed if meconium staining of the amniotic fluid is accompanied by neonatal oxygen dependency and a consistent radiographic picture. Figure 55.4 shows the classic radiographic findings of MAS namely, atelectasis, pneumothorax, and hyperexpanded areas of the lung. Presence of meconium-stained liquor, especially that with thick meconium along with abnormal foetal heart

Flow chart 55.1: Development of foetal asphyxia and acidosis due to aspiration of meconium

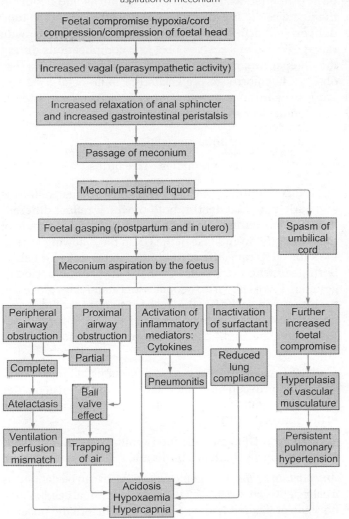

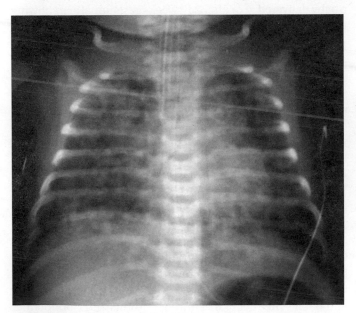

Fig. 55.4: Chest X-ray of a 2-day-old infant showing signs of meconium aspiration syndrome

Table 55.3: Therapies for management of meconium aspiration syndrome

Time period of instituting therapy	Methods
Antenatal therapies	• Amnioinfusion • Delivery by caesarean section • Maternal sedation
Intrapartum/postpartum management	• Oropharyngeal suctioning • Physical manoeuvres
Postnatal intervention	Intratracheal suctioning

tracing on electronic foetal monitor must be treated as an emergency. On the other hand, thin meconium-stained liquor and reassuring foetal heart pattern on electronic monitoring can be treated conservatively. Various therapies for management of MAS based on the time period of instituting the therapy are enlisted in Table 55.3.

Necrotising Enterocolitis

Necrotising enterocolitis is a disorder encountered in very premature infants and involves injury to the inner surface of the intestines. Newborns with NEC may develop abdominal swelling, bloodstained stools and vomiting of greenish, yellow, bile-stained intestinal fluid. The newborn may appear very sick and lethargic and develop hypothermia and/or apnoea.[18] The diagnosis of NEC is confirmed by abdominal X-rays, which may show pneumatosis intestinalis (gas in the intestinal walls) or free air is in the abdominal cavity in case of intestinal perforation. Approximately 60–80% of newborns with this disorder are able to survive.

To prevent the occurrence of NEC, premature newborns should be preferably fed with their mother's breast milk rather than formula milk. Treatment of NEC involves stopping feedings, passing a suction tube into the stomach to relieve pressure from swallowed air and milk, thereby decompressing the intestines and administration of IV fluids and antibiotics.[19] About 70% of newborns with NEC do not require surgery. However, surgery may be required if there is intestinal perforation with peritonitis or there is progressive worsening of the condition despite treatment. Surgery involves resection of the non-viable portion of intestine along with a colostomy. Peritoneal drains may be placed into the abdominal cavity on each side of the lower abdomen in extremely sick infants, who would not be able to survive extensive surgery.

Group B Streptococcal Infection in the Baby

Infants of mother who are carriers of Group B Streptococcus (GBS) are at a risk of acquiring this infection at the time of childbirth. Babies, which are particularly at an increased risk of acquiring GBS disease, include those whose mothers had spontaneous rupture of membranes, prolonged rupture of membrane, evidence of invasive GBS disease in the mother, etc. There are two main types of GBS infection: early-onset (occurs during the 1st week of life) and late-onset (occurs from the 1st week through 3 months of life). Early-onset disease is caused by the passage of infant through the genital tract of an infected mother and can cause perinatal asphyxia, sepsis, respiratory failure, meningitis and/or pneumonia. Late-onset

CHAPTER 55

GBS disease occurs due to acquisition of infection after birth from a carrier mother. Meningitis is more common with late-onset GBS disease than with early-onset GBS disease. GBS disease in the infant is a life-threatening emergency. The most important ways of preventing early-onset GBS infection in the infant include testing all women for GBS bacteria late in pregnancy between 35 weeks to 37 weeks of gestation and administration of antibiotics during labour to mothers, who have tested positive for GBS.[20]

❖ Hypoxic ischaemic encephalopathy [refer to Chapter 49 for details (Antepartum and Intrapartum Foetal Asphyxia)]

❖ Blood or pus coming out from the umbilical stump.

CLINICAL PEARLS

❖ Appropriate breastfeeding support should be provided to the woman for initiation and continuation of breastfeeding regardless of the location of care.

❖ Presence of hydrocele, vaginal bleeding or mastitis in the neonate during the 1st week of life is no cause of concern and usually disappears on its own.

❖ A neonate which has been delivered vaginally, has a gestational age greater than 38 weeks, is a singleton birth having birthweight appropriate for gestational age, has normal vitals, has passed stools and urine, feeds successfully and is normal on general physical examination, can be discharged by 48 hours of birth.

EVIDENCE-BASED MEDICINE

❖ Presently, the use of invasive measures such as reheating with warm plasma expanders or exchange transfusion with warmed blood remains controversial in newborns with hypothermia. The benefit of using these strategies is yet not known.[21]

❖ Treatment with dextrose gel is an inexpensive and simple to administer strategy for treatment of neonatal hypoglycaemia. Massage of dextrose gel 200 mg/kg over the buccal mucosa is more effective than feeding alone, and should be considered for first-line therapy of hypoglycaemia in late-preterm and term infants. Dextrose gel should be considered for first-line treatment to manage hypoglycaemia in late preterm and term babies in the first 48 hours after birth.[7]

PERINATAL MORTALITY

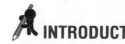

INTRODUCTION

Death of the babies during the antenatal period or within a few days of birth is reflective of obstetric complications or inadequate care during the antepartum/intrapartum or postpartum period. Perinatal mortality rate (PMR) can be considered as an indicator of the quality of obstetric care. PMR is defined as the number of stillbirths and deaths in the first week of life (early neonatal deaths) per 1,000 total deliveries. Perinatal mortality can be related to a wide range of problems such as obstetric complications during the antepartum, intrapartum and postpartum periods (e.g. obstetric haemorrhage, pre-eclampsia, multifoetal gestation, etc.), congenital anomalies, preterm labour, etc. PMR is calculated, using the following formula:

$$PMR = \frac{\text{Total mortalities}}{\text{Total mortalities} + \text{Live births}} \times 1,000$$

Perinatal mortality includes two components: stillbirths and early neonatal deaths, both of which reflect different aspects of obstetric care. The WHO criteria for calculation of the PMR differ from those of the UK in the following aspect: PMR for WHO ranges from stillbirths at 22 weeks (or babies born dead who are weighing >500 g in case the period of gestation is not known) to neonates less than 7 days of age. On the other hand, in the UK, the legal definition of a stillbirth was altered to 24 weeks' gestation instead of 28 weeks or more in 1992. Therefore, in UK, the following definitions for stillbirths and neonatal deaths are followed.

Stillbirths: According to the legal definitions in England and Wales, stillbirth can be defined as a baby delivered at or after 24^{+0} weeks gestational age showing no signs of life, irrespective of the time of death.

Stillbirth rate: This can be defined as number of stillbirths per 1,000 total births (both live births and stillbirths).

Antepartum stillbirth: Antepartum stillbirth can be defined as a baby delivered at or after 24^{+0} weeks gestational age showing no signs of life and known to have died before the onset of labour.

Intrapartum stillbirth: Intrapartum stillbirth can be defined as a baby delivered at or after 24^{+0} weeks gestational age showing no signs of life and known to be alive at the onset of labour.

Neonatal deaths: Neonatal death can be defined as deaths (per 1,000 live births) occurring within 28 days of birth in a live born baby (born at 20^{+0} weeks gestational age or later), or with a birth weight of 400 g or more (where an accurate estimate of gestational age is not available). Early neonatal deaths are deaths occurring in less than 7 completed days of birth (first week of life or 168 hours). Late neonatal deaths, on the other hand, are deaths occurring after 7 completed days but before 28 completed days of life.

Infant mortality rate: Infant mortality rate can be defined as number of infant death (deaths during first year of life) per 1,000 live births.

In the UK, PMR is calculated on an annual basis by the Confidential Enquiry into Stillbirths and Deaths in Infancy (CESDI), set up in 1992. Similar to CEMD, since June 2012, CESDI is carried out by MBRRACE-UK collaboration (Mothers and Babies: Reducing Risk through Audits and Confidential Enquiries across the UK).[22] For details related to MBRRACE-UK, kindly refer to Chapter 33 (Maternal Mortality).

PART II

According to the Perinatal Mortality Surveillance Report by MBRRACE-UK (2016), 4,722 perinatal deaths occurred between January to December 2014 in the UK amongst the babies, born at 24 or greater than 24 weeks of gestation in 2013. Of these, there were 3,286 stillbirths and 1,436 neonatal deaths. This is equivalent to the PMR of approximately 6 (5.92 to be exact) per 1,000 births, which is less than the rest of the world (50–60/1,000 in 2013). However, this rate still needs to be reduced further because it is still higher than those reported by the best performing countries in Europe. Nearly two-thirds of these total perinatal deaths were stillbirths. Though there has been a fall in the rate of neonatal deaths over last 15 years, there has been no change in the rate of stillbirths. According to the MBRRACE-UK (2016), the various causes for neonatal deaths and stillbirths have been described, respectively, in Tables 55.4 and 55.5.[23]

The MBRRACE report (2016) also revealed the following issues:

❖ The percentage of perinatal deaths as a result of an underlying congenital anomaly varied from 0% to 53% for Trusts and Health Boards depending upon the place of birth. Complications occurring during the neonatal period, followed by the congenital anomalies, were the most important causes of neonatal deaths. Preterm birth is another important cause of neonatal deaths, which can be reduced by maternal administration of corticosteroids prior to the delivery. On the other hand, in approximately half the cases of stillbirths, the cause remained unknown. Rate of stillbirths in the antepartum period can be reduced by well-defined antenatal services, focussing on the diagnosis and management of compromised foetuses.

❖ Perinatal postpartum examination, which needs to be conducted in all cases of perinatal deaths, has been described in details in Chapter 28 (Intrauterine Death). According to the MBRRACE (2016) report, postmortem examination was offered to over 90% of the families who experienced a stillbirth or neonatal death. However, only 45% of NHS Trusts and Health Boards were identified to be offering postmortem examination for all the cases of stillbirths and neonatal deaths within their organisation. On the other hand, nearly 22% of organisations offered a postmortem for less than 90% cases of neonatal deaths.

Overall, parental consent for a postmortem was received for only 40% of all stillbirths and neonatal deaths.

❖ Significant variation in the PMRs was observed across the UK and particular areas have been identified where the mortality rates are more than 10% of the average. Detailed local review of stillbirth and neonatal death rates is required in these areas.

❖ This report also identified that the rate of perinatal mortality was higher amongst pregnant women living in areas with the highest levels of social deprivation in the UK in comparison to the births from the least deprived areas of the UK. Mortality rates were identified to be higher amongst the babies of Black or Black British (9.9 per 1,000 women) and those with Asian or Asian British ethnicity (8.7 per 1,000 total births). The risk of perinatal deaths is also increased in cases of multifoetal gestation (due to an increased incidence of prematurity) and mothers in extremes of age (mothers over the age of 40 years or teenage pregnancy).

RECOMMENDATIONS

The report has made several recommendations with the vision of improving healthcare services, thereby bringing down the PMR further. These include the following:

❖ *Local review*: Local reviews must be conducted in the organisations where PMRs are up to 10% and more than 10% higher than the UK average. This comprises of checking the data for case validation and data quality. This should be followed by a complete review of the healthcare services provided in all cases of perinatal deaths. This would help in assessing the quality of care for each individual death by identifying any local factors, which might be responsible for the reported high rates of perinatal mortality. The review would also help in highlighting if the healthcare providers need to make any changes to improve their quality of obstetric care.

❖ *Investigation into each individual case*: Each individual case of stillbirth and neonatal death must be investigated using a standardized process and an independent, multidisciplinary peer review. All organisations, irrespective of their individual PMR, should investigate each case of stillbirth and neonatal death. This process of assessment

Table 55.4: Causes of neonatal deaths[23]

Underlying causes	Percentage of cases (%)
Complications after birth (in the neonatal period)	31
Congenital anomalies	28
Preterm births	13
Infection	7
Complications before labour	5
Complications during labour	5
Unknown causes	5
Not reported	4
Placental problems	2

Table 55.5: Causes of stillbirths[23]

Underlying causes	Percentage of cases (%)
Unknown causes	46
Placental problems	22
Congenital anomalies	6
Complications during labour	6
Complications before labour	5
Not reported	4
Mother's health	4
Umbilical cord abnormalities	4
Infection	3

CHAPTER 55

PART II

should be based on the recommendations provided by the Report of the Morecambe Bay Investigation.[24] This report is an independent investigation into the management, delivery and outcomes of care provided by the maternity and neonatal services at the University Hospitals of Morecambe Bay NHS Foundation Trust from January 2004 to June 2013.

❖ *Reporting of cases of perinatal mortality to MBRRACE-UK*: All organisations responsible for maternity services should have systematic processes in place in order to ensure that all the stillbirths and neonatal deaths are reported to MBRRACE-UK. This would help in ensuring the international consistency of the reporting of PMRs. All Trusts and Health Boards should work closely with MBRRACE-UK to improve their coding of the cause of death, based on the CODAC (Cause of Death and Associated Conditions) classification system.

❖ *Postmortem examination*: A postmortem examination should be offered in all cases of stillbirth and neonatal death in order to identify the cause of death where possible. This helps in excluding the potential contributory factors, particularly those that might affect future pregnancies. This is likely to play an important role in the future counselling of the parents, especially when they plan their next child. In cases of stillbirths, regardless of whether the parents provide consent for postmortem examination, the placenta must be always sent for histological examination, preferably by a specialist pathologist.

❖ *Accurate reporting of data in NHS Trusts and Health Boards*: It is essential that all Trusts and Health Boards provide data, which is complete and accurate, in a timely manner to ensure quality assurance. This can be achieved by reporting all relevant perinatal deaths to MBRRACE-UK, including those cases where the baby was discharged home or to a hospice for palliative care.

❖ *Setting up of national targets*: Nationally aspired targets for stillbirth, neonatal deaths and perinatal deaths need to be established against services, which can be assessed in future.

NATIONAL INITIATIVES

Some initiatives taken by the government to help decrease the rate of perinatal mortality are described next.

Saving Babies' Lives Care Bundle

'Saving babies lives' is an initiative designed by the government to bring down the rates of stillbirth and early neonatal death. It brings together the following four components of care which can be documented as evidence-based and/or best practice:[25]
1. Reducing smoking in pregnancy
2. Risk assessment and surveillance for foetal growth restriction
3. Raising maternal awareness of reduced foetal movement
4. Effective foetal monitoring during labour.

Each Baby Counts

'Each Baby Counts' is the national quality improvement programme launched by the RCOG to reduce the number of perinatal deaths or the number of babies which are left severely disabled as a result of events occurring at the time of pregnancy and labour.[26]

1,000 Lives Improvement

'1,000 Lives Improvement' is a national improvement service initiated by Public Health Wales for NHS Wales.[27] This program aims at working with NHS Wales and its partner organisations to help achieve sustainable, measurable improvements in the quality of healthcare services for people using these services in Wales.

Maternity and Children Quality Improvement Collaborative

The overall aim of this program, launched in March 2013, is to help improve healthcare outcomes and reduce inequalities in healthcare services by providing a safe, high quality care experience for all women, babies and families in Scotland.[28]

Northern Ireland Maternal and Infant Loss Steering Group

Northern Ireland Maternal and Infant Loss (NIMI) steering group has adopted a strategy to help reduce the number of stillbirths and neonatal deaths in North Ireland.[23]

REFERENCES

1. The National Collaborating Centre for Primary Care, UK (NCCPC). Postnatal Care: Routine Postnatal Care of Women and Their Babies. NICE Clinical Guidelines No. 37. London: Royal College of General Practitioners (UK); 2006.
2. Kasap B, Duman N, Ozer E, Tatli M, Kumral A, Ozkan H. Transient tachypnea of the newborn: predictive factor for prolonged tachypnea. Pediatr Int. 2008;50(1):81-4.
3. Silasi M, Coonrod DV, Kim M, Drachman D. Transient tachypnea of the newborn: is labor prior to cesarean delivery protective? Am J Perinatol. 2010;27(10):797-802.
4. Milner AD, Saunders RA, Hopkin IE. Effects of delivery by caesarean section on lung mechanics and lung volume in the human neonate. Arch Dis Child. 1978;53(7):545-8.
5. McGowan JE. Neonatal hypoglycemia. Pediatr Rev. 1999;20(7): 6e-15.
6. American Academy of Paediatrics. Postnatal glucose homeostasis in late-preterm and term infants. Pediatrics. 2011; 127(3):575-9.
7. Harris DL, Weston PJ, Signal M, Chase JG, Harding JE. Dextrose gel for neonatal hypoglycaemia (the Sugar Babies Study): a randomised, double-blind, placebo-controlled trial. Lancet. 2013;382(9910):2077-83.
8. Lunze K, Bloom DE, Jamison DT, Hamer DH. The global burden of neonatal hypothermia: systematic review of a major challenge for newborn survival. BMC Med. 2013;11:24.
9. Saigal S, Doyle LW. An overview of mortality and sequelae of preterm birth from infancy to adulthood. Lancet. 2008;371 (9608):261-9.

10. Christensen RD, Yaish HM. Hemolytic disorders causing severe neonatal hyperbilirubinemia. Clin Perinatol. 2015;42(3):515-27.

11. Woodgate P, Jardine LA. Neonatal jaundice: phototherapy. BMJ Clin Evid. 2015;2015.

12. Huang MJ, Kua KE, Teng HC, Tang KS, Weng HW, Huang CS. Risk factors for severe hyperbilirubinemia in neonates. Pediatr Res. 2004;56(5):682-9.

13. Torday J, Carson L, Lawson RE. Saturated phosphatidylcholine in amniotic fluid and prediction of the respiratory distress syndrome. N Engl J Med. 1979;301:913-18.

14. Rodriguez RJ, Martin RJ, Fanaroff AA. Respiratory distress syndrome and its management. In: Martin RJ, Fanaroff AA (Eds). Fanaroff & Martin's Neonatal-perinatal Medicine: Diseases of the Fetus and Infant, 7th edition. St. Louis: Mosby; 2002. pp. 1001-11.

15. Lucas A, Adrian TE, Aynsley-Green A, Bloom SR. Gut hormones in fetal distress. Lancet. 1979;2:968.

16. Lucas A, Christofides ND, Adrian TE, Bloom SR, Aynsley-Green A. Fetal distress, meconium, and motilin. Lancet. 1979;1:718.

17. Mahmoud EL, Benirschke K, Vaucher YE, Poitras P. Motilin levels in term neonates who have passed meconium prior to birth. J Pediatr Gastroenterol Nutr. 1988;7:95-9.

18. Lin PW, Stoll BJ. Necrotising enterocolitis. Lancet. 2006;368 (9543):1271-83.

19. Panigrahi P. Necrotizing enterocolitis: a practical guide to its prevention and management. Paediatr Drugs. 2006;8(3):151-65.

20. National Center for Immunization and Respiratory Diseases, Division of Bacterial Diseases. Preventing Early-Onset Group B Strep Disease (GBS). USA: CDC; 2016.

21. American Heart Association. Part 13: Neonatal Resuscitation Guidelines. Circulation. 2005;112:IV-188-95.

22. Knight M. How will the new confidential enquiries into maternal and infant death in the UK operate? The work of MBRRACE-UK. Obstet Gynaecol. 2012;15:65.

23. Manktelow BN, Smith LK, Seaton SE, Hyman-Taylor P, Kurinczuk JJ, Field DJ, et al; MBRRACE-UK Perinatal Mortality Surveillance Report, UK Perinatal Deaths for Births from January to December 2014. Leicester: The Infant Mortality and Morbidity Studies, Department of Health Sciences, University of Leicester; 2016.

24. Kirkup B. (2016). The Report of the Morecambe Bay Investigation: An independent investigation into the management, delivery and outcomes of care provided by the maternity and neonatal services at the University Hospitals of Morecambe Bay NHS Foundation Trust from January 2004 to June 2013. [online] Available from www.gov.uk/government/publications. [Accessed December, 2016].

25. NHS England. (2016). NHS England's Saving Babies' Lives Care: A care bundle for reducing stillbirth. [online] Available from www.england.nhs.uk/2016/03/stillbirths. [Accessed December, 2016].

26. The Royal College of Obstetricians and Gynaecologists (RCOG). (2016). Each Baby Counts. [online] Available from www.rcog.org.uk/eachbabycounts. [Accessed December, 2016].

27. NHS Wales. (2016). 1000 Lives Improvement, National Stillbirth Working Group. [online] Available from www.1000livesplus.wales.nhs.uk. [Accessed December, 2016].

28. Scottish Patient Safety Programme. (2016). Maternity and Children's Quality Improvement Collaborative. [online] Available from http://www.scottishpatientsafetyprogramme.scot.nhs.uk/programmes/mcqic. [Accessed December, 2016].

CHAPTER 55

SECTION 11

General Gynaecology

GYNAECOLOGY

Normal and Abnormal Embryological Development

NORMAL EMBRYOLOGICAL DEVELOPMENT

DEVELOPMENT OF GONADS AND INTERNAL GENITALIA

The sexual identity of individuals depends on their genetic, gonadal and phenotypic sex. Genetic or chromosomal sex is determined by the sex chromosomes, with XX karyotype being a genetic female and XY karyotype being a genetic male. Chromosomal sex is determined at the time of fertilisation and is dependent on the presence of Y chromosome. SRY gene located on the short branch of Y chromosome, directs the gonad to become testis. In the absence of Y chromosome, the bipotential gonad differentiates into an ovary about 2 weeks later than when testicular development begins in the male.[1] Gonadal sex, which is determined by the genetic sex, is established next. Gonadal sex is dependent on the presence of gonads: testes in males and ovaries in females. It controls the development of both internal and external genitalia. Internal genitalia in males comprises of testes, epididymis and vas deferens, while in females, it comprises of fallopian tubes, uterus and cervix.[2] Phenotypic sex is determined by the appearance of external genitalia and secondary sexual characteristics, which develop at the time of puberty. The development of gonads begin during the 5th week of gestation in the human embryos with the development of a protuberance known as the genital or gonadal ridge. The primordial germ cells migrate into the developing gonad between 4th and 6th weeks of gestation, simultaneously proliferating at the same time. Initially, the germ cells begin to divide by mitosis so that their number increases and they contain a diploid number of chromosomes. Soon thereafter, these cells undergo meiotic division, a process called gametogenesis, in which the number of chromosomes gets halved (haploid number). The mesonephric ducts (Wolffian

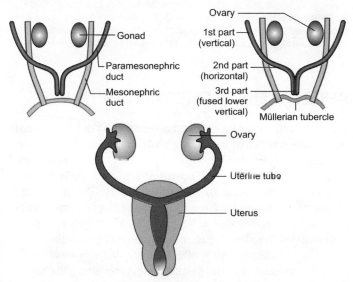

Fig. 56.1: Formation of uterus and uterine tubes by the fusion of paramesonephric ducts

ducts) and paramesonephric ducts (Müllerian ducts) are two discreet duct systems, which coexist in all embryos during the ambisexual period of development (i.e. up to 8 weeks of gestation). Under the influence of testosterone from the Leydig cells of testes, the Wolffian ducts form the epididymis, vas deferens and seminal vesicles (male internal genitalia).[3] In the absence of gonadal testosterone production, regression of the Wolffian ducts occurs. The sertoli cells of testis produce a substance called Müllerian inhibiting substance (MIS) or anti-Müllerian hormone (AMH), which suppresses the development of female internal genitalia from Müllerian ducts in males. In the absence of MIS in females, Müllerian ducts develop passively to form fallopian tubes, uterus and upper vagina (Fig. 56.1). Development of vagina is described in Figures 56.2A to D. Differentiation of Müllerian ducts occurs in a cephalocaudal direction to form the female internal genital organs.[4]

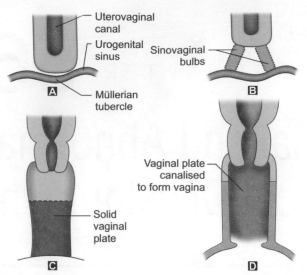

Figs 56.2A to D: Formation of vagina. (A) Mesoderm of uterovaginal canal pressing on the posterior wall of the endodermal urogenital sinus (UGS) forming Müllerian tubercle; (B) Sinovaginal bulbs formed by proliferation of the endoderm of UGS; (C) Solid vaginal plate formed by fusion of mesodermal uterovaginal canal and endodermal sinovaginal bulbs; (D) Vagina formed by canalisation of vagina plate (part derived from mesoderm is purple; part derived from endoderm is grey)

DEVELOPMENT OF EXTERNAL GENITALIA

The external genitalia can be recognised as male or female by the 16th week of foetal life with the help of ultrasound examination. External genitalia persists in the bipotential state until 9 weeks of gestation at which time it consists of a genital tubercle, urogenital sinus (UGS) and lateral labioscrotal folds or swellings (Fig. 56.3). Dihydrotestosterone, produced by the testes acting via the androgen receptors, determines the development of external genitalia. In the absence of masculinising effect of dihydrotestosterone, the undifferentiated external genitalia develop along the female lines. The genital tubercle develops into the clitoris and genital folds into labia majora. Under the influence of testosterone, the genital tubercle forms the penis, the edges of the UGS fuse to form the penile urethra and the labioscrotal folds fuse to form the scrotum. This process is complete by 12–14 weeks of gestation. The UGS, which is of endodermal origin, is derived from the cloaca. It gives rise to caudal two-thirds of vagina in females and forms prostate, bulbourethral glands and urethra in males.

 CLINICAL PEARLS

❖ The uterus and upper one-third of the vagina develop from the paramesonephric ducts, while the lower two-thirds of the vagina develops from the UGS. By the 5th month, the vagina is usually completely canalised.
❖ The Wolffian duct degenerates in female foetus. It can sometimes still be traced in adult females, when it is known as Gartner's duct, which runs medially through the broad ligament and down the side of the vagina.

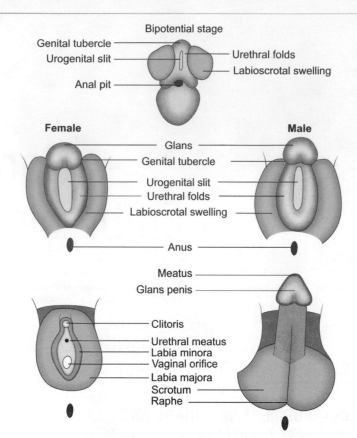

Fig. 56.3: Development of external genitalia

❖ The genital and urinary systems are closely associated. Therefore, abnormalities of the Müllerian duct system can commonly affect the urinary system.

SEX AND INTERSEXUALITY

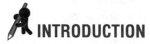 **INTRODUCTION**

Intersexuality refers to individuals whose biological sex cannot be classified clearly as male or female. Previously used terms such as intersex, pseudohermaphroditism and hermaphroditism have particularly become controversial in the modern day clinical practice. These terms are interpreted as possibly derogatory by patients.[5] Moreover, they can be confusing to both the practitioners and the parents. The new terminology in use is 'disorders of sex development' (DSD) and basically comprises of three conditions: (1) sex chromosome DSD, (2) 46,XY DSD and (3) 46,XX DSD. The new classification system now encompasses a wide range of disorders such as Turner's syndrome, having the chromosomal composition 45X [Chapter 57 (Karyotypic Abnormalities)], Klinefelter's syndrome (47,XXY), and congenital adrenal hyperplasia (CAH), which were previously not considered as intersex conditions. DSD can be defined as congenital conditions in which development of chromosomal, gonadal, or anatomical sex is atypical. The proposed revised nomenclature changes in terminology are described in Table 56.1.[6,7] In a normal individual, sexual differentiation involves the following

Table 56.1: Proposed changes in terminology[6,7]

Previous	Proposed
Intersex	Disorders of sex development (DSD)
• Male pseudohermaphrodite • Undervirilisation of an XY male • Undermasculinisation of an XY male	46,XY DSD
• Female pseudohermaphrodite • Overvirilisation of an XX female • Masculinisation of an XX female	46,XX DSD
True hermaphrodite	Ovotesticular DSD
XX male or XX sex reversal	46,XX testicular DSD
XY sex reversal	46,XY complete gonadal dysgenesis

aspects: gonadal development, genital development and behavioural differentiation, and has been described in details previously in this chapter. On the other hand, DSD is characterised by the presence of intermediate or atypical combinations of physical features which distinguish male and female genders from each other. DSD comprises a wide range of conditions including individuals having standard male or female genitalia, but an amalgam of internal genital organs and karyotype as well as those with ambiguous external genitalia. Features of some commonly encountered DSD are described in Table 56.2.[8-10]

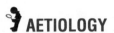

AETIOLOGY

Disorders of sex development commonly occur either due to disruption of gonadal differentiation or abnormal production or action of foetal sex steroids. This can frequently occur due to the abnormal development of chromosomal, gonadal or anatomical sex (e.g. masculinisation of female, or partial or incomplete masculinisation in a male). Some of the causes are as follows:

Disorders of Gender Identity Associated with Normal Constitution of Sex Chromosomes

❖ *Female pseudohermaphroditism*: Female pseudohermaphrodites have a chromosomal sex of a female, but have external genitalia of a male. This can occur due to adrenogenital syndrome (associated with excessive testosterone production), etc.

❖ *Male pseudohermaphroditism*: Male pseudohermaphrodites have chromosomal sex of a male, but have external genitalia of a female. This can occur due to causes such as primary gonadal deficit, testicular regression syndrome; Leydig cell agenesis, defects in testosterone synthesis; deficiency of 17-α-hydroxylase, defect in Müllerian inhibiting system, end-organ defects such as androgen insensitivity syndrome (testicular feminisation), incomplete androgen insensitivity syndrome (Reifenstein's syndrome); disorders of testosterone metabolism such as 5-α-reductase deficiency.

❖ *Hormonal influences*: Excessive exposure to androgens (e.g. virilising tumours of ovaries, etc.) can cause masculinisation of female external genitalia. Presence of oestrogens in males can cause gynaecomastia.

Disorders of Gender Identity Associated with Abnormal Constitution of Sex Chromosomes

❖ *Infrequently associated with ambiguous genitalia*: Klinefelter's syndrome, Turner's syndrome, pure gonadal dysgenesis, etc.

❖ *Frequently associated with ambiguous genitalia*: Mixed gonadal dysgenesis, true hermaphroditism [an individual containing both male gonadal tissue (testes) and female gonadal tissue (ovaries)].

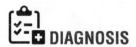 **DIAGNOSIS**

Clinical Presentation

❖ *Ambiguous genitalia*: An intersex individual may have biological characteristics of both male and the female sexes. Signs of feminism in a male child include apparent male genitalia with hypospadias (opening of urethra below the phallus), underdevelopment of the phallus (micropenis), split scrotum and bilateral undescended testicles. Signs of masculinisation in females include apparent female genitalia with an enlarged clitoris, posterior labial fusion, hirsutism or an inguinal or labial mass.

❖ *Clinical presentation in older children*: Clinical presentations in older children and young adults include: previously unrecognised genital ambiguity; inguinal hernia in a girl; delayed or incomplete puberty in both boys and girls; virilisation in a girl; primary amenorrhoea in a girl; breast development in a boy; and rarely cyclical haematuria in a boy.

❖ *External anatomical sex*: This is determined from features such as body contours, development of musculature, bone (pelvis), distribution of hair on the face, chest, etc., breast development and appearance of external genitalia.

❖ *Internal anatomical sex*: Presence of internal genitalia, such as uterus, fallopian tubes and ovary is an evidence of the individual being a female.

❖ *Gonadal sex*: This is evident on the biopsy of the gonadal structure.

❖ *Psychological sex*: This is determined by one's behaviour, speech, dress and sexual inclination.

Table 56.2: Features of some commonly encountered disorders of sex development[8-10]

Disorder	Cause	Karyotype	External genitalia	Internal genitalia
Congenital adrenal hyperplasia: This is the most common DSD having a prevalence of 1 in 10,000.	This disorder is related to the deficiency of the enzyme 21 hydroxylase, resulting in the deficiency of the hormone, cortisol. This causes adrenal gland to undergo hyperplasia in an effort to produce sufficient amounts of cortisol. In the process, large amounts of androgens are produced, which cause masculinisation of the female external genitalia.	46,XX	Virilised or masculinised external genitalia. In the past, usual practice was to cosmetically feminise the appearance with help of genital surgery. However, now there is much controversy regarding the usefulness of this procedure. In fact, this surgery is likely to be associated with the risk of damage to clitoral orgasm.	Uterus and ovaries are present. Gender assignment is that of a female due to the presence of uterus and ovaries. There is a potential of fertility.
Complete androgen insensitivity syndrome	There is disruption of the androgen receptor gene on the long arm of X-chromosome due to which the body cells are unable to respond to androgens.	46,XY	The external genitalia are of female type with variable degree of vaginal hypoplasia because the body cells are unable to respond to androgens. There is normal breast development along with normal female behaviour and gender identity because oestradiol is produced from the circulating testosterone levels in the body. The pubic and axillary hairs are absent because body cells are unable to respond to androgens.	Testes are present. Due to the presence of SRY gene, the foetus initially starts developing along the male pathway and normal development of both the testicles occurs. Both AMH and testosterone are normally produced which cause the regression of Müllerian ducts. Testes are present as intra-abdominal organs and they produce high levels of circulating testosterone. Intra-abdominal gonads are associated with a small risk of malignancy until after the age of 50 years.
Partial androgen insensitivity syndrome	There is incomplete response to androgens	46,XY	Due to partial response to androgens, the presentation of external genitalia may vary from ambiguous genitalia to normal male genitalia with infertility. Physical growth of external genitalia is unpredictable. Therefore, future sexual function as male or female remains unknown. There is lack of sufficient information regarding development of sexual orientation and gender identity.	Testes are present
Swyer's syndrome (gonadal dysgenesis)	There is a defect in SRY gene due to which gonadal/testicular development does not occur. In the absence of SRY gene, ovarian development probably occurs. This, however, cannot be sustained due to the lack of second X (sex) chromosome. As a result, there is formation of dysgenetic streak gonads	46,XY	There is presence of female external genitalia, poor breast development and normal pubic and axillary hair. Since the dysgenetic streak gonads are not capable of producing testosterone or AMH, there is development of Müllerian duct which forms vagina and cervix. Since the streak gonads are not capable of producing sex hormones during puberty, there is poor breast development with primary amenorrhoea.	There is presence of female streak gonads and uterus. Development of the Müllerian duct results in the formation of uterus. Due to presence of uterus, menstruation can be commenced using HRT (both oestrogen and progestogens). Pregnancy is possible with the use of donor oocytes. Gonadectomy of streak gonads is recommended due to high risk of malignancy in dysgenetic gonads.
Deficiency of 5-α reductase or deficiency of type 3-β-hydroxysteroid dehydrogenase	Both the conditions are autosomal recessive disorders associated with the deficiency of enzymes involved in the synthesis of androgen	46,XY	Initially, an XY foetus starts development along the male pathway. However, due to deficiency of androgens, there is development of female or ambiguous genitalia, which may undergo virilisation at the time of puberty. Secondary sexual development is usually along the male lines with poor breast development and normal pubic and axillary hair.	• There is presence of testis in situ. Due to the presence of the functioning testis, nearly 60–80% individuals undergo change in gender from female to male at some point of life from late childhood onwards. • Testes are usually intra-abdominal during childhood and may migrate into the inguinal canal or into the labioscrotal folds after puberty.

Contd...

Contd...

Ovotesticular DSD (rarest DSD)	There is combination of ovary and/or testis and/or ovotestis. Due to presence of both the gonads, there may be a variable clinical presentation	46,XX 46,XY	Often ambiguous	A combination of uterus and/or male ducts may be present.
Müllerian agenesis (Mayer-Rokitansky Küster-Hauser syndrome)	This syndrome occurs due to defect in fusion of the Müllerian ducts resulting in absence of proximal one-third of vagina with or without the uterus. Since the ovaries are not Müllerian structures, they are normal. The cause of this syndrome is unknown and is probably related to the mutations in the gene for anti-Müllerian hormones or the gene for anti-Müllerian hormone receptor	46,XX	There is usually an absence or hypoplasia of the internal vagina. The vagina may be shortened and present as a blind pouch. There is normal development of secondary sexual characteristics, including breasts and pubic hair	Usually there is absence of fallopian tubes and uterus. In case the uterus is not present, pregnancy is possible through surrogacy and IVF

Investigations

- *Karyotyping*: This may involve study of buccal smear (presence of Barr bodies), skin biopsy or a neutrophil examination (drumstick-like projection).
- *Examination of external genitalia*: Detailed examination of external genitalia preferably under general anaesthesia must be performed.
- *Gonadal biopsy*: This helps in identifying either male or female genitalia and may also reveal the presence of degenerated testis or streak gonads.
- *Imaging studies*: This includes abdominopelvic ultrasound examination, which may help in identifying ovarian neoplasms and adrenal tumours. MRI to check for suspected adrenal neoplasms, radiography of pituitary fossa and the skeleton may also be performed in some cases. Intravenous pyelography may be done to check for any renal anomalies.
- *Hormone estimation*: This includes determination of the serum levels of hormones such as oestrogens, gonadotropins, anti-Müllerian hormone, 17-ketosteroids, testosterone, and 17-hydroxyprogesterone in urine. Decision-making algorithms are available in most units to direct further investigations.[11] These include hCG and adrenocorticotropic hormone (ACTH) stimulation tests (synacthen test) to assess testicular and adrenal steroid biosynthesis respectively.
- Serum electrolyte levels.
- Psychological assessment of the patient's sexuality.

Though substantial progress has been made in understanding the genetic basis of human sexual development,[12] a specific molecular diagnosis is established in only about 20% of cases of DSD. CAH is likely to be present in the majority of virilised infants with chromosomal configuration 46,XX. In contrast, a definitive diagnosis would be established in only 50% of children with DSD having a chromosomal configuration 46,XY.[13,14]

MANAGEMENT

- An experienced multidisciplinary team comprising paediatric subspecialists in endocrinology, surgery or urology or both, psychologists or psychiatrists, gynaecologists, genetic counsellor, neonatologist, social worker, and nursing and medical ethics professionals, must be involved in the evaluation and long-term management of such patients. This team should develop a plan for clinical management with respect to diagnosis, gender assignment, and treatment options of the patient. The diagnosis must be disclosed to the patients and their parents. They must also be provided appropriate information related to the condition.
- *Gender assignment in newborn infants*: Uncertainty in gender assessment may be disturbing and stressful for families. Therefore, a specific gender must be assigned to all individuals. However, gender assignment must be avoided before expert evaluation has been performed in the newborns. Factors, which may influence gender assignment, include the diagnosis, genital appearance, surgical options, requirement for life-long replacement therapy, the likely potential for fertility, opinion of the family, and the circumstances relating to the cultural practices. For example, most of the patients with complete androgen insensitivity, having a chromosomal composition of 46,XY, who are assigned as females during infancy identify as females later in life.[15]
- *Disclosure of information*: Open communication with patients and families is essential and they must be involved in the clinical decision-making. Over the past decade, the major change in management of these patients has been to sensitively disclose all the relevant information to the patient in a supported environment rather than withholding details from the patients. Concerns of the patients and their families must be respected and shared in strict confidence. The parents should be counselled that the DSD child has the potential to become a well-adjusted, functional member of society and DSD is in no way shameful. It should be emphasised to the parents that initially the best course of action may not be clear. However, the healthcare team would work with the family to reach the best possible set of decisions in the given circumstances. Options for vaginal enlargement in case of vaginal agenesis or hypoplasia and future fertility options must be discussed with the patients and their families. If there is a probable risk for development of gonadal malignancy in the future, it should also be discussed with the patient.

❖ *Screening for associated medical conditions*: This is important because patients with DSD may commonly have coexisting medical conditions.

❖ *Access to peer support*: Support groups have an important role in the delivery of care to DSD patients and their families. All patients should have an access to peer support via national support organisations.[16]

Surgical Management

Cosmetic vaginal surgery must be considered where relevant. Surgery should only be undertaken by those surgeons having an expertise in the care of children and have received specific training in the surgery of DSD. During surgery, emphasis should be on the maintenance of functional outcome rather than a strictly cosmetic appearance. Surgical management of intersex can be categorised into one of the following two:

1. Restoration of functionality (or potential functionality)
2. *Enhancement surgery*: Enhancement surgery to enable the individual to identify with a particular sex, e.g. breast enlargement surgery, may be required in some cases.
   - While deciding surgery in cases of DSD, those surgical management options should be preferably considered which are likely to facilitate the chances of fertility.
   - In patients with complete androgen insensitivity and those with partial androgen insensitivity, raised as females, the testes should be removed to prevent the development of malignancy in the adulthood.[12] With the availability of oestrogen replacement therapy, early removal of the testes at the time of diagnosis can be attempted, which also takes care of the associated hernia and psychological problems in the patient.
   - The streak gonads in a patient with mixed gonadal dysgenesis raised as male should be removed either via laparoscope or by laparotomy during the early childhood.[12] Bilateral gonadectomy must also be performed during early childhood in females with bilateral streak gonads having gonadal dysgenesis and Y-chromosome material.

Sex Steroid Replacement Therapy

Hypogonadism may commonly occur in patients with dysgenetic gonads, those having defects in the biosynthesis of sex steroids or those who are resistant to androgens. Hormonal therapy can be considered at the time the puberty is initiated in the patient. Commencement of hormonal therapy during this time helps in replicating the normal pubertal maturation, helps in inducing the development of secondary sexual characteristics, causing a pubertal growth spurt, optimal accumulation of bone mineral and provision of psychosocial support, which helps in psychosexual maturation.[17] In males, intramuscular depot injections of testosterone esters are commonly administered.[18-20] Patients with partial androgen insensitivity syndrome may require supraphysiological doses of testosterone for optimal effect.[21]

Oestrogen supplementation may be required in the females with hypogonadism to help induce pubertal changes

and menses. A progestin is usually added after the patient experiences breakthrough bleeding or within 1–2 years of continuous oestrogen therapy to prevent unopposed action of oestrogen on the uterine endometrium.

Psychosocial Management

Psychosocial care is an essential component of management, which helps in promoting positive adaptation and must be provided by mental health staff having an expertise in DSD.

CLINICAL PEARLS

❖ Presence of one Barr body suggests presence of two X-chromosomes.
❖ Treatment should be best deferred until puberty when the pragmatic sex of the individual becomes apparent.

EVIDENCE-BASED MEDICINE

❖ Available evidence supports the current recommendation that markedly virilised 46,XX infants with CAH must be raised as females.[22]
❖ There is no evidence to indicate that the addition of cyclic progesterone is beneficial for women without a uterus, who are being administered oestrogen therapy.[23]

AMBIGUOUS GENITALIA

INTRODUCTION

Ambiguous genitalia refer to the sexual anatomy of external genitalia, which cannot be classified as typically female or male.

AETIOLOGY

Ambiguous genitalia occur due to variation in any of the processes of development of sexual organs. Some important causes are:

❖ *Virilisation*: This could be due to adrenogenital syndrome which causes hyperplasia of adrenal cortex and can be of two types: (1) congenital or intrauterine adrenogenital syndrome (deficiency of 21-hydroxylase) and (2) postnatal adrenogenital syndrome (due to excessive production of ACTH from a basophil adenoma of anterior pituitary). Other causes of virilisation include virilising tumours and conditions of ovary (arrhenoblastoma, hilus cell tumour, PCOS, hyperthecosis, etc.)
❖ *Exposure to maternal androgens*: Virilisation of a female foetus may occur if progestational agents or androgens are used during the first trimester of pregnancy.

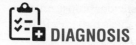

DIAGNOSIS

Clinical Presentation

❖ A family history of genital ambiguity, infertility or unexpected changes at puberty may suggest a genetically transmitted trait.

❖ *Physical examination*: Virilism may be associated with hirsutism, male appearance and breast atrophy.

❖ *External genitalia examination*: This may show the following features:
  • External genitalia may show a feminine appearance with larger than-average clitoris (clitoral hypertrophy) and partially fused labia, giving appearance of scrotum

  OR
  • External genitalia may appear masculine with a smaller-than average penis that is open along the under-side (hypospadic). The scrotum may be empty without the presence of testicles.
  • The position of urethral meatus must be noted.

❖ *Gonadal examination*: Documentation of palpable gonads is important.

❖ *Rectal examination*: This may reveal the cervix and uterus, confirming internal Müllerian structures.

Investigations

Logical work-up in infants with ambiguous genitalia includes the following:

❖ Chromosomal analysis
❖ Endocrine screening
❖ Serum chemistry or electrolyte tests
❖ Androgen-receptor levels
❖ 5-α reductase type II levels
❖ *Imaging studies:* Renal or bladder ultrasonography can be performed at the bedside in the neonatal ICU. Ultrasonography usually allows visualisation of a neonate's adrenal glands, which may be enlarged and show a cribriform appearance in infants with CAH.
  • Ultrasonography also helps in identifying Müllerian structures. CT scanning and MRI are usually not indicated but may help identify internal anatomy.

MANAGEMENT

❖ Gynaecologists may be involved in the care of older children who may develop ambiguous genitalia at the time of puberty. Vaginal hypoplasia or agenesis may be present in many individuals with ambiguous genitalia. The treatment options, surgical vaginoplasty and vaginal self-dilatation, need to be discussed with the patient.[23]

❖ Gynaecologists may also be involved in the care of adults who underwent feminising genital surgery during their childhood and have come for a follow-up visit. Repeat surgery may be required in these cases for vaginal stenosis, vaginal hypoplasia or genital cosmesis. Though treatment in these cases is likely to improve the psychological and sexual outcomes, there is no definite evidence to prove this.

❖ There has been a lot of controversy regarding both the optimal timing for surgery and the type of surgical intervention to be done. Presently, it is recommended that the surgery should be preferably performed during or after adolescence.[24,25] Currently, there is also considerable consensus that vaginal dilatation therapy is the treatment of choice for vaginal hypoplasia.[26] Vaginal dilatation therapy must be preferably reserved for adolescents and adult patients. Vaginal dilatation is favoured over vaginoplasty because this procedure is not associated with any surgical risks such as stenosis of the introitus; loss of vaginal length; vaginal prolapse; dryness of the vagina; excessive vaginal discharge; risk of malignancy in the vaginal graft material, etc. The vaginal self-dilation therapy is associated with success rates as high as 80% in achieving appropriate vaginal length. Moreover, the outcome of vaginoplasty is largely related to patient's motivation, genital configuration and surgeon's expertise.

❖ *Exploratory laparotomy or gonadal biopsy*: Open exploration may help in the identification of internal duct anatomy and allow gonadal tissue to be obtained for histologic characterisation.

❖ *Diagnostic laparoscopy or gonadal biopsy*: Laparoscopic examination under general anaesthesia may allow rapid identification and delineation of the internal duct anatomy. Biopsy of gonads may also be performed laparoscopically.

❖ *Male pseudohermaphroditism*: These individuals look like females, are therefore reared as women and must be continued to be reared as such. In cases of complete androgen insensitivity, gonadectomy (removal of undescended testis) must be performed after completion of puberty due to high chances of development of malignancy in an undescended male gonad.[27] However, in cases of incomplete androgen insensitivity, earlier surgery may be required to prevent hirsutism and/or virilisation at the time of puberty. Administration of oestrogens near puberty helps in the growth of breasts. Surgical correction of external genitalia and creation of an artificial vagina is required for sexual functioning.

❖ *Female pseudohermaphroditism*: In cases of congenital adrenogenital syndrome, administration of synthetic cortisone or synthetic corticosteroids (glucocorticoids, hydrocortisone, etc.) may help to control the excessive production of ACTH and may also help in restoring menstruation. Restoration of external genitalia to a feminine pattern can be done with help of plastic surgery. McIndoe's vaginoplasty to create an artificial vagina can be considered if the patient is engaged and married.

Outcomes of Infant Genital Surgery

While some studies have suggested satisfactory outcomes from early surgery,[22,28,29] evidence from small cohort studies has indicated that early surgery may require repeat genital surgeries or vaginal dilatation for a majority of patients.[30,31] Repeat surgery is usually required at or after puberty and is usually required for the stenosis of vaginal introitus. Sometimes, it may also be required for cosmesis. Clitoroplasty has been identified to be associated with problems related to reduced sexual sensitivity, loss of clitoral tissue, and cosmetic issues.[32,33] Small observation studies have shown that orgasm may be reduced in adults who had undergone clitoroplasty in the childhood.[34,35]

Currently, the role of performing vaginoplasty in the child is less clear. Scarring at the vaginal introitus may occur based on the technique used at the time of vaginoplasty. This may necessitate repeated surgical modification before reliable sexual function can be obtained. Therefore, this procedure is usually deferred until adolescence when the procedure can be performed after obtaining appropriate informed consent. Moreover, surgery to construct a neo-vagina is associated with the risk of neoplasia.[36]

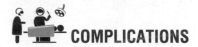

COMPLICATIONS

In the cases where non-functional testes are present (e.g. androgen insensitivity syndrome), there is a risk of development of malignancy later in life.

CLINICAL PEARLS

❖ Congenital adrenal hyperplasia is the most common cause of ambiguous genitalia in the newborn.
❖ Different graft materials such as peritoneum, amnion, skin, bowel, muscle flaps, labial expansion flaps, etc. can be used during vaginoplasty.
❖ Feminising genitoplasty is associated with a smaller amount of surgical intervention and therefore fewer urological difficulties in comparison to masculinising genitoplasty.[28]

EVIDENCE-BASED MEDICINE

❖ Sexual function in the patients with DSD has been found to be impaired in comparison to that of normal population.[37,38] However, it still remains controversial whether this impairment occurs as a result of surgery or is due to DSD per se.
❖ Intra-abdominal gonads, often encountered in patients with DSD may be associated with a high risk of malignancy. The highest risk of tumours is found in testis-specific protein Y encoded (TSPY) positive gonadal dysgenesis and partial androgen insensitivity syndrome with intra-abdominal gonads. On the other hand, the lowest risk of malignancy is associated with ovotestis and complete androgen insensitivity.[39-41] A scrotal testis in patients with gonadal dysgenesis is at a risk for malignancy. The

present evidence indicates that a testicular biopsy must be performed at the time of puberty in these patients. If there are any signs of a premalignant lesions, sperm banking must be done before treating the patient with low-dose radiotherapy, which may be curative.[42]

REFERENCES

1. Baker TG. A quantitative and cytological study of germ cells in the human ovaries. Proc R Soc Lond B Biol Sci. 1963;158:417-33.
2. Moore KL, Persaud TV, Torchia MG. The Developing Human: Clinically Oriented Embryology, 10th edition. Philadelphia: Elsevier Health Sciences; 2015.
3. Moore KL, Persaud TV. The urogenital system. In: Moore KL, Persaud TVN (Eds). The Developing Human: Clinically Oriented Embryology, 6th edition. Philadelphia: WB Saunders; 1998. pp. 303-47.
4. Acién P. Embryological observations on the female genital tract. Hum Reprod. 1992;7(4):437-45.
5. Conn J, Gillam L, Conway G. Revealing the diagnosis of androgen insensitivity syndrome in adulthood. BMJ. 2005; 331(7517):628-30.
6. Dreger AD, Chase C, Sousa A, Gruppuso PA, Frader J. Changing the nomenclature/taxonomy for intersex: A scientific and clinical rationale. J Pediatr Endocrinol Metab. 2005;18(8):729-33.
7. Brown J, Warne G. Practical management of the intersex infant. J Pediatr Endocrinol Metab. 2005;18(1):3-23.
8. Hughes IA, Houk C, Ahmed SF, Lee PA, LWPES Consensus Group; ESPE Consensus Group. Consensus statement on management of intersex disorders. Arch Dis Child. 2006;91(7): 554-63.
9. Houk CP, Hughes IA, Ahmed SF, Lee PA; Writing Committee for the International Intersex Consensus Conference Participants. Summary of consensus statement on intersex disorders and their management. International Intersex Consensus Conference. Pediatrics. 2006;118(2):753-7.
10. Creighton S, Minto C. Managing intersex. BMJ. 2001;323(7324): 1264-5.
11. Ogilvy-Stuart AL, Brain CE. Early assessment of ambiguous genitalia. Arch Dis Child. 2004;89(5):401-7.
12. Grumbach MM, Hughes IA, Conte FA. Disorders of sex differentiation. In: Larsen PR, Kronenberg HM, Melmed S, Polonsky KM (Eds). Williams Textbook of Endocrinology, 10th edition. Philadelphia: WB Saunders; 2003. pp. 842-1002.
13. Ahmed SF, Cheng A, Dovey L, Hawkins JR, Martin H, Rowland J, et al. Phenotypic features, androgen receptor binding, and mutational analysis in 278 clinical cases reported as androgen insensitivity syndrome. J Clin Endocrinol Metab. 2000;85 (2):658-65.
14. Morel Y, Rey R, Teinturier C, Nicolino M, Michel-Calemard L, Mowszowicz I, et al. Aetiological diagnosis of male sex ambiguity: a collaborative study. Eur J Pediatr. 2002;161(1):49-59.
15. Mazur T. Gender dysphoria and gender change in androgen insensitivity or micropenis. Arch Sex Behav. 2005;34(4):411-21.
16. Warne G. Support groups for CAH and AIS. Endocrinologist. 2003;13:175-8.
17. Warne GL, Grover S, Zajac JD. Hormonal therapies for individuals with intersex conditions: protocol for use. Treat Endocrinol. 2005;4(1):19-29.

18. Rogol AD. New facets of androgen replacement therapy during childhood and adolescence. Expert Opin Pharmacother. 2005;6(8):1319-36.

19. Ahmed SF, Tucker P, Mayo A, Wallace AM, Hughes IA. Randomized, crossover comparison study of the short-term effect of oral testosterone undecanoate and intramuscular testosterone depot on linear growth and serum bone alkaline phosphatase. J Pediatr Endocrinol Metab. 2004;17(7):941-50.

20. Mayo A, Macintyre H, Wallace AM, Ahmed SF. Transdermal testosterone application: pharmacokinetics and effects on pubertal status, short-term growth, and bone turnover. J Clin Endocrinol Metab. 2004;89(2):681-7.

21. Weidemann W, Peters B, Romalo G, Spindler KD, Schweikert HU. Response to androgen treatment in a patient with partial androgen insensitivity and a mutation in the deoxyribonucleic acid binding domain of the androgen receptor. J Clin Endocrinol Metab. 1998;83(4):1173-6.

22. Clayton PE, Miller WL, Oberfield SE, Ritzen EM, Speisser PW, ESPE/LWPES CAH Working Group. Consensus statement on 21-hydroxylase deficiency from the Lawson Wilkins Pediatric Endocrine Society and the European Society for Paediatric Endocrinology. Horm Res. 2002;58(4):188-95.

23. Robson S, Oliver GD. Management of vaginal agenesis: review of 10 years practice at a tertiary referral centre. Aust NZ J Obstet Gynaecol. 2000;40(4):430-3.

24. British Association of Paediatric Surgeons Working Party. (2001). Statement of the British Association of Paediatric Surgeons Working Party on the Surgical Management of Children Born with Ambiguous Genitalia. [online] Available from www.baps.org.uk/documents/Intersex%20statement.htm. [Accessed September, 2016].

25. Creighton SM, Minto CL, Steele SJ. Objective cosmetic and anatomical outcomes at adolescence of feminising surgery for ambiguous genitalia done in childhood. Lancet. 2001;358(9276):124-5.

26. Ismail-Pratt IS, Bikoo M, Liao LM, Conway GS, Creighton SM. Normalization of the vagina by dilator treatment alone in Complete Androgen Insensitivity Syndrome and Mayer-Rokitansky-Kuster-Hauser Syndrome. Hum Reprod. 2007;22(7):2020-4.

27. Alizai NK, Thomas DF, Lilford RJ, Batchelor AG, Johnson N. Feminizing genitoplasty for CAH: what happens at puberty? J Urol. 1999;161(5):1588-91.

28. Migeon CJ, Wisniewski AB, Gearhart JP, Meyer-Bahlburg HF, Rock JA, Brown TR, et al. Ambiguous genitalia with perineoscrotal hypospadias in 46,XY individuals: long-term medical, surgical, and psychosexual outcome. Pediatrics. 2002;110(3):e31.

29. Lee PA, Witchel SF. Genital surgery among females with congenital adrenal hyperplasias: changes over the past five decades. J Pediatr Endocrinol Metab. 2002;15(9):1473-7.

30. Warne G, Grover S, Hutson J, Sinclair A, Metcalfe S, Northam E, et al. A long-term outcome study of the intersex conditions. J Pediatr Endocrinol Metab. 2005;18(6):555-67.

31. Crouch NS, Minto CL, Laio LM, Woodhouse CR, Creighton SM. Genital sensation after feminizing genitoplasty for congenital adrenal hyperplasia: a pilot study. BJU Int. 2004;93(1):135-8.

32. Creighton SM. Long-term outcome of feminization surgery: the London experience. BJU Int. 2004;93(Suppl 3):44-6.

33. Gastaud F, Bouvattier C, Duranteau L, Brauner R, Thibaud E, Kutten F, et al. Impaired sexual and reproductive outcomes in women with classical forms of congenital adrenal hyperplasia. J Clin Endocrinol Metab. 2007;92(4):1391-6.

34. Randolph J, Hung W, Rathlev MC. Clitoroplasty for females born with ambiguous genitalia: a long-term study of 37 patients. J Pediatr Surg. 1981;16(6):882-7.

35. Newman K, Randolph J, Parson S. Functional results in young women having clitoral reconstruction as infants. J Pediatr Surg. 1992;27(2):180-3.

36. Steiner E, Woernie F, Kuhn W, Beckmann K, Schmidt M, Pilch H, et al. Carcinoma of the neovagina: case report and review of the literature. Gynecol Oncol. 2002;84(1):171-5.

37. Köhler B, Kleinemeier E, Lux A, Hiort O, Grüters A, Thyen U. Satisfaction with genital surgery and sexual life of adults with XY disorders of sex development: results from the German clinical evaluation study. J Clin Endocrinol Metab. 2012;97(2):577-88.

38. Callens N, van der Zwan YG, Drop SL, Cools M, Beerendonk CM, Wolffenbuttel KP, et al. Do surgical interventions influence psychosexual and cosmetic outcomes in women with disorders of sex development? ISRN Endocrinol. 2012; 2012:276742.

39. Cools M, van Aerde K, Kersemaekers AM, Boter M, Drop SL, Wolffenbuttel KP, et al. Morphological and immuno-histochemical differences between gonadal maturation delay and early germ cell neoplasia in patients with undervirilization syndromes. J Clin Endocrinol Metab. 2005;90(9):5295-303.

40. Ramani P, Yeung CK, Habeebu SS. Testicular intratubular germ cell neoplasia in children and adults with intersex. Am J Surg Pathol. 1993;17(11):1124-33.

41. Hannema SE, Scott IS, Rajpert-De Meyts E, Skakkebaek NE, Coleman N, Hughes IA. Testicular development in the complete androgen insensitivity syndrome. J Pathol. 2006; 208(4):518-27.

42. Rørth M, Rajpert-De Meyts E, Andersson L, Dieckmann KP, Fosså SD, Grigor KM, et al. Carcinoma in situ in testis. Scand J Urol Nephrol Suppl. 2000;205:166-86.

Karyotypic Abnormalities

Karyotypic abnormalities are a common cause of primary amenorrhoea. The most common karyotypic abnormality associated with an aberration of one of the sex chromosomes is Turner's syndrome. It is not only an important cause of primary amenorrhoea in young girls, but can also be considered as a disorder of sex development. This syndrome would be discussed in details in this chapter.

GONADAL DYSGENESIS (TURNER'S SYNDROME)

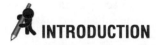

INTRODUCTION

Turner's syndrome is a condition affecting only young girls and women wherein one of the sex chromosomes, the X chromosome is partially or completely missing. This can be considered as the most common karyotypic abnormality, which affects women. Due to the missing sex chromosome, the gonads are largely dysgenetic. The ovaries are represented by streak gonads, which are characteristically composed of connective tissue with no follicles or only a few atretic follicles. Although the uterus and vagina are present, there is complete amenorrhoea because the gonads do not produce any hormones. In approximately one-third of the women, the ovaries can be imaged with the help of pelvic sonography. This syndrome occurs with a frequency of 1 in 2,500 live female births and can affect up to 3% of all conceptions.[1] Approximately 97–98% of the affected pregnancies land up in a miscarriage and fail to reach term. Nearly 10% of all miscarriages are likely to have a 45X karyotype.

At puberty, there is no appearance of secondary sexual characteristics and the external genitalia and breasts remain infantile. Among these patients, the spontaneous conceptions are rare and if occur, they are associated with a high risk for sex chromosome aneuploidy and spontaneous abortions.

There is a much higher incidence of hypothyroidism associated with Turner's syndrome although the cause for this is not completely known. It is supposed to be due to autoimmune causes.

AETIOLOGY

This disorder results from the loss of an entire or a part of X chromosome. Thus, their karyotype is 45,XO. Nearly 50% of the patients may be mosaics (45,X; 46,XX).[2] Only a part of the X chromosome may be missing in some patients. This may be associated with a number of structural abnormalities of X chromosome such as ring chromosome, isochromosome and terminal deletions.

Most patients with Turner's syndrome experience the loss of X chromosome of paternal origin and retain the X chromosome of maternal origin. Since the Y chromosome is absent, this syndrome occurs only in the females. Modern genotyping techniques have revealed a subgroup of cases with Turner's syndrome having a mosaic genotype expressing a Y chromosome. In some of these cases, fragments of the missing sex chromosome may be still present. If this happens to be a Y chromosome, there is a 10–12% risk of development of gonadoblastoma. Gonadectomy is usually advised in these cases.

DIAGNOSIS

Clinical Presentation

Clinical presentation in these conditions comprises of the following characteristics:[3]

❖ Primary hypogonadism and presence of streak gonads
❖ *Primary amenorrhoea and delayed or absent pubertal development*: Though most patients with Turner's syndrome present with primary amenorrhoea due to ovarian failure and do not experience any pubertal

development, some patients (especially the mosaics) may develop normally and present with secondary amenorrhoea later in life. These patients may have experienced some amount of pubertal development.

❖ *Intelligence*: It usually remains unaffected. Normal intelligence is a typical feature of Turner's syndrome. However, there may be an increased risk of impairment of non-verbal skills such as arithmetic and visuospatial skills. Severe mental retardation may be present in a rare patient with small ring chromosome because the ring chromosome does not undergo X-inactivation. Attention-deficit hyperactivity disorders and visual-spatial organisation disorders are also common in patients with Turner's syndrome.

❖ *Cancer risk*: Though the overall risk of developing a cancer in a patient with Turner's syndrome is similar to that of general population, the incidence of CNS tumours, bladder cancer and endometrial cancer is increased. On the other hand, the incidence of breast cancer is decreased.

❖ *A characteristic phenotype*: It may be present, which includes the following features:
  • Short stature: Growth failure resulting in low birth-weight at birth and short stature during childhood and adolescence is an important feature of Turner's syndrome. Pubertal growth spurt fails to occur and adult height is usually between 1.25 metres to 1.5 metres. The average height is approximately 1.42 metres. Short stature is the most commonly present abnormality, which is virtually present in all the patients with this type of chromosomal abnormality.
  • Female phenotype with webbed neck
  • Wide carrying angle (cubitus valgus)
  • Shield chest with widely spaced nipples
  • A low occipital hairline
  • High-arched palate, micrognathia and defective dental development
  • A short fourth metacarpal and hypoplastic nails
  • Low set ears may be present in up to 80% of cases
  • It may be associated with cystic hygroma
  • Infantile lymphoedema: At birth, there may be lympho-edema, especially, in the dorsum of the hand and foot, resulting in puffy hand and feet.
  • Abnormalities of cardiovascular, renal, ocular and organ systems can commonly occur and have been described under the heading of 'complications'.

Investigations

❖ *Karyotype analysis*: This is recommended for all girls with unexplained short stature, delayed puberty and other features suggestive of Turner's syndrome. Karyotype analysis must comprise of examination of at least 30 cells in order to detect significant mosaicism. If the clinician is clinically suspecting Turner's syndrome, but the karyotype analysis comes out as normal, a second tissue such as skin biopsy must be considered.

❖ *Fluorescence in situ hybridisation*: Individuals having chromosomes of uncertain origin or those with any evidence of virilisation also must be evaluated using FISH and Y-chromosome specific probes because those having all or part of a Y chromosome are at an increased risk of development of a gonadoblastoma. In these cases, removal of the gonads may be required.

❖ *Early pregnancy screening*: The incidence of this abnormality is not likely to increase with maternal age. However, these cases are likely to be linked with increased nuchal thickness due to an increased association of Turner's syndrome with cystic hygroma and non-immune foetal hydrops.[4]

❖ *Serum gonadotropin levels*: These cases are likely to be associated with hypergonadotropic hypogonadism. Therefore, they are likely to be associated with raised levels of gonadotropins (FSH and LH) and reduced levels of serum oestradiol.

DIFFERENTIAL DIAGNOSIS

Noonan syndrome: This is associated with a phenotypic appearance similar to Turner's syndrome. However, this is an autosomal dominant condition, which does not affect the sex chromosome. Therefore, there is no abnormality of ovarian function. Moreover, Noonan syndrome can also affect both males and females in comparison to the Turner's syndrome, which affects only the females.[5]

MANAGEMENT

❖ *Growth hormones*: They must be prescribed to the patients as soon as the height falls below the 5th percentile for age. This usually occurs between the ages from 2 years to 5 years.[6] Early treatment with growth hormone can help in increasing the lean body mass, which helps the patient achieve a normal adult height.

❖ *Hormone replacement therapy*: After optimal growth has been achieved using growth hormones, the girls are referred to a gynaecologist for advice related to HRT, which may be required in cases of ovarian failure. In these cases, women fail to achieve growth of secondary sexual characters at the time of puberty. A low dose of oestrogens is initially administered to encourage the growth of breasts.[7,8] Oestrogen therapy is initially started in the dosage of 0.25–0.5 mg micronised oestradiol and later gradually increased to 2.0 mg of micronised oestradiol over a period of 2 years. Oestrogen can also be delivered via transdermal route, starting at the dosage of 6.25 µg/h and gradually increasing the dosage.[9] They can be initially administered at a higher dosage if the girl presents at an older age. After nearly 2 years of therapy with oestradiol, cyclical progestins must be added to cause endometrial shedding at regular intervals, thereby preventing endometrial hyperplasia by suppressing endometrial development. HRT should be preferably continued until the age of 50 years to help maintain the bone density.[10] Since oestrogen therapy reduces height velocity by causing closure of the epiphysis, its use is not recommended before the age of 13–14 years.

❖ *Removal of gonads*: This is usually not required unless the person is a mosaic having 46,XY karyotype.[11]

❖ *Pregnancy and fertility*: Pregnancy may be possible in such patients given the option of oocyte donation.[12] Ovarian tissue can be cryopreserved as an option for future fertility, because many girls with Turner's syndrome may have development of follicles in their ovaries during adolescence, particularly the girls with mosaicism.[13,14] However, the patient must be counselled regarding the increased risk of mortality during the pregnancy mainly due to the complications such as aortic dissection or rupture. The patient must undergo a complete cardiovascular assessment before being referred to the assisted conception unit for conception using donor oocytes. Pregnancy rates with Turner's syndrome are similar to those achieved with other causes of premature ovarian failure. However, pregnancies in women with Turner's syndrome are likely to be associated with an increased risk of complications such as hypertension and diabetes during pregnancy.[15] Caesarean deliveries may be required in these cases due to the patient's short stature.

COMPLICATIONS

Turner's syndrome has long-term health implications and may be associated with a high premature mortality rate (nearly three times higher in comparison to the normal population). Due to the increased risk of complications, these patients should regularly undergo the following tests: BP measurement; thyroid function tests; LFTs; lipid profile and glucose levels (every yearly) and tests such as Echo; bone densitometry and audiogram (every 3–5 years).[16] According to the recommendations by the Turner Syndrome Consensus Study Group (2007), magnetic resonance angiography, rather than Echo should be used for the assessment of the structural cardiovascular abnormalities (especially aortic dilatation) in these women.[17] The patients diagnosed with well-defined cardiovascular defects must be cautioned in regards to pregnancy. The following complications are likely to occur in cases of Turner's syndrome:[18]

❖ *Osteoporosis*: This is due to oestrogen deficiency. It is responsible for an increased incidence of bone fractures.

❖ *Congenital anomalies*: Turner's syndrome may be associated with some cardiac, renal or ocular abnormalities.

❖ *Cardiac anomalies*: The overall mortality rate is increased by three-folds primarily due to the cardiovascular diseases. Some of the cardiac anomalies are as follows:[19,20]

  • Aortic valve disease: This is the most common cardiac anomaly, which may occur in 20–30% cases and includes defects such as bicuspid aortic valve, aortic root dilatation, etc.

  • Coarctation of the aorta: This is the most common serious cardiac anomaly, which may be found in up to 3–10% of the cases. This may be responsible for producing secondary hypertension and ejection systolic murmur. This may be commonly associated with bicuspid aortic valves (11% cases) and dissecting aortic aneurysm (16% cases).

  • Other cardiac anomalies: Other associated cardiac anomalies, which may be sometimes present, include elongation of the transverse aortic arch, persistent left superior vena cava, anomalous pulmonary venous return and an aberrant right subclavian artery. Even young children with Turner's syndrome may have a prolonged QT interval.

❖ *Renal anomalies*: Approximately 30–50% patients with Turner's syndrome may have an associated renal anomaly. Horseshoe kidney is the most common anomaly amongst them.

❖ *Ocular anomalies*: Some individuals may have ocular abnormalities such as amblyopia, strabismus, ptosis, hypertelorism, epicanthus, red-green colour blindness, etc.[21]

❖ *Endocrine anomalies*: Endocrine abnormalities may include hypothyroidism and diabetes mellitus, which may develop in nearly 25% individuals.

❖ *Other anomalies*: Other abnormalities may include celiac disease, sensorineural hearing loss due to disruption of the Eustachian tube and otitis media,[22] and abnormality of liver function.

❖ *Hypertension*: It is common in this condition; it may be idiopathic or secondary to some causes such as coarctation of aorta.

CLINICAL PEARLS

❖ Karyotype analysis must be done in all cases with elevated gonadotropin levels.[23]

❖ Due to presence of streak gonads, which lack ovarian follicles, no gonadal sex hormones are produced at the time of puberty and the patients present with primary amenorrhoea.

EVIDENCE-BASED MEDICINE

Though HRT is commonly prescribed in cases of Turner's syndrome for achieving feminisation and for the maintenance of bone health during the adult years, there is little published evidence regarding the long-term effects of using HRT in these cases. Presently, there is also limited evidence regarding the optimal HRT preparation, which must be used in these cases.[7-10]

PART III

REFERENCES

1. Nielsen J, Wohlert M. Chromosome abnormalities found among 34,910 newborn children: results from a 13-year incidence study in Arhus, Denmark. Hum Genet. 1991;87(1):81-3.

2. Ferguson-Smith MA. Karyotype-phenotype correlations in gonadal dysgenesis and their bearing on the pathogenesis of malformations. J Med Genet. 1965;2:142-55.

3. Turner HH. A syndrome of infantilism, congenital webbed neck, and cubitus valgus. Endocrinology. 1938;23:566-74.

4. Nicolaides KH, Azar G, Snijders RJ, Gosden CM. Fetal nuchal oedema: associated malformations and chromosomal defects. Fetal Diagn Ther. 1992;7(2):123-31.

5. Chacko E, Graber E, Regelmann MO, Wallach E, Costin G, Rapaport R. Update on Turner and Noonan syndromes. Endocrinol Metab Clin North Am. 2012;41(4):713-34.

6. Chernausek SD, Attie KM, Cara JF, Rosenfeld RG, Frane J. Growth hormone therapy of Turner syndrome: the impact of age of estrogen replacement on final height. Genentech, Inc., Collaborative Study Group. J Clin Endocrinol Metab. 2000;85(7):2439-45.

7. Rosenfield RL, Devine N, Hunold JJ, Mauras N, Moshang Jr T, Root AW. Salutary effects of combining early very low-dose systemic estradiol with growth hormone therapy in girls with Turner syndrome. J Clin Endocrinol Metab. 2005;90:6424-30.

8. Royal College of Obstetricians and Gynaecologists (RCOG). (2013). Sex steroid treatment for pubertal induction and replacement in the adolescent girl. Scientific Impact Paper No. 40. London: RCOG Press; 2013.

9. Ankarberg-Lindgren C, Elfving M, Wikland KA, Norjavaara E. Nocturnal application of transdermal estradiol patches produces levels of estradiol that mimic those seen at the onset of spontaneous puberty in girls. J Clin Endocrinol Metab. 2001;86(7):3039-44.

10. Hogler W, Briody J, Moore B, Garnett S, Lu PW, Cowell CT. Importance of estrogen on bone health in Turner syndrome: a cross-sectional and longitudinal study using dual-energy x-ray absorptiometry. J Clin Endocrinol Metab. 2004;89(1):193-9.

11. Cools M, Drop SL, Wolffenbuttel KP, Oosterhuis JW, Looijenga LH. Germ cell tumors in the intersex gonad: old paths, new directions, moving frontiers. Endocr Rev. 2006;27(5):468-84.

12. Alvaro Mercadal B, Imbert R, Demeestere I, Englert Y, Delbaere A. Pregnancy outcome after oocyte donation in patients with Turner›s syndrome and partial X monosomy. Hum Reprod. 2011;26(8):2061-8.

13. Hreinsson JG, Otala M, Fridstrom M, Borgstrom B, Rasmussen C, Lundqvist M, et al. Follicles are found in the ovaries of adolescent girls with Turner's syndrome. J Clin Endocrinol Metab. 2002;87(8):3618-23.

14. Oktay K, Bedoschi G, Berkowitz K, Bronson R, Kashani B, McGovern P, et al. Fertility Preservation in Women with Turner Syndrome: A Comprehensive Review and Practical Guidelines. J Pediatr Adolesc Gynecol. 2016;29(5):409-16.

15. Hovatta O. Pregnancies in women with Turner's syndrome. Ann Med. 1999;31(2):106-10.

16. Conway GS, Band M, Doyle J, Davies MC. How do you monitor the patient with Turner›s syndrome in adulthood? Clin Endocrinol (Oxf). 2010;73(6):696-9.

17. Bondy CA; Turner Syndrome Study Group. Care of girls and women with Turner syndrome: a guideline of the Turner Syndrome Study Group. J Clin Endocrinol Metab. 2007;92(1):10-25.

18. Elsheikh M, Conway GS, Wass JA. Medical problems in adult women with Turner's syndrome. Ann Med. 1999;31(2):99-105.

19. Practice Committee of American Society for Reproductive Medicine. Increased maternal cardiovascular mortality associated with pregnancy in women with Turner syndrome. Fertil Steril. 2012;97(2):282-4.

20. Gotzsche CO, Krag-Olsen B, Nielsen J, Sørensen KE, Kristensen BO. Prevalence of cardiovascular malformations and association with karyotypes in Turner's syndrome. Arch Dis Child. 1994;71(5):433-6.

21. Denniston AK, Butler L. Ophthalmic features of Turner's syndrome. Eye. 2004;18(7):680-4.

22. Barrenasa M, Landin-Wilhelmsenb K, Hansonc C. Ear and hearing in relation to genotype and growth in Turner syndrome. Hear Res. 2000;144(1-2):21-8.

23. Pinsker JE. Clinical review: Turner syndrome: Updating the paradigm of clinical care. J Clin Endocrinol Metab. 2012;97(6):E994-1003.

Menstrual Cycle

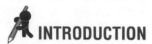 **INTRODUCTION**

In every normal women belonging to the reproductive age group, the uterine endometrium undergoes regular cyclic changes under the influence of hormones oestrogens and progesterone produced by the ovaries. This causes the uterine endometrium to become receptive to implantation of the early embryo at the correct time of the cycle in coordination with the arrival of newly fertilised embryo in the uterine cavity. In case the fertilisation has occurred, the embryo implants. In the event, fertilisation does not occur, the overgrown uterine endometrium sloughs off resulting in menses. This constitutes the menstrual cycle, which would now be discussed at length. The events of the normal menstrual cycle are shown in Figure 58.1. The menstrual cycle is due to synchronous and interrelated events occurring in the ovaries as well as the uterine endometrium: the ovarian cycle (oogenesis) as well as the uterine cycle (endometrial preparation). In a normal adult woman, menstrual cycle lasts between 28 days and 35 days. The duration of luteal phase is fixed at 14 days, whereas the duration of follicular phase can vary between 14 days to 21 days.[1]

OVARIAN CYCLE

The primordial germ cells arrive in the female gonad at about 9 weeks of gestation, following which they differentiate into oogonia, resulting in the formation of several clusters of oogonia. It is assumed that each cluster of oogonia is formed by one primordial cell. These clusters get surrounded by flat epithelial cells which are derived from epithelial covering of the ovary. These represent the follicular cells. Starting from 6 weeks to 8 weeks of gestation, rapid mitotic division occurs so that the number of oogonia reaches 6–7 million by 16–20 weeks (4–5 months) of gestation. This represents the maximal oogonal content of the gonads. From this point onwards, germ

cell content reduces irretrievably. By the 7th month, a large number of oogonia have degenerated except for those that are present near the surface of the ovary. At birth, the cortical content of germ cells is about 500,000–2,000,000 as a result of prenatal oocyte depletion. Also, during this time, the division of ovary into cortex and medulla has been achieved.

At the onset of puberty, the germ cell mass has been further reduced to 300,000–500,000 units. Out of these, only about 500 would actually ovulate. The remaining oocytes would fail to ovulate and become atretic within the ovary to the point of menopause. These follicles undergo depletion as a result of programmed cell death or apoptosis. The rate of loss of

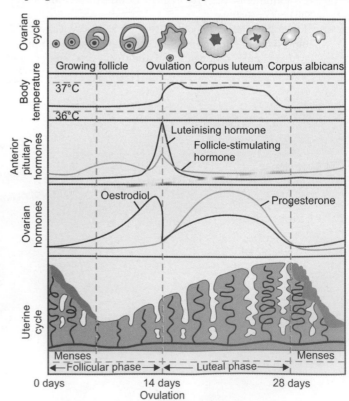

Fig. 58.1: Events taking place during the normal menstrual cycle

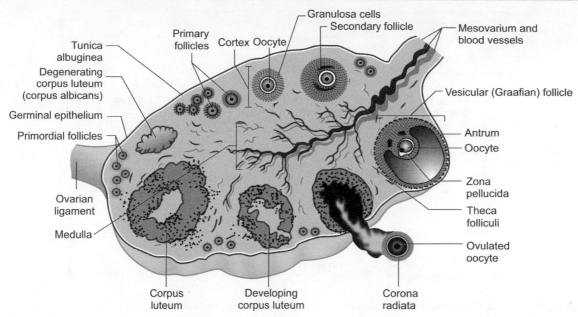

Fig. 58.2: Stages of development of ovarian follicles

primordial follicle pool is variable amongst individuals, with the age of loss of fertility and menopause varying amongst individuals between 40 years to 55 years.[2] After attainment of puberty, each month about 15–20 oocytes would get selected to mature, out of which eventually only one would ovulate.

The ovarian cortex comprises of 1,000 primordial follicles. Primordial follicle comprises a primary oocyte arrested in the prophase of meiosis. It is enveloped by a layer of spindle-shaped pregranulosa cells, surrounded by a basement membrane and measures about 30–60 µm in diameter. This unit is known as the primordial follicle, which gets converted into a primary follicle as the pregranulosa cells become cuboidal in nature, proliferate and gets converted into the granulosa cells (Fig. 58.2). In the primary follicle, granulosa cells multiply to form multiple layers and may acquire a diameter between 40 µm to 54 µm. The cells of the granulosa and the oocyte secrete a layer of glycoproteins on the surface of the oocyte, which forms a tough covering, the zona pellucida around the oocyte. As the follicle grows, the cells of the theca folliculi get arranged into an inner layer of secretory cells called as theca interna and an outer fibrous layer—the theca externa that is derived from the ovary. With further growth, the primary follicle gets converted into preantral follicle (secondary follicle) and then into antral follicle (tertiary follicle). In the absence of further stimulation by gonadotropins, the secondary follicles undergo atresia and apoptosis. The preantral follicle comprises of a fully developed oocyte surrounded by a zona pellucida, granulosa cells, a basal lamina and theca cells (which have been differentiated into two layers, theca interna and externa by a capillary network). It measures about 120 µm in diameter. The preantral follicle still lacks the fluid filled cavity or the antrum. Soon small fluid-filled cavities start appearing in the preantral follicle. These small cavities eventually join together to form a single large cavity, converting the preantral follicle into the antral follicle.

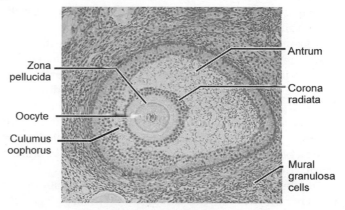

Fig. 58.3: Dominant follicle

Prior to ovulation, the antral follicle forms the Graafian follicle (Fig. 58.3). In the Graafian follicle (dominant follicle), due to the accumulation of large amount of fluid (liquor folliculi), the oocyte, along with its covering of the follicular cells gets pushed eccentrically towards one side. As a result of the fluid accumulation in the dominant follicle, the granulosa cells become organised into three compartments: (1) mural granulosa cells, surrounding the antrum; (2) cumulus oophorus, the stalk of granulosa cells connecting the oocyte to the mural granulosa cells; and (3) corona radiata, layer of granulosa cells in direct contact with the oocyte.[3] The mature follicle may be 25 mm in diameter, which projects for about 15 mm on the surface of ovary.

The earliest phase of development of follicles is independent of the gonadotropins, FSH and LH and lasts for about 74–80 days. These are probably regulated by the interplay between local autocrine and paracrine factors including locally released growth factors within the ovary such as bone morphogenic proteins (BMPs) also known as cytokines or metabologens, activins or GDF-9.[4]

CHAPTER 58

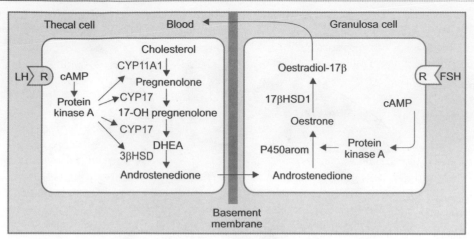

Fig. 58.4: Two-cell two-gonadotropin theory

Abbreviations: 3βHSD, 3 beta-hydroxysteroid dehydrogenase; 17βHSD1, 17 beta-hydroxysteroid dehydrogenase type 1; cAMP, cyclic adenosine monophosphate; CYP11A1, cytochrome P450 family 11 subfamily A member 1; CYP17, cytochrome P450 17 alpha hydroxylase/17, 20 lyase; P450 arom, aromatase

As previously described, the germ cells give rise to oogonia around 9th week of foetal life. These enter the first meiotic division and are converted into oocytes. Progression of meiosis to the diplotene stage is accomplished throughout the pregnancy and completed by birth. In the last week before birth, all the primary oocytes complete the diplotene stage but do not progress further. Instead, they get arrested in the diplotene stage of prophase. During this phase, the chromatin network becomes lacy. The primary oocytes remain arrested at this stage and do not undergo the completion of first meiotic division till the age of puberty, when the completion of first meiotic division occurs at the time of ovulation. Second meiotic division starts but gets arrested in the metaphase, which is completed only at the time of fertilisation. Primordial follicle comprises a primary oocyte arrested in the prophase of meiosis.

The theca or granulosa cell layers of the ovarian follicle act as per the 'two cell-two gonadotropin theory' (Fig. 58.4). The outer theca cell layer of the ovarian follicle has receptors for LH and the necessary enzymes to synthesise androgens. On the other hand, the granulosa cell layer, which is in close contact with the ovarian follicle, has enzyme aromatase, which converts the androgens produced by the outer theca layer into oestrogen under the effect of the hormone FSH.

As the growing ovarian follicle secretes oestradiol into the circulation, the circulating level of FSH is reduced by negative feedback inhibition over the hypothalamus and the ovary. As a result, other follicles in the cohort are not exposed to sufficient high levels of FSH to allow their development. This causes them to become atretic and die off. Also, with the progression of the follicular phase, activity of inhibin A predominates over that of activin. This facilitates the selection of the dominant follicle, which is able to maintain steroidogenesis in the face, of declining FSH levels.

Initial follicular development is independent of hormonal influence. However, soon FSH takes control and stimulates a cohort of follicles encouraging them to develop into preantral stage. FSH causes aromatisation of the androgens present in the theca cells into oestrogen in the granulosa cells. Out of the various follicles, only one single follicle is destined to develop into a dominant follicle, which undergoes ovulation. Oestrogen exerts a negative feedback effect on FSH as a result of which growth of all the follicles except dominant follicle is inhibited. Oestradiol levels derived from the dominant follicle increase rapidly and exert a negative feedback effect on FSH release. While causing a decline in FSH levels, the mid-follicular rise in oestradiol levels exert a positive feedback influence on LH secretion. The presence of LH in the follicle prior to ovulation is important for optimal follicular development, which ultimately results in formation of a healthy oocyte. A surge of LH takes place just prior to ovulation. LH levels rise steadily during the late follicular phase. LH initiates luteinisation and progesterone production in the granulosa layer. A preovulatory rise in progesterone facilitates the positive feedback action of oestrogen and may be required to induce the mid-cycle FSH peak. Ovulation occurs about 10–12 hours after the LH peak and 24–36 hours after the peak oestradiol levels have been attained. The onset of LH surge is the most reliable indicator of impending ovulation. Ovulation usually occurs within 36 hours (34–39 hours) of the onset of LH surge.

OVULATION

Every month, a cohort of antral follicles begins to develop from the stage of primary follicle. As previously described, the initial stages of follicular development are independent of FSH. The preantral follicles produce glycoprotein substances such as inhibin B and anti-Müllerian hormone (AMH) into the circulation. Soon under the influence of the GnRH, produced by the hypothalamus, the anterior pituitary is stimulated to produce FSH and LH hormones. Under the influence of FSH, the secretion of AMH declines. However, the leading follicle continues to secrete inhibin B. The growth of the leading antral follicle under the influence of FSH coincides with the intercycle rise of FSH. Only one follicle eventually develops near the surface of the ovary to the stage of full maturity. As the follicular diameter becomes approximately 18 mm, the rising oestradiol concentration triggers a coordinated secretion of LH from the anterior pituitary. This is known as the 'LH surge'. This LH surge triggers the final maturation of the oocyte with the completion of meiosis I. This causes extrusion of first polar body, containing one of the two haploid sets of chromosome from the oocyte. At the same time, LH surge also initiates an inflammatory reaction with the walls of follicle adjacent to the fimbrial end of fallopian tube. Release of various cytokines, interleukins, prostaglandins, etc. and formation of new blood vessels eventually result in rupture of the follicle and extrusion of ovum about 38 hours following LH surge. While ovulation occurs from the dominant follicle, other oocytes, which are not destined to ovulate, die and eventually get converted into fibrous tissue, the corpus atreticum. Ovulation takes place as the ovarian follicle ruptures and the discharged oocyte is carried into the peritoneal cavity via the uterine tube. Another important event preceding ovulation is as follows: oestrogen production peaks (must be >200 pg/mL for >24 hours) and is responsible for triggering the FSH and LH surge. During this time, the follicle increases in size to about 18–20 mm.

Once the oocyte has been extruded out, the cells of the empty ovarian follicle get converted into the corpus luteum (CL) which produces progesterone for about 14 days, in the absence of fertilisation. Production of progesterone from the CL induces secretory changes in the endometrium. Progesterone secretion also suppresses secretion of FSH from the anterior pituitary, preventing the development of further dominant follicles. If the fertilisation does occur, progesterone is produced for further 3–4 months by the CL under the effect of β-hCG produced by the trophoblasts, following which it eventually dies off. In the absence of 'rescue' by β-hCG, the CL involutes after 2 weeks, resulting in a decline in the concentration of progesterone in the circulation. Progesterone withdrawal ultimately causes sloughing off of the uterine endometrium resulting in menstruation.

The released oocyte moves from the ovary into the uterine tube and may get fertilised by the male gamete in the ampulla of the uterine tube. Even though many spermatozoa may approach the oocyte, only one spermatozoon is allowed to enter the oocyte. It passes the zona pellucida by capacitation and acrosome reaction. The process of fertilisation between two haploid gametes results in the formation of a diploid zygote, thereby restoring the number of chromosomes to that of the normal somatic cell. The sperms remain viable for up to 4–5 days after reaching the female reproductive tract. On the other hand, the ovum may remain viable for 12–24 hours. Therefore, there is a 'window' of about 24 hours during which the ovum can be fertilised. On fertilisation, the chromosomal configuration can be of two types, either 44 (XY), i.e. a male child or 44 (XX), i.e. a female child. Fertilisation of the sperm and egg occurs in the fimbrial or ampullary end of the fallopian tube and transport between this region and implantation in the endometrium takes between 5 to 7 days. The fertilised ovum implants, well past the 16-cell stage.

ROLE OF VARIOUS HORMONES IN REGULATION OF MENSTRUAL CYCLES

The hypothalamic-pituitary axis, by producing GnRH is responsible for the optimal reproductive function:

spermatogenesis and ejaculatory function in males and menstrual cycle (process of coordinated endometrial preparation and oogenesis) in females. The nocturnal release of GnRH from the hypothalamus at the time of puberty is responsible for stimulating the release of gonadotropins (FSH and LH) from the pituitary gland. GnRH is a decapeptide which passes via the portal veins from the hypothalamus to the anterior pituitary gland and controls the pulsatile release of FSH and LH. Neurons secreting GnRH are located in the ventromedial nucleus of the hypothalamus to which they migrate from the olfactory area of the brain.[5] Pulsatile release of GnRH at the time of puberty is responsible for pulsatile secretion of gonadotropins from the anterior pituitary which helps in the initiation of ovarian activity and the menstrual cycles.[6] On the other hand, sustained continuous administration of exogenous GnRH analogues in the artificial IVF cycles has an initial flare-up effect (increased production of LH and FSH) followed by downregulation associated with decreased production of LH and FSH.

ROLE OF INHIBINS, ACTIVIN AND FOLLISTATIN

Inhibins, activins and follistatin are protein molecules involved in the autocrine or paracrine regulation of the menstrual function. Inhibins are glycoprotein molecules secreted by the granulosa cells of the ovarian follicle as well as the theca or granulosa cells of the CL. Activin and inhibin molecules produce almost directly opposite biological effects. FSH induces granulosa cells to secrete both activin and inhibin A. Inhibin molecules comprise of α and β chains linked by disulphide bonds. Inhibin A comprises an α and a β A subunit. It is primarily secreted by mature dominant follicle and CL. On the other hand, inhibin B comprises of an α and a β B subunit and is released by the cohort of antral follicles in the early follicular phase and the early dominant follicle. Both inhibin A and B suppress FSH secretion eventually causing inhibition of FSH.[7] Also, inhibin B produced by the early dominant follicle acts with oestradiol to inhibit the growth of other members of the activated cohort of follicles. Secretion of inhibin is reduced by GnRH and increased by IGF1. Inhibin A reaches a peak in the mid-luteal phase. Inhibin B reaches a peak in the early to mid-follicular phase. Second peak is achieved at the time of ovulation.

On the other hand, activin supplements FSH action by increasing its receptors. It also increases the proliferation of granulosa cells and production of the enzyme aromatase. It also inhibits production of androgens by the theca cells. The granulosa cells also secrete follistatin, which bears no significant resemblance to the α- and β-subunits of the inhibin or activin family. Follistatin combines with activin, thereby inhibiting its action. It also directly suppresses the synthesis and secretion of FSH by the pituitary.[8]

MENSTRUAL CYCLE

The first day of a typical menstrual cycle (day 1) corresponds to the first day of menses. The menstrual phase usually lasts for 5 days and involves the disintegration and sloughing of the functionalis layer of the endometrium. Interplay of various prostaglandins (e.g. prostaglandin $F_{2\alpha}$ and prostaglandin E_2) is involved in regulation of menstrual cycle. Prostaglandin $F_{2\alpha}$ causes myometrial contractions and vasoconstriction, whereas prostaglandin E_2 causes vasodilatation and muscle relaxation. A typical menstrual cycle comprises of 28 days. Ovulation occurs in the middle of the menstrual cycle, i.e. day 14 of a typical cycle. The first 14 days of the cycle, before the menstruation occurs form the proliferative phase, while the next 14 days of the cycle form the secretory phase. During the follicular phase of normal ovarian cycle (equivalent to the proliferative phase of endometrial cycle), there is an increase in the blood levels of the hormone oestrogen. During this phase, the maturation of the dominant follicle takes place. At the mid-point of the cycle, ovulation occurs. Following the process of ovulation, the ruptured ovarian follicle gets converted into CL, the main hormone produced by CL being progesterone. During the luteal phase of the ovarian cycle (corresponding to the secretory phase of endometrial cycle) as the CL matures, the main hormone produced is progesterone. The endometrium during this phase gets transformed for implantation of conceptus in anticipation of the pregnancy. If pregnancy occurs, the rising levels of hCG stimulate and rescue the endometrium. In case the pregnancy does not occur, the CL undergoes regression. As a result, the levels of oestrogen and progesterone rapidly decline causing withdrawal of the functional support of the endometrium. This results in menstrual bleeding, marking the end of one endometrial cycle and the beginning of the other.

Proliferative (Follicular) Phase

The proliferative (follicular) phase extends from day 5 to day 14 of the typical cycle. In this phase, the endometrial proliferation occurs under oestrogen stimulation. The oestrogen is produced by the developing ovarian follicles under the influence of FSH. This causes marked cellular proliferation of the endometrium and an increase in the length and tortuosity of the spiral arteries. Endometrial glands develop and contain some glycogen. This phase ends as ovulation occurs.

The following changes take place during the proliferative phase (Fig. 58.5):
❖ The functional and the basal layers of endometrium become well defined. The proliferation mainly occurs in the functional layer. The basal layer measures 1 mm in thickness, while the functional layer reaches a maximum thickness of about 3.5–5 mm by 14th day.
❖ The glands become elongated and slightly sinuous and the columnar epithelium lining them becomes taller. In the beginning, the glands are narrow and tubular, lined by low columnar epithelial cells. Mitosis becomes prominent and the areas of pseudostratification are observed.
❖ There is an increase in ciliated and microvillous cells in the endometrial glands.
❖ Endometrial stroma becomes oedematous with wide separation of the individual cells. The stroma gets

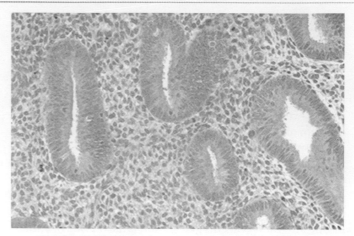

Fig. 58.5: Proliferative endometrium *(For colour version, see Plate 4)*

infiltrated with numerous cells including macrophages, leucocytes, etc.
❖ In the initial phase, the spiral vessels are uncoiled and unbranched. However, soon the growth of the straight vessels occurs so that they start becoming more coiled and spiral.

Secretory (Luteal) Phase

This phase is marked by production of progesterone and less potent oestrogens by the CL. It extends from day 15 to day 28 of the typical cycle. The peak of secretory changes in the endometrium occurs 7–9 days after ovulation when the endometrium is most receptive to implantation by the free-lying blastocyst.[9] This time period is also known as the implantation window and can be considered as the optimal time for embryo transfer in the IVF cycles.

The functionalis layer of the endometrium increases in thickness and the stroma becomes oedematous. The glands become tortuous with dilated lumens and store glycogen. If pregnancy occurs, the placenta produces hCG to replace progesterone, and the endometrium (and the accompanying pregnancy) are maintained. If pregnancy does not occur, the oestrogen and progesterone levels cause negative feedback at the hypothalamus, resulting in the fall in the levels of the hormones FSH and LH. The spiral arteries become less coiled and have decreased blood flow. At the end of this period, they alternately contract and relax, causing disintegration of the functionalis layer and eventually menses. The proliferative phase of the endometrium starts when the regeneration of the menstruating endometrium (which had been sloughed off) begins. The endometrial features of the secretory phase include the following (Fig. 58.6):
❖ The most characteristic feature of this phase is development of subnuclear vacuolation in the glandular epithelial cells. In this, the glycogen-filled vacuoles develop between the nuclei and the basement membrane (by the day 17–18). This is the first evidence that ovulation has taken place.
❖ The endometrium measures about 8–10 mm in the secretory phase. The secretory phase reaches its peak activity by the 22nd day of the cycle after which no growth occurs.

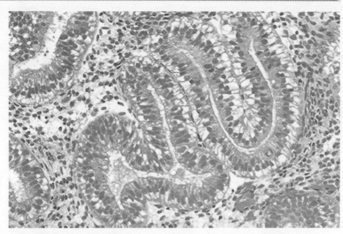

Fig. 58.6: The secretory phase endometrium *(For colour version, see Plate 4)*

- The glands become crenated and tortuous to assume a characteristic corkscrew-shaped appearance. The corkscrew pattern of the glands becomes saw-toothed in the later part of the secretory phase.
- The stroma of the functional layer becomes oedematous further.
- The functional layer of the endometrium can be divided into two layers:
  1. Superficial or compact layer
  2. Deep spongy layer
- The spiral vessels become dense and deeply coiled.

CLINICAL PEARLS

- It is the duty of the clinician to identify abnormal menstrual patterns, in women starting right from adolescence, which may result in potential health concerns during adulthood.
- Abnormal uterine bleeding could occur due to causes such as ovulatory dysfunction (anovulation), endocrinological disturbances of hypothalamic-pituitary axis, disorders of coagulation (von Willebrand's disease, platelet disorders, etc.) and rarely malignancy (e.g. oestrogen-producing ovarian tumours, androgen-producing tumours, etc.).[10]

REFERENCES

1. Sherman BM, Korenman SG. Hormonal characteristics of the human menstrual cycle throughout reproductive life. J Clin Invest. 1975;55(4):699-706.
2. Ecochard R, Gougeon A. Side of ovulation and cycle characteristics in normally fertile women. Hum Reprod. 2000;15(4):752-5.
3. Tsafriri A, Chun SY, Reich R. Follicular rupture and ovulation. In: Adashi EY, Leung PC (Eds). The Ovary, 1st edition. New York: Raven Press; 1993. p. 227.
4. van der Merwe JV. Contemporary physiology of the menstrual cycle. Part II. The reproductive hormones, regulatory mechanisms and cyclical hormonal changes. S Afr Med J. 1981;59(23):834-8.
5. Van Look PF, Baird DT. Regulatory mechanisms during the menstrual cycle. Eur J Obstet Gynecol Reprod Biol. 1980;11(2):121-44.
6. Diaz A, Laufer MR, Breech LL. Menstruation in girls and adolescents: using the menstrual cycle as a vital sign. Pediatrics. 2006;118(5):2245-50.
7. de Kretser DM, Hedger MP, Loveland KL, Phillips DJ. Inhibins, activins and follistatin in reproduction. Hum Reprod Update. 2002;8(6):529-41.
8. Muttukrishna S, Tannetta D, Groome N, Sargent I. Activin and follistatin in female reproduction. Mol Cell Endocrinol. 2004;225(1-2):45-56.
9. Harper MJ. The implantation window. Baillieres Clin Obstet Gynaecol. 1992;6(2):351-71.
10. American College of Obstetricians and Gynaecologists. Menstruation in girls and adolescents: using the menstrual cycle as a vital sign (Committee opinion No. 65). Obstet Gynecol. 2015;126:e143-6.

Adolescent and Paediatric Gynaecology

PUBERTY

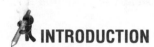

INTRODUCTION

Puberty is the process of physical changes, which causes transformation of the child's body into that of an adult, capable of reproduction. It can be defined as progression from appearance of sexual characteristics to sexual, reproductive and mental maturity. Before puberty, body differences between boys and girls are almost entirely restricted to the genitalia. During puberty, there is development of secondary sexual characteristics which lead to development of major differences in size, shape, composition and function in many body structures and systems.

Puberty tends to begin from the age of 10 years. The age of onset of puberty has been declining in the US over the past century by approximately 6–12 months.[1] On an average, African-American girls begin puberty between the ages of 8 to 9 years, while European-American girls experience it by the age of 10 years. Mean age of occurrence of menarche is 12.9 years with a range of 11–15 years. In the beginning when the menstrual cycles first start, they may be anovular in nature with no follicular development due to irregular GnRH pulse frequency In general, the four signs of puberty in most adolescent girls are an acceleration of growth, followed by breast budding (thelarche), followed by the appearance of pubic hair (pubarche) and finally the onset of menses (menarche).[2] This sequence of events occurs over a period of 1–6 years (average 4–5 years). Pubarche usually occurs as a result of adrenal androgen secretion (adrenarche). In a substantial number of cases, the sequence of events may be reversed with pubarche preceding thelarche.

The peak height velocity in females occurs just before menarche. The peak height velocity is 6–11 cm/year in females but 7–13 cm/year in males. If peak height velocity is reached earlier than 8 years in females, investigations should be undertaken. On the other hand, testicular enlargement is the first sign of puberty in males and the growth spurt occurs at the final phase in males.

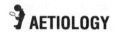

AETIOLOGY

Puberty is initiated as a result of hormone signals sent from the brain to the gonads (the ovaries and testes). The hormonal signals are responsible for stimulating the growth and function of a variety of organs such as brain, bones, muscles, skin, breast and sex organs. The principal hormone involved in males is testosterone, while that in females is oestradiol. Interaction of various hormones secreted through the hypothalamus-pituitary-ovarian axis and other endocrine organs, such as adrenals and thyroid glands, plays a role. Other factors, such as genetic, environmental (nutrition, emotional stress and childhood illnesses), etc. may also play a role. Binding of G-protein coupled receptor, KISS1R (also known as GPR54) with its ligand, 'kisspeptin' has been identified to generate neuroendocrine signals for controlling the GnRH pulse generator at the onset of puberty. Genetic mechanisms related to single gene mutations, environmental factors, nutritional factors and endocrine disruptors have also been implicated in abnormal timing of puberty.

The first event of puberty is thought to be the nocturnal release of GnRH from the hypothalamus. The reactivation of hypothalamic-pituitary-gonadal axis at the time of puberty can cause a rise in the levels of FSH and LH. This in turn, stimulates the synthesis of oestrogen and testosterone in the ovaries and testes of young girls and boys respectively.

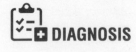

DIAGNOSIS

Clinical Presentation

The process of puberty typically begins by the age of 10 or 11 years in girls and by the age of 12 or 13 years in boys.[3]

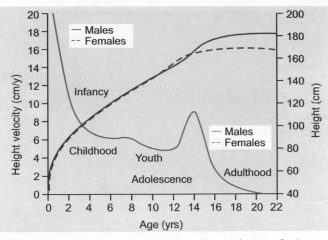

Fig. 59.1: Changes in height in both girls and boys at the time of puberty

Table 59.1: Tanner stages of breast development[4]

Stage	Characteristic features
Stage 1	Prepubertal stage
Stage 2	Breast budding: Enlargement and widening of the areolae
Stage 3	Breast enlargement beyond the areolae
Stage 4	Further enlargement of the breasts with the areolae and nipples forming the secondary mounds
Stage 5	Adult breast contour

Table 59.2: Tanner stages of pubic hair development[4]

Stage	Characteristic features
Stage 1	Prepubertal hair
Stage 2	Presexual hair: Occurrence of long, relatively straight hair on labia majora
Stage 3	Sexual hair: The hair becomes curly, coarser and there is an outwards extension
Stage 4	Mid-escutcheon: Further extension of the hair to cover the labia
Stage 5	Female escutcheon: Extension of hair over the medial thighs

During the period of puberty, there are anatomical (development of secondary sexual and genital organs), physical, endocrinological, psychological and emotional changes. The sequence of occurrence of pubertal changes in females is as follows: physical growth (Fig. 59.1) followed by development of secondary sexual characters and thelarche (by 10–12 years). Pubarche occurs after approximately 1 year and lastly there is development of ovaries and genital organs followed by occurrence of menarche.

❖ *Thelarche*: This refers to the breast development and occurs at the average age of 10.5 years. The first physical sign of puberty in girls is appearance of a firm, tender lump under the centre of the areola in one or both the breasts.

❖ *Pubarche*: The next noticeable change of puberty is development of pubic hair, usually occurring within a few months of thelarche.

❖ *Menarche*: This refers to the occurrence of first menstrual bleeding and typically occurs about 2 years after thelarche. The average age of menarche in girls is 11.75 years.

❖ *Vagina, uterus, and ovaries*: The mucosal surface of the vagina also responds to the increasing levels of oestrogen, changing from a thin, bright red prepubertal vaginal mucosa to a thicker, dull-pink colour postpuberty. There also occurs keratinisation of skin and transformation of the vaginal epithelium into a multilayered squamous epithelium under the influence of oestrogen. Vaginal epithelium turns acidic with the appearance of Doderlein's bacilli. There is development of labia majora with deposition of fat. Rapid growth of the uterus occurs so that the prepubertal uterus to cervix ratio changes from 1:1 to 2:1 or 3:1. There is also enlargement of ovaries and occurrence of ovulation.

❖ *Body shape, fat distribution and physical development*: There is an increase in the girl's height and weight, which is usually completed by 14 years of age. There is broadening of the lower half of the pelvis and hips, thereby resulting in a wider birth canal. Fat deposition occurs in a typical female distribution in the areas of breasts, hips, buttocks, thighs, upper arms and pubis.

Physical Examination

Breast enlargement: This may initially be unilateral or asymmetric. Gradually, the breast diameter increases, the areola darkens and thickens, and the nipple becomes more prominent. Staging system for describing the physical changes of puberty were first described by Marshall and Tanner and is known as the Tanner staging system. There are five Tanner stages of breast and pubic hair development in girls, described respectively, in Tables 59.1 and 59.2.[4]

❖ Examination of the external genitalia: This may reveal the presence of pubic hair or enlargement of the clitoris. The vaginal mucosa, which is a deep-red colour in prepubertal girls, becomes pastel-pink in appearance as oestrogen exposure increases.

Investigations

X-ray of the non-dominant hand, elbow and knees is done in order to assess the bone age.

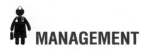

MANAGEMENT

Sex Education

Although puberty is a natural physiological process, sex education regarding the pubertal changes helps in allaying stress and anxiety from the minds of young girls. Young girls need to be educated about sex and STDs. In case of possibility of sexual intercourse at young age, contraception (barrier methods, initially) must be prescribed. Extra nutrition (especially proteins, iron and calcium) may be required to support their growth.

COMPLICATIONS

Some commonly occurring gynaecological problems during this period are:

❖ Precocious puberty
❖ Delayed puberty
❖ Menstrual abnormalities
❖ Dysmenorrhoea
❖ Vaginal discharge
❖ Teenage or unwanted pregnancies
❖ Cryptomenorrhoea (occurrence of menstruation without any external flow of blood, e.g. in cases of imperforate hymen).

CLINICAL PEARLS

❖ While puberty refers to an individual's sexual and physical maturation rather than the psychosocial and cultural aspects of development, adolescence is the period of psychological and social transition between childhood and adulthood.
❖ Although the growth and maturation of Graafian follicles occur at the time of puberty, ovulation may not occur as late as 1–2 years after menarche. Due to this, menstrual periods largely remain anovular and may be irregular, prolonged, scanty or excessive.
❖ Occurrence of menstruation before the development of secondary sexual characteristics can be considered as abnormal and is usually due to the feminising ovarian tumours or the malignancy of the genital tract.

EVIDENCE-BASED MEDICINE

❖ Early pubertal development is associated with a slightly reduced adult height and an increased risk for obesity in comparison to a late menarche.[2]
❖ Low BMI in adolescent women may result in delayed menarche as occurring in the cases of anorexia nervosa.[2]

PRECOCIOUS PUBERTY

INTRODUCTION

Precocious puberty refers to the appearance of physical and hormonal signs of pubertal development at an earlier age than is considered normal. This can be characterised by the development of both breasts and pubic hair in girls and by the development of pubic hair and testicular enlargement in boys (testicular enlargement can be defined as an increase in the volume of >4 mL or a diameter of 2.5 cm).[5,6] Precocious puberty is defined as pubertal development occurring more

PART III

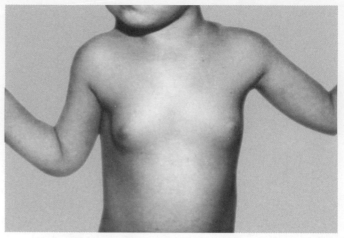

Fig. 59.2: Precocious breast development in a 7-year-old girl

than 2.5 standard deviation (SD) earlier than the average age. If the average age of puberty was considered to be 10 years, the development of secondary sexual characteristics before 8 years in females (Fig. 59.2) or onset of menses before the age of 10 years (chronological age) would be defined as precocious puberty. Development of secondary sexual characteristics before 9 years in males is also considered precocious.

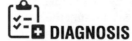

AETIOLOGY

Precocious puberty can be of two types:
1. Central precocious puberty (CPP) (constitutional/true/complete precocious puberty), which is gonadotropin dependent
2. Precocious pseudopuberty, which is gonadotropin independent. Difference between CPP and precocious pseudopuberty is described in Table 59.3.[7]

DIAGNOSIS

Clinical Presentation

The diagnosis is made with the help of a careful history and physical examination in conjunction with the use of radiologic and laboratory evaluations. The clinician must differentiate CPP from precocious pseudopuberty at the time of examination. In CPP, the secondary sexual characteristics appear in a chronological order and eventually regular menstrual cycles are established. Due to exposure to oestrogens, there is an initial spurt of height followed by premature closure of epiphysis due to which the ultimate height remains stunted.[8]

Investigations

Following investigations are required in cases of precocious puberty:
❖ *Radiography*: After taking complete history and performing physical examination, radiography of the hand and wrist must be performed in order to determine the bone age.

Table 59.3: Differences between gonadotropin-dependent and gonadotropin-independent precocious puberty

Characteristics	Gonadotropin-dependent precocious puberty	Gonadotropin-independent precocious puberty
Alternative name	Also known as central precocious puberty or true precocious puberty	Also known as peripheral precocious puberty or pseudo-precocious puberty
Aetiology	It is characterised by early maturation and activation of the hypothalamic-pituitary-gonadal axis. However, the sequence of pubertal events is normal and proceeds at a normal pace	It is independent of GnRH and gonadotropins. It usually results from exposure to sex-steroid hormones which may be derived from the gonads, adrenals or the environment
Consistency of sexual characteristics with the child's gender	It is isosexual in nature, i.e. developing sexual characteristics are consistent with the child's gender	It could be either isosexual or contrasexual in nature, where sexual characteristics are inconsistent with the child's gender (e.g. virilisation in girls or feminisation in boys)
Levels of gonadotropins	Levels of gonadotropins, particularly FSH and LH are increased	Levels of gonadotropins are low
Causes	<ul><li>Idiopathic (70–80%)</li><li>*CNS lesions*: Congenital such as hydrocephalus, acquired such as post-irradiation, infection, surgery, cysts, or tumours (such as microscopic hamartomas, astrocytomas, ependymomas, pineal tumours, optic and hypothalamic gliomas)</li><li>Hypothyroidism</li></ul>	<ul><li>McCune-Albright syndrome</li><li>Ovarian tumours (granulosa tumour, malignant teratoma or arrhenoblastoma of ovary)</li><li>Adrenal cortical lesions (tumour or hyperplasia)</li><li>Testicular disorders (Leydig cell tumours) and administration of exogenous sex steroids</li></ul>

The individuals who require further endocrine evaluation and imaging include the following:

- Children with advanced bone age
- Children with normal bone age accompanied by the development of both breasts and pubic hair
- Children with normal bone age associated with accelerated growth and breast or pubic hair development.

❖ *Measurement of gonadotropin levels*: Measurement of GnRH-stimulated serum gonadotropin levels helps in differentiating between the two types of precocious puberties. Measurement of the stimulated serum LH concentration can be considered as the most useful diagnostic parameter. In case of gonadotropin-dependent precocious puberty, there are elevated basal or stimulated serum LH levels. Other tests which may be required to evaluate the cause of CPP include the following:

- *MRI*: In cases of CPP, MRI head is indicated to exclude an intracranial lesion[9]
- *Thyroid function tests*: Thyroid function tests are not a routine requirement in the evaluation of precocious puberty. These may be required in case of clinical suspicion of thyroid dysfunction.

❖ *Evaluation of the causes of precocious pseudopuberty*: In case of gonadotropin-independent precocious puberty (as evidenced by normal basal and stimulated LH levels), other tests which need to be done include:

- Serum concentration of oestradiol, testosterone and hCG (for detection of functional ovarian cysts, tumours and functional adrenal tumours)
- Late afternoon cortisol levels (Cushing's syndrome)
- Dehydroepiandrosterone (DHEA), dehydroepiandrosterone sulphate (DHEA-S; premature adrenarche)
- 17-hydroxyprogesterone (congenital adrenal hyperplasia).

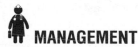

MANAGEMENT

Surgical Management

When CPP is caused by a CNS tumour other than a hamartoma, surgical resection may be attempted. Radiation therapy is often indicated if surgical resection is incomplete.

Medical Management

Gonadotropin-releasing hormone analogue: Continuous administration of luteinising hormone releasing hormone (LHRH) and GnRH agonists provides negative feedback and results in decreased levels of LH and FSH, 2–4 weeks after initiating treatment. GnRH analogues in the dosage of 100 µg intranasally BD for 6 months can be used to suppress menstruation because the young girls might not be capable of managing menstrual hygiene.[10]

COMPLICATIONS

- ❖ Rapid bone maturation can cause linear growth to cease too early and can result in an ultimate short adult stature.
- ❖ The early appearance of breasts or menses in girls and increased libido in boys can cause emotional distress for some children.
- ❖ Young girls with precocious puberty may be stressed, may become withdrawn, may exhibit behavioural problems (such as poor self-esteem and higher anxiety, irritability or withdrawal) and may have difficulty adjusting to wearing and changing pads.

CLINICAL PEARLS

A history of early puberty in a parent or sibling is relevant and decreases the likelihood that early puberty has an organic cause.

EVIDENCE-BASED MEDICINE

Future reproductive capacity is usually not compromised in cases of true precocious puberty.[11]

DELAYED PUBERTY

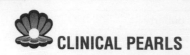

INTRODUCTION

Delayed puberty can be defined as the failure to begin sexual maturation at an age which is 2.5 SD above the mean age of onset of puberty. Delayed puberty in girls can be described if there is no occurrence of breast development by the age of 13 years, or no menarche by 3 years after breast development or by the age of 16 years. In boys, delayed puberty can be defined as no testicular enlargement by 14 years, or delay in development for 5 years or more after onset of genitalia enlargement. In the US, the evaluation of delayed puberty is recommended at 13 years in girls and 14 years or older in boys who do not demonstrate any signs of sexual maturation. However, if other secondary sexual characteristics have developed normally in a girl with primary amenorrhoea, an expectant approach can be adopted until the age of 16 years, following which the girl must be investigated.

AETIOLOGY

The main cause of delayed puberty is hypogonadism, which could be either hypogonadotropic hypogonadism (inactive hypothalamic-pituitary axis) or hypergonadotropic hypogonadism (primary gonadal failure) (Table 59.4). In these cases there is absence of breast and pubic hair development. In cases of hypogonadotropic hypogonadism, there is absent or reduced level of gonadotropins. In hypergonadotropic hypogonadism, there is normal release of gonadotropins, but there is no response from the gonads. As a result, there is no negative feedback to control gonadotropin levels. Another important cause of delayed puberty is constitutional delay of growth and puberty.

Constitutional Growth Delay

Constitutional growth delay is a temporary delay in skeletal growth and height of a child with no other physical abnormality causing the delay.[12] This can be considered as one of the most important causes of delayed puberty and short stature. In cases of constitutional delay of puberty, normal prepubertal growth nadir is prolonged and pulsatile GnRH secretion is slow to

Table 59.4: Various causes of delayed puberty

Absence of breast and pubic hair development	
Hypogonadotropic hypogonadism	**Hypergonadotropic hypogonadism**
• Functional GnRH deficiency, reflecting a constitutional delay in the reactivation of hypothalamic-gonadal axis • Normal variation, sometimes familial • Suppressive effects of chronic stress due to illness, malnutrition or excessive exercise • Systemic disease, e.g. malnutrition, cystic fibrosis, renal failure, heart disease and malabsorption • Genetic defects (Kallman's syndrome) • Anatomic abnormalities (hypothalamic and pituitary tumours, e.g. cranio-pharyngioma) • Thyroid deficiency (hypothyroidism) • Hyperprolactinaemia • Pituitary failure • Androgen receptor defect, e.g. testicular feminisation (complete or partial defects) • Anorexia nervosa • Emotional deprivation • Excessive exercise	• Primary gonadal failure (primary testicular failure, e.g. Klinefelter's syndrome or primary ovarian failure, e.g. Turner's syndrome) • Previous treatment of malignancy (gonadectomy, chemotherapy, gonadal irradiation, etc.) • Galactosaemia (in association with ovarian failure) • Autoimmune ovarian failure (may be associated with abnormalities such as Addison's disease, vitiligo, hypothyroidism, etc.) • Congenital adrenal hyperplasia (due to the deficiency of 17-α hydroxylase)
Normal breast and pubic hair development: Normal progression of puberty, but failure of menstruation	
• Anatomical abnormalities (e.g. Müllerian agenesis) • Imperforate hymen or transverse vaginal septum • Hyperprolactinaemia • Congenital adrenal hyperplasia	
Normal breast development, but scanty or absent pubic hair	
• Androgen insensitivity syndrome (failure of pubic hair development due to end-organ insensitivity to androgens)	

develop. Family history is often positive with the siblings or parents also giving a history of delayed puberty. X-ray of left hand and wrist demonstrates the bone age to be delayed. If the bone age reaches 13 years in girls or 14 years in boys without the evidence of puberty, the patient is more likely to have GnRH deficiency rather than constitutional delay of puberty. Also, in cases of constitutional delay of puberty, laboratory evaluation reveals prepubertal testosterone levels and low or normal gonadotropin levels. In cases of constitutional delay of puberty, even though the puberty is delayed, it begins before the bone age of 13 years in girls or 14 years in boys. Height is often less than 5th percentile, but growth rate is normal for the skeletal age.[13] Onset of adrenarche is delayed.

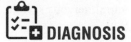

DIAGNOSIS

Clinical Presentation

A detailed history must be taken from the girl as well as her mother to determine if puberty itself is delayed or just the onset of menstruation is delayed. The age at the onset of breast and pubic hair development and the age at which she had a growth spurt, if she experienced any, must be enquired.

General Physical Examination

This should include accurate measurement of the patient's height and assessment of the stage of breast and pubic hair development. An internal vaginal examination is usually not required and should be avoided in young girls. An inspection of the external genitalia usually proves to be sufficient.

Investigations

The investigations which are performed in cases of delayed puberty include the following:[14]

- ❖ *Radiology*: An X-ray of the hand to assess bone age helps in revealing whether the child has reached a stage of physical maturation at which puberty should be occurring. Visible secondary sexual development usually begins when girls achieve a bone age of 10.5–11 years.
- ❖ *Gonadotropin levels*: Measurement of gonadotropin levels helps in revealing if the cause is due to the defect of the gonads (elevated gonadotropin levels) or due to the deficiency of the sex steroids (reduced gonadotropin levels).
- ❖ *Serum prolactin levels*: In cases of raised serum prolactin levels, imaging by MRI is indicated to rule out a pituitary lactotrophic adenoma, except in cases where hyperprolactinaemia can be attributed to be secondary to medications.
- ❖ *Measurement of serum TSH and free thyroxine levels*: Measurement of these can help in identifying the cases of primary and secondary hypothyroidism.
- ❖ *Measurement of serum DHEA-S concentration*: Measurement of serum DHEA-S levels is important to differentiate between constitutional growth delay and GnRH deficiency.

Patients with congenital GnRH deficiency are likely to have normal adrenarche and therefore normal levels of DHEA-S.

- ❖ *Karyotype analysis*: In cases of hypergonadotropic hypogonadism, karyotype analysis must be performed, which helps in ruling out chromosomal abnormalities (especially Turner's syndrome and Klinefelter's syndrome). In a short-female chromosome analysis should be performed to rule out Turner's syndrome.
- ❖ *Serum testosterone levels*: High serum testosterone levels indicate androgen insensitivity (male pseudohermaphroditism) which comprises a normal male karyotype (46 XY) with an abnormality in the androgen receptor. This results in unresponsiveness to androgens, which prevents masculinisation of male genitalia. As a result, there is development of female external genitalia. The person is phenotypically a female with normal breasts, but absent pubic hair. There may be presence of intra-abdominal testes.
- ❖ *Ultrasound examination*: This may be required to confirm the presence of uterus and ovaries.
- ❖ *Other tests*: Other tests, such as CBC, ESR, LFT, etc., help in ruling out chronic illnesses.

MANAGEMENT

- ❖ If no obvious cause of delayed puberty can be detected, reassurance and prediction of puberty based on bone age works in most cases. If on radiological assessment, bone age is less than the chronological age, wait and watch policy must be adopted. Most of these girls eventually develop secondary sexual characteristics and menarche over a period of time.
- ❖ *Therapy with sex hormones*: Pubertal delay due to gonadotropin deficiency may be treated with testosterone replacement or hCG. The treatment most commonly involves administration of testosterone or related compounds to boys and oestrogens to girls in extreme cases. Growth hormone can also be sometimes prescribed. Treatment with pulsatile gonadotropins has also been used. However, this treatment is difficult to sustain because subcutaneous injection attached to a portable pump may be required for several months. The more widely used approach involves the administration of low doses of ethinyl oestradiol in the dosage of 1–2 µg per day for 3–6 months.

  Hormone therapy can also be initiated in patients with congenital GnRH deficiency or constitutional delay of puberty over 12 years having no signs of spontaneous sexual maturation and causing significant distress or anxiety.
- ❖ *Treatment of the underlying cause*: This comprises of treating the underlying cause such as thyroid HRT for hypothyroidism, therapy with dopamine agonists for hyperprolactinaemia, excision of craniopharyngioma, etc.

COMPLICATIONS

Delayed puberty may cause anxiety or stress to the girls as well as her parents.

CLINICAL PEARLS

❖ Ovarian failure is the most common cause of delayed puberty. In suspected cases, karyotyping and estimation of gonadotropin levels are essential investigations.

❖ Pathologies such as imperforate hymen and congenital absence of uterus do not cause delayed puberty. They, however, may cause absence of menstruation.

❖ Careful clinical assessment and appreciation of the normal physiology remain the important approaches to the patients with delayed puberty.

EVIDENCE-BASED MEDICINE

❖ The present evidence indicates that girls who are not treated for delayed puberty may experience considerable distress which may significantly affect their school as well as social performance. According to the statistics by the American Academy of Paediatrics nearly 50% of girls, who were not given any treatment, would have preferred to receive treatment.[15]

❖ Novel therapies with a more physiological basis such as gonadotropins or kisspeptin-agonist are being investigated for the management of delayed puberty due to hypogonadotropic hypogonadism.[16]

REFERENCES

1. Anderson SE, Must A. Interpreting the continued decline in the average age at menarche: results from two nationally representative surveys of U.S. girls studied 10 years apart. J Pediatr. 2005;147(6):753-60.

2. DiVall SA, Radovick S. Endocrinology of female puberty. Curr Opin Endocrinol Diabetes Obes. 2009;16(1):1-4.

3. Coleman L, Coleman J. The measurement of puberty: a review. J Adolesc. 2002;25(5):535-50.

4. Marshall WA, Tanner JM. Variations in pattern of pubertal changes in girls. Arch Dis Child. 1969;44(235):291-303.

5. Parent AS, Teilmann G, Juul A, Skakkebaek NE, Toppari J, Bourguignon JP. The timing of normal puberty and the age limits of sexual precocity: variations around the world, secular trends, and changes after migration. Endocr Rev. 2003;24(5):668-93.

6. Bridges NA, Christopher JA, Hindmarsh PC, Brook CG. Sexual precocity: sex incidence and aetiology. Arch Dis Child. 1994;70(2):116-8.

7. Chalumeau M, Chemaitilly W, Trivin C, Adan L, Bréart G, Brauner R. Central precocious puberty in girls: an evidence-based diagnosis tree to predict central nervous system abnormalities. Pediatrics. 2002;109(1):61-7.

8. Cesario SK, Hughes LA. Precocious puberty: a comprehensive review of literature. J Obstet Gynecol Neonatal Nurs. 2007;36(3):263-74.

9. Ng SM, Kumar Y, Cody D, Smith CS, Didi M. Cranial MRI scans are indicated in all girls with central precocious puberty. Arch Dis Child. 2003;88(5):414-8.

10. Kaplowitz PB, Oberfield SE. Reexamination of the age limit for defining when puberty is precocious in girls in the United States: implications for evaluation and treatment. Drug and Therapeutics and Executive Committees of the Lawson Wilkins Pediatric Endocrine Society. Pediatrics. 1999;104(4 Pt 1):936-41.

11. Lazar L, Padoa A, Phillip M. Growth pattern and final height after cessation of gonadotropin-suppressive therapy in girls with central sexual precocity. J Clin Endocrinol Metab. 2007;92(9):3483-9.

12. Trotman GE. Delayed puberty in the female patient. Curr Opin Obstet Gynecol. 2016;28(5):366-72.

13. Crowne EC, Shalet SM, Wallace WH, Eminson DM, Price DA. Final height in girls with untreated constitutional delay in growth and puberty. Eur J Pediatr. 1991;150(10):708-12.

14. Albanese A, Stanhope R. Investigation of delayed puberty. Clin Endocrinol (Oxf). 1995;43(1):105-10.

15. American Academy of Pediatrics. Sexuality education for children and adolescents: Committee on Psychosocial Aspects of Child and Family Health and Committee on Adolescence. Pediatrics. 2001;108(2):498-502.

16. Wei C, Crowne EC. Recent advances in the understanding and management of delayed puberty. Arch Dis Child. 2016; 101(5):481-8.

PART III

CHAPTER **60**

Menopause and Hormone Replacement Therapy

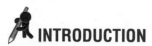 **INTRODUCTION**

Menopause can be defined as the cessation of ovarian function resulting in permanent amenorrhoea (lasting for at least 1 year). The onset of menopause involves physical, sexual and psychological adjustments. Menopause normally occurs between the age of 45 to 50 years, with the average being about 47 years. Climacteric (perimenopause or the menopausal transition) is the phase of waning ovarian activity, which may begin 2–3 years before menopause and may continue 2–5 years after it. This can be regarded as the phase of transition between the active and inactive ovarian function. The period of menopausal transition varies from 2 years to 8 years. The period following menopause is known as postmenopause. The first 4 years following menopause are the early postmenopause and the later years are the late postmenopause.

Hormone therapy is generally prescribed for treating troublesome menopausal symptoms such as hot flushes or vaginal dryness. HRT refers to the intake of supplements of hormones such as oestrogen alone or oestrogen in combination with progesterone (progestin in its synthetic form). Short-term use of hormones (<5 years) is usually not associated with an increased risk of complications (e.g. increased risk for breast cancer). HRT is not prescribed to all menopausal women. The hormones must be consumed for the shortest period of time possible.[1] They must be selectively prescribed to women who are at high risk for menopausal abnormalities. Indications for the use of HRT are as follows:

Menopausal and postmenopausal patients: Symptomatic patients suffering from vasomotor, urinary symptoms or symptoms related to genital atrophy, such as dryness, itching, dysuria, dyspareunia, etc., require HRT. Individuals at high risk for cardiovascular diseases, osteoporosis, Alzheimer's disease, etc. may also require HRT. Oestrogen exerts a cardio-protective effect by maintaining high levels of high-density lipoprotein (HDL) and lowering the levels of low-density lipoprotein (LDL).

Premature menopause: Women suffering from premature menopause, such as premature ovarian failure, or those who have undergone surgical oophorectomy.

 AETIOLOGY

Menopause occurs due to a decline in ovarian activity resulting in a gradual depletion in the number of oocytes produced by the ovary. As a result, there is a decline in the levels of hormones, oestrogen and inhibin. There is nearly 50% reduction in androgen production and approximately 90% reduction in oestrogen production at the time of menopause.[2] Oestrogen levels may become as low as 10–20 pg/mL. There is failure of ovulation, failure of formation of corpus luteum and failure of secretion of progesterone by the ovaries. Oestrogenic activity is reduced and there occurs endometrial atrophy, resulting in amenorrhoea. Initially, there is a rebound increase in the secretion of FSH and LH by the anterior pituitary due to the removal of negative feedback inhibition of gonadotropin production, resulting in an increase in the levels of FSH [>40 international units (IU)/L] and LH (>20 IU/L). However, with further advancing years, the gonadotropic activity of pituitary glands also ceases and a fall in FSH levels eventually occurs (Fig. 60.1). The cycles eventually become anovulatory and there is no progesterone production. The ovarian stroma does continue to produce oestrogens and androgens. The adrenal androgen production also continues though at a lower level. These androgens are converted into oestrone in the peripheral tissues. Unopposed action of oestrone on the endometrium eventually results in proliferative changes, hyperplasia and sometimes even carcinoma.

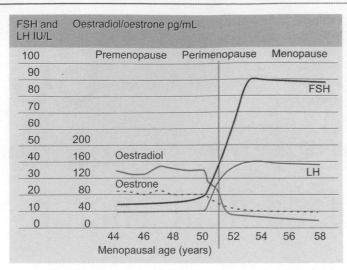

Fig. 60.1: Changes in the levels of various hormones at the time of menopause

Immediate effects	Intermediate effects	Long-term effects

Table 60.1: Various effects of menopause

Immediate effects	Intermediate effects	Long-term effects
• Vasomotor symptoms (hot flushes, sweating, palpitations) • Mood swings (depression, anxiety, irritability) • Sexual dysfunction (dyspareunia and reduced libido) • Urinary symptoms (dysuria, lower recurrent urinary tract infection, urgency, etc.) • Insomnia • Sexual dysfunction • Cognitive dysfunction (memory loss, poor concentration, tiredness, loss of motivation, etc.)	• *Genital atrophy*: Thinning of the vaginal mucosa, loss of superficial keratinised cells, reduced secretions from the glands and an increase in the vaginal pH • *Reduction in collagen support and atrophy*: Skin changes, easy bruising and an increased vulnerability to trauma and infection • *Urodynamic changes*: Stress incontinence, urgency and an increased frequency of urination • Pelvic organ prolapse	• *Osteoporosis*: It is due to oestrogen deficiency and affects the trabecular bone • Cardiovascular effects • Dementia

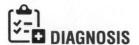 **DIAGNOSIS**

Clinical Presentation

Menopause is a hypo-oestrogenic state, which can result in the various effects enlisted in Table 60.1.

Anatomical Changes

Anatomical changes occurring during menopause include atrophy and retrogression of the genital organs. Moreover, there are aberrations in the endocrine balance maintained during the child-bearing period.

Symptoms: Nearly 60–70% of women remain asymptomatic; others may experience various symptoms, which are described next. These need to be elicited at the time of taking history:

❖ *Vaginal dryness*: Signs and symptoms of vaginal dryness include dryness, itching, burning, pain or light bleeding with sexual intercourse, increased urinary frequency or urgency.

❖ *Cessation of periods*: This could be a sudden cessation or gradual diminution in the amount of blood loss for each successive menstrual period, until the menstrual flow eventually ceases.

❖ *Hot flushes*: Hot flushes and sweating commonly occur as a result of vasomotor disturbances and may be present in nearly 85% of women. These may be preceded by a headache. A hot flush can be defined as an acute sensation of heat and skin changes, which may be followed with profuse perspiration and sweating. Skin changes may be in the form of reddening of the skin over neck, chest and head accompanied by an increase in heart rate and a feeling of intense body heat. It is mediated by noradrenaline and serotonin. There is an increase in the core body temperature and vasodilatation during hot flushes.

❖ *Osteoporosis*: There is likely to be a reduction in bone mineral mass, resulting in osteopenia and/or osteoporosis, which may predispose to fracture development.

❖ *Mental symptoms*: Mental depression may occur due to disturbed sleep and inability to cope up with the body changes. There may also be irritability and loss of concentration. Pseudocyesis (fear of pregnancy) and cancer phobia may develop in some women.

❖ *Neurological symptoms*: These may include paraesthesia (sensation of pins and needles).

❖ *Libido*: Although many women experience reduced libido, some women may also experience an increase in libido due to riddance of menstruation and fear of pregnancy.

❖ *Urinary symptoms*: These may include symptoms such as dysuria, stress and urge incontinence and recurrent vaginal infections. Genital symptoms, such as dryness of vagina, dyspareunia, genital prolapse and urinary and/or faecal incontinence may also occur.

❖ *Long-term effects*: In the long term, menopause is likely to result in complications such as arthritis, osteoporosis, fractures, cerebrovascular accidents, ischaemic heart disease, myocardial infarction (MI), atherosclerosis, stroke, skin changes, Alzheimer's disease, etc.

General Physical Examination

❖ *Vulva*: Atrophic changes in vulva are the natural sequelae of oestrogen deficiency characterised by loss of normal architecture and thinning of the skin. Vulvar atrophy may also occur.

❖ *Vagina*: There may be loss of thick keratinised mucosa and reduction in the amount of glycogen produced by the vaginal epithelium. There is an increase in the vaginal pH. A vaginal pH of greater than 4.5 is almost always associated with oestrogen deficiency. These changes are clinically visible in the form of thinning of the vaginal walls, loss of rugae, narrowing of the vaginal orifice and may result in symptoms such as dyspareunia.

PART III

❖ *Features suggestive of atrophy*: There may be thinning of the skin of labia minora and vestibule, and reduction in the amount of fat in labia majora. There is also reduction of pubic hair. Red patches around the urethra and introitus caused by senile vulvitis may occur.

❖ *Uterus*: There is reduction in the size of the fundus relative to the cervix, a decrease in myometrial thickness and thinning of the endometrium. Laxity of the pelvic cellular tissues and ligaments predispose to the development of uterovaginal prolapse.

❖ *Ovaries*: The postmenopausal ovary decreases in size even during use of HRT and should not be palpable by routine pelvic examination. Any enlargement of the ovary should be considered as malignancy until proven otherwise.

Investigations

Menopause can be easily diagnosed on the basis of clinical presentation (e.g. amenorrhoea, night sweats, hot flushes, etc.), when the patient is at least 1 year postmenopausal. A triad of hot flushes, amenorrhoea for 1 year and raised serum FSH levels more than 15 IU/L helps in establishing the diagnosis of menopause. Prior to the initiation of HRT, the following investigations need to be performed:

History and physical examination: A complete history and physical examination including blood pressure measurement, assessment of breasts, pelvic and rectal examination must be done.

Routine investigations: These include estimation of blood sugar, lipid profile, electrocardiogram, mammography, Pap smear and pelvic ultrasound.

Endometrial sampling and/or biopsy: This may be required in cases with high-risk factors for endometrial cancer (e.g. morbid obesity, diabetes and hypertension), history of abnormal uterine bleeding, history of PCOS or prior use of oestrogenic medications.

Dual energy X-ray absorptiometry (DEXA): This helps in determining the level of osteopenia and osteoporosis and the propensity for fracture development.

Hormone levels: Measurement of levels of oestrogen and FSH helps in deciding the requirement for HRT.

 MANAGEMENT

Gynaecological management comprises of the following steps:

❖ *Counselling*: This involves explaining the normal menopause-related changes to the patient, giving her advice related to contraception and asking her to eat a well-balanced nutritious diet (rich in vitamin A, C, D and E). She must be advised to regularly do weight-bearing exercises, which may help to prevent or delay osteoporosis.

❖ *Antidepressants or antianxiety agents*: These may be prescribed to relieve the woman of her anxiety and depression.

❖ *Lifestyle modifications*: These help in reducing the risk of osteoporosis and in improving the quality of life. Some of the strategies for lifestyle modification are as follows:
  • Weight-bearing exercises (walking, jogging, etc.)
  • Exposure to sunlight
  • Increasing the intake of food rich in calcium and vitamin D: These women must receive 1–1.5 g of elemental calcium and 1,000–1,500 IU of vitamin D daily.

❖ *Hormone replacement therapy*: HRT helps in providing relief from immediate postmenopausal symptoms. This therapy has been described in details later in the chapter.

❖ *Alternative therapy*: This may involve the use of naturally available substances such as black cohosh, phytoestrogens, red clover, oil of evening primrose, vitamin E, etc.[3]

❖ *Treatment of hot flushes*: Low doses of certain antidepressants [selective serotonin reuptake inhibitors (SSRIs), e.g. paroxetine, fluoxetine, citalopram, etc.,] and [serotonin and norepinephrine reuptake inhibitors (SNRIs), such as venlafaxine, desvenlafaxine, etc.] may decrease hot flushes. Though unlicensed, both SSRIs and SNRIs have been found to be more effective than placebo in reducing the symptoms of hot flushes.[4,5] Drugs, such as gabapentin (Neurontin)[6] and clonidine (a centrally acting α-agonist), can also be used for the treatment of hot flushes. Clonidine is a licensed nonhormonal treatment for vasomotor symptoms such as hot flushes.

❖ *Transdermal skin patches*: Their use helps in avoiding first-pass effect and liver metabolism. Hormonal implants and Mirena have also been recently introduced in HRT.

❖ *Osteoporosis treatment*: Medicines, such as bisphosphonates (etidronate, tiludronate, etc.), hormones, such as oestrogen, and selective oestrogen receptor modulators (SERMs) (e.g. raloxifene) play an important role in osteoporosis treatment.

❖ *Tibolone*: This is a synthetic derivative of 19-nortestosterone, which has weak oestrogenic, progestogenic and androgenic action. In the dosage of 2.5 mg daily, tibolone is cardioprotective, helps in improving bone resorption and relieving vasomotor symptoms. This drug may however cause irregular bleeding in nearly 15% of individuals.

❖ *Other treatment options*: These include nonhormonal alternatives such as SERMs, selective tissue oestrogen activity regulator (STEAR), etc.[7]

Hormone Replacement Therapy

Hormone replacement therapy refers to a woman taking supplements of hormones such as oestrogen alone or oestrogen in combination with progesterone (progestin in its synthetic form). HRT can be taken in the form of an oral pill, transdermal patch, gel and vaginal preparations (cream or slow-releasing suppository). [8-11]

Different Types of Hormone Replacement Therapy Preparations

There are three routes of oestrogen administration available: (1) oral; (2) transdermal; and (3) vaginal. Some commonly available HRT preparations are described next.

❖ *Pills containing conjugated oestrogen and progesterone*: One of the most commonly used brands of conjugated oestrogens is Premarin˙, manufactured from the urine of pregnant horses (mares). Most clinicians recommend starting with a low dose of oral conjugated oestrogen, i.e. 0.45 mg or 0.625 mg. If the lowest dose does not improve patient's symptoms, a higher dose option can be considered. Natural equine conjugated oestrogen must be prescribed in the dosage of 0.625 mg for days 1–25 each month and progestogen, such as medroxyprogesterone acetate (5–10 mg), dydrogesterone (5–10 mg), norethisterone N (2.5 mg), norethindrone or norgestrel, etc., must also be administered daily for days 13–25 each month in order to prevent endometrial hyperplasia and/or cancer. No hormones are given during the remainder of the month. Most patients demonstrate withdrawal bleeding during the hormone-free interval. To prevent withdrawal bleeding, these hormones can also be prescribed continuously. Many patients may have irregular bleeding, but 95% are likely to become amenorrhoeic within 1 year.

In order to reduce the inherent risks related to hormone therapy, lowest effective dose of HRT must be prescribed for the shortest amount of time. All types of oestrogen can provide relief from the menopausal symptoms. Birth control pills containing very low-dose oestrogen can be considered as a good option for women in their 40s who experience troublesome symptoms of climacteric (e.g. hot flushes, irregular bleeding, etc.) and who still require a dependable form of contraception. However, birth control pills are generally not recommended for postmenopausal women because the dose of oestrogen is higher than that required to provide relief against hot flushes.

❖ *Vaginal oestrogen preparations (creams, ring and tablets)*: Very low doses of vaginal oestrogen in form of vaginal creams, vaginal ring, or vaginal oestrogen tablets can be used for treating women with vaginal dryness. Such low-dose vaginal oestrogens do not usually require concurrent use of a progestin pill. Oestrogen vaginal cream (Ovestin cream containing the active hormone oestriol) can be used in the dosage of 1–2 g everyday for days 10–12 each month, for a period of 3–6 months until the symptoms disappear.

❖ *Transdermal skin patches*: Oestrogen patches are effective for increasing bone density and treating menopausal symptoms. Women with an intact uterus who use an oestrogen patch must also take progestins simultaneously in order to reduce the risk of uterine cancer. Oestrogen patch treatment may be associated with fewer complications in comparison to treatment with oral oestrogen preparations.

Uses of Hormone Replacement Therapy

Various uses of HRT are enlisted in Table 60.2. Currently oestrogen therapy is not considered to be a first-line therapy for prevention of osteoporosis. Presently, bisphosphonates and/or raloxifene have been recommended as the first-line treatment for prevention of osteoporosis.

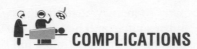

COMPLICATIONS

Osteoporosis

Osteoporosis is defined as a disease characterised by reduced bone mass and microarchitectural deterioration of bone tissue, resulting in enhanced bone fragility and an increased fracture risk. Osteoporotic fractures are a significant cause of mortality and morbidity in the UK.[12] Oestrogen appears to control the function of both osteoclasts and osteoblasts in bone, and this influences the rate of absorption and deposition of calcium. Remodelling of bone continues throughout life. However, following menopause, due to oestrogen deprivation, the osteoclastic activity far exceeds the osteoblast's ability to lay down calcium. Low levels of natural oestrogen around and after menopause diminish the body's ability to absorb calcium and to metabolise vitamin D. This results in the thinning of trabecular bone and eventually osteoporosis. Various other risk factors for the occurrence of osteoporosis are enumerated in Box 60.1.

The risk of fractures due to osteoporosis depends on the bone mass at the time of menopause and rate of bone loss following menopause. Peak bone density in women normally occurs at about 25 years of age, following which the bone loss starts to occur. After the age of 35 years, men and women normally lose 0.3–0.5% of their bone density per year as a part of normal aging process (Fig. 60.2). Menopause results in falling oestrogen levels, which may result in the development of primary osteoporosis. As the regulatory effect of oestrogen on bone resorption is lost, it is accelerated and not adequately balanced by compensatory bone formation.

Table 60.2: Various uses of hormone replacement therapy

Menopausal symptoms	Treatment
Depression	Oestrogen therapy with or without anti-depressants
Sleep problems	Oestrogen therapy
Migraine headaches	Continuous hormone regimens should be used. Cyclic regimens must be avoided to prevent initiating the oestrogen withdrawal headaches
Moderate-to-severe vasomotor symptoms without any history of breast cancer or cardiovascular disease	Short-term oestrogen therapy
Vaginal atrophy	Vaginal oestrogens can be used in almost all postmenopausal women with symptoms of vaginal atrophy except for those with a history of breast cancer
Mild urogenital atrophy	Vaginal moisturising agents on a regular basis and vaginal lubricants at the time of intercourse
Moderate-to-severe urogenital atrophy	Low-dose vaginal oestrogen

Box 60.1: Risk factors for development of osteoporosis

❏ Female gender
❏ Genetic predisposition: Family history of osteoporosis
❏ Age >65 years
❏ Vertebral compression fractures
❏ Fragility fractures after the age of 40 years
❏ Caucasian or Asian race
❏ Thin or small body frames (low BMI)
❏ Multiparity
❏ Excessive alcohol consumption, cigarette smoking
❏ Lack of exercise, sedentary lifestyle
❏ Diet low in calcium and vitamin D (poor exposure to sunlight)
❏ Low oestrogen levels, amenorrhoea, etc.
❏ Drugs [corticosteroids, anticonvulsants (phenytoin), etc.]
❏ Other endocrine disorders (Cushing's syndrome, hyperpara-thyroidism, hyperthyroidism, etc.)
❏ Rheumatoid arthritis

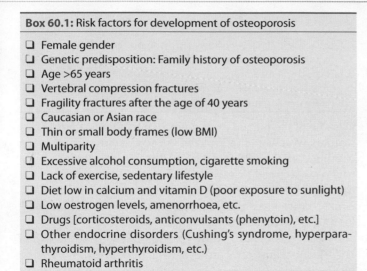
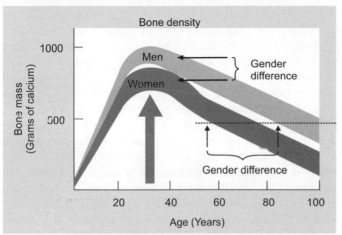

Fig. 60.2: Changes in bone marrow density with age and gender

This is often associated with an increased risk of fractures of the hip and wrist. Compression fractures of the vertebrae can often occur resulting in the development of a dowager hump. Recurrent compression fractures often result in back pain. Due to osteoporotic changes in the vertebral bones, they are likely to become weaker and thinner. The intervertebral discs also lose their fluid content, undergo degeneration and become compressed. As a result, the spine loses its normal S-shape and becomes kyphotic.

An approach combining the assessment of bone mineral density (BMD) and estimation of the patient's clinical risk factors for fracture development with use of the fracture risk assessment tool (FRAX) is likely to improve the evaluation of patients with osteoporosis.[13] Assessment of BMD using DEXA is the gold standard for the diagnosis of osteoporosis.[14] Using a DEXA scan, the patient's bone density is compared to the average bone density in young adults of same sex and race. The score is called the T-score and it expresses the bone density in terms of standard deviations (SDs) below the peak young adult bone mass. Osteoporosis can be defined as the bone density score of –2.5 SD or below. Osteopenia, on the other hand, can be defined as a bone density T-score between –1 SD and –2.5 SD amongst all women who are aged 65 years or older. Severe osteoporosis is used to describe those patients

who have a T-score below –2.5 SD and have suffered a fragility fracture. Normal BMD is defined as a T-score between +2.5 SD and –1.0 SD. There is another score, called the Z-score which is sometimes used in cases of severe osteoporosis and is based on the comparison to the age-matched normal individuals.

The FRAX tool developed by the WHO helps in assessing an individual's 10 years risk for developing fractures (spine, forearm, hip or shoulder).[15] This tool is accessible online. It incorporates 11 risk factors and femoral neck raw BMD in g/cm². This helps in calculating the 10 years fracture risk probability. This tool also helps in identifying the patients who may benefit from pharmacotherapy.

In order to reduce the risk for development of osteoporosis later in life, lifestyle modifications such as regular weight-bearing exercises and high intake of vitamin D and calcium must begin during adolescence. For prevention of osteoporosis-related fractures, the following therapeutic options are available:

❖ *Hormone replacement therapy*: While postmenopausal HRT helps in preventing the onset of osteoporosis, it has little effect in the treatment of established osteoporosis. HRT provides additional hormones, which help in locking the receptors on cell surface and repairing the balance between the minerals absorbed and minerals retained in the bloodstream. Due to lack of oestrogen, minerals such as calcium are not retained inside the bone. As a result, the bone is not able to retain its strength and it wastes away. Calcium supplementation is valuable in elderly postmenopausal women. However, it may be less effective in younger, physically active patients. Physical exercise is also likely to be important in prevention of the osteoporotic fractures mainly through improvement of posture, mobility and muscular functioning.

❖ *Selective oestrogen receptor modulators*: SERMs such as raloxifene (Evista) have been approved by the United States Food and Drug Administration (USFDA) for the prevention and treatment of osteoporosis in postmenopausal women. Results from the MORE (Multiple Outcomes of Raloxifene Evaluation) study have indicated that raloxifene helps in maintaining BMD by acting as an oestrogen agonist in the skeleton and preventing new vertebral fractures in postmenopausal women.[16] Moreover, raloxifene also helps in reducing the risk of breast cancer by nearly 65% in postmenopausal women with osteoporosis. However, the main concern with the use of raloxifene therapy is the increased incidence of venous thromboembolism. Previous history of venous thromboembolism is a contraindication for use of raloxifene.[17]

❖ *Bisphosphonates*: Presently, the most effective medications for treatment of osteoporosis are bisphosphonates and include alendronate, risedronate and ibandronate. These drugs reduce the risk of fracture development by suppressing bone resorption by osteoclasts. They however do not reduce osteoblast formation. Bisphosphonates can be used both for prevention and treatment of osteoporosis. It can be considered as the drugs of choice for treatment of established osteoporosis. This can be in the form of weekly alendronate, monthly ibandronate or yearly IV zoledronic

Table 60.3: Dosage of some commonly used bisphosphonates

Various preparations of bisphosphonates	For prevention	For treatment
Alendronate	5 mg daily 35 mg weekly	10 mg daily 70 mg weekly
Risedronate	5 mg daily 35 mg weekly 150 mg monthly	5 mg daily 35 mg weekly 150 mg monthly
Ibandronate	2.5 mg daily	2.5 mg daily 150 mg monthly
Zoledronic acid	5 mg IV every 2 years	5 mg IV every year

acid. Dosages of some commonly used bisphosphonates are enlisted in Table 60.3.

❖ *Tibolone*: This drug has been described in details previously in the text.

❖ *Novel therapies*: New therapeutic agents such as calcitonin nasal spray (useful for treatment of painful vertebral crush fractures), injectable recombinant parathyroid hormone and a monoclonal antibody (denosumab) have also been approved for the treatment of osteoporosis. Denosumab is a human monoclonal antibody to receptor activator of nuclear factor kappa-B ligand (RANKL). RANKL is secreted by osteoblasts and binds to its receptor RANK on the surface of osteoclasts, thereby stimulating its activity. Denosumab binds with great affinity to RANKL, thereby preventing the activation of RANK. Thus, it prevents both the maturation and survival of osteoclasts as well as active bone resorption by osteoclasts.

Cardiovascular Disease

Premenopausal women are likely to be protected against cardiovascular heart diseases (CHD) in comparison to the men belonging to the same age groups. This could be partly related to high HDL and low LDL levels in premenopausal women. Various other mechanisms through which oestrogen exerts a protective effect are described in Box 60.2. Therefore, coronary heart disease is uncommon amongst premenopausal women, especially if they do not smoke. However, there is a rapid rise in the risk of coronary heart disease following menopause and presently cardiovascular disease has become a leading cause of death amongst postmenopausal women in the UK.

Initially, it was believed that prescription of HRT is likely to result in protection against the development of CHD. There had been lack of clear guidelines regarding the use of postmenopausal hormone therapy since the past decade. However, now oestrogen replacement therapy is no longer indicated for the prevention of CHD in postmenopausal women. This recommendation initially made by the American Heart Association (AHA)[18] in 2001 had been further strengthened by the results of the Women's Health Initiative (WHI)[19] and Heart and Estrogen/Progestin Replacement (HERS and HERS-II) trials.[20,21] WHI was initiated in 1991 by the US National Institute of Health and comprised of three clinical trials and an observation study, which were directed to address the major health-related problems causing mortality and morbidity amongst postmenopausal women.[19] This

Box 60.2: Cardioprotective mechanisms of oestrogen

❑ Decrease in the level of low-density lipoproteins (LDLs)
❑ Increase in the level of high-density lipoproteins (HDLs)
❑ Nitric oxide mediated coronary vasodilatation
❑ Direct vasodilatatory effect on the endometrium
❑ Reduction in the atheroma volume

was one of the largest trials comprising of more than 16,000 women, who were randomized to receive either continuous combined HRT or placebo. The WHI (oestrogen plus progestin trial) was stopped in July 2002, after investigators found that the combination hormone therapy resulted in health risks, which outweighed the benefits. Participants were followed for an average of 5.6 years.

The results of WHI study (2002) showed that the use of HRT did not cause any cardiovascular benefits. Moreover, the results of this study also showed that the use of HRT might also be associated with an increased risk of stroke, venous thromboembolism and breast cancer. These conflicting findings have raised speculation regarding the effect of HRT on the woman's cardiovascular risk. Before 2002, prior to the publication of results of this study, use of HRT was characterised as providing significant cardiovascular and skeletal benefits, with minimal or no adverse effects. The results of WHI study were interpreted in various ways; many societies and health organisations now started claiming that HRT was dangerous. Some health authorities started recommending that HRT must be prescribed only in cases where the vasomotor symptoms were severe and could not be managed with alternative therapies. This led to holdup of the previous consensus, which stated, "all menopausal women should consider HRT". This was replaced with a new consensus statement, "the prescription of smallest dose of HRT for the shortest duration of time". As a result, clinicians now started prescribing HRT for a few weeks only, and then stopping it because of potential risks.

However, all the authorities did not accept the conflicting results of WHI study. The European Menopause and Andropause Society (EMAS) stood firmly against these conceptual changes in their practical guidelines.[22] The situation changed again following the reappraisal of the WHI study, which has disclosed that age acts as a major factor in the benefit-risk balance for hormone users.

Subsequent analysis of the WHI study published in 2007 identified that the timing of administration of HRT is likely to be significant. Little cardiovascular harm is observed when HRT is commenced in the immediate postmenopausal period in comparison to the administration of HRT many years after menopause.

In contrast to the results of the WHI study (2002), outcomes of the RCT (published in the BMJ, 2012), which took its data from the Danish Osteoporosis Prevention Study (DOPS), have shown that continued use of HRT amongst the menopausal women for a period of 10 years has been found to be associated with a significant reduction in the risk of MI, heart failure or death with no increased risk of venous thromboembolism or stroke.[23] According to the authors of this study, long-term use of HRT, when started soon after menopause for a prolonged duration of time, does not increase the risk of adverse cardiovascular events. Moreover, in this study, synthetic 17-β-oestradiol was used, while in the WHI study, conjugated equine oestrogens were used. This difference in medication, along with variations in patient characteristics, probably was the cause of disparity in the results between this study and the WHI study.[24,25]

Present evidence indicates that the benefits outweigh the risks of the HRT treatment started for most women near the menopause. For such women, HRT not just provides relief from hot flushes, night sweats and vaginal dryness, but also helps in reducing the risks for heart disease and fracture. The results of WHI study are now interpreted as high risk of cardiovascular disease due to HRT in older women who are on an average 10–12 years past menopause. In older women, HRT may be associated with an increased risk of CHD, venous thromboembolism and stroke. The emerging evidence suggests that the risk of CHD events with HRT is majorly limited to older postmenopausal women, with younger postmenopausal women at very low risk for CHD-related events. This increase is more in women having pre-existing risk factors for cardiovascular disease.

Breast Cancer

Women's Health Initiative trial and the Million Women study have shown that there is a small increased risk of breast cancer in women who take combined oestrogen-progestin therapy in comparison to those taking oestrogen only preparations or tibolone.[26,27] A critique of the Million Woman study has shown that this study could have suffered from detection bias because the women participating in this study were recruited from the National Breast Screening Programme.[28]

Early menopause often occurs in women undergoing treatment for breast cancer. In these women, hormone therapy (oestrogen only or combined oestrogen and progestogens) by any route is not recommended. The hormones could increase the chance of the cancer recurrence. These recommendations are based on the results from the WHI and the HABITS (Hormonal replacement therapy after Breast Cancer-Is It Safe?) trial. The HABITS trial had to be terminated midway in the year 2003 due to an unacceptable risk of breast cancer for the women (having a previous history of breast cancer) exposed to HRT.[29]

Even if HRT is prescribed for short term, mammograms and breast examinations must be routinely performed. According to the recommendations by the USFDA, labels describing the warnings related to the possible risk of heart disease, stroke and cancer must be added to all oestrogen and oestrogen-progestin containing HRT preparations.

Dementia

Based on the results of WHI study, postmenopausal hormone therapy should also not be prescribed after the age of 65 years for prevention of dementia. However, some clinicians feel that oestrogen treatment might be helpful in preventing dementia if prescribed in the early years after menopause.

Stroke

Women's Health Initiative trial has shown that the combination of oestrogen with progestins increases the risk of ischaemic stroke in generally healthy postmenopausal women.[30,31] This increased risk does not appear to be related to the timing of the initiation of HRT.[31]

On the other hand, HERS, the first large RCT examining the effect of hormone therapy on risk of strokes, has not indicated any significant association between postmenopausal hormone therapy and risk of stroke among postmenopausal women followed up for a mean of 4.1 years.[20]

Endometrial Hyperplasia and Endometrial Cancer

Unopposed oestrogen therapy at any dose and duration between 1 to 3 years is likely to increase the risk for endometrial hyperplasia and endometrial cancer.[32] WHI trial has shown that hormone therapy with oestrogens alone is likely to result in an increased risk of endometrial cancer. Cancer can occur even after 6 months of unopposed oestrogen therapy in women having an intact uterus. In such women, progestin preparations, either sequentially or in a low-dose regimen, should be added along with oestrogens. Women who have undergone hysterectomy do not require progestins. In women who have undergone subtotal hysterectomy, it is important to establish that there is no residual endometrium before prescribing oestrogen only HRT.

Other Complications due to Hormone Replacement Therapy

Absolute contraindications to HRT are described in Box 60.3.

 CLINICAL PEARLS

❖ There is 50% reduction in androgen production and 66% reduction in oestrogen production at the time of menopause. Oestrogen levels may become as low as 10–20 pg/mL.
❖ Continuous bleeding, menorrhagia or irregular bleeding during the perimenopausal or menopausal period must be considered as abnormal and warrant investigations to rule out any potential malignancies.

Box 60.3: Contraindications for consuming hormone replacement therapy

❑ Current or past history of breast cancer
❑ Family history of breast cancer
❑ Coronary heart disease
❑ Thromboembolism, heart attack or stroke
❑ Hypertriglyceridaemia
❑ Familial hyperlipidaemia
❑ Undiagnosed genital bleeding
❑ Active intrinsic liver disease
❑ Oestrogen-dependent tumours
❑ History of uterine cancer

CHAPTER 60

❖ Chronic vulvar puritis or irritation which does not respond to oestrogen therapy must be fully evaluated to rule out underlying malignancy.

❖ In order to reduce the inherent risks of hormone therapy, lowest effective dose of HRT must be used for the shortest amount of time required to treat symptoms.

❖ Before prescribing HRT, women must be informed about the risks and benefits of prescribing HRT.

❖ Hormone replacement therapy can be considered as the best treatment option for vasomotor symptoms, mood changes, vaginal symptoms and prevention of osteoporosis.

EVIDENCE-BASED MEDICINE

❖ Hormone replacement therapy does not appear to increase the risk of cardiovascular disease in women in whom HRT is started within 10 years of menopause.[19-25] Women who are not at an increased risk of heart attacks related to HRT include women who became menopausal less than 10 years before starting HRT and women who are between the age of 50 to 59 years at the time of taking the hormone therapy. The risk of having a heart attack related to the use of HRT is increased in the following women: Women who had become menopausal more than 10 years previously and women over the age of 60 years.

❖ There is significant evidence to support the use of oestrogens for the treatment of urogenital symptoms. Oestrogen therapy is likely to cause an increase in the lactobacilli in the vagina, prevent recurrent urinary tract infections and cause alleviation of the symptoms such as urge incontinence, increased urinary frequency and nocturia. Oestrogens are also likely to cause an improvement in stress incontinence when administered in combination with α-adrenergic agonists.[8-11]

REFERENCES

1. American College of Obstetricians and Gynecologists Women's Health Care Physicians. Executive summary. Hormone therapy. Obstet Gynecol. 2004;104(4 Suppl):1S-4S.
2. Myers LS, Dixen J, Morrissette D, Carmichael M, Davidson JM. Effects of estrogen, androgen, and progestin on sexual psychophysiology and behavior in postmenopausal women. J Clin Endocrinol Metab. 1990;70(4):1124-31.
3. Nedrow A, Miller J, Walker M, Nygren P, Huffman LH, Nelson HD. Complementary and alternative therapies for the management of menopause-related symptoms: a systematic evidence review. Arch Intern Med. 2006;166(14):1453-65.
4. Stearns V. Clinical update: new treatment for hot flushes. Lancet. 2007;369(9579):2062-4.
5. Nelson HD. Commonly used types of postmenopausal estrogen for treatment of hot flushes: scientific review. JAMA. 2004;291(13):1610-20.
6. Pandya KJ, Morrow GR, Roscoe JA, Zhao H, Hickok JT, Pajon E, et al. Gabapentin for hot flushes in 420 women with breast cancer: a randomized double-blind placebo control trial. Lancet. 2005;366(9488):818-24.
7. Rees M, Mander T. Managing the Menopause without Oestrogen. London: Royal Society of Medicine Press; 2004.
8. North American Menopause Society. Estrogen and progestogen use in postmenopausal women: 2010 position statement of The North American Menopause Society. Menopause. 2010;17(2):242-55.
9. North American Menopause Society. The 2012 hormone therapy position statement of: The North American Menopause Society. Menopause. 2012;19(3):257-71.
10. Practice Committee of American Society for Reproductive Medicine. Estrogen and progestogen therapy in post-menopausal women. Fertil Steril. 2008;90(5 Suppl): S88-102.
11. Shifren JL, Schiff I. Role of hormone therapy in the management of menopause. Obstet Gynecol. 2010;115(4):839-55.
12. Ström O, Borgström F, Kanis JA, Compston J, Cooper C, McCloskey EV, et al. Osteoporosis: burden, healthcare provision and the opportunities in the EU. a report prepared in collaboration with the International Osteoporosis Foundation (IOF) and the European Federation of Pharmaceutical Industry Associations (EFPIA). Arch Osteoporos. 2011;6(1):59-155.
13. Unnanuntana A, Gladnick BP, Donnelly E, Lane JM. The assessment of fracture risk. J Bone Joint Surg Am. 2010;92(3): 743-53.
14. Kanis JA, McCloskey EV, Johansson H, Oden A, Melton LJ, Khaltaev N. A reference standard for the description of osteoporosis. Bone. 2008;42(3):467-75.
15. Kanis JA, Melton LJ, Christiansen C, Johnston CC, Khaltaev N. The diagnosis of osteoporosis. J Bone Miner Res. 1994;9(8):1137-41.
16. Agnusdei D, Iori N. Raloxifene: results from the MORE study. J Musculoskelet Neuronal Interact. 2000;1(2):127-32.
17. Hansdóttir H. Raloxifene for older women: a review of the literature. Clin Interv Aging. 2008;3(1):45-50.
18. Mosca L, Collins P, Herrington DM, Mendelsohn ME, Pasternak RC, Robertson RM, et al. Hormone replacement therapy and cardiovascular disease: a statement for healthcare professionals from the American Heart Association. Circulation. 2001;104(4):499-503.
19. Hsia J, Langer RD, Manson JE, Kuller L, Johnson KC, Hendrix SL, et al. Conjugated equine estrogens and coronary heart disease: the Women's Health Initiative. Arch Intern Med. 2006;166(3):357-65.
20. Hulley S, Grady D, Bush T, Furberg C, Herrington D, Riggs B, et al. Randomized trial of estrogen plus progestin for secondary prevention of coronary heart disease in postmenopausal women. Heart and Estrogen/progestin Replacement Study (HERS) Research Group. JAMA. 1998;280(7):605-13.
21. Grady D, Herrington D, Bittner V, Blumenthal R, Davidson M, Hlatky M, et al. Cardiovascular disease outcomes during 6.8 years of hormone therapy: Heart and Estrogen/progestin Replacement Study follow-up (HERS II). JAMA. 2002; 288(1):49-57.
22. Gompel A, Rozenberg S, Barlow DH, EMAS board members. The EMAS 2008 update on clinical recommendations on postmenopausal hormone replacement therapy. Maturitas. 2008;61(3):227-32.
23. Schierbeck LL, Rejnmark L, Tofteng CL, Stilgren L, Eiken P, Mosekilde L, et al. Effect of hormone replacement therapy on cardiovascular events in recently postmenopausal women: randomised trial. BMJ. 2012;345:e6409.
24. Dubey RK, Imthurn B, Barton M, Jackson EK. Vascular consequences of menopause and hormone therapy: importance of timing of treatment and type of estrogen. Cardiovasc Res. 2005;66(2):295-306.

25. Hodis HN, Mack WJ. A "window of opportunity:" the reduction of coronary heart disease and total mortality with menopausal therapies is age and time dependent. Brain Res. 2011;1379:244-52.

26. Rossouw JE, Anderson GL, Prentice RL, LaCroix AZ, Kooperberg C, Stefanick ML, et al. Risks and benefits of oestrogen plus progestin's in healthy postmenopausal women. JAMA. 2002;288(3):321-33.

27. Beral V, Million Women Study Collaborators. Breast cancer and hormone-replacement therapy in Million Women Study. Lancet. 2003;362(9382):419-27.

28. Panay N. Commentary regarding recent Million Women Study critique and subsequent publicity. Menopause Int. 2012;18(1):33-5.

29. Holmberg L, Anderson H, HABITS steering and data monitoring committees. HABITS (hormonal replacement therapy after breast cancer--is it safe?), a randomised comparison: trial stopped. Lancet. 2004;363(9407):453-5.

30. Wassertheil-Smoller S, Hendrix SL, Limacher M, Heiss G, Kooperberg C, Baird A, et al. Effect of oestrogen plus progestogen on stroke in postmenopausal women: the Women's Health Initiative: a randomized trial. JAMA. 2003; 289(20):2673-84.

31. Grodstein F, Manson JE, Stampfer MJ, Rexrode K. Post-menopausal hormone therapy and stroke: role of time since menopause and age at the initiation of hormone therapy. Arch Intern Med. 2008;168(8):861-6.

32. Furness S, Roberts H, Marjoribanks J, Lethaby A, Hickey M, Farquhar C. Hormone therapy in postmenopausal women and risk of endometrial hyperplasia. Cochrane Database Syst Rev. 2009;(2):CD000402.

CHAPTER 60

Injuries of the Female Genital Tract and Female Genital Mutilation

INJURIES OF THE FEMALE GENITAL TRACT

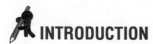 **INTRODUCTION**

A genital injury can be defined as an injury occurring to the genitals or perineum. Genital injuries can be very painful and can bleed heavily. It can affect the reproductive organs as well as the bladder and urethra. The amount of damage can range from minimal to severe.

AETIOLOGY

Injury to the genitals can occur due to the following causes:[1,2]
- *Obstetric causes*: Most injuries to the genital tract occur during childbirth and delivery, especially in cases of abnormal labour and/or obstetric manipulation.
- *Rape or sexual assault*: Violent intercourse or an alleged rape in young girls is a frequent cause of injury to the genital tract.
- *Vaginal atrophy*: Forceful penetration in postmenopausal women having vaginal atrophy is another important cause of injury to the genital tract.
- *Malformations*: Presence of malformations, such as imperforate hymen, presence of vaginal septum, etc., may be responsible for producing injury with unintentional causes of trauma (e.g. sexual intercourse).
- *Trauma*: Vulvar injuries due to direct trauma (e.g. falling astride sharp objects, etc.).
- *Criminal abortion*: Insertion of foreign bodies in the vagina for attempting criminal abortion.
- *Female genital mutilation (FGM)*: In some regions of the world, injuries to the genital tract can occur as a result of FGM. This has been described in details later in the text.

- *Placement of foreign bodies in the vagina*: Young girls (usually <4 years of age) may insert foreign objects into the vagina as part of a developmentally normal exploration of the body.
- *Perforation of uterus*: This can occur during the procedures such as suction evacuation, dilatation and curettage, transcervical resection of endometrium, etc.

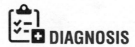 **DIAGNOSIS**

Clinical Presentation

- A per speculum examination must be conducted to examine the vaginal walls, fornices and the cervix in order to check for any associated injuries. Anaesthesia may be required to perform a thorough examination and to repair severe injuries.
- Information about the nature of the object, which has caused injury, must be obtained; sharp objects may have penetrated the adjacent organs as well.
- In case of insertion of a foreign body, there may be persistent and malodorous discharge from the vagina.[3]

Investigations

Ultrasound, CT and MRI may be required to evaluate the affected area for additional injuries.

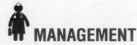 **MANAGEMENT**

Management of genital tract injuries comprises of the following steps:[4]
- If the patient has urinary retention, bladder may be catheterised.

❖ The area of injury must thoroughly be cleaned with soap, water and antiseptic solution. Lacerations must be irrigated with saline.

❖ Haemostasis must be maintained and bleeding vessels must be ligated. All devitalised tissues must be excised.

❖ All deep lacerations must be repaired with absorbable sutures without tension and the skin be repaired with non-absorbable sutures.

❖ A laparotomy with complete exploration of the genital and gastrointestinal tract may be required, if the peritoneum has been penetrated.

❖ *Haematomas*: Small haematomas respond to bed rest, sitz bath, hot fomentation and magnesium sulphate ointment. For large haematomas, incision of the swelling under general anaesthesia for evacuation of clots may be required.

❖ *Rape*: All the alleged cases of rape must be treated like medicolegal cases and police must also be informed. A dose of penicillin should be administered in order to protect the patient against bacterial infection (especially STDs). The patient can be protected against pregnancy by using emergency contraception. Psychological counselling must be arranged.

❖ *Foreign bodies*: The foreign body in the vagina must be removed on a per speculum examination followed by application of local antiseptic douches. Uterine foreign bodies must be removed under anaesthesia and antibiotics be prescribed based on the results of culture and sensitivity.

❖ *Perforation*: In case of perforation, antibiotics need to be prescribed. If signs of peritoneal infection are present, laparotomy may be required.

❖ *Injury to the external genitalia*: Sexual abuse must be ruled out in case of injury to the external genitalia. The most common sign of trauma to the genital tract is presence of blood at the vaginal introitus.

❖ Primary closure of the penetrating vaginal injuries is recommended to prevent fistula formation.[5] In case there are no tears or lacerations; conservative management with NSAIDs and ice packs is usually sufficient.

COMPLICATIONS

❖ *Extensive haemorrhage*: This may result in the development of shock. There may be the development of subsequent anaemia and local infection.

❖ Haematoma in the parametrium

❖ Rectovaginal fistula

❖ Fibrosis and atresia of vaginal or cervical lacerations can result in dyspareunia or even apareunia.

❖ Injury to the cervix may result in cervical incompetence or cervical stenosis.

CLINICAL PEARLS

❖ It is important to rule out sexual abuse, rape, and assault, especially in cases of young girls.

❖ Even the minor injuries to the genital area are likely to bleed excessively due to the presence of rich blood supply in this area.

❖ An important cause of vulvovaginal haematoma is inadequate haemostasis during repair of an episiotomy or a perineal tear.

FEMALE GENITAL MUTILATION

INTRODUCTION

Female genital mutilation, also known as 'female genital cutting', or 'cutting', or 'female circumcision' refers to 'all procedures involving partial or total removal of the external female genitalia or causing injury to the female genital organs for non-medical reasons'.[3,5] FGM has been practiced since early 450 BC and was widely performed throughout ancient Egypt in many other societies and cultures.[6] In early 1800s to the mid-1950s, surgeries such as clitoridectomy, hysterectomy and oophorectomy were commonly performed in the United States and Great Britain for the treatment of various disorders such as masturbation, lesbianism, falling of the womb, floating womb, emaciation, debility, nymphomania, seizures, hysteria, etc.[6,7]

The procedure of FGM is usually performed by traditional practitioners, who have received no formal medical training. As a result, the procedure is performed without the use of anaesthetics, using crude instruments such as knives, scissors or razor blades. However, there has been a global trend towards medicalisation of FGM.[8] In some countries, a significant number of FGM procedures are performed by the health professionals. These include countries such as Egypt, Sudan and Kenya. FGM is likely to occur amongst all socioeconomic groups. However, daughters of urban and educated women are less likely to undergo FGM in comparison to the daughters of rural and less educated women.[9]

Female genital mutilation is almost always carried out on girls between infancy and the age of 15 years. However, the age at which the procedure is performed significantly varies between countries. It is estimated that in over half of the countries practising FGM, the procedure is performed under the age of 5 years. In some communities reinfibulation may be performed in an adult woman following childbirth.

Classification of Female Genital Mutilation

The widely accepted classification of FGM developed by the WHO in 1995 and updated in 2007 is shown in Table 61.1 and Figures 61.1A to D.[10]

Prevalence of Female Genital Mutilation

As per the estimates by UNICEF, over 130 million women and girls have undergone FGM worldwide.[4] It is considered as a traditional cultural practice in several African countries.

Table 61.1: World Health Organization's classification of female genital mutilation (2007)[10]

Type 1	Partial or total excision of the clitoris and/or the prepuce (clitoridectomy)
Type 2	Partial or total removal of the clitoris and the labia minora, with or without excision of the labia majora
Type 3	Infibulation or narrowing of the vaginal orifice by cutting and appositioning the labia minora and/or the labia majora, with or without excision of the clitoris
Type 4	Any other procedure which is performed for non-medical reasons and causes injures to the female genital organs such as pricking, piercing or incision of the clitoris and/or labia; stretching of the clitoris and/or labia; cauterisation by burning of the clitoris and surrounding tissues; scraping of tissue surrounding the vaginal orifice; introduction of corrosive substances or herbs into the vagina for the purpose of tightening or narrowing it, etc.

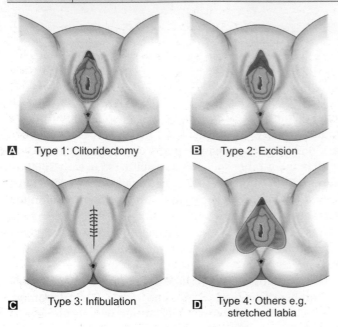

A Type 1: Clitoridectomy

B Type 2: Excision

C Type 3: Infibulation

D Type 4: Others e.g. stretched labia

Figs 61.1A to D: World Health Organization's classification of female genital mutilation

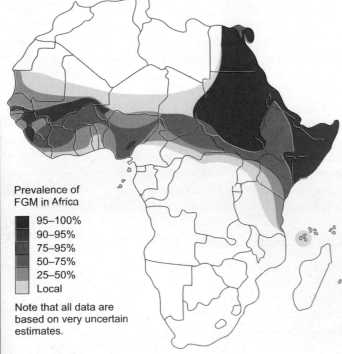

Prevalence of FGM in Africa

- 95–100%
- 90–95%
- 75–95%
- 50–75%
- 25–50%
- Local

Note that all data are based on very uncertain estimates.

Fig. 61.2: Map of Africa showing prevalence of female genital mutilation in the country

Abbreviation: FGM, female genital multilation

Prevalence of FGM in various African countries is demonstrated in Figure 61.2.[11] Outside Africa, FGM is also practised in Yemen, Iraqi Kurdistan, and parts of Indonesia and Malaysia.

The type of FGM varies between countries. Type 3 FGM is practised almost entirely in Africa, with the highest prevalence in north-eastern Africa, including Somalia, Sudan, Ethiopia, Eritrea and Djibouti. Prevalence of FGM is also likely to vary within a particular country, where it may be associated with particular ethnic groups.

As a result of migration, there has been a substantial increase in the number of girls and women with FGM living in North America, Australia, New Zealand and Europe.[8] It has been estimated that there are nearly 137,000 women and girls in England and Wales, who were born in countries where FGM is traditionally practiced and had undergone FGM.[12] This figure is inclusive of nearly 10,000 girls under the age of 15 years. There is circumstantial evidence indicating that girls are taken from the UK to their country of origin to undergo FGM and some cases of FGM may also take place in the UK. The Health and Social Care Information Centre (HSCIC), implemented by the Department of Health, is involved in collection of data related to numbers of women with FGM receiving care from the National Health Service in England.

INDICATIONS

Female genital mutilation is not performed for any medical or health-related reasons. FGM is practised for various complex reasons, with the belief that it is likely to be beneficial for the girl.[8] On the contrary, it has no health-related benefits and may harm the girls and women in many ways. FGM is a practice which violates human rights and is a form of child abuse. It can be considered as a severe form of violence against women and girls. The likely reasons given for FGM include the following:

- *Psychosexual causes*:
  - Maintenance of a woman's chastity and virginity before marriage
  - Maintenance of her fidelity during marriage
  - Promotion of morally appropriate fertility
- *Sociologic causes*:
  - Initiation into womanhood
  - Maintenance of cultural heritage and social cohesion
  - Protection against spells
- *Outright myths*: Bizarre traditions are prevalent in certain communities, which consider the clitoris as dangerous and can cause damage to a penis.[13]

DIAGNOSIS

Clinical Presentation

❖ *Antenatal examination*: All women, especially those coming from communities where FGM is traditionally practiced should be asked for a history of FGM at their booking antenatal visit so that this can be identified early in the pregnancy. This should be documented in the woman's maternity case notes.

❖ *Gynaecological examination*: Sometimes women with FGM may present with symptoms directly associated with FGM or with coexisting gynaecological morbidity, e.g. dyspareunia, menstrual abnormalities, etc. The vulva should be inspected to determine the type of FGM. External examination would also help in determining if deinfibulation is indicated, so as to enable vaginal examination and carrying out gynaecological tests (e.g. Pap smear, genital infection screening, etc.). External examination would also be useful in identifying any other FGM-related morbidity, e.g. epidermoid inclusion cysts.

Investigations

❖ *Psychological referral*: All women who have undergone FGM in the past should be referred for psychological and/or psychosexual assessment and treatment.

❖ *Screening for blood-transmitted infections*: These women should be tested for infections such as HIV, hepatitis B and C.

❖ *Sexual health screening*: Screening for sexually transmitted infections should be done.

❖ *Gynaecological referral*: Where suitable, women should be referred to gynaecological subspecialties.

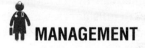

MANAGEMENT

Laws in the UK Pertaining to Female Genital Mutilation

According to the Female Genital Mutilation Act 2003 in England, Wales and Northern Ireland and the Prohibition of Female Genital Mutilation (Scotland) Act 2005 in Scotland, FGM is illegal in the UK. If FGM is confirmed in a girl under the age of 18 years, it is compulsory to report this to the police within 1 month of its confirmation.[14]

Female genital cosmetic surgery is also barred in the UK unless it is essential for the maintenance of the patient's physical or mental health. Surgeons undertaking such surgery must take appropriate measures for ensuring compliance with the FGM Acts. Reinfibulation is an illegal procedure. There is no clinical justification for this procedure and it should not be undertaken under any circumstances.

Management in Obstetric and Gynaecological Practice

❖ All acute trusts or health boards should appoint selected consultant-obstetricians and midwives responsible for the care of women with FGM.

❖ All gynaecologists, obstetricians and midwives should receive mandatory training on FGM and its management, including the technique of deinfibulation. They should complete the programme of FGM e-modules developed by Health Education, England. Healthcare professionals should be cautious regarding the clinical signs and symptoms of recent FGM, such as pain, haemorrhage, infection, urinary retention, etc.

❖ Most specialist FGM services in the UK are available in the major cities. They are usually located in a hospital or community clinic (e.g. GP surgery or sexual health clinics). Consultant obstetrician and/or gynaecologist must lead the specialist multidisciplinary FGM services, which may offer the following services: information and advice about FGM; risk assessment tools for safeguarding children; gynaecological assessment; deinfibulation; access to other services, etc. Healthcare professionals must adopt a sensitive and non-judgemental approach towards such patients and carry out consultation with them in a safe and private environment. In case the healthcare professional is unable to understand the woman's language, professional interpreters must be used; family members should not be used as interpreters.

❖ Specialist FGM services should offer access to services such as psychological assessment and treatment, psychosexual services, screening and treatment of sexual health related diseases and services pertaining to gynaecological subspecialties such as urogynaecology, infertility, etc.

❖ Specialist FGM services should work in collaboration with other healthcare providers, including GPs and acute trusts, voluntary sector organisations, the police, social services and schools.

Management of Recently Diagnosed Cases of Female Genital Mutilation

❖ Women detected with the evidence of recent FGM must be referred by their GP to the hospital-based specialist FGM services.

❖ An accurate record of the findings at the time of clinical examination should be maintained in the patient's clinical records. This could be supported by photographic record of the lesions where appropriate.

❖ All women and girls with acute or recent FGM must be referred to the police and social services.

Management of Female Genital Mutilation during Pregnancy

Women with FGM are at an increased risk of obstetric complications. Therefore, consultant-led care is generally recommended in these cases. However, some women with previous uncomplicated vaginal deliveries may be suitable for

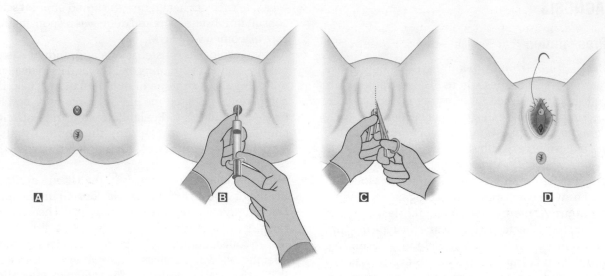

Figs 61.3A to D: Technique of deinfibulation: (A) Infibulation of the vaginal introitus, resulting in the formation of midline scarred tissue; (B) Infiltration of midline scar with local anaesthetic agent; (C) Incision of midline scar until the external urethral meatus is visible; (D) Suturing of cut edges with absorbable sutures

midwifery-led care in labour. In the UK, vaginal examination is not performed in the pregnant women until the onset of labour, unless there is a clinical indication. Therefore, early identification of FGM in pregnancy is best attained by taking the history of exposure to FGM from the women, especially those belonging to ethnic groups with high prevalence of FGM, at the time of their booking antenatal visit.[15]

Management during the Antenatal Period

❖ The woman should be referred for psychological assessment and treatment.
❖ Besides the routine antenatal screening tests such as hepatitis B, HIV and syphilis, screening for hepatitis C should also be offered.
❖ The appropriate plan of care must be discussed and recorded by the midwife or obstetrician.
❖ *Requirement for deinfibulation*: Deinfibulation is the surgical procedure which aims at the division of the scarred tissue sealing the vaginal introitus in type 3 FGM. This helps in opening up the closed vaginal introitus (Figs 61.3A to D). This is an elective procedure which must be performed by an appropriately trained midwife or an obstetrician. During the antenatal visit, vulva must be inspected to determine the type of FGM and to assess if there is any requirement for deinfibulation. If the introitus is sufficiently open to permit vaginal examination and the urethral meatus is visible, deinfibulation may not be required. However, adequate vaginal assessment during labour may be impossible for women with type 3 FGM. In these cases, deinfibulation is recommended during the antenatal period, typically at around 20 weeks of gestation.

If there is requirement for deinfibulation, it may be performed antenatally, in the first stage of labour, at the time of delivery or perioperatively after caesarean section. It is usually performed under local anaesthetic in a delivery suite. The procedures of deinfibulation (when the introitus is narrowed) and selective episiotomy (based on assessment at the time of delivery) may help in improving the clinical outcomes in these women.[16]

❖ Women should be informed that reinfibulation would not be undertaken under any circumstances.

Management during the Intrapartum Period

❖ Women with FGM should be preferably delivered in units having immediate access to emergency obstetric care.
❖ Intravenous access must be established in labour and blood sample should be taken for CBC, blood group-and-save.
❖ Most cases of FGM should be provided care by a consultant obstetrician. However, in certain circumstances, women with FGM may be considered low risk and midwifery-led care may be provided during labour.
❖ The impact of FGM on labour and delivery should be sensitively discussed with the patient and a plan of care must be agreed upon.
❖ *Deinfibulation in the intrapartum period*: If during the intrapartum period, vaginal examination is not possible or it is not possible to perform various intrapartum procedures such as urinary catheterisation, etc., then deinfibulation is recommended during the first stage of labour. This is usually performed after administration of an epidural, which not only covers the procedure, but also subsequent vaginal examinations and delivery. If vaginal access is adequate during the intrapartum period, then deinfibulation can be performed at the time of delivery under local anaesthetic.

The technique and principle of deinfibulation at the time of delivery is similar to deinfibulation performed during the antenatal or postpartum period. However,

PART III

when deinfibulation is performed prepregnancy, during the antenatal period or during the first stage of labour, either a scalpel or scissors may be used for making the incision. In contrast, when deinfibulation is performed at the time of delivery, the incision should be preferably made with scissors (rather than a scalpel) just prior to the crowning of the foetal head. Local anaesthesia in the form of local infiltration with lidocaine without adrenaline should be used. Once the procedure has been performed, the requirement for episiotomy may be assessed. Nevertheless, episiotomy is commonly required (irrespective of FGM type) because skin of the introitus is usually scarred and has reduced elasticity in these cases.

❖ *Emergency caesarean delivery*: If the woman for whom deinfibulation was planned at the time of delivery has to undergo an emergency caesarean delivery, there remains an on-going requirement for deinfibulation during the subsequent pregnancy to permit safe vaginal delivery. Such woman can be given the option of undergoing perioperative deinfibulation, after safe caesarean delivery of the baby, once the maternal and neonatal well-being has been confirmed. This option should be discussed with the mother before she is transferred to the operation theatre.

❖ Labial tears in women with FGM should be managed in the manner similar to the women without FGM. Repairs should be performed where clinically indicated, after discussion with the woman. Appropriate materials and techniques should be used for suturing.

Postnatal Care

❖ If a planned deinfibulation could not be performed due to delivery by an emergency caesarean section, the woman should be followed-up in the gynaecology outpatient department or FGM clinic so that deinfibulation can be offered to her before a subsequent pregnancy.

❖ The discharging midwife should ensure that before the patient is discharged, all documentation is complete and all legal and regulatory processes have been adhered.

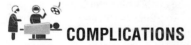

COMPLICATIONS

Short-Term Complications

The most common short-term complications related to FGM include haemorrhage, urinary retention, genital swelling, infection, fever, etc.[17] Excessive haemorrhage is the most important cause of death in these women.

Long-term Complications

Reported long-term complications of FGM are as follows:

❖ *Genital scarring*: Female genital mutilation can result in unsightly and painful genital scarring. Keloid scarring has been reported in up to 3% of women. There may be a formation of epidermoid inclusion cysts and sebaceous cysts, which may require surgical excision. Infibulation cysts and neuromas can also occur.

❖ *Urinary tract complications*: Complications of the lower urinary tract are particularly more common in women with type 2 or type 3 FGM. Various urinary tract complications, which can occur, are as described next:

• *Urinary tract infection*: Female genital mutilation can be associated with complications such as urinary tract infection, dyspareunia and bacterial vaginosis.

• *Urinary obstruction*: Poor flow of urine beneath the infibulation scar may result in symptoms of urinary obstruction. Stasis of urine due to obstruction may result in recurrent urinary tract infection and urinary or vaginal calculi.[18] The recommended treatment in these cases of urinary obstruction is deinfibulation. Damage to the urethra during FGM of any type may result in the development of a urinary stricture or fistulae. These may require assessment by a urologist or urogynaecologist.

❖ *Impaired sexual function*: Female genital mutilation may be associated with several consequences related to sexual health including dyspareunia, apareunia, impaired sexual functioning, etc. Dyspareunia may occur as a result of vaginal narrowing and formation of painful scar tissue. Sometimes, complete inability to perform sexual intercourse or apareunia and vulvovaginal lacerations may also result. The removal of sexually sensitive tissue of clitoris and labia minora may reduce sexual sensation. This may be associated with numerous sexual consequences such as reduction in sexual desire and arousal, reduced frequency of orgasm or anorgasmia, decreased lubrication and poor sexual satisfaction.[19-21]

❖ *Psychological sequelae*: Female genital mutilation is likely to have several psychological effects, such as panic attacks, anxiety, post-traumatic stress disorder, etc.[22] FGM has been linked to an increased incidence of domestic violence in Africa.[23,24]

❖ *Menstrual difficulties*: Female genital mutilation is likely to result in haematocolpos. Dysmenorrhoea has also been reported amongst women with FGM. However, the underlying mechanisms behind this presently remain unclear.[13]

❖ *Genital infection and pelvic inflammatory disease*: Female genital mutilation has been associated with an increased risk of genital infections such as bacterial vaginosis and herpes simplex (especially type 2).[25] However, currently there is no conclusive evidence to show that FGM is associated with an increased risk of pelvic inflammatory disease.[26]

❖ *Infertility*: Female genital mutilation is likely to cause infertility by causing complications such as apareunia, dyspareunia, impaired sexual function, ascending infections, etc. However, presently, there is limited evidence to indicate that FGM might result in infertility. While no such link has been demonstrated by any randomised trials, one case-control study has shown a positive association between primary infertility and FGM.[27]

- *HIV and hepatitis B infection*: Although, it is believed that FGM may increase the risk of transmission of viruses, such as hepatitis B, hepatitis C and HIV, probably due to the sharing of non-sterile instruments when FGM is performed in groups, there is presently no definite epidemiological evidence to support this.
- *Obstetric complications*: Various obstetric complications are likely to occur with various types of FGM. However, the risk is greater with greater tissue damage. A meta-analysis by Berg et al.[28] reviewed maternal outcomes in women with FGM. Though this meta-analysis included some studies from the US and Europe, majority of the studies were from Africa. This meta-analysis reported an increased risk of complications such as prolonged labour, PPH and perineal trauma in association with FGM. A large prospective study by the WHO, which investigated both maternal and perinatal outcomes amongst 28,000 women belonging to 6 African countries, has shown an increased risk of caesarean delivery, low birth weight, an increased requirement for neonatal resuscitations, and risk of stillbirths and early neonatal deaths.[29] No good quality study from UK or Europe investigating the effect of FGM on maternal and perinatal outcomes is presently available. However, evidence from epidemiological studies has shown a higher incidence of poor neonatal outcome and deaths amongst non-European migrant women in the UK from FGM-practising countries.[30,31]

  Other obstetric consequences that have been described with FGM include fear of childbirth, difficulty in performance of simple obstetric procedures such as application of foetal scalp electrodes and foetal blood sampling, difficulty in catheterisation during labour, wound infection and retention of lochia.[29] FGM is also likely to increase the risk for development of subsequent obstetric fistulae in future as a result of obstructed labour.[32]
- *Complications in the male partner*: History of FGM in the female can result in the following complications in the male partner: difficulty in penetration, wounds and infections on the penis, and psychological problems.[33]

CLINICAL PEARLS

- Deinfibulation is sometimes described as the reversal of FGM. However, this is not completely correct because this procedure does not replace genital tissue nor does it restore the normal genital anatomy and function.
- Reinfibulation refers to the resuturing (usually after childbirth) of the incised scar tissue in a woman with FGM type 2 or 3. Previously there was uncertainty as to whether reinfibulation was covered by the FGM Acts.[34] However, it is now accepted that reinfibulation is illegal and should not be performed under any circumstances.
- Clinicians should be aware of the psychological sequelae and other complications associated with various types of FGM.

EVIDENCE-BASED MEDICINE

- *Role of clitoral reconstruction*: Reconstructive clitoral surgery is believed to restore clitoral function. However, according to the available evidence, clitoral reconstruction should not be performed because it is associated with unacceptable complications without any conclusive evidence of benefit.[35] Surgery is unlikely to replace clitoral tissue removed at the time of FGM. Moreover, surgical exploration of the clitoral area may result in further damage to the clitoral nerves and vasculature, resulting in the loss of sensation.

  Also, the existing studies are retrospective with poor follow-up. There is no standardised method for the assessment of sexual function. Presently, there is requirement for well-designed clinical trials in future to investigate the safety and effectiveness of this procedure.
- Though narrowing of vagina as a result of FGM may cause abnormalities in urodynamic function, presently, there is no evidence that FGM directly increases the long-term risk of genital prolapse or urinary incontinence.[36]

REFERENCES

1. Shannon RD. Management of genitourinary trauma. Surg Clin North Am. 1979;59(3):395-409.
2. McAleer IM, Kaplan GW, Scherz HC, Packer MG, Lynch FP. Genitourinary trauma in the pediatric patient. Urology. 1993;42(5):563-7.
3. Bryk DJ, Zhao LC. Guideline of guidelines: a review of urological trauma guidelines. BJU Int. 2016;117(2):226-34.
4. Zou Q, Fu Q. Diagnosis and treatment of acute urogenital and genitalia tract traumas: 10-year clinical experience. Pak J Med Sci. 2015;31(4):925-9.
5. Phonsombat S, Master VA, McAninch JW. Penetrating external genital trauma: a 30-year single institution experience. J Urol. 2008;180(1):192-6
6. Barstow DG. Female genital mutilation: the penultimate gender abuse. Child Abuse Neglect. 1999;23(5):501-10.
7. Morris JG, Donohoe M. The history of hysteria. Pharos Alpha Omega Alpha Honor Med Soc. 2004;67(2):40-3.
8. United Nations Children's Fund. Female Genital Mutilation/Cutting: A statistical overview and exploration of the dynamics of change. New York: UNICEF; 2013.
9. Cook RJ, Dickens BM, Fathalla MF. Female genital cutting (mutilation/circumcision): ethical and legal dimensions. Intl J Gynecol Obstet. 2002;79(3):281-7.
10. World Health Organization (WHO). Eliminating female genital mutilation: an interagency statement. Geneva: WHO; 2008.
11. Blatant World. (2010). Map showing approximate prevalence of FGM across Africa. [online] Available from www.flickr.com/photos/blatantworld/5052042739/in/set-72157622910728412. [Accessed September, 2016].
12. Female Genital Mutilation in England and Wales. (2014). Updated statistical estimates of the numbers of affected women living in England and Wales and girls at risk: Interim report on provisional estimates. [online] Available from www.trustforlondon.org.uk/wp-content/uploads/2014/07/

FGM-statistics-report-21-07-14-no-embargo.pdf. [Accessed September, 2016].

13. World Health Organization (WHO). Female genital mutilation: A joint WHO/UNICEF/UNFPA statement. Geneva: WHO; 1997.

14. Royal College of Obstetricians and Gynaecologists (RCOG). Female Genital Mutilation and its Management. Green-top Guideline No. 53. London: RCOG Press; 2015.

15. Health and Social Care Information Centre (HSCIC). Female Genital Mutilation (FGM) Enhanced Dataset. Requirements Specification. Leeds: HSCIC; 2015.

16. Balogun OO, Hirayama F, Wariki WM, Koyanagi A, Mori R. Interventions for improving outcomes for pregnant women who have experienced genital cutting. Cochrane Database Syst Rev. 2013;(2):CD009872.

17. Berg RC, Underland V, Odgaard-Jensen J, Fretheim A, Vist GE. Effects of female genital cutting on physical health outcomes: a systematic review and meta-analysis. BMJ Open. 2014;4(11):e006316.

18. Yusuf L, Negash S. Vaginal calculus following severe form of female genital mutilation: a case report. Ethiop Med J. 2008;46(2):185-8.

19. Berg RC, Denison E. Does female genital mutilation/cutting (FGM/C) affect women's sexual functioning? A systematic review of the sexual consequences of FGM/C. Sex Res Soc Policy. 2012;9(1):41-56.

20. Andersson SH, Rymer J, Joyce DW, Momoh C, Gayle CM. Sexual quality of life in women who have undergone female genital mutilation: a case–control study. BJOG. 2012;119(13):1606-11.

21. Alsibiani SA, Rouzi AA. Sexual function in women with female genital mutilation. Fertil Steril. 2010;93(3):722-4.

22. Behrendt A, Moritz S. Post-traumatic stress disorder and memory problems after female genital mutilation. Am J Psychiatry. 2005;162(5):1000-2.

23. Salihu HM, August EM, Salemi JL, Weldeselasse H, Sarro YS, Alio AP. The association between female genital mutilation and intimate partner violence. BJOG. 2012;119(13):1597-605.

24. Peltzer K, Pengpid S. Female genital mutilation and intimate partner violence in the Ivory Coast. BMC Womens Health. 2014;14:13.

25. Morison L, Scherf C, Ekpo G, Paine K, West B, Coleman R, et al. The long-term reproductive health consequences of female genital cutting in rural Gambia: a community-based survey. Trop Med Int Health. 2001;6(8):643-53.

26. Elmusharaf S, Elkhidir I, Hoffmann S, Almroth L. A case-control study on the association between female genital mutilation and sexually transmitted infections in Sudan. BJOG. 2006;113(4):469-74.

27. Almroth L, Elmusharaf S, El Hadi N, Obeid A, El Sheikh MA, Elfadil SM, et al. Primary infertility after genital mutilation in girlhood in Sudan: a case-control study. Lancet. 2005;366(9483):385-91.

28. Berg RC, Odgaard-Jensen J, Fretheim A, Underland V, Vist G. An updated systematic review and meta-analysis of the obstetric consequences of female genital mutilation/ cutting. Obstet Gynecol Int. 2014;2014:542859.

29. WHO study group on female genital mutilation and obstetric outcome, Banks E, Meirik O, Farley T, Akande O, Bathija H, et al. Female genital mutilation and obstetric outcome: WHO collaborative prospective study in six African countries. Lancet. 2006;367(9525):1835-41.

30. Gissler M, Alexander S, Macfarlane A, Small R, Stray-Pedersen B, Zeitlin J, et al. Stillbirths and infant deaths among migrants in industrialized countries. Acta Obstet Gynecol Scand. 2009;88(2):134-48.

31. Small R, Gagnon A, Gissler M, Zeitlin J, Bennis M, Glazier R, et al. Somali women and their pregnancy outcomes postmigration: data from six receiving countries. BJOG. 2008;115(13):1630-40.

32. Browning A, Allsworth JE, Wall LL. The relationship between female genital cutting and obstetric fistulae. Obstet Gynecol. 2010;115(3):578-83.

33. Almroth L, Almroth-Berggren V, Hassanein OM, Al-Said SS, Hasan SS, Lithell UB, et al. Male complications of female genital mutilation. Soc Sci Med. 2001;53(11):1455-60.

34. Royal College of Midwives (RCM), Royal College of Nursing, Royal College of Obstetricians and Gynaecologists (RCOG), Equality Now, Unite. Tackling FGM in the UK: Intercollegiate recommendations for identifying, recording and reporting. London: RCM; 2013.

35. Foldès P, Cuzin B, Andro A. Reconstructive surgery after female genital mutilation: a prospective cohort study. Lancet. 2012;380(9837):134-41.

36. Peterman A, Johnson K. Incontinence and trauma: sexual violence, female genital cutting and proxy measures of gynecological fistula. Soc Sci Med. 2009;68(5):971-9.

Child Abuse, Sexual Assault and Rape

CHILD ABUSE

INTRODUCTION

Abuse can be defined as a form of maltreatment of a child.[1] A child can be abused when someone either inflicts harm upon them or by failing to act to prevent harm. Children may be abused by someone from the family, or someone whom they know. Sometimes, they may be abused in an institutional or community setting by their acquaintances. Rarely, they may be abused by someone whom they do not know (e.g. via the internet). A child may be abused by an adult or a group of adults, or another child or children. Various forms in which abuse can be inflicted upon the child include psychological, physical, sexual, financial and emotional.

A child can be defined as an individual who has not yet reached his or her 18th birthday.[1] The facts that a child has reached 16 years of age, is living independently or is in further education, is a member of the armed forces, is in hospital or in custody or in the secure estate, does not change his or her status or rights to services or protection.

AETIOLOGY

Some of the risk factors for child abuse are as follows:

* *Homelessness*: Childhood physical and sexual abuse is more prevalent amongst the homeless children in Western countries in comparison to the global population.
* *Age group*: Physical abuse is likely to be more prevalent amongst the younger children in comparison to the older ones.
* *Gender*: Rates of sexual abuse are higher amongst the female population.

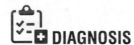

DIAGNOSIS

Clinical Presentation

Many children may not directly disclose the event of abuse. Instead, they may present with indirect complaints suggestive of sexual abuse such as bleeding through the vagina, soreness in the genital region, and STDs, behavioural changes, and bruises or abrasions on the body (especially in cases of domestic violence), etc. Typical clinical presentation in cases of child abuse is presence of unexplained injuries over the body.

Investigations

* Collection and preservation of the forensic specimen from the plaintiffs and suspects.
* *Documentation of the allegations by the plaintiff*: This should be done in a manner to ensure that the evidence is admissible in the court.
* *Forensic documentation of the injuries*: All the injuries must be accurately documented. Photographic documentation of the injuries should be also done wherever possible.

MANAGEMENT

Management of cases of child abuse needs to be individualised, depending upon the child's age, nature of abuse, and the wishes of the children and their parents. The child should be given a full opportunity to provide complete details about the event related to abuse in an environment in which he or she feels safe.

Ensuring the Victim's Safety

The most important step of management when the victim presents with an episode of abuse is ensuring the victim's safety and safety of any third party, if any, (e.g. children, dependents, etc.). The clinicians should also ensure their own safety.

Safeguarding the Children

Safeguarding issues are important for both children and vulnerable adults.[2] Provision of early help is more effective in promoting the welfare of children than reacting later. Early help means providing support as soon as a problem emerges, at any point in a child's life, from the foundation years through to the teenage years.

Provision of effective early help involves the close working of local authorities, under Section 10 of the Children Act 2004, to identify children and families who are likely to get benefitted from early help.[3] Children and families may require support from a wide range of local agencies, e.g. education, health, housing, police, etc. In cases where multiple agencies are involved, an interagency assessment must be conducted.

An assessment for evaluating the requirement for early help must be undertaken by a lead professional who could be a General Practitioner (GP), family support worker, teacher, health visitor and/or special educational needs coordinator. Thus, it is the responsibility of every healthcare worker and not just the specialist to be alert regarding the safeguarding issues. This lead professional should provide support to the child and their family by coordinating the delivery of support services to them. These activities are likely to help in significantly improving the outcomes for the child and their overall welfare.

Healthcare professionals need to identify and respond early to the needs of all vulnerable children, including unborn children, babies, older children, young carers (particularly those, showing signs of engaging in antisocial or criminal behaviour), disabled children having specific additional requirements and/or special educational needs, and children in a challenging family circumstance, such as substance abuse, adult mental health problems and domestic violence.

These services must focus towards improving functioning of the family and building up the family's own capability to solve problems. This should be done within a structured, evidence-based framework involving regular review of the progress. Under the Children Act 1989, a child in need is defined as a child who is unlikely to achieve a reasonable level of health or development; or whose health and development is likely to be significantly or further impaired, without the provision of services; or a child who is disabled. Under this act, local authorities are required to provide assessment and services for children in need in order to safeguard and promote their welfare.[4]

According to Section 13 of the Children Act (2004), each local authority is required to establish a Local Safeguarding Children Board (LSCB) for the purpose of safeguarding and promoting the welfare and safety of children in their area of the authority.[3] This especially includes vulnerable children and families, with respect of abuse.

Consent and Capacity

The concept of taking consent in the victims of sexual abuse and the concept of capacity has been discussed in the section of rape and sexual abuse described later in the chapter.

Medical Care

Assessment and medical treatment of the injuries must be undertaken.

Medical Aftercare

Medical aftercare in victims of sexual abuse has been discussed in the section of rape and sexual abuse described later in the chapter.

Psychological Care

Any episode of abuse, especially sexual abuse can be particularly disturbing for the child. The clinician must therefore care for the psychological needs of the victim, including the risk of suicide and self-harm.

COMPLICATIONS

Child abuse can be associated with massive health-related consequences.[5-7] Some of them are described next in details. Consequences particularly associated with child sexual abuse are described in the section of rape and sexual abuse discussed later in the chapter.

❖ *Emotional or psychological complications*: Child abuse can be associated with long-term psychological problems such as low self-esteem, poor performance at school, self-harm or suicide.

❖ *Problems related to interpersonal relationships*: Children may frequently develop feelings of shame and guilt, which can have devastating effects on their ability to develop strong interpersonal relationships when they reach adulthood.

❖ *Problems related to social functioning*: Feeling of guilt and shame related to abuse early in life may have an adverse effect on the social functioning of these women later in life.

CLINICAL PEARLS

❖ Since long-term consequences of child abuse can be massive, prevention and early detection is an important aspect of management of these patients.

❖ Someone who already knows the child/children is more likely to abuse them. Therefore, educating the children about these issues is likely to empower them.

EVIDENCE-BASED MEDICINE

* Presence of limited evidence indicates that the children with disabilities are more likely to be victims of abuse in comparison to their peers who are not disabled. However, there is requirement for further well-designed controlled trials in the future due to paucity of robust evidence, and lack of well-designed research studies.[8]
* Provision of help during the early phases of life for safeguarding the children can help prevent development of further problems in the future.[2]

CHILD SEXUAL ABUSE AND RAPE

INTRODUCTION

Sexual abuse involves forcing or alluring a child or a young person to take part in sexual activities. This act may not necessarily involve a high level of violence. Also, child may or may not be aware of what is happening. The activities may involve physical contact, including sexual assault by penetration (e.g. rape or oral sex). It may also include non-penetrative activities such as masturbation, kissing, rubbing, touching outside of clothing and non-contact activities, such as forcing the child to look at sexual images or produce sexual images, or watch sexual activities. Encouraging children to behave in sexually inappropriate ways, or training a child in preparation for abuse (including via the internet) can also be considered as forms of sexual abuse.

Sexual assault has been defined by Section 3 of the Sexual Offences Act (2003) as an act when a person (A):[9]

* Intentionally touches another person (B)
* The touching is sexual
* B does not consent to the touching, and
* A does not reasonably believe that B consents.

Rape has been defined by Section 1 of the Sexual Offences Act (2003)[9] as an act when a person (A):

* Intentionally penetrates the vagina, anus or mouth of another person (B) with his penis,
* B does not consent to the penetration, and
* A does not reasonably believe that B consents.

AETIOLOGY

Some children are at an increased risk of sexual abuse in comparison to the others. Some such risk factors are as follows:

* *Victim's sex*: Girls are likely to be at an increased risk of sexual abuse in comparison to the boys
* *Mental health status*: Children with mental or intellectual impairment are more prone to abuse
* *Presence of disability*: Children with disability are at an increased risk of abuse

* *Homelessness*: Childhood sexual abuse is more prevalent amongst the homeless children in Western countries.

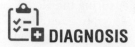

DIAGNOSIS

Clinical Presentation

* Patients with rape or sexual abuse may either present immediately or at a late stage (after a time interval from the episode). Besides the time interval of presentation, the clinical presentation can also vary dependent on whether or not the patient directly discloses the episode of abuse to the clinician.
* Many children may not directly reveal the event of sexual abuse or rape. Instead they may present with indirect complaints such as bleeding through the vagina, soreness in the genital region, STDs, unplanned pregnancy, request for emergency contraception, etc. The clinician conducting physical examination in such cases must be fully aware of the normal gynaecological anatomy of a prepubertal girl.
* Sometimes the victims of sexual abuse may present late (several days after the event) with psychological compliant such as depression, self-harm, substance abuse, sexual dysfunction, etc.
* The forensic physician should preferably take the history related to the event of sexual assault or rape. Wherever possible, history should be taken by asking open rather than closed questions.
* Before proceeding with the clinical examination, the clinician needs to have a careful discussion with the child and his or her carer regarding various issues such as consent for examination, limitations of confidentiality, nature of the examination, and disclosure of information for safeguarding purposes. Since sexual abuse is related to the disregard of consent and abuse of power, the examining clinician must exert a great deal of care in not repeating the procedure again unintentionally while examining the patient.

Anogenital Examination

Sexual assault may be commonly associated with injury to the anogenital tract. However, all cases of sexual assault may not be associated with injury to the anogenital tract. Even if such injuries do occur, they tend to heal rapidly. Thus, if the victim is examined a few days after the episode, the injuries may have completely healed. A lack of injuries, therefore, does not counteract their allegations. A forensic physician trained in sexual assault should preferably do the accurate documentation of the injuries, including the photographic documentation. In majority of cases, none or minor injuries may be recognised. No matter how small an injury is, it must be definitely documented. Various injuries, which can be identified, include abrasions, incisions, lacerations, burns, etc.

The Royal College of Paediatrics and Child Health (RCPCH) and the Faculty of Forensic and Legal Medicine (FFLM, 2012) have provided guidelines on paediatric forensic examinations to be performed in relation to possible child sexual abuse: when it is suspected, witnessed or whenever a child has made an allegation of sexual abuse.[10] According to these guidelines, a single doctor can conduct a paediatric forensic examination provided that he or she has all the necessary skills. If a single doctor does not appear to have all the necessary knowledge, skills and experience for a particular paediatric forensic examination, two doctors with complementary skills should conduct a joint examination.

Examination of External Genitalia

According to the evidence-based review and guidance for best practice regarding the physical signs of sexual abuse provided by RCPCH and FFLM (2015), the external genitalia must be inspected for the signs suggestive of sexual abuse such as presence of erythema, oedema, bruising, abrasions and/or lacerations.[11]

Investigations

The investigations which are conducted during child sexual abuse and rape are similar to those which are carried out in case of child abuse and have been discussed previously in the text.

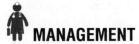

MANAGEMENT

Ensuring the Victim's Safety

The most important step of management when the victim presents with an episode of rape or assault is ensuring the victim's safety and safety of any third party, if present (e.g. children, dependents, etc.). The clinicians should also ensure their own safety.

Safeguarding

It is the responsibility of all the healthcare professionals to safeguard the interests of all children who have been victimised. Knowledge of the local safeguarding process (described previously in the text) is of vital importance for all healthcare professionals involved in the care of such individuals. The clinician should make any safeguarding referrals, if required.

Not Replicating the Event of Sexual Abuse

One of the most important aspects of management in cases of sexual abuse or rape, which the clinician needs to understand is that any episode of sexual violence is associated with the loss of power and control by the victim and forceful exertion of the power and control by the assailant. It is important for the clinician not to replicate this wherever possible by taking appropriate consent from the victim.[12] The clinician should try as far as possible to give back the power and control to the patient. The clinician must explain various treatment options to the victim and highlight the advantages and disadvantages of each. The victim should be encouraged to make a choice and their decision should be respected.

Consent and Capacity

Before performing physical examination and treatment in these patients, appropriate consent must be taken from the patient. The term 'capacity' implies that the person should be capable of giving consent, i.e. they should be able to understand the implication of the information provided to them.[13] Individuals with parental responsibility may be required to give consent for a child up to the age of 16 years to have treatment or to undergo physical examination.[14] The term, 'capacity' is of special significance in cases of child sexual abuse and rape because the victims would be of 16 years or younger. To understand the concept of consent and capacity, a thorough understanding of the Mental Capacity Act (2005) is essential.

The Mental Capacity Act 2005

The main aim of this act is to provide a legal framework for making decisions on behalf of those adults who lack the capacity for making a particular decision by themselves. This act relates to all individuals aged 16 years or more, and applies to the process of making decision and not to the outcome of decision. The five important principles of the Mental Capacity Act (2005) are as follows:[15]

1. All the adults are recognised to have capacity unless there is evidence to the contrary.
2. Every possible step to confirm capacity must be taken before deciding that someone lacks capacity.
3. A person must not be assumed to be incapable of making a decision because he or she makes an unwise decision.
4. A decision made under the 'Mental Capacity Act, 2005' on behalf of the individuals lacking capacity must be done considering the patient's best interests.
5. While making decisions on behalf of the individuals lacking capacity, the clinician must ensure that it is minimally restrictive of the person's right and freedom of action.

If there is doubt about whether the patients have capacity or not, the health professional must get expert opinions from consultant psychiatrist or psychologist having a background in dealing with patients having learning difficulties. Regarding the level of capacity of young girls to make autonomous decisions independent of those with parental responsibility, there are two terms, (1) Gillick's competence and (2) Fraser's competence, which are commonly used in clinical practice.

❖ *Gillick's competence*: In the early 1980s, the Department of Health issued a circular, which stated that a doctor could provide contraceptive advice or treatment to a girl under the age of 16 years without parental knowledge or consent. Many parents were not happy about this because they thought that such policy might encourage their children to engage in sexual activity. One such parent was Victoria Gillick, who was a mother of a 10 year old, Roman Catholic and 'pro-life activist', filed a case/legal challenge against the NHS for providing contraceptive advice to the girls under the age of 16 years'. The spokesman for the judges was Lord Fraser. Their view was that a child under the age of 16 years could be competent to give consent without involving their parents, provided they are capable of assessing the advantages and disadvantages of the proposed treatment.[16-18] The concept of 'Gillick competence' was derived from this, i.e. Gillick's competence can be described as the ability of an under-age child to give valid consent.

❖ *Fraser guidelines*: According to the Fraser guidelines, there are five conditions, which must be met for a child to be 'competent'. Fraser's competence is in preference to saying a child is 'Gillick competent'. This means that a doctor can provide contraceptive advice and treatment to a child under the age of 16 years without parental consent. However, one of the following conditions needs to be fulfilled. These five conditions came to be known as the 'Fraser Guidelines'.[19]

1. The young person must understand the advice being given.
2. The young person cannot be convinced to involve parents or carers or allow the medical practitioner to do so on their behalf.
3. It is likely that the young person will begin or continue having intercourse with or without treatment or contraception.
4. The young person's physical or mental health (or both) is likely to suffer unless he or she receives treatment or contraception.
5. The young person's best interests require administration of contraceptive advice, treatment or supplies without parental consent.

Gillick and Fraser are originally related to contraception only. However, now they have tended to extend to cover other areas. In 1990, the Access to Health Records Act stated that a 'Gillick competent' child could deny parental access to their health records.

Referral to Sexual Assault Referral Centres

The rape victims must be given the option of being referred to the Sexual Assault Referral Centres (SARCs). These centres can provide holistic, medical, forensic, emotional and psychological care of the victims.[2] Here there are specifically trained doctors, support workers and counsellors to take care of the victims. Besides taking care of the victims of sexual assault and rape who have reported to the police, SARCs also provide the option of seeing the victims who do not wish to report to the police.

Most SARCs and voluntary organisations also have an access to independent sexual violence advisors (ISVA), who are victim-focussed advocates helping people, who have experienced sexual abuse or assault, to access the services (e.g. police services) and support (e.g. emotional and practical support) they require.

Medical Care

Assessment and medical treatment of the injuries must be undertaken.

Medical Aftercare

❖ *Assessment of the risk of STDs*: The victim should be assessed for the risk of STDs. Keeping in mind the incubation period of most STIs, the usual practice is to screen the patients 2 weeks after the assault and then again at 3 months for the bloodborne viruses.

❖ *Postexposure prophylaxis against infection*: Advice related to HIV postexposure prophylaxis and hepatitis B postexposure prophylaxis is available from the British Association for Sexual Health and HIV (BASHH).[20] HIV postexposure prophylaxis must preferably be administered within 72 hours of exposure and hepatitis B postexposure prophylaxis within 6 weeks of exposure. Flow chart 62.1 highlights the algorithm for immediate management in cases of exposure of HIV or HBV.[20]

❖ *Advice related to emergency contraception*: This may be especially important in cases of rape. Emergency contraception can be prescribed using a copper coil. While inserting a copper coil, use of prophylactic antibiotics is usually recommended.

❖ *Pregnancy testing*: This may be required in some cases, especially, those presenting late after the episode.

❖ *Paternity testing*: If pregnancy occurs after rape or sexual assault, paternity analysis can be carried out if there is a doubt about the father's identity. Paternity testing can be either carried out when the child is born or using the products of conception in case of termination.

❖ *Psychological follow-up*: This may vary from child to child depending upon the severity of the crime and the child's temperament. Some sexual assault units have dedicated staff committed towards the follow-up care of these patients.

❖ *Appropriate specialist's referral*: Referral to appropriate specialists must be made following the risk assessment for safeguarding the child's best interests.

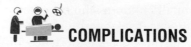

COMPLICATIONS

Child sexual abuse can be associated with massive health-related consequences. Some of them are described next in details:

❖ *Emotional or psychological complications*: Sexual abuse during the childhood can be associated with long-term psychological problems such as low self-esteem, poor performance at school, depression, self-harm or suicide.[5,21,22]

❖ *Problems related to sexual adjustment*: Children who have faced abuse early during their lives may find it difficult to build up healthy sexual relationship with their partners later in life.[5]

Flow chart 62.1: Algorithm for immediate management in cases of exposure of HIV or HBV[20]

Assess risk of exposure

No risk

Criteria:
- Intact skin visibly contaminated with blood or body fluids
- Kissing
- Casual touching

Action:
- Reassure parents and child
- Discharge

Low risk

Criteria:
- Mucous membrane or conjuictval contact with blood or body fluids
- Superficial injury that does not draw blood
- Associated with needle/instrument not visibly contaminated with blood or body fluid

Action:
- Counsel family about risks of HIV/HBV/HCV transmission
- *Recommend standard HBV immunisation:* Day 0, 1 month, 6 months (or booster if already immunised)
- *PEP not recommended:* Explain risks of HIV PEP (drug side effects which outweigh the extremely low risk of HIV transmission)

Moderate risk

Criteria:
- Skin penetrating injury that draws blood by needle/instrument contaminated with blood or body fluid
- Wound causing bleeding and produced by a sharp instrument visibly contaminated with blood
- Sexual contact with individual of unknown HIV status

Action:
- Counsel family about risk of HIV/HBV/HCV transmission
- *Recommend accelerated HBV immunisation:* Day 0, 1 month and 2 months (or booster if already immunised)
- Discuss risks of HIV PEP
- *Consider HIV PEP*: It is generally considered that transmission of HIV is likely to be increased following aggravated sexual intercourse, such as that experienced during sexual assault. Clinicians may therefore consider recommending PEP more readily in such situations

High risk

Criteria:
- Significant exposure to blood or body fluids from source known to be HIV, HCV or HBV infected

Action:
- Counsel family about risk of HIV/HBV/HCV transmission
- *Recommend accelerated HBV immunisation:* Day 0, 1 month, 2 months (or booster if already immunised) Consider HBV Ig if source is a highly infectious HBV carrier and child is susceptible
- Discuss risks of HIV PEP
- Recommend starting HIV PEP

Abbreviations: HBV, hepatitis B virus; PEP, postexposure prophylaxis; HCV, hepatitis C virus

❖ *Problems related to interpersonal relationships*: Children may frequently develop the feelings of shame and guilt, which can have devastating effects on their ability to develop strong sexual relationships when they reach adulthood.[5]

❖ *Problems related to social functioning*: Feeling of guilt and shame related to sexual abuse early in life may have an adverse effect on the social functioning of these women later in life.[5]

❖ *Physical illness*: Severe sexual abuse may be related to the development of physical problems later in life, e.g. cardiovascular disease, type 2 diabetes, hypertension, etc.[6,7,23]

CLINICAL PEARLS

❖ Sexual abuse is not solely committed by adult males. Acts of sexual abuse can also be committed by women and other children.

❖ It is important for the clinician to remain highly vigilant regarding the diagnosis of child sexual abuse or rape

if the child presents with any of the indirect problems suggestive of child sexual abuse, e.g. vaginal bleeding, genital soreness, etc. Disclosure about sexual assault or rape must be facilitated by empowering the child. Senior colleagues should be preferably involved at an early stage.

❖ Absence of injury to the anogenital tract does not rule out the possibility of sexual abuse.

❖ Healthcare professionals must remember that persons cannot be assumed to lack of capacity on the basis of their physical appearance, age, or behaviour.

EVIDENCE-BASED MEDICINE

The clinician must not get involved in the practice of performing virginity test or confirming the virginity of a particular patient. Not only are there several ethical issues related to this practice, presently there is no evidence to define the accuracy of this test in determining whether the person is sexually active or not.[24-26]

CHAPTER 62

REFERENCES

1. Her Majesty' Government. Working together to safeguard children. A guide to inter-agency working to safeguard and promote the welfare of children. London: HMSO; 2015.
2. Royal College of Paediatrics and Child Health (RCPCH). Safeguarding Children and Young people: roles and competences for health care staff. London: RCPCH; 2014.
3. Her Majesty's Stationery Office (HMSO). The Children Act 2004. London: HMSO; 2004.
4. Her Majesty's Stationery Office (HMSO). The Children Act 1989. London: HMSO; 1989.
5. Ahmad S. Adult psychosexual dysfunction as a sequel of child sexual abuse. Sexual and Relationship Therapy. 2006;21(4):405-18.
6. Riley EH, Wright RJ, Jun HJ, Hibert EN, Rich-Edwards JW. Hypertension in adult survivors of child abuse: Observations from the Nurses' Health Study II. J Epidemiol Community Health. 2010;64(5):413-8.
7. Rich-Edwards JW, Spiegelman D, Lividoti Hibert EN, Jun HJ, Todd TJ, Kawachi I, et al. Abuse in childhood and adolescence as a predictor of type 2 diabetes in adult women. Am J Prev Med. 2010;39(6):529-36.
8. Jones L, Bellis MA, Wood S, Hughes K, McCoy E, Eckley L, et al. Prevalence and risk of violence against children with disabilities: a systemic review and meta-analysis of observational studies. Lancet. 2012;380(9845):899-907.
9. Her Majesty's Stationery Office (HMSO). Sexual Offences Act 2003. London: HMSO; 2003.
10. Royal College of Paediatrics and Child Health and Forensic and Legal Medicine (FFLM). (2012). Guidelines on paediatric forensic examinations in relation to possible child sexual abuse. [online] Available from www.fflm.ac.uk/wp-content/uploads/documentstore/1352802061.pdf. [Accessed September, 2016].
11. The Royal College of Paediatrics and Child Health (RCPCH), the Faculty of Forensic and legal medicine (FFLM). (2015).The physical signs of child sexual abuse. An evidence-based review and guidance for best practice. [online] Available from www.rcpch.ac.uk/physical-signs-child-sexual-abuse. [Accessed September, 2016].
12. National Society for Prevention of Cruelty to Children (NSPCC). Child sexual abuse research briefing. London: NSPCC; 2013.
13. Gilmore S, Herring J. 'No' is the hardest word: consent and children's autonomy. Child and Family Law Quarterly. 2011; 23(1):3-25.
14. British Medical Association Consent, Rights and Choices in Health Care for Children and Young People. London: BMJ Publishing Group; 2001.
15. McFarlane A. Mental capacity: One standard for all ages. Family Law. 2011;41(5):479-85.
16. British and Irish Legal Information Institute. (1985). Gillick Vs West Norfolk & Wisbech Area Health Authority, UKHL 7. [online] Available from www.bailii.org/uk/cases/UKHL/1985/7.html. [Accessed September, 2016].
17. De Cruz SP. Parents, doctors and children: The Gillick case and beyond. J Soc Welfare Law. 1987;9(2):93-108.
18. Taylor R. Reversing the retreat from Gillick? R (Axon) vs Secretary of State for Health. Child and Family Law Quarterly. 2007;19(1):81-97.
19. Wheeler R. Gillick or Fraser? A plea for consistency over competence in children: Gillick and Fraser are not interchangeable. BMJ. 2006;332(7545):807.
20. Foster C, Tudor-Williams G, Bamford A. (2015). Post-Exposure Prophylaxis (PEP) Guidelines for children and adolescents potentially exposed to blood-borne viruses. [online] Available from www.bashh.org. [Accessed September, 2016].
21. Sheldrick C. Adult sequelae of child sexual abuse. Br J Psychiatry Suppl. 1991;(10):55-62.
22. Roosa MW, Reinholtz C, Angelini PJ. The relation of child sexual abuse and depression in young women: Comparisons across four ethnic groups. J Abnorm Child Psychol. 1999;27(1):65-76.
23. Rich-Edwards JW, Mason S, Rexrode K, Spiegelman D, Hibert E, Kawachi I, et al. Physical and sexual abuse in childhood as predictors of early onset cardiovascular events in women. Circulation. 2012;126(8):920-7.
24. Herrmann B, Eydam AK. Guidelines and evidence. Recent developments in medical child protection. Bundesgesundheitsblatt Gesundheitsforschung Gesundheitsschutz. 2010; 53(11):1173-9.
25. Berkoff MC, Zolotor AJ, Makoroff KL, Thackeray JD, Shapiro RA, Runyan DK. Has this prepubertal girl been sexually abused? JAMA. 2008;300(23):2779-92.
26. Pillai M. Genital findings in prepubertal girls: what can be concluded from an examination? J Pediatr Adolesc Gynecol. 2008;21(4):177-85.

Dyspareunia and Other Psychosexual Problems

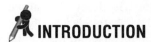 INTRODUCTION

Dyspareunia can be defined as recurrent or persistent genital pain associated with sexual activity, which usually occurs at the time of penetration during sexual intercourse. It is likely to be associated with significant distress or interpersonal conflict.[1] It is not a condition in itself but a symptom caused by several medical or psychosocial problems. While dyspareunia occurs almost exclusively in women, it can rarely also affect men. True dyspareunia in women frequently occurs along with vaginismus, a condition that causes the vaginal muscles to tense up during penetration. Dyspareunia can be classified as primary or secondary based on whether it always occurs (primary) or occurs following a period of pain-free sexual activity (secondary). It can be also classified as superficial or deep depending upon the site of pain. It is often associated with other disorders of female sexual dysfunction including reduced libido and arousal, anorgasmia, problems related to arousal, etc., and can have a significant impact on the woman's mental and physical health, relationships with her partners and efforts to conceive. Problems related to sexual arousal in association with dyspareunia are likely to result in further sexual pain and avoidance of sexual activity.

Diagnostic and Statistical Manual of Mental Disorders, 4th edition (DSM-IV) has classified disorders of female sexual function into four categories: (1) disorders of sexual desire [hypoactive sexual desire disorders (HSDDs), aversion disorders]; (2) disorders of sexual arousal; (3) orgasmic disorders; and (4) disorders of sexual pain (dyspareunia, vaginismus, etc.).[2] DSM-IV had defined HSDD as all disorders associated with persistent deficient or absent sexual fantasies, thoughts and desire for or receptivity to sexual activity. For this condition to be regarded as a disorder, it must cause marked distress or interpersonal difficulties to the patient. Also, it should not be better accounted for by another mental disorder, a drug (legal or illegal), or some other medical condition.[3] Recently, this definition has been broadened and

is termed as Women's Sexual Interest or Desire Disorder.[4] It is defined as the absent or diminished feelings of sexual interest or desire, absent sexual thoughts or fantasies, and a lack of responsive desire. Deficiency of testosterone can be considered as the underlying cause for HSDD amongst postmenopausal women. Disorders of sexual arousal, which are also commonly encountered amongst women, are different from disorders of sexual desire. However, there occurs a significant overlap between these two.

AETIOLOGY

Causes of dyspareunia are listed in Table 63.1.[5] Some significant risk factors for dyspareunia are as follows: younger age, lower level of education, urinary tract symptoms, poor health, emotional problems or stress, etc.[6]

Female sexual dysfunction occurs due to complex interplay between physiological; psychological (relationship problems, poor body image, reduced self-esteem, mood disorders, adverse effect of psychotropic medication use, etc.); emotional; musculogenic (hyper or hypotonicity of pelvic floor muscles); neurogenic (spinal cord injury, disorders of the central or peripheral nervous system, etc.); vasculogenic (reduced blood flow to genitals as a result of atherosclerosis, hormonal influences, trauma, etc.) and

Table 63.1: Causes of dyspareunia

Superficial dyspareunia	Deep dyspareunia
• Vulvitis and vulvovaginitis (due to infection, hypoestrogenism, etc.) • Vestibulodynia • Vulvodynia • Urethral disorders and cystitis • Difficulty in arousal (e.g. lack of vaginal lubrication) • Perineal injury due to obstetric trauma (e.g. episiotomy) • Radiation vaginitis	• Pelvic inflammatory disease • Endometriosis • Pelvic masses (e.g. ovarian cysts) • Pelvic congestion syndrome • Retroverted uterus • Irritable bowel syndrome • Psychosexual issues

endocrinological causes (dysfunction of hypothalamic-pituitary axis , menopause, chronic oral contraceptive use, premature ovarian failure components, etc.).

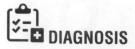

DIAGNOSIS

Clinical Presentation

The history, including a focussed sexual history and physical examination, is usually sufficient to reach a specific diagnosis. Asking the patient details related to the characteristics of pain can help identify the cause of dyspareunia. In case of secondary dyspareunia, the physician should ask about the specific events, which could have triggered the pain, e.g. psychosocial trauma or exposure to infection. The type of pain experienced by the patient can also help determine the underlying cause for pain. If penetration is difficult to achieve, it could be related to vulvodynia or accompanying vaginismus. Lack of arousal may be an ongoing reaction to pain. Concomitant presence of other psychosexual disorders (e.g. arousal disorders) is likely to result in lack of lubrication. Positional pain is likely to be associated with pelvic structural problems, e.g. uterine retroversion.[7] Pain at the time of penile entry is likely to occur with conditions such as presence of dermatological lesions over the vulva (e.g. lichen planus, lichen sclerosus, psoriasis, etc.), vulvodynia, vaginismus, etc. On the other hand, deep dyspareunia is likely to be associated with pathologies such as endometriosis, adnexal pathologies, pelvic inflammatory diseases, interstitial cystitis, pelvic adhesions, retroverted uterus, uterine myomas, etc. There are some conditions which are likely to be associated with both pain at the time of entry and deep pain, e.g. dyspareunia due to vaginal atrophy, postpartum dyspareunia, etc.

Clinical presentation in various disorders of sexual function is described in Table 63.2.

Physical Examination

In cases of dyspareunia, an educational pelvic examination is usually performed during which the patient is given the opportunity to participate by holding a mirror while the physician explains the findings at the time of conducting the pelvic examination.[7,9] Besides clarifying the normal and abnormal findings and the correlation of the abnormal pathology with pain, an educational pelvic examination also helps in increasing the patient's perception of pain-control and improving her self-image. Physical examination should also involve visual inspection of the external genitalia and examination of the internal genitalia. The mucosal surfaces should be inspected for areas of erythema or discolouration, abrasions or signs of trauma, lesions indicative of dermatological diseases (e.g. lichen sclerosus, lichen planus, etc.), etc. Abnormal vaginal discharge could be suggestive of infection. For women who describe localised pain, a cotton swab should be used to accurately identify the source of the pain. Pain that can be localised to the vagina and supporting structures may be indicative of vulvodynia or vaginitis. Pain that localises to the bladder, ovaries, etc. is suggestive of likely pathology within these structures.

Internal examination should be performed with a single finger to help minimise the patient's discomfort. In the single-finger vaginal examination, a single well-lubricated finger is gently inserted through the vaginal introitus. A patient with significant vaginismus may not be able to tolerate even this. Each internal organ is gently palpated with the help of a finger to make an effort for isolating the source of the pain. Tightness or tenderness of muscles, or difficulty with voluntary contraction or relaxation of the muscles of the pelvic floor is

Table 63.2: Revised definitions for female sexual dysfunction from the Second International Consensus of Sexual Medicine[8]

Disorders	Characteristics
Sexual desire or interest disorder	Absent or diminished feelings of sexual interest or desire, absent sexual thoughts or fantasies, and a lack of responsive desire, all of which are considered to be beyond the normal decrease experienced with increasing age and duration of relationship
Subjective sexual arousal disorder	Absent or diminished feelings of sexual arousal from any type of sexual stimulation. However, vaginal lubrication and/or other signs of physical response do occur
Genital sexual arousal disorder	Complaints of impaired genital sexual arousal, which may include minimal vulvar swelling or vaginal lubrication from any type of sexual stimulation and reduced sexual sensations from caressing genitalia. However, subjective sexual excitement occurs with non-genital sexual stimuli
Combined genital and subjective arousal disorder	Absent or diminished feelings of sexual arousal from any type of sexual stimuli plus complaints of absent or impaired genital sexual arousal
Persistent genital arousal disorder	Spontaneous, intrusive, and unwanted genital arousal in the absence of sexual interest and desire. Arousal is not relieved by orgasms and may persist for hours or days
Women's orgasmic disorder	Despite self-report of high sexual arousal or excitement, there is lack of orgasm, markedly diminished intensity of orgasmic sensations, or marked delay of orgasm from any kind of stimulation
Dyspareunia	Persistent or recurrent pain with attempted or completed vaginal entry and/or penile vaginal intercourse
Vaginismus	Persistent or recurrent difficulties with vaginal entry of a penis, finger, or other object. This difficulty occurs despite the woman's expressed desire to participate
Sexual aversion disorder	Extreme anxiety or disgust at the anticipation of or attempt at any sexual activity

suggestive of the pelvic floor muscle dysfunction.[10] Palpation of structures such as the urethra, bladder, and cervix must also be done for evaluation of the causes of dyspareunia associated with these organs. Once the single-finger examination has been comfortably done, a gentle bimanual examination must be performed for evaluation of pelvic and adnexal structures, if it is not too uncomfortable for the patient.[9]

Investigations

The investigations, which may be required in these cases, include the following:

❖ Pelvic ultrasound
❖ Microbiological swabs
❖ Laparoscopy
❖ Vulval biopsy.

DIFFERENTIAL DIAGNOSIS

Common diagnoses include provoked vulvodynia, inadequate lubrication, postpartum dyspareunia and vaginal atrophy. Vaginismus may be identified as a contributing factor. Several of the most common causes of dyspareunia are described next in details.

Vaginismus

Vaginismus can be described as an involuntary spasm of the pelvic floor muscles (pubococcygeus and other muscles), resulting in painful and difficult penetration of vagina at the time of sexual intercourse. It also results in difficulty at the time of insertion of the tampon or at the time of clinical examination. The relative roles of various factors such as pain, muscular dysfunction and psychological factors in determining the aetiopathogenesis of vaginismus presently remain controversial. Vaginismus can be described as primary (experience of vaginismus with first-time intercourse attempts) or secondary (development of vaginismus after a period of pain-free sexual intercourse). There is a significant clinical overlap between vaginismus and dyspareunia.[10] Therefore, the Diagnostic and Statistical Manual of Mental Disorders, 5th edition (DSM-V), now regards dyspareunia and vaginismus as a single entity, characterised by pain, anxiety and problems with penetration.[11] Vaginismus can be frequently associated with organic vulvar disorders such as vulvar vestibulitis. Management, therefore, typically focuses on finding out whether vaginismus is the primary problem or as a result of an underlying organic vulvar disease. Treatment involves medical care of the underlying causes of pain in combination with pelvic floor physical therapy. Cognitive behaviour therapy or psychotherapy, also involving systemic desensitisation, training of the pubococcygeal muscles and the use of vaginal trainers may also be included in the treatment regimen.[12] Injections of OnabotulinumtoxinA (Botox®) are emerging as a promising new therapy for vaginismus, but are not within the scope of the primary care physician.[13]

Vulvodynia

'International Society for the Study of Vulvovaginal Disease' has described vulvodynia as chronic vulvar discomfort or pain, usually described as a burning pain, which occurs in the absence of clinical findings indicative of a specific, neurologic disorder.[14] Vulvodynia is likely to be associated with psychiatric disorders (e.g. anxiety, depression, etc.). Vulvodynia can be classified as provoked, unprovoked, or mixed. In unprovoked vulvodynia, the pain usually occurs continuously. In provoked vulvodynia, on the other hand, the pain is triggered by touch, e.g. with the insertion of tampon or sexual intercourse. Vulvodynia can also be categorised as generalised (pain is experienced in multiple areas, e.g. in the labia, vestibule and clitoris, perineum, inner thighs, etc.) or localised (pain is localised to one area of vulva).[14] If the pain is localised in the vestibule, this is known as vestibulodynia (formerly known as 'vulvar vestibulitis syndrome'). For details related to vulvodynia, kindly refer to Chapter 88 (Vulvar Cancer and Vulval Pain Syndromes).

In cases of provoked vulvodynia, light touching with a moist cotton swab may reveal localised areas of highly intense pain. A multidisciplinary team approach is required for treating vulvodynia. Combination of multiple therapies is often required.

Inadequate Lubrication

Inadequate lubrication could be related to disorders of sexual arousal or disorders resulting in chronic vaginal dryness. Chronic vaginal dryness may be associated with the following causes: endocrinological causes (e.g. hypothalamic-pituitary dysfunction, premature ovarian failure, menopause, etc.), vascular cause (e.g. peripheral atherosclerosis, anaemia, etc.), neurological causes (e.g. diabetic neuropathy, spinal cord injury, surgery of the spinal cord, etc.), or iatrogenic (e.g. hormonal contraceptive use, chemotherapy, radiation). Inadequate lubrication often leads to friction and microtrauma of the vulvar and vaginal epithelium. Management involves treatment of the underlying disorders.[15]

Postpartum Dyspareunia

Common problems during the postpartum period such as stretching of perineal tissues, sutured lacerations or episiotomy wounds, perineal injuries as a result of operative vaginal delivery, etc., are likely to result in sclerotic healing and resultant dyspareunia (both entry and deep). Also, the postpartum period, especially in breastfeeding women, is associated with a significant decline in the levels of circulating oestrogen, thereby further aggravating vaginal dryness and dyspareunia. Moreover, the postpartum period can be associated with psychosexual problems such as decreased arousal and lubrication, which further contribute to dyspareunia.[16] Vaginal lubricants are typically used as the first-line therapy for cases of postpartum dyspareunia. Women having identifiable perineal defects, scarring or significant anatomical distortion may benefit from revision perineoplasty.[17]

MANAGEMENT

❖ *Patient education:* Clinicians can help alleviate the patient's sexual concerns by educating them about normal sexual functioning and normal female anatomy. An educational pelvic examination (previously described in the text) forms an important component of patient education. Therapy highlighting lifestyle changes such as stress management, adequate rest and regular exercise must be emphasised upon the patient.

❖ Treatment must be directed towards the underlying gynaecological or urogenital cause of dyspareunia.

❖ Depending on the diagnosis, various treatment options include physical therapy of the pelvic floor, use of lubricants, surgical intervention, etc.

❖ An adjunctive course of cognitive behavioural therapy, which focuses on the relationship of pain to anxiety, and that of muscle contractions to pain perception helps in alleviation of psychological problems.

❖ Psychotherapy, which addresses the patient's own fears about vaginal penetration and allows her to gain increasing degree of comfort with her own genitals as well as that of her partner and eventually vaginal penetration, is helpful in alleviation of symptoms related to vaginismus.

❖ Medical therapies such as amitriptyline and topical analgesics prove to be effective for treating vulvodynia.

❖ Phosphodiesterase inhibitors (e.g. bupropion) have been shown to have some degree of benefit in a small subgroup of women having sexual dysfunction, typically orgasmic disorders.[18]

Dyspareunia Associated with Vaginal Atrophy in Postmenopausal Women

Dyspareunia is a common presenting symptom amongst postmenopausal women with vaginal atrophy.[19,20] Both natural and iatrogenic menopause by causing a reduction in oestradiol levels can cause changes in sexual function including loss of libido. In case of vaginal atrophy, the vaginal mucosa becomes thinner, paler, drier, and loses its elasticity. There is a loss of vaginal rugae. Also, the vagina shortens in length and narrows down. This is likely to cause vaginal dryness, resulting in painful sexual intercourse or dyspareunia. The most effective treatment for vaginal atrophy and dryness is oestrogen replacement. Various oestrogen preparations: cream, ring, or tablet, have been found to be associated with a statistically significant reduction in symptoms of vaginal atrophy in comparison with the placebo.[21] Ospemifene (Osphena®), a novel selective oestrogen receptor modulator which increases vaginal epithelial cells (thereby increasing the thickness of vaginal epithelium) and reduces the vaginal pH has been approved by the USFDA for the treatment of postmenopausal dyspareunia.[22] Testosterone can also be used in case of vaginal atrophy. However, it should be used in conjunction with systemic oestradiol.

Role of Testosterone Therapy on Sexual Function

Though testosterone has been commonly used for the treatment of women with various sexual disorders, the use of testosterone therapy is still considered controversial in clinical practice. In normal women, testosterone is produced by the ovaries and adrenal glands. While no relationship between endogenous testosterone levels and sexual dysfunction has yet been evidently established in premenopausal women, low levels of testosterone due to menopause or other causes is likely to result in reduced libido, reduced sexual well-being and sexual activity in women.[23] Besides the age-related decline in the levels of testosterone, other potential causes of low androgen levels in women include premature ovarian failure, iatrogenic menopause (due to chemotherapy, radiation therapy to the pelvis or bilateral oophorectomy), etc. Low-dose testosterone therapy is efficacious for the treatment of low libido in postmenopausal women who are adequately oestrogenised or women with low androgen levels.[24] Though no androgen preparation has been currently approved by the FDA for the treatment of disorders related to sexual interest or desire in women, androgen therapy has been used off-label to treat low libido and sexual dysfunction in women for over 40 years. Testosterone therapy is administered via multiple routes including oral pills (methyltestosterone and testosterone undecanoate); subcutaneous pellets; intramuscular injection (cypionate, propionate and enanthate); testosterone transdermal matrix patches, gels, creams and sprays; and sublingual drops. Women should be prescribed androgen therapy following a discussion regarding the risks and benefits of therapy. Testosterone therapy is likely to result in side effects such as acne, hirsutism, lowering of high-density lipoprotein (HDL) levels, etc.

CLINICAL PEARLS

❖ The PLISSIT (Permission, Limited Information, Specific Suggestions, Intensive Therapy) or ALLOW (Ask, Legitimise, Limitations, Open up, Work together) methods can be used by the clinicians to enable them to carry out discussions related to sexual problems with their patient.[25]

❖ If dyspareunia has negatively affected the patient's relationship with her partner or her self-esteem, she is likely to derive some benefit from support groups, individual therapy, or couple's therapy.

❖ Even if the woman is using systemic oestradiol therapy in case of vaginal atrophy, she should also be prescribed local oestrogens in form of creams and pessaries.

❖ Tibolone is a selective tissue-oestrogenic-activity regulator (STEAR), which is likely to be effective for the treatment of problems related to reduced libido in postmenopausal women.[26]

❖ Hypoactive sexual desire disorder can be considered as the most common type of female sexual dysfunction and is often related to a psychological or physiological cause.

EVIDENCE-BASED MEDICINE

❖ Oestrogen formulations in form of cream, ring, or tablet are useful for effectively providing relief from symptoms of vaginal atrophy in comparison to placebo or non-hormonal gels.[20-22]

❖ Though there is limited evidence in the form of small trials, drugs such as amitriptyline and lidocaine ointment are commonly used for treating the cases of vulvodynia.[27-29]

❖ Surgical excision of painful areas (e.g. vestibulectomy for vestibulodynia) can be offered to the patients with provoked vulvodynia, which is unresponsive to conservative management.[27]

REFERENCES

1. Lewis RW, Fugl-Meyer KS, Corona G, Hayes RD, Laumann EO, Moreira ED, et al. Definitions/epidemiology/risk factors for sexual dysfunction. J Sex Med. 2010;7(4 Pt 2):1598-607.

2. Sexual and gender identity disorders. In: American Psychiatric Association. Diagnostic and Statistical Manual of Mental Disorders, 4th edition. Washington, DC: American Psychiatric Association; 2000, pp. 493-538.

3. Basson R, Berman J, Burnett A, Derogatis L, Ferguson D, Fourcroy J, et al. Report of the international consensus development conference on female sexual dysfunction: definitions and classifications. J Urol. 2000;163(3):888-93.

4. Basson R, Leiblum S, Brotto L, Derogatis L, Fourcroy J, Fugl-Meyer K, et al. Definitions of women's sexual dysfunction reconsidered: advocating expansion and revision. J Psychosom Obstet Gynaecol. 2003;24(4):221-29.

5. Ferrero S, Ragni N, Remorgida V. Deep dyspareunia: causes, treatments, and results. Curr Opin Obstet Gynecol. 2008;20(4): 394-9.

6. Laumann EO, Paik A, Rosen RC. Sexual dysfunction in the United States: prevalence and predictors. JAMA. 1999;281 (6):537-44.

7. Basson R, Wierman ME, van Lankveld J, Brotto L. Summary of the recommendations on sexual dysfunctions in women. J Sex Med. 2010;7(1 Pt 2):314-26.

8. Basson R, Althof S, Davis S, Fugl-Meyer K, Goldstein I, Leiblum S, et al. Summary of the recommendations on sexual dysfunctions in women. J Sex Med. 2004;1(1):24-34.

9. Huber JD, Pukall CF, Boyer SC, Reissing ED, Chamberlain SM. "Just relax": physicians' experiences with women who are difficult or impossible to examine gynecologically. J Sex Med. 2009;6(3):791-9.

10. Faubion SS, Shuster LT, Bharucha AE. Recognition and management of nonrelaxing pelvic floor dysfunction. Mayo Clin Proc. 2012;87(2):187-93.

11. American Psychiatric Association. Diagnostic and Statistical Manual of Mental Disorders, 5th edition. Arlington, VA: American Psychiatric Association; 2013.

12. Frank JE, Mistretta P, Will J. Diagnosis and treatment of female sexual dysfunction. Am Fam Physician. 2008;77(5):635-42.

13. Bertolasi L, Frasson E, Cappelletti JY, Vicentini S, Bordignon M, Graziottin A. Botulinum neurotoxin type A injections for vaginismus secondary to vulvar vestibulitis syndrome. Obstet Gynecol. 2009;114(5):1008-16.

14. Moyal-Barracco M, Lynch PJ. 2003 ISSVD terminology and classification of vulvodynia. J Reprod Med. 2004;49(10):772-7.

15. Stika CS. Atrophic vaginitis. Dermatol Ther. 2010;23(5):514-22.

16. Leeman LM, Rogers RG. Sex after childbirth: postpartum sexual function. Obstet Gynecol. 2012;119(3):647-55.

17. Woodward AP, Matthews CA. Outcomes of revision perineoplasty for persistent postpartum dyspareunia. Female Pelvic Med Reconstr Surg. 2010;16(2):135-9.

18. Segraves RT, Clayton A, Croft H, Wolf A, Warnock J. Bupropion sustained release for the treatment of hypoactive sexual desire disorder in premenopausal women. J Clin Psychopharmacol. 2004;24(3):339-42.

19. Mac Bride MB, Rhodes DJ, Shuster LT. Vulvovaginal atrophy. Mayo Clin Proc. 2010;85(1):87-94.

20. Krychman ML. Vaginal estrogens for the treatment of dyspareunia. J Sex Med. 2011;8(3):666-74.

21. Suckling J, Lethaby A, Kennedy R. Local oestrogen for vaginal atrophy in postmenopausal women. Cochrane Database Syst Rev. 2006;(4):CD001500.

22. Soe LH, Wurz GT, Kao CJ, DeGregorio MW. Ospemifene for the treatment of dyspareunia associated with vulvar and vaginal atrophy: potential benefits in bone and breast. Int J Womans Health. 2013;5:605-11.

23. Davis SR, Davison SL, Donath S, Bell RJ. Circulating androgen levels and self-reported sexual function in women. JAMA. 2005;294(1):91-6.

24. Bolour S, Braunstein G. Testosterone therapy in women: a review. Int J Impot Res. 2005;17(5):399-408.

25. Feldman J, Striepe M. Women's sexual health. Clin Fam Pract. 2004;6(4):839-61.

26. Davis SR. The effects of tibolone on mood and libido. Menopause. 2002;9(3):162-70.

27. Andrews JC. Vulvodynia interventions—systematic review and evidence grading. Obstet Gynecol Surv. 2011;66(5):299-315.

28. Reed BD, Caron AM, Gorenflo DW, Haefner HK. Treatment of vulvodynia with tricyclic antidepressants: efficacy and associated factors. J Low Genit Tract Dis. 2006;10(4):245-51.

29. Zolnoun DA, Hartmann KE, Steege JF. Overnight 5% lidocaine ointment for treatment of vulvar vestibulitis. Obstet Gynecol. 2003;102(1):84-7.

SECTION 12

Abnormalities of Menstruation

GYNAECOLOGY

Abnormal Uterine Bleeding

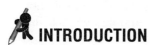 **INTRODUCTION**

Abnormal uterine bleeding (AUB) is defined by ACOG (2013) as bleeding from the uterine corpus, which is abnormal in regularity, volume, frequency, or duration, occurring in the absence of pregnancy.[1] AUB may be acute or chronic. Acute AUB refers to an episode of heavy bleeding of sufficient quantity, requiring immediate clinical intervention to prevent further blood loss. Chronic AUB, on the other hand, refers to AUB present for most of the previous 6 months. The term 'menorrhagia', previously considered as the most important cause of AUB has now been replaced by the term, 'heavy menstrual bleeding (HMB)' as per the NICE guidelines (2007). HMB should be defined as excessive menstrual blood loss which interferes with the woman's physical, emotional, social and material quality of life. This can occur alone or in combination with other symptoms. Any interventions should aim to improve quality of life measures. The previous definition of HMB based on the measured blood loss of more than 60–80 mL per period is no longer in clinical use. Other patterns of AUB can include intermenstrual bleeding (IMB) and postcoital bleeding (PCB). Prevalence of HMB varies between 4% to 50%.[2]

AETIOLOGY

There has been general inconsistency in the nomenclature used for describing AUB in the women of reproductive age group and there is a plethora of potential causes. The FIGO has approved a new classification system (PALM-COEIN) for causes of AUB in non-gravid women of reproductive age (Flow chart 64.1).[3] Of the nine categories in the new FIGO classification system (PALM-COEIN), the first four are defined as visually objective structural criteria (PALM: **p**olyp, **a**denomyosis, **l**eiomyoma, and **m**alignancy and hyperplasia), the pathologies that can be measured visually with imaging

Flow chart 64.1: Basic PALM-COEIN classification system for the causes of abnormal uterine bleeding (AUB) in non-gravid women of reproductive age group (system approved by the International Federation of Gynecology and Obstetrics)[3]

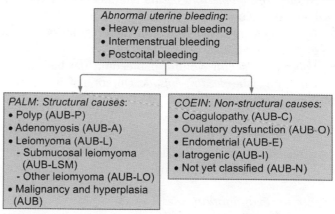

techniques, such as sonography and/or histopathology testing. Leiomyomas are the most common structural cause of painless HMB. Painful heavy bleeding may be due to adenomyosis. Endometrial polyps are often associated with IMB. Histological abnormalities of the endometrium, ranging from simple and complex endometrial hyperplasia to severe atypia and malignancy, are often linked to perimenopause. The incidence of malignancy increases with age and is rare in premenopausal women.

The next four are unrelated to structural abnormalities (COEI: **c**oagulopathy, **o**vulatory dysfunction, **e**ndometrial and **i**atrogenic), which are the non-structural entities that are not defined on imaging or histopathology testing. The 'iatrogenic' category refers to AUB associated with the use of exogenous gonadal steroids, intrauterine systems or devices, or other systemic or local agents. The final category stands for the entities that are (N) **n**ot yet classified. This classification system for the causes of AUB is likely to facilitate clinical care and treatment of such patients. Taking the patient's medical history should be guided by the PALM-COEIN classification system in order to exclude various pathologies and reach a specific diagnosis regarding the cause for AUB.

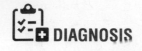 **DIAGNOSIS**

Clinical Presentation

History-taking should define the nature of the bleeding and related symptoms that might suggest structural or histological abnormality, impact on the patient's quality of life and well-being, and other factors which may determine treatment options (such as presence of comorbidity). A detailed and accurate family history is essential for detecting the underlying medical problems, especially coagulation defects (Box 64.1)[4] and assessing the impact of the problem in each individual case. Use of simple menstrual calendars may be useful in establishing the pattern of bleeding. She should be asked about the following characteristics related to the episode of bleeding:

❖ *Intermenstrual intervals*: Intermenstrual intervals between the episodes of bleeding may be shortened due to the prolonged duration of bleeding
❖ *Number of days bleeding occurs*: Number of days when the bleeding occurs may be increased
❖ *Cycle regularity*: Cycles may lose their regularity because of the irregular episodes of bleeding
❖ *Volume of bleeding*: Volume of bleeding may be heavy
❖ *Duration of the bleeding episode*: Duration of the bleeding episode may be prolonged.

General Physical Examination

Signs related to excessive blood loss (tachycardia, hypotension, etc.) may be evident on the general physical examination.

Abdominal Examination

In some cases of AUB, due to structural causes (e.g. leiomyoma) the uterus may be so enlarged that it can be palpated on per abdominal examination.

Pelvic Examination

Per speculum examination: Per speculum examination helps in identifying trauma to the genital tract as well as vaginal or cervical cause of bleeding.

Bimanual examination: Pelvic examination must not be done in young girls presenting with the history of menorrhagia, who are not sexually active. However, it may be useful in women belonging to reproductive age group, presenting with dysfunctional uterine bleeding (DUB).

Gynaecological examination helps in excluding the various conditions described in Box 64.2, which may be responsible for producing abnormal bleeding.

Investigations

If the history is suggestive of HMB without any underlying structural or histological abnormality, pharmaceutical treatment can be started without carrying out a physical examination or other investigations at initial consultation in primary care. However, if the chosen treatment is levonor-gestrel-releasing intrauterine system (LNG-IUS), internal examination may be required.

On the other hand, if the history is suggestive of HMB with structural or histological abnormality or there is presence of symptoms such as IMB, PCB, pelvic pain and/or pressure symptoms, a physical examination and/or other investigations must be performed. Some of the investigations which need to be performed are as follows:

❖ *Ultrasound examination*: Ultrasound is the first-line diagnostic tool for identifying structural abnormalities (e.g. endometrial polyps, submucous fibroids, etc.). It is especially important in cases where the uterus appears to be enlarged on pelvic and/or abdominal examination. Ultrasound examination can be supplemented with additional investigations such as biopsy and/or hystero-scopy, if required.[5,6] Imaging should be undertaken in the

---

Box 64.1: Clinical screening for a patient with heavy menstrual bleeding (HMB) having an underlying disorder of haemostasis[4]

A positive screening result* comprises the following circumstances:
❑ HMB since menarche
❑ One of the following conditions:
  – PPH
  – Surgery-related bleeding
  – Bleeding associated with dental work
❑ Two or more of the following conditions:
  – Bruising, one to two times per month
  – Epistaxis, one to two times per month
  – Frequent gum bleeding
  – Family history of bleeding symptoms

*Patients with a positive screening result should be considered for further evaluation, including consultation with a haematologist and testing for von Willebrand factor and ristocetin cofactor.

Box 64.2: Differential diagnosis of dysfunctional uterine bleeding

Postmenopausal women
❑ Cervical cancer, cervicitis, atrophic vaginitis, endometrial atrophy
❑ Submucous fibroids, endometrial hyperplasia and endometrial polyps
❑ HRT

Premenopausal women
❑ *Infection, trauma*: Cervicitis, PID, endometritis, laceration, abrasion, foreign body, IUCD
❑ *Benign pelvic pathology*: Cervical polyp, endometrial polyp, leiomyoma, adenomyosis, etc.
❑ *Malignancy, neoplasm*: Cervical, endometrial or ovarian malignancy
❑ *Premalignant lesions*: Cervical lesions, endometrial hyperplasia
❑ *Trauma*: Foreign bodies, abrasions, lacerations, sexual abuse or assault
❑ *Medications/iatrogenic*: Intrauterine device, hormones (oral contraceptives, oestrogen, progesterone)
❑ *Systemic diseases*: Hepatic disease, renal disease, coagulopathy, thrombocytopenia, von Willebrand's disease, leukaemia

following circumstances: when the uterus is palpable on per abdominal examination; a mass whose origin cannot be determined is felt on vaginal examination; and there is a failure of pharmaceutical treatment (NSAIDs, hormonal therapy, etc.). TVS helps in the evaluation of endometrial thickness, uterine shape, size and contour and adnexa, and helps in ruling out different pelvic pathologies (leiomyomas, endometriosis, etc.).

❖ *Endometrial biopsy*: If appropriate, a biopsy should be taken to exclude endometrial cancer or atypical hyperplasia. Indications for a biopsy include persistent or prolonged IMB, women with specific risk factors for endometrial cancer (e.g. women aged 45 years or more, obesity and tamoxifen therapy), treatment failure or ineffective treatment. Endometrial biopsy is also recommended in women over the age of 45 years if the previous treatment strategies have failed. Various endometrial sampling devices are available, e.g. Pipelle® sampler, which has been shown to have high sensitivity in the detection of both endometrial cancer and atypical hyperplasia. However, it is not possible to detect polyps or fibroids on biopsy.

❖ *Complete blood count*: A full blood count test should be carried out on all women with HMB. Testing for coagulation disorders (e.g. von Willebrand's disease) should be considered in young women experiencing HMB since menarche or having personal or family history suggestive of a coagulation disorder.

❖ *Additional tests*: Tests such as serum ferritin levels and levels of female hormones (e.g. oestradiol, progestin, etc.) are not routinely required in women with HMB. They may be required in the presence of specific clinical circumstances.

❖ *Thyroid function tests*: Testing for thyroid functions is also not routinely required and should only be carried out in circumstances where clinical signs and symptoms of thyroid disease are present.

❖ *Hysteroscopy*: It provides accurate visualisation of the uterine cavity (Fig. 64.1). It has greater accuracy than TVS

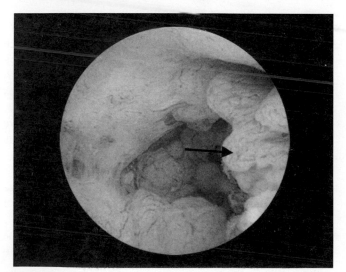

Fig. 64.1: Hysteroscopic appearance of an exophytic endometrial cancer growth (indicated by arrow) *(For colour version, see Plate 4)*

in the diagnosis of endometrial polyps and submucous fibroids. However, due to its invasive nature and high cost, hysteroscopy should be used as a diagnostic tool only when the results on ultrasound are inconclusive.

Where dilatation is required for non-hysteroscopic ablative procedures, hysteroscopy should be used immediately prior to the procedure to ensure correct placement of the device.

❖ *Saline infusion sonography*: Saline infusion sonography (SIS) is an investigation which helps in delineating the uterine cavity. However, it should not be used as a first-line diagnostic tool except in centres where there is limited provision of outpatient hysteroscopy.[7]

❖ *Dilatation and curettage*: Dilatation and curettage alone should not be used as a diagnostic tool. Presently, this investigation has been largely replaced by clinic-based investigations. According to the current guidelines, TVS along with endometrial biopsy should be used as an initial investigation in cases of AUB.[5,6] Hysteroscopy should be used as a back-up investigation in case of non-conclusive findings on TVS and endometrial biopsy.

❖ *Magnetic resonance imaging*: This investigation is normally not used as a first-line diagnostic tool for investigation of cases with AUB.

❖ *Colposcopy*: In cases of IMB and PCB, careful examination of cervix is essential. If there is a presence of suspicious findings on cervical examination, colposcopic examination may be required. In cases of IMB and PCB, it is also essential to exclude chlamydial infection. No further investigations are required in cases of midcycle IMB.

 # MANAGEMENT

Numerous factors are likely to influence the decisions regarding investigations and treatment of AUB, including factors such as the patient's age, her reproductive wishes for the future, menstrual pattern, severity of her symptoms and the degree of social disruption caused by her symptoms.

Management of patients with AUB comprises of the following:[8]

❖ Assessment of the patient's clinical condition and maintenance of her haemodynamic stability (especially in cases of an acute episode)

❖ Determining the most likely aetiology of bleeding

❖ Selecting the most appropriate treatment for the patient.

Pharmaceutical Treatments for Heavy Menstrual Bleeding

❖ Pharmaceutical treatment should be considered in cases where there is no structural or histological abnormality, fibroids are less than 3 cm in diameter, and there is no distortion of the uterine cavity.

❖ Before recommending treatment, the clinician needs to determine if the hormonal or non-hormonal treatment options would be acceptable to her (i.e. whether she is wishing to conceive in future or not).

CHAPTER 64

- If the prescription of pharmaceutical treatment appears as an appropriate option, various treatment options must be considered in the order described as follows: LNG-IUS; tranexamic acid or NSAIDs; combined OCPs (COCPs); long-acting oral or injectable progestogens.[8]

- Cases of HMB are initially dealt with in the primary-care settings following abdominal and/or pelvic examination and measurement of CBC. If the first pharmaceutical treatment option proves to be ineffective, a second pharmaceutical treatment option can be considered rather than immediately referring the patient to the secondary care.

- Various pharmaceutical treatment options are described next in detail:

  - *Levonorgestrel-releasing intrauterine system*: Women offered an LNG-IUS should be advised that they need to wait for at least 6 cycles to observe the benefits of the treatment.[9]

  - *Progestogens*: Norethisterone in the dosage of 15 mg daily from days 5 to 26 of the menstrual cycle, or injectable long-acting progestogens can be administered for controlling HMB.[10] Administration of oral progestogens only during the luteal phase should not be used for the treatment of HMB. Cyclical progestogens are effective for controlling HMB related to ovulatory dysfunction when they are administered for at least 21 days out of 28 days. Continuous high-dose progestogens (e.g. depot preparations) may be useful if they induce amenorrhoea.

  - *Tranexamic acid or NSAIDs*: If hormonal treatments are not acceptable to the woman, then either tranexamic acid or NSAIDs can be used.[11] Etamsylate, however, should not be used for the treatment of HMB. These treatment options must be used for as long as they appear to be clinically useful to the woman. They should be stopped if there is no improvement in the symptoms within three menstrual cycles. Use of NSAIDs appears preferable to tranexamic acid when HMB coexists with dysmenorrhoea.

  - *Gonadotropin-releasing hormone agonists*: Use of a GnRH analogue could be considered prior to surgery or as a therapeutic option when all other treatment options for uterine fibroids, including surgery or uterine artery embolisation (UAE), are contraindicated. If this treatment is to be prescribed for more than 6 months or if adverse effects are experienced, then the use of add-back therapy (HRT or tibolone) is recommended to prevent complications related to the prolonged use of GnRH agonists.

  - *Danazol*: Use of danazol is not recommended for the management of HMB.

Surgical Treatments for Heavy Menstrual Bleeding

Non-hysterectomy Surgery (Endometrial Ablation)

- Methods for endometrial ablation help in treating AUB by destroying the endometrial lining. These methods for endometrial ablation are mainly of two types: First-generation (hysteroscopic) methods and second-generation (non-hysteroscopic) methods (Box 64.3).[12]

Box 64.3: Procedures for endometrial ablation[12]

First-generation procedures
- ❑ Hysteroscopic laser ablation
- ❑ Transcervical resection of the endometrium
- ❑ Roller ball ablation of the endometrium

Second-generation procedures
- ❑ Cryoablation
- ❑ Hydrothermal ablation
- ❑ Laser thermoablation
- ❑ Microwave ablation
- ❑ Thermal balloon ablation
- ❑ Electrosurgical ablation
- ❑ Photodynamic ablation
- ❑ Radiofrequency-induced thermal ablation

- Second-generation methods of endometrial ablation are favoured over the first-generation methods of endometrial ablation for the control of HMB because these methods are likely to be quicker, safer, simpler and more cost-effective in comparison to the first-generation methods.[13-16]

- Repeat ablation is not done for second-generation methods. Also, endometrial thinning agents are not required in these cases in comparison to the first-generation methods.[17] Alternatively, the surgery can be scheduled in the postmenstrual phase, thereby avoiding the use of endometrial thinning agents.

- Endometrial ablation should be considered as a therapeutic option in the women experiencing bleeding which is likely to have a severe impact on their quality of life. Moreover, before using this option, the clinician should make sure that the woman is not desirous of future childbearing.

- Endometrial ablation may be offered as an initial treatment option for HMB after having a full discussion with the woman regarding the risks and benefits of using other treatment options.

- Patient preparation for endometrial ablation is described in Box 64.4. Women undergoing endometrial ablation must be counselled to avoid subsequent pregnancy in future. They must also be advised to use effective contraception, if required, after endometrial ablation.

- Endometrial ablation should be considered in women with HMB who have a normal uterus (no >10 weeks in absence of any abnormality) and also those with small uterine fibroids (<3 cm in diameter). Some contraindications to the use of endometrial ablation are described in the Box 64.5.

- All women considering endometrial ablation should have an access to a second-generation ablation technique. This technique should be preferably used in cases where no structural or histological abnormality is present.

- *Dilatation and curettage*: Use of dilatation and curettage is not recommended as a therapeutic option in cases of HMB.

- *Uterine fibroids associated with HMB*: Further interventions for uterine fibroids associated with HMB include the following:

  - Symptomatic endometrial polyps and small submucous fibroids should be removed via hysteroscopic route.

Box 64.4: Patient preparation for endometrial ablation

Preoperative evaluation
❏ Taking informed consent after adequate counselling
❏ Urine pregnancy test (to rule out pregnancy)
❏ Performing cervical cultures (to rule out infection)
❏ *Uterine evaluation*:
   – Endometrial sampling (to exclude endometrial hyperplasia or cancer)
   – Assessment of the uterine cavity for the presence of intracavitary myomas, endometrial polyps, or other abnormalities (e.g. uterine septum), using saline infusion sonography or office hysteroscopy to assess the uterine cavity
   – Sounding of the uterus (>10 weeks in size)
   – Removal of an IUCD (if present)
   – Endometrial preparation using GnRH agonists initiated 30–60 days prior to the procedure (to be used only with non-resectoscopic ablation devices with the exception of Thermachoice® device and NovaSure®)

Operative setup
❏ *Antibiotic prophylaxis*: Not routinely administered prior to endometrial ablation
❏ *Anaesthesia*: Resectoscopic ablation may be performed with regional or general anaesthesia. Non-resectoscopic endometrial ablation can be performed using local, regional, or general anaesthesia
❏ *NSAIDs*: Administration of an oral NSAID at least 1 hour preoperatively to inhibit uterine contractions

Follow-up
❏ *Counselling regarding contraception*: Women who have undergone endometrial ablation must be counselled about the need for contraception
❏ *Exclusion of endometrial neoplasia*: Women with recurrent abnormal uterine bleeding after the procedure must be evaluated with endometrial sampling to exclude endometrial neoplasia
❏ *Use of postmenopausal hormone therapy*: Women with endometrial ablation who want to use postmenopausal hormone therapy should be prescribed progestins along with oestrogen for protection against development of endometrial cancer in the residual tissue

Box 64.5: Contraindications for using endometrial ablation techniques

❏ Presence of endometrial carcinoma or premalignant change of the endometrium (e.g. adenomatous hyperplasia)
❏ Patient with any anatomical or pathological condition associated with weakness of the myometrium (e.g. history of previous classical caesarean section or transmural myomectomy)
❏ A patient with active genital or urinary tract infection at the time of procedure (e.g. cervicitis, vaginitis, endometritis, salpingitis, or cystitis)
❏ A patient with an intrauterine device currently in place
❏ A patient who is pregnant or who wants to become pregnant in the future
❏ Postmenopausal women
❏ Women having congenital uterine anomalies (e.g. bicornuate uterus)
❏ A uterine cavity length , i.e. >10–12 cm

Box 64.6: Indications for hysterectomy in the presence of heavy menstrual bleeding

❏ Failure or non-suitability or denial of other treatment options by the woman
❏ Patient wishes for amenorrhoea
❏ Woman specifically requests hysterectomy
❏ Woman no longer wishes to retain her uterus and fertility

- In cases of HMB having significant impact on the woman's quality of life, due to presence of large fibroids (>3 cm in diameter), surgical procedures such as UAE, myomectomy or hysterectomy can be considered. For details kindly refer to Chapter 65 (Uterine Leiomyoma).

Hysterectomy

Hysterectomy should not be used as a first-line treatment specifically for HMB. It should be considered in the presence of indications listed in Box 64.6.

❖ While deciding the route of hysterectomy, the following factors need to be taken into account:[18] Presence of other gynaecological conditions or disease (e.g. endometriosis, fibroids, etc.), size and the number of fibroids if present, uterine size and mobility, descent of the uterus and vaginal access, size and shape of the vagina, history of previous surgery, skills and experience of the individual surgeon, etc.

❖ *Counselling related to the impact of surgery*: Though long-term satisfaction rates are higher with abdominal hysterectomy, it may be associated with significant mortality and morbidity.[19] This procedure should therefore be used only when the simpler less invasive alternatives have failed. Women offered hysterectomy should be fully counselled regarding the impact of surgery on their sexual feelings, expectations, fertility, psychological behaviour and bladder function, requirement for further treatment, probable complications of surgery, alternative options, etc. Women offered hysterectomy should also be informed about the increased risk of serious complications associated with hysterectomy in the presence of uterine fibroids, e.g. intraoperative haemorrhage, damage to adjacent abdominal organs, etc. Women should also be informed about the threat of likely loss of ovarian function and its consequences, even if their ovaries are retained at the time of hysterectomy.

❖ *Route of hysterectomy*: Following individual assessment of each patient for deciding the route of hysterectomy, the following order for the route should be considered: First choice of hysterectomy via vaginal route and second choice of hysterectomy via abdominal route. Vaginal hysterectomy is more cost-effective than the abdominal route and therefore must be preferred over abdominal hysterectomy wherever possible.[20,21] Vaginal hysterectomy is also likely to result in a quicker return to normal activities in comparison to abdominal hysterectomy. Laparoscopic hysterectomy serves as a lucrative alternative to the abdominal route. Laparoscopic approach proves useful in the presence of conditions such as morbid obesity or requirement for

CHAPTER 64

oophorectomy during vaginal hysterectomy. In these cases, laparoscopic approach should be considered and suitable expertise be sought.

However, laparoscopic hysterectomy may be associated with a greater risk of serious complications (e.g. risk of damaging the bladder or ureter) if the surgeon is not adequately trained in the technique. Therefore, surgeons embarking upon the procedure of laparoscopic hysterectomy should have acquired additional specialist training.

When the decision for abdominal hysterectomy has been taken, both the total method (removal of the uterus and the cervix) and subtotal method (removal of the uterus and preservation of the cervix) should be discussed with the woman. She should be counselled that subtotal hysterectomy is not likely to offer any long-term advantage over total hysterectomy. In fact, subtotal hysterectomy may be associated with continued menstrual bleeding even though there is a reduction in short-term morbidity.[22]

❖ *Removal of ovaries (oophorectomy) with hysterectomy*: Removal of healthy ovaries at the time of hysterectomy should not be undertaken. Removal of ovaries should only be undertaken with the express wish and consent of the woman after discussing with her the possible pros and cons of the procedure. If removal of ovaries is being considered, the impact of this on the woman's wellbeing and, e.g. the possible requirement for HRT in future should be discussed.

Women having a significant family history of breast or ovarian cancer should be referred for genetic counselling before taking a decision about oophorectomy. Women considering bilateral oophorectomy should be informed that this procedure is likely to reduce the risk of ovarian and breast cancer.

In women under the age of 45 years considering hysterectomy for HMB in the presence of symptoms related to ovarian dysfunction (e.g. premenstrual syndrome), a trial of pharmaceutical ovarian suppression for at least 3 months can be used as a guide to direct the requirement for oophorectomy.

COMPLICATIONS

Some complications associated with HMB per se are tabulated below:

❖ Severe anaemia
❖ Infertility (due to anovulatory HMB)
❖ *Social consequences*: Adverse effect on school or work performance
❖ Chronic pelvic pain (resulting from infection due to prolonged use of tampons)

❖ Depression
❖ Haemorrhagic shock (rarely due to massive bleeding)
❖ *Side effects related to endometrial ablation*: Uterine perforation, fluid overload, haemorrhage, infection, etc.

Complications associated with the particular methods used for management of HMB are tabulated in Table 64.1.

CLINICAL PEARLS

❖ All perimenopausal patients with persistent AUB should be evaluated with endometrial studies in order to exclude the presence of endometrial hyperplasia or carcinoma.
❖ Endometrial aspiration is a commonly used method of endometrial sampling, which can be performed as an outpatient procedure without any anaesthetic requirements.
❖ Measuring menstrual blood loss either directly (alkaline haematin) or indirectly (pictorial blood loss assessment chart) is not routinely recommended for HMB.
❖ Whether menstrual blood loss is a problem, should be determined not by measuring blood loss but by the woman herself.
❖ Use of endometrial ablation in women over the age of 45 years is associated with a reduced risk of further surgical intervention in future.
❖ Complications are more likely to occur with hysterectomy when it is performed in the presence of fibroids.
❖ Oophorectomy at the time of hysterectomy may result in menopausal-like symptoms.

EVIDENCE-BASED MEDICINE

❖ Though the second-generation methods of endometrial ablation are associated with a reduced risk of complications, there have been a few reports indicative of uterine perforation and thermal damage to the surrounding tissues. The available evidence indicates that such procedures must be carried out under TVS or hysteroscopic guidance, to ensure correct placement of the device. Additionally, myometrial thickness must be preassessed by ultrasound, especially in women with previous history of uterine surgery.[12-17]
❖ The available evidence supports the use of vaginal and laparoscopic routes over the abdominal route for hysterectomy. Nevertheless, appropriate individual assessment and skills and experience of the gynaecologist involved in the surgery must be considered before deciding the method of hysterectomy: laparoscopic, vaginal or abdominal.[18-21]

Table 64.1: Complications associated with the treatment method for heavy menstrual bleeding

Treatment method	Common (1 in 100 chance)	Rare (1 in 1,000 to 1 in 10,000 chance)
Levonorgestrel-releasing intrauterine system	Irregular bleeding (may last for >6 months), breast tenderness, acne or minor and transient headaches	Amenorrhoea, uterine perforation at the time of insertion
Tranexamic acid	Tiredness, stuffy nose, joint pain	Indigestion, diarrhoea, headaches
Non-steroidal anti-inflammatory drugs	Indigestion, diarrhoea	Worsening of asthma in sensitive individuals, peptic ulcers with possible bleeding and peritonitis
Combined oral contraceptives	Mood changes, headaches, nausea, fluid retention, breast tenderness	Deep vein thrombosis, stroke, heart attacks
Oral progestogen (norethisterone)	Weight gain, bloating, breast tenderness, headaches and acne. However, most of these side-effects are usually minor and transient	Depression
Injected progestogen	Weight gain, irregular bleeding, amenorrhoea, premenstrual-like syndrome (including bloating, fluid retention, breast tenderness)	Small loss of bone mineral density can occur. This is largely recovered when treatment is discontinued
Gonadotropin-releasing hormone analogue	Menopausal-like symptoms (such as hot flushes, increased sweating, vaginal dryness)	Osteoporosis, particularly trabecular bone with the use of >6 months
Endometrial ablation	Vaginal discharge, increased cramping, requirement for additional surgery	Perforation (very rare with second-generation techniques), uterine haemorrhage, haematometra, infection, urinary tract injuries, bowel injuries, perioperative hysterectomy, uterine cavity occlusion, cervical stenosis and postablation tubal sterilisation syndrome
Uterine artery embolisation	Persistent vaginal discharge, postembolisation syndrome, pain, nausea, vomiting and fever (not involving hospitalisation)	Haemorrhage; non-target embolisation causing tissue necrosis; infection causing septicaemia, requirement for additional surgery; premature ovarian failure particularly in women >45 years old; haematoma; etc.
Myomectomy	Excessive blood loss, resulting in anaemia (in an already compromised patient)	Haemorrhage, adhesions (which may lead to pain and/or impaired fertility); requirement for additional surgery; recurrence of fibroids; perforation (hysteroscopic route); infection, etc.
Hysterectomy	Infection	• Thrombosis (DVT and pulmonary embolism), intraoperative haemorrhage; damage to other abdominal organs, such as the urinary tract or bowel; urinary dysfunction (increased urinary frequency and incontinence) • Very rarely, death can also occur

REFERENCES

1. American College of Obstetricians and Gynecologists. ACOG committee opinion no. 557: Management of acute abnormal uterine bleeding in nonpregnant reproductive-aged women. Obstet Gynecol. 2013;121(4):891-6.
2. Committee on Practice Bulletins–Gynecology. Practice bulletin no. 128: Diagnosis of abnormal uterine bleeding in reproductive-aged women. Obstet Gynecol. 2012;120(1):197-206.
3. Munro MG, Critchley HO, Broder MS, Fraser IS, FIGO Working Group on Menstrual Disorders. FIGO classification system (PALM-COEIN) for causes of abnormal uterine bleeding in nongravid women of reproductive age. Int J Gynaecol Obstet. 2011;113(1):3-13.
4. Kouides PA, Conard J, Peyvandi F, Lukes A, Kadir R. Hemostasis and menstruation: appropriate investigation for underlying disorders of hemostasis in women with excessive menstrual bleeding. Fertil Steril. 2005;84(5):1345-51.
5. Farquhar C, Ekeroma A, Furness S, Arroll B. A systematic review of transvaginal ultrasonography, sonohysterography and hysteroscopy for investigation of abnormal uterine bleeding in premenopausal women. Acta Obstet Gynecol Scand. 2003;82(6):493-504.
6. Critchley HO, Warner P, Lee AJ, Brechin S, Guise J, Graham B. Evaluation of abnormal uterine bleeding: comparison of three outpatient procedures within cohorts defined by age and menopausal status. Health Technol Assess. 2004;8(34):1-139.
7. Cooper NA, Barton PM, Breijer M, Caffrey O, Opmeer BC, Timmermans A, et al. Cost-effectiveness of diagnostic strategies for the management of abnormal uterine bleeding (heavy menstrual bleeding and post-menopausal bleeding): a decision analysis. Health Technol Assess. 2014;18(24):1-201.
8. Lethaby A, Farquhar C. Treatments for heavy menstrual bleeding. BMJ. 2003;327(7426):1243-4.
9. National Institute of Clinical Excellence (NICE). (2014). Long-acting reversible contraception. [online] Available from www.nice.org.uk/guidance/cg30?unlid= 98242427720151231135. [Accessed September, 2016].
10. Munro MG, Mainor N, Basu R, Brisinger M, Barreda L. Oral medroxyprogesterone acetate and combination oral contraceptives for acute uterine bleeding: a randomized controlled trial. Obstet Gynecol. 2006;108(4):924-9.
11. James AH, Kouides PA, Abdul-Kadir R, Dietrich JE, Edlund M, Federici AB, et al. Evaluation and management of acute menorrhagia in women with and without underlying bleeding disorders: consensus from an international expert panel. Eur J Obstet Gynecol Reprod Biol. 2011;158(2):124-34.
12. Daniels JP, Middleton LJ, Champaneria R, Khan KS, Cooper K, Mol BWJ, et al. Second generation endometrial ablation

techniques for heavy menstrual bleeding: network meta-analysis. BMJ. 2012;344:e2564.

13. Madhu CK, Nattey J, Naeem T. Second generation endometrial ablation techniques: an audit of clinical practice. Arch Gynaecol Obstet. 2009;280(4):599-602.

14. Nichols CM, Gill EJ. Thermal balloon endometrial ablation for management of acute uterine hemorrhage. Obstet Gynecol. 2002;100(5 Pt 2):1092-4.

15. Loffer FD, Grainger D. Five-year follow-up of patients participating in a randomised trial of uterine balloon therapy versus rollerball ablation for treatment of menorrhagia. J Am Assoc Gynecol Laparosc. 2002;9(4):429-35.

16. Cooper KG, Bain C, Parkin DE. Comparison of microwave endometrial ablation and transcervical resection of the endometrium for treatment of heavy menstrual loss: a randomised trial. Lancet. 1999;354(9193):1859-63.

17. Overton C, Hargreaves J, Maresh M. A national survey of the complications of endometrial destruction for menstrual disorders: the MISTLETOE study. Minimally Invasive Surgical

Techniques--Laser, EndoThermal or Endorescetion. Br J Obstet Gynaecol. 1997;104(12):1351-9.

18. Kovac SR, Barhan S, Lister M, Tucker L, Bishop M, Das A. Guidelines for the selection of the route of hysterectomy: application in a resident clinic population. Am J Obstet Gynecol. 2002;187(6):1521-7.

19. Aarts JW, Nieboer TE, Johnson N, Tavender E, Garry R, Mol BJ, et al. Surgical approach to hysterectomy for benign gynaecological disease. Cochrane Database Syst Rev. 2015;(8):CD003677.

20. Dorsey JH, Holtz PM, Griffiths RI, McGrath MM, Steinberg EP. Costs and charges associated with three alternative techniques of hysterectomy. N Engl J Med. 1996;335(7):476-82.

21. ACOG Committee Opinion No. 444: choosing the route of hysterectomy for benign disease. Obstet Gynecol. 2009;114(5):1156-8.

22. American College of Obstetricians and Gynecologists. ACOG Committee Opinion No. 388: supracervical hysterectomy. Obstet Gynecol. 2007;110(5):1215-7.

Uterine Leiomyomas

INTRODUCTION

Uterine leiomyomas (uterine myomas, fibromyomas or fibroids) are well-circumscribed benign tumours developing from uterine myometrium, most commonly encountered amongst women of reproductive age group (30–44 years). A typical myoma is a pale, firm, rubbery, well-circumscribed mass distinct from neighbouring tissues and has a whorled appearance due to presence of interlacing fibres of myometrial muscle, surrounded by a connective tissue capsule. There are three types of fibroids (Fig. 65.1). Of the different types of fibroids, the most common are intramural or interstitial fibroids (which are present within the uterine myometrium), followed by submucosal fibroids (which grow beneath the uterine endometrial lining) and subserosal fibroids (which grow beneath the uterine serosa).[1]

AETIOLOGY

Though the process through which fibroid formation is initiated is yet not clear, it is believed that this process is dependent on hormones. Also the presence of increased levels of receptors for both oestrogen and progesterone in the uterine myometrium are likely to trigger the development of fibroids. Several growth factors are also likely to have a role in mediating the growth of fibroids. Various risk factors, which can result in the development of fibroids, are as follows:

❖ *Heredity*: Patient with a positive family history of fibroid, especially in the first-degree relatives (mother or sister) is at an increased risk of developing fibroids.
❖ *Race*: Black women are more likely to have fibroids than the women of other racial groups.
❖ *High oestrogen levels*: Some factors, which may be responsible for an increased risk of fibroids related to hyper-oestrogenism, are described next.

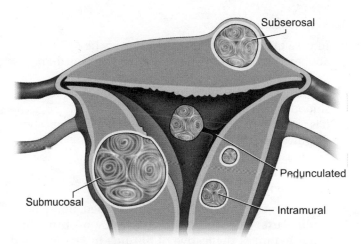

Fig. 65.1: Different types of fibroids

• *Long-term use of OCPs and Depo-Provera*: Exposure to OCPs at the age of 13–16 years is likely to be associated with an increased risk.
• Obesity increases the risk probably due to higher levels of endogenous oestrogens.
• *Parity*: Child-bearing during the reproductive years (24–29 years) provides the greatest protection against myoma development by producing amenorrhoea (thereby reduced oestrogen levels) during pregnancy. Nulliparity is, therefore, associated with an increased risk of fibroids.
❖ *Pelvic inflammatory disease*: There is a positive association between fibroids and pelvic inflammatory disease.
❖ Smoking.

DIAGNOSIS

Clinical Presentation

❖ *Heavy menstrual bleeding*: The main symptom attributable to leiomyomas is heavy menstrual bleeding (HMB), which has replaced the previously used term, menorrhagia. The blood loss is usually heaviest on day 2nd or 3rd of the menstrual periods. Submucosal and intramural fibroids, which cause distortion of the uterine cavity, are likely to result in HMB. There is little evidence that subserosal or pedunculated fibroids can also contribute to heavy menstrual loss. For details, kindly refer to Chapter 64 (Abnormal Uterine Bleeding).

❖ *Anaemia*: Excessive bleeding, if remains untreated over a long period of time, can result in the development of anaemia.[2]

❖ *Other symptoms*: These may include symptoms such as urinary symptoms, low backache, rectal tenesmus and constipation.

❖ *Abdominal pain*: Fibroids are usually not painful.

❖ *Infertility*: Uterine fibroids could be responsible for infertility by interfering with the implantation of the fertilised ovum, due to distortion of the endometrial cavity and disturbances of ovulation.

Abdominal Examination

❖ In case of a large fibroid, the mass may be palpable per abdomen and usually appears to be arising from the pelvis, i.e. it may be difficult to get below the mass.

❖ It is usually well defined, having a firm consistency and a smooth surface.

❖ It is usually movable from side to side, but not from above downwards.

❖ The mass is nearly always dull to percussion.

Pelvic Examination

❖ Presence of an enlarged, irregularly shaped, non-tender, mobile uterus with firm consistency on bimanual examination is suggestive of fibroids in women aged 30–40 years.

❖ The tumour is found to either replace the uterus or be attached to the cervix.

Investigations

The following investigations are required in a patient presenting with leiomyomas:

❖ *Complete blood count along with platelet count and a peripheral smear*: To rule out anaemia and coagulation disorder

❖ *Ultrasound examination*: Ultrasound examination (both TVS and TAS) has become the investigation of choice for diagnosing myomas. Ultrasound examination can help in assessing the size, location and number of uterine fibroids (Figs 65.2 to 65.4). TVS is the gold standard investigation in the presence of fibroids.[3] TAS may be required in cases where the uterus is palpable per abdominally (uterine size >12 weeks).[4] It is important to note the number, position and the size of each individual fibroid. It is also important to document the overall uterine dimensions and the condition of the ovaries and adjacent adnexa.

❖ *Magnetic resonance imaging*: Though the use of MRI is not routinely recommended due to its high cost, it is useful in mapping the size and location of leiomyomas and in

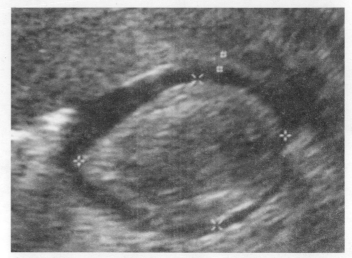

Fig. 65.2: Visualisation of intracavitary fibroids on saline infusion sonography

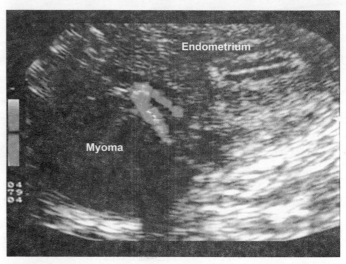

Fig. 65.3: Colour Doppler shows presence of subserosal fibroids with peripheral vascularisation *(For colour version, see Plate 4)*

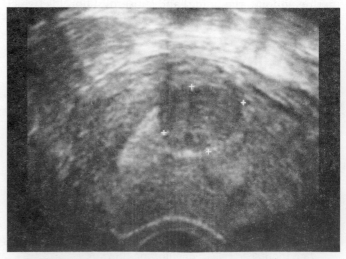

Fig. 65.4: Submucous fibroid protruding inside the endometrial cavity

accurately identifying adenomyosis. MRI may be used in cases where the clinician is doubtful about the nature of fibroid mass or to assess its suitability for performing uterine artery embolisation (UAE).

❖ *Ruling out presence of malignancy*: In case the patient has risk factors for endometrial cancer or she is in the peri-menopausal age group or gives history of intermenstrual and postcoital bleeding, endometrial biopsy and Pap smear are required to rule out carcinoma endometrium and carcinoma cervix, respectively.

❖ *Hysteroscopy and saline infusion sonography*: These investigations may be useful in cases of submucosal fibroids for improving the diagnostic accuracy.[5]

DIFFERENTIAL DIAGNOSIS

❖ Various causes of HMB, which need to be excluded, have been described previously in Chapter 64 (Abnormal Uterine Bleeding).

❖ Various causes of uterine enlargement, which may be mistaken for fibroids and need to be excluded, include pregnancy, adenomyosis, benign ovarian tumour, etc.

MANAGEMENT

Women with asymptomatic uterine fibroids do not require any treatment. Treatment options for symptomatic fibroids are listed in Flow chart 65.1.[6]

Conservative Treatment

Most women with uterine fibroids do not require any treatment. These tumours are usually less than 3 cm in size and do not cause distortion of the uterine cavity. These fibroids are either asymptomatic or associated with symptoms (such as pelvic pain or HMB), which can be controlled with common medications such as over-the-counter pain medication for control of pain and iron supplements in presence of symptoms related to anaemia. Patient counselling and education forms an important component of the conservative management and comprises the following:

❖ The patient must be reassured that the bleeding related to fibroids is a common, benign cause of bleeding and nothing to worry about.

❖ Patient must be provided information regarding various treatment options, including the probable expectations and adverse effects. They must be reassured that in case she experiences failure with one treatment option, other options are available, which can be used.

❖ Patient must be periodically assessed with either pelvic examination or ultrasound examination to determine whether fibroids are changing in size or if she is developing symptoms that would require surgical treatment. Periodic assessment is especially important if the patient is planning a pregnancy.

❖ *Advice to maintain a menstrual calendar*: Women who have abnormal blood loss must be encouraged to chart their menstrual blood loss every month. Amount of bleeding (scanty, moderate and heavy) and occurrence of menstrual cramps and pain must also be noted.

Medical Management

Though the definitive treatment for uterine fibroids is surgery, medical therapy is sometimes instituted with the following aims:

❖ Alleviation of symptoms

Flow chart 65.1: Treatment options for a patient diagnosed with fibroid uterus

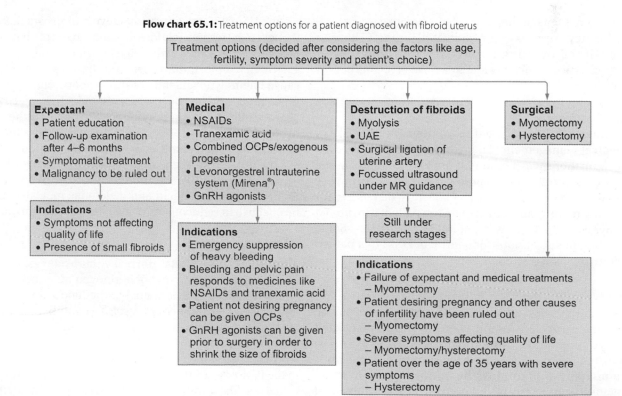

Abbreviations: GnRH, genadotropin-releasing hormone; NSAIDs, non-steroidal anti-inflammatory drugs; OCPs, oral contraceptive pills; UAE, uterine artery embolisation

CHAPTER 65

Flow chart 65.2: Management plan of a patient with fibroid uterus presenting with heavy menstrual bleeding (HMB)

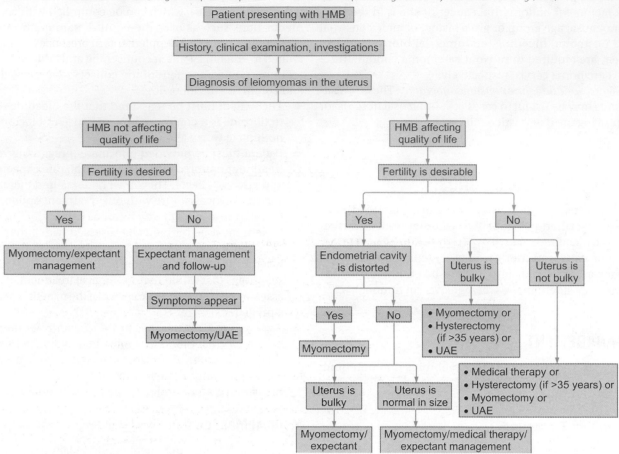

Abbreviation: UAE, uterine artery embolisation

- ❖ Improvement of haemoglobin status before surgery
- ❖ Emergency suppression of heavy bleeding (This can be achieved by using norethisterone 15 mg/day or medroxyprogesterone acetate in a dose of 30 mg/day for 3 weeks)
- ❖ Minimising the size and vascularity of uterine fibroids prior to surgery.

If the uterus is not enlarged more than 10–12 weeks in size, medical management can be initiated in primary care. However, further investigations must be initiated. On the other hand, if there is no response to medical therapy or uterus is more than 12 weeks in size, she must be referred for further assessment. Management plan in a patient with fibroid presenting with HMB is described in Flow chart 65.2. Some medical therapeutic options for control of HMB in a patient with leiomyoma are discussed next.

Prostaglandin Synthetase Inhibitors

Non-steroidal anti-inflammatory drugs (typically mefenamic acid) may be particularly useful when bleeding is associated with pelvic pain and dysmenorrhoea. Various NSAIDs, including mefenamic acid, have been shown to significantly reduce menstrual blood loss by inhibiting the enzyme prostaglandin synthetase, which is involved in production of prostaglandins.

Imbalance between various levels of prostaglandins is thought to be responsible for the pathogenesis of menorrhagia. Side effects associated with their use include nausea, vomiting, gastric discomfort, diarrhoea and dizziness. Rarely, it can cause haemolytic anaemia or thrombocytopenia. However, mefenamic acid has been observed to be less effective than haemostatic agents (tranexamic acid) in reducing the amount of blood loss (20% vs 54%), but in general, it has a lower side effect profile. Mefenamic acid is administered in the dose of 500 mg TDS during menses. Other analgesic drugs belonging to the class of NSAIDs, including drugs like naprosyn, ibuprofen, indomethacin and diclofenac may also prove to be effective in reducing pelvic pain and dysmenorrhoea.

Haemostatic Agents

Tranexamic acid: Under normal circumstances, clotting of blood requires conversion of fibrinogen into fibrin. Fibrinolytic substances (fibrinolysins) in the blood are responsible for breakdown of blood clot, resulting in prolonged bleeding. Haemostatic agents like tranexamic acid help in reducing the blood loss by inhibiting this fibrinolytic activity, thereby sealing the bleeding vessels. Tranexamic acid is administered in the IV dosage of 10–15 mg/kg body weight, 2–3 times a day or 0.5–1 g/day orally in divided doses, leading to a total of 3–6 g/day for the first 3 days of the cycle. Side effects due to tranexamic acid are dose-related and may include symptoms like nausea, vomiting, diarrhoea and dizziness. Rarely, there may be transient colour vision disturbance or intracranial thrombosis. This drug has now been approved by the United States Food and Drug Administration (USFDA) for treatment of heavy bleeding. In the UK, tranexamic acid is used in preference to NSAIDs for the first-line management of patients with fibroids with HMB.

Etamsylate: This is another haemostatic drug, which helps in achieving haemostasis by reducing capillary bleeding. It helps in increasing the capillary wall strength and increasing platelet adhesion. It is used orally in the dosage of 250–500 mg three times a day.

Gonadotropin-releasing Hormone Agonists

Gonadotropin-releasing hormone agonists can be considered as the most effective medical therapy for uterine myomas.

Mode of action: GnRH is produced by the hypothalamus and stimulates the release of the gonadotropins like FSH and LH by the pituitary gland. These hormones then trigger the ovary to secrete hormones like oestrogen and progesterone, which in turn stimulate ovarian follicular development. Administration of GnRH agonists simulate the action of GnRH in the body. However, continuous exposure to GnRH agonists desensitise the pituitary gonadotrophs resulting in loss of gonadotropin release, thereby causing a reduction in oestrogen production. Therefore, following an initial gonadotropin release associated with rising oestradiol levels, gonadotropin levels eventually fall off to castrate levels, with resultant hypogonadism. As a result, due to the use of GnRH agonists, medical oophorectomy or medical menopause is produced. Most women with fibroids will develop amenorrhoea, improvement in anaemia (if present) and a significant reduction in uterine size within 3 months of initiating this therapy.

Treatment with GnRH agonists, by reducing oestrogen production may cause nearly 50% reduction in the initial volume of the myoma within 3 months of therapy.[7] Maximum fibroid shrinkage usually occurs after 3 months of treatment. Therefore, GnRH agonist treatment should be restricted to a 3–6-month interval. GnRH agonists are at times prescribed before surgery for uterine fibroids. They help in reducing the blood loss at the time of surgery by shrinking the tumour size, thereby eliminating the need for blood transfusions at the time of surgery. This form of medical castration is also effective in inducing amenorrhoea in patients with dysfunctional uterine bleeding by breaking the ongoing cycle of abnormal bleeding in many anovulatory patients. Use of GnRH agonists in woman of childbearing age can help to shrink the size of fibroid tumours, thereby eliminating the need for a hysterectomy, thus preserving fertility. Alternatively, their use may allow a simpler surgical procedure like laparoscopic hysterectomy, thereby avoiding abdominal surgery. Long-term use of GnRH therapy is likely to have an adverse effect on bones resulting in bone loss. There is a scope for the long-term use of GnRH agonists with the use of hormone add-back therapy. GnRH agonists in combination with low-dose HRT can be used for obtaining long-term relief from HMB related to fibroids in women in whom surgery is contraindicated or declined, and other medical methods have failed.[8] Before the administration of HRT is begun, the clinician must ensure that GnRH agonists had been administered alone for 3 months to ensure the shrinkage of fibroids. Various options of HRT, which have been tried, include low-dose combination of oral oestrogens and progestogens; progestogens alone and tibolone.[9]

Exogenous Progestins and Oral Contraceptive Agents

Use of exogenous progestins is not likely to bring about a reduction in the size of fibroids. Exogenous progestins, however, may help in providing relief against the HMB associated with leiomyomas, especially if administered continuously for 21 out of 28 days. Progestogen-releasing intrauterine devices [levonorgestrel-releasing intrauterine system (LNG-IUS)] may be beneficial for controlling HMB associated with fibroids. However, there is an associated risk of expulsion with the use of this device. The LNG-IUS is described in details later in the text. Long-term use of depot medroxyprogesterone acetate is likely to provide some protection against the development of fibroids.[10] However, its role in the protection against fibroid-associated HMB presently remains unclear.

Some studies continue to suggest that oestrogen-progestin contraceptive pills are contraindicated in women with uterine leiomyomas because these pills are likely to cause uterine enlargement. However, most clinicians feel that use of OCPs can partially suppress oestrogen stimulation, reducing the growth of uterine fibroids resulting in long-term protection. It is difficult to determine the effectiveness of both exogenous progestins and OCPs in the treatment of leiomyoma-associated symptoms. This might serve as a useful option for women with fibroids desiring contraception.

Levonorgestrel Intrauterine System

Levonorgestrel intrauterine system (Mirena®) was initially developed as a highly effective and reversible method of contraception. However, its use has also been observed to provide excellent reduction in the amount of menstrual blood loss.[11,12] LNG-IUS helps in reducing the amount of menstrual blood loss by causing the local release of the progestogen, levonorgestrel within the uterine cavity. However, use of LNG-IUS is likely to be associated with a high expulsion rate (6–13%) in comparison to the rate of 3% in the general population.[13] Women should be warned about this risk before they start using LNG-IUS. The dose of progestogen released within the uterine cavity is equivalent to two progestogen only tablets each week (which is approximately equivalent to 15–20 µg of levonorgestrel per day). This dose of progesterone helps in thinning the endometrial lining, thereby helping in considerably reducing the volume of menstrual blood loss. Menstrual bleeding may eventually stop while the IUS is in place. The device has now been approved by the FDA for control of HMB. Another added advantage of using IUS is that it provides effective contraception for a period of 5 years and must be removed or replaced after the expiry of this period. However, IUS should not be used in presence of large uterine fibroids (>3 cm), which cause distortion of the uterine cavity.

CHAPTER 65

Use of IUS can result in the development of side effects like change in menstrual bleeding pattern such as frequent, prolonged or heavy bleeding; spotting, light, scanty bleeding, irregular bleeding or cessation of bleeding; development of ovarian cysts; weight gain; oedema; headache; depression; nervousness; mood swings; nausea; pain including lower abdominal pain, back pain, breast pain, dysmenorrhoea; acne; and vaginal discharge including cervicitis, genital infections, etc. Other side effects related to the use of IUS include the following:

❖ Breakthrough bleeding in the first few cycles
❖ 20% develop amenorrhoea within 1 year
❖ Presence of functional ovarian cysts
❖ High risk of expulsion.

Antiprogestins and Progesterone Receptor Modulators

Since progesterone appears to be capable of stimulating growth of the uterine fibroids, antiprogestins like mifepristone and progesterone receptor modulators can help in reducing fibroid growth. Mifepristone is the most widely used antiprogestin and is thought to cause a reduction in the size of leiomyomas comparable to that caused by GnRH.[14] It is administered in the dose of 5–50 mg once a day for a period of 3–6 months and is not currently approved by the USFDA for the treatment of myomas. The main impediment to its off-label use is that currently available doses (200 mg) are not appropriate. The primary concern with the use of both these agents is the potential for an increased risk for endometrial cancer or hyperplasia. Ulipristal acetate is a selective progesterone receptor modulator that inhibits ovulation, but has little impact on serum oestradiol levels. It is thought to cause a reduction in uterine size in cases of fibroid uterus.[15-17] However, the available dose is the main impediment to its off-label treatment.

Selective Oestrogen Receptor Modulators

Some studies have shown that the use of selective oestrogen receptor modulators (SERMs) (e.g. raloxifene) help in reducing the size of fibroids and improving clinical outcomes.[18] However, well-designed, randomised studies in future are required to establish definite evidence regarding the benefit of SERMs in treating women with uterine fibroids.

Danazol

This is an androgenic agonist, with strong antigonadotropic activity, due to which it can inhibit LH and FSH. As a result, it can suppress fibroid growth but is also associated with a high rate of adverse effects such as weight gain, acne, hirsutism, oedema, hair loss, deepening of voice, flushing, sweating, vaginal dryness, etc. and is thus often less acceptable to patients. Another androgenic drug, gestrinone decreases myoma volume and induces amenorrhoea in women with leiomyomas. Androgenic side effects with gestrinone are fewer in comparison with danazol. An advantage of this drug is that there is a carry-over effect after it is discontinued. Gestrinone can be considered as a potentially useful short-term management option.

Surgical Treatment

Presently, the main modality of curative treatment in a patient with leiomyomas is surgery and acts as a definitive cure. Indications for surgery in patients with myomas are tabulated in Box 65.1. If the woman has completed her family and does not wish to preserve her uterus, hysterectomy can be done.[19] Myomectomy is an option for women who desire future pregnancy or wish to preserve their uterus.

❖ Hysterectomy: It can be performed in three ways: (1) abdominally, (2) vaginally, and in some cases (3) laparo-scopically.
❖ Myomectomy: Surgical removal of myomas from the uterine cavity is termed as myomectomy. Myomectomy can be performed abdominally, laparoscopically or hysteroscopically.[20] Laparotomy remains the preferred route for myomectomies performed in specialist centres and is associated with low morbidity and favourable outcomes for subsequent pregnancies.[21]
❖ The advantages of hysteroscopic and laparoscopic myo-mectomy are that they can be performed as an outpatient procedure and allow faster recovery in comparison to conventional abdominal laparotomy.
❖ Hysteroscopic myomectomy (Figs 65.5A to C) forms the procedure of choice for completely submucosal myomas (T-0) or those myomas having less than 50% extension into the myometrium (T-I myomas).[22] However, hysteroscopic resection should not normally be attempted in fibromyomas belonging to T-II category (Fig. 65.6).[23] This is so because, when submucous myomas have intramural extensions greater than 50%, hysteroscopic resection may be associated with a higher rate of complications (Box 65.2), including increased rate of conversion to laparotomy, higher rates of intravascular extravasation of distending media, prolonged operating times and increased requirement for repeat surgery. This procedure serves as an effective approach for providing relief from HMB associated with submucous fibroids. Effectiveness of treatment, especially in cases of HMB can be further increased by concurrent endometrial ablation in cases not desiring future fertility.

Uterine Artery Embolisation

Uterine artery embolisation is a relatively new, novel technique for the treatment of uterine fibroids, which was first performed by Ravina, a French gynaecologist in 1995.[24]

> **Box 65.1:** Indications for surgery in patients with myomas
>
> ❑ Presence of large fibroids (>3 cm in diameter)
> ❑ Severe bleeding, having a significant impact on a woman's quality of life, which is refractory to drug therapy
> ❑ Persistent or intolerable pain or pressure
> ❑ Urinary or intestinal symptoms due to presence of a large myoma
> ❑ History of infertility and future pregnancy is desired
> ❑ History of recurrent spontaneous abortions and future pregnancy is desired
> ❑ Rapid enlargement of a myoma (especially after menopause) raising the suspicion of leiomyosarcoma (a rare cause)

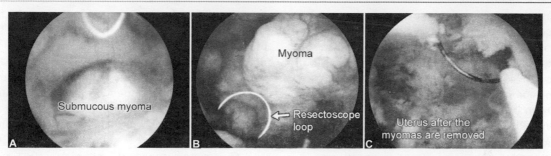

Figs 65.5A to C: Hysteroscopic myomectomy: (A) Hysteroscopic view showing presence of a submucous fibroid; (B) Beginning of the hysteroscopic resection of submucous fibroid; (C) Completion of the hysteroscopic resection of submucous fibroid *(For colour version, see Plate 4)*

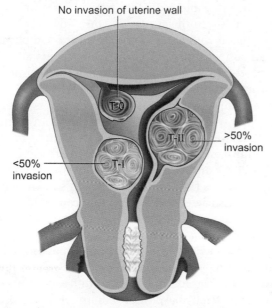

Fig. 65.6: European Society of Hysteroscopy classification of myomas

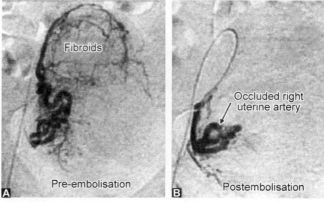

Figs 65.7A and B: Arteriogram showing embolisation of the right uterine vessels: (A) Pre-embolisation arteriogram showing increased blood supply to the fibroids; (B) Postembolisation arteriogram showing occluded blood supply to the fibroids (indicated by the arrow)

Box 65.2: Complications related to hysteroscopic myomectomy

❑ Severe intraoperative bleeding, requiring an emergency hysterectomy
❑ Electrical burns to the genital tract, bowel, etc.
❑ Hyponatraemia, blindness, coma and death from excessive absorption of irrigant fluid have also been reported
❑ Fluid imbalance may occur with prolonged surgical procedures. Therefore, careful monitoring of irrigant fluid balance is required
❑ The fertility and pregnancy outcomes following hysteroscopic myomectomy appear to be similar to those following laparoscopic and abdominal myomectomies

---

UAE is a non-hysterectomy surgical technique, which helps in reducing the size of the uterine fibroids by shrinking them, without actually removing them. Besides uterine fibroids, the technique of embolisation has been used to treat various other medical pathologies like inoperable cancers, brain aneurysms, arteriovenous shunts in the lung, etc. The procedure of UAE itself lasts between 1 hour and 2 hours. Though general anaesthesia is usually not required, the procedure is usually performed under sedation or local anaesthesia. In this technique, the interventional radiologist introduces and manipulates a catheter through the femoral artery into the internal iliac and uterine arteries (Figs 65.7A and B).[25] Once the fibroids are visualised on X-ray, an embolising agent [gelatin microspheres (trisacryl gelatin) or polyvinyl alcohol] is injected, which helps in blocking both the uterine arteries, thereby cutting off the blood supply to the fibroids. Compared to normal uterine cells, fibroid cells are much more sensitive to low oxygen saturation. Thus, due to the lack of sufficient blood supply, the fibroids become avascular and shrink, ultimately resulting in cell death, their degeneration and eventual absorption by the myometrium. Within a period of 6 months, there is nearly 60% shrinkage in the size of fibroid. The normal myometrium, on the other hand, receives new blood supply from vaginal and ovarian vasculature. As fibroids begin to undergo necrosis, any active bleeding commonly subsides. The dying cells of the fibroids may release toxins, which may cause irritation to the surrounding tissues, thereby causing pain and inflammation in the first few days following the procedure. Though the rate of recovery usually varies from one woman to the other, it usually takes a few months for the fibroids to fully shrink and the full effect of the procedure to be evident. Nearly 6–9 months after UAE, there is 50% reduction in the median measured menstrual blood loss.[26]

Complications associated with UAE are usually minor and may include complications such as local haematomas at the puncture site, urinary retention, postembolisation syndrome

CHAPTER 65

(low-grade fever, leucocytosis, increasing pelvic pain and a vaginal discharge following UAE) malaise, nausea and exhaustion, infection, transcervical fibroid tissue passage, etc.

Total radiation exposure following UAE is similar to that of one to two CT scans or barium enemas. Management of pain following the procedure may require a 1-day hospital stay, followed by 1–2 weeks of NSAIDs medications. Most women return to normal activity within 1–3 weeks. Major complications such as pulmonary embolism, arterial thrombosis, groin haematomas, local infections, guidewire perforation of arteries, allergic reaction to contrast medium, endometritis, ischaemia of pelvic organs, sepsis and death are rare events with UAE. The 3-month complication rate following UAE may result in the requirement for hysterectomy in a small group of women.[27] These may occur in approximately 0.5% cases of embolisation performed for symptomatic fibroids. UAE has been found to be associated with numerous fertility-related complications including increased rate of miscarriage and abnormal placentation during pregnancy.

Effect on fertility: The ovaries may stop functioning in about 5% of the women following embolisation and early menopause may result. This may be a particularly devastating complication for young patients who wish to conceive in future. The ovarian function may cease due to reduced blood supply. The blood supply to the ovaries may be blocked off due to misembolisation or as a result of the blockage of uterine artery in women in whom the main blood vessels supplying the ovaries branches off from the uterine artery. As a result, if the uterine artery is blocked, the blood supply to the ovary is also blocked off and the ovaries may cease functioning.

Pregnancy outcomes: Though this procedure helps in preserving the uterus, pregnancies following UAE have been reported to be at higher risk in comparison to the general population. Till date, there have been limited number of pregnancies following UAE. Therefore, there is limited evidence regarding the pregnancy outcomes following UAE. UAE is likely to be associated with a live birth rate of 57.8% in comparison to the birth rate of 77.4% after myomectomy.[28] The risk of various complications such as miscarriages, placenta praevia, placental abruption and pre-eclampsia has been found to be similar with both the procedures. However, the risk of complications such as preterm delivery and PPH was significantly increased in women who conceived after UAE. More evidence from randomised trials is required before UAE can be offered as a choice of treatment for fibroids in women wishing to preserve their fertility.[28] As a result, the women who wish to conceive in future are not recommended to use UAE as treatment option for their fibroids.

Risk of underlying malignancy: No samples are sent for biopsy in UAE; therefore, any underlying malignancy is likely to remain undetected. However, this is unlikely to cause any problem because the chances of malignancy in cases of fibroids are extremely low.

Presently, there is limited evidence regarding the safety and efficacy of the procedure. The worldwide success rate of the procedure in causing improvement of symptoms has been considered to be approximately 85%. UAE may be the right treatment choice for women in whom the symptomatic relief may be obtained by shrinking the fibroids to a little more than half their present size. However, UAE may not be very helpful for women with extremely large fibroids because they may not shrink enough to make a significant difference in the symptoms. The women with larger uteri and/or more number of leiomyomas are likely to be associated with high failure rates.

A Cochrane review by Gupta et al. (2012) including five randomised control trials comparing UAE with surgery (abdominal hysterectomy or myomectomy) has shown that the procedure of UAE is associated with shorter duration of hospital stay and a quicker return to routine activities in comparison to the surgery.[29] UAE, however, is likely to be associated with a higher rate of minor complications in comparison with surgery. Moreover, there is an increased likelihood for requirement of surgical intervention within 2–5 years of the initial procedure of UAE. There is limited evidence suggesting that myomectomy is likely to be associated with better fertility outcomes in comparison to UAE. However, further research is required in this area. A UK multicentre retrospective cohort study comparing hysterectomy and UAE for the treatment of symptomatic uterine fibroids (HOPEFUL study) has shown that UAE is likely to be associated with fewer complications in comparison to hysterectomy. Nevertheless, minor side effects are likely to occur following embolisation. However, hysterectomy is likely to be associated with better symptomatic improvement. Nearly 25% of women having UAE were likely to require further treatment for fibroid symptoms. Both treatments appear to be safe and effective over the medium term, and the choice of treatment depends on the clinical circumstances and personal preference for each individual woman.[30] In women of reproductive age groups, choice between myomectomy and UAE is related to the prospects for future pregnancy.

While the procedure of UAE, due to its non-invasive nature, is associated with several advantages such as a significant reduction in the length of the hospital stay and 24-hour pain level, and a rapid return to normal activities, its use needs to be weighed against the several disadvantages associated with the procedure. This mainly includes the risk for the requirement of a second intervention in almost one-third of patients. The choice should therefore be based on the clinical circumstances and the patient's decision.[31-33]

Focussed Ultrasound for Treatment of Fibroids

This is another new technique for destruction of fibroids, which is still under the research stages. In this technique, ultrasound energy, which uses high-frequency energy in the form of sound waves, is used for destroying fibroids.[34] This energy can be focussed on a single point inside a patient's body (e.g. on a fibroid) so that the heat created by the energy is able to destroy the fibroid cells by causing coagulative necrosis. Since the technique uses MRI to focus the ultrasound waves, hence the term 'magnetic resonance-guided focussed ultrasound (MRgFUS)' is used to describe this technique.

Still in its early stages of development, focussed ultrasound is a non-invasive alternative to treat fibroids. The use of focussed ultrasound is associated with very low risk and rapid recovery. However, presently, there is limited evidence regarding the safety and efficacy of the procedure; therefore, it is not recommended for women desiring future fertility.[35] In future, with the improvement in technology, MRgFUS would probably serve as a proven alternative for women with symptomatic fibroids.

ExAblate 2000 system is a new device, approved by the FDA, based on MRgFUS technique, which serves as a non-invasive method for treating fibroids, while retaining the uterus. Though the device has been shown to successfully treat fibroid related HMB in nearly 70% of the women within 6 months of treatment, the remaining 30% have been observed to require an alternative surgical treatment for fibroids within a year.[36] This implies that while the ExAblate treatment may succeed in reducing the symptoms from the treated fibroids, there may be a recurrence of fibroids in some women, thereby requiring an additional treatment with either ExAblate or an alternative treatment modality. The device labelling indicates that no more than two treatments should be performed in a 2-week period. The maximum size of fibroids that can be treated with this method is not yet known. Symptomatic improvement is observed within the first 3 months following this procedure and this improvement has been found to be maintained at least through 24–36-month follow-up. Increasing amount of experience with this method has been found to be associated with a lower incidence of adverse events. The procedure is time-consuming and costly, but short-term morbidity is low and recovery is rapid. Good quality trials are required in the future to determine long-term outcome and optimal candidates for this procedure.

COMPLICATIONS

❖ Heavy menstrual bleeding [For details, kindly refer to Chapter 64 (Abdominal Uterine Bleeding)]
❖ Severe pain, anaemia
❖ Infertility
❖ Toxic shock syndrome
❖ *Torsion*: Torsion of the pedicle of a subserous pedunculated leiomyoma may interfere first with venous, then with the arterial supply.
❖ *Ascites or pseudo-Meigs syndrome*: Very mobile, pedunculated subserous tumours may produce ascites by causing mechanical irritation of the peritoneum. Sometimes, ascites may be accompanied by a right-sided hydrothorax, resulting in pseudo-Meigs syndrome.
❖ *Infection*: A submucous leiomyoma may sometimes become infected and ulcerated at its lower pole.
❖ *Complications related to treatment options*: Treatment options by themselves [medication or surgery (hysterectomy or myomectomy) or UAE may be associated with their own inherent complications].[37]

❖ *Secondary changes (degenerative changes)*:
  • *Atrophy*: Shrinkage of the fibroid can occur as a result of reduced blood supply of the fibroid, usually following menopause.
  • *Hyaline degeneration*: This is the most common type of degeneration in which a homogeneous substance that stains pink with eosin replaces the fibrous tissue cells.
  • *Calcification*: This is characterised by the deposition of phosphates and carbonates of calcium along the course of blood vessels, usually starting at the periphery.
  • Myxomatous or cystic degeneration
  • *Red or carneous degeneration*: This type of degeneration of uterine fibroid usually develops during pregnancy and must be managed conservatively. It may be associated with constitutional symptoms like malaise, nausea, vomiting, fever and severe abdominal pain.
  • *Sarcomatous change*: Occurrence of malignant changes in a leiomyoma is an extremely rare occurrence, occurring in only about 0.2% of tumours.

CLINICAL PEARLS

❖ Women suffering from leiomyomas, especially those in the perimenopausal group, who have continuous or irregular bleeding, should be subjected to a thorough endometrial evaluation in order to rule out the presence of endometrial cancer.
❖ The nearer the leiomyomas are to the endometrial cavity, the more likely are they to produce HMB.
❖ Conservative management is offered to perimenopausal women with symptomatic fibroids. This treatment strategy is based on the assumption that these symptoms are likely to resolve on their own as the woman reaches menopause.
❖ Most fibroids remain uncomplicated during pregnancy. Some possible adverse effects related to the presence of fibroids during pregnancy include abortion, preterm labour, PPROM, placental abruption, IUGR, malpresentation, obstructed labour, caesarean section, caesarean hysterectomy, PPH, etc.

EVIDENCE-BASED MEDICINE

❖ Presently, there are no randomised trials regarding the use of OCPs for controlling HMB associated with fibroids. One observation study, however, has demonstrated nearly 50% reduction in the amount of menstrual blood loss with the use of high-dose OCPs in a woman with clinically diagnosed fibroids. This reduction in blood loss was statistically significant.[38]
❖ There is limited evidence to indicate that both the continuous combined HRT preparations and tibolone serve as an effective add-back therapy, which helps in reducing bone loss in women with fibroids undergoing long-term treatment with GnRH agonists.[8] Similar treatment strategy involving the use of oral combined HRT preparations or tibolone and conservative management of fibroids can be employed in postmenopausal women with fibroids.[9]

REFERENCES

1. DeCherney AH, Nathan L. Current Obstetric and Gynecologic Diagnosis and Treatment, 9th edition. New York: McGraw-Hill Medical; 2003.
2. Cohen BJ, Gibor Y. Anemia and menstrual blood loss. Obstet Gynecol Surv. 1980;35(10):597-618.
3. Mendelson EB, Bohm-Velez M, Joseph N, Neiman HL. Endometrial abnormalities: evaluation with transvaginal sonography. AJR Am J Roentgenol. 1988;150(1):139-42.
4. Cicinelli E, Romano F, Anastastio PS. Transabdominal sonohysterography, transvaginal sonography and hysteroscopy in the evaluation of submucous myomas. Obstet Gynecol. 1995;85(1):42-7.
5. Towbin NA, Gviazda IM, March CM. Office hysteroscopy versus transvaginal ultrasound in the evaluation of patients with excessive uterine bleeding. Am J Obstet Gynecol. 1996;174(6):1678-82.
6. Farquhar C, Arroll B, Ekeroma A, Fentiman G, Lethaby A, Rademaker L, et al. An evidence-based guideline for the management of uterine fibroids. Aust N Z J Obstet Gynaecol. 2001;41(2):125-40.
7. Lethaby A, Vollenhoven B, Sowter M. Preoperative GnRH analogue therapy before hysterectomy or myomectomy for uterine fibroids. Cochrane Database Syst Rev. 2001;(2): CD000547.
8. de Aloysio D, Altieri P, Penacchioni P, Salgarello M, Ventura V. Bleeding patterns in a recent postmenopausal patient with uterine myomas: comparison between two regimens of HRT. Maturitas. 1998;29(3):261-4.
9. Palomba S, Affinito P, Tommaselli GA, Nappi C. Clinical trial of the effects of tibolone administered with GnRh analogues for the treatment of uterine leiomyomata. Fertil Steril. 1998;70(1):111-8.
10. Perino A, Chianchiano N, Petronio M, Cittadini E. Role of leuprolide acetate depot in hysteroscopic surgery: a controlled study. Fertil Steril. 1993;59(3):507-10.
11. Reid PC, Virtanen-Kari S. Randomised comparative trial of the levonorgestrel intrauterine system and mefenamic acid for the treatment of idiopathic menorrhagia: A multiple analysis using total menstrual fluid loss, menstrual blood loss and pictorial blood loss assessment charts. BJOG. 2005;112(8):1121-5.
12. Soysal S, Soysal M. The efficacy of levonorgestrel-releasing intrauterine device in selected cases of myoma-related menorrhagia: a prospective controlled trial. Gynecol Obstet Invest. 2005;59(1):29-35.
13. Stewart A, Cummins C, Gold L, Jordan R, Phillips W. The effectiveness of the levonorgestrel-releasing intrauterine system in menorrhagia: a systematic review. BJOG. 2001;108(1):74-86.
14. Tristan M, Orozco LJ, Steed A, Ramírez-Morera A, Stone P. Mifepristone for uterine fibroids. Cochrane Database Syst Rev. 2012;(8):CD007687.
15. Croxtall JD. Ulipristal acetate: in uterine fibroids. Drugs. 2012;72(8):1075-85.
16. Donnez J, Tatarchuk TF, Bouchard P, Puscasiu L, Zakharenko NF, Ivanova T, et al. Ulipristal Acetate versus Placebo for Fibroid Treatment before Surgery. N Engl J Med. 2012;366(5):409-20.
17. Donnez J, Tomaszewski J, Vázquez F, Bouchard P, Lemieszczuk B, Baró F, et al. Ulipristal acetate versus leuprolide acetate for uterine fibroids. N Engl J Med. 2012;366(5):421-32.

18. Wu T, Chen X, Xie L. Selective estrogen receptor modulators (SERMs) for uterine leiomyomas. Cochrane Database Syst Rev. 2007;(4):CD005287.
19. Hillis SD, Marchbanks PA, Peterson HB. Uterine size and risk of complications among women undergoing abdominal hysterectomy for leiomyomas. Obstet Gynecol. 1996;87(4): 539-43.
20. Nezhat C, Nezhat F, Silfen SL, Schaffer N, Evans D. Laparoscopic myomectomy. Int J Fertil. 1991;36(5):275-80.
21. Jin C, Hu Y, Chen XC, Zheng FY, Lin F, Zhou K, et al. Laparoscopic versus open myomectomy—a meta-analysis of randomized controlled trials. Eur J Obstet Gynecol Reprod Biol. 2009;145(1):14-21.
22. Neuwirth RS, Amin HK. Excision of submucous fibroids with hysteroscopic control. Am J Obstet Gynecol. 1976;126(1):95-9.
23. Wamsteker K, Emanuel MH, de Kruif JH. Transcervical hysteroscopic resection of submucous fibroids for abnormal uterine bleeding: results regarding the degree of intramural extension. Obstet Gynecol. 1993;82(5):736-40.
24. Ravina JH, Herbreteau D, Ciraru-Vigneron N, Bouret JM, Houdart E, Aymard A, et al. Arterial embolization to treat uterine myomas. Lancet. 1995;346(8976):671-2.
25. Royal College of Obstetricians and Gynaecologists (RCOG), Royal College of Radiologists (RCR). (2013). Clinical recommendations on the use of uterine artery embolization (UAE) in the management of uterine fibroids. [online]. Available from www.rcog.org.uk/globalassets/documents/ guidelines/23-12-2013_rcog_rcr_uae.pdf. [Accessed October, 2016].
26. Khaund A, Moss JG, McMillan N, Lumsden MA. Evaluation of the effect of uterine artery embolization on the menstrual blood loss and uterine volume. BJOG. 2004;111(7):700-5.
27. Pron G, Mocarski E, Cohen M, Colgan T, Bennett J, Common A, et al. Hysterectomy for complications after uterine artery embolisation for leiomyoma: results of a Canadian multicentric clinical trial. J Am Assoc Gynecol Laparosc. 2003;10(1):99-106.
28. Sud S, Maheshwari A, Bhattacharya S. Obstetric outcomes after treatment of fibroids by uterine artery embolization: a systematic review. Expert Rev Obstet Gynecol. 2009;4(4): 429-41.
29. Gupta JK, Sinha A, Lumsden MA, Hickey M. Uterine artery embolization for symptomatic uterine fibroids. Cochrane Database Syst Rev. 2012;(5):CD005073.
30. Dutton S, Hirst A, McPherson K, Nicholson T, Maresh M. A UK multicentre retrospective cohort study comparing hysterectomy and uterine artery embolisation for the treatment of symptomatic uterine fibroids (HOPEFUL study). main results on medium-term safety and efficacy. BJOG. 2007;114(11):1340-51.
31. Edwards RD, Moss JG, Lumsden MA, Wu O, Murray LS, Twaddle S, et al. Uterine artery embolization versus surgery for symptomatic uterine fibroids. N Engl J Med. 2007;356(4): 360-70.
32. Moss JG, Cooper KG, Khaund A, Murray LS, Murray GD, Wu O, et al. Randomised comparison of uterine artery embolisation (UAE) with surgical treatment in patients with symptomatic uterine fibroids (REST trial): 5-year results. BJOG. 2011;118(8):936-44.
33. You JH, Sahota DS, Yuen PM. Uterine artery embolisation or myomectomy for symptomatic uterine fibroids: a cost utility analysis. Fertil Steril. 2009;91(2):580-8.

34. Stewart EA, Gedroyc WM, Tempany CM, Quade BJ, Inbar Y, Ehrenstein T, et al. Focused ultrasound treatment of uterine fibroid tumors: safety and feasibility of a noninvasive thermoablative technique. Am J Obstet Gynecol. 2003; 189(1):48-54.

35. Stewart EA, Rabinovici J, Tempany CM, Inbar Y, Regan L, Gostout B, et al. Clinical outcomes of focused ultrasound surgery for the treatment of uterine fibroids. Fertil Steril. 2006;85:22-9.

36. Roberts A. MR-guided focussed ultrasound for the treatment of uterine fibroids. Semin Intervent Radiol. 2008;25(4): 394-405.

37. McPherson K, Metcalfe MA, Herbert A, Maresh M, Casbard A, Hargreaves J, et al. Severe complications of hysterectomy: the VALUE study. BJOG. 2004;111(7):688-94.

38. Orsini G, Laricchia L, Fanelli M. Low-dose combination oral contraceptives use in women with uterine leiomyomas. Minerva Ginecol. 2002;54(3):253-61.

Dysmenorrhoea and Pelvic Pain

INTRODUCTION

Dysmenorrhoea has been defined by the ACOG as a gynaecological medical condition characterised by presence of pain during the menstrual phase. The pain may be severe enough to interfere with normal activities of daily living. The pain could be sharp, throbbing, dull, nauseating, burning or shooting in nature. It may either precede menstruation by several days or may accompany it. However, it usually subsides as the menstrual bleeding ceases.[1] Dysmenorrhoea can be of two types: primary (spasmodic or the first day pain) and secondary (congestive type).[2] Dysmenorrhoea is labelled as primary in the absence of underlying medical disease or pathology. Secondary dysmenorrhoea, on the other hand, is associated with an underlying medical disease or pathology. Some of the common causes of secondary dysmenorrhoea include endometriosis, leiomyomas, adenomyosis, ovarian cysts, pelvic congestion, copper IUCDs, etc. Another type of dysmenorrhoea is the membranous type, where the endometrium is shed off in form of casts at the time of menstruation. The passage of casts is accompanied by painful uterine cramps. Primary dysmenorrhoea is widely prevalent, present in about 70% of teenagers and 30–40% of menstruating women.[3] According to the recent study by Ju et al., based on the review of 15 primary studies, published between 2002 and 2011, the prevalence of dysmenorrhoea has been found to vary between 16% to 91%.[4] Of these, nearly 2–29% women suffered from severe pain.

AETIOLOGY

Primary Dysmenorrhoea

The pathophysiology of primary dysmenorrhoea is not yet understood. Some of the probable factors are described next.

- *Behavioural and psychological factors*: Primary dysmenorrhoea is regarded as a physiological variant of the normal response to the ovarian hormone withdrawal. Therefore, onset of menstrual bleeding cannot be considered as a pathological variation. However, various behavioural, social, psychological and emotional factors may influence the overall impact of dysmenorrhoea over an individual.

- *Muscular incoordination and uterine hyperactivity*: Uterine myometrial hyperactivity due to increased production of prostaglandins during menstruation is likely to cause reduced blood flow through the myometrium, thereby resulting in uterine ischaemia.

- *Hormonal imbalance*: Stimulation of the uterus by progesterone could be another factor involved in its pathogenesis because dysmenorrhoea usually occurs only with the ovulatory cycles.

- *Prostaglandins*: Excessive amounts of prostaglandin $F_{2\alpha}$ could be responsible because they cause myometrial contraction and constriction of small endometrial vessels to produce ischaemia and breakdown of endometrium causing bleeding and pain.

- *Other factors*: High levels of vasopressin may stimulate uterine activity.

Secondary Dysmenorrhoea

Most important cause of secondary dysmenorrhoea is endometriosis, which is also an important cause of chronic pelvic pain.[4] Adenomyosis is another important cause for secondary dysmenorrhoea typically in older, multiparous women. Symptoms and signs of adenomyosis include dysmenorrhoea, menorrhagia (heavy menstrual bleeding) and a uniformly enlarged uterus. Presence of uterine fibroids can sometimes cause dysmenorrhoea with the passage of clots. Degeneration of fibroids or expulsion of the fibroid through cervical canal may at times result in acute pain. Other causes of secondary dysmenorrhoea include cervical stenosis, intrauterine adhesions, residual or trapped ovaries, pelvic inflammatory disease (PID), pelvic venous congestion, and rarely congenital müllerian abnormalities, which cause obstruction of the menstrual flow.

Risk Factors

The condition is more prevalent amongst younger or teen-aged girls. Parity is inversely related to the incidence of dysmenorrhoea, with nulliparous women being at an increased risk of dysmenorrhoea.[5] There is usually an association with the family history and stressful lifestyle. Use of OCPs, exercise and high intake of fruits and vegetables is likely to have a protective effect. Other risk factors associated with development of dysmenorrhoea include heavy menstrual blood loss, premenstrual symptoms, irregular cycles, clinically suspected PID, sexual abuse, menarche before the age of 12 years, etc.[5]

DIAGNOSIS

Diagnosis is mainly based on the medical history of typical spasmodic, cramping, subrapubic pain and menstrual history (relation to the first day of periods). Also, there is absence of any clinical features suggestive of underlying gynaecological problems in cases of primary dysmenorrhoea. On the other hand, signs and symptoms suggestive of underlying gynaecological pathology can be observed in cases of secondary dysmenorrhoea. This can be backed by clinical examination, if required, and usually does not require any investigations. A pelvic examination should be performed in adolescents who have had vaginal intercourse due to a high risk of PID in this group of population. Pelvic examination is not indicated in a teenager who is not sexually active.

Clinical Presentation

❖ *Relationship with the periods*: Pain is usually present a few hours before and after the onset of menstruation. It rarely lasts for more than 12 hours even in its severest form.
❖ *Region*: Pain is usually present in the lower abdomen or umbilical or suprapubic regions.
❖ *Character*: Pain is usually colicky in nature.
❖ *Radiation of pain*: Radiation of the pain occurs towards the front and inner aspect of the thighs or lower back.
❖ *Associated symptoms*: It may be often associated with symptoms such as nausea or vomiting, diarrhoea, constipation, headache, dizziness, disorientation, fainting, fatigue, etc.
❖ *Age of onset*: Pain reaches its maximum during the age of 18–24 years and then diminishes in severity.
❖ *Relation with the ovulatory cycles*: Pain usually occurs in association with ovulation.

Pelvic Examination

Pelvic examination is within normal limits in cases of primary dysmenorrhoea. On the other hand, in the cases of secondary dysmenorrhoea, the underlying gynaecological pathology can be detected on pelvic examination. Abdominal and/or pelvic examination must be performed to assess tenderness, uterine size and presence of any mass. Reduced uterine mobility along with tenderness and thickness or nodularity in the pouch of Douglas is suggestive of endometriosis. Adenomyosis, on the other hand, may be associated with uniform, tender uterine enlargement. Localised tender trigger points may be identified in the muscles of abdominal wall or the pelvic floor.

Investigations

In cases of secondary dysmenorrhoea, the following investigations may be required to diagnose the underlying pathology:
❖ Pap smear
❖ *Imaging*: Ultrasound examination may be required if there is presence of an abnormality on the clinical examination. In case imaging investigations are required, TAS is the investigation of choice. TAS is a cheap and non-invasive investigation, which helps in establishing the diagnosis of uterine fibroids, adenomyosis, ovarian cysts and endometriosis. It also helps in ruling out congenital uterine abnormalities or significant ovarian pathology. CT scan and/or MRI may follow gynaecological ultrasound, especially if the findings on the ultrasound are equivocal.
❖ *Hysterosalpingography*: This helps in the identification of intrauterine adhesions
❖ *Endocervical swabs and culture of peritoneal fluid*: This helps in diagnosing or screening for PID
❖ *Diagnostic laparoscopy or hysteroscopy*: This may be useful for diagnostic as well as curative purposes, especially in cases of endometriosis. However, laparoscopy is an invasive procedure and it is associated with its own inherent risks. It should preferably not be performed before therapeutic trial of medical therapy.

DIFFERENTIAL DIAGNOSIS

❖ *Corpus luteum haematoma*: This can be defined as haemorrhage into and from the corpus luteum. Patient experiences acute onset of sharp pain in the lower abdomen, moving from one side to the other, often accompanied by feeling of faintness and uterine bleeding. The main differentiating feature is that the pain occurs during the second half of a previously normal cycle.
❖ *Ovulation pain (Mittelschmerz)*: This usually occurs during the 10th to 14th day of the menstrual cycle. The pain is usually localised to the hypogastrium or one of the two iliac fossae and may be at times accompanied by ovulation bleeding.
❖ *Orthopaedic conditions*: Orthopaedic conditions such as disc lesions and arthritic changes in the spine may at times mimic dysmenorrhoeal pain.

MANAGEMENT

Cases of dysmenorrhoea are usually managed by a GP or a primary care physician. Referral to the gynaecologist may be required if there is lack of response to standard therapies or there is an atypical presentation or there is a suspicion of underlying pelvic abnormality. The management of cases of dysmenorrhoea is described in Flow chart 66.1.[6,7]

Some of the most commonly used drugs for dysmenorrhoea are described next.

Flow chart 66.1: Management of cases of dysmenorrhoea

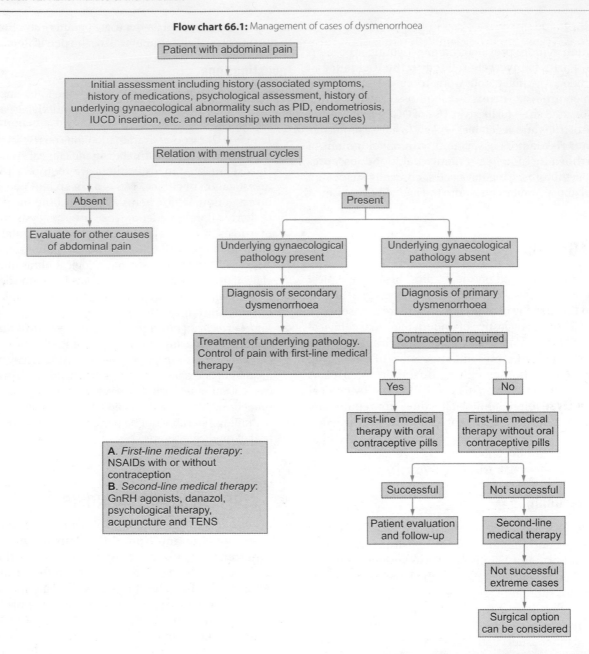

Non-steroidal Anti-inflammatory Drugs

Non-steroidal anti-inflammatory drugs are the most commonly used medicines and their use is restricted to the symptomatic days. They do not interfere with ovulation. Rather, they exert their action by preventing the synthesis of prostaglandins due to inhibition of the enzyme cyclooxygenase. The following NSAIDs may be used: indomethacin 24 mg TDS or QID; ibuprofen 400 mg TDS; naproxen sodium 240 mg TDS; ketoprofen 40 mg TDS and mefenamic acid 240–400 mg BD or QID. There does not appear to be any significant discrepancy in the efficacy or side-effects of various NSAIDs.[8] Use of NSAIDs forms an effective treatment option for dysmenorrhoea, and these drugs can be used in combination with other analgesics such as paracetamol or codeine. However, the women who are prescribed these drugs must be made aware of the significant risk of adverse effects associated with their use.[8]

Combined Oral Contraceptive Pills

Combined oral contraceptive pills (COCPs) are commonly used for the treatment of primary dysmenorrhoea, especially in the women desiring contraception. The efficacy of OCPs is related to the inhibition of ovulation. Cochrane review by Wong et al. (2009) has shown limited evidence regarding the efficacy of OCPs for treatment of the cases of primary dysmenorrhoea.[9] However, smaller RCTs have shown the response rates of OCPs to be as high as 80%.[10] Despite the lack of high-quality evidence, COCPs can be considered as a safe and effective therapy for the treatment of primary dysmenorrhoea. No particular type of OCP pill has been found to be more effective than the others.[9] Both 28-day and extended-cycle oral contraceptives can be used in women with primary dysmenorrhoea who also desire contraception.[11] The second- and third-generation formulations are likely to be more expensive and carry a marginally high risk of thrombotic complications. Transdermal or vaginal preparations are also available. Both the types of OCP regimens, continuous versus cyclic administration of OCPs, have been found to be equally effective in cases of dysmenorrhoea.[12]

Other Hormonal Preparations

Ovulation suppression using various hormonal formulations is used for the treatment of dysmenorrhoea, particularly that secondary to endometriosis. These include the second-line formulations such as continuous high dosage of progestogens, androgens and GnRH analogues (preferably with add-back therapy). Low-dose progestogens can also be used. However, their use can be associated with side-effects such as irregular or non-cyclic bleeding. Levonorgestrel-releasing intrauterine system is an effective modality for the treatment of dysmenorrhoea secondary to endometriosis and adenomyosis. This may also serve as a useful option in women with primary dysmenorrhoea looking for contraception.

Second-line formulations are used in women whose symptoms are incompletely relieved with first-line therapies.

Alternative Therapies for Primary and Secondary Dysmenorrhoea

Physical therapies such as transcutaneous electric nerve stimulation (TENS), acupuncture and topical heat application appear to be useful. Acupuncture, exercise and behavioural therapies (focusing on both physical and psychological coping strategies for symptom alleviation) have also been found to be useful for the treatment of dysmenorrhoea, especially in those individuals where NSAIDs or oral contraceptives are contraindicated or refused.[13-17] However, there is a requirement of further well-controlled randomised trials in future to prove this. Presently there is not enough evidence to support the use of yoga, acupuncture, or massage.

Though various dietary and herbal therapies have been tried, only thiamine or B_1 (in the dosage of 100 mg daily) and magnesium have been found to be more effective than placebo. Dosage of magnesium to be used for the treatment of dysmenorrhoea is yet not clear. Presently, there is no evidence regarding the beneficial action of herbal or dietary therapy for the management of primary or secondary dysmenorrhoea.[18] Chinese herbal medicine may be a suitable alternative in cases where the conventional treatment for primary dysmenorrhoea has failed, not tolerated or is contraindicated. The Cochrane review by Zhu et al. (2008) has shown that there is good evidence supporting the use of Chinese herbal medicine for the treatment of primary dysmenorrhoea.[19] However, some of the trials included in the review were limited due to the poor methodological quality.

CLINICAL PEARLS

❖ Symptoms of dysmenorrhoea are likely to improve with increased age, parity and use of oral contraceptives.

❖ Though endometriosis and adenomyosis can both occur in young women, it is rarely a cause of dysmenorrhoea in these cases.

❖ Hormonal therapy is the treatment of choice for those women who desire contraception.

❖ An ultrasound scan is useful for identifying the underlying pathology associated with secondary dysmenorrhoea.

❖ The mainstay for treatment of primary dysmenorrhoea is the NSAIDs with or without the OCPs.

❖ Gonadotropin-releasing hormone analogues, through abolition of ovarian function may produce bone loss, so they do not serve as a very practical option.

EVIDENCE-BASED MEDICINE

❖ Presently, there is inconclusive evidence related to the association of modifiable factors such as cigarette smoking, diet, obesity, depression and drug abuse with dysmenorrhoea.[4,5]

❖ Present evidence indicates that alternative therapies including physical and behavioural therapies, dietary supplements and Chinese herbal medicines may have a role in the management of dysmenorrhoea.[14-19]

❖ There is insufficient evidence to support the use of pelvic nerve interruption for the relief of primary or secondary dysmenorrhoea.[20]

REFERENCES

1. Lentz GM, Lobo RA, Gershenson DM, Katz VL. Comprehensive Gynecology, 6th edition. Philadelphia, PA, USA: Mosby Elsevier; 2012.
2. Impey L, Child T. Obstetrics and Gynaecology, 4th edition. Chichester, UK: Wiley Blackwell; 2012.
3. Zondervan KT, Yudkin PL, Vessey MP, Dawes MG, Barlow DH, Kennedy SH. The prevalence of chronic pelvic pain in women in the United Kingdom: a systematic review. Br J Obstet Gynaecol. 1998;105(1):93-9.
4. Ju H, Jones M, Mishra G. The prevalence and risk factors of dysmenorrhea. Epidemiol Rev. 2014;36:104-13.
5. Patel V, Tanksale V, Sahasrabhojanee M, Gupte S, Nevrekar P. The burden and determinants of dysmenorrhoea: a population-based survey of 2262 women in Goa, India. BJOG. 2006;113(4):453-63.
6. Proctor M, Farquhar C. Diagnosis and management of dysmenorrhoea. BMJ. 2006;332(7550):1134-8.
7. Won HR, Abbott J. Optimum management of chronic cyclical pelvic pain: an evidence-based and systematic approach. Int J Womens Health. 2010;2:263-77.
8. Marjoribanks J, Ayeleke RO, Farquhar C, Proctor M. Non-steroidal anti-inflammatory drugs for dysmenorrhoea. Cochrane Database of Syst Rev. 2015;(7):CD001751.
9. Wong CL, Farquhar C, Roberts H, Proctor M. Oral contraceptive pill for primary dysmenorrhoea. Cochrane Database Syst Rev. 2009;(4):CD002120.
10. ACOG practice bulletin no. 110: noncontraceptive uses of hormonal contraceptives. Obstet Gynecol. 2010;115(1):206-18.

11. Morrow C, Naumburg EH. Dysmenorrhea. Prim Care. 2009; 36(1):19-32.

12. Dmitrovic R, Kunselman AR, Legro RS. Continuous compared with cyclic oral contraceptives for the treatment of primary dysmenorrhea: a randomized controlled trial. Obstet Gynecol. 2012;119(6):1143-50.

13. Khan KS, Champaneria R, Latthe PM. How effective are non-drug, non-surgical treatments for primary dysmenorrhoea? BMJ. 2012;344:e3011.

14. Proctor ML, Murphy PA, Pattison HM, Suckling J, Farquhar C. Behavioural interventions for primary and secondary dysmenorrhoea. Cochrane Database Syst Rev. 2007;(3):CD002248.

15. Brown J, Brown S. Exercise for dysmenorrhoea. Cochrane Database Syst Rev. 2010;(2):CD004142.

16. Smith CA, Zhu X, He L, Song J. Acupuncture for primary dysmenorrhoea. Cochrane Database Syst Rev. 2011;(1): CD007854.

17. Iorno V, Burani R, Bianchini B, Minelli E, Martinelli F, Ciatto S. Acupuncture treatment of dysmenorrhoea resistant to conventional medical treatment. Evid Based Complement Alternat Med. 2008;5(2):227-30.

18. Proctor ML, Murphy PA. Herbal and dietary therapies for primary and secondary dysmenorrhoea. Cochrane Database Syst Rev. 2008;(2):CD005288.

19. Zhu X, Proctor M, Bensoussan A, Wu E, Smith CA. Chinese herbal medicine for primary dysmenorrhoea. Cochrane Database Syst Rev. 2008;(2):CD005288.

20. Proctor ML, Latthe PM, Farquhar CM, Khan KS, Johnson NP. Surgical interruption of pelvic nerve pathways for primary and secondary dysmenorrhoea. Cochrane Database Syst Rev. 2005;(4):CD001896.

Premenstrual Syndrome

INTRODUCTION

Premenstrual syndrome (PMS) or premenstrual tension includes a combination of physical, psychological and emotional symptoms, which the women experience for a few days (usually 7–10 days) preceding menstruation. The symptoms typically recur during the luteal phase of each menstrual (ovarian) cycle and significantly regress by the end of menstruation. There is an absence of an underlying organic or psychiatric disease.[1] The main features, which point towards the diagnosis of PMS, are presence of symptoms consistent with PMS, occurrence of these symptoms only during the luteal phase of the cycle and negative impact of these symptoms on patient's functions and lifestyle. Grading of PMS is described in Table 67.1. The prevalence of severe PMS varies between 3% to 30%.[2,3] Prevalence of PMS appears to be higher amongst women who are obese, do not exercise and have low levels of academic achievement. On the other hand, use of hormonal contraception is likely to be associated with a lower incidence of PMS.

Table 67.1: Grading of premenstrual syndrome (PMS)

Grades	Characteristics
Mild	Symptoms of PMS do not interfere with personal/social and professional life
Moderate	Symptoms of PMS interfere with personal/social and professional life. However, she is able to function and interact, although this may be at a suboptimal level
Severe	She is unable to interact at personal/social/professional levels and withdraws from social and professional activities. This is usually resistant to treatment
Premenstrual dysphoric disorder (PMDD)	This is a severe, sometimes disabling extension of PMS. It comprises of cluster of affective, behavioural and somatic symptoms

AETIOLOGY

❖ The causes of PMS are not completely understood and may be multifactorial
❖ It is commonly linked to the luteal (ovarian) phase of the menstrual cycle because premenstrual symptoms are typically absent before puberty, during pregnancy and after menopause
❖ The effect of hormones such as oestradiol and progesterone on the neurotransmitters like serotonin and gamma-aminobutyric acid (GABA) appear to be important factors in the aetiopathogenesis of PMS.

DIAGNOSIS

Diagnostic criteria for PMS devised by National Institute of Mental Health is described in Box 67.1.[4]

Clinical Presentation

While assessing women with PMS, symptoms over at least two cycles must be recorded using a symptom diary in a prospective manner because retrospective recall of symptoms is unreliable. Some of the symptoms of PMS, which are commonly observed, include the following:
❖ Abdominal bloating, breast tenderness
❖ Headache
❖ Sleeplessness, fatigue

Box 67.1: Diagnostic criteria for premenstrual syndrome (PMS)[4]

❑ A 30% increase in the intensity of symptoms of PMS (measured using a standardised instrument) from cycle days 4th to 10th in comparison with the 6-day interval before the onset of menses
❑ Documentation of these changes in a daily symptom diary for at least two consecutive cycles

Box 67.2: Differential diagnosis of premenstrual syndrome

Psychiatric disorders
❑ Anxiety and mood disorders (e.g. depression, anxiety, dysthymia, panic)
❑ Personality disorder
❑ Anorexia or bulimia

Chronic medical disorders
❑ Diabetes mellitus
❑ Hypothyroidism
❑ Anaemia

Gynaecological conditions
❑ Dysmenorrhoea
❑ Perimenopause
❑ Use of OCPs
❑ Substance abuse

❖ Emotional liability and emotional outbursts
❖ Mood swings, depression, irritability, lassitude, insomnia
❖ Fluid retention
❖ Increase in appetite, craving for sweet foods
❖ Intestinal distension, colonic spasm, congestive dysmenorrhoea.

DIFFERENTIAL DIAGNOSIS

Premenstrual syndrome is a diagnosis of exclusion, usually established after excluding a variety of psychiatric and medical disorders described in Box 67.2.

MANAGEMENT

Management of PMS is summarised in Flow chart 67.1. Reassurance, counselling, psychotherapy and selective use of medicines are useful in most of the cases. These various options are described next in details.

Lifestyle Changes

When treating women with PMS, she should be advised to make certain changes in her lifestyle including general advice about exercise, dietary changes and stress reduction. Various dietary supplements, which are likely to prove useful in the cases of PMS, include evening primrose oil, isoflavones, calcium, magnesium, vitamin E, vitamin B_6, etc. Results of a systematic review has shown that vitamin B_6 in the dosage of up to 100 mg/day (and possibly 50 mg/day) are likely to be beneficial in the treatment of premenstrual symptoms and premenstrual depression.[5] There is no conclusive evidence regarding the neurological side effects with this dosage of vitamin B_6. She should be asked to maintain a diary of her symptoms over several cycles to evaluate the effect of treatment. She should be advised to have a diet with low glycaemic index. Evidence from non-randomised trials indicate that regular exercising helps in improving the symptoms of PMS.[6] It is important to avoid prescribing complex gynaecological and hormonal interventions and

Flow chart. 67.1: Management of premenstrual syndrome (PMS)

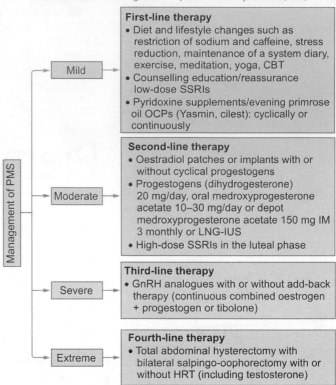

Abbreviations: CBT, cognitive behavioural therapy; LNG-IUS, levonorgestrel -intrauterine system; SSRIs, selective serotonin reuptake inhibitors

referral to the gynaecologist at the beginning of symptoms. These options should be considered when simple measures have been tried and not worked or the symptoms of PMS are extremely severe. Initially, the GPs should deal with most cases of PMS.

Complementary Therapies

An integrated approach must be adopted for treating the women with PMS. This may include complementary medicines most of which may not be evidence-based. Nevertheless, they are commonly used for the treatment of PMS. When treating women with PMS using complementary medicines, the clinicians need to consider that presently there is unavailability of good evidence to support the use of various complementary therapies for the treatment of symptoms related to PMS. Moreover, the legal responsibility for the patient's well-being rests with the referring clinician. Also, interactions with conventional medicines should be considered. Herbal medicines [e.g. fruit of chaste tree (*Vitex agnus castus*)] containing dopaminergic compounds, helps in effectively improving premenstrual mastodynia and possibly other symptoms of the PMS as well.[6,7] Treatment with this drug is also well accepted.

Other alternative approaches such as massage therapy, self-help, relaxation and aromatherapy are popular therapies used for treatment of symptoms related to PMS.[8] The beneficial effect of these therapies is likely to outweigh any possible harm. However, there is concern regarding the risk of side effects of these herbal preparations, particularly St John's wort, due to interactions with other drugs.

PART III

Traditional Chinese herbal medicines (e.g. ginkgo biloba, pollen extract, etc.) are also frequently used for the treatment of PMS. However, presently there is insufficient evidence to support the use of Chinese herbal medicine for PMS. There is requirement of further well-controlled trials in future before any final conclusions could be drawn.[9]

Cognitive Behavioural Therapy

When treating women with severe PMS, cognitive behavioural therapy (CBT) should be considered routinely as a treatment option. A clinical psychology referral is usually required for this patient group. A recent RCT has shown that though the antidepressant, fluoxetine is likely to be associated with a more rapid improvement, CBT is likely to be associated with better maintenance of treatment effects in comparison with fluoxetine.[10] There appears to be no additional benefit of combining fluoxetine with CBT.

Selective Serotonin Reuptake Inhibitors and Selective Serotonin and Noradrenaline Reuptake Inhibitors

There is increasing evidence that serotonin may be involved in the pathogenesis of PMS. A number of selective serotonin reuptake inhibitors (SSRIs) have been used to treat severe PMS or premenstrual dysphoric disorder (PMDD). Fluoxetine in the dosage of 20 or 60 mg has been found to significantly reduce symptoms of tension, irritability and dysphoria, as well as physical symptoms. The adverse effects of these drugs are likely to be dose related, with significantly fewer events occurring in the women receiving 20 mg fluoxetine per day in comparison to the women receiving 60 mg fluoxetine per day.[10] A meta-analysis of all available RCTs involving SSRIs used in PMS has established superior efficacy of SSRIs in comparison with placebo.[11] Daily treatment with fluoxetine is likely to significantly improve physical symptoms such as breast tenderness, bloating and headache in women with PMDD.[12] Physical and psychological symptoms of PMS also improve with SSRIs.

Selective serotonin reuptake inhibitors and selective serotonin and noradrenaline reuptake inhibitors (SNRIs) should be considered as the first-line pharmaceutical management options for treatment of severe PMS in view of their proven efficacy and safety in adults.

As per the notification of Medicines and Healthcare products Regulatory Agency (MHRA), prescription of these drugs should be particularly restricted to the healthcare professionals (gynaecologists, psychiatrists or GPs) having a particular expertise in this area. Before prescription, the clinician needs to maintain a balance between the risks and benefits of these drugs in adults.[13]

Dosing

When treating women with PMS, either luteal phase or continuous dosing with SSRIs can be recommended. There is increasing strong evidence demonstrating the increased efficacy of SSRIs in the symptomatic luteal phase in comparison to their use throughout the cycle.[14] When treating women with PMS, it is recommended that SSRI therapy should be withdrawn gradually and tapered over a few weeks to avoid withdrawal symptoms, which may occur, if SSRIs have been administered continuously. Abrupt withdrawal of an SSRI may result in side effects such as gastrointestinal disturbances, headache, anxiety, dizziness, paraesthesia, sleep disturbances, fatigue, influenza-like symptoms, sweating, etc.

Adverse Effects

Women with PMS treated with SSRIs should be warned about the possible adverse effects such as nausea, insomnia and reduction in libido.

Newer SSRI/SNRI Regimens

When treating women with PMS, use of newer agents during the luteal phase may help in optimising the efficacy and minimising the adverse effects of SSRIs. The use of newer SSRIs, such as citalopram, may help in producing resolution of symptoms in cases where other conventional SSRIs have failed.[15]

Ovulation Suppression Using Hormonal Regimens

Since the symptoms of PMS occur in the postovulatory phase of menstrual cycle, anovulation due to the use of ovarian suppression drugs is likely to cause disappearance of the cyclical symptoms in women with PMS. A number of hormonal therapies are available, which help in suppressing ovulation, thereby alleviating the symptoms of PMS. However, they may have significant adverse effects which may influence the efficacy of the treatment or the duration for which they may be given. Some of the ovulation suppressing therapies are discussed next.

Combined Oral Contraceptive Pill

When treating women with PMS, newer contraceptive pill types, especially those containing the third-generation progestogens are likely to act as an effective treatment for PMS. They are usually considered as one of the first-line pharmaceutical interventions. However, the benefits of these combined pills have not been shown in the randomised prospective trials.[16] This is probably due to the fact that most of these studies were based on OCPs containing second-generation progestogens (i.e. levonorgestrel or norethisterone), which are likely to reinforce PMS-type symptoms. On the other hand, the new combined contraceptive pill (Yasmin®) contains a third-generation progestogen, drospirenone, having antimineralocorticoid and antiandrogenic properties. Data from observational and small randomised trials has indicated that a lower dose variety of Yasmin® (Yaz®, containing 20 μg ethinyl oestradiol in combination with 3 mg drospirenone) is effective for treating PMDD.[17,18] This OCP, however, is not yet available in the UK. Presently, it is only licensed for treatment of PMDD in the USA.

Continuous versus cyclical use of combined oral contraceptive pills: When treating women with PMS, emerging data suggest that consideration should be given to the use of the contraceptive pill continuously rather than cyclically.[19] Further evidence related to the efficacy and safety of this regimen is required in future to allow its recommendation.

Percutaneous Oestradiol Patch and Implant

Percutaneous oestradiol, either in the form of an implant or as a patch, in combination with cyclical progestogen, has been shown to be effective for the management of physical and psychological symptoms of severe PMS. When oestradiol patches or implants are used for suppressing ovulation in women with PMS, alternative barrier or intrauterine methods of contraception should be used.[20] Since the availability of patches, implants are less commonly used for PMS. In a randomised, double-blind, placebo-controlled trial, use of transdermal oestradiol patches (200 μg) was found to be highly effective.[21] Use of 100-μg oestradiol patches twice weekly were found to be as effective as 200-μg patches in reducing the level of symptoms related to PMS. Moreover, the lower dosage was better tolerated by the patient.[22]

Use of progestogens: When treating women with PMS using oestradiol, treatment with the lowest possible dose of progestogen is recommended to minimise adverse effects. Levonorgestrel-releasing intrauterine system (LNG-IUS) helps in releasing small amounts of progestogens to avoid endometrial hyperplasia related to uninterrupted used of oestradiol. However, women should be informed that low systemic levels of levonorgestrel released by the LNG-IUS could initially produce PMS-type adverse effects. Nevertheless, intrauterine administration of progestogen has the potential to avoid systemic absorption and, thereby avoiding progestogenic effects.[23,24]

Danazol

Danazol is an androgenic steroid used for cycle suppression. Women with PMS should be advised that, although treatment with low-dose danazol (in the dosage of 200 mg twice daily) is effective, its use should be considered after keeping in mind its potential irreversible virilising side effects. Women treated with danazol for PMS should be advised to use contraception during treatment. A randomised trial by Mansel et al. demonstrated the beneficial effects of danazol in reducing breast tenderness, but not other PMS-related symptoms.[25] Other studies have demonstrated greater benefit of danazol in providing relief from severe PMS during the premenstrual period in comparison to the placebo.[26] However, this benefit may be muffled or even reversed when the entire cycle is considered because danazol therapy may cause some bothersome side effects, which may interfere with the usual symptom-free late follicular phase of women with PMS. This can be prevented by limiting danazol treatment to the luteal phase only.[27]

Gonadotropin-releasing Analogues

Gonadotropin-releasing hormone therapy must be prescribed only as a last resort in case the woman experiences severe PMS-associated symptoms. GnRH analogue therapy causes profound cycle suppression, thereby inhibiting the production of ovarian steroids, resulting in the elimination of premenstrual symptoms. However, prolonged use of GnRH therapy can result in hypo-oestrogenic symptoms. Therapy with GnRH analogues should be rarely used as a first-line therapy for alleviation of symptoms related to PMS. Rather, it can be recommended as second- or even third-line treatment. Add-back hormone therapy is recommended to prevent the hypo-oestrogenic symptoms related to gonadotropin therapy. A recent meta-analysis of GnRH analogues has confirmed their efficacy in comparison with the placebo.[28] Efficacy of symptom relief was found to be greater for physical than for behavioural symptoms. However, this result was not statistically significant.

Add-back therapy: When treating women with PMS where add-back hormone therapy is required, continuous combined HRT or tibolone should be recommended, because they help in reducing menopausal symptoms, particularly reduced bone density, without causing reappearance of PMS-like progestogenic effects.[29,30]

When treating women with PMS, with GnRH agonist therapy, treatment should only be continued for 6 months when used alone. Treatment should be combined with add-back therapy to reduce trabecular bone density loss in women undergoing long-term treatment with GnRH agonists. Women on long-term treatment should have annual measurement of bone mineral density (ideally by dual energy X-ray absorptiometry). Treatment should be stopped if bone density declines significantly in a scan performed 1 year apart. General advice about how exercise, diet and smoking affect bone mineral density should be administered to help reduce bone loss.[31]

Surgical Approach

This comprises of total abdominal hysterectomy with bilateral salpingo-oophorectomy (TAH-BSO). This is a permanent form of ovulation suppression because this helps in removing the ovarian cycle completely. The procedure is only rarely performed for cases of very severe PMS where no other alternative therapeutic option has been found to be effective. However, the surgery has been observed to be highly beneficial in providing relief from the symptoms of PMS.[32] When treating women with PMS, surgery should not be planned without preoperative use of GnRH analogues as a test of cure and to ensure that HRT is tolerated.

Role of Hormone Replacement Therapy

When treating women with PMS, HRT should be considered in women undergoing surgical oophorectomy before the age of 50 years. Without adequate hormone therapy, PMS symptoms are likely to be replaced by those of the menopause. Consideration should also be given towards the replacement of testosterone, because the ovaries are responsible for nearly 50% production of testosterone and its deficiency could result in low levels of libido, which may be very distressing for the patient.[33]

COMPLICATIONS

Premenstrual syndrome may be a cause of individual misery, marital disharmony, absenteeism and even crimes such as murder and suicide.

CLINICAL PEARLS

❖ A psychiatric referral may be required in women with marked underlying psychopathology.

❖ Progestogens such as norethisterone and levonorgestrel can produce PMS-like effects by competing for the mineralocorticoid, androgen and CNS receptors.

❖ Women who have had a hysterectomy with ovarian conservation are likely to experience the cyclical symptoms even in the absence of menstruation (ovarian cycle syndrome).

EVIDENCE-BASED MEDICINE

❖ When treating PMS with oestradiol, women should be informed that there is insufficient data to advise on the long-term effects of oestradiol on the breast and endometrial tissue. There is insufficient evidence to determine whether there is an increased risk of endometrial or breast carcinoma in premenopausal women using percutaneous oestrogen patches without using cyclical progestogen or LNG-IUS. There is requirement of randomised placebo-controlled trials evaluating such outcomes in large population groups.[34]

❖ Presently, there is insufficient evidence to recommend the routine use of progesterone or progestogens for treatment of PMS symptoms. The use of progesterone or progestogens has not been found to be better than placebo for alleviation of symptoms related to PMS.[35,36]

REFERENCES

1. Magos AL, Studd JW. The premenstrual syndrome. In: Studd J (Ed). Progress in Obstetrics and Gynaecology, Volume 4. London: Churchill Livingstone; 1984. pp. 334-50.
2. Reid RL. Premenstrual syndrome. N Engl J Med. 1991;324: 1208-10.
3. Sadler C, Inskip H, Smith H, Panay N. A study to investigate the relationship between lifestyle factors and premenstrual symptoms. J Br Menopause Soc. 2004;10(Suppl 2):15.
4. ACOG Practice Bulletin. Clinical management guidelines for obstetrician-gynecologists, Number 14, April 2000. Premenstrual syndrome. Obstet Gynecol. 2000;94:1-9.
5. Wyatt KM, Dimmock PW, Jones PW, O'Brien PMS. Efficacy of vitamin B-6 in the treatment of premenstrual syndrome: systematic review. BMJ. 1999;318(7195):1375-81.
6. Schellenberg R. Treatment for the premenstrual syndrome with agnus castus fruit extract: prospective, randomised, placebo controlled study. BMJ. 2001;322(7279):134-7.
7. Wuttke W, Jarry H, Christoffel V, Spengler B, Seidlová-Wuttke D. Chaste tree (Vitex agnus-castus)—pharmacology and clinical indications. Phytomedicine. 2003;10(4):348-57.
8. Carter J, Verhoef MJ. Efficacy of self-help and alternative treatments of premenstrual syndrome. Womens Health Issues. 1994;4(3):130-7.
9. Jing Z, Yang X, Ismail KM, Chen X, Wu T. Chinese herbal medicine for premenstrual syndrome. Cochrane Database Syst Rev. 2009;(1):CD006414.
10. Steiner M, Steinberg S, Stewart D, Carter D, Berger C, Reid R, et al. Fluoxetine in the treatment of premenstrual dysphoria. Canadian Fluoxetine/Premenstrual Dysphoria Collaborative Study Group. New Engl J Med. 1995;332(23):1529-34.
11. Dimmock PW, Wyatt KM, Jones PW, O'Brien PM. Efficacy of selective serotonin-reuptake inhibitors in premenstrual syndrome: a systematic review. Lancet. 2000;356(9236):1131-6.
12. Steiner M, Romano SJ, Babcock S, Dillon J, Shuler C, Berger C, et al. The efficacy of fluoxetine in improving physical symptoms associated with premenstrual dysphoric disorder. BJOG. 2001;108(5):462-8.
13. Medicines and Healthcare products Regulatory Agency. (2014). SSRIs and SNRIs: use and safety. [online] Available from www.gov.uk/government/publications/ssris-and-snris-use-and-safety. [Accessed September, 2016].
14. Freeman EW, Rickels K, Arredondo F, Kao LC, Pollack S, Sondheimer S. Full or half-cycle treatment of severe premenstrual syndrome with a serotonergic antidepressant. J Clin Psychopharmacol. 1999;19(1):3-8.
15. Freeman EW, Jabara S, Sondheimer SJ, Auletto R. Citalopram in PMS patients with prior SSRI treatment failure: a preliminary study. J Women's Health Gend Based Med. 2002;11(5):459-64.
16. Graham CA, Sherwin BB. A prospective treatment study of premenstrual symptoms using a triphasic oral contraceptive. J Psychosom Res. 1992;36(3):257-66.
17. Freeman EW, Kroll R, Rapkin A, Pearlstein T, Brown C, Parsey K, et al. Evaluation of a unique oral contraceptive in the treatment of premenstrual dysphoric disorder. J Womens Health Gend Based Med. 2001;10(6):561-9.
18. Pearlstein TB, Bachmann GA, Zacur HA, Yonkers KA. Treatment of premenstrual dysphoric disorder with a new drospirenone containing oral contraceptive formulation. Contraception. 2005;72(6):414-21.
19. Coffee AL, Kuehl TJ, Willis S, Sulak PJ. Oral contraceptives and premenstrual symptoms: Comparison of a 21/7 and extended regimen. Am J Obstet Gynecol. 2006;195(5):1311-9.
20. Magos AL, Brincat M, Studd JW. Treatment of the premenstrual syndrome by subcutaneous estradiol implants and cyclical oral norethisterone: placebo controlled study. Br Med J (Clin Res Ed). 1986;292(6536):1629-33.
21. Watson NR, Studd JW, Savvas M, Garnett T, Baber RJ. Treatment of severe premenstrual syndrome with oestradiol patches and cyclical oral norethisterone. Lancet. 1989;2(8665):730-2.
22. Smith RN, Studd JW, Zamblera D, Holland EF. A randomised comparison over 8 months of 100 mg and 200 mg twice weekly doses of transdermal estradiol in the treatment of severe premenstrual syndrome. Br J Obstet Gynaecol. 1995;102(6):475-84.
23. Panay N, Studd J. Progestogen intolerance and compliance with hormone replacement therapy in menopausal women. Hum Reprod Update. 1997;3(2):159-71.

24. Faculty of Family Planning and Reproductive Health Clinical Effectiveness Unit. FFPRHC Guidance (April 2004). The levonorgestrel-releasing intrauterine system (LNG-IUS) in contraception and reproductive health. J Fam Plann Reprod Health Care. 2004;30(2):99-108.

25. Mansel RE, Wisbey JR, Hughes LE. Controlled trial of the antigonadotropin danazol in painful nodular benign breast disease. Lancet. 1982;1(8278):928-30.

26. Watts JF, Butt WR, Logan Edwards R. A clinical trial using danazol for the treatment of premenstrual tension. Br J Obstet Gynaecol. 1987;94(1):30-4.

27. O'Brien PM, Abukhalil IE. Randomized controlled trial of the management of premenstrual syndrome and premenstrual mastalgia using luteal phase-only danazol. Am J Obstet Gynecol. 1999;180(1 Pt 1):18-23.

28. Wyatt KM, Dimmock PW, Ismail KM, Jones PW, O'Brien PM. The effectiveness of GnRHa with and without 'add-back' therapy in treating premenstrual syndrome: a meta-analysis. BJOG. 2004;111(6):585-93.

29. Leather AT, Studd JW, Watson NR, Holland EF. The prevention of bone loss in young women treated with GnRH analogues with 'add back' estrogen therapy. Obstet Gynecol. 1993;81(1):104-7.

30. Di Carlo C, Palomba S, Tommaselli GA, Guida M, Di Spiezio Sardo A, Nappi C. Use of leuprolide acetate plus tibolone in the treatment of severe premenstrual syndrome. Fertil Steril. 2001;75(2):380-4.

31. Sagsveen M, Farmer JE, Prentice A, Breeze A. Gonadotrophin releasing analogues for endometriosis: bone mineral density. Cochrane Database Syst Rev. 2003;(4):CD001297.

32. Cronje WH, Vashisht A, Studd JW. Hysterectomy and bilateral oophorectomy for severe premenstrual syndrome. Hum Reprod. 2004;19(9):2152-5.

33. Nappi RE, Wawra K, Schmitt S. Hypoactive sexual desire disorder in postmenopausal women. Gynecol Endocrinol. 2006;22(6):318-23.

34. Royal College of Obstetricians and Gynaecologists (RCOG). (2007). Green top guideline No 48: Management of Premenstrual Syndrome. [online] Available from www.rcog.org.uk/globalassets/documents/guidelines/gt48managementpremensturalsyndrome.pdf. [Accessed September, 2016].

35. Wyatt K, Dimmock P, Jones P, Obhrai M, O'Brien S. Efficacy of progesterone and progestogens in management of premenstrual syndrome: systematic review. BMJ. 2001;323 (7316):776–80.

36. Ford O, Lethaby A, Mol BW, Roberts H. Progesterone for premenstrual syndrome. Cochrane Database Syst Rev. 2009;(2):CD003415.

Chronic Pelvic Pain and Endometriosis

CHRONIC PELVIC PAIN

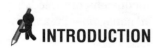 INTRODUCTION

The ACOG has defined chronic pelvic pain (CPP) as cyclic or non-cyclic pain, emanating from the pelvic area, which has been present for 6 months or more.[1] The pain often results in functional disability. It may also be present in the perineal region and cause discomfort in the anus, rectum, coccyx and sacrum. It is often associated with symptoms such as premenstrual pain, dysmenorrhoea, dyspareunia, exercise-related pain, or cramping, with or without menstrual exacerbation of sufficient severity to cause functional disability or require medical care.

Chronic pelvic pain is not a disease, but a symptom, which rarely reflects a single pathologic process. Though its aetiology remains unclear, it is believed to be multifactorial in nature. Different neurophysiological mechanisms may be involved in the pathophysiology of CPP.

AETIOLOGY

Identifying the Cause of Pelvic Pain

The most important question for the patient and the clinician is to identify the cause of pain. In general, the three most common sources of pain include:
1. *Pain of somatic origin*: This type of pain arises from skin, muscles and bone tissue and is commonly described by the patients as throbbing, stabbing or burning type of pain.
2. *Visceral origin*: This type of pain arises from internal organs and tends to be diffuse and more generalised.
3. *Neuropathic origin*: The pain of neuropathic origin arises from damaged nerve fibres and may be described as numbness, pins and needles, and may produce electric

current-like sensations. The main contributing factors in women with CPP are identified by history and physical examination in most cases. Many disorders of the reproductive tract, urological organs, gastrointestinal (GI), musculoskeletal and psychoneurological systems may be associated with CPP. Psychological problems (depression and sleep disorders) and social issues may commonly occur in association with CPP. Resolving these issues may be important in determining the management plan. The various gynaecological and non-gynaecological causes for CPP have been enumerated in Box 68.1.[2]

DIAGNOSIS

Clinical Presentation

❖ The pain often localises to the pelvis, infraumbilical part of the anterior abdominal wall, lumbosacral area of the back or buttocks and often leads to functional disability.
❖ It is often associated with symptoms such as premenstrual pain, dysmenorrhoea, dyspareunia, exercise-related pain or cramping, with or without menstrual exacerbation of sufficient severity to cause functional disability.
❖ The pain may be steady, or it may come and go. It can feel like a dull ache, or it can be sharp and may be generalised or localised.
❖ The pain may be mild, or it may be severe enough to negatively affect health-related quality of life.
❖ Patients with CPP may often present with the symptoms suggestive of irritable bowel syndrome (IBS) or interstitial cystitis.
❖ The most important gynaecological cause of CPP is endometriosis and is discussed in details later in this chapter. The most common symptoms related to endometriosis are dysmenorrhoea, dyspareunia and low back pain, which worsen during menses.

Box 68.1: Causes of chronic pelvic pain

Gynaecological causes
- ❑ Endometriosis
- ❑ Chocolate cyst of ovary
- ❑ Ovarian adhesions
- ❑ Polycystic ovarian disease
- ❑ Chronic pelvic inflammatory disease
- ❑ Pelvic and tubal adhesions
- ❑ Pelvic tuberculosis
- ❑ Uterine fibroids and adenomyosis
- ❑ Benign or malignant ovarian tumours

Gastrointestinal causes
- ❑ Irritable bowel syndrome
- ❑ Chronic intermittent bowel obstruction
- ❑ Diverticulitis, colitis, appendicitis
- ❑ Carcinoma rectum

Renal causes
- ❑ Ureteric or bladder stones
- ❑ UTI, interstitial cystitis, radiation cystitis
- ❑ Bladder malignancy

Musculoskeletal disease
- ❑ Abdominal wall myofascial pain
- ❑ Degenerative joint disease including muscle strains and pain
- ❑ Disc herniation, rupture or spondylosis

Psychiatric/neurological cause
- ❑ Abdominal epilepsy, abdominal migraines
- ❑ Depression, sleep disturbances, somatisation
- ❑ Nerve entrapment, neurologic dysfunction

Miscellaneous causes
- ❑ Familial Mediterranean fever
- ❑ Herpes zoster
- ❑ Porphyria

Abdominal Examination

The findings on abdominal examination vary with the cause and have been discussed in various chapters.

Pelvic Examination

The findings on pelvic examination vary with the cause and have been discussed in various chapters.

Investigations

❖ *Screening for sexually transmitted infections*: In case of suspicion of pelvic inflammatory disease (PID), suitable samples to screen for infection, particularly *Chlamydia trachomatis* and gonorrhoea, should be taken.[3]

❖ *Transvaginal sonography*: This is a useful investigation for identification of adnexal masses. It can also be useful in cases of adenomyosis and endometriosis.[4]

❖ *Magnetic resonance imaging*: Magnetic resonance imaging may serve as a useful test for diagnosis of adenomyosis and endometriosis in presence of uncertain findings on ultrasound.

❖ *Diagnostic laparoscopy*: Diagnostic laparoscopy had been regarded in the past as the 'gold standard' investigation for diagnosis of CPP. However, due to its invasive nature and potential complications, it is now considered as

the second-line investigation in case other therapeutic interventions fail.[5-7] Microlaparoscopy or 'conscious pain mapping' has been proposed as an alternative to diagnostic laparoscopy under general anaesthesia.[8] Presently, this technique is not widely adopted.

MANAGEMENT

Management of cases of CPP is described in Flow chart 68.1. The discovery of exact pelvic pathology or cause of pain helps the clinician in instituting therapy appropriate to the aetiology. The treatment needs to be individualised and must be decided after taking various parameters into consideration. In many women with CPP, treatment begins with identification of source of pain. Treatment should be directed at treating the underlying cause of pelvic pain.

Non-gynaecological Management

❖ If no therapeutic cause of pain is identified, women should be offered appropriate analgesia to control their pain.

❖ If the symptoms of pain are not adequately controlled, the patient may be referred to a pain management team or a specialist pelvic pain clinic.

❖ Women with IBS should be offered trial with antispasmodics (e.g. mebeverine hydrochloride) and should be encouraged to modify their diet in an attempt to control the symptoms. The most commonly used dietary restriction includes limitation of grains and dairy products.[9]

❖ The efficacy of bulking agents in cases of IBS has yet not been established but they are commonly used.[10,11]

❖ In case of a non-gynaecological cause of pelvic pain, the patient should be instructed to follow a course of proper bowel hygiene for at least 2 months.[9]

Gynaecological Management

❖ The patient should be given a menstrual calendar to document correlation of pain with menstrual cycle, following which she should be advised to return after 2 months for a follow-up review.

❖ Women with cyclical pain should be offered a therapeutic trial using suppression with hormonal treatment (e.g. combined oral contraceptive, progestogens, danazol or GnRH analogues) for a period of 3–6 months before undergoing a diagnostic laparoscopy.[12-14]

❖ In case of suspected endometriosis as a cause of pelvic pain, diagnostic laparoscopy may be performed.

COMPLICATIONS

Complications related to endometriosis and PID, the two most important gynaecological causes of pelvic pain, have been discussed in this chapter and Chapter 91 (Pelvic Inflammatory Disease) respectively.

Flow chart 68.1: Algorithm for the management of chronic pelvic pain in women

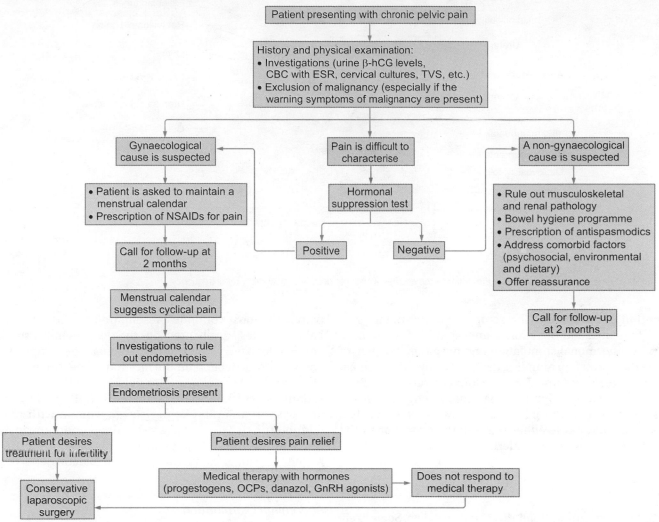

CLINICAL PEARLS

❖ Endometriosis and PID are the two most common causes of CPP in women belonging to the reproductive age groups and may be associated with infertility in nearly 30–40% cases.

❖ The occurrence of pelvic venous congestion as a cause of CPP presently remains controversial.

EVIDENCE-BASED MEDICINE

❖ Adhesions may occur due to causes such as endometriosis, previous surgery or previous infection. Adhesions, especially dense adhesions, may be a cause of chronic pain in women, mostly when the organ gets distended or stretched. Presently, there is little evidence to show that the division of fine adhesions in women with CPP is likely to provide pain relief. On the other hand, division of dense vascular adhesion is likely to be associated with pain relief.[15,16]

❖ Diagnostic laparoscopy should be performed only in case of CPP where there is a high index of clinical suspicion regarding presence of adhesive disease or endometriosis, requiring surgical intervention. Though diagnostic laparoscopy is the only test capable of reliably diagnosing peritoneal endometriosis, its use in all cases of CPP is best avoided due to the risk of potential complications with laparoscopy, e.g. injury to bowel, bladder or blood vessel and even death.[5-7,17,18]

ENDOMETRIOSIS

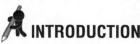 INTRODUCTION

Endometriosis is characterised by the occurrence of endometrial stroma and glands outside the uterus in the pelvic cavity, including all the reproductive organs as well as on the bladder, bowel, intestines, colon, appendix and rectum (Fig. 68.1). Endometrial lesions have been identified in virtually all tissues and organs of the female body with the

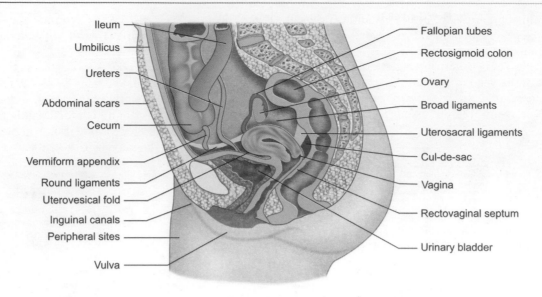

Ileum
Umbilicus
Ureters
Abdominal scars
Cecum
Vermiform appendix
Round ligaments
Uterovesical fold
Inguinal canals
Peripheral sites
Vulva

Fallopian tubes
Rectosigmoid colon
Ovary
Broad ligaments
Uterosacral ligaments
Cul-de-sac
Vagina
Rectovaginal septum
Urinary bladder

Fig. 68.1: Common sites of endometriosis in decreasing order of frequency

exception of the spleen. The ectopic endometrial tissues, both the glands and the stroma, are capable of responding to cyclical hormonal stimulation and have the tendency to invade the normal surrounding tissues. The ovary is the most common site for endometriosis. Lesions can vary in size from tiny spots to large endometriomas. Endometriomas or the retention cysts of the ovary are also known as the chocolate cysts. They may cause adhesions and the distortion of the fallopian tubes resulting in infertility.

AETIOLOGY

The pathogenesis of endometriosis is yet not clear. Some likely mechanisms for its pathogenesis are as follows:

- *Retrograde menstruation*: Retrograde menstrual flux can be considered as an essential element in the pathogenesis of endometriosis.
- *Theory of coelomic metaplasia*: Peritoneal epithelium can get 'transformed' into endometrial tissue under the influence of some unknown stimulus.
- *Metastatic theory of lymphatic and vascular spread*: Metastatic deposition of endometrial tissues at ectopic sites can occur via lymphatic and vascular routes.
- *Immunological defects and genetic factors*.

Pain during endometriosis is mainly due to the release of inflammatory mediators such as prostaglandins from the superficial lesions. Pain in cases of deep lesions may be related to infiltration, constriction of nerves or secondary to adhesions.

DIAGNOSIS

Clinical Presentation

The patients with endometriosis typically present with dysmenorrhoea, CPP, deep dyspareunia, cyclical intestinal complaints, fatigue or weariness and infertility.[19] Cyclic pelvic pain is the most common presentation of endometriosis. Pain characteristically precedes the onset of menstruation and is associated with deep dyspareunia. The symptoms of endometriosis depend on the location of the disease. Deep endometriosis of the posterior pelvis and the rectovaginal septum is associated with increased severity of dyschezia and dyspareunia, in comparison to women with pelvic endometriosis without posterior deep endometriosis.[20] Some of the unrecognised symptoms of endometriosis include intestinal complaints: periodic bloating, diarrhoea or constipation.[19,21]

Abdominal Examination

The abdominal examination can help identify areas of tenderness and the presence of masses or other anatomical findings, which may help in reaching accurate diagnosis. Carnett's sign can be performed to distinguish whether the pain is due to an intra-abdominal pathology or pathology in the anterior abdominal wall.

Per Speculum Examination

Deep endometriotic lesions can be visualised on the posterior fornix of the vaginal wall.[22]

Bimanual Pelvic Examination

Vaginal examination must be performed in all women suspected of endometriosis. However, vaginal examination may be inappropriate for adolescents and/or women without a previous history of sexual intercourse. In such cases, rectal examination can be helpful for the diagnosis of endometriosis. The following findings may be observed on the vaginal examination:

- *Tenderness upon pelvic examination*: This is best detected at the time of menses when the endometrial implants are likely to be largest and most tender. A moistened cotton swab can be used to elicit point tenderness in the vulva and vagina. The bimanual examination may reveal nodularity and thickening of uterosacral ligaments and cul-de-sac, which may be present in moderate to severe cases.

❖ The uterus may be fixed in retroversion, owing to adhesions.

❖ A bluish nodule may be seen in the vagina due to infiltration from the posterior vaginal wall.

❖ On vaginal examination, there may be infiltration or nodules of the vagina, uterosacral ligaments or pouch of Douglas.

❖ Adnexal tenderness with or without adnexal enlargement (endometriomas) may indicate ovarian endometriosis.

Rectal Examination

A rectal examination may reveal rectal or posterior uterine masses, presence of nodules in the uterosacral ligaments, cul-de-sac or rectovaginal septum and/or pelvic floor point tenderness.

Investigations

Investigations which may facilitate diagnosis are:

❖ *Urine β-hCG levels*: This helps in ruling out pregnancy-related complications.

❖ *Complete blood count*: Elevated leucocyte count points towards infection, whereas reduced haemoglobin level suggests anaemia, which could be the result of chronic or acute blood loss.

❖ *Urine analysis/urine culture*: This helps in excluding out the presence of possible urolithiasis, cystitis and UTI.

❖ *Cervical cultures*: This may help in detecting infection such as gonorrhoea and chlamydia.

❖ *Serum cancer antigen 125 (CA-125) test*: Serum CA-125 has been proposed as a biomarker for endometriosis. Presently, serum CA-125 measurement has limited potential for the diagnosis of endometriosis.[23] CA-125 levels may be increased to values greater than 35 IU/mL in nearly 80% cases of endometriosis.

❖ *Imaging studies*: Ultrasound examination (both trans-abdominal and transvaginal) is the most commonly used investigation which may help in revealing the pelvic pathology responsible for producing pain. Imaging investigations such as CT and MRI may be helpful in some cases.

❖ *Transvaginal sonography*: Transvaginal sonography serves as a useful method for both identifying and ruling out deep rectal endometriosis and or an ovarian endometrioma.[4,24] The following ultrasound characteristics are helpful in diagnosing an ovarian endometrioma in premenopausal women: Unilocular mass with ground glass echogenicity, one to four compartments (locules) and no papillary structures with detectable blood flow. Clinicians in many institutions across Europe are not experienced in performing TVS for the diagnosis of rectal endometriosis. Therefore, TVS cannot be recommended for the diagnosis of rectal endometriosis unless it is performed by clinicians who are highly experienced in TVS.

❖ *Magnetic resonance imaging*: Presently, the usefulness of MRI for diagnosing peritoneal endometriosis is not well established.[25] It may be, however, useful in the assessment of deep lesions.

❖ *Diagnostic laparoscopy*: Laparoscopy, backed by biopsy, remains the gold standard for the diagnosis of endometriosis. However, the patient must be appropriately counselled prior to surgery. Laparoscopy can help in identifying the following lesions: endometriotic nodules or lesions having blue-black or a powder-burned appearance (Figs 68.2 and 68.3). However, the lesions can be red, white or non-pigmented. Laparoscopy can also detect presence of blood (Fig. 68.4) or endometriotic deposits in cul-de-sac and its obliteration. Where appropriate, therapeutic treatment such as adhesiolysis or ablative surgical therapy of endometriotic lesions (Fig. 68.5) should be carried out in the same sitting. The operator must stage the disease on the basis of revised American Fertility classification of endometriosis (Table 68.1).[26] Though this classification system is often used for deciding the disease management, it shows poor correlation with the symptom of pain.

A good quality laparoscopic procedure must involve a two-port approach and must include systematic inspection

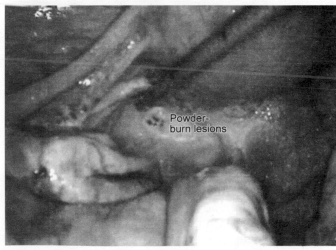

Fig. 68.2: Powder-burn lesions over endometrial surface
(*For colour version, see Plate 5*)

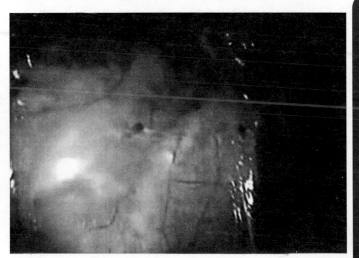

Fig. 68.3: Nodular endometrial lesions (*For colour version, see Plate 5*)

CHAPTER 68

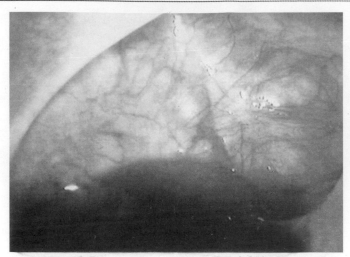

Fig. 68.4: Presence of blood in cul-de-sac *(For colour version, see Plate 5)*

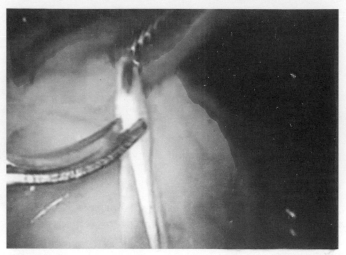

Fig. 68.5: Laparoscopic excision of nodular endometrial lesions overlying the round ligament *(For colour version, see Plate 5)*

of the uterus and adnexa, peritoneum of ovarian fossae, vesicouterine fold, pouch of Douglas, pararectal spaces, the rectum and sigmoid, uterosacral ligaments, pelvic sidewalls, the appendix and caecum, and the diaphragm. Speculum examination and palpation of the vagina and cervix under laparoscopic control must also be done to look for any 'buried' nodules. At the time of laparoscopic examination, the ovaries must be carefully mobilised in order to inspect their anterior surface for the presence of adhesions, which is strongly suggestive of endometriosis. Biopsy may be performed to confirm the nature of the lesions in case of doubt. However, this is associated with a risk and therefore, there is no need for routine biopsy in all cases. Biopsy is typically recommended if the size of the lesions is greater than 3 cm. The ureters, bladder and bowel involvement must also be evaluated by additional imaging techniques if there is clinical suspicion of deep endometriosis.

A negative diagnostic laparoscopy (i.e. a laparoscopy during which no lesions of endometriosis are identified) appears to be highly accurate for exclusion of endometriosis. A woman with a negative laparoscopy can be adequately reassured that she does not require further testing or treatment. However, a positive laparoscopy (presence of visual changes suggestive of endometriosis) lacks specificity and is less informative. A positive laparoscopy is of limited value when used in isolation without histology.[27] It presently remains controversial, whether medical treatment should be started first before embarking on an invasive procedure like a laparoscopy in women with symptoms and signs of endometriosis.

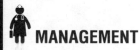 **MANAGEMENT**

Management of patients with endometriosis may be expectant, medical or surgical and is usually based on the presenting complaints and the disease staging (Table 68.1). One of the main criteria, which help the gynaecologist decide whether to consider medical or surgical management, is whether

Table 68.1: Revised American Fertility Society classification of endometriosis[26]

Peritoneum			
Endometriosis lesion	*<1 cm*	*1–3 cm*	*>3 cm*
Superficial	1	2	4
Deep	2	4	6
Ovary			
Right superficial	1	2	4
Right deep	4	16	20
Left superficial	1	2	4
Left deep	4	16	20
Posterior cul-de-sac obliteration			
Partial		*Complete*	
4		40	
Ovary			
Adhesions	*<1/3 enclosure*	*1/3–2/3 enclosure*	*>2/3 enclosure*
Right filmy	1	2	4
Right dense	4	8	16
Left filmy	1	2	4
Left dense	4	8	16
Tube			
Right filmy	1	2	4
Right dense	4"	8*	16
Left filmy	1	2	4
Left dense	4*	8*	16

* If the fimbriated end of the fallopian tube is completely enclosed, the point assignment is changed to 16.

Disease staging: Stage I (minimal): 1–5; stage II (mild): 6–15; stage III (moderate): 16–40; stage IV (severe): >40

the patient's main complaint is infertility or pelvic pain. The algorithm for treatment of endometriosis is described in Flow chart 68.2. While medical therapy has a role in the symptomatic management of endometriosis, it has no role in the management of endometriosis-associated infertility. In fact, hormonal therapy may rather enhance infertility.

Flow chart 68.2: Algorithm for treatment of patients with endometriosis

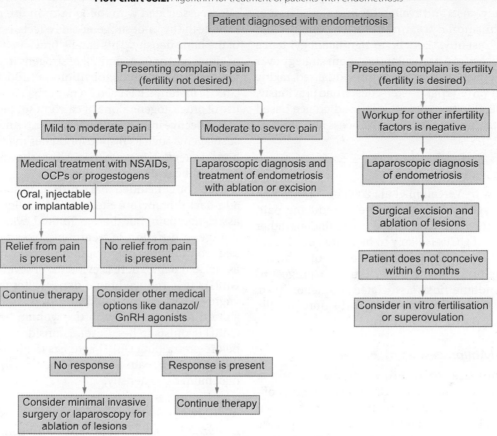

MANAGEMENT WHEN PAIN IS THE MAIN PRESENTING COMPLAINT

Before starting empirical treatment, other causes of pelvic pain should be ruled out, as far as possible. Initial treatment comprises of using analgesic drugs, especially NSAIDs or combined oral contraceptives pills (COCPs). Use of levonorgestrel-releasing intrauterine system (LNG-IUS) or continuous progestogens can be considered if oestrogenic preparations are contraindicated or give rise to side effects. These therapies can be used for long term if effective and well tolerated. Patients in whom the initial therapies (NSAIDs, OCPs, progestins) do not prove to be successful can be considered for GnRH agonists. The use of GnRH agonists is preferred over androgenic agents such as danazol and gestrinone because the latter drugs can cause unacceptable androgenic side-effects. Initially, a trial of GnRH agonists is tried for 2–3 months. This can be further continued for 6 months if the patient experiences relief from pain. This is likely to be more cost-effective than initial laparoscopy with local ablation in case of clinically suspected endometriosis given that the incidence of long-term symptom recurrence is similar for both the strategies.

Majority of medical therapies act by suppression of the ovaries and induction of amenorrhoea. This merely inactivates and does not remove the local disease. Symptoms, therefore, may recur following the cessation of therapy in a high proportion of patients. Since both medical and surgical treatments are associated with a high risk of recurrence following the interruption of therapy, medical treatment may be required to be instituted on an intermittent basis in the long term. These treatment strategies are described next.

Analgesics for Treatment of Endometriosis-associated Pain

Pain is a cardinal symptom of endometriosis. Studies have demonstrated elevated prostaglandin levels in peritoneal fluid and endometriotic tissue in women with endometriosis. As a result, NSAIDs are widely used analgesics in clinical practice.[28] Before prescribing NSAIDs to the patient, clinicians must discuss the role of NSAIDs in provision of pain relief along with its side-effects profile, including risk of gastric ulceration and cardiovascular disease.

In conclusion, the effectiveness of NSAIDs (naproxen) in treating endometriosis-associated dysmenorrhoea is not well established owing to a lack of studies.

Use of Hormonal Therapies

Endometriosis is considered a predominantly oestrogen-dependent disease. Thus, hormonal suppression might be an attractive medical approach to treat the disease and its symptoms. Currently, hormonal contraceptives, progestogens, antiprogestogens, GnRH agonists and aromatase inhibitors are in clinical use.[29-31] The guideline development group (GDG)

CHAPTER 68

recommends that clinicians must take patient preferences, side-effects, efficacy, costs and availability into consideration when choosing hormonal treatment for endometriosis-associated pain. Presently, there is no significant evidence supporting the efficacy of a particular treatment strategy over the others. Management plans must be individualised, taking into consideration various parameters, described previously. Woman should be able to make an informed choice based on a good understanding of the disease process and its effect on her body.

Hormonal Contraceptives

A systematic review by Vercellini et al., 2003 has shown that use of low-dose cyclic OCPs is effective in reducing pain symptoms in patients with endometriosis.[32] Continuous rather than the cyclic use of OCPs is likely to be more effective for pain control. Clinicians may consider the use of a vaginal contraceptive ring or a transdermal (oestrogen/progestin) patch to reduce endometriosis-associated dysmenorrhoea, dyspareunia and CPP.[33] Due to their good safety profile, combined OCPs are useful for long-term use.

Progestogens and Antiprogestogens

Continuous administration of progestogens is likely to cause inhibition of ovulation. They also exert an anti-proliferative effect on the endometriotic implants, causing their decidualisation and eventual atrophy. A recent systematic Cochrane review by Brown et al., (2012) determined that there was no evidence to suggest a benefit of progestogens over other treatments.[30] However, continuous progestogens serve as an effective therapy for the alleviation of painful symptoms associated with endometriosis. Nevertheless, progestogens must be used with caution due to the scarcity of data and absence of placebo-controlled studies. Also, progestogens may be associated with certain side effects, which can limit its use. The most common side effect of progestogens is breakthrough bleeding. Other side effects reported with the use of progestogens include weight gain, breast tenderness, bloating, headache, nausea, etc.

Levonorgestrel-releasing Intrauterine System

Levonorgestrel-releasing intrauterine system does not suppress ovulation but acts locally on the endometrium. Due to its locally mediated action, LNG-IUS is likely to serve useful for the management of endometriosis-associated pain. Three studies (Petta et al., 2005; Gomes et al., 2007 and Ferreira et al., 2010) have investigated the potential of a LNG-IUS for management of endometriosis-associated symptoms.[34-36] These studies have concluded that LNG-IUS is effective for the management of endometriosis-associated pain as well for the maintenance of pain control following surgical treatment.

Gonadotropin-releasing Hormone Agonist

The results from the Cochrane review by Brown et al. (2010) suggest that GnRHa is more effective than placebo but inferior to the LNG-IUS or oral danazol in providing relief from the endometriosis-associated pain.[31] The most common side effects associated with the long-term use of GnRH agonists include the hypo-oestrogenic side effects, especially reduction of the bone density. This can be prevented through addition of either oral or transdermal oestrogens in combination with various progestogens, or tibolone (add-back therapy) to GnRHa therapy if it is used for more than 6 months.[37] However, use of progestogens alone or calcium supplements is unlikely to be effective in preventing bone loss.[38] Antiresorptive agents such agents such as bisphosphonates may help in providing bone protection in women in whom the add-back therapy is contraindicated or is not tolerated.

It can be concluded that GnRH agonists, with and without add-back therapy, are effective in the relief of endometriosis-associated pain, but there is limited evidence regarding its dosage or duration of treatment. No specific GnRHa can be recommended over another in relieving endometriosis-associated pain. There is evidence of severe side effects with GnRHa (e.g. reduced bone density, hot flushes, insomnia, vaginal dryness, reduced libido, headache, etc.) which should be discussed with the woman before prescribing GnRH agonists to her. Careful consideration must be given before prescribing GnRH agonists to the young women and adolescents, because these women may not have reached maximum bone density.

Androgenic Agents

Danazol: Danazol, a synthetic androgen, is the derivative of ethinyl testosterone, which has been shown to be highly effective in relieving the symptoms of endometriosis by inhibiting pituitary gonadotropins (FSH and LH). This may result in the development of a relative hypo-oestrogenic state. Danazol probably provides pain relief by producing endometrial atrophy. A Cochrane review by Farquhar et al., 2007 has shown that Danazol in the dosage of 400-600 mg daily is effective in treating the symptoms and signs of endometriosis.[39] However, its use is limited by the occurrence of androgenic side effects. Recent studies indicate that vaginal danazol may be better tolerated.[40] According to the ESHRE recommendations (2013), danazol should not be used if any other medical therapy is available, due to occurrence of severe side effects (acne, greasy skin, deepening of voice, hirsutism, vaginal spotting, weight gain, muscle cramps, etc.).[41] Atherogenic effects on the lipid profile have also been reported. However, neither danazol nor gestrinone cause any adverse effect on the bone density. Therefore, these serve as beneficial alternatives to GnRH analogues in women who are susceptible to bone loss or those in whom oestrogenic add-back preparations are contraindicated.

Gestrinone: Gestrinone is a 19-norsteroid derivative having antioestrogenic, antiprogestogenic, antigonadotropic and androgenic properties. It has a long half-life and is therefore administered twice weekly orally in a dose of 1.25–2.5 mg. The consumption of this drug induces amenorrhoea in 50–100% of women with endometriosis. Resumption of menses occurs after cessation of treatment. Though the use of gestrinone can cause androgenic side effects, these are less intense in comparison to danazol. Gestrinone has been found to be as effective as GnRH agonists for providing relief from pelvic pain associated with endometriosis for up to 6 months after cessation of therapy.

Aromatase Inhibitors

The most common third-generation aromatase inhibitors letrozole and anastrozole are reversible inhibitors of the enzyme aromatase, which compete with androgens for aromatase-binding sites. Even though the evidence for increased expression of aromatase P450 in endometriotic tissue still remains controversial; aromatase inhibitors have been studied for treatment of pain in women with endometriosis. Two systematic reviews evaluating the potential of aromatase inhibitors for the treatment of endometriosis-associated pain (Ferrero et al., 2011; Nawathe et al., 2008) have concluded that future studies are required to assess if aromatase inhibitors would be useful in long term for improvement of pain symptoms in comparison to the conventional therapy.[42,43]

Use of these agents is likely to result in hypo-oestrogenic side effects, such as vaginal dryness, hot flushes and reduced bone mineral density.

Adjuvant Therapy

This includes the use of tricyclic antidepressants such as amitriptyline and antiepileptics such as gabapentin for the management of chronic pain of endometriosis in patients who are resistant to the conventional therapies.

Surgery for Treatment of Endometriosis-associated Pain

Surgical treatment involving elimination of endometriotic lesions (through excision, diathermy or ablation/evaporation), division of adhesions (for restoring pelvic anatomy) and interruption of nerve pathways for alleviation of pain has long been used for the management of endometriosis. Surgical treatment of endometriomas must preferably be via laparoscopic cystectomy.

Laparotomy and laparoscopy are equally effective in the treatment of endometriosis-associated pain. Operative laparoscopy (excision/ablation) is more effective for the treatment of pelvic pain associated with all stages of endometriosis, compared to diagnostic laparoscopy only. Laparoscopic surgery is usually associated with less pain, shorter duration of hospital stay, quicker recovery and better cosmesis, in comparison to laparotomy. Therefore, laparoscopic surgery is usually preferred to open surgery. If the clinician having relevant experience with laparoscopy is not available, the patient should be referred to a centre of expertise because operative laparoscopy for advanced disease may be associated with a significant risk. When the lesions of endometriosis are identified at the time of diagnostic laparoscopy, clinicians are recommended to surgically treat these for reducing endometriosis-associated pain.[44] While laparoscopic surgery is effective for the treatment of pain secondary to endometriosis, long-term recurrence of pain can occur in nearly 50% individuals.

Ablation versus Excision of Endometriosis

Clinicians may consider using either ablation or excision of peritoneal endometriosis for reducing endometriosis-associated pain because both the procedures have been found to be equally effective.[45,46]

Laparoscopic Uterosacral Nerve Ablation versus Presacral Neurectomy

The minimally invasive procedure, laparoscopic uterosacral nerve ablation (LUNA), has not been found to be useful for alleviation of pain related to endometriosis.[47] Presacral neurectomy (PSN), on the other hand, has been found to be beneficial for treatment of endometriosis-associated midline pain as an adjunct to conservative laparoscopic surgery. However, PSN is a procedure requiring high degree of skill. Moreover, it may be associated with an increased risk of adverse effects such as bleeding, constipation, urinary urgency, etc.

Hysterectomy for Endometriosis-associated Pain

Hysterectomy with removal of the ovaries and all visible endometriosis lesions can be considered as a treatment option in women who are not desirous of future childbearing and have failed to respond to more conservative treatments. Prior to the surgery, women should be informed that hysterectomy might not necessarily cure the symptoms or the disease because disease excision may be incomplete.[48]

Prevention of Adhesions following Endometriosis Surgery

Clinical evidence: There are a number of barrier, fluid and pharmacological agents, which have been used for prevention of adhesions at the time of gynaecological surgery. Some such agents include oxidised regenerated cellulose (Interceed®), polytetrafluoroethylene surgical membrane (Gore-Tex®), fibrin sheet, sodium hyaluronate and carboxymethylcellulose combination (Seprafilm®), polyethylene oxide and carboxymethylcellulose gel (Oxiplex/AP®), icodextrin 4% (Adept®), hyaluronic acid products and polyethylene glycol hydrogel (SprayGel®), etc. Studies have shown that the use of oxidised regenerated cellulose helps in preventing adhesion formation during operative laparoscopy for endometriosis. On the other hand, use of icodextrin after operative laparoscopy for endometriosis is not likely to prevent adhesion formation. Therefore, its use is not recommended.[49,50] Clinicians should also be aware that other antiadhesion agents such as polytetrafluoroethylene surgical membrane, hyaluronic acid products, etc. have been studied and found to be effective for adhesion prevention in the perspective of pelvic surgery and not specifically in women with endometriosis.

TREATMENT OF ENDOMETRIOSIS-ASSOCIATED INFERTILITY

Various treatment options (medical, surgical, medical adjunct to surgery and alternative treatments) are used for improving fertility in women with endometriosis.

CHAPTER 68

Hormonal Therapies for Treatment of Endometriosis-associated Infertility

Use of hormonal treatment (e.g. danazol, GnRH analogues, OCPs, etc.) for suppression of ovarian function is unlikely to improve fertility in cases of minimal to mild endometriosis.[51]

Surgery for Treatment of Endometriosis-associated Infertility

Jacobson et al. (2010) have shown that operative laparoscopy including adhesiolysis is effective in increasing the pregnancy or live birth rate in comparison to diagnostic laparoscopy alone in women with minimal to mild endometriosis.[52] If the patient does not conceive after 6 months of operative laparoscopy or in cases of severe endometriosis lesions, assisted reproductive techniques (in vitro fertilisation and superovulation) can be considered. For details related to such techniques, kindly refer to Chapter 76 (Assisted Reproductive Techniques).

CLINICAL PEARLS

❖ Endometriosis is an oestrogen-dependent disease, characterised by the regression of lesions following treatment with drugs that block oestradiol synthesis.

❖ Hormone therapy and GnRH agonists help in providing pain relief but they delay fertility.

❖ Both laparoscopy and laparotomy are associated with similar pregnancy rates. However, laparoscopy is associated with reduced postoperative morbidity.

❖ Self-help and support groups can play an important role in pain management by helping the women better adapt to living with a chronic painful condition.

EVIDENCE-BASED MEDICINE

Presently, there is limited evidence regarding the efficacy of complementary and alternative therapy (acupuncture, meditation, massage, antioxidant and herbal medicine) for treatment of infertility in patients with endometriosis. Future RCTs of good quality are needed to investigate a possible role for complementary and alternative medicine in the treatment of endometriosis-related infertility.[53-57]

REFERENCES

1. ACOG Committee on Practice Bulletins-Gynecology. ACOG Practice Bulletin No. 51. Chronic pelvic pain. Obstet Gynecol. 2004;103(3):589-605.
2. Royal College of Obstetricians and Gynaecologists. The Initial Management of Chronic Pelvic Pain. Green-top Guideline No. 41. London: RCOG; 2012.
3. Royal College of Obstetricians and Gynaecologists. Management of acute pelvic inflammatory disease. Green-top Guideline No. 32. London: RCOG; 2008.
4. Moore J, Copley S, Morris J, Lindsell D, Golding S, Kennedy S. A systematic review of the accuracy of ultrasound in the diagnosis of endometriosis. Ultrasound Obstet Gynecol. 2002;20(6):630-4.
5. Jansen FW, Kapiteyn K, Trimbos-Kemper T, Hermans J, Trimbos JB. Complications of laparoscopy: a prospective multicentre observational study. Br J Obstet Gynaecol. 1997;104(5):595-600.
6. Chapron C, Querleu D, Bruhat M, Madelenat P, Fernandez H, Pierre F, et al. Surgical complications of diagnostic and operative gynaecological laparoscopy: a series of 29,966 cases. Hum Reprod. 1998;13(4):867-72.
7. Royal College of Obstetricians and Gynaecologists. Preventing entry-related gynaecological laparoscopic injuries. Greentop Guideline No. 49. London: RCOG; 2008.
8. Swanton A, Iyer L, Reginald PW. Diagnosis, treatment and follow up of women undergoing conscious pain mapping for chronic pelvic pain: a prospective cohort study. BJOG. 2006;113(7):792-6.
9. Nanda R, James R, Smith H, Dudley CR, Jewell DP. Food intolerance and the irritable bowel syndrome. Gut. 1989;30(8): 1099-104.
10. Spiller R, Aziz Q, Creed F, Emmanuel A, Houghton L, Hungin P, et al. Clinical Services Committee of The British Society of Gastroenterology. Guidelines on the irritable bowel syndrome: mechanisms and practical management. Gut. 2007;56(12):1770-98.
11. Jaiwala J, Imperiale TF, Kroenke K. Pharmacologic treatment of the irritable bowel syndrome: a systematic review of randomized, controlled trials. Ann Intern Med. 2000;133(2): 136-47.
12. Soysal ME, Soysal S, Kubilay V, Ozer S. A randomized controlled trial of goserelin and medroxyprogesterone acetate in the treatment of pelvic congestion. Hum Reprod. 2001;16(5):931-9.
13. Shokeir T, Amr M, Abdelshaheed M. The efficacy of Implanon for the treatment of chronic pelvic pain associated with pelvic congestion: 1-year randomized controlled pilot study. Arch Gynecol Obstet. 2009;280(3):437-43.
14. Ling FW. Randomized controlled trial of depot leuprolide in patients with chronic pelvic pain and clinically suspected endometriosis. Pelvic Pain Study Group. Obstet Gynecol. 1999;93(1):51-8.
15. Swank DJ, Swank-Bordewijk SC, Hop WC, van Erp WF, Janssen IM, Bonjer HJ, et al. Laparoscopic adhesiolysis in patients with chronic abdominal pain: a blinded randomised controlled multi-centre trial. Lancet. 2003;361(9365):1247-51.
16. Prior A, Wilson K, Whorwell PJ, Faragher EB. Irritable bowel syndrome in the gynecological clinic. Survey of 798 new referrals. Dig Dis Sci. 1989;34(12):1820-4.
17. Howard FM. The role of laparoscopy as a diagnostic tool in chronic pelvic pain. Baillieres Best Pract Res Clin Obstet Gynaecol. 2000;14(3):467-94.
18. Moore J, Ziebland S, Kennedy S. "People sometimes react funny if they're not told enough": women's views about the risks of diagnostic laparoscopy. Health Expect. 2002;5(4):302-9.
19. Davis GD, Thillet E, Lindemann J. Clinical characteristics of adolescent endometriosis. J Adolesc Health. 1993;14(5):362-8.
20. Seracchioli R, Mabrouk M, Guerrini M, Manuzzi L, Savelli L, Frascà C, et al. Dyschezia and posterior deep infiltrating endometriosis: analysis of 360 cases. J Minim Invasive Gynecol. 2008;15(6):695-9.
21. Bellelis P, Dias JA, Podgaec S, Gonzales M, Baracat EC, Abrão MS. Epidemiological and clinical aspects of pelvic endometriosis—a case series. Rev Assoc Med Bras. 2010;56(4): 467-71.

22. Bazot M, Lafont C, Rouzier R, Roseau G, Thomassin-Naggara I, Daraï E. Diagnostic accuracy of physical examination, transvaginal sonography, rectal endoscopic sonography, and magnetic resonance imaging to diagnose deep infiltrating endometriosis. Fertil Steril. 2009;92(6):1825-33.

23. Mol BW, Bayram N, Lijmer JG, Wiegerinck MA, Bongers MY, van der Veen F, et al. The performance of CA-125 measurement in the detection of endometriosis: a meta-analysis. Fertil Steril. 1998;70(6):1101-08.

24. Hudelist G, Fritzer N, Thomas A, Niehues C, Oppelt P, Haas D, et al. Diagnostic delay for endometriosis in Austria and Germany: causes and possible consequences. Hum Reprod. 2012;27(12):3412-6.

25. Stratton P, Winkel C, Premkumar A, Chow C, Wilson J, Hearns-Stokes R, et al. Diagnostic accuracy of laparoscopy, magnetic resonance imaging, and histopathologic examination for the detection of endometriosis. Fertil Steril. 2003;79(5):1078-85.

26. Revised American Society for Reproductive Medicine classification of endometriosis: 1996. Fertil Steril. 1997;67(5):817-21.

27. Wykes CB, Clark TJ, Khan KS. Accuracy of laparoscopy in the diagnosis of endometriosis: a systematic quantitative review. BJOG. 2004;111(11):1204-12.

28. Marjoribanks J, Proctor M, Farquhar C, Derks RS. Nonsteroidal anti-inflammatory drugs for dysmenorrhoea. Cochrane Database Syst Rev. 2010;(1):CD001751.

29. Vercellini P, Trespidi L, Colombo A, Vendola N, Marchini M, Crosignani PG. A gonadotropin-releasing hormone agonist versus a low-dose oral contraceptive for pelvic pain associated with endometriosis. Fertil Steril. 1993;60(1):75-9.

30. Brown J, Kives S, Akhtar M. Progestagens and anti-progestagens for pain associated with endometriosis. Cochrane Database Syst Rev. 2012;(3):CD002122.

31. Brown J, Pan A, Hart RJ. Gonadotrophin-releasing hormone analogues for pain associated with endometriosis. Cochrane Database Syst Rev. 2010;(12):CD008475.

32. Vercellini P, Frontino G, De Giorgi O, Pietropaolo G, Pasin R, Crosignani PG. Continuous use of an oral contraceptive for endometriosis-associated recurrent dysmenorrhea that does not respond to a cyclic pill regimen. Fertil Steril. 2003;80(3):560-3.

33. Vercellini P, Barbara G, Somigliana E, Bianchi S, Abbiati A, Fedele L. Comparison of contraceptive ring and patch for the treatment of symptomatic endometriosis. Fertil Steril. 2010;93(7):2150-61.

34. Petta CA, Ferriani RA, Abrao MS, Hassan D, Rosa E Silva JC, Podgaec S, et al. Randomized clinical trial of a levonorgestrel-releasing intrauterine system and a depot GnRH analogue for the treatment of chronic pelvic pain in women with endometriosis. Hum Reprod. 2005;20(7):1993-8.

35. Gomes MK, Ferriani RA, Rosa e Silva JC, Japur de Sá Rosa e Silva AC, Vieira CS, Cândido dos Reis FJ. The levonorgestrel-releasing intrauterine system and endometriosis staging. Fertil Steril. 2007;87(5):1231-4.

36. Ferreira RA, Vieira CS, Rosa-E-Silva JC, Rosa-e-Silva AC, Nogueira AA, Ferriani RA. Effects of the levonorgestrelreleasing intrauterine system on cardiovascular risk markers in patients with endometriosis: a comparative study with the GnRH analogue. Contraception. 2010;81(2):117-22.

37. Barbieri RL. Hormone treatment of endometriosis: the estrogen threshold hypothesis. Am J Obstet Gynecol. 1992;166(2):740-5.

38. Sagsveen M, Farmer JE, Prentice A, Breeze A. Gonadotrophin-releasing hormone analogues for endometriosis: bone mineral density. Cochrane Database Syst Rev. 2003;(4):CD001297.

39. Farquhar C, Prentice A, Singla A, Selak V. Danazol for pelvic pain associated with endometriosis. Cochrane Database Syst Rev. 2007;(4):CD000068.

40. Bhattacharya SM, Tolasaria A, Khan B. Vaginal danazol for the treatment of endometriosis-related pelvic pain. Int J Gynecol Obstet. 2011;115(3):294-5.

41. Dunselman GA, Vermeulen N, Becker C, Calhaz-Jorge C, D'Hooghe T, De Bie B, et al. ESHRE guideline: management of women with endometriosis. Hum Reprod. 2014;29(3):400-12.

42. Ferrero S, Gillott DJ, Venturini PL, Remorgida V. Use of aromatase inhibitors to treat endometriosis-related pain symptoms: a systematic review. Reprod Biol Endocrinol. 2011;9:89.

43. Nawathe A, Patwardhan S, Yates D, Harrison GR, Khan KS. Systematic review of the effects of aromatase inhibitors on pain associated with endometriosis. BJOG. 2008;115(7):818-22.

44. Jacobson TZ, Duffy JM, Barlow D, Koninckx PR, Garry R. Laparo-scopic surgery for pelvic pain associated with endometriosis. Cochrane Database Syst Rev. 2009;(4): CD001300.

45. Healey M, Ang WC, Cheng C. Surgical treatment of endo-metriosis: a prospective randomized double-blinded trial comparing excision and ablation. Fertil Steril. 2010;94(7):2536-40.

46. Wright J, Lotfallah H, Jones K, Lovell D. A randomized trial of excision versus ablation for mild endometriosis. Fertil Steril. 2005;83(6):1830-6.

47. Proctor M, Latthe PM, Farquhar CM, Khan KS, Johnson NP. Surgical interruption of pelvic nerve pathways for primary and secondary dysmenorrhoea. Cochrane Database Syst Rev. 2005;(4):CD001896.

48. Martin DC. Hysterectomy for treatment of pain associated with endometriosis. J Minim Invasive Gynecol. 2006;13(6):566-72.

49. Brown CB, Luciano AA, Martin D, Peers E, Scrimgeour A, diZerega GS, et al. Adept (icodextrin 4% solution) reduces adhesions after laparoscopic surgery for adhesiolysis: a double blind, randomized, controlled study. Fertil Steril. 2007;88(5):1413-26.

50. Trew G, Pistofidis G, Pados G, Lower A, Mettler L, Wallwiener D, et al. Gynaecological endoscopic evaluation of 4% icodextrin solution: a European, multicentre, double-blind, randomized study of the efficacy and safety in the reduction of de novo adhesions after laparoscopic gynaecological surgery. Hum Reprod. 2011;26(8):2015-27.

51. Hughes E, Brown J, Collins JJ, Farquhar C, Fedorkow DM, Vandekerckhove P. Ovulation suppression for endometriosis for women with subfertility. Cochrane Database Syst Rev. 2007;(3):CD000155.

52. Jacobson TZ, Duffy JM, Barlow D, Farquhar C, Koninckx PR, Olive D. Laparoscopic surgery for subfertility associated with endometriosis. Cochrane Database Syst Rev. 2010;(1):CD001398.

53. Agarwal A, Gupta S, Sharma RK. Role of oxidative stress in female reproduction. Reprod Biol Endocrinol. 2005;3:28.

54. Burks-Wicks C, Cohen M, Fallbacher J, Taylor RN, Wieser F. A Western primer of Chinese herbal therapy in endometriosis and infertility. Womens Health (Lond Engl). 2005;1(3):447-63.

55. Xu X, Yin H, Tang D, Zhang L, Gosden RG. Application of traditional Chinese medicine in the treatment of infertility. Human Fertil (Camb). 2003;6(4):161-8.

56. Gerhard I, Postneek F. Auricular acupuncture in the treatment of female infertility. Gynecol Endocrinol. 1992;6(3):171-81.

57. Wurn BF, Wurn LJ, King CR, Heuer MA, Roscow AS, Hornberger K, et al. Treating fallopian tube occlusion with a manual pelvic physical therapy. Altern Ther Health Med. 2008;14(1):18-23.

CHAPTER 68

Adenomyosis

INTRODUCTION

Adenomyosis is a condition in which there is a growth of endometrial cells inside the uterine myometrium (usually >2.5 mm beneath the basal endometrium).[1] It is associated with myometrial hypertrophy and may be either diffuse or focal (adenomyoma). Microscopically, there are ectopic, non-neoplastic endometrial glands and stroma, surrounded by hypertrophic and hyperplastic myometrium.[2]

The majority of cases of adenomyosis are diagnosed following histological examination of hysterectomy specimens showing a prevalence varying between 5% to 70%.[3] The prevalence in general population, however, remains unclear. The majority of cases are reported amongst women in the age groups of 40–50 years and there is a positive association with parity. No association has been observed with age at menarche, menopausal status, or age at hysterectomy or its indication.

Associated Pathology

Nearly 80% of women with adenomyomas may also have other lesions, most common being the leiomyomas. Other lesions which may frequently occur in these cases include endometrial polyps, endometrial hyperplasia (with or without atypia), adenocarcinoma and pelvic endometriosis.[4] Presence of adenomyosis, however, has no adverse effect on cancer survival.[5]

AETIOLOGY

Abnormal ingrowth and invagination of the basal endometrium into the subendometrial myometrium at the endometrial-myometrial interface is likely to result in development of adenomyosis.[6] Though the exact cause of adenomyosis remains unknown, various factors, such as hormonal, genetic and immunological, are likely to play a role in the pathogenesis of adenomyosis. Some likely causes are as follows:

- *Uterine trauma*: Various causes of uterine trauma that may break the barrier between the endometrium and myometrium include surgical procedures such as caesarean section, tubal ligation, and pregnancy termination. Pregnancy is another factor which can break this barrier.
- *Oestrogen dominance*: Conditions associated with the localised production of excessive oestrogens may predispose the woman to develop adenomyosis.
- *Abnormal level of various cytokines*: Increased levels of IL-18 (interleukin 18) receptor mRNA (messenger RNA) and the ratio of IL-18 binding protein to IL-18, and dysregulation of leukaemia inhibitory factor.

DIAGNOSIS

Clinical Presentation

Nearly 35% of women with adenomyosis uteri are asymptomatic. Commonly occurring symptoms include menorrhagia (unresponsive to hormonal therapy or uterine curettage) and progressively increasing dysmenorrhoea. Menorrhagia can occur in nearly 40–50% cases, dysmenorrhoea in 10–30% cases and metrorrhagia in 10–12% cases.[7,8] Menorrhagia may be due to dysfunctional contractility of the myometrium, endometrial hyperplasia and anovulation. Other symptoms may include pelvic pain, backache, dyspareunia, dyschezia and subfertility. Older women tend to be more symptomatic in comparison to younger women.

Pelvic Examination

- Uterus may become diffuse and enlarged in cases of diffuse adenomyosis. Uterus may be enlarged to about 12–14 weeks in size and may be tender to touch, soft and boggy.
- Adenomyosis is associated with uterine fibroids in about 6–20% cases.

Investigations

Presently, there is lack of a reliable, non-invasive diagnostic test for diagnosing adenomyosis. No serum markers for the diagnosis of adenomyosis are currently available. Some investigations, which are commonly performed, include the following:

❖ *Ultrasound examination*: Transvaginal sonography (TVS) is better than transabdominal sonography (TAS) in demonstrating the subtle features suggestive of adenomyosis uteri. Some features suggestive of adenomyosis on TVS are enlisted in Box 69.1.[9-16] Presently, there is no consensus regarding whether one or some of these criteria should be used for making the diagnosis of adenomyosis. Most authorities presently use three or more of these criteria for making the diagnosis of adenomyosis.[17] A recent meta-analysis has indicated that ultrasound features such as presence of myometrial cysts, linear myometrial striations, poor delineation of the endomyometrial junction and a heterogenous myometrium are associated with an increased probability of the presence of disease (Fig. 69.1).[18]

In the normal woman, the myometrium has three distinct sonographic layers of which the middle layer is the most echogenic and the inner layer is hypoechoic relative to the middle and outer layers. This hypoechogenicity is responsible for producing the subendometrial or myometrial halo. The presence of adenomyosis uteri can cause alterations in the sonographic appearance of these zones. Studies regarding the accuracy of TVS for detection of adenomyosis have reported the rates of sensitivity varying between 53% to 89% and specificity varying between 50% to 99%. Three-dimensional ultrasonography is likely to offer higher accuracy in determining uterine volume and pathology.

❖ *Magnetic resonance imaging*: This is superior to ultrasound for the diagnosis of adenomyosis. There has been growing evidence to support the use of MRI in the diagnosis of

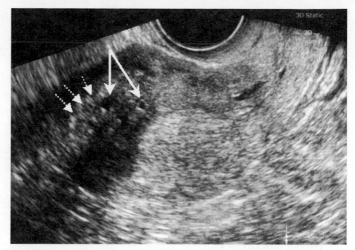

Fig. 69.1: Ultrasound showing mottled texture of the myometrium and presence of hypoechoic areas within the hyperechoic area in the fundal region which is suggestive of adenomyosis

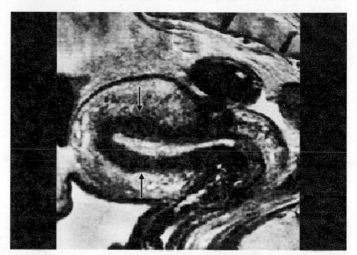

Fig. 69.2: Sagittal T_2-weighted MR image showing diffuse, even thickening of the junctional zone (as depicted by arrows) which is consistent with the diagnosis of diffuse adenomyosis

adenomyosis uteri. MRI may be considered when findings on TVS appear to be inconclusive. However, its high cost and limited availability may impede its routine use. The presence of heterotopic endometrial glands and stroma in the myometrium appear as bright foci within the myometrium on T_2-weighted MR images (Fig. 69.2). Adjacent smooth muscle hyperplasia may present as areas of reduced signal intensity on MRI. On MRI examination, there is considerable variation in the thickness of junctional zone, ranging from 2 mm to 8 mm.[19,20] The appearance of diffuse or focal widening of the junctional zone on MRI is suggestive of adenomyosis uteri. Several studies which have compared the accuracy of TVS and MRI have found both these techniques to have comparable sensitivities and specificities. Nevertheless, MRI is less observer-dependent. MRI has proved to be superior to TVS in the presence of associated leiomyomas or additional pathologies.[21] MRI is more useful in distinguishing adenomyosis from fibroids in an enlarged uterus.

❖ *CA-125*: Level of CA-125 in the peripheral blood may be raised.

Box 69.1: Criteria used to diagnose adenomyosis using TVS[9-16]

❑ Globular uterine enlargement in the absence of leiomyomas
❑ Asymmetric enlargement of the anterior or posterior myometrial wall
❑ Heterogeneous, poorly circumscribed anechoic areas within the myometrium
❑ Hyperechoic islands or nodules, finger-like projections or linear striations, indistinct endometrial stripe
❑ Anechoic lacunae or cystic spaces of varying size, which may be blood-filled
❑ Focal or diffuse thickening of the junctional zone
❑ Low-signal intensity uterine mass with ill-defined border
❑ Junctional zone thickness: 12 mm
❑ Indistinct endometrial-myometrial border
❑ Localised high signal foci within an area of low signal intensity
❑ Myometrial linear striations
❑ Parallel shadowing
❑ Bright foci in endometrium of similar intensity to the myometrium (T_1-weighted)
❑ Ratio of maximal junctional zone thickness to myometrium thickness: 40%
❑ Subendometrial halo thickening

❖ *Histopathological examination*: The final diagnosis is established by histopathological examination of the hysterectomy specimen.

DIFFERENTIAL DIAGNOSIS

Leiomyomas: Adenomyosis is most commonly confused with leiomyomas. Transvaginal ultrasonography is an effective, non-invasive and relatively inexpensive procedure for establishing the diagnosis of adenomyoma preoperatively.

MANAGEMENT

Different surgical and medical modalities of treatment have been used for the management of cases of adenomyosis uteri. Management is often directed at the treatment of symptoms.

MEDICAL THERAPY

Medical treatment for cases of adenomyosis comprises of NSAIDs, hormone therapy, danazol, GnRH agonists and Mirena® IUCD Medical non-hormonal therapy, including mefenamic and tranexamic acid, may be effective for the symptomatic relief of menorrhagia in patients with uterine adenomyosis.[22] Symptomatic relief is also obtained using hormonal treatment including progestogens, the combined OCPs and GnRH analogues.

Combined oral contraceptive pills: Use of low-dose, continuous combined oral contraceptives with withdrawal bleeding after every 4–6 months may be effective in relieving menorrhagia and dysmenorrhoea associated with adenomyosis.[23] However, there is no specific study related to this therapy in cases with adenomyosis.

Gonadotropin-releasing hormone analogues: Use of GnRH analogues is also likely to be useful for the treatment of adenomyosis uteri by reducing uterine volume and providing symptomatic relief.[24] However, these benefits are rapidly reversed following the cessation of treatment. Moreover, they are also likely to cause skeletal and general side-effects. There could be a role for long term use of GnRH therapy in association with add-back therapy as described with uterine fibroids and endometriosis [Chapters 65 (Uterine Leiomyoma) and 68 (Chronic Pelvic Pain and Endometriosis)].

Danazol: The use of danazol has largely become out-dated due to its androgenic side-effects. Danazol-loaded intra-uterine device has been used as a non-invasive method for the treatment of infertile women with adenomyosis uteri.[25,26] This method is likely to result in pregnancy following the discontinuation of treatment. Moreover, it is associated with preservation of both menstrual and ovulatory functions and a significant decrease in dysmenorrhoea.

Levonorgestrel-intrauterine system: LNG-IUS has been tried as the treatment option of moderate or severe dysmenorrhoea and/or menorrhagia associated with adenomyosis.[27] There is some evidence that the presence of deep lesions of adenomyosis is associated with the failure of endometrial ablation.[28,29] In these situations, LNG-IUS has also been successfully used for the treatment of adenomyosis-associated menorrhagia, especially when inserted immediately after endometrial ablation.

SURGICAL MANAGEMENT

Hysterectomy

Total hysterectomy with or without bilateral salpingo-oophorectomy is the treatment of choice in elderly patients who are past their childbearing age or those who have completed their childbearing.[10] Decision to perform a hysterectomy is usually based on the presence of other pathologies such as leiomyomas or failure of medical or conservative management in cases of menorrhagia. Conservative surgery may be performed in the younger patients.

Conservative Surgery

Uterine Artery Embolisation

Uterine artery embolisation (UAE) is presently developing as an effective and safe method for the treatment of adenomyosis. UAE, by causing reduction of the uterine blood flow by blocking the uterine artery, has been shown to reduce the symptoms associated with adenomyosis uteri and to improve the quality of life.[30] However, the recurrence rate of adenomyosis following the procedure has yet not been evaluated. UAE can be considered as a recognised treatment option for women with adenomyosis having concurrent fibroids.[31] However, all patients undergoing UAE should be counselled regarding the chances of treatment failure, recurrence rates and the requirement for hysterectomy in future.[32] The chances of a subsequent successful pregnancy following the procedure are unclear. For details related to UAE, kindly refer to Chapter 65 (Uterine Leiomyoma).

Endomyometrial Ablation

Endometrial ablation or resection can be considered as an option for women with superficial adenomyosis, presenting with the complaints of menorrhagia. However, the option of endometrial ablation cannot be used in women desiring future pregnancy.[33] Moreover, this procedure is likely to be associated with an increased failure rate in patients with deep adenomyosis.

Magnetic Resonance-guided Focussed Ultrasound

Magnetic resonance-guided focussed ultrasound (MRgFUS) has also been tried as a non-invasive option for the treatment of adenomyosis.[34] However, further studies are required in future for assessment of the overall safety and long-term effectiveness of MRgFUS for the treatment of adenomyosis.

PART III

COMPLICATIONS

- Adenomyosis can be associated with considerable morbidity due to the presence of debilitating symptoms such as menorrhágia, dysmenorrhoea, chronic pelvic pain, etc.
- Reduced fertility
- Coexistence of pelvic abnormalities such as uterine fibroids, endometrial hyperplasia and endometrial adenocarcinoma.

CLINICAL PEARLS

- Multiparas between the ages of 30 to 50 years are most commonly affected with this disease.
- The margins of adenomyosis are poorly defined because the endometrial glands and stroma are in direct contact with the myometrium. Hence, these lesions cannot be enucleated.
- The diagnosis of adenomyosis can only be confirmed by a pathologist.
- Magnetic resonance imaging has a higher specificity than TVS, but similar sensitivity regarding the diagnosis of adenomyosis.
- Endometrial ablation for the treatment of heavy menstrual bleeding in cases of adenomyosis is likely to be associated with a high failure rate.
- The role of invasive hysteroscopic or laparoscopic biopsy for diagnosing adenomyosis remains limited.

EVIDENCE-BASED MEDICINE

- Presently, there is limited evidence regarding the use of medical, non-hormonal therapy for the treatment of cases of adenomyosis. These treatment strategies are likely to result in a variable and unpredictable degree of symptomatic relief, which is usually limited to the duration of treatment.[10]
- Uterine artery embolisation is used in women with adenomyosis alone or in combination with uterine fibroids. The present evidence indicates that this procedure may be effective in cases where adenomyosis is present in association with uterine fibroids.[30,31] However, there is limited evidence regarding the efficacy of UAE in cases where the predominant lesion is adenomyosis.[32]

REFERENCES

1. Uduwela AS, Perera MA, Aiqing L, Fraser IS. Endometrial–myometrial interface: relationship to adenomyosis and changes in pregnancy. Obstet Gynecol Surv. 2000;55(6):390-400.

2. Maheshwari A, Gurunath S, Fatima F, Bhattacharya S. Adenomyosis and subfertility: a systematic review of prevalence, diagnosis, treatment and fertility outcomes. Hum Reprod Update. 2012;18(4):374-92.

3. Azziz R. Adenomyosis: current perspectives. Obstet Gynecol Clin North Am. 1989;16(1):221-35.

4. Bergholt T, Eriksen L, Berendt N, Jacobsen M, Hertz JB. Prevalence and risk factors of adenomyosis at hysterectomy. Hum Reprod. 2001;16(11):2418-21.

5. Hall JB, Young RH, Nelson JH. The prognostic significance of adenomyosis in endometrial carcinoma. Gynecol Oncol. 1984;17(1):32-40.

6. Mehasseb MK, Habiba MA. Adenomyosis uteri: an update. Obstet Gynaecol. 2009;11(1):41-7.

7. Parazzini F, Vercellini P, Panazza S, Chatenoud L, Oldani S, Crosignani PG. Risk factors for adenomyosis. Hum Reprod. 1997;12(6):1275-9.

8. Vavilis D, Agorastos T, Tzafetas J, Loufopoulos A, Vakiani M, Constantinidis T, et al. Adenomyosis at hysterectomy: prevalence and relationship to operative findings and reproductive and menstrual factors. Clin Exp Obstet Gynecol. 1997;24(1):36-8.

9. Ascher SM, Arnold LL, Patt RH, Schruefer JJ, Bagley AS, Semelka RC, et al. Adenomyosis: prospective comparison of MR imaging and transvaginal sonography. Radiology. 1994;190(3):803-6.

10. Reinhold C, McCarthy S, Bret PM, Mehio A, Atri M, Zakarian R, et al. Diffuse adenomyosis: comparison of endovaginal US and MR imaging with histopathologic correlation. Radiology. 1996;199(1):151-8.

11. Brosens JJ, de Souza NM, Barker FG, Paraschos T, Winston RM. Endovaginal ultrasonography in the diagnosis of adenomyosis uteri: identifying the predictive characteristics. Br J Obstet Gynaecol. 1995;102(6):471-4.

12. Reinhold C, Atri M, Mehio A, Zakarian R, Aldis AE, Bret PM. Diffuse uterine adenomyosis: morphologic criteria and diagnostic accuracy of endovaginal sonography. Radiology. 1995;197(3):609-14.

13. Fedele L, Bianchi S, Dorta M, Zanotti F, Brioschi D, Carinelli S. Transvaginal ultrasonography in the differential diagnosis of adenomyoma versus leiomyoma. Am J Obstet Gynecol. 1992;167(3):603-6.

14. Hirai M, Shibata K, Sagai H, Sekiya S, Goldberg BB. Transvaginal pulsed and color Doppler sonography for the evaluation of adenomyosis. J Ultrasound Med. 1995;14(7):529-32.

15. Atri M, Reinhold C, Mehio AR, Chapman WB, Bret PM. Adenomyosis: US features with histologic correlation in an in-vitro study. Radiology. 2000;215(3):783-90.

16. Fedele L, Bianchi S, Raffaelli R, Portuese A, Dorta M. Treatment of adenomyosis-associated menorrhagia with a levonorgestrel-releasing intrauterine device. Fertil Steril. 1997;68(3):426-9.

17. Dueholm M. Transvaginal ultrasound for diagnosis of adenomyosis: a review. Best Pract Res Clin Obstet Gynaecol. 2006;20(4):569-82.

18. Dartmouth K. A systematic review with meta-analysis: the common sonographic characteristics of adenomyosis. Ultrasound. 2014;22(3):148-57.

19. Hauth EA, Jaeger HJ, Libera H, Lange S, Forsting M. MR imaging of the uterus and cervix in healthy women: determination of normal values. Eur Radiol. 2007;17(3):734-42.

20. Lee JK, Gersell DJ, Balfe DM, Worthington JL, Picus D, Gapp G. The uterus: in vitro MR-anatomic correlation of normal and abnormal specimens. Radiology. 1985;157(1):175-9.

21. Bazot M, Cortez A, Darai E, Rouger J, Chopier J, Antoine JM, et al. Ultrasonography compared with magnetic resonance imaging for the diagnosis of adenomyosis: correlation with histopathology. Hum Reprod. 2001;16(11):2427-33.

22. Azziz R. Adenomyosis: current perspectives. Obstet Gynecol Clin North Am. 1989;16(1):221-35.

23. Moghissi KS. Treatment of endometriosis with estrogen-progestin combination and progestogens alone. Clin Obstet Gynecol. 1988;31(4):823-8.

24. Grow DR, Filer RB. Treatment of adenomyosis with long-term GnRH analogues: a case report. Obstet Gynecol. 1991;78(3 Pt 2):538-9.

25. Igarashi M, Abe Y, Fukuda M, Ando A, Miyasaka M, Yoshida M, et al. Novel conservative medical therapy for uterine adenomyosis with a danazol-loaded intrauterine device. Fertil Steril. 2000;74(2):412-3.

26. Tamaoka Y, Orikasa H, Sakakura K, Kamei K, Nagatani M, Ezawa S. Direct effect of danazol on endometrial hyperplasia in adenomyotic women: treatment with danazol containing intrauterine device. Hum Cell. 2000;13(3):127-33.

27. Sheng J, Zhang WY, Zhang JP, Lu D. The LNG-IUS study on adenomyosis: a 3-year follow-up study on the efficacy and side effects of the use of levonorgestrel intrauterine system for the treatment of dysmenorrhea associated with adenomyosis. Contraception. 2009;79(3):189-93.

28. Maia H, Maltez A, Coelho G, Athayde C, Coutinho EM. Insertion of mirena after endometrial resection in patients with adenomyosis. J Am Assoc Gynecol Laparosc. 2003;10(4):512-6.

29. Rabinovici J, Stewart EA. New interventional techniques for adenomyosis. Best Pract Res Clin Obstet Gynaecol. 2006;20(4):617-36.

30. Siskin GP, Tublin ME, Stainken BF, Dowling K, Dolen EG. Uterine artery embolization for the treatment of adenomyosis: clinical response and evaluation with MR imaging. AJR Am J Roentgenol. 2001;177(2):297-302.

31. Kim MD, Kim S, Kim NK, Lee MH, Ahn EH, Kim HJ, et al. Long-term results of uterine artery embolization for symptomatic adenomyosis. AJR Am J Roentgenol. 2007;188(1):176-81.

32. Lohle PN, De Vries J, Klazen CA, Boekkooi PF, Vervest HA, Smeets AJ, et al. Uterine artery embolization for symptomatic adenomyosis with or without uterine leiomyomas with the use of calibrated tris-acryl gelatin microspheres: midterm clinical and MR imaging follow-up. J Vasc Interv Radiol. 2007;18(7):835-41.

33. McCausland AM, McCausland VM. Depth of endometrial penetration in adenomyosis helps determine outcome of rollerball ablation. Am J Obstet Gynecol. 1996;174(6):1786-94.

34. Rabinovici J, Inbar Y, Eylon SC, Schiff E, Hananel A, Freundlich D. Pregnancy and live birth after focused ultrasound surgery for symptomatic focal adenomyosis: a case report. Hum Reprod. 2006;21(5):1255-9.

SECTION 13

Reproductive Medicine

GYNAECOLOGY

Normal Conception

EMBRYOLOGY AND EARLY FOETAL DEVELOPMENT

Gametogenesis

Gametogenesis comprises of spermatogenesis (in males) and oogenesis (in females).

Spermatogenesis

The process in which spermatogonia gets transformed into spermatozoon is known as spermatogenesis. The testes are responsible for producing sperms and male hormone, mainly testosterone. Spermatogenesis is primarily under the control of FSH and testosterone.[1] FSH is bound to Sertoli cells and stimulates the production of testicular fluid. The LH also has a role in the regulation of spermatogenesis and influences production of testosterone. The rate of testosterone synthesis and secretion is dependent on LH. In the testes, LH binds to receptors on Leydig cells and stimulates synthesis and secretion of testosterone. Besides producing testosterone, testes are also involved in the production of small amounts of other hormones such as oestrone and oestradiol in men. However, the major portions of these hormones, oestrone and oestradiol, are derived by peripheral aromatisation of androstenedione and testosterone, respectively. Sertoli cells in testis are equivalent to the granulosa cells of the ovary and respond primarily to FSH. Sertoli cells are responsible for producing inhibin. On the other hand, Leydig cells have receptors for LH and therefore mainly respond to this hormone. Testosterone is synthesised in the interstitial Leydig cells from where it diffuses into the seminiferous tubules and plays an important role in the facilitation of the process of spermatogenesis, which involves the production of sperms. The process of spermatogenesis takes place in the space between the Sertoli cells, with Leydig cells releasing testosterone to stimulate the process. Testosterone gets converted into dihydrotestosterone in the peripheral tissues with help of an enzyme 5-α reductase in males.

Dihydrotestosterone is more potent than testosterone. Besides spermatogenesis, testosterone also induces the development of secondary sexual characteristics in males such as deepening of voice, growth of body hair, penile growth, etc. Androgens also stimulate the activity of sebaceous glands.

The time required for the completion of the entire process of development of spermatozoon from the spermatogonium is about 70–75 days. Stages of spermatogenesis are described in Figure 70.1. Initial process of spermatogenesis involves mitotic division, which is responsible for converting spermatogonia to primary spermatocytes. The spermatozoa then develop through a process of meiosis so that eventually diploid spermatocytes get converted into four haploid spermatids. The spermatogonia, up to the stage of spermatids, are situated in the deep recesses of Sertoli cells which not only provide support to the germ cells during spermatogenesis, but also provide nourishment during their development. The spermatids eventually transform into spermatozoa, by a process known as spermiogenesis.

Oogenesis

The various stages of oogenesis have been described in Figure 70.2. The primordial germ cells, after arriving in the female gonad, differentiate into oogonia around 9th week of gestation. These enter the first meiotic division and are converted into oocytes. Progression of meiosis to the diplotene stage is accomplished throughout the pregnancy and is completed by birth. In the last week before birth, all the primary oocytes complete the diplotene stage, but do not progress further. Instead, they get arrested in the diplotene stage of prophase. The primary oocytes remain arrested at this stage and do not undergo the completion of first meiotic division till the age of puberty, when the completion of first meiotic division occurs at the time of ovulation.[2] Second meiotic division starts, but gets arrested in the metaphase, which is completed only at the time of fertilisation.

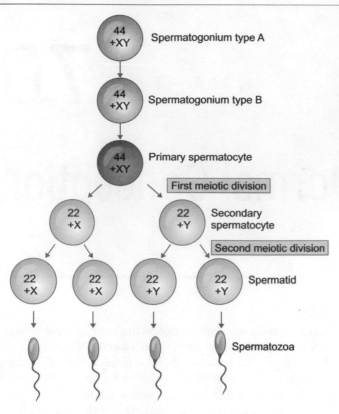

Fig. 70.1: Stages of spermatogenesis

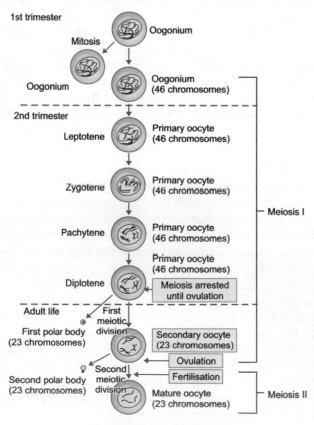

Fig. 70.2: Stages of oogenesis

OVULATION-FERTILISATION

Ovulation takes place as the ovarian follicle ruptures and the discharged oocyte is carried into the peritoneal cavity via the uterine tube. The fertilisation life span of the released ovum varies from 24 hours to 36 hours. Details related to ovulation are described in Chapter 58 (Menstrual Cycle). Once the oocyte has been extruded out, the cells of the empty ovarian follicle get converted into the corpus luteum which produces progesterone for about 14 days, in absence of fertilisation and for 3–4 months if fertilisation has taken place, after which it eventually dies off.[3] The oocyte moves from the ovary to the uterine tube and may get fertilised by the male gamete in the ampulla of the uterine tube. Even though many spermatozoa may approach the oocyte, only one spermatozoon is allowed to enter the oocyte. The mechanism through which the zona pellucida (surrounding the ovum) precludes more than one sperm from entering the oocyte is known as the zona reaction. The sperm passes the zona pellucida by capacitation and acrosome reaction. The process of fertilisation between two haploid gametes results in the formation of a diploid zygote, thereby restoring the number of chromosomes to that of the normal somatic cell. On fertilisation, the chromosomal configuration can be of two types, either 44 (XY), i.e. a male child or 44 (XX), i.e. a female child. The process of ovulation and fertilisation has been summarised in Figure 70.3.

CLEAVAGE DIVISION AND FORMATION OF MORULA

The zygote, a diploid cell with 46 chromosomes, formed as a result of fertilisation of mature egg with a sperm, undergoes numerous cleavage divisions to produce cells known as blastomeres (Fig. 70.4). At this stage, the zygote is present inside the fallopian tube and is surrounded by a thick zona pellucida. For 3 days as the blastomeres continue to divide, they produce a solid, mulberry-like ball of cells. This 16-celled ball is called morula. The morula enters the uterine cavity approximately 3 days after fertilisation, and floats around in the cavity for a few more days. During this time, fluid gradually accumulates between the morula's cells, transforming the morula into a blastocyst.

FORMATION OF BLASTOCYST

As the fluid begins to pass through the zona pellucida and gets accumulated between the cells, the morula looks like a cyst and becomes the blastocyst. When the blastocyst reaches 58-celled stage at about 4th to 5th day of fertilisation, it gets transformed into two types of cells: (1) trophoblast cells and (2) an inner cell mass, which forms the embryo proper (Fig. 70.5). The cells of the inner cell mass get displaced to one side. This side of the blastocyst is known as embryonic pole and the opposite side as the abembryonic pole. The inner cell mass (consisting of blastomeres) is destined to form the various tissues of the embryo. The trophoblast comprises of outer single layer of flattened cells, which later get converted into the future placenta. The cavity of the blastocyst is called the blastocoele.

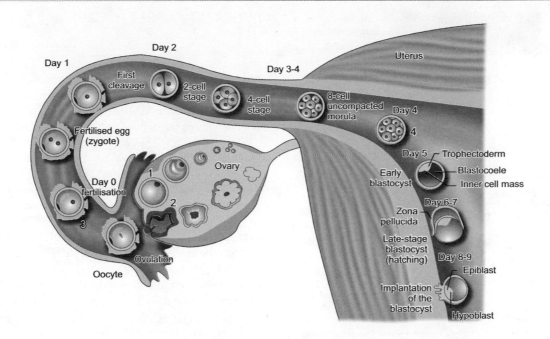

Fig. 70.3: Process of ovulation, fertilisation and implantation

Key: 1, Maturation of ovarian follicle; 2, Ovulation and formation of corpus luteum; 3, fertilisation in the ampulla of uterine tube; 4, Formation of morula

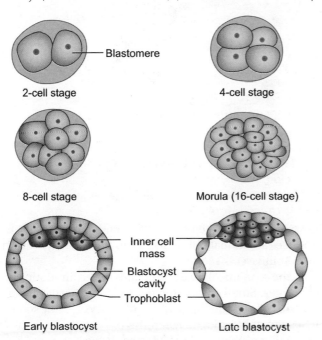

Fig. 70.4: Conversion of embryo from 2-celled stage to the late blastocyst stage

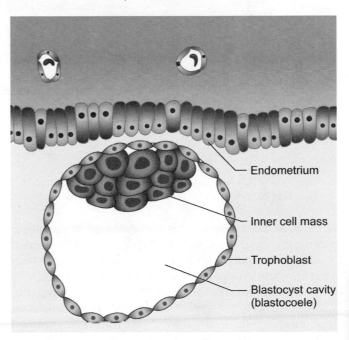

Fig. 70.5: Blastocyst at a later stage with inner cell mass shifted to one side

The function of zona pellucida which is still surrounding the blastocyst is mainly protective. Its presence prevents implantation of the blastocyst in the uterine wall. As the fluid gets imbibed into the blastocyst and it increases in size, the tough layer of zona pellucida eventually ruptures. Once in the uterus, as the zona pellucida ruptures and gets casted off, the trophoblast comes in direct contact with the endometrium to begin the implantation. Implantation begins with the burrowing of the blastocyst into the endometrium. At this stage, there are about 100–250 cells in the blastocyst. The blastocyst begins to implant at about 6–7 days after fertilisation.[4] The most common site of implantation is upper posterior wall of the uterine cavity. The prerequisite for successful implantation requires an endometrium which has been primed with oestrogen and progesterone. The process of implantation involves the destruction of maternal tissue, following which the blastocyst sticks to the uterine wall, gradually eroding the uterine lining. The invasiveness of trophoblast helps in attachment of the blastocyst to the decidua and helps in deriving nutrition for the growth of the embryo.[5] Moreover, once inside the uterine wall, the blastocyst invades the mother's blood vessels, and destroys

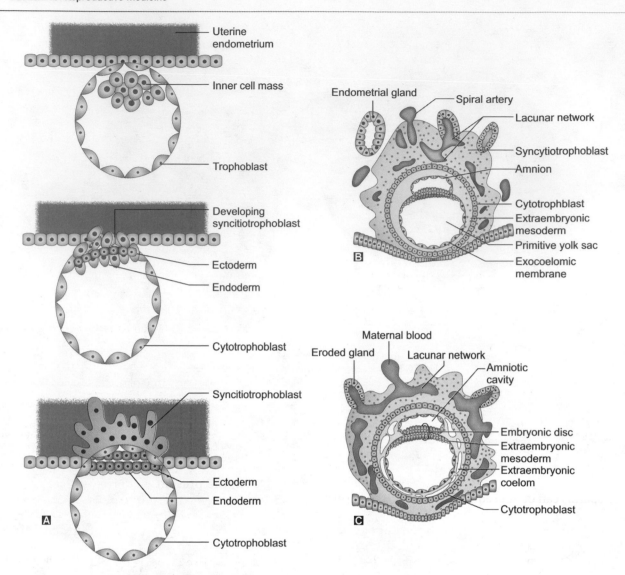

Figs 70.6A to C: (A) Stages of implantation of blastocyst; (B) Blastocyst at the time of implantation; (C) Blastocyst at 12th day after fertilisation

the walls of these vessels. This process helps in establishing an uteroplacental blood flow. By 8th day postfertilisation, the trophoblast gets differentiated into an outer multinucleated syncytium known as syncytiotrophoblast and an inner layer of cytotrophoblasts. In the multinucleated syncytium, there is absence of cell borders within the individual cells. As the trophoblastic cells invade deeper into the endometrium, by 10th day postfertilisation, the blastocyst gets totally embedded within the endometrium (Figs 70.6A and B). As the blastocyst implants into the uterine wall, simultaneously it also prepares its cells and surrounding endometrium to develop into a placenta.[6] The blastocyst consists of two groups of cells: (1) the inner cell mass, which become the embryo, and (2) the trophoblast cells, which are crucial in producing the chorion (the embryonic portion of the placenta). As early as 7–8 days after fertilisation, the inner cell mass or the embryonic disc gets differentiated into a top layer, ectoderm (epiblast) and an underlying layer of endoderm (hypoblast). Small cells appear between the embryonic disc and trophoblast enclosing a space that later gets transformed into amniotic cavity. The ectoderm forms the floor of the amniotic cavity while the roof

is formed by amniogenic cells. The endodermal germ layer produces additional cells which form a new cavity, known as the definitive yolk sac.

As the amniotic fluid accumulates in the amniotic cavity, it enlarges. Small embryonic mesenchymal cells appear as isolated cells within the cavity of blastocyst.[7] They soon line the cavity of blastocyst. When the blastocyst is completely lined with mesoderm, it is termed as chorionic vesicle. This is surrounded by a membrane called chorion which is composed of trophoblasts and mesenchyme.

Soon numerous small cavities appear within the extraembryonic mesoderm. These cavities shortly become confluent and form the extraembryonic coelom (Fig. 70.6C). The extraembryonic coelom splits the extraembryonic mesoderm into two layers: (1) the extraembryonic somatopleuric mesoderm, lining the trophoblast and amnion, and (2) the extraembryonic splanchnopleuric mesoderm, covering the yolk sac. The extraembryonic somatic mesoderm and the two layers of trophoblast constitute the chorion. The membrane called amnion is composed of amniogenic cells along with somatopleuric extraembryonic mesoderm. As the

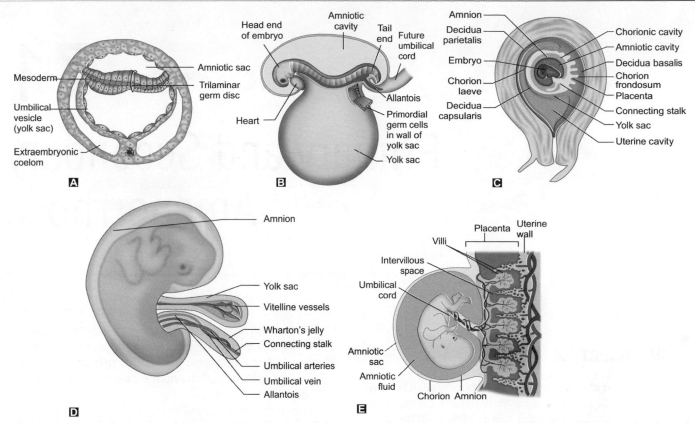

Figs 70.7A to E: Early development of the embryo: (A) Development of trilaminar germ disc; (B) Development of early stage embryo; (C) Uterus with embryo of 6-weeks size; (D) 6-weeks old embryo; (E) Development of foetus

folding of the embryo takes place, amniotic cavity completely surrounds the embryo (Figs 70.7A to C). With the development of extraembryonic coelom, the yolk sac becomes much smaller and is known as the secondary yolk sac. Around the amniotic cavity is the extraembryonic coelom. Outside the embryonic coelom is the chorion. As the foetus grows, there is enlargement of the amniotic cavity, resulting in progressive reduction in the size of extraembryonic coelom. Eventually, the extraembryonic coelom completely disappears, causing the amnion to come in contact with chorion and fuse with it to form the chorioamniotic membrane.

The mesodermal cells, in which extraembryonic coelom has not extended, eventually condense to form the body stalk. This connects the embryo to the chorion, and is responsible for supplying the nutrients. Connecting stalk later forms the umbilical cord.

As previously described, in the early stages, the embryo acquires the form of a three layered disc. This disc may be known by various names such as the germ disc, the embryonic area, embryonic shield or embryonic disc. The three layers also called as germ layers, from outside inwards are: (1) ectoderm (outer layer), (2) mesoderm (middle layer) and (3) endoderm (inner layer). These three layers of embryo are responsible for formation of different organ systems and

tissues giving the embryo more 'human-like' appearance (Figs 70.7D and E). When the embryo becomes 7 or 8 weeks old, it is known as a 'foetus'.

REFERENCES

1. Speroff L, Glass RH, Kase NG (Eds). Clinical Gynecologic Endocrinology and Infertility, 5th edition. Baltimore: Williams and Wilkins; 1994.
2. Fortune JE. Ovarian follicular growth and development in mammals. Biol Reprod. 1994;50(2):225-32.
3. Westergaard L, Christensen IJ, McNatty KP. Steroid levels in ovarian follicular fluid related to follicle size and health status during the normal menstrual cycle in women. Hum Reprod. 1986;1(4):227-32.
4. Rogers PA. Current studies on human implantation: a brief overview. Reprod Fertil Dev. 1995;7(6):1395-99.
5. Yoshinaga K. Uterine receptivity for blastocyst implantation. Ann NY Acad Sci. 1988;541:424-31.
6. Ringler GE, Strauss JF. Recent advances in understanding the process of implantation. Curr Opin Obstet Gynecol. 1990;2(5):703-8.
7. England MA (Ed). Life Before Birth, 2nd edition. St. Louis, MO: Mosby-Wolfe; 1996.

CHAPTER 70

Primary and Secondary Amenorrhoea

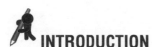

INTRODUCTION

Amenorrhoea or absence of menstrual periods can be of two types: primary (woman has never experienced menstrual cycles) and secondary (woman had experienced menstrual bleeding previously before experiencing cessation for at least 6 months). Primary amenorrhoea can be defined as follows:[1]

❖ Absence of menses by the age of 14 years with the absence of growth or development of secondary sexual characteristics or
❖ Absence of menses by the age of 16 years with normal development of secondary sexual characteristics.

AETIOLOGY

Pathophysiology of Menstrual Bleeding

As previously described in Chapter 58 (Menstrual Cycle), circulating oestradiol levels in the body stimulate the growth of uterine endometrium. Progesterone, which is produced by the corpus luteum, is formed after ovulation. It transforms proliferating endometrium into a secretory one. If pregnancy does not occur, this secretory endometrium breaks down and sheds in the form of menstrual bleeding. A complex interaction between the hypothalamic-pituitary ovarian axis and the outflow tract (uterus, cervix and vagina) is required for the normal menstrual bleeding to take place. For menstrual cycles to occur normally, the following are required:

❖ *An intact outflow tract*: An intact outflow tract, which connects the bleeding occurring in the internal genitalia with the outside, is essential for normal menstrual flow. This requires a patent outflow tract and continuity of the vaginal orifice, vaginal canal and endocervix with the uterine cavity.
❖ *Normal endometrial development*: Normal development of endometrial lining which responds cyclically to stimulation by oestrogen and progesterone.

❖ *Normal functioning ovaries*: Proper functioning of the ovaries is required for secretion and synthesis of oestrogens and progesterone. The entire spectrum of follicle development, ovulation and formation of corpus luteum occurs here.
❖ *Normal functioning pituitary glands*: The stimulus for the production of ovarian hormones and ovarian follicles is provided by the hormones secreted from anterior pituitary including hormones such as FSH and LH.
❖ *Normal functioning hypothalamus*: The secretion of these hormones by the pituitary is dependent on secretion of GnRH by the hypothalamus.

Any disruption of the interaction in aforementioned compartments can result in amenorrhoea. The causes of primary amenorrhoea are related to defects in any of the four compartments as shown in Figure 71.1 and are described here:[2]

1. *Compartment I*: Outflow tract and the uterus
2. *Compartment II*: Defect in ovulation
3. *Compartment III*: Defect at the level of pituitary gland
4. *Compartment IV*: Defect at the level of hypothalamus and CNS.

The various causes of primary amenorrhoea are mentioned in Box 71.1.

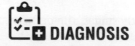

DIAGNOSIS

Clinical Presentation

❖ Absence of periods.
❖ *Body mass index*: Increased BMI could be associated with PCOD.
❖ *Anthropomorphic measurements and growth chart*: These measurements may detect abnormalities, such as constitutional delay of growth and puberty.
❖ *Signs of androgen excess*: Signs such as hirsutism or acne could be associated with PCOS.

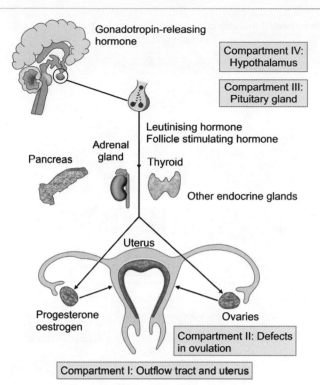

Fig. 71.1: Causes of primary amenorrhoea related to defects in either of the four compartments

Box 71.1: Causes of primary amenorrhoea

Defects in compartment I (outflow tract and uterus)
❑ Müllerian agenesis (Mayer-Rokitansky-Küster-Hauser syndrome)
❑ Androgen insensitivity syndrome
❑ 5-alpha reductase deficiency
❑ Asherman's syndrome
❑ Imperforate hymen

Defects in compartment II (ovulation)
❑ Gonadal dysgenesis (Turner's syndrome)
❑ Premature ovarian failure
❑ Polycystic ovarian syndrome
❑ Postpill amenorrhoea

Defects in compartment III (disorders of anterior pituitary)
❑ Hyperprolactinaemia
❑ Gonadotropin deficiency, e.g. Kallmann's syndrome
❑ Tumours of the hypothalamus or pituitary
❑ Hypopituitarism

Defects in compartment IV (hypothalamus)
❑ Anorexia nervosa
❑ Chronic illness, anorexia, weight loss, stress
❑ Hyperprolactinaemia

❖ *Signs of virilisation*: Signs such as deepening of voice, clitoromegaly, etc. could be related to the presence of androgen-secreting tumours.
❖ *Clitoral measurement*: A clitoral index greater than 35 mm² is an evidence of increased androgen effect.
❖ *Dysmorphic features*: Features such as webbed neck, short stature and widely spaced nipples could be suggestive of Turner's syndrome.

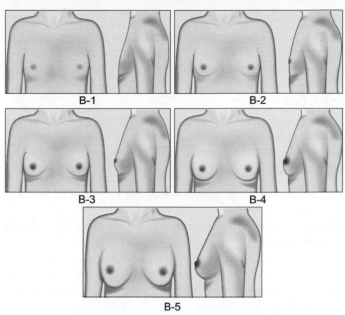

Fig. 71.2: Tanner staging for breast development

B-1: Prepubertal; B-2: Breast bud; B-3: Enlargement of breast and areola with no separation of the contour; B-4: Projection of areola and papilla to form a secondary mound above the level of the breast; B-5: Recession of the areola to the general contour of the breast with projection of the papilla only

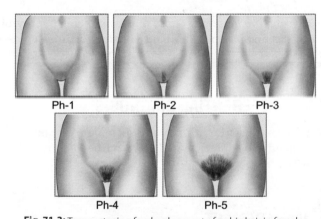

Fig. 71.3: Tanner staging for development of pubic hair in females

Ph-1: Prepubertal; Ph-2: Sparse growth of long slightly pigmented hair usually slightly curly mainly along the labia; Ph-3: The hair is darker, coarser and curlier and spreads over the junction of the pubes; Ph-4: The hair spreads covering the pubes; Ph-5: The hair extends to the medial surface of the thighs and is distributed as an inverse triangle

❖ *Symptoms suggestive of Cushing's disease*: These include features such as striae, buffalo hump, central obesity, easy bruising, hypertension or proximal muscle weakness
❖ *Thyroid examination*: This is especially essential because thyroid diseases serve as an important cause of amenorrhoea and menstrual irregularities
❖ *Breast examination*: This helps in ruling out galactorrhoea
❖ *Fundoscopy and assessment of visual fields*: This must be done if there is suspicion of pituitary tumour
❖ *Pubertal development*: Tanner stage of development of breast and pubic hair has been described in Figures 71.2 and 71.3, respectively and has been previously discussed in Chapter 59 (Adolescent and Paediatric Gynaecology).

CHAPTER 71

Per Speculum Examination

❖ Detection of outflow tract abnormalities, such as transverse vaginal septum, imperforate hymen, etc.
❖ Distribution of pubic hair pattern.

Pelvic Examination

Rudimentary or absent uterus can be detected on bimanual examination.

Investigations

The following investigations may be required in cases of amenorrhoea:[3]

❖ *Karyotyping*: This is important for identifying the patient's genetic sex
❖ *Serum testosterone or androgen level*: May be mildly raised in women with PCOS or may be highly raised in women with androgen-secreting tumours of the ovary or adrenal gland
❖ *Gonadotropin levels*: Low level of gonadotropins is associated with hypogonadotropic hypogonadism, while high level of gonadotropins is associated with hypergonadotropic hypogonadism
❖ *Serum prolactin levels*: This may be raised in women with prolactinomas
❖ *Thyroid function tests*: These may be indicative of thyroid dysfunction as a possible cause of amenorrhoea.

DIFFERENTIAL DIAGNOSIS

The various causes for primary and secondary amenorrhoea, which need to be differentiated are described in Box 71.1 and Table 71.1, respectively.[4]

MANAGEMENT

The treatment of primary and secondary amenorrhoea is based on the causative factor.

Management of Primary Amenorrhoea

The first step of management in case of primary amenorrhoea is to determine whether the patient has developed secondary

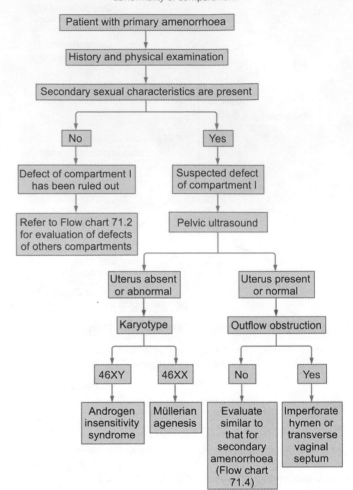

Flow chart 71.1: Evaluation of primary amenorrhoea in cases with suspected abnormality of compartment I

sexual characteristics or not. In these patients, the presence or absence of secondary sexual development directs further course of evaluation. Evaluation of the patient with primary amenorrhoea is described in Flow charts 71.1 and 71.2.[5]

Secondary Sexual Characteristics Have Developed

If a patient with amenorrhoea has experienced normal breast development, but minimal or no pubic hair, the usual diagnosis is androgen insensitivity syndrome (i.e. patient is phenotypically a female, but genetically a male with undescended testes). If testes are present, they should be removed because of the high risk of malignant transformation

Table 71.1: Various causes of secondary amenorrhoea

No features of androgen excess are present	Features of androgen excess
• Physiological, e.g. pregnancy, lactation, menopause	• Polycystic ovary syndrome
• Iatrogenic, e.g. depot medroxyprogesterone acetate, contraceptive injection, radiotherapy, chemotherapy	• Cushing's syndrome
• Systemic disease, e.g. chronic illness, hypo- or hyperthyroidism	• Late-onset congenital adrenal hyperplasia
• Uterine causes, e.g. cervical stenosis, Asherman's syndrome	• Adrenal or ovarian androgen-producing tumour
• Ovarian causes, e.g. premature ovarian failure, resistant ovary syndrome	
• Hypothalamic causes, e.g. weight loss, exercise, psychological distress, chronic illness, idiopathic	
• Pituitary causes, e.g. hyperprolactinaemia, hypopituitarism, Sheehan's syndrome	
• Hypothalamic/pituitary damage, e.g. tumours, cranial irradiation, head injuries, sarcoidosis, tuberculosis	

Flow chart 71.2: Evaluation of primary amenorrhoea in cases with suspected abnormality of compartment II to IV

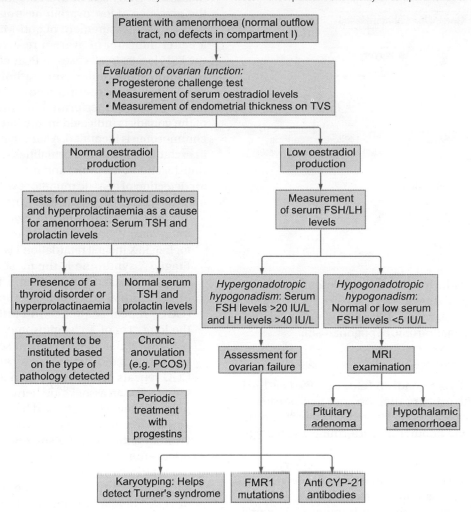

after puberty. In case of genital tract abnormalities, a karyotype analysis is required in order to determine proper treatment (Flow chart 71.3).[5]

If a patient has normal secondary sexual characteristics, including pubic hair, the clinician should perform MRI or ultrasonography to determine if a uterus is present. If the ultrasound examination shows presence of a normal uterus, outflow tract obstruction should be considered. An imperforate hymen or a transverse vaginal septum can cause congenital outflow tract obstruction. Imperforate hymen typically results in cyclic abdominal pain due to accumulation of the blood in the uterus and vagina.

If the outflow tract is patent, the physician should continue an evaluation similar to that for secondary amenorrhoea. If the uterus is absent or abnormal, a karyotype analysis should be performed to determine if the patient is genetically female. If the patient is genetically a female (46XX), the cause of amenorrhoea could be Müllerian agenesis, where there is congenital absence of vagina and abnormal (usually rudimentary) uterine development. If the karyotype is that of a genetic male (46XY), the patient could be probably suffering from androgen insensitivity syndrome.[6]

Secondary Sexual Characteristics Have Not Developed

If there is absence of secondary sexual characteristics, estimation for serum gonadotropin levels must be performed. This test helps in diagnosis of two causes of amenorrhoea: (1) hypogonadotropic hypogonadism and (2) hypergonadotropic hypogonadism. In cases of hypergonadotropic hypogonadism, a karyotype analysis must be performed to determine whether the cause of amenorrhoea is related to POF (46XX), or to Turner's syndrome (45XO).

Hypogonadotropic Hypogonadism

Hypogonadotropic hypogonadism is associated with low levels of FSH and LH, usually less than 5 IU/L. This could be related to the abnormalities in the secretion of GnRH, which is commonly due to disruption of the hypothalamic-pituitary-ovarian axis. The important causes for this include constitutional delay of growth and puberty and hypothalamic or pituitary failure. Hypothalamic amenorrhoea is often caused by excessive weight loss, exercise or stress. BMI of less than 19 kg/m² (normal range 20–25 kg/m²) has been found to be associated with amenorrhoea.

CHAPTER 71

Flow chart 71.3: Management protocol in case of genital tract abnormalities

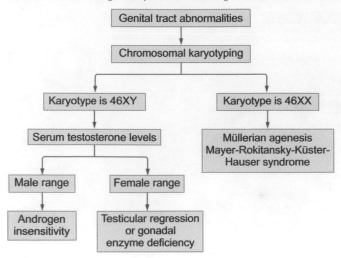

The mechanism by which stress or weight loss affects GnRH secretion is presently unknown.

Kallmann's syndrome, which is associated with anosmia, can also cause hypogonadotropic hypogonadism.

Hypergonadotropic Hypogonadism

Hypergonadotropic hypogonadism (elevated FSH and LH levels) in patients with primary amenorrhoea may be caused by gonadal dysgenesis or POF. These two causes can be differentiated from one another by performing a karyotype analysis.

1. *Gonadal dysgenesis*: Turner's syndrome (45,XO karyotype) is the most common cause for female gonadal dysgenesis. About 50% have mosaic forms such as 45X/46XX or 45X/46XY. Characteristic physical findings of Turner's syndrome include webbing of the neck, lymphoedema, shield chest with widely spaced nipples, scoliosis, wide carrying angle, coarctation of the aorta, streak ovaries and short stature. Individuals with the various forms of gonadal dysgenesis typically present with hypergonadotropic amenorrhoea regardless of the extent of pubertal development and the presence or absence of associated anomalies or stigmata. It is well known that cytogenetic abnormalities of the X chromosome can impair ovarian development and function.

2. *Premature ovarian failure*: Normally, menopause occurs at about 50 years of age and is caused by ovarian follicle depletion. Sometimes, ovarian failure can occur prematurely. POF is characterised by amenorrhoea, hypo-oestrogenism, and increased gonadotropin levels occurring before 40 years of age.[7] Women with POF are at an increased risk of osteoporosis and heart disease. Two types of inherited enzymatic defects also may be associated with POF. These include 17α-hydroxylase deficiency and deficiency of the enzyme galactose-1-phosphate uridylyltransferase. POF can also be sometimes associated with autoimmune endocrine disorders such as hypothyroidism, Addison's disease and diabetes mellitus. Therefore, fasting glucose levels, TSH, and, if clinically appropriate, morning cortisol levels should be

measured. Diagnosis of ovarian failure is established in the presence of low ovarian oestrogen and high serum FSH levels. Measurement of anti-Müllerian hormone is a better indicator of ovarian reserve in comparison to the FSH levels. In all cases of POF, efforts must be made to evaluate the underlying pathology. Nevertheless, most cases may remain unexplained. A karyotype analysis must be performed because surgical removal of the gonads is indicated in any individual in whom a Y chromosome is identified. A karyotype analysis also helps in excluding genetic abnormalities such as chromosomal translocations, deletions and mosaicism, etc. Some tests for detection of genetic mutation, which need to be done in these cases, include the following:

- *Testing for Fragile X mental retardation (FMR1) pre-mutations*: Women with POF must be offered testing for fragile X mental retardation 1 (FMR1) premutations. Fragile X syndrome is the most common cause for mental retardation and autism. This syndrome results from abnormal expansion of an unstable trinucleotide (CGG) repeat sequence in FMR1 gene located on the long arm of X chromosome. The gene normally contains about 30 CGG repeat sequences. However, in presence of fragile X syndrome, the number of CGG repeats can be more than 200. There has been found to be an association between POF and fragile X premutations, characterised by 55–200 CGG repeats.

- *Testing for antiadrenal antibodies (anti-CYP 21)*: Ovarian failure may be sometimes due to Addison's disease (autoimmune adrenal insufficiency). Presence of antiadrenal antibodies (anti-CYP 21) is strongly suggestive of autoimmune oophoritis as the cause of POF. Therefore, women with POF require careful evaluation to exclude adrenal insufficiency.

Management of Secondary Amenorrhoea

The management plan of a patient with secondary amenorrhoea is described in Flow chart 71.4.[8] The first step in the management of patients with secondary amenorrhoea is to rule out pregnancy because that is the most common cause of secondary amenorrhoea. Once the pregnancy has been ruled out, the initial workup involves measurement of TSH and prolactin levels and a progestin challenge test. In case, the patient with amenorrhoea also presents with galactorrhoea, imaging of sella turcica may also be required. Hypothyroidism may also produce galactorrhoea by reducing the levels of dopamine (a prolactin inhibitory substance). Hypothyroidism also causes unopposed thyrotropin-releasing hormone (TRH) production, resulting in stimulation of pituitary cells, which produce prolactin.

The progestin challenge test can be performed using the following:

- 200 mg of parenteral progesterone in oil
- Oral micronised progesterone in the dose of 300 mg daily
- Medroxyprogesterone in the dosage of 10 mg daily for 5 days
- *Micronised progesterone gel (4–8%)*: Intravaginal application for at least six times.

Flow chart 71.4: Management plan of a patient with secondary amenorrhoea

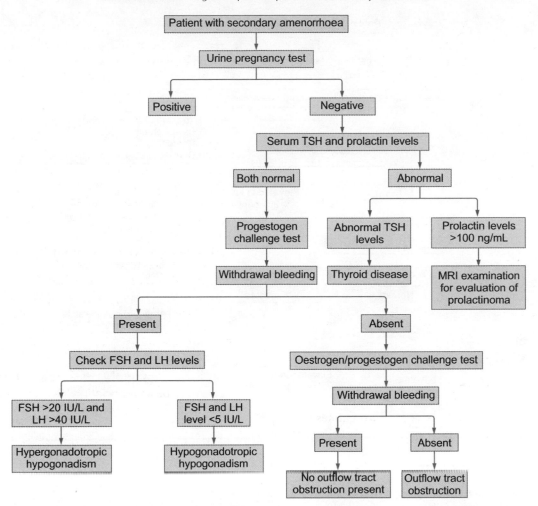

Following 2–7 days of conclusion of a progestin challenge test, the patient either does or does not bleed. If the patient bleeds, the diagnosis of anovulation can be established. Presence of bleeding confirms the presence of a functional outflow tract and a uterus lined by reactive endometrium prepared by endogenous oestrogens. Significant hyper-androgenaemia associated with anovulation and PCOS is an important cause of amenorrhoea, which responds to the progestin challenge test. Chronic unopposed exposure of the endometrium to endogenous oestrogens can serve as a risk factor for the development of endometrial cancer. At the minimum, these women must be prescribed a progestational agent (5 mg daily) for first 2 weeks of each month in order to reduce the risk of the development of endometrial cancer. OCPs can be given in case the contraception is desired.

If withdrawal bleeding does not occur in response to progestational medications, there can be two causes: (1) either the outflow tract is not patent or (2) the endometrium has not been adequately prepared by endogenous oestrogens. In order to differentiate between the two, orally active oestrogens (1.25 mg of conjugated oestrogens) must be administered for at least 21 days. An orally active progestational agent (10 mg of medroxyprogesterone) can be added in the last 5 days to achieve withdrawal bleeding. If no withdrawal bleeding

occurs even after the addition of oestrogens, amenorrhoea is probably related to a defect in compartment I (outflow tract and uterine endometrium). If withdrawal bleeding occurs, there is no defect in compartment I. It also implies that compartment I has normal functional activities if properly stimulated by oestrogens.

If withdrawal bleeding occurs, the next step aims at finding if the ovaries and the pituitary gland are functioning normally or not. This involves the assay of serum gonadotropin levels. In normal adult females, FSH ranges between 5 IU/L to 20 IU/L, with ovulatory mid-cycle peak of about two times the baseline level, whereas the LH levels vary between 5 IU/L and 40 IU/L, with an ovulatory mid-cycle peak of about three times the baseline level. Hypogonadotropic hypogonadism which is associated with levels of both FSH and LH less than 5 IU/L, could be due to prepubertal state and hypothalamic or pituitary dysfunction. Hypergonadotropic hypogonadism, on the other hand, could be due to postmenopausal state, castrate females and ovarian failure. In these cases, FSH levels are greater than 20 IU/L and LH levels are greater than 40 IU/L.

Chronic Anovulation

When the results of various investigations reveal normal ovarian oestrogen production and normal FSH levels,

CHAPTER 71

Flow chart 71.5: Management of galactorrhoea in an amenorrhoeic patient

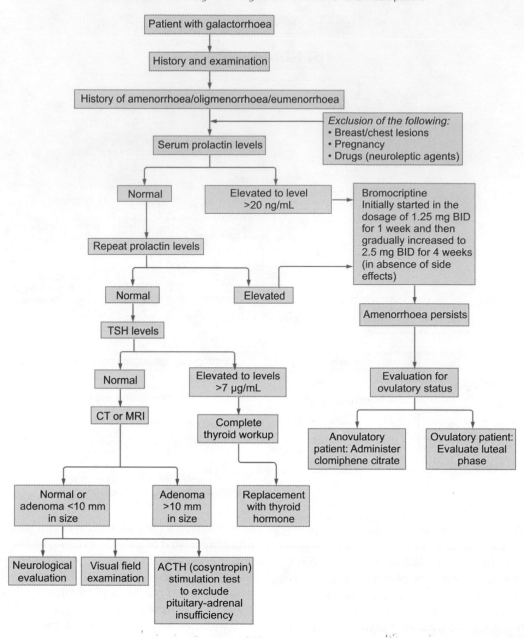

Abbreviation: ACTH, adrenocorticotropic hormone

diagnosis of chronic anovulation is established. Since hyper-prolactinaemia is one of the most common causes of anovulation and amenorrhoea, measurement of serum prolactin levels is done. Measurement of serum prolactin levels is especially important in cases with galactorrhoea. Management of an amenorrhoeic patient with galactorrhoea is described in Flow chart 71.5.[9]

Since thyroid disorders are also easily identifiable and treatable, measurement of serum TSH concentration is also justified in all women with amenorrhoea. Other likely causes of anovulation, besides thyroid and prolactin disorders, include PCOS and obesity. Women with PCOS usually have signs of hyperandrogenism due to which they can easily be identified.

A normal random prolactin measurement of 15–20 ng/mL is helpful in excluding hyperprolactinaemia. Mildly elevated prolactin levels (20–40 ng/mL) are best repeated and confirmed before the diagnosis of hyperprolactinaemia is made. Once intake of some medicines (causing galactorrhoea) have been ruled out as a cause of hyperprolactinaemia, further evaluation with MRI is required in women with amenorrhoea and hyperprolactinaemia to exclude pituitary tumours or hypothalamic mass lesions.

Women with chronic anovulation are likely to progress to hyperplasia, atypia and cancer within a short duration of time due to unopposed oestrogen stimulation. At the minimum, these women require periodic treatment with progestins to induce menstruation and provide protection against the risk of developing endometrial cancer.

Table 71.2: Interpretation of serum gonadotropin levels

Clinical state	Serum FSH	Serum LH
Normal adult woman	5–20 IU/L	5–40 IU/L
Hypogonadotropic state	<5 IU/L	<5 IU/L
Hypergonadotropic state	>20 IU/L	>40 IU/L

Specific Treatment

The treatment of primary and secondary amenorrhoea is based on the causative factor. Evaluation of serum gonadotropin levels (Table 71.2) helps in deciding the underlying pathology and hence further management. Treatment goals include prevention of complications such as osteoporosis, endometrial hyperplasia, heart disease, etc.; preservation of fertility; and, in case of primary amenorrhoea, progression of normal pubertal development.

Disorders of Sexual Development

Management of disorders of sexual development (Müllerian agenesis, androgen insensitivity syndrome) has been described in details in Chapter 56 (Normal and Abnormal Embryological Development).

Turner's Syndrome

Management of cases of amenorrhoea due to Turner's syndrome is described in Chapter 57 (Karyotypic Abnormalities).

Hypothalamic Amenorrhoea

Treatment of hypothalamic amenorrhoea depends on the underlying aetiology.

Anorexia nervosa: Women with excessive weight loss should be screened for eating disorders and treated accordingly if anorexia nervosa or bulimia nervosa is diagnosed. Menstrual cycles usually return after a healthy body weight has been achieved.

In patients with amenorrhoea caused by eating disorders or excessive exercise, the use of OCPs or menopausal hormone therapy may decrease bone turnover and partially reverse bone loss. However, neither therapy has been shown to significantly increase the bone mass. Adequate calcium and vitamin D intake are recommended for these patients.

Hyperprolactinaemia: Microadenomas are slow growing and rarely malignant. Treatment of microadenomas should focus on management of infertility, galactorrhoea and breast discomfort. A prolactin-producing microadenoma usually responds to treatment with dopamine agonists. A dopamine agonist can help improve the symptom of amenorrhoea and fertility. Bromocriptine, a dopamine agonist, is the most commonly used drug for treatment. Trans-sphenoidal surgery may be an option for women with large macroadenomas (>3 cm) or those who are resistant to treatment with dopamine agonists.

Polycystic Ovarian Syndrome

Treatment of PCOS has been discussed in detail in Chapter 74 (Polycystic Ovarian Disease).

Thyroid Dysfunction

Hypothyroidism is treated using thyroid preparations such as levothyroxine sodium (e.g. eltroxin).

Hypopituitarism

Hypopituitarism is associated with generalised deficiency of various hormones. In these cases, thyroid replacement therapy should not be instituted until adrenal function has been assessed and treated. Serum gonadotropin and gonadal steroid levels are typically low in cases of hypopituitarism. In cases with hypopituitarism where oocytes are still present, ovulation can be induced with exogenous gonadotropins (FSH or LH) when pregnancy is desired. Human menopausal gonadotropin (hMG) is the treatment of choice for patients with primary amenorrhoea due to hypopituitarism. In order to prevent the risk of ovarian hyperstimulation syndrome, hMG should be started at the minimal dose (75 IU SC QD for 7 days). Exogenous pulsatile GnRH using a subcutaneous pump may also be used to induce ovulation if the disorder is hypothalamic. When pregnancy is not desired, signs and symptoms of oestrogen deficiency can be prevented by instituting maintenance therapy with cyclic oestrogen and progestogens.

Premature Ovarian Failure

The treatment in women with POF comprises the following:

❖ Psychological and emotional support
❖ Appropriate genetic counselling (especially in cases of FMR1 premutations)
❖ Appropriate monitoring in patients with autoimmune diseases
❖ If pregnancy is desired, use of donor oocytes with in vitro fertilisation is most likely to result in pregnancy.[10]
❖ Spontaneous pregnancy can rarely occur in cases of POF, especially in women who have been administered ethinyl oestradiol to suppress high endogenous FSH levels.[11] Therefore, women with POF must be prescribed some form of contraception. A threshold of FSH levels of less than or equal to 15 mIU/mL should be preferably attained before commencing ovarian stimulation in these patients.

Treatment with exogenous oestrogens: In absence of endogenous oestrogens, women with POF are at an increased risk for developing complications such as osteopenia, osteoporosis and early coronary heart disease. They may also develop symptoms of oestrogen deficiency such as vasomotor flushes and genitourinary atrophy. Treatment with oral oestrogens (micronised oestradiol, 1–2 mg daily or conjugated equine oestrogens 0.625–1.25 mg daily) or transdermal oestrogens must be undertaken in these women. Since most of these women also have an intact uterus, cyclical treatment with progestogens (micronised progesterone, 200 mg daily or medroxyprogesterone acetate 10 mg daily) for 12–14 days each month serves as useful option for prevention of endometrial hyperplasia or malignancy, etc.

CHAPTER 71

COMPLICATIONS

❖ *Osteoporosis*: Use of hormone replacement therapy, calcium and vitamin D preparations may prove to be useful in these patients.

❖ *Cardiovascular disease*: Young women having amenorrhoea associated with oestrogen deficiency may also be at an increased risk of developing cardiovascular disease, hypertension and type 2 diabetes in future.

❖ *Endometrial hyperplasia*: Women with amenorrhoea having unopposed oestrogen secretion are at an increased risk of developing endometrial hyperplasia and endometrial carcinoma in future.

❖ *Infertility*: Women with amenorrhoea generally do not ovulate and are usually infertile.

❖ *Psychological distress*: Amenorrhoea may cause women to start having concerns regarding the loss of fertility or loss of femininity, thereby resulting in anxiety.

CLINICAL PEARLS

❖ Treatment goals in these cases include prevention of complications, such as osteoporosis, endometrial hyperplasia, heart disease; preservation of fertility; and progression of normal pubertal development (in case of primary amenorrhoea).

❖ Pregnancy should definitely be excluded in women presenting with secondary amenorrhoea.

❖ In cases of androgen insensitivity syndrome, due to high incidence of malignancy in the gonads with Y chromosomes, the testes must be removed at the age of 16–18 years, once full development has been attained after puberty.

EVIDENCE-BASED MEDICINE

❖ *Role of leptin in regulation of menstrual cycle*: Leptin is a protein secreted by adipocytes and acts as the critical link between adipose tissues and the reproductive system.[12] Leptin binds to specific receptors and modifies the expression of several hypothalamic neuropeptides, thereby regulating the neuroendocrine function. Leptins in association with gonadotropins and the growth hormone are likely to interact with the reproductive axis at multiple sites, with stimulatory effects at the hypothalamus and pituitary and inhibitory actions at the gonads.[13] Leptins are likely to play a role in target reproductive organs, such as the endometrium, placenta and mammary gland, thereby influencing important physiologic processes such as menstruation, pregnancy and lactation.[14]

Leptins also regulate energy intake and expenditure. Increasing amount of evidence has suggested that leptin helps in signalling information to the brain regarding the critical amount of fat stores which are required for luteinising hormone-releasing hormone (LHRH) secretion and activation of the hypothalamic-pituitary-gonadal axis. Initiation of puberty in animals and humans has been found to be associated with rising leptin levels. Normal levels of leptin are required for the maintenance of menstrual cycles and normal reproductive function in women.[13] Moreover, circadian and ultradian variations of leptin levels may be associated with minute-to-minute variations in the levels of LH and oestradiol in normal women. Falling levels of leptin in response to starvation may result in reduced levels of oestradiol and amenorrhoea in individuals with anorexia nervosa or strenuously exercising athletes. Additionally, leptin has a potentially important role during pregnancy and in the physiology of the neonate and may influence ovarian steroidogenesis. Recently, leptin has been shown to be a marker of adequate nutritional stores.[15] Conditions with suboptimal nutritional status, such as anorexia nervosa, exercise-induced amenorrhoea, and functional hypothalamic amenorrhoea, may be associated with low serum levels of leptin. On the other hand, conditions with excessive energy stores or metabolic disturbances, such as obesity and PCOS may be associated with elevated serum or follicular fluid leptin levels. Relative leptin deficiency or resistance is likely to be responsible for the reproductive abnormalities occurring with these conditions.

Therefore, administration of leptin is likely to provide new therapeutic options for the reproductive dysfunction associated with relative leptin deficiency or resistance. Understanding the role of leptin might be useful for new treatments in reproductive pathologies. Replacement with exogenous recombinant leptin is likely to improve reproductive and neuroendocrine function in women with hypothalamic amenorrhoea.[16]

❖ Natural conception sometimes can rarely occur in cases of POF. This probably occurs due to erratic recommencement of ovarian activity later in life. Present evidence has also indicated successful induction of ovulation after suppression of FSH using ethinyl oestradiol.[10,11]

REFERENCES

1. Speroff L, Fritz MA. Clinical Gynecologic Endocrinology and Infertility. Lippincott Williams and Wilkins; 2005. p. 403.

2. Master-Hunter T, Heiman DL. Amenorrhea: evaluation and treatment. Am Fam Physician. 2006;73(8):1374-82.

3. Practice Committee of the American Society for Reproductive Medicine. Current evaluation of amenorrhea. Fertil Steril. 2004;82(Suppl 1):S33-9.

4. Practice Committee of the American Society for Reproductive Medicine. Current evaluation of amenorrhea. Fertil Steril. 2006;86(5 Suppl 1):S148-55.

5. Gardner DG, Shoback D (Eds). Greenspan's Basic and Clinical Endocrinology, 9th edition. New York: McGraw-Hill; 2011.

6. Hughes IA, Deeb A. Androgen resistance. Best Pract Res Clin Endocrinol Metab. 2006;20(4):577-98.

7. Rebar RW. Premature ovarian failure. Obstet Gynecol. 2009; 113(6):1355-63.

8. Pletcher JR, Slap GB. Menstrual disorders. Amenorrhea. Pediatr Clin North Am. 1999;46(3):505-18.

9. Crosignani PG. Current treatment issues in female hyper-prolactinaemia. Eur J Obstet Gynecol Reprod Biol. 2006;125(2): 152-64.

10. Check JH. Pharmacological options in resistant ovary syndrome and premature ovarian failure. Clin Exp Obstet Gynecol. 2006;33(2):71-7.

11. Tartagni M, Cicinelli E, De Pergola G, De Salvia MA, Lavopa C, Loverro G. Effects of pretreatment with estrogens on ovarian stimulation with gonadotropins in women with premature ovarian failure: a randomized, placebo-controlled trial. Fertil Steril. 2007;87(4):858-61.

12. Mantzoros CS. Role of leptin in reproduction. Ann NY Acad Sci. 2000;900:174-83.

13. Moschos S, Chan JL, Mantzoros CS. Leptin and reproduction: a review. Fertil Steril. 2002;77(3):433-4.

14. Cervero A, Domínguez F, Horcajadas JA, Quiñonero A, Pellicer A, Simón C. The role of the leptin in reproduction. Curr Opin Obstet Gynecol. 2006;18(3):297-303.

15. Thong FS, Graham TE. Leptin and reproduction: is it a critical link between adipose tissue, nutrition, and reproduction? Can J Appl Physiol. 1999;24(4):317-36.

16. Welt CK, Chan JL, Bullen J, Murphy R, Smith P, DePaoli AM, et al. Recombinant human leptin in women with hypothalamic amenorrhea. N Engl J Med. 2004;351(10):987-97.

Male Infertility

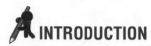 INTRODUCTION

Infertility is defined as the inability to conceive even after trying with unprotected intercourse for a period of 1 year for couples in which the woman is under 35 years and 6 months of trying for couples in which the woman is over 35 years of age. In nearly 30% of cases, the cause can be attributed to the male partner, which would be primarily discussed in this chapter. Infertility in males is commonly due to abnormal semen quality or sexual dysfunction.[1]

AETIOLOGY

Some of the important causes of male infertility are described in Table 72.1.

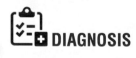 DIAGNOSIS

Clinical Presentation

A great deal of tact and sensitivity must be observed by the clinician at the time of taking the history and examination, and while discussing the abnormal results obtained during investigations with them. History, which needs to be obtained from the male partner, comprises of the following:

Sexual History

❖ *History of presenting complaints*: The history should include several points specific to the patient's sexual functioning including history of impotence, erectile dysfunction, premature ejaculation, change in libido, etc., and precise nature of the dysfunction, for example, whether the problem is in attaining or sustaining an erection, or whether there is difficulty with penetration due to insufficient rigidity, etc. The presence or absence of nocturnal and morning erections and their quality must be asked. The patient must be enquired if he is taking any treatment, both pharmacologic and non-pharmacologic for his problem. Complaints of reduced libido may also be associated with depression, loss of interest in daily activities, a decline in erectile function, fatigue, etc. Thus, history related to these symptoms must also be elicited. Determination of the period of infertility at the time of taking history is most important.

❖ History related to the frequency of intercourse or use of any lubricants, which may be toxic to sperms, must be enquired.

❖ History of pain both at the time of ejaculation and erection must be enquired. The time of pain onset, its localisation to any specific organ and the quality of pain must also be asked.

❖ History of testicular trauma, previous sexual relationships, history of any previous pregnancy and the existence of offspring from previous partners must also be asked.

❖ History of undergoing previous treatment for infertility including semen analysis must also be asked.

❖ Any complaints specific to the genitourinary structures, such as complaints of a dull ache or fullness in the scrotum, or non-radiating pain on one side, dysuria, dyspareunia, etc. must also be asked.

❖ History of exposure to environmental toxins, such as excessive heat, radiation, and chemicals such as heavy metals, and glycol ethers or other organic solvents needs to be asked.

Medical History

❖ History of treatment for malignancy (especially chemo-therapy or radiotherapy), regardless of site, should be documented.

❖ History of medical disorders such as diabetes, chronic obstructive pulmonary disease, renal insufficiency, haemochromatosis, hepatic insufficiency, etc. which may contribute to male subfertility, must be asked.

Table 72.1: Causes of male infertility

Cause	Prevalence (%)
Hypothalamic pituitary disease (secondary hypogonadism)	1–2
• *Congenital disorders*: Kallmann's syndrome, Laurence-Moon-Biedl syndrome, Prader-Willi syndrome, lower oculocerebral syndrome, familial cerebellar ataxia, etc.	
• *Acquired diseases*:	
– *Tumours*: Pituitary macroadenomas (macroprolactinomas and non-functioning adenomas)	
– *Infiltrative diseases*: Sarcoidosis, histiocytosis, tuberculosis, fungal infections, transfusion siderosis, haemochromatosis, etc.	
– *Vascular lesions*: Pituitary infarction and carotid aneurysm	
– *Hormonal*: Hyperprolactinaemia, oestrogen excess, glucocorticoid excess and androgen excess	
– *Drugs*: Opioid-like or other CNS-activating drugs, including many psychotropic drugs, GnRH analogues (agonists and antagonists), etc.	
– *Systemic illness*: Any serious systemic illness: acute systemic infections (e.g. smallpox, mumps, other viral infections, etc.) and chronic systemic infections (e.g. tuberculosis, leprosy, filariasis, prostatitis, renal, hepatic diseases, diabetic neuropathy, etc.)[2]	
– Chronic nutritional deficiency	
Testicular disease	30–40
• *Congenital or developmental disorders of the testes*:	
– Klinefelter's syndrome[3]	
– Autosomal and X chromosome defects	
– Y chromosome microdeletions	
– *Defective androgen receptor or synthesis*: Men with congenital androgen insensitivity due to androgen receptor or postreceptor abnormalities[4] and those with 5-α-reductase deficiency are nearly always infertile	
– Disorders of the oestrogen receptor or oestrogen synthesis	
– Inactivating mutation in FSH receptor gene	
– Myotonic dystrophy	
– Cryptorchidism, varicoceles and other less common disorders	
• *Acquired disorders of the testes*:	
– *Drugs*: Cyclophosphamide, chlorambucil, antiandrogens (flutamide, cyproterone, spironolactone), ketoconazole, cimetidine, antihypertensive drugs (reserpine, methyldopa, guanethidine, etc.), propranolol, corticosteroids, anabolic steroids, antipsychotics, etc.	
– Radiation	
– *Environmental factors*: Environmental toxins such as lead, cadmium and mercury; exposure of testes to high temperature (e.g. workers in blast furnace)[5]	
– Antisperm antibodies	
– *Systemic disorders*: Chronic renal insufficiency, cirrhosis, or malnutrition	
– *STDs*: Chlamydia, gonorrhoea and syphilis	
– Substance abuse (excessive intake of alcohol and/or drugs)	
– *Environmental factors*: Exposure to chemicals, such as lead, nickel, mercury, anaesthetic agents, pesticides, tobacco smoking, excessive alcohol intake, etc.	
– *Previous surgery*: Inguinal, scrotal, retroperitoneal, bladder neck, vasectomy, hernia repair	
• *Post-testicular defects (disorders of sperm transport)*	10–20
– *Abnormalities of the epididymis*: Absence, dysfunction or obstruction of the epididymis	
– *Abnormalities of the vas*: Bilateral obstruction, ligation or altered peristalsis of the vas deferens results in infertility, infection (gonorrhoea, Chlamydia, tuberculosis) resulting in the development of obstruction	
– *Defective ejaculation*: Spinal cord disease or trauma, sympathectomy, or autonomic disease (e.g. diabetes mellitus), erectile dysfunction, mechanical obstruction (condoms and diaphragm use), premature ejaculation, infrequency of intercourse, etc.	
• *Idiopathic*: Failure to conceive with an apparently normal female partner despite of having repeatedly normal semen analyses	40–50

❖ History of systemic illness, particularly a febrile illness and any recent weight gain or loss in last 6 months must be asked.

Surgical History

History of any surgery related to genitourinary organs such as orchidopexy, repair of inguinal hernia, epispadias or hypospadias repair, prostate surgery, bladder reconstructions, bladder or testicular surgeries needs to be asked. The patient should be asked specifically if there is a history of a vasectomy.

Treatment History

The dose and duration of use of certain prescription drugs, which can affect sperm count, motility and morphology, must be documented. Some of the drugs, which can commonly affect semen parameters by reducing spermatogenesis, include calcium channel blockers, spironolactone, chemotherapy drugs, anabolic steroids, etc. The patient must also be asked about the ingestion of herbal drugs or drugs belonging to other alternative systems of medicine and other over-the-counter medications. Many times, the patient may not disclose this history unless specifically enquired. Any of these substances may be responsible for affecting spermatogenesis.

Social History

Cigarette smoking, excessive alcohol consumption and consistent marijuana use are all known to be gonadotoxins. A careful history of the use of these agents and other illicit drug use must be part of the complete male infertility evaluation. Cigarette smoking has been thought to cause changes in sperm morphology, production and motility while chronic alcohol use may contribute to infertility by causing erectile dysfunction and hypogonadism. Simply eliminating these agents can improve semen parameters in the absence of other physical findings. Patients should be asked about recreational activities, as some activities, such as long-distance cycling, may put pressure on the perineal area and result in possible impairment of erectile function. Certain occupations which result in exposure of male genital organs to high temperatures such as men working in blast furnaces may be the reason behind the patient's infertility.

Family History

It is important to elicit the family history of birth defects or reproductive failure. The family history must include a discussion regarding the presence of testicular or other genitourinary malignancies specifically related to prostate or bladder in other family members. The patient should be queried regarding siblings or extended family members who may have had similar fertility problems. It is especially important to ask about the family history of cystic fibrosis because this genetic disease could be responsible for producing infertility by causing congenital absence of vas deferens. According to the ACOG recommendations, screening for cystic fibrosis should be made available to all the couples seeking preconceptional care and not just to those with a personal or family history of cystic fibrosis. The screening should be specifically offered to couples belonging to racial or ethnic groups with a high risk for cystic fibrosis (e.g. Caucasians, particularly those of Ashkenazi Jewish descent).

Examination of Male Partner

The patient should be examined for age-appropriate development of male secondary sex characteristics, gynaecomastia, or hirsutism. The structures of male external genitalia, which must be evaluated, include the penis, scrotum, testes, epididymis, spermatic cord and vas deferens. The clinician must examine the external genitalia for the presence of following abnormalities:

❖ The scrotum must be carefully and thoroughly palpated, and the presence of all scrotal structures should be confirmed, along with their size and consistency.
❖ Presence of congenital abnormalities of the genital tract, e.g. hypospadias, cryptorchidism (undescended testes), absence of the vas deferens (unilateral or bilateral), etc. must be assessed.
❖ Testicular size, presence of tenderness on palpation of testicle and presence of any associated mass must be assessed. If any mass is palpated, it must be verified whether the mass is arising from the testicles or is separate from it.

❖ Urethra must be assessed for presence of any stenosis, diverticulum, etc.
❖ *Presence of an inguinal hernia or varicocele*: A varicocele can be exaggerated during physical examination by asking the patient to perform the Valsalva manoeuvre while standing. The varicocele normally disappears when the patient lies down. A long-standing varicocele may result in testicular atrophy. If the varicocele is large, it may be visible during inspection resulting in 'bag of worms' appearance.
❖ The complete physical examination should also include a digital rectal examination.

Investigation

Semen Analysis

Semen analysis is the most important investigation and acts as a starting point in investigation of the male infertility. A comprehensive semen analysis must be performed in a certified andrology laboratory, which must be subjected to external and internal quality assessments at regular intervals. Male patient should be instructed well in advance that they must provide a semen sample after a period of abstinence of 2–5 days. This sample is collected through masturbation, and must be collected into a container, which is non-toxic to the sperms. The semen is usually not collected from condom samples because it may be containing a spermicidal agent. The patient is discouraged from attempting to collect a sample through intercourse, as coitus interruptus is not a reliable means for sample collection. Ideally, the specimen must be collected at the same andrology laboratory which would conduct the test. If the sample is collected at home, it should be transported to the laboratory within 30 minutes to ensure the accuracy of the results. The primary values that are evaluated at the time of semen analysis include the volume of the ejaculate, sperm motility, total sperm concentration, sperm morphology, motility and viability. The odds of male infertility increase with the number of major semen parameters (sperm concentration, mobility and morphology) in the subfertile range. The probability is 2–3 times higher in presence of one abnormal parameter; 5–7 times higher in presence of two abnormal parameters and nearly 16 times higher in presence of all three abnormal parameters. Normal parameters for semen analysis described by WHO are given in Table 72.2.[6] In 2010, the WHO published revised lower reference limits for semen analysis, which represented the 5th percentile in a population of over 1,900 men (whose partners conceived within 12 months) from eight countries, belonging to three continents. The results of semen analysis conducted as part of an initial assessment should be compared with WHO (2010) lower reference values as described in Table 72.3.[7]

Spermatogenesis takes approximately 72 days. Therefore, the sperm analysis must be repeated after 3 months if any of the parameters appear abnormal or as soon as possible in case of gross sperm deficiency. Morphology has become an important parameter for evaluation of the quality of sperm and their capability for fertilisation. Kruger reported a new classification based on strict sperm morphology after fixing

Table 72.2: Normal parameters for semen analysis (WHO, 4th edition, 1999)[6]

Parameter	Normal range
Volume	1.5–5.0 mL
Liquefaction time	Within 60 minutes
Viscosity	<3 (scale 0–4)
pH level	7.2–7.8
Sperm concentration	20 million or greater
Total sperm number	40 million spermatozoa per ejaculate or more
Motility	50%, forward progression; 50% or more motile (grades a* and b†) or 25% or more with progressive motility (grade a) within 60 minutes of ejaculation
Morphology	>50% normal (WHO, 1987, 2nd edition) >30% normal (WHO, 1992, 3rd edition) >14% normal (WHO, 1999, 4th edition)
Vitality	75% or more live
Round cells	<5 million cells/mL
Sperm agglutination	<2 (scale of 0–3)

*Grade a: Rapid progressive motility (sperm moving swiftly, usually in a straight line)
†Grade b: Slow or sluggish progressive motility (sperms may be less linear in their progression)

Table 72.3: Parameters for semen analysis: Lower reference limits (95% CI) in fertile men (WHO, 5th edition, 2010)[7]

Parameter	Normal range
Volume	1.5 mL (1.4–1.7 mL)
Sperm concentration	15 (12–16) million/mL or greater
Total sperm number	39 (33–46) million spermatozoa per ejaculate or more
Motility	32%, forward progression; 40% total motility (progressive + non-progressive motility)
Morphology	Normal sperms (>4%) using 'strict' Tygerberg method
Vitality	58 (55–63)% or more live

and staining the sperm. According to this criterion, sperm morphology of greater than 14% is considered as normal. Morphology of less than 4% is associated with severe infertility and is an indication for assisted reproduction technology/intracytoplasmic sperm injection (ICSI).

Strict criteria of normal sperm morphology as established by Kruger et al. have been defined as spermatozoa having an oval configuration with a smooth contour, with head length varying from 5 μm to 6 μm, the width varying from 2.5 μm to 3.5 μm and the width/length ratio varying between 1/2 to 3/5. The acrosome must be well defined, comprising 40–70% of the distal part of the head. No abnormalities of the neck, mid-piece or tail are accepted. Borderline forms are also considered abnormal. In Kruger's practice, only the normal forms are considered and are known as the 'percentage of ideal forms (PIF)'. A PIF of greater than 4% is considered favourable and less than 4% is considered as unfavourable.[8]

The strict sperm morphology remains the best available predictor of sperm function (the capacity to fertilise a mature oocyte).

Since relatively few laboratories performing routine semen analysis have sufficient test volume and highly trained and experienced personnel to provide a valid assessment of strict sperm morphology, the earlier WHO standards for sperm morphology (2nd to 4th edition), which classified more sperms as normal are still being widely used in most hospital laboratories.

Interpretation of semen analysis: Abnormal semen analysis results can be attributed to various unknown reasons such as short period of sexual abstinence, poor sexual stimulus, etc. Therefore, it is important to repeat the semen analysis at least 1 month later before reaching a diagnosis. Terminology associated with abnormal results of semen analysis is described in Table 72.4. To establish the diagnosis of azoospermia, the semen specimen must be centrifuged at high speed (3,000 g for 15 minutes) following which the pellet must be examined under high magnification (400×). Absence of sperms must be documented on at least two separate occasions.

A low semen volume (<1.5 mL) in association with azoospermia or severe oligozoospermia is suggestive of genital tract obstruction, which is commonly due to two causes. These include either congenital absence of the vas deferens or obstruction of ejaculatory ducts. Low semen pH is indicative of congenital absence of vas deferens. In presence of normal pH of seminal fluid, transrectal ultrasound (TRU) examination must be performed. In case TRU shows dilated seminal vesicles, this is indicative of ejaculatory duct obstruction.

According to the new reference limits set for semen analysis by the WHO (2010), the lower reference limit for sperm concentration is 15 million/mL. Certain studies have shown that some men can be fertile even with sperm counts lower than this, while some men with sperm counts higher than this can be subfertile. For the purposes of IVF, sperm concentration of 10 million/mL or even less can be satisfactory.

White blood cells are normally not present in the seminal fluid. Increased WBC in the seminal fluid ejaculate is an indicator of genital infection or inflammation. Leucocytes in the seminal fluid may release reactive oxygen species, which may be related with poor quality of semen. Though presently, there is no evidence-based cut-off limit for the diagnosis of possible infection, clinically accepted cut-off value is considered as 1 million leucocytes/mL of ejaculate. When the round cell count exceeds 5 million cells/mL, additional tests must be performed to differentiate leucocytes from immature sperms and to identify those men having true leucocytospermia (>1 million leucocytes/mL). These individuals may require additional evaluation for genital tract infections or inflammation.

Determination of Serum Testosterone Levels

Serum testosterone levels particularly that of total testosterone, free testosterone, LH and FSH must be measured if hypogonadism is suspected as a cause for infertility. Morning values are preferred to afternoon blood samples because

CHAPTER 72

Table 72.4: Terminology associated with abnormal results of semen analysis

Terminology	Interpretation	Causes
Normozoospermia	Normal ejaculate as defined by the WHO reference values	
Hypospermia	Decrease in semen volume to <2 mL per ejaculation	
Hyperspermia	Increase in semen volume to >8 mL per ejaculation	
Aspermia	No ejaculate	
Azoospermia	Absence of sperms in the semen	Congenital absence or bilateral obstruction of the vas deferens or ejaculatory ducts
Oligozoospermia	Concentration of sperms <20 million sperms/mL	Ejaculatory dysfunction such as retrograde ejaculation, genetic conditions, or hormonal disturbances
Asthenozoospermia	Sperm motility of <50%	Extreme temperatures
Teratospermia	An increased number of sperms with abnormal morphology at the head, neck or tail level	
Teratozoospermia	Sperm morphology less than the WHO reference	
Oligoasthenoteratozoospermia	Disturbance of all three variables: (1) Motility, (2) morphology and (3) sperm concentration	
Cryptozoospermia	Few spermatozoa recovered after centrifugation	

testosterone is secreted in the morning. Hypogonadism is the only cause of male infertility that can successfully be treated with hormone therapy.

Zona-free Hamster Oocyte Penetration Test

Also known as the sperm penetration assay, this test is not routinely done because the results would not influence the clinical management.

Other Investigations

These may include investigations, such as semen culture, antisperm antibody estimation, scrotal ultrasound, hormonal assays, karyotyping, vasography, etc.

Karyotyping: Routine karyotyping is usually not required. It may be performed in the following circumstances:
- ❖ Karyotyping the male partner in presence of severe oligo-spermia
- ❖ Karyotyping the women in case of very early premature menopause (prior to the age of 40 years)
- ❖ Karyotyping both partners in case of recurrent pregnancy losses.

MANAGEMENT

- ❖ *Lifestyle modification:* The patient must be advised to discontinue smoking, stop consumption of excessive alcohol and/or intake of drugs, such as bodybuilding steroids and illicit drugs, wear loose fitting underwear and cool clothes and avoid high-temperature baths like saunas, etc. Coital frequency should also be increased in order to improve the chances of conception.
- ❖ *Assisted reproductive techniques:* Assisted reproductive techniques (ART) and micromanipulation of sperms have become the most important treatment strategies in case

of male infertility due to primary testicular dysfunction or obstructive azoospermia. The various ART procedures, which can be used, include procedures such as sperm washing or capacitation, intrauterine insemination, gamete intrafallopian transfer, IVF and micromanipulation (ICSI). The various ART procedures have been described in details in Chapter 76 (Assisted Reproductive Techniques).

- ❖ *Medical therapy:* Some of these include clomiphene citrate, tamoxifen, gonadotropins, aromatase inhibitors, antibiotics (for treatment of infection), steroids, etc.[9-12] However, there is no definite evidence to prove the efficacy of these therapeutic regimens in improving the pregnancy rate or sperm concentration. Vitamin E and selenium can help counter oxidative stress, which is associated with sperm DNA damage.[13] Oxidative stress is likely to produce a damaging effect over the sperms. Therefore, supplementation with antioxidants is likely to improve the sperm quality by reducing the oxidative stress. Low-quality evidence from four small RCTs has shown that supplementation with antioxidant therapy in subfertile males is likely to improve the rate of live births.[14] A hormone-antioxidant combination may improve sperm count and motility. Phosphodiesterase type 5 inhibitors, e.g. sildenafil, can be used in the patients with ejaculatory sexual dysfunction. Administration of ubiquinol (a reduced form of coenzyme Q10) has also been observed to significantly improve semen parameters such as sperm density, sperm motility and sperm morphology.[15]
- ❖ *Hormonal therapy:* Pulsatile secretion of gonadotropin-releasing hormone or human menopausal gonadotropins and hCGs has been successfully used for the treatment of hypogonadotropic hypogonadism. This treatment is likely to restore the spermatogenic drive. However, such treatment can become quite expensive because initiation of spermatogenesis can take several months.

❖ *Treatment of antisperm antibodies*: Many empirical therapies, e.g. condoms, corticosteroids, intrauterine insemination of washed spermatozoa, etc. have been suggested for treatment of infertile men with antisperm antibodies. The value of these treatment modalities largely remains controversial. Currently, treatment modalities like IVF and ICSI are employed in these cases. Donor insemination can be used as an option in cases where ICSI cannot be used due to financial constraints.

❖ *Surgical therapy*: Surgery may be employed for treatment of conditions, such as duct obstruction, varicoceles, undescended testes, etc. Varicocelectomy or ligation of varicocele, which had been practiced in the past, has now become largely uncalled-for because it does not improve pregnancy rates. Therefore, varicocelectomy should not be offered as a form of fertility treatment.[16] Modern microsurgical and robotic-assisted microsurgery techniques can also prove to be useful for procedures such as vasectomy reversal, with success rate being as high as 80%.[17] The chances of success of surgery usually depend upon the length of time since vasectomy was carried out, with the success rates being higher if the length of time since the surgery was carried out is less.[18] In some cases of vasectomy, there may be a formation of antisperm antibodies, which may interfere with the reversal process. In these cases where there is presence of antisperm antibodies and in cases where vasectomy has failed, the clinician can resort to IVF with ICSI. Many centres are now offering collection and cryopreservation of sperms from the epididymis at the time of vasectomy reversal. These frozen sperms can be subsequently used for ICSI in case there is a failure of the reversal operation.[19]

In men with obstructive azoospermia, surgical correction of epididymal blockage should be offered at centres where appropriate surgical expertise is available. According to NICE guidelines (2013), surgical correction should be considered as an alternative to surgical sperm recovery and IVF because it is more likely to improve the fertility rates.[20]

❖ *Management of ejaculatory failure:* Intracytoplasmic sperm injection serves as a viable alternative for a patient with an ejaculation in whom intrauterine insemination or IVF has failed.[21]

❖ *Incurable cases*: In cases where none of the treatment modalities seem to work, the only options may be donor insemination or adoption.

CLINICAL PEARLS

❖ The first test in the evaluation of the infertile couple is the semen analysis. A perfectly normal semen analysis report generally precludes a significant male factor component. Therefore, treatment should be more appropriately targeted towards the woman.

❖ Ideally, the semen analysis should be performed at least twice to confirm results because there can be a considerable variability in the sperm quality when assessed over time in the same individual.

❖ Semen analysis is an investigation whose results are largely operator dependent. Therefore, adequate training of the operator is essential for minimising both intraobserver and interobserver variations.

❖ Reversal of vasectomy serves as an effective treatment option for men with infertility due to vasectomy.

EVIDENCE-BASED MEDICINE

❖ Presently, there is no evidence to indicate that use of therapeutic modalities such as antioestrogens, androgens, hCG, human growth hormone, insulin-like growth factor-1, aromatase inhibitors, kinin-enhancing drugs and bromocriptine are effective in improving the sperm quality. Bromocriptine, however, proves to be useful in men with sexual dysfunction as a result of hyperprolactinaemia.[22-24]

❖ There is limited evidence to indicate that antioestrogenic preparations (e.g. clomiphene and tamoxifen) are likely to have a beneficial effect on endocrinal outcomes (e.g. increase in testosterone levels) and sperm concentration and motility in infertile males with idiopathic oligoasthenospermia. However, future well-designed trials are required for evaluating the use of antioestrogens for increasing the fertility of males with idiopathic oligoasthenospermia.[25,26]

❖ Testosterone replacement therapy and anabolic androgenic steroids are commonly being used in clinical practice for treatment of younger men with infertility.[27-29] However, the present evidence indicates that both of these therapeutic strategies are likely to suppress the hypothalamus-pituitary-gonadal axis, resulting in attenuation of spermatogenesis, thereby causing oligozoospermia and/or reversible azoospermia. Therefore, the use of these treatment modalities should be preferably avoided.

❖ Presently, there is no evidence to indicate that the use of antibiotics in men having leucocytes in their semen is likely to improve the pregnancy rates unless there is an identified infection.[20]

REFERENCES

1. Hirsh A. Male subfertility. BMJ. 2003;327(7416):669-72.
2. Baker HW. Reproductive effects of nontesticular illness. Endocrinol Metab Clin North Am. 1998;27(4):831-50.
3. Yoshida A, Miura K, Nagao K, Hara H, Ishii N, Shirai M. Sexual function and clinical features of patients with Klinefelter's syndrome with the chief complaint of male infertility. Int J Androl. 1997;20(2):80-5.
4. Wang C, McDonald V, Leung A, Superlano L, Berman N, Hull L, et al. Effect of increased scrotal temperature on sperm production in normal men. Fertil Steril. 1997;68(2):334-9.
5. Aiman J, Griffin JE, Gazak JM, Wilson JD, MacDonald PC. Androgen insensitivity as a cause of infertility in otherwise normal men. N Engl J Med. 1979;300(5):223-7.
6. World Health Organization. WHO Laboratory Manual for the Examination of Human Semen and Sperm Cervical Mucus Interaction, 4th edition. Cambridge, UK: Cambridge University Press; 1999.

CHAPTER 72

7. Cooper TG, Noonan E, von Eckardstein S, Auger J, Baker HW, Behre HM, et al. World Health Organization reference values for human semen characteristics. Hum Reprod Update. 2010;16(3):231-45.

8. Rowe PJ, Comhaire FH, Hargreave TB, Mahmoud AM. WHO manual for the standardized investigation, diagnosis and management of the infertile male. Cambridge, UK: Cambridge University Press; 2000.

9. Pavlovich CP, King P, Goldstein M, Schlegel PN. Evidence of a treatable endocrinopathy in infertile men. J Urol. 2001;165(3):837-41.

10. Finkel DM, Phillips JL, Snyder PJ. Stimulation of spermatogenesis by gonadotropins in men with hypogonadotropic hypogonadism. N Engl J Med. 1985;313(11):651-5.

11. Santi D, Granata AR, Simoni M. FSH treatment of male idiopathic infertility improves pregnancy rate: a meta-analysis. Endocr Connect. 2015;4(3):R46-58.

12. Whitten SJ, Nangia AK, Kolettis PN. Select patients with hypogonadotropic hypogonadism may respond to treatment with clomiphene citrate. Fertil Steril. 2006;86(6):1664-8.

13. Scott R, MacPherson A, Yates RW, Hussain B, Dixon J. The effect of oral selenium supplementation on human sperm motility. Br J Urol. 1998;82(1):76-80.

14. Showell MG, Mackenzie-Proctor R, Brown J, Yazdani A, Stankiewicz MT, Hart RJ. Antioxidants for male subfertility. Cochrane Database Syst Rev. 2014;(12):CD007411.

15. Safarinejad MR, Safarinejad S, Shafiei N, Safarinejad S. Effects of the reduced form of coenzyme q(10) (ubiquinol) on semen parameters in men with idiopathic infertility: a double-blind, placebo controlled, randomized study. J Urol. 2012;188(2):526-31.

16. Cocuzza M, Cocuzza MA, Bragais FM, Agarwal A. The role of varicocele repair in the new era of assisted reproductive technology. Clinics (Sao Paulo). 2008;63(3):395-404.

17. Gudeloglu A, Brahmbhatt JV, Parekattil SJ. Robotic microsurgery in male infertility and urology-taking robotics to the next level. Transl Androl Urol. 2014;3(1):102-12.

18. Belker AM, Thomas AJ, Fuchs EF. Results of 1,469 microsurgical vasectomy reversals by the Vasovasostomy Study Group. J Urol. 1991;145(3):505-11.

19. Lewis R. Freezing sperm a viable option in azoospermic men. Medscape Medical News. August 12, 2013.

20. National Institute of Clinical Excellence (NICE). Fertility problems: assessment and treatment. Clinical guidelines CG156. UK: NICE; 2013.

21. Schatte EC, Orejuela FJ, Lipshultz LI, Kim ED, Lamb DJ. Treatment of infertility due to anejaculation in the male with electroejaculation and intracytoplasmic sperm injection. J Urol. 2000;163(6):1717-20.

22. Vandekerckhove P, Lilford R, Vail A, Hughes E. Bromocriptine for idiopathic oligo/asthenospermia. Cochrane Database Syst Rev. 2000;(2):CD000152.

23. Vandekerckhove P, Lilford R, Vail A, Hughes E. Androgens versus placebo or no treatment for idiopathic oligo/asthenospermia. Cochrane Database Syst Rev. 2000;(2):CD000150.

24. Laufer N, Yaffe H, Margalioth EJ, Livshin J, Ben-David M, Schenker JG. Effect of bromocriptine treatment on male infertility associated with hyperprolactinemia. Arch Androl. 1981;6(4):343-6.

25. Vandekerckhove P, Lilford R, Vail A, Hughes E. Clomiphene or tamoxifen for idiopathic oligo/asthenospermia. Cochrane Database Syst Rev. 2000;(2):CD000151.

26. Chua ME, Escusa KG, Luna S, Tapia LC, Dofitas B, Morales M. Revisiting oestrogen antagonists (clomiphene or tamoxifen) as medical empiric therapy for idiopathic male infertility: a meta-analysis. Andrology. 2013;1(5):749-57.

27. McBride JA, Coward RM. Recovery of spermatogenesis following testosterone replacement therapy or anabolic-androgenic steroid use. Asian J Androl. 2016;18(3):373-80.

28. Moss JL, Crosnoe LE, Kim ED. Effect of rejuvenation hormones on spermatogenesis. Fertil Steril. 2013;99(7):1814-20.

29. Rahnema CD, Lipshultz LI, Crosnoe LE, Kovac JR, Kim ED. Anabolic steroid-induced hypogonadism: diagnosis and treatment. Fertil Steril. 2014;101(5):1271-9.

Female Infertility

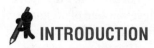 **INTRODUCTION**

Infertility is defined as the inability to conceive even after trying with unprotected intercourse for a period of 1 year for couples in which the woman is under 35 years and 6 months of trying for couples in which the woman is over 35 years of age. Investigations may be started earlier in a women with irregular menstrual cycles or in presence of known risk factors for infertility, such as endometriosis, history of pelvic inflammatory disease (PID), reproductive tract malformations, etc. or having a male partner with known or suspected poor semen quality. Infertility commonly results due to the disease of the reproductive system, in either a male or a female, which inhibits the ability to conceive and deliver a child. In the UK, roughly 9% of the couples belonging to the reproductive age group are affected by infertility.[1] Of these, nearly 50% seek help. Approximately, one in six couples is affected by infertility, and there are a number of factors, both male and female, that can cause the condition. In fact, in nearly 35% of cases, the cause is attributed to the male; in 50%, the cause can be attributed to female; 5% of cases can be attributed to unusual causes; and in remaining 10% of cases, the causes are unknown. Though both male and female factors are responsible for producing infertility, female factor infertility would primarily be discussed in this chapter. Amongst the female causes of infertility, the ovulatory dysfunction (most commonly PCOD) followed by tubal pathology (most commonly PID) is the most common cause of infertility. Nearly 15–30% cases of female infertility are due to an unexplained pathology. The remainder cases are due to relatively uncommon/unusual problems such as uterine pathology. Nevertheless, the evaluation for infertility must focus on the couple as a whole and not on one or the other partner. Both the partners must be encouraged to attend the clinic at the time of each appointment.

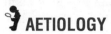 **AETIOLOGY**

FACTORS AFFECTING FERTILITY IN FEMALES

Various causes for female infertility are tabulated in Box 73.1 and described below in details.[2]

Cervical Factor Infertility

The uterine cervix plays an important role in capturing, nurturing, and then transportation and capacitation of the sperms after intercourse. The cervix ultimately releases the mature sperms into uterus and fallopian tube. Cervical factors account for 5–10% cases of infertility. Cervical factor infertility can most commonly result due to abnormalities of the cervical mucus-sperm interaction and narrowing of the cervical canal due to cervical stenosis.

Box 73.1: Causes of female infertility

❑ *Cervical factor infertility*
  - Abnormalities of the mucus-sperm interaction
  - Narrowing of the cervical canal due to cervical stenosis
❑ *Uterine factor infertility*
  - Total absence of the uterus and vagina (Mayer-Rokitansky-Küster-Hauser syndrome)
  - Diethylstilbestrol-induced uterine malformations
  - Asherman's syndrome, endometritis (due to tuberculosis)
  - Leiomyomas
❑ *Ovarian factor infertility*
  - Polycystic ovarian syndrome
❑ *Tubal factors*
  - Pelvic inflammatory disease associated with gonorrhoeal and chlamydial infection
❑ *Peritoneal factors*
  - Infection
  - Adhesions and adnexal masses
  - Endometriosis

Uterine Factor Infertility

The uterus is the ultimate destination for the fertilised egg and the site for embryo implantation and foetal growth. Therefore, uterine factors may be associated with primary infertility or with recurrent pregnancy wastage and premature delivery. Uterine factors may affect either the endometrium or myometrium and are responsible for nearly 2–5% cases of infertility. Uterine factors can be congenital or acquired and would be discussed below.

Congenital Defects

Abnormalities in the development of the Müllerian ducts may result in a spectrum of congenital or Müllerian duct abnormalities varying from total absence of the uterus and vagina (Mayer-Rokitansky-Küster-Hauser syndrome) to minor defects such as arcuate uterus and vaginal septa (transverse or longitudinal). The classification of Müllerian anomalies by the American Fertility Society (AFS, 1988) is described in Figure 73.1.[3] The relationship between Müllerian anomalies and infertility is not entirely clear, except when there is absolute absence of the uterus, cervix or vagina.

Acquired Causes

Drug-induced uterine malformations: The drug diethyl-stilbestrol (DES), used for treating patients with a history of recurrent miscarriages during 1950s was found to be responsible for producing numerous defects such as malformations of the uterine cervix, irregularities of the endometrial cavity (e.g. T-shaped uterus), malfunction of the fallopian tubes, menstrual irregularities and development of clear cell carcinoma of the vagina.

Asherman's syndrome: Development of adhesions or synechiae within the endometrial cavity may result in its partial or total obliteration. This could be due to Asherman's syndrome, which may develop following a vigorous dilatation and curettage procedure.

Endometritis: Endometritis or inflammation of the uterine cavity due to infections such as tuberculosis could be associated with an increased risk of infertility.

Leiomyomas: The impact of fibroids on fertility presently remains controversial and has been a subject of extensive debate. Uterine fibroids have been covered in details in Chapter 65 (Uterine Leiomyoma). As a sole factor, fibroids probably account for only 2–3% of infertility cases.[4] Leiomyomas are more common in nulliparous or relatively infertile women, but it is not known whether infertility causes myomas or vice versa or whether both the conditions have a common cause. The general view is that the uterus which is deprived of pregnancy consoles itself with myomas. This has been aptly summed up by the saying, 'Fibroids are rewards of virtue, babies the fruit of sin'. Postponement of pregnancy results in an uninterrupted oestrogenic stimulation of the uterus, which can act as a predisposing factor for development of myoma. Presence of myomas may then discourage the development of pregnancy. However, mere presence of myomas in an infertile patient should not be considered as a cause of her infertility. First, she should be investigated for all the common causes of infertility (including the tubal factor, the ovarian factor, male factor, etc.). Only after all the other common causes of infertility in a woman have been ruled out, presence of myomas may be considered as a cause for infertility in a woman. The extent to which presence of myomas can influence fertility in a woman depends upon the position of fibroids inside the uterus, the number of fibroids and their size. Myomas can cause infertility through the following mechanisms:

❖ Distortion of the endometrial cavity: Presence of sub-mucous myomas may distort the endometrial cavity, thereby interfering with normal implantation. Thus, submucous myomas are most likely to affect the woman's

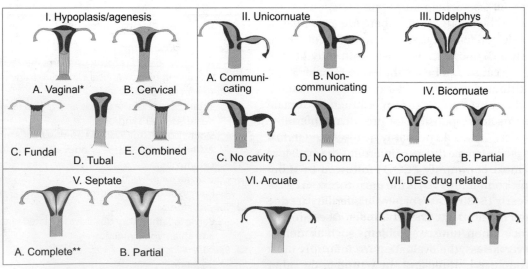

Fig. 73.1: Classification of the uterine anomalies by the American Society for Reproductive Medicine[3]
Abbreviation: DES, diethylstilbestrol
*Uterus may be normal or may take a variety of abnormal forms.
**May have two distinct cervices.

fertility followed by the interstitial myomas and lastly the subserosal myomas. Subserosal myomas are located farthest from the endometrial cavity; as a result, they are associated with minimum effect on fertility. Removal of fibroids that distort the uterine cavity may be indicated in infertile women, where no other factors have been identified, and in women about to undergo IVF. Besides causing distortion of the uterine cavity, myomas may also cause dysfunctional uterine contractions, which may interfere with sperm migration, ovum transport or nidation. Furthermore, the growth of myoma is dependent on oestrogen production. Thus, uterine myomas in a woman are often associated with anovulation, which may play a role in producing infertility. Also, menorrhagia and dyspareunia associated with uterine myomas can cause infertility to some extent.

- ❖ *Anatomical location of the fibroid*: The anatomical location of myoma inside the uterus can affect fertility. For example, presence of large submucous fibroids in the vicinity of cervix may result in displacement of cervix, which can prevent normal deposition of sperms at the cervical os or a submucosal myoma impinging on the intramural portion of the fallopian tube can interfere with the proper transportation of ovum.
- ❖ *Inflammation*: Biological factors like infiltration of inflammatory cells (macrophages) and production of inflammatory mediators [cytokines, monocyte chemo-attractant protein-1 (MCP-1), prostaglandin $F_{2\alpha}$, etc.] due to presence of fibroids may be responsible for producing infertility.
- ❖ *Indirect evidence*: Since there is very limited direct evidence in form of prospective randomised controlled trials regarding the role of myoma in producing infertility, we have to depend on indirect evidence. The indirect evidence is mainly available in two forms: the first one is studying the effect of fibroids based on the outcomes of assisted reproductive techniques (IVF, gamete intra-fallopian transfer, etc.). The second is assessing the outcome of fertility following removal of myomas. Various studies have indicated pregnancy rates of 44–62% following myomectomy.[5]

Ovarian Factor Infertility

Oogenesis occurs in the ovary from the first trimester of embryonic life and is completed by 28–30 weeks of gestation. By then, approximately 6–7 million oogonia are present. This can be considered as the maximal oogonial content of the gonad. They are arrested at the prophase stage of the first meiosis division. Subsequently, the number of oocytes irretrievably decreases until the menopause is attained because of a continuous process of atresia. At birth, the pool of oocytes is reduced to approximately 2 million. By menarche, approximately 500,000 oocytes are present. These oocytes are used throughout the reproductive years until menopause. The ovulatory process begins after the maturation of hypothalamus-pituitary-ovarian axis and there occurs production of gonadotropins (FSH and LH),

under the regulation of GnRH. Though a cohort of follicles is recruited every month, only a single oocyte ultimately gets selected, develops to the preovulatory stage and is known as the dominant follicle. LH surge occurring during the midpoint of the menstrual cycle triggers the ovulatory process and stimulates the formation of the corpus luteum. Following ovulation, the luteal phase begins under the influence of progesterone secreted by corpus luteum. Furthermore, ovulation induces the resumption of meiosis by the oocyte, which had been arrested at the prophase stage.

Causes of Ovulatory Dysfunction

Ovulatory dysfunction results in an alteration in the frequency and duration of the menstrual cycle. Anovulation or failure to ovulate is one of the most common causes for infertility. Absence of ovulation can also be associated with primary or secondary amenorrhoea or oligomenorrhoea. Amenorrhoea as a cause of infertility has been discussed in details in Chapter 71 (Primary and Secondary Amenorrhoea). The rise in prevalence of infertility with increase in woman's age could be related to reduction in the ovarian reservoir. Female fertility is likely to decline after the age of 35 years and even more rapidly after the age of 40 years. Besides a decline in female fertility, increase in woman's age is also likely to be associated with an increased rate of miscarriage. PCOS, a common endocrine disorder in women, frequently results in infertility by causing ovulatory dysfunction. Classification of various ovulatory disorders as devised by the World Health Organization (WHO) is described in Table 73.1.

Polycystic ovarian syndrome: Polycystic ovarian syndrome is the most common cause of hyperandrogenic chronic anovulation. It is an endocrine disorder associated with oligmenorrhoea or anovulation and hyperandrogenism. Besides ovulatory dysfunction, PCOS is also associated with metabolic disturbances such as peripheral insulin resistance and compensatory hyperinsulinaemia.[6,7] For details related to PCOS, kindly refer to Chapter 74 (Polycystic Ovarian Disease).

Tubal Factors

The fallopian tubes play an important role in reproduction. After ovulation, the fimbriae pick up oocyte from the peritoneal fluid that has accumulated in the cul de sac. The epithelial cilia in the tubal epithelium then transport the oocyte up to the ampulla. The capacitated spermatozoa are transported from the cervix through the endometrial cavity into the ampulla of fallopian tube, where ultimately fertilisation occurs. Fallopian tube abnormalities, tubal damage or obstruction may result in either infertility or abnormal implantation or ectopic pregnancy.

Causes of Tubal Obstruction

Pelvic inflammatory disease: Pelvic inflammatory disease is typically associated with gonorrhoeal and chlamydial infection. Formation of peritoneal adhesions secondary to PID can compromise the motility of the fallopian tubes. Furthermore, obstruction of the distal end of the fallopian

Table 73.1: WHO classification of ovulatory disorders

WHO class	Pathology	Causes	Incidence	Treatment strategy
WHO class 1: Hypogonadotropic hypogonadal anovulation	Low or low-normal levels of serum FSH and low serum oestradiol concentrations	• Destruction of anterior pituitary by a tumour (benign non-functioning adenoma or craniopharyngioma) • Pituitary infection (tuberculosis) • Ischaemia (Sheehan's syndrome) • Excessive exercise or low body weight • Congenital causes (Laurence-Moon syndrome, Kallmann's syndrome, Prader-Willi syndrome, etc.)	5–10% of women	Lifestyle modification
WHO class 2: Normogonadotropic normo-oestrogenic anovulation	Normal levels of gonadotropins and oestrogens. However, FSH secretion during the follicular phase of the cycle is subnormal	Women with PCOS	Most common, accounting for 70–85% of cases	• Weight modulation • Clomiphene citrate or other selective oestrogen receptor modulators • Metformin or other insulin-sensitising agents • Gonadotropin therapy • Aromatase inhibitors • Laparoscopic ovarian diathermy • Assisted reproductive technology
WHO class 3: Hypergonadotropic hypo-oestrogenic anovulation	High to normal levels of gonadotropins and low levels of oestrogen	• Primary gonadal failure (premature ovarian failure) or gonadal dysgenesis • Resistant ovary syndrome	Accounts for 10–30% cases	Gonadotropin therapy and in vitro fertilisation
Hyperprolactinaemic anovulation	Inhibition of gonadotropin and oestrogen secretion due to hyperprolactinaemia; gonadotropin concentrations in this condition are usually normal or decreased	Prolactin-secreting adenoma	Accounts for 1–2% cases	Bromocriptine or other dopamine agonist (only in cases of hyperprolactinaemia and anovulation)

tubes results in accumulation of the normally secreted tubal fluid, creating distension of the tube. This subsequently causes damage to the epithelial cilia and may result in development of hydrosalpinx.[8]

Other causes of tubal obstruction: Tubal obstruction can commonly result due to formation of scar tissue and adhesions due to infections (especially chlamydia and gonorrhoea), endometriosis, pelvic tuberculosis, salpingitis isthmica nodosa (i.e. diverticulosis of the fallopian tube), and abdominal or gynaecological surgery (e.g. tubal ligation for sterilisation). Tubal obstruction prevents the ovum from entering or travelling down the fallopian tube and meeting the sperm. Damage to the ciliary epithelium of the fallopian tube as a result of infection can result in the development of abnormal implantation or an ectopic pregnancy. Ectopic pregnancy has been discussed in details in Chapter 35 (Ectopic Pregnancy).

Peritoneal Factors

The uterus, ovaries and fallopian tubes are all present in the same space within the peritoneal cavity. The released ovum from the ovary often gets extruded into the peritoneal cavity into the cul-de-sac from where it is picked up by the fimbriae. Anatomical defects or physiological dysfunctions of the peritoneal cavity, including infection, adhesions and adnexal masses, may cause infertility.

Peritoneal Defects

Endometriosis: Endometriosis is an enigmatic disease characterised by the growth of endometrial tissue outside the uterus, which may affect a woman's fertility. Detailed description of endometriosis has been done in Chapter 68 (Chronic Pelvic Pain and Endometriosis). Endometriotic lesions vary from microscopic to macroscopic size. Classic endometriosis appears as bluish-black pigments (i.e.

Table 73.2: Different mechanisms through which endometriosis results in infertility[9]

Types of endometriosis	Cause for infertility
Severe endometriosis	• Damage to the fallopian tubes due to presence of adhesions • Damage to the ovaries due to presence of endo-metriomas
Minimal and mild endometriosis	• Increased peritoneal macrophages that increase phagocytosis of the sperms, reduced sperm binding to the zona pellucida, proliferation of peritoneal lymphocytes, increased production of cytokinin and immunoglobulins and defective activity of natural killer cells • Ovulatory disorders such as luteal phase deficiency, oligo-ovulation and luteinised unruptured follicle syndrome

'powder-burn lesions') that affect the peritoneal surfaces of the bladder, ovary, fallopian tubes, cul-de-sac and bowel. Non-classic endometriosis may appear as red, tan or white-coloured lesions and vesicles. Medical treatment of minimal or mild endometriosis has not been shown to increase the pregnancy rates. Moderate-to-severe endometriosis should be treated surgically. Different mechanisms through which endometriosis may result in infertility are described in Table 73.2.[9]

FACTORS AFFECTING FERTILITY IN BOTH SEXES

Environmental and Occupational Factors

Excessive radiation may damage the germinal cells. It has yet not been proven whether exposure to heavy metals, such as lead, excessive heat, microwave radiation, ultrasonography, etc. may also be responsible for inducing infertility.

Toxic Effects Related to Tobacco, Marijuana and Other Drugs

Smoking has been associated with infertility in both males and females. Various chemical substances in tobacco such as nicotine and polycyclic aromatic hydrocarbons have been observed to block spermatogenesis and decrease testicular size. In women, various chemicals present in the tobacco smoke are thought to affect the transportation of sperm and ova across the fallopian tube by altering the cervical mucus and the cilial epithelium, respectively.[10] Marijuana and its metabolite, delta-9 tetrahydrocannabinol, inhibit the secretion of LH and FSH in women, thereby inducing ovulatory and luteal phase dysfunction. Also, marijuana use affects male fertility by reducing the sperm count and the quality of the sperm. Use of heroin, cocaine and crack cocaine may produce similar effects. Chronic alcoholism in women may induce ovulatory dysfunction, thereby producing infertility. Alcohol use by males interferes with the synthesis of testosterone and may reduce sperm concentration. Alcoholism may also inhibit sexual response and cause impotence.

Exercise

Exercise should be encouraged as part of normal activity. However, compulsive exercise is deleterious, especially for long-distance runners, athletes, dancers, etc. In these women, excessive exercise could also result in amenorrhoea. In males, excessive exercise has been associated with oligospermia.

Inadequate Diet Associated with Extreme Weight Loss or Gain

Both excessive weight gain and loss may have an impact on the woman's fertility. Although weight loss associated with anorexia nervosa or bulimia induces hypothalamic amenorrhoea, obesity may be associated with anovulation and oligomenorrhoea. In men, obesity has been associated with decreased sperm quality.

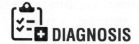 **DIAGNOSIS**

Clinical Presentation

During the consultation, the following history should be taken from the woman.

History of Presenting Complaints

❖ *Type of infertility*: A detailed medical history regarding the type of infertility (primary or secondary), its duration and if any treatment for this had been sought in the past. Primary infertility implies that woman had never been able to conceive in the past. Secondary infertility implies that the woman had conceived in the past (irrespective of the outcome of pregnancy, whether she progressed till term or had a miscarriage), but is presently not being able to conceive.

❖ *Patient's age*: It is important to know the woman's age because increasing age of women (>35 years) is associated with reduced fertility. The present evidence indicates that age-related decline in female fertility is largely due to progressive follicular depletion and a high rate of abnormalities (particularly aneuploidy) in the aging oocytes.[11] The available evidence also indicates a decrease in the pregnancy rate and an increase in the time to conception with an increase in the age of the male partner.[11] However, since this decline is rarely observed before the age of 45–50 years, male factors contribute very little towards the overall age-related decline in fertility.

❖ *Duration of infertility*: Duration of the couple's attempts for becoming pregnant, whether or not they have ever had children or a positive pregnancy test together with same or a different partner in the past needs to be asked. Number and outcome of any previous pregnancies including ectopic pregnancy and/or miscarriages also needs to be determined.

❖ *Thyroid dysfunction or galactorrhoea*: Symptoms suggestive of thyroid disease, pelvic or abdominal pain and galactorrhoea must be asked. Thyroid dysfunction is commonly associated with menstrual abnormalities and reduced fertility. Galactorrhoea or milk secretion from the breasts is often a manifestation of pineal gland tumour and may be associated with amenorrhoea.

- ❖ *Previous history of Pap smears*: Previous history of abnormal Pap smears or undergoing treatment for cervical intra-epithelial neoplasia could be responsible for causing cervical stenosis.
- ❖ *History of vaginal or cervical discharge*: This must be enquired. The infections could be at times responsible for producing infertility, e.g. infection with *chlamydia* can cause PID and tubal blockage resulting in subsequent infertility.

Sexual History

Sexual history must be taken in details in order to enquire about the frequency of sexual intercourse, use of lubricants (e.g. K-Y gel) that could be spermicidal, use of vaginal douches after intercourse and history of any sexual dysfunction. History of sexual dysfunction such as absence of orgasm or painful intercourse (dyspareunia) must be enquired. History related to the frequency of intercourse and presence of deep dyspareunia (suggestive of endometriosis), also needs to be enquired. Use of any form of contraception including natural methods, medical methods and surgical form of contraception (e.g. vasectomy, tubal ligation) needs to be asked. Overall pattern of sexual activity during the period of time the couple has been trying to conceive, specifically in relation to ovulation, needs to be asked. The patient should also be asked if she had ever used ovulation-predictor kits or has been prescribed ovulation-promoting medications such as clomiphene citrate (CC). The patient should be explained about the period of fertility. The optimal chances for pregnancy occur if the patient has intercourse in the 6 days before ovulation, with day 6 being the actual day of ovulation. Sometimes, simply advising the patients to adjust the timing of their intercourse can result in a significantly increased chance for pregnancy.

Patient's Lifestyle

Detailed history regarding the patient's lifestyle; consumption of alcohol, tobacco; use of recreational drugs of abuse (amount and frequency); occupation; and physical activities must be asked.

Menstrual History

The age of attaining menarche and puberty must be asked. The woman should be questioned in details about her menstrual history and asked about the frequency, cycle length, patterns since menarche and history of dysmenorrhoea. Regular menstrual cycles are usually ovulatory in nature, while irregular cycles may be anovulatory in nature. A history of weight changes, hirsutism, frontal balding, and acne should also be addressed. History of progressively worsening dysmenorrhoea, newly developed dyspareunia and physical findings of focal tenderness or nodularity of cul-de-sac point towards endometriosis. Irregular or infrequent menstrual cycles are usually indicative of ovulatory dysfunction.

Obstetric History

The patient should be enquired about details regarding previous pregnancies (including miscarriages or medical terminations of pregnancy and previous history of live births), dead babies or stillborn children. She should also be asked if she has ever undergone evaluation regarding infertility issues and any medical or surgical management that had been instituted. The patient should be asked about outcome of each of the previous pregnancies; interval between successive pregnancies and presence of some other complications associated with any pregnancy. If the patient has ever experienced pregnancy losses, she should be asked about the duration of pregnancy at the time of miscarriage, hCG levels, if they were done, ultrasonographic data, if available, and the presence or absence of foetal heartbeat as documented on the ultrasound report. History of previous pregnancy is particularly important because couples who have conceived before usually have a better prognosis in comparison to those who have never conceived. A history of past obstetric haemorrhage suggesting postpartum pituitary necrosis (i.e. Sheehan's syndrome) must be asked.

Past History

A previous history of pelvic infection, endometriosis, fibroids, cervical dysplasia, septic abortion, ruptured appendix, ectopic pregnancy and gynaecological surgery, e.g. abdominal myomectomy, adnexal surgery, surgery of cervix, fallopian tube, pelvis, abdomen, etc. raises the suspicion for tubal or peritoneal disease. Past or current episodes of STDs or PIDs must also be enquired. The patient must be asked if she is currently receiving any medical treatment, the reason for treatment and if she has any history of allergies. Past treatment history is also important because drugs such as NSAIDs can interfere with ovulation and antidepressants can raise prolactin levels. History of use of contraception also needs to be asked because use of OCPs and long-acting progestogens can be associated with period of amenorrhoea.

Family History

Family history of birth defects, mental retardation, early menopause or reproductive failure needs to be taken.

General Physical Examination

This requires routine measurement of the patient's vital signs including pulse rate, blood pressure and temperature. Other important aspects of the general physical examination include measurement of the following parameters:

Body mass index: Measurement of the patient's height and weight to calculate the BMI. Calculation of BMI is important because extremely low (<19) or extremely high BMI (>30) may be associated with reduced fertility.[12] Moreover, abdominal obesity may be associated with insulin resistance.

Thyroid examination: Note for thyroid enlargement, nodule or tenderness.

Eye examination: Eye examination must be performed in order to establish the presence of exophthalmos, which may be associated with hyperthyroidism.

Stigmata of Turner's syndrome: The presence of epicanthus, low set ears and hairline, and webbed neck can be associated with chromosomal abnormality such as Turner's syndrome.

Breast examination: A breast examination must be performed in order to evaluate breast development and to assess the breasts for the presence of abnormal masses or secretions, especially galactorrhoea. This opportunity must be taken by the gynaecologist to educate patients about breast self-examination during the early days of their menstrual cycles.

Signs of androgen excess: Signs of androgen excess such as hirsutism, acne, deepening of the voice, hypertrichosis, etc. must be looked for.

Examination of extremities: The extremities must be examined in order to rule out malformations, such as shortness of the fourth finger or cubitus valgus, which can be associated with chromosomal abnormalities and other congenital defects.

Examination of the skin: The skin must be examined for the presence of acne, hypertrichosis and hirsutism, which are indicative of androgen excess.

Examination of the secondary sexual characteristics: Failure of development of secondary sexual characteristics must always prompt a workup for hypopituitarism. Loss of axillary and pubic hair and atrophy of the external genitalia should lead the physician to suspect hypopituitarism in a previously menstruating young woman who develops amenorrhoea. Tanner stages of development of breasts and pubic hair have been described in Chapter 59 (Adolescent and Paediatric Gynaecology).

Specific Systemic Examination

Abdominal Examination

The abdominal examination should be done to detect the presence of abnormal masses in the abdomen. Masses felt in the hypogastrium could be arising from the pelvic region.

Pelvic Examination

Per speculum examination: The distribution of hair pattern on the external genitalia should be particularly noted before the per speculum examination. The inspection of the vaginal mucosa may indicate a deficiency of oestrogens or the presence of infection. Cervical stenosis can be diagnosed during a speculum examination. Complete cervical stenosis is confirmed by the inability to pass a 1–2 mm probe into the uterine cavity.

Bimanual examination: Bimanual examination should be performed to establish the direction of the cervix and the size and position of the uterus. The gynaecologist should look for presence of any mass, tenderness or nodularity in adnexa or cul-de-sac. Various pelvic pathologies, such as fibroids, adnexal masses, tenderness or pelvic nodules indicative of infection or endometriosis, can be detected on bimanual examination. Many uterine defects related to infertility such as absence of the vagina and uterus, presence of vaginal

---

> **Box 73.2:** Work-up of an infertile couple
>
> ❑ *Minimal investigations (required in most couples)*
> - Semen analysis to assess male factors
> - Menstrual history, assessment of LH surge in urine prior to ovulation, and/or luteal phase progesterone level to assess ovulatory function and endometrial receptivity
> - Hysterosalpingography to assess tubal patency and the uterine cavity
> - Day 3 serum FSH and oestradiol levels to assess ovarian reserve (following clomiphene citrate challenge)
>
> ❑ *Additional tests required in select couples*
> - Pelvic ultrasound to assess for uterine myomas and ovarian cysts
> - Laparoscopy to diagnose endometriosis or other pelvic pathology
>
> ❑ *Additional tests for assessment of ovarian reserve in women >35 years of age*
> - Clomiphene citrate challenge test, ultrasound for early follicular antral follicle count, day 3 serum inhibin B level, or anti-Müllerian hormone measurement
> - Assessment of thyroid function

septum, etc. can be detected during the pelvic examination. Tenderness or masses in the adnexae or posterior cul-de-sac (pouch of Douglas) are suggestive of chronic PID or endometriosis. Palpable tender nodules in the posterior cul-de-sac, uterosacral ligaments, or rectovaginal septum are additional signs of endometriosis.

Investigations

Investigations, which need to be performed in an infertile couple, are enumerated in Box 73.2 and are described next in details.

Routine Investigations

These include thyroid function tests (particularly TSH levels) and serum prolactin levels.

Tests for Ovarian Factors

Assessment of ovarian function can be done with help of tests such as clomiphene citrate challenge test (CCCT), estimation of serum progesterone levels on day 21, ultrasound examination to confirm follicular rupture or ovulation, and/or establish the diagnosis of PCOD.[13]

Checking the Ovarian Reserve

Diminished ovarian reserve can refer to a reduction in quality or quantity of oocytes, or a reduction in reproductive potential. Since a large number of patients nowadays are presenting for diagnostic evaluation later in their lifespans, identification of diminished ovarian reserve is becoming increasingly important. The level of ovarian reserve and the age of the female partner are the most important prognostic factors in the fertility work-up. The level of ovarian reserve is supposed to decrease with age. Checking for ovarian reserve is specifically indicated in patients 35 years or older.[14] Other circumstances where testing for ovarian reserve may also be required include the following conditions: unexplained infertility; family history of early menopause; history of some ovarian surgery in the past (e.g. ovarian cystectomy or drilling, unilateral oophorectomy, chemotherapy or radiation therapy); poor response to exogenous gonadotropin secretion, etc.

Presently, there is no ideal test for assessing ovarian reserve. Though a number of screening tests are being used, none of the tests has been found to be extremely accurate in predicting the fertility potential. For women over 35 years of age and younger women having risk factors for premature ovarian failure, the test commonly used for testing ovarian reserve is determination of day 3 FSH level. Other tests which are being used include the CCCT, antral follicle count (AFC), and the levels of anti-Müllerian hormone (AMH).

❖ *Clomiphene citrate challenge test*: This test involves oral administration of 100 mg CC on days 5 through nine of the menstrual cycle, followed by measurement of oestradiol and FSH levels on day 3 and measurement of FSH levels on day 10. Women with good ovarian reserve usually produce sufficient amount of oestradiol from small follicles early in the menstrual cycle, thereby maintaining FSH at a low level. In contrast, women with a reduced pool of follicles and oocytes are unable to produce sufficient amount of ovarian hormones, which is unable to inhibit the pituitary secretion of FSH, causing the FSH levels to rise early in the cycle.

❖ *Day 3 FSH concentration*: A day 3 FSH concentration less than 10 mIU/mL is suggestive of adequate ovarian reserve, whereas FSH levels varying between 10 mIU/mL and 15 mIU/mL can be considered as borderline. The upper threshold for a normal FSH concentration varies from laboratory to laboratory due to the use of different FSH assay reference standards and various methodologies for assay. An elevated FSH level (>10 IU/L) on day 3 is suggestive of reduced ovarian reserve. Such patients may respond poorly to ovulation-inducing drugs and may eventually require egg donation. If the day 3 FSH or CCCT is abnormal, the patient should be referred to a reproductive endocrinologist to discuss further treatment options such as aggressive ovulation induction, IVF, or use of donor oocytes.

❖ *Antral follicle count*: The number of antral follicles (defined as follicles measuring 2–10 mm in diameter) can be measured with the help of ultrasound examination. In a normal woman, number of antral follicles in the ovary is proportional to the number of primordial follicles remaining. Therefore, as the number of primordial follicles decreases, the number of visible small antral follicles also declines. On transvaginal ultrasound, a low AFC ranging from 4 antral follicles to 10 antral follicles between days 2 and 4 of a regular menstrual cycle is suggestive of poor ovarian reserve.[15] Although AFC is a good predictor of ovarian reserve and response, it is less predictive of oocyte quality, the ability to conceive with IVF, and pregnancy outcome. Low AFC has, however, high specificity for predicting poor response to ovarian stimulation and treatment failure.

❖ *AntiMüllerian hormone*: Since AMH is usually derived from the granulosa cells of the small (<8 mm) preantral and early antral follicles, its levels are independent of gonadotropins and exhibit very little variation within and between the cycles. AMH levels reflect the size of the primordial follicle pool. Therefore, in a normal adult woman, levels of this hormone progressively reduce with the gradual decline in the pool of primordial follicle with age. AMH levels are almost undetectable at the time of menopause. Low AMH values (0.2–0.7 ng/mL) have a high sensitivity and specificity for predicting poor response to stimulation protocols, but not for predicting pregnancy.[16] Measurement of AMH helps identify reduced ovarian follicle pool in some patients (e.g. those receiving chemotherapy or radiotherapy for cancer).

❖ *Inhibin B levels*: Inhibin is secreted by the granulosa cells of smaller antral follicles. However, its concentration is likely to increase in response to exogenous GnRH stimulation. Therefore, levels of inhibin B are usually not regarded as a reliable measure of ovarian reserve.

❖ *Ovarian volume*: Progressive follicular depletion is associated with a reduction in ovarian volume. Therefore, ovarian volume (L × W × 0.52) shows a good correlation with the number of oocytes retrieved, but poorly with the pregnancy rates.

❖ *Serum progesterone levels in the mid-luteal phase*: In a normal woman, serum progesterone levels generally remain below 1 ng/mL during the follicular phase. These levels rise slightly on the day of LH surge (1–2 ng/mL) and steadily thereafter. The levels of this hormone peak 7–8 days following ovulation and decline again. Serum progesterone levels in the mid-luteal phase (7 days before the date of next expected period) greater than 10 ng/mL are indicative of ovulation.[17,18] Serum progesterone levels in the mid-luteal phase less than 3 ng/mL indicate that ovulation has probably not occurred. This could be related to the incorrect timing for withdrawing the blood sample or luteinised unruptured follicle. Such patients must be evaluated for polycystic ovaries and may require ovulation induction. Measurement of serum progesterone levels is the simplest, most common, objective and reliable test of ovulatory function as long as it is appropriately timed. A properly timed serum progesterone concentration can be considered as the simplest and most reliable method when the clinician's aim is to confirm ovulatory function in a woman with regular monthly menses.

❖ *Ovulation prediction kit*: An over-the-counter urinary ovulation prediction kit helps in detecting mid-cycle LH surge in the urine. Therefore, this test is highly effective for calculating the timing of the LH surge that consistently indicates ovulation. LH surge is a brief event and typically lasts between 48 hours to 50 hours from start to finish. This test is usually positive on a single day and occasionally on two consecutive days. To detect the LH surge, testing is done daily, beginning 2–3 days before the day of expected LH surge based on the overall cycle length. Ovulation usually occurs 14–26 hours after detection of LH surge (and indicative colour change in the kit) and almost always within 48 hours. Therefore, the interval of greatest fertility includes the day LH surge is detected and the following 2 days.[19] However, there is no evidence to indicate that the use of commercially available ovulation prediction kits is likely to increase the rate of fecundability.[20] Furthermore, the use of these kits may increase the couple's psychological stress, thereby further delaying fertility.

❖ *Ultrasound*: Serial ultrasonographic examination can be performed to confirm follicular rupture or ovulation. Ultrasound examination is also helpful in diagnosing PCOS.

Tests for Uterine Factor

The commonly used investigations include hysterosalpingography (HSG), pelvic ultrasonography, saline infusion sonography (SIS) and endometrial biopsy or operative procedures, such as laparoscopy and hysteroscopy.

Ultrasonography

Pelvic ultrasonography (both transabdominal and transvaginal) has become an important tool in the evaluation and monitoring of infertile patients, especially during ovulation induction. Pelvic ultrasonography allows precise evaluation of the uterus, endometrial cavity and adnexa (especially the ovaries). Pelvic sonograms help in the early detection of uterine fibroids, endometrial polyps, ovarian cysts, adnexal masses and endometriomas. Ultrasonography can also help in diagnosing conditions such as ectopic pregnancy, polycystic ovaries and persistent corpus luteum cysts. In the diagnostic evaluation of the infertile couple, ultrasound examination of the endometrium has no proven value. Although ultrasound examination cannot be used to evaluate endometrial receptivity, it does help in the identification of important uterine pathology in infertile women (e.g. presence of congenital malformations, septate uterus and bicornuate uterus).

Hysteroscopy

Hysteroscopy is a method for direct visualisation of the endometrial cavity, which is commonly performed as an outpatient procedure using local anaesthesia (i.e. paracervical block). Hysteroscopy is a definitive method used for both the diagnosis and treatment of intrauterine pathology, which is likely to have an effect on the fertility. While performing hysteroscopy, solutions such as Hyskon (previously used), glycine and sorbitol (used nowadays) are used for intrauterine instillation. Hysteroscopic examination helps in evaluation of tubal ostia and the diagnosis and treatment of endometrial pathology. Hysteroscopic surgery can also be used for the treatment of intrauterine pathologies such as uterine synechiae, endometrial polyps, submucous myomas, removal of foreign bodies (e.g. intrauterine devices) and lysis of intrauterine adhesions produced by Asherman's syndrome.

In patients undergoing hysteroscopy, performing laparoscopy simultaneously helps in avoiding the requirement for HSG.

Tests for Tubal and Peritoneal Factors

The two most frequent tests used for diagnosis of tubal pathology are laparoscopy and HSG. Non-invasive or minimally invasive investigations, which may serve as an alternative to HSG for testing tubal patency, include chlamydia antibody testing and/or hysterosalpingo-contrast sonography (HyCoSy). More invasive tests such as laparoscopy with chromotubation and fluoroscopic/hysteroscopic selective tubal cannulation may be required to confirm the diagnosis of suspected tubal pathology. An endoscopic procedure known as falloposcopy is sometimes used for delineating fallopian tube pathology.

Hysterosalpingogram

The HSG is the most frequently used diagnostic tool for evaluation of the endometrial cavity as well as the tubal pathology. If performed meticulously under fluoroscopic guidance, HSG helps in providing accurate information about the endocervical canal, endometrial cavity, cornual ostium, patency of the fallopian tubes and status of the fimbriae. Tubal patency is indicated by spillage of dye into the endometrial cavity. HSG is able to accurately define the shape and size of the uterine cavity. It can help diagnose uterine developmental anomalies (e.g. unicornuate uterus, septate uterus, bicornuate uterus and uterus didelphys), submucous myomas, adnexal masses, intrauterine adhesions and endometrial polyps.[21] Furthermore, the HSG also provides indirect evidence regarding the presence of pelvic adhesions and uterine, ovarian, or adnexal masses. Normal uterine cavity is symmetrical and triangular in shape. It is widest at the level of cornual orifices near the fundus. HSG is best performed during the 2–5-day interval period immediately following end of menses.

Laparoscopy

Gynaecological laparoscopy is used for diagnosis as well as treatment of pelvic pathology. During laparoscopic examination, a laparoscope is used for visualising the pelvic area, uterine surface, anterior and posterior cul-de-sac, fallopian tubes and ovaries. Gynaecological laparoscopy is commonly used for diagnosing and treating endometriosis, PID, ectopic pregnancy and removal of adhesions and scar tissue.[22] Laparoscopy can be used for monitoring the effects of ovulation induction medicines on the ovaries, and taking biopsies from ovarian cysts. Diagnostic laparoscopy may be performed under deep sedation and local anaesthesia, while operative laparoscopy typically requires general anaesthesia. The process of chromotubation involves injection of a dye solution through the cannula inserted inside the cervix so as to enable the evaluation of tubal patency. For this procedure, indigo carmine dye is usually preferred over the dye methylene blue due to the possible risk of acute methaemoglobinaemia. Laparoscopy is an invasive and expensive procedure.

CHAPTER 73

Moreover, findings at laparoscopy usually do not change the initial management of the infertile couple when the initial investigations performed for evaluation of infertility were either normal or there was severe male factor infertility. Laparoscopy is contraindicated in patients with probable bowel obstruction, bowel distension, cardiopulmonary disease or shock due to internal bleeding.

Laparoscopy is associated with the risk of complications such as bowel perforation, uterine and pelvic vessel injury, bladder trauma, etc. Therefore, the procedure must be preferably performed by a skilled and an experienced surgeon. Currently, laparoscopy has become the gold standard method for detection of tubal patency. In suspected cases of endo-metriosis or pelvic adhesions, diagnostic laparoscopy and chromotubation is preferred. Ablation of implants and lysis of adhesions can also be performed at the time of laparoscopy.[22]

Falloposcopy

Falloposcopy is defined as transvaginal microendoscopy of the fallopian tubes and enables the gynaecologist to directly visualise the entire lumen of the fallopian tube.

Chlamydia Antibodies

Chlamydia trachomatis: IgG antibody testing is a simple, inexpensive, non-invasive test with some evidence supporting its use as a method for predicting the presence of tubal disease. Studies suggest that antibodies to *Chlamydia* are more predictive of infertility due to tubal factor than an abnormal HSG or a history of previous use of a copper intrauterine device.[23]

Hysterosalpingo-contrast Sonography

In this method, echogenic contrast media is injected transcervically, following which ultrasound is used for visualising the uterus, tubes and adnexa. It is a safe, well-tolerated, quick and easy method for obtaining information related to tubal status, the uterine cavity, ovaries and the myometrium.

Evaluation of Cervical Factor

This aims at testing the characteristics of the cervical mucus with the help of postcoital test (Sim's or Huhner's test).[24] However, presently the routine use of postcoital testing of cervical mucus for investigating the fertility problems is not recommended by NICE (2013) because it has no predictive value on pregnancy rate.[25]

MANAGEMENT

A treatment plan should be generated based on the diagnosis established through the findings of laboratory investigations, clinical examination, duration of infertility and the woman's age. Following this, the treatment can comprise the following:

❖ *Patient counselling*: The couple must be instructed that for conception to occur, they must have intercourse every 2–3 days.

❖ *Lifestyle changes*: For couples attempting conception, it is recommended that the BMI between 20 to 25 is achieved. Alcohol consumption must be limited to one or two units, once or twice a week for women. Women who smoke should be advised to quit smoking.

❖ *Treatment of cervical factors*: Chronic cervicitis may be treated with antibiotics. The most successful treatment option for infertility related to cervical factors is artificial intrauterine insemination (IUI). This can be performed by depositing the sperms at the level of internal cervical os (cervical insemination) or inside the endometrial cavity.

❖ *Treatment of uterine factors*: This involves lysis of uterine septae and uterine synechiae, surgical treatment of uterine anomalies (e.g. bicornuate uterus, etc.), hysteroscopic removal of endometrial polyps, etc. Treatment of fibroids has been described in Chapter 65 (Uterine Leiomyoma).

❖ *Treatment of tubal factors of infertility*: This may include microsurgery and laparoscopy. Tubal obstruction due to elective sterilisation is usually repaired using microsurgical techniques. The pregnancy rate following a tubal reanastomosis performed by surgeons skilled in microsurgery varies from 70% to 80%.[26] Nowadays, laparoscopic surgical approach is widely being used for the treatment of multiple tuboperitoneal pathologies, especially endometriosis, using techniques, such as electrocautery, endocoagulation, lasers, etc.[27] Treatment of endometriosis has been discussed in details in Chapter 68 (Chronic Pelvic Pain and Endometriosis). For women with proximal tubal obstruction, selective salpingography plus tubal catheterisation, or hysteroscopic tubal cannulation, may serve as effective treatment options. Various surgical procedures for improving tubal patency are enlisted in Table 73.3.[28]

❖ *Treatment of ovarian factors*: Some commonly used treatment options for PCOS include weight loss through diet and exercise, ovulation-inducing medicines, such as CC, insulin-sensitizing agents (such as glucophage®/metformin), dietary changes (low glycaemic diet) and surgery (ovarian drilling). Ovulation-inducing drugs, which are commonly used, include CC, hMGs and synthetic GnRH analogues.[29,30] If no treatment option seems to work, the last option for the clinician to consider is assisted reproductive techniques, which have been discussed in Chapter 76 (Assisted Reproductive Techniques).

Table 73.3: Surgical procedures for improving tubal patency[28]

Types of tubal pathology	Surgical procedure
Distal obstruction	• Fimbrioplasty: The lysis of fimbrial adhesions or dilatation of fimbrial strictures • Neosalpingostomy: Creation of a new tubal opening in a distally occluded tube
Proximal obstruction	• Selective salpingography plus tubal catheterisation • Hysteroscopic or fluoroscopic tubal catheterisation • Tubocornual anastomosis by laparotomy

❖ *Unexplained infertility*: Couples with a diagnosis of unexplained infertility must typically undergo a trial of ovarian stimulation with or without IUI.[31] With such treatment strategy, most couples are likely to conceive without any further intervention.

❖ *Male factor infertility*: Couples with male factor infertility are typically offered IVF as one of their treatment options.

❖ *Susceptibility to rubella*: Women who are concerned about their fertility should be offered testing for their rubella status. Women who are found susceptible to rubella should be offered vaccination and contraception for at least 1 month following vaccination.

CLINICAL PEARLS

❖ The age of the female partner is the most important determinant of the couple's fertility.

❖ Ovulatory disorders are the most common cause of female infertility. Of the various ovulatory disorders, anovulation due to PCOS is the most common cause of female infertility.

❖ Pelvic inflammatory disease is the major cause of infertility due to tubal factors in the Western world. *Chlamydia trachomatis* is the main pathogen involved in these cases.

EVIDENCE-BASED MEDICINE

❖ There is no evidence to indicate that ovulation detection kits and basal body temperature charts help in increasing the chance of conception.[20]

❖ Moderate to severe endometriosis is an important cause for infertility. The available evidence indicates that treatment with drugs is ineffective in the treatment of endometriosis-related infertility. Surgical ablation of minimal to mild endometriosis at the time of diagnostic laparoscopy helps in the treatment of infertility. Surgical treatment also helps in improving pregnancy rates amongst women with moderate to severe endometriosis.[25]

❖ Women should not be offered an endometrial biopsy for evaluation of the luteal phase as part of the investigation of their fertility problems because presently, there is no evidence that medical treatment of luteal phase defect is likely to improve the pregnancy rates.[32]

REFERENCES

1. Boivin J, Bunting L, Collins JA, Nygren KG. International estimates of infertility prevalence and treatment-seeking: potential need and demand for infertility medical care. Hum Reprod. 2007;22(6):1506-12.
2. Speroff L, Fritz M. Clinical Gynecologic Endocrinology and Infertility, 7th edition. Baltimore, MD: Lippincott Williams & Wilkins; 2004. pp. 547-71.
3. The American Fertility Society classifications of adnexal adhesions, distal tubal occlusion, tubal occlusion secondary to tubal ligation, tubal pregnancies, Müllerian anomalies and intrauterine adhesions. Fertil Steril. 1988;49(6):944-55.
4. Donnez J, Jadoul P. What are the implications of myomas on fertility? A need for a debate? Hum Reprod. 2002;17(6):1424-30.
5. Sudik R, Hüsch K, Steller J, Daume E. Fertility and pregnancy outcome after myomectomy in sterility patients. Eur J Obstet Gynecol Reprod Biol. 1996;65(2):209-14.
6. Franks S, Stark J, Hardy K. Follicle dynamics and anovulation in polycystic ovary syndrome. Hum Reprod Update. 2008;14(4):367-78.
7. Goldzieher JW. Polycystic ovarian disease. Fertil Steril. 1981;35(4):371-94.
8. Weström L. Effect of acute pelvic inflammatory disease on fertility. Am J Obstet Gynecol. 1975;121(5):707-13.
9. Strathy JH, Molgaard CA, Coulam CB, Melton LJ. Endometriosis and infertility: a laparoscopic study of endometriosis among fertile and infertile women. Fertil Steril. 1982;38(6):667-72.
10. Phipps WR, Cramer DW, Schiff I, Belisle S, Stillman R, Albrecht B, et al. The association between smoking and female infertility as influenced by cause of the infertility. Fertil Steril. 1987;48(3):377-82.
11. Female age-related fertility decline. Committee Opinion No. 589. American College of Obstetricians and Gynecologists. Obstet Gynecol. 2014;123:719-21.
12. Pandey S, Maheshwari A, Bhattacharya S. Should access to fertility treatment be determined by female body mass index? Hum Reprod. 2010;25(4):815-20.
13. Guermandi E, Vegetti W, Bianchi MM, Uglietti A, Ragni G, Crosignani P. Reliability of ovulation tests in infertile women. Obstet Gynecol. 2001;97(1):92-6.
14. Johnson NP, Bagrie EM, Coomarasamy A, Bhattacharya S, Shelling AN, Jessop S, et al. Ovarian reserve tests for predicting fertility outcomes for assisted reproductive technology: the International Systematic Collaboration of Ovarian Reserve Evaluation protocol for a systematic review of ovarian reserve test accuracy. BJOG. 2006;113(12):1472-80.
15. Jones GE. Some newer aspects of the management of infertility. J Am Med Assoc. 1949;141:1123-9.
16. Visser JA, de Jong FH, Laven JS, Themmen AP. AntiMüllerian hormone: a new marker for ovarian function. Reproduction. 2006;131(1):1-9.
17. Warne DW, Tredway D, Schertz JC, Schnieper-Samec S, Alam V, Eshkol A. Midluteal serum progesterone levels and pregnancy following ovulation induction with human follicle-stimulating hormone: results of a combined-data analysis. J Reprod Med. 2011;56(1-2):31-8.
18. Jones GS. The clinical evaluation of ovulation and the luteal phase. J Reprod Med. 1977;18(3):139-42.
19. Balen AH, Rutherford AJ. Management of infertility. BMJ. 2007;335:608.
20. Stanford JB, White GL, Hatasaka H. Timing intercourse to achieve pregnancy: current evidence. Obstet Gynecol. 2002;100(6):1333-41.
21. Hunt RB, Siegler AM. Hysterosalpingography: Techniques and Interpretations. St. Louis, MO: Mosby-Year Book; 1990.
22. Mettler L, Giesel H, Semm K. Treatment of female infertility due to tubal obstruction by operative laparoscopy. Fertil Steril. 1979;32(4):384-8.
23. Veenemans LM, van der Linden PJ. The value of Chlamydia trachomatis antibody testing in predicting tubal factor infertility. Hum Reprod. 2002;17(3):695-8.
24. Giner J, Merino G, Luna J, Aznar R. Evaluation of the Sims-Huhner postcoital test in fertile couples. Fertil Steril. 1974;25(2):145-8.

25. National Institute for Health and Care Excellence NICE. Fertility problems: assessment and treatment. NICE clinical guidelines (CG156). London: NICE; 2013.

26. Gomel V, Yarali H. Infertility surgery: microsurgery. Curr Opin Obstet Gynecol. 1992;4(3):390-9.

27. Olive DL. Conservative surgery. In: Schenken RS (Ed). Endometriosis: Contemporary Concepts in Clinical Management. Philadelphia, PA: Lippincott Williams & Wilkins; 1989. pp. 213-49.

28. Winston RM. Reversal of tubal sterilization. Clin Obstet Gynecol. 1980;23(4):1261-8.

29. Shirai E, Iizuka R, Notake Y. Clomiphene citrate and its effects upon ovulation and estrogen. Fertil Steril. 1972;23(5):331-8.

30. Garcia J, Jones GS, Wentz AC. The use of clomiphene citrate. Fertil Steril. 1977;28(7):707-17.

31. Dodson WC, Haney AF. Controlled ovarian hyperstimulation and intrauterine insemination for treatment of infertility. Fertil Steril. 1991;55(3):457-67.

32. Balasch J, Fábregues F, Creus M, Vanrell JA. The usefulness of endometrial biopsy for luteal phase evaluation in infertility. Hum Reprod. 1992;7(7):973-7.

Polycystic Ovarian Disease

INTRODUCTION

The condition, polycystic ovarian disease, also known as PCOD, is a relatively common endocrine disorder amongst nearly 10% of women in the reproductive age group.[1] It is a disorder associated with anovulation, features of androgen excess, obesity, infertility and hypersecretion of LH. It is characterised by the presence of many minute cysts in the ovaries and excessive production of androgens. In cases of PCOD, acceptable rates of ovulation and pregnancy can be achieved using clomiphene citrate (CC), metformin and gonadotropins. However, some women remain anovulatory or cannot be successfully treated medically and in these cases ovarian surgery serves as a useful alternative option.

AETIOLOGY

Despite of many years of research, the pathophysiology of PCOD has not been completely understood. The probable pathophysiology of PCOD is described in Flow chart 74.1. Common endocrine abnormalities in PCOD include chronically high levels of LH, thereby resulting in an elevated LH/FSH ratio (usually 2.5 or greater), hyperandrogenism, hyperinsulinaemia, insulin resistance and dyslipidaemia.[2] These endocrine disturbances interfere with ovarian folliculogenesis and result in anovulation. Moreover, these endocrine disturbances are likely to constitute towards an increased risk for development of cardiovascular diseases and diabetes. Elevated LH levels in patients with PCOD result in the hyperplasia of stromal and thecal cells in the ovarian follicles. This ultimately results in an increased androgen production by the adrenal glands [dehydroepiandrosterone (DHEA) and dehydroepiandrosterone sulphate (DHEAS)] and ovarian stroma (androstenedione). High intraovarian androgen levels may further contribute to follicular atresia.

This also results in an increased peripheral availability of ovarian testosterone (androstenedione), which gets converted in the skin to dihydrotestosterone, with the help of the enzyme 5α-reductase, thereby accounting for acne and hirsutism in these women. Moreover, increased androstenedione secretion results in an increased production of a type of oestrogen, principally oestrone, by aromatisation in the peripheral tissues. These chronically elevated oestrogen levels produce a negative feedback at the level of the hypothalamo-pituitary axis, further resulting in reduced FSH production, which causes an increase in the LH/FSH ratio by 2.5 or more. Thus, the inappropriate gonadotropin secretion is secondary to the abnormal steroid feedback, rather than a primary abnormality at the level of the hypothalamus-pituitary. Low levels of FSH in the follicle prevent induction of aromatase activity and result in the lack of ovarian oestrogen production. As granulosa cell mitosis and follicular growth requires an oestrogenic follicular microenvironment, follicular maturation gets arrested. This is responsible for producing anovulation.

DIAGNOSIS

Clinical Presentation

Women with polycystic ovarian disease are frequently associated with weight gain, excessive hair growth on the face and body, oligomenorrhoea or amenorrhoea, infrequent or absent ovulation, miscarriage and infertility. According to the American Society of Reproductive Medicine (ASRM) and the ESHRE joint consensus meeting in November 2003, the diagnosis of PCOD should be made, when two of the following three criteria are met:[3]
1. Infrequent or absent ovulation (anovulation)
2. Clinical or biochemical features of hyperandrogenism, such as excessive hair growth, acne, raised LH and raised androgen levels

Flow chart 74.1: Pathophysiology of polycystic ovarian disease

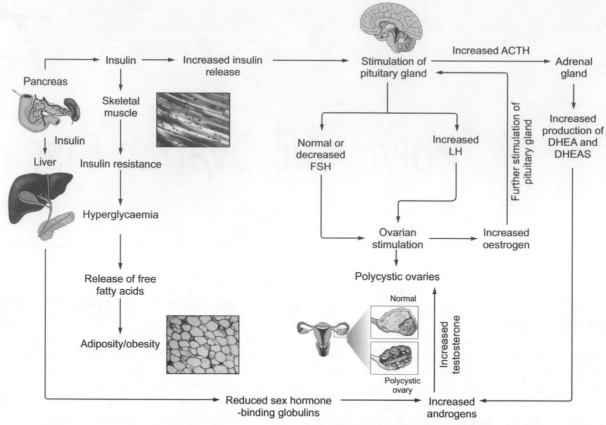

Abbreviations: ACTH, adrenocorticotrophic hormone; DHEA, dehydroepiandrosterone; DHEAS, dehydroepiandrosterone sulphate

3. *Polycystic ovaries*: Morphologically there is bilateral enlargement, thickened ovarian capsule, multiple follicular cysts (usually ranging between 2 mm and 8 mm in diameter) and an increased amount of stroma. Features of polycystic ovarian morphology on ultrasound scan are as follows (Fig. 74.1):[4]

- Greater than 12 follicles measuring between 2 mm to 9 mm in diameter, located peripherally, resulting in a pearl necklace appearance.
- Increased echogenicity of ovarian stroma and/or ovarian volume greater than 10 mL. The distribution of the follicles is not required, with one ovary being sufficient for the diagnosis.

Other aetiologies (e.g. congenital adrenal hyperplasias, androgen-secreting tumours, Cushing's syndrome, etc.) which can cause hyperandrogenism and/or similar ultrasound and biochemical features should be excluded.

Investigations

Diagnosis of PCOD is made through ultrasound examination or diagnostic laparoscopy. Blood levels of hormones, such as LH, FSH, androgens and sex hormone-binding globulins (SHBGs), must also be performed in these patients. FSH levels are low or normal and LH levels are often raised, resulting in a raised LH/FSH ratio. The levels of androgens and testosterone may also be raised. Various serum parameters altered in

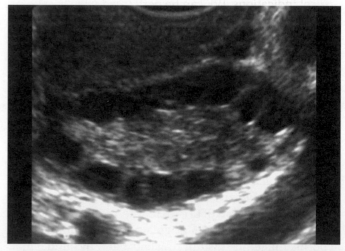

Fig. 74.1: Ultrasound features of polycystic ovarian morphology

cases of PCOD are summarised in Table 74.1.[5] There is a reduction in the levels of SHBGs, resulting in an elevation of free androgen index. Though fasting insulin levels are increased in cases of PCOD, this parameter is not routinely assessed. Instead the insulin resistance is assessed with the help of 75 g oral glucose tolerance test (OGTT) in women with PCOD and a BMI more than 30 kg/m². Due to a higher risk of insulin resistance amongst South Asian women, assessment for glucose tolerance must be undertaken when BMI is more than 25 kg/m².

Table 74.1: Serum parameters which are altered in cases of PCOD[5]

Normal levels	Levels in PCOD
Serum testosterone (0.5–1.8 nmol/L)	Increased levels of androgens (testosterone and androstenedione)
Sex hormone-binding globulins [SHBG (16–119 nmol/L)]	Reduced levels of SHBG
Free androgen index (testosterone levels × 100 / SHBG) < 5	Increased free androgen index
FSH (2–8 IU/L)	Reduced/normal FSH levels
LH (2–10 IU/L)	Increased LH levels
Anti-müllerian hormone (35 pmol/L)	Increased
Serum oestradiol/oesterone levels	Increased
Fasting insulin levels (<30 mU/L)	Increased

Table 74.2: Criteria for the metabolic syndrome in women with PCOD[3,6]

Risk factor	Cut-off
Abdominal obesity (waist circumference)	>88 cm (>35 inch)
Triglycerides	>150 mg/dL
HDL-C	<50 mg/dL
Blood pressure	>130 mmHg systolic and >85 mmHg dystolic
Fasting and 2 h glucose from OGTT	110–126 mg/dL and/or 2 h glucose 140–199 mg/dL

Abbreviations: HDL-C, high-density lipoprotein-cholesterol; OGTT, oral glucose tolerance test

Many patients with PCOD are at an increased risk of having features of metabolic syndrome (Table 74.2) such as insulin resistance, obesity, hyperinsulinaemia, dyslipidaemia, etc. due to which they may be at an increased risk for cardiovascular disease.[6]

MANAGEMENT

Algorithm for treatment of patients with PCOD is described in Flow chart 74.2. Some commonly used treatment options for PCOD include ovulation-inducing medicines such as CC, insulin-sensitising agents (such as Glucophage®/metformin), dietary changes (low-glycaemic diet) and surgery (ovarian drilling). The primary treatment for PCOD is weight loss through lifestyle changes such as dietary changes and exercise.[7] This line of therapy helps in improving the insulin sensitivity. Modest weight loss also helps in lowering the androgen levels, improving hirsutism, normalisation of menstrual cycles, resumption of ovulation and reduction of insulin resistance. However, it may take months before these results become apparent. Besides facilitating fertility, the aims of treatment in women with PCOD are to control hirsutism, to prevent endometrial hyperplasia from unopposed acyclic oestrogen secretion, and to prevent the long-term consequences of insulin resistance. The treatment must be individualised according to the needs and desires of each patient. Use of OCPs or cyclic progestational agents can help maintain a normal endometrium and also reduce the increased risk of endometrial hyperplasia and carcinoma.

For the women with PCOD who want to conceive, CC is used initially because of its high success rate and relative simplicity and inexpensiveness. CC is able to induce ovulation in nearly 80% of the individuals and 40% are able to conceive. Other possible therapeutic approaches for ovulation induction include the use of insulin-sensitising agents, gonadotropins (perhaps preceded by GnRH analogues), FSH alone, pulsatile GnRH and wedge resection of the ovaries at laparotomy. Management of patients with PCOD suffering from hirsutism is described in Chapter 75 (Hirsutism).

MEDICAL MANAGEMENT

Menstrual Irregularities

First-line medical therapy for managing menstrual irregularities is cases of PCOD consist of using an oral contraceptive. According to the recommendations by ACOG, low-dose hormonal contraceptive agents must be used for the management of menstrual dysfunction in cases of patients with PCOD.[8] The contraceptive agents help in controlling endocrinological abnormalities related to PCOD by inhibiting ovarian androgen production as well as by increasing the production of SHBG. In presence of hirsutism, OCPs containing antiandrogens, e.g. Dianette® (containing 35 µg of ethinyl oestradiol and 2 mg cyproterone acetate) and Yasmin® (containing drospirenone) can be prescribed. They help in alleviating hirsutism by supressing free androgen levels. The clinician should ensure that the patient is not pregnant before starting therapy with oral contraceptive agents or androgen-blocking agents because of the risk associated with transplacental passage of these agents. Progestogens, e.g. 3-monthly injections of depot medroxyprogesterone acetate (DMPA) or Mirena® intrauterine system can be sometimes used as an alternative to OCPs.

Induction of Ovulation

Presently, ovulation induction using CC is the treatment of choice in patients with PCOD. Pregnancy rate with CC is approximately 40–50% and the abortion rate is about 30–40%.[9] In patients with hyperinsulinaemia, resistant to CC, insulin-sensitising agents, such as metformin can be prescribed. Metformin has now become the first-line of management in cases of CC-resistant women with PCOD. If ovulation does not occur within several months after treatment with metformin, surgical method [laparoscopic ovarian drilling (LOD)] or gonadotropins can be considered as effective options depending upon patient's choice. Usually, the surgical approach is chosen when a patient has already failed to ovulate on CC at maximal doses and has not responded to insulin-sensitising agents. Before undertaking surgery, the patient must be explained all pros and cons related with the procedure. It has been reported that the procedure can result in high rate of spontaneous postoperative ovulation and conception. Moreover, the subsequent ovulation induction using medicines becomes easier.

Flow chart 74.2: Treatment of patients with polycystic ovarian disease (PCOD)

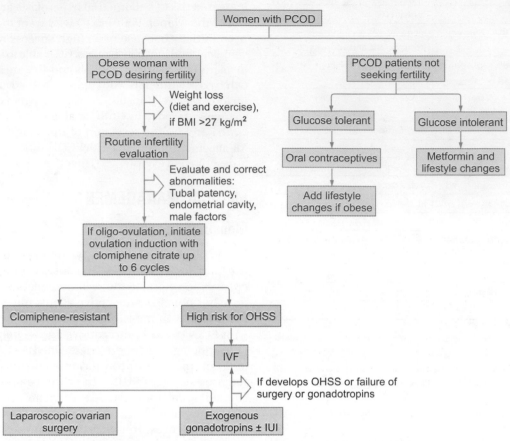

Abbreviations: IUI, intrauterine insemination; OHSS, ovarian hyperstimulation syndrome

Clomiphene Citrate

Clomiphene citrate is a non-steroidal selective oestrogen receptor modulator (SERM) with both oestrogen antagonist and agonist effects. It is largely believed to exert its anti-oestrogen effect by competing with the oestrogen receptors at the level of hypothalamus, pituitary and ovaries. By blocking the oestrogen receptors within the hypothalamus, CC alleviates the negative feedback effect exerted by endogenous oestrogens. As a result, the GnRH release gets normalised. Therefore, the secretion of FSH and LH is able to re-establish the normal process of ovulation and is capable of normalising follicular recruitment, selection and development. CC can also be prescribed to the women with unexplained fertility problems.

The standard dose of CC is 50 mg PO once a day for 5 days, starting on the day 3–5 of the menstrual cycle or after progestin-induced bleeding. The response to CC is monitored using pelvic ultrasonography starting on the day 12 of the menstrual cycle. The follicle should develop to a diameter of 23–24 mm before a spontaneous LH surge occurs.

Anovulatory women with PCOD, having a BMI of more than 25 kg/m² who have not responded to CC alone, should be offered metformin in combination with CC. Women who are prescribed metformin should be informed about the side effects, such as nausea, vomiting and other gastrointestinal disturbances, associated with its use.

Human Menopausal Gonadotropins

Human menopausal gonadotropin (hMG) and its derivatives are indicated for ovulation induction in patients with primary amenorrhoea and/or infertility, who did not respond to ovulation induction with CC. hMG (Menopur®) contains 75 U of FSH and 75 U of LH per mL, although the concentration may vary in the range of 60–90 U for FSH and for LH in the range of 60–120 U. The new generations of available gonadotropins are produced by genetically engineered mammalian cells, i.e. Chinese hamster ovary cells. Gonadotropins such as hMG, urinary FSH and recombinant FSH are equally effective in achieving pregnancy.

Tamoxifen

Tamoxifen citrate is a SERM, which is extensively used for the secondary chemoprevention of hormone-responsive breast cancer. It is now also being used for ovulation induction in PCOD. Tamoxifen has lower antioestrogenic effects on the endometrium and cervix in comparison to clomiphene.

Aromatase Inhibitors

Aromatase inhibitors, such as letrozole and anastrozole, inhibit the action of the enzyme aromatase, which is responsible for the process of aromatisation (conversion of androgens into

PART III

oestrogens). As a result, oestrogen levels are dramatically reduced, releasing the hypothalamic-pituitary axis from its negative feedback. Though the FDA has not approved the use of aromatase inhibitors for induction of ovulation in cases of PCOD, use of aromatase inhibitors in combination with gonadotropins have also emerged as novel ovarian stimulants for performing IVF in women with breast cancer.

Metformin

Patients with PCOD, having a BMI of more than 25 kg/m² are often resistant to treatment with CC alone. These patients commonly have other problems, such as hyperinsulinism and hyperandrogenism, associated with acanthosis nigricans. This group is amenable to metformin treatment in combination with CC. Metformin improves insulin sensitivity and decreases hepatic gluconeogenesis and, therefore, reduces hyperinsulinism, basal and stimulated LH levels, and free testosterone concentration. Consequently, the patient with PCOD becomes responsive to CC ovulation induction. Metformin is used as an insulin sensitiser. It helps in treating the root cause of PCOD and improves fertility by rectifying endocrine and metabolic functions.

Adverse effects of metformin include gastrointestinal intolerance, nausea, vomiting and abdominal cramps. Weight loss has also been observed. The initial dose is 500 mg PO once a day for 7 days, then 500 mg BID for another 7 days, and finally 500 mg TID. Since patients can ovulate while on metformin treatment, pelvic ultrasonography is required for documentation of ovulation. In case ovulation does not occur, CC is started at the initial dose of 50 mg/day for 5 days.

SURGICAL MANAGEMENT

Laparoscopic ovarian drilling is a surgical treatment that can trigger ovulation in women with PCOD. In this method, different techniques, such as electrocauterisation, laser, electrocoagulation, biopsy, etc. are used for destroying ovarian follicles. Destroying part of the ovaries has been reported to restore regular ovulation cycles.

Laparoscopic Ovarian Drilling

Women with PCOD who have not responded to CC should be offered LOD because it is as effective as gonadotropin treatment and is not associated with an increased risk of multiple pregnancy. This procedure involves creation of approximately 4–20 holes, having a size of 3 mm diameter and 3 mm depth to be made in each ovary, preferably on the antimesenteric side (Figs 74.2A to D). Women who are unable to conceive naturally following the previously mentioned therapeutic options often respond to assisted reproductive technologies (ARTs), including IVF.

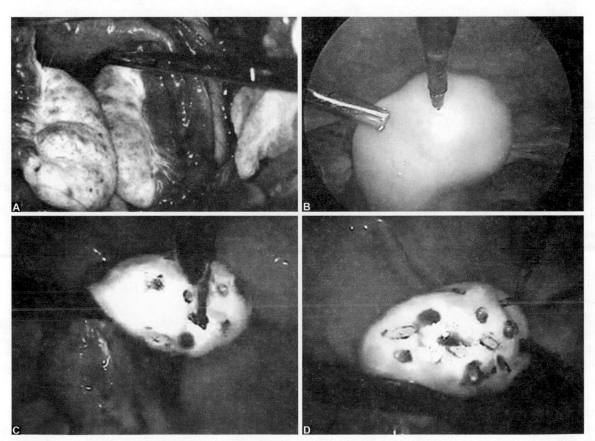

Figs 74.2A to D: Laparoscopic ovarian drilling. (A) Laparoscopic visualisation of the pelvis in an effort to locate the ovaries; (B) Lifting the ovaries out of the ovarian fossa and placing them over the cervicouterine junction; (C) The procedure of laparoscopic ovarian drilling using electrocauterisation; (D) Appearance of the ovary following the procedure (*For colour version, see Plate 5*)

When PCOD was first described by Stein and Leventhal in 1935, the first line of management of these patients comprised of bilateral ovarian wedge resection.[10] Though the procedure resulted in high rate of ovulation, this was soon abandoned due to the high risk of postoperative adhesion formation. As a result, this procedure was soon replaced with ovulation induction, using medicines, such as CC, tamoxifen, bromocriptine and gonadotropins. The preferred treatment of choice at present in patients with PCOD is ovulation induction with CC. This treatment is associated with nearly 70% rate of ovulation after the first treatment. Recent studies have also suggested a possible linkage between the use of ovulation-inducing drugs and long-term risk of ovarian cancer.

As a result, a new mode of surgical therapy known as LOD has gained popularity because this procedure is associated with none or minimal requirement of gonadotropins for inducing ovulation.[11] Moreover, it can be performed as an outpatient procedure and is associated with reduced amount of surgical trauma and postoperative adhesion formation.[12] It has now been recognised that LOD is an effective treatment option for CC resistance and anovulatory infertility associated with PCOD.[13]

Advantages

The main advantages associated with the procedure of LOD are as follows:

- ❖ There is no additional risk of multiple pregnancy or ovarian hyperstimulation syndrome (OHSS), as reported with the use of gonadotropins
- ❖ The procedure is considered to be associated with fewer postoperative adhesions in comparison to laparotomy
- ❖ It is associated with minimum morbidity and no requirement for cyclic monitoring as required with the ovulation-inducing drugs
- ❖ Laparoscopic ovarian drilling yields a better ovulation and pregnancy rate in comparison to other surgical modalities for ovulation induction. Studies of women with PCOD have shown that ovarian drilling results in an ovulation rate ranging between 53% and 92% and a pregnancy rate of 70–80%.[11,13]
- ❖ Laparoscopic ovarian drilling is associated with a low miscarriage rate (14%) in comparison to that associated with ovulation induction, using gonadotropins (50%).[13]

Mechanism of Action of Laparoscopic Ovarian Drilling

Several surgical approaches for restoring ovulation in women with PCOD have been studied over the years, e.g. classical wedge resection, multiple ovarian biopsies, laser vaporisation and electrocautery. All types of ovarian surgeries share a common goal of creating ovarian damage and from an endocrine point of view can be seen as equivalent procedures. Mechanism of action of any of these surgical procedures, whether using wedge resection, cautery or laser vaporisation in cases of PCOD is yet not understood. Stein and Leventhal[10] were the first ones to propose bilateral wedge resection, as a method of choice for the induction of ovulation in clomiphene

resistant PCOD patients. According to Stein and Leventhal, the procedure of wedge resection worked by reducing the mechanical crowding of the cortex by cysts, which facilitated the normal movement of graafian follicle to the surface of the ovary. Gjönnaess in his study postulated that ovulation ensues in cases of LOD due to extensive capsular destruction, resulting in the discharge of contents of a number of follicular cysts.[11] Ovulation probably occurs due to a reduction in stromal mass or disruption of parenchymal blood flow leading to a reduction in production of ovarian androgens and the levels of LH. Gadir et al.[13] in their study found that the procedure of LOD resulted in a reduced concentration of LH after the procedure. On the other hand, the effect of this procedure on FSH levels was found to be variable. The FSH concentration increases rapidly and thereafter demonstrates a cyclical rise as the ovulatory function gets restored. The increase in the FSH levels is likely to result in the normalisation of LH/FSH ratio, causing recruitment of new cohort of follicles, thereby bringing the resumption of ovarian function. The procedure has also been found to be associated with a marked reduction in the circulating levels of androgens, i.e. androstenedione, testosterone and DHEAS. Moreover, LOD in a young woman is supposed to improve intraovarian stromal blood flow, so that the risk of OHSS in the subsequent ovarian induction cycles may be avoided. Daniell and Miller (1989) have suggested that physical opening of the subcapsular cysts during the process of LOD is likely to cause release of androgen containing follicular fluid, thereby lowering the androgen content of the ovary.[14] Other likely mechanism for the success of LOD could be related to the fact that follicular destruction causes a reduction in the number of atretic follicles and thereby reduced androgen production. There is a reduction in the level of free and total testosterone by about 40–50% of the preoperative levels.[15] Destruction of ovarian stromal elements and release of androgen-rich follicular fluid from the puncture of subcapsular cysts causes a fall in the circulating levels of androgens. Reduction in the level of substrate for follicular aromatase produces a fall in the circulating oestradiol levels. This releases the pituitary from the negative feedback inhibition, thereby resulting in an increased production of FSH by the pituitary. Furthermore, there is a fall in the LH levels.[16-19] All these changes result in the normalisation of LH/FSH ratio, leading to follicular development followed by ovulation. In summary, the procedure of LOD is able to normalise the hormonal imbalance occurring as a result of PCOD.

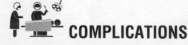

COMPLICATIONS

Complications Related to Polycystic Ovarian Disease Per Se

The possible late sequela of PCOD includes development of complications such as type 2 diabetes mellitus, dyslipidaemia, hypertension, cardiovascular disease, endometrial cancer, etc. in future.

Complications Related to Medical Management

Complications related to the use of various medicines for PCOD are described next.

Clomiphene Citrate

Multiple pregnancy: Women who are being prescribed CC should be informed that this drug might be associated with the risk of multiple gestation. Women undergoing treatment with CC should be offered ultrasound monitoring during at least the first cycle of treatment to ensure that they receive a dose that minimises the risk of multiple pregnancy.

Thickening of cervical mucus: Another important adverse effect associated with the use of this drug is the thickening of the cervical mucus under the antioestrogenic effect of CC. This may create an iatrogenic cervical factor, which may be responsible for producing infertility in a patient who has otherwise ovulated.

Other adverse effects: Other side effects, which may be rarely associated with CC, include hot flashes, scotomas, dryness of the vagina, headache and ovarian hyperstimulation. The use of CC is contraindicated in cases of ovarian cyst, pregnancy and liver disease. Its use is also controversial in patients with a history of breast cancer.

Gonadotropins

Side effects associated with the use of gonadotropins are as follows:

❖ Multiple adverse effects and complications that may occur following the use of the gonadotropins, include polyfollicular response, multiple pregnancy, ectopic pregnancy, miscarriages, ovarian torsion and rupture, and OHSS.[20] Due to the risk of various side effects, especially OHSS, the administration of hMG and its derivatives should be directly supervised by a reproductive endocrinologist under ultrasound guidance and daily determinations of oestradiol, FSH and LH levels. Moreover, it is expensive, stressful and time-consuming form of treatment, which usually needs intensive monitoring.

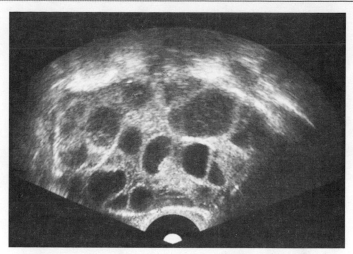

Fig. 74.3: Ovarian hyperstimulation syndrome showing 'wheel-spoke appearance' on transvaginal examination

❖ *Ovarian hyperstimulation syndrome*: OHSS is an iatrogenic condition that occurs in patients undergoing ovulation induction with hMG or controlled ovarian hyperstimulation for ARTs (Fig. 74.3). The incidence rate fluctuates from 0.1% to 30%. The pathophysiology of the disease is not well understood, but is associated with massive extravascular accumulation of fluid. This causes severe depletion of the intravascular volume resulting in dehydration, haemoconcentration and electrolyte imbalance (i.e. hyponatraemia, hyperkalaemia, etc.). Schenker and Weinstein have classified OHSS into three main categories: (1) mild, (2) moderate and (3) severe (Table 74.3).[21]

Risk factors for development of OHSS: Various risk factors for the development of OHSS include young age of the patient (<35 years), polycystic ovary-like appearance of ovaries, asthenic habitus, pregnancy and hCG luteal supplementation.[22] Exogenous hCG administration is critical for the development of OHSS. Severe OHSS is dependent on both exogenous administration of hCG or endogenous pregnancy-derived hCG. hCG is administered exogenously during ovarian stimulation for both triggering ovulation and for luteal support.

Table 74.3: Classification of ovarian hyperstimulation syndrome [21]

Degree	Symptoms and signs
Mild form	
Stage A	Symptoms such as abdominal heaviness, abdominal swelling and pain. Chemical hyperstimulation: 17β-oestradiol levels of 1,000–1,500 pg/mL
Stage B	Chemical hyperstimulation: ovaries enlarged up to 6 cm in diameter. Each ovary is characterised by presence of multiple follicular and corpus luteum cysts
Moderate form	
Stage A	17β-oestradiol levels >4,000 pg/mL; ovaries enlarged up to 6–12 cm
Stage B	Presence of ascites on ultrasound examination, findings as in stage A with gastrointestinal symptoms such as vomiting and diarrhoea
Severe form	
Stage A	17β-oestradiol levels >4,000 pg/mL; ovaries enlarged to >12 cm plus clinical manifestations including pleural effusion, pericardial effusion, breathing difficulties, hypovolaemia, impairment of renal function, electrolyte imbalance, disturbance in liver function, thromboembolic phenomena, shock, tension ascites and acute respiratory distress syndrome
Stage B	Presence of all the above plus change in the blood volume, increased blood viscosity due to haemoconcentration, coagulation abnormalities and diminished renal perfusion and function

CHAPTER 74

Moreover, different protocols used for stimulation of ovaries in ART cycles may also affect the incidence and the severity of OHSS. Stimulation of ovaries is likely to result in high serum oestradiol levels and development of multiple follicles.

Pathogenesis: The exact pathogenesis of OHSS is yet not clear. It is thought to occur as a result of increased vascular permeability.[23] The exact substances responsible for this have yet not been identified. Mechanism of fluid shift occurring in cases of OHSS is shown in Flow chart 74.3.

Management of OHSS: No active form of treatment is required for mild OHSS. Patient observation and maintenance of hydration by the oral route usually works for such patients. Close observation and hospitalisation is usually required for moderate grade OHSS, since these patients may rapidly undergo a change of status, particularly when conception occurs. Patients with severe OHSS may require immediate hospitalisation and treatment. During hospitalisation, careful monitoring of haemodynamic stability is required. Large volume crystalloid infusion is recommended for renewal of the depleted intravascular volume. However, these patients must be closely monitored, as this can result in sequestration of fluid in the third space. Management of OHSS is summarised in Flow chart 74.4. Monitoring of induction of ovulation is the most reliable method in the prevention of OHSS. When the peak plasma oestradiol levels are greater than 2,000 pg/mL, or an abnormal increase in the serum oestradiol levels (doubling during 2 or 3 days) occurs, hCG should be withheld.

Complications of OHSS: The most serious complications of OHSS are both arterial and venous thromboembolic phenomena.[24] Arterial thromboembolic phenomena may result in cardiovascular accidents and sometimes even death.

Complications Related to Surgical Management

Complications associated with LOD are enumerated here:

❖ Accidental injury to internal organs or major blood vessels from the laparoscope or other surgical instruments.
❖ Internal bleeding
❖ Pain after the procedure as a result of pneumoperitoneum
❖ Problems caused by anaesthesia
❖ *Adhesions*: Adhesion formation was a significant complication of bilateral ovarian wedge resection, which occurred as a result of tissue handling and serosal trauma at the time of laparotomy. Adhesions lead to non-availability of ovarian surface for ovulation, thereby resulting in anovulation. Moreover, presence of adhesions may interfere with peritoneal ovum transport as well. As a result, the procedure, which had been performed with the intention of resolving the problem of infertility, may itself become responsible for producing infertility. On the other hand, LOD has a small but definite potential for causing tubal adhesions. The definite aetiology of pelvic adhesion formation is not yet clearly known. However, there are some factors which are associated with an increased risk for the development of pelvic adhesions.

Flow chart 74.3: Mechanism of fluid shift occurring in ovarian hyperstimulation syndrome

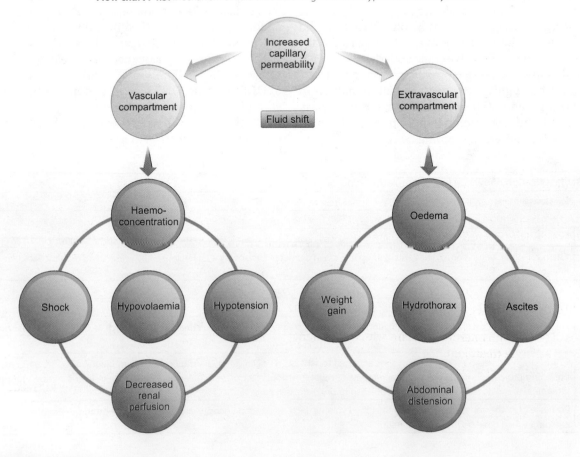

Flow chart 74.4: Management of ovarian hyperstimulation syndrome (OHSS)

Management of a patient with OHSS

Patient monitoring
Monitoring of the following:
- Vital signs
- *Fluid balance*: Fluid intake, urinary output
- Daily measurement of the patient's weight and abdominal girth
- Central venous pressure monitoring
- *Blood tests*: Complete blood count, haematocrit, serum electrolytes and proteins, liver function tests, coagulation profile, acid-base balance, blood gases
- Urine osmolarity
- *Imaging*: Ultrasonography (abdomen, chest), computed tomography (abdomen, chest)

Patient treatment
- *Maintenance of blood volume*: Plasma expanders
- *Reduction of capillary permeability*: Indomethacin, angiotensin converting enzyme inhibitors
- *Prevention of thromboembolic phenomenon*: Heparin
- *Surgery*: Only in cases of torsion/rupture of ovarian cysts

Some of these factors include intra-abdominal infection, tissue hypoxia or ischaemia, tissue drying, manipulation of tissues during surgery, presence of a reactive foreign body or intraperitoneal blood.

❖ *Atrophy*: Ovarian atrophy and failure is a rare complication of LOD. Rarely, the ovaries can undergo irreparable damage and experience atrophy.[17] It appears that application of seven or more punctures per ovary represent an excessive amount of thermal energy used and therefore must be discouraged. Despite the absence of strong evidence, regarding the association of premature ovarian failure with LOD, precautions should be taken to minimise the chances of causing irreversible damage to the ovaries. These include keeping the dose of ovarian cautery to the minimum effective level and avoiding putting any cautery points close to the ovarian hilum.

❖ *Hyperprolactinaemia*: Hyperprolactinaemia after ovarian cauterisation can be considered as a possible cause of anovulation in women with polycystic ovaries and improved gonadotropin and androgen levels. The cause of hyperprolactinaemia remains unknown. Therefore, determination of levels of prolactin in anovulatory patients after LOD is recommended.

CLINICAL PEARLS

❖ In cases of PCOD with infertility, therapy with clomiphene forms the first-line treatment.
❖ The use of LOD appears to be as effective as the use of CC in the treatment of PCOD with a lower risk of complications. Moreover, the correction of hormonal levels as a result of LOD helps in preventing miscarriages. LOD is now considered as a treatment of choice in patients with PCOD, who are resistant to CC.

❖ Hyperandrogenism can be managed with combined OCPs like Dianette® and Yasmin®. Spironolactone can be used as an alternative in case COCPs are not used. Drugs like ketoconazole, flutamide and finasteride are not widely used in the UK for hirsutism.

❖ Management of cases of PCOD and metabolic syndrome requires a combination of medical therapy, psychological support and lifestyle modifications. Management of psychological parameters is important in cases of PCOD because such women are likely to suffer from low self-esteem and altered body image.

EVIDENCE-BASED MEDICINE

❖ Bariatric surgery is likely to serve as an effective option for weight loss in women with PCOD. Bariatric surgery is likely to prevent or reverse metabolic syndrome and reduce the cardiovascular risk in women with PCOD.[25] Bariatric surgery may also have reproductive benefits in PCOD patients by restoring the hypothalamic-pituitary axis and improving pregnancy outcomes. According to the Cochrane review by Colquitt et al., individuals with BMI more than 40 kg/m² should be considered for bariatric surgery.[26] In presence of co-morbidities such as diabetes, the cut-off limit for BMI must be lowered to 30–35 kg/m².

❖ Presently, there is limited evidence regarding the use of statins for reducing cardiovascular mortality and morbidity in cases of PCOD.[27]

REFERENCES

1. Hart R, Hickey M, Franks S. Definitions, prevalence and symptoms of polycystic ovaries and polycystic ovary syndrome. Best Pract Res Clin Obstet Gynaecol. 2004;18(5):671-83.
2. Holte J. Disturbances in insulin secretion and sensitivity in women with the polycystic ovary syndrome. Baillieres Clin Endocrinol Metab. 1996;10(2):221-47.
3. Rotterdam ESHRE/ASRM-Sponsored PCOS consensus workshop group. Revised 2003 consensus on diagnostic criteria and long-term health risks related to polycystic ovary syndrome (PCOS). Hum Reprod. 2004;19(1):41-7.
4. Michelmore KF, Balen AH, Dunger DB, Vessey MP. Polycystic ovaries and associated clinical and biochemical features in young women. Clin Endocrinol (Oxf). 1999;51(6):779-86.
5. Balen AH, Laven JS, Tan SL, Dewailly D. Ultrasound assessment of polycystic ovaries: international consensus definitions. Hum Reprod Update. 2003;9(6):505-14.
6. Sharpless JL. Polycystic Ovary Syndrome and the Metabolic Syndrome. Clinical Diabetes. 2003;21(4):154-61.
7. Moran LJ, Hutchison SK, Norman RJ, Teede HJ. Lifestyle changes in women with polycystic ovary syndrome. Cochrane Database Syst Rev. 2011;(7):CD007506.

8. ACOG Committee on Practice Bulletins-Gynecology. ACOG Practice Bulletin. Clinical management guidelines for obstetrician-gynecologists number 34, February 2002. Management of infertility caused by ovulatory dysfunction. American College of Obstetricians and Gynecologists. Obstet Gynecol. 2002;99(2):347-58.

9. Clark JH, Markaverich BM. The agonistic antagonistic properties of clomiphene: a review. Pharmacol Ther. 1981; 15(3):467-519.

10. Stein FI, Leventhal ML. Amenorrhea associated with bilateral polycystic ovaries. Am J Obstet Gynecol. 1935;29:181-91.

11. Gjönnaess H. Polycystic ovarian syndrome treated by ovarian cautery through the laparoscope. Fertil Steril. 1984;41(1):20-5.

12. Pirwany I, Tulandi T. Laparoscopic treatment of polycystic ovaries: is it time to relinquish the procedure. Fertil Steril. 2003;80(2):241-51.

13. Gadir AA, Alnaser HMI, Mowafi RS, Shaw RW. The response of patients with polycystic ovarian disease to human menopausal gonadotropin therapy after ovarian electrocautery or a luteinizing hormone-releasing hormone agonist. Fertil Steril. 1992;57(2):309-13.

14. Daniell JF, Miller W. Polycystic ovaries treated by laparoscopic laser vaporization. Fertil Steril. 1989;51(2):232-6.

15. Campo S, Felli A, Lamanna MA, Barini A, Garcea N. Endocrine changes and clinical outcome after Laparoscopic ovarian resection in with polycystic ovaries. Hum Reprod. 1993; 8(3):359-63.

16. Stegmann BJ, Craig HR, Bay RC, Coonrod DV, Brady MJ, Garbaciak JA. Characteristics predictive of response to ovarian diathermy in women with polycystic ovarian syndrome. Am J Obstet Gynecol. 2003;188(5):1171-3.

17. Sumioki H, Utsunomyiya T, Matsuoka K, Korenaga M, Kadota T. The effect of laparoscopic multiple punch resection of the ovary on hypothalamo-pituitary axis in polycystic ovary syndrome. Fertil Steril. 1988;50(4):567-72.

18. Kucuk M, Kilic-Okman T. Hormonal profiles and clinical outcome after laparoscopic ovarian drilling in women with polycystic ovarian syndrome. Med Sci Monit. 2005;11(1): CR29-34.

19. Kovacs G, Buckler H, Bangah M, Outch K, Burger H, Healy D. Treatment of anovulation due to polycystic ovarian syndrome by laparoscopic ovarian cautery. Br J Obstet Gynaecol. 1991;98(1):30-5.

20. Gadir AA, Mowafi RS, Alnaser HMI, Alonezi OM, Shaw RW Ovarian electrocautery versus human menopausal gonadotropins and pure follicle stimulating hormone therapy in the treatment of patients with polycystic ovarian disease. Clin Endocrinol (Oxf). 1990;33(5):585-92.

21. Schenker JG, Weinstein D. Ovarian hyperstimulation syndrome: a current survey. Fertil Steril. 1978;30(3):255-68.

22. Polishuk WZ, Schenker JG. Ovarian overstimulation syndrome. Fertil Steril. 1969;20(3):443-50.

23. Elchalal U, Schenker JG. The pathophysiology of ovarian hyperstimulation syndrome--views and ideas. Hum Reprod. 1997;12(6):1129-37.

24. Hansen AT, Kesmodel US, Juul S, Hvas AM. Increased venous thrombosis incidence in pregnancies after in vitro fertilization. Hum Reprod. 2014;29(3):611-7.

25. Malik SM, Traub ML. Defining the role of bariatric surgery in polycystic ovarian syndrome patients. World J Diabetes. 2012;3(4):71-9.

26. Colquitt JL, Picot J, Loveman E, Clegg AJ. Surgery for obesity. Cochrane Database Syst Rev. 2009;(2):CD003641.

27. Sathyapalan T, Atkin SL. Evidence for statin therapy in polycystic ovary syndrome. Ther Adv Endocrinol Metab. 2010;1(1):15-22.

Hirsutism

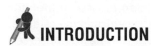

INTRODUCTION

Hirsutism is defined as the presence of coarse, dark, terminal hair in a male pattern in a woman. The most common areas where increased hair growth is apparent are upper lips, chin, side burns, chest and linea alba of abdomen. Hirsutism only affects women. Approximately 10–15% of the women are likely to suffer from some degree of hirsutism.[1] Excessive hair in cases of hirsutism is 'terminal' hair, coarse and pigmented as opposed to 'vellus' hair, the fine hair that covers much of the body. Hirsutism can be scored using the modified Ferriman-Gallwey system. A score of greater than 8 is considered as diagnostic.[2,3]

Hirsutism is in contrast to virilisation, which reflects very high levels of androgens and manifests in form of features such as deepening of the voice, enlargement of the clitoris, male pattern hair loss, e.g. temporal recession, breast atrophy, increased muscle mass, etc. Women with virilism will have hirsutism, but vice versa is usually not true.

AETIOLOGY

Hirsutism is usually an end result of the underlying adrenal-ovarian or central endocrine imbalance.[4] Various causes of hirsutism are tabulated in Box 75.1.

Before puberty, vellus hairs which are lightly fine pigmented cover most of the body. At the time of puberty, increased androgen production promotes conversion of these villus hairs into terminal hairs. Dihydrotestosterone (DHT) is the androgen which acts on the hair follicle to produce terminal pigmented hair. The local production of DHT is determined by the activity of the enzyme 5-α-reductase in the skin because this enzyme is responsible for converting testosterone to DHT.

In women, the androgens are primarily produced by the adrenal glands and the ovaries (Flow chart 75.1). Androgens

Box 75.1: Causes of hirsutism

- ❏ Polycystic ovary syndrome (up to 80% of all cases)
- ❏ Idiopathic hirsutism (up to 15% of all cases)
- ❏ Other causes (up to 5% of all cases)
- ❏ *Conditions associated with raised androgen levels*
  - HAIR-AN syndrome [hyperandrogenism (HA), insulin resistance (IR) and acanthosis nigricans (AN): Usually due to defect of the insulin receptor]
  - Late-onset congenital adrenal hyperplasia
  - Androgen-secreting tumours (adrenal and ovarian)
  - Cushing's syndrome
  - Hypothyroidism (increased concentration of SHBG, resulting in high levels of free testosterone)
- ❏ *Conditions associated with normal androgen levels*
  - Acromegaly
  - Drugs (androgenic agents: danazol, 19-nortestosterone-derived progestogens, e.g. 'Primolut-N', norethisterone, anabolic steroids, etc., and non-androgenic agents: methyldopa, metoclopramide, phenothiazines, phenytoin, valproate, etc.)

Abbreviation: SHBG, sex hormone-binding globulin

such as testosterone and androstenedione are produced by the ovaries, whereas adrenal glands are responsible for producing androgens such as androstenedione and dehydro-epiandrosterone (DHEA). Testosterone is produced by the theca cells of the ovary under the influence of LH and insulin acting through insulin-like growth factor-1 (IGF-1). Testosterone is then converted into oestradiol by the granulosa cells. The transition of the ovarian environment from an androgen-dominant to an oestrogen-dominant one is essential for normal ovulation and ovarian function. Increased androgen production occurring in conditions such as PCOS is likely to disrupt this process resulting in anovulation. Increased androgen production as a result of the disturbed ovarian-endocrinological balance is also responsible for hirsutism.

Flow chart 75.1: Production of androgens from various sources

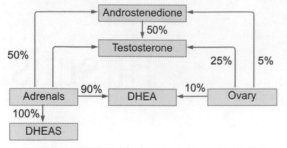

Abbreviations: DHEAS, dehydroepiandrosterone sulphate; DHEA, dehydroepiandrosterone

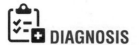

DIAGNOSIS

Clinical Presentation

Points to be elicited at the time of taking history and performing clinical examination in cases of hirsutism are tabulated in Box 75.2. While taking the history, clinician must enquire about the duration of the condition, its progression and severity. Recent onset of hirsutism associated with rapid progression and high grade of severity is likely to be associated with a more ominous cause such as adrenal or ovarian tumours.

General Physical Examination

Calculation of BMI: Height and weight should be measured in these cases to calculate BMI. PCOS patients with an increased BMI may be commonly associated with hirsutism.

The Ferriman-Gallwey scoring system for evaluation of hirsutism: The physical examination in cases of hirsutism involves use of the Ferriman-Gallwey hirsutism scoring system, which helps categorise the severity and distribution of excess hair growth. The Ferriman-Gallwey scoring system was developed in 1961 by Dr D Ferriman and Dr JD Gallwey to quantify the degree of hirsutism, and it was later modified in 1981.[2,3] In the modified system, the abnormal distribution of hair is assessed in nine areas of the body as explained in Figures 75.1A to I and given a score ranging from 0 to 4. The score increases with the increasing hair density and include the following areas: upper lip, chin, chest, upper abdomen, lower abdomen, upper arms, thighs, buttocks and back. Therefore, total score can vary from a minimum of 0 to a maximum of 36. In the original method, 11 areas of the body were assessed (two extra regions being forearm and legs). A Ferriman-Gallwey score of 8 or higher is considered to be diagnostic of hirsutism.

PART III

Box 75.2: Points to be elicited at the time of taking history and performing clinical examination in cases of hirsutism

- ❑ Onset of hirsutism (recent or late)
- ❑ Type of progression (rapid or slow)
- ❑ Degree of hirsutism (mild or severe)
- ❑ Signs suggestive of other medical disorders (e.g. acromegaly, Cushing's disease, hypothyroidism, etc.)
- ❑ Signs suggestive of chronic anovulation or PCOS (e.g. menstrual irregularity, infertility, etc.)
- ❑ Signs of virilisation
- ❑ Deepening of the voice
- ❑ Enlargement of the clitoris
- ❑ Reduction in breast volume
- ❑ Hair loss (male pattern balding)
- ❑ Acne
- ❑ Family history of hirsutism
- ❑ Ethnicity (hair distribution is associated with huge racial variation)
- ❑ Drugs (e.g. androgen therapy, danazol, etc.)

Presence of other cutaneous signs: During physical examination of cases with hirsutism, the clinician must also look for other cutaneous signs of hyperandrogenism such as acne, seborrhoea, etc. Acanthosis nigricans may be also observed in cases of PCOS and is a sign of insulin resistance. It is a skin disorder characterised by skin, which becomes thicker, hyperpigmented and acquires a velvety texture.

Pelvic Examination

A pelvic mass may be sometimes detected on pelvic examination. This may be due to androgen-producing ovarian tumours.

Investigations

The following investigations must be ordered:[5]

❖ *An ultrasound scan of the pelvis:* This helps in diagnosis of conditions such as PCOS, ovarian tumours, etc.

❖ *A basic hormone profile:* These include the following:

- Androgen levels: Measurement of androgens such as early-morning total or free testosterone levels, dehydroepiandrosterone sulphate (DHEAS), and androstenedione needs to be done. Total testosterone levels more than 5 mmol/L indicate possible androgen-producing tumour either of adrenal or ovarian origin. Dehydroepiandrosterone levels are also measured in these cases to differentiate between the adrenal or ovarian cause because its levels may be particularly elevated in presence of an adrenal cause.

- Levels of sex hormone-binding globulins (SHBG): In order to evaluate changes in SHBG levels, measurement of free androgen index is particularly useful, especially if testosterone levels are within normal limits. Reduced SHBG levels in presence of normal testosterone levels may be associated with an increase in the free androgen index.

- Gonadotropin levels: Ratio of LH:FSH greater than 2 has been considered indicative but is not diagnostic of PCOS.

- ❖ *Metabolic profile*: A fasting lipid profile and fasting serum glucose are usually recommended. If the fasting serum glucose is normal, a 75-g oral glucose tolerance test and insulin concentration is recommended, particularly in cases of PCOS.
- ❖ *Other investigations*: These might be added on an individual basis, such as tests for acromegaly, Cushing's disease, congenital adrenal hyperplasia, etc. For example, 17-hydroxyprogesterone (OHP) levels may be raised in cases of congenital adrenal hyperplasia (Flow chart 75.2). Dexamethasone suppression test and 24-hour free urinary cortisol levels can be measured in cases of Cushing's syndrome.

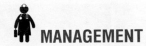

MANAGEMENT

Management of hirsutism is summarised in Flow chart 75.3.

General Therapy

Psychological therapy: Since the condition is likely to be associated with a feeling of low self-esteem and an altered body image, she needs to be carefully explained about the cause of hirsutism and must be counselled that she is not losing her femininity. She must also be advised that treatment for hirsutism is likely to prevent further hair growth.

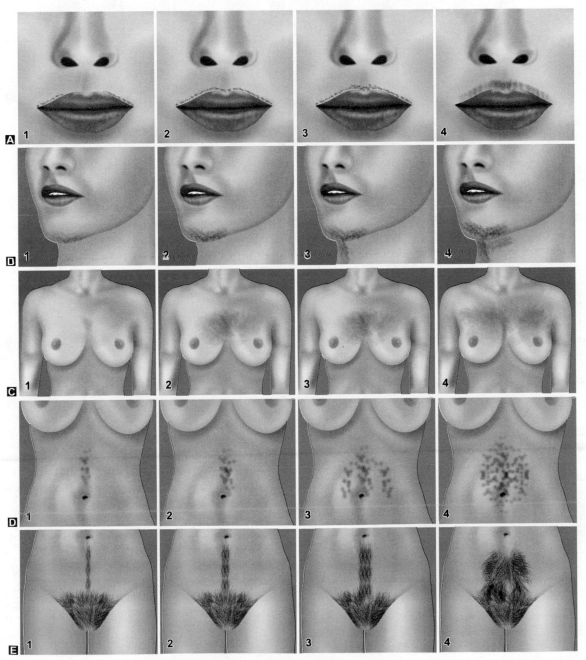

Figs 75.1A to E

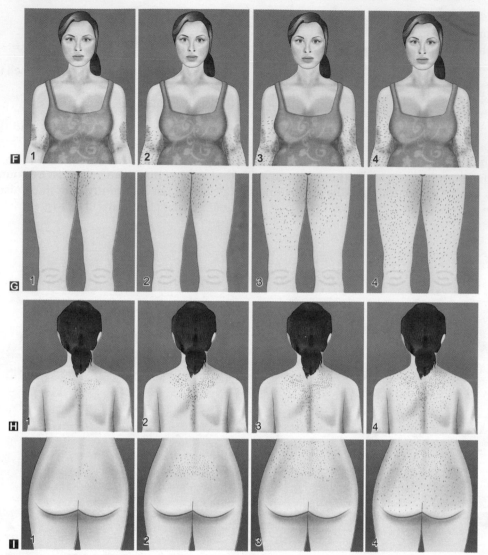

Figs 75.1F to I

Figs 75.1A to I: Scoring the extent of hirsutism using the modified Ferriman-Gallwey scoring system: hair growth on (A) Upper lip, (B) Chin, (C) Chest, (D) Upper abdomen and (E) Lower abdomen. Hair growth over (F) Arms, (G) Thighs, (H) Upper back and (I) Buttocks (lower back)

Flow chart 75.2: Diagnosis of congenital adrenal hyperplasia

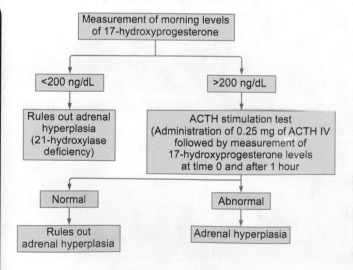

Abbreviation: ACTH, adrenocorticotropic hormone

It is unlikely to affect the existent hair growth. She may be, therefore, required to remove the current hair growth using physical means. Also, there may be hair regrowth following the use of physical or cosmetic methods.

Treatment of the underlying cause: Besides dealing with excessive hair growth, treatment must also be directed towards treatment of the underlying cause, e.g. weight loss in an obese patient with PCOS. This is one of the most effective approaches, which increases SHBG, thereby reducing the level of androgens. It can help restore ovulatory cycles and fertility in the absence of any other treatment.

Physical therapy: The mainstay of treatment of hirsutism is removal of excessive hair using mechanical or cosmetic methods such as plucking, shaving, waxing, using depilatory creams, bleaching, etc. and clinic-based treatments such as clinic-based waxing, electrolysis, light-based (laser or pulsed-light) hair removal, etc.[6] These methods can also be combined with drug therapy if they do not prove to be sufficient on their own.

Flow chart 75.3: Management of hirsutism

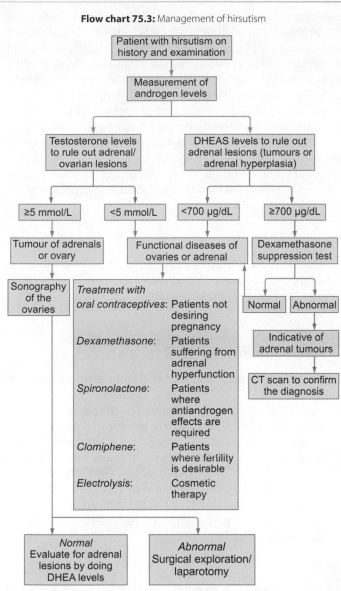

Abbreviations: DHEAS, dehydroepiandrosterone sulphate; DHEA, dehydro-epiandrosterone

Systemic Therapy

Systemic therapy can prove useful if cosmetic therapy does not prove to be sufficient on its own. Numerous pharmacological agents are available for treatment of hirsutism. However, none can be considered to be perfect. Therefore, therapy must be initiated only in those patients who have given an informed consent following complete explanation about the possible benefits and risks of a particular treatment strategy. Alternative treatment approaches must be also be explained to the patient. The drugs most commonly used for treatment of hirsutism include OCPs containing low-androgenic progestins; antiandrogenic drugs, such as spironolactone, cyproterone, flutamide, etc.; insulin sensitisers, such as metformin (Glucophage®), GnRH analogues, etc.

Oral Contraceptive Agents

The drugs most commonly used for suppressing ovarian androgen production include OCPs, especially amongst young women with menstrual irregularities also desiring contraception. OCPs act by reducing the fraction of free testosterone by increasing the serum levels of SHBG. They also help in opposing the production of androgens by theca cells and in reducing the adrenal androgen production.

Low-dose OCPs and progestin-only mini pills fail to suppress ovulation in as many as 50% of women, resulting in the production of ovarian androgens at an irregular rate. OCPs containing progestogens such as levonorgestrel and norethisterone should be preferably avoided because they are likely to result in an increased androgenic effect in the tissues.[7] On the other hand, OCPs containing third-generation progestins with low androgenic activity, e.g., drospirenone, gestodene, norgestimate, etc. are more useful in cases of hirsutism.[8]

Hyperandrogenism can be managed with combined OCPs containing antiandrogenic compounds like Dianette® (2 mg cyproterone acetate and ethinyl oestradiol) and Yasmin® (drospirenone and ethinyl oestradiol).[9] Cyproterone acetate is a progestational agent, which inhibits gonadotropin secretion, blocks androgen action and results in an increased hepatic clearance of androgens. It is used in combined oral contraceptives (Dianette®) or in a reverse sequential regimen.[10] The combination of cyproterone acetate and ethinyl oestradiol is also known as co-cyprindiol tablets, which is available as generic medicine in the UK. The reverse sequential regimen involves the administration of cyproterone acetate in the dosage of 50–100 mg/day for the first 10 days (day 5–15) and ethinyl oestradiol in the dosage of 25–50 μg/day from day 5 to day 25 of the cycle. Dianette® is available in a pack of 21 pills, which are to be taken once every day for a period of 21 days followed by a pill-free interval of 1 week. Following the pill-free interval, a new pack must be started if the patient is still experiencing the symptoms. If improvement occurs, dosage of cyproterone acetate can be reduced to 5 mg/day. The pills can be stopped completely following 3–4 months of complete symptomatic improvement. When cyproterone is administered in high doses (50–100 mg), an effective contraception should be simultaneously used in sexually active women of childbearing age group due to the risk of feminisation of the male foetus in case pregnancy occurs.

Antiandrogens

Antiandrogens are medications which help in cases of hirsutism by reducing androgen production or blocking the action of androgens on the hair follicle. Since these medications are likely to cause birth defects and feminisation of the male foetus, an effective form of contraception is required for sexually active premenopausal women taking antiandrogens.[11]

❖ *Spironolactone*: Spironolactone is the most commonly used antiandrogen due to its relative safety and demonstrated effectiveness. Spironolactone in the dosage of 25–200 mg/day can effectively help suppress hirsutism.[12] If the usage of OCPs is unable to control the growth of excessive hair, spironolactone may be recommended. It can also be used as an alternative in cases where combined OCPs are not used. It acts by the blockage of the androgen receptors and inhibition of the enzyme 5-α-reductase. If the initial dose is not effective after several months of treatment, a higher dose may be recommended. It may be associated with side effects such as diuresis, postural hypotension, menstrual irregularities and rarely hyperkalaemia. However, its antimineralocorticoid and diuretic properties rarely manifest in young women. The most bothersome limiting side effect of spironolactone in women of childbearing age group is menorrhagia or unscheduled menstrual bleeding.[13]

❖ *Flutamide*: Flutamide, used in the dosage of 250–500 mg, is a potent androgen-receptor antagonist. However, it is relatively contraindicated because of its relatively high hepatotoxicity.[14] Therefore, it must be used cautiously and its use must be restricted to tertiary-care settings.

❖ *Finasteride*: If the above-mentioned treatment options do not appear to control hirsutism, finasteride (in the dose of 5 mg/day) appears to be a useful treatment option because it has a different mode of action. Finasteride acts by suppressing the enzyme 5-α-reductase, which converts testosterone to the more potent DHT. It can result in mild side effects such as gastrointestinal disturbances, dryness of skin, reduced libido, teratogenic effects, etc.

Insulin Sensitisers

High levels of insulin are likely to lower the production of SHBG, thereby increasing the free fraction of androgen. Therefore, use of insulin sensitising agents, e.g. metformin or thiazolidinediones, is likely to help control hirsutism. Treatment of insulin resistance is likely to improve hyper-androgenaemia and ovulatory function in many women with PCOS. However, the present evidence regarding the effectiveness of insulin sensitising agents in the treatment of PCOS-associated hirsutism has presented with conflicting evidence.[15,16]

Gonadotropin-releasing Hormone Agonists

In severe resistant cases, GnRH agonists can be used for suppressing the production of gonadotropins from the pituitary gland. However, use of GnRH analogues for the treatment of hirsutism is associated with inconsistent results. Initial administration of GnRH agonists stimulates the release of FSH and LH. This is followed by the eventual downregulation of pituitary gland, thereby producing a hypogonadotropic-hypogonadic state. These drugs are effective in hirsutism because of the 'downregulation' of FSH and LH production. The limiting factors are its high cost and risks of long-term treatment (e.g. loss of bone mass, menopausal-like symptoms, etc.). However, they can be used with 'add back' therapy, e.g. the oral contraceptives.

Eflornithine

The FDA has approved the drug, eflornithine hydrochloride (13.9% cream), Vaniqa® as a topical treatment therapy for unwanted facial hair growth. This drug is an irreversible inhibitor of L-ornithine decarboxylase, a rate-limiting enzyme involved in the synthesis of polyamines, which is critical for the proliferation of the matrix cells in the hair follicle and hence may be important for controlling hair growth and proliferation.[17] It, therefore, serves as an alternative therapy in women who wish to avoid the use of hormones. Treatment with eflornithine hydrochloride 13.9% cream does not remove hairs. Rather, it slows down and reduces their size so that the hairs that are already present become less visible and coarse. Though the use of this drug is likely to result in visual improvement within a few weeks, the hair growth is likely to reappear upon discontinuation of this drug.[18] Eflornithine may cause side effects such as skin irritation and acne in a small number of patients.

Surgical Therapy

Surgical approach may be required in cases of tumours of adrenal glands or ovary. Hypophysectomy may be sometimes required in cases of cranial lesions.

COMPLICATIONS

The main problems associated with hirsutism include the following:

❖ *Psychological disorders*: Hirsutism can be perceived as loss of femininity by some women, resulting in development of feeling of lowered self-esteem and altered body image, which may further lead to psychological disturbances (e.g. depression), mental trauma and emotional anguish.

❖ *Social difficulty*: The woman may tend to avoid social situations due to her altered body image, resulting in the development of psychological disorders such as anxiety, depression, etc.

CLINICAL PEARLS

❖ The hair cycle comprises of two phases; period of active growth (the anagen phase) and the resting phase (the telogen phase).

❖ Polycystic ovarian syndrome is the most common cause of hirsutism.

❖ Combined OCPs are the most commonly used single therapy in cases of hirsutism.

❖ Since drug therapy may take nearly 8–9 months to show visible results in cases of hirsutism, physical cosmetic treatment measures such as electrolysis, waxing, bleaching, etc. may be simultaneously used along with medical therapy to produce immediate results.

❖ According to the recommendations by the British National Formulary, all antiandrogenic drugs are potentially teratogenic, so clinicians must prescribe these drugs to only those women belonging to the reproductive age group, who are using some reliable form of contraception.

❖ Drugs such as ketoconazole, flutamide and finasteride are not commonly used in the UK for treatment of hirsutism.

EVIDENCE-BASED MEDICINE

❖ Present evidence shows that spironolactone is an effective treatment for hirsutism.[12,13]

❖ Use of metformin is likely to be beneficial in women with PCOS by improving the rate of ovulation. It is also likely to reduce hair growth by improving insulin resistance. Low quality, imprecise and inconsistent evidence suggests that insulin sensitisers are likely to provide limited benefits for women with hirsutism.[15,16] However, a recent meta-analysis has shown that metformin is likely to have an efficacy similar to that of an OCP containing 2 mg of cyproterone acetate and 35 µg of ethinyl oestradiol.[19]

REFERENCES

1. Azziz R. The evaluation and management of hirsutism. Obstet Gynaecol. 2003;101(5 Pt 1):995-1007.
2. Ferriman D, Gallwey JD. Clinical assessment of body hair growth in women. J Clin Endocrinol Metab. 1961;21:1440-7.
3. Yildiz BO. Assessment, diagnosis and treatment of a patient with hirsutism. Nat Clin Pract Endocrinol Metab. 2008;4(5): 294-300.
4. Blume-Peytavi U, Hahn S. Medical treatment of hirsutism. Dermatol Ther. 2008;21(5):329-39.
5. Koulouri O, Conway GS. Management of hirsutism. BMJ. 2009;338:b847.
6. van Zuuren EJ, Fedorowicz Z, Carter B, Pandis N. Interventions for hirsutism (excluding laser and photoepilation therapy alone). Cochrane Database Syst Rev. 2015;(4):CD010334.
7. Darney PD. The androgenicity of progestins. Am J Med. 1995;98(1A):104S-10S.
8. Kaplan B. Desogestrel, norgestimate, and gestodene: the newer progestins. Ann Pharmacother. 1995;29(7-8):736-42.
9. Batukan C, Muderris II, Ozcelik B, Ozturk A. Comparison of two oral contraceptives containing either drospirenone or cyproterone acetate in the treatment of hirsutism. Gynecol Endocrinol. 2007;23(1):38-44.
10. Van der Spuy ZM, le Roux PA. Cyproterone acetate for hirsutism. Cochrane Database Syst Rev. 2003;(4):CD001125.
11. Swiglo BA, Cosma M, Flynn DN, Kurtz DM, Labella ML, MullanRJ, et al. Clinical review: antiandrogens for the treatment of hirsutism: a systematic review and metaanalyses of randomized controlled trials. J Clin Endocrinol Metab. 2008;93(4):1153-60.
12. Brown J, Farquhar C, Lee O, Toomath R, Jepson RG. Spironolactone versus placebo or in combination with steroids for hirsutism and/or acne. Cochrane Database Syst Rev. 2009; (2):CD000194.
13. Helfer EL, Miller JL, Rose LI. Side-effects of spironolactone therapy in the hirsute woman. J Clin Endocrinol Metab. 1988;66(1):208-11.
14. Andrade RJ, Lucena MI, Fernandez MC, Suarez F, Montero JL, Fraga E, et al. Fulminant liver failure associated with flutamide therapy for hirsutism. Lancet. 1999;353(9157):983.
15. Cosma M, Swiglo BA, Flynn DN, Kurtz DM, Labella ML, Mullan RJ, et al. Clinical review: insulin sensitizers for the treatment of hirsutism: a systematic review and meta-analyses of randomized controlled trials. J Clin Endocrinol Metab. 2008;93(4):1135-42.
16. Costello M, Shrestha B, Eden J, Sjoblom P, Johnson N. Insulin-sensitising drugs versus the combined oral contraceptive pill for hirsutism, acne and risk of diabetes, cardiovascular disease, and endometrial cancer in polycystic ovary syndrome. Cochrane Database Syst Rev. 2007;(1):CD005552.
17. Balfour JA, McClellan K. Topical eflornithine. Am J Clin Dermatol. 2001;2(3):197-201.
18. Wolf JE, Shander D, Huber F, Jackson J, Lin CS, Mathes BM, et al. Randomized, double-blind clinical evaluation of the efficacy and safety of topical eflornithine HCl 13.9% cream in the treatment of women with facial hair. Int J Dermatol. 2007;46(1):94-8.
19. Jing Z, Liang-Zhi X, Tai-Xiang W, Ying T, Yu-Jian J. The effect of Diane-35 and metformin in the treatment of polycystic ovary syndrome: an updated systemic review. Gynecol Endocrinol. 2008;24(10):590-600.

Assisted Reproductive Techniques

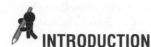

INTRODUCTION

With increasing developments in the field of science and technology, IVF is now being recognised as an established treatment for infertility. The various techniques of IVF and its modifications are together termed as assisted reproductive techniques (ARTs). According to the data by Human Fertilisation and Embryology Authority (HFEA), UK, approximately 14,000 babies were born in the year 2010 as a result of IVF treatment using a woman's own eggs, including those born as multiples.[1] IVF is the result of scientific developments and advancements in the field of obstetrics and gynaecology. In this process, the ovaries are stimulated by the use of fertility medicines, following which one or more oocytes are aspirated from the ovarian follicle. The fertilisation of male and female gametes occurs in the laboratory after which one or more embryos are transferred inside the uterine cavity. The process of IVF comprises the following steps: suppression of pituitary glands; stimulation of ovaries to initiate superovulation; oocyte maturation; retrieving a preovulatory oocyte from the ovary; fertilising it with a sperm in the laboratory; and subsequently transferring the embryo within the endometrial cavity. Following the first IVF pregnancy, which was reported by Steptoe and Edwards in 1976, more than 4 million pregnancies have been achieved worldwide due to IVF.[2] The results of IVF now slightly exceed the fecundability of natural conception cycles in general population. The most important factors affecting the success rate of IVF are number of oocytes retrieved from the ovary and the number of high-quality embryos derived from them in the laboratory. Embryos obtained in excess can be cryopreserved for future use.

Three full cycles of IVF (either self or NHS-funded), with or without intracytoplasmic sperm injection (ICSI) must be offered to the women below the age of 40 years, if she has not conceived even after 2 years of regular unprotected intercourse or 12 cycles of artificial insemination [where six

or more are by intrauterine insemination (IUI)].[3] If the woman reaches the age of 40 years during treatment, the ongoing full cycle must be completed, but remaining ones must be abandoned.

Women aged 40–42 years who have not conceived after 2 years of regular unprotected intercourse or 12 cycles of artificial insemination (where six or more are by IUI) must be offered one full cycle of IVF, with or without ICSI in presence of following conditions:[3]

❖ They have never previously had IVF treatment
❖ There is no evidence of low ovarian reserve
❖ They have been counselled regarding the added consequences of IVF and pregnancy at the age above 40 years.

OTHER ASSISTED REPRODUCTIVE TECHNIQUES

Though IVF is the most commonly used ART, its various modifications are employed in the clinical practice. IVF-related procedures such as gamete intrafallopian transfer (GIFT) and zygote intrafallopian transfer (ZIFT) are sometimes used as alternatives to IVF. In the procedure of GIFT, retrieved oocytes and sperms are placed via laparoscopic route inside the fallopian tube. ZIFT, on the other hand, involves placement of the fertilised embryo via laparoscopic route inside the fallopian tube. Both the techniques are not presently in much use due to their invasive nature, risks and low success rate. Some techniques which help in facilitating fertilisation include partial zona dissection (PZD), subzonal sperm injection (SUZI), ICSI and assisted hatching (AH). Currently, only ICSI is being used clinically. ICSI involves injection of a single live sperm directly into the ovum. It is commonly used in cases of male factor infertility such as severe deficits in semen quality, obstructive azoospermia and non-obstructive azoospermia. Intracytoplasmic morphologically selected sperm injection (IMSI), a modification of ICSI, was introduced in 2001.[4] It involves selection of the spermatozoon at a higher magnification, e.g. the spermatozoon can be evaluated for fine integrity of its nucleus or selection of a normal spermatozoon with a vacuole-free head. IMSI is usually indicated in cases of severe male infertility.

Another ART, which is being commonly employed nowadays, is in vitro maturation (IVM), where immature oocytes are retrieved from the antral follicles of unstimulated or minimally stimulated ovaries.[5] This new technology is likely to offer several advantages over controlled ovarian stimulation such as reduced costs, simplicity of the procedure and elimination of ovarian hyperstimulation syndrome (OHSS). IVM is commonly used in cases of polycystic ovaries in order to reduce the risk of OHSS. Another emerging technique is frozen embryo transfer (FET), in which frozen embryos from the previous IVF cycle are thawed and transferred into the woman's uterus. This technique can be used in cases where embryos were electively frozen. Frozen embryos can remain frozen for up to 10 years. This technique helps in reducing the risk of ovarian hyperstimulation. Women with regular ovulatory cycles should be informed that the likelihood of a live birth after replacement of frozen-thawed embryos is similar for embryos replaced during natural cycles and hormone-supplemented cycles.

The ART procedures can also be done by using donors. In case of women with premature ovarian failure or low ovarian reserve, IVF using oocytes from the donor and sperms from the husband or partner can be employed. In male partner with aspermia, IVF can be performed using sperms from the donor and oocytes from the wife or partner. In cases where there is combined female and male factor infertility or in cases with repeated IVF failures, IVF can be done using donor embryos. If the woman has underlying anatomical abnormalities or medical indications, IVF can be performed using surrogacy where the embryos (using the couple's sperms and oocyte) are transferred into the uterus of a surrogate mother.

INDICATIONS

Indications for IVF include the following:
* Tubal factor infertility (in case of completely blocked tubes, IVF serves as the primary therapy)[6]
* Damage or absence of fallopian tubes
* Uterine factor infertility (severe cases of Asherman's syndrome, irreparable distortion of the uterine cavity, etc.)
* Uterine malformations (e.g. unicornuate uterus)
* Severe pelvic adhesions
* Severe endometriosis which is unresponsive to medical or surgical treatment
* *Male factor infertility*: Severe oligospermia or a history of obstructive azoospermia in the male partner (IUI can work in mild to moderate cases. However, in severe cases the primary therapy is IVF)
* Diminished ovarian reserve or premature ovarian failure
* Gonadal dysgenesis including Turner's syndrome
* Bilateral oophorectomy
* Ovarian failure following chemotherapy or radiotherapy.
* All other cases of infertility where less invasive therapy has failed (e.g. endometriosis, ovulatory dysfunction, unexplained infertility).

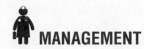

MANAGEMENT

PREPARATION PRIOR TO THE PROCEDURE

Following steps must be undertaken prior to ART procedure:
* A complete evaluation of infertility (both male and female) must be performed on both the partners before embarking upon ART.
* Treatable causes of subfertility must be treated prior to initiating IVF
* In the absence of any absolute indication for IVF (bilateral blocked tubes and severe male factor infertility), the couple must be offered 3–6 cycles of superovulation and IUI before proceeding to IVF.
* Young couples having no obvious cause of infertility must be advised to have 1 complete year of unprotected intercourse and conventional therapy since 88% of the couples are expected to conceive within 1 year and a further 50% during the 2nd year. A shorter time period is preferred in older couples. Infertile couples where the woman is greater than 40 years of age may be offered IVF as the primary treatment option.
* Alternative treatment options must be considered first before resorting to IVF while counselling the woman with male factor infertility and tubal factor infertility (where tubes are not completely blocked).
* *Patient counselling*: Prior to considering IVF as a treatment option for patients with infertility, the couple should be counselled regarding the risks and benefits of IVF in accordance with the Code of Practice by the HFEA. Woman should be informed that the chances of a live birth following IVF treatment reduce with an increase in the woman's age and that the optimal female age range for achieving a successful IVF treatment is 23–39 years. Chances of a live birth per treatment cycle are greater than 20% for women aged 23–35 years, 15% for women aged 36–38 years, 10% for women aged 39 years, and 6% for women aged 40 years or older. IVF does not reverse the age-dependent decline in infertility in the older women, particularly those above the age of 40 years.[7]

The chances of conception greatly reduce after three cycles of IVF. Also, treatment is more effective in women who have previously been pregnant and/or had a live birth. Couples should be informed that maternal and paternal smoking can adversely affect the success rate of assisted reproduction procedures, including IVF treatment.[8] Therefore, the couple should be asked to abstain from alcohol and smoking. Women should also be informed that a BMI outside the normal range (19–30) is likely to reduce the success rate of assisted reproduction procedures. Therefore, they should be counselled to maintain a BMI within the normal range. Women should be informed that lack of success in the previous IVF cycles does not reduce the success rate during subsequent treatment cycles until approximately the fourth IVF cycle.

❖ *Woman's FSH and oestradiol levels*: The success rate of IVF procedure can be predicted by the concentrations of FSH and oestradiol levels. High day 3 levels of FSH and oestradiol serve as poor prognostic factors because they may be associated with rapid premature follicle recruitment and reduced oocyte numbers.[9]

STEPS OF THE PROCEDURE

In vitro fertilisation consists of retrieving preovulatory oocytes from the ovary and fertilising them with sperms in the laboratory, with subsequent embryo transfer within the endometrial cavity. The procedure of IVF comprises of following steps:

1. Ovarian stimulation for IVF
2. Follicular aspiration
3. Oocyte classification
4. Sperm preparation and oocyte insemination
5. Embryo culture
6. Embryo transfer.

Ovarian Stimulation for In Vitro Fertilisation

The success of IVF is related to the patient's age and the number of embryos transferred into the endometrial cavity. Without the use of stimulating medications, the ovaries can create and release only one mature egg per menstrual cycle. Therefore, nowadays, most clinicians use ovarian stimulation strategies to obtain synchronous development of multiple follicles. The strategy of transferring multiple embryos at one time is likely to ensure that at least one of them implants and produces a live birth. IVF stimulation protocols generally involve the use of drugs for the three following purposes:[10]

1. *Prevention of the endogenous luteinising hormone surge*: Downregulation and other regimens help in avoiding premature LH surges in IVF cycles. There are mainly two classes of medications used for preventing the endogenous surge and ovulation until the developing eggs are ready: (1) GnRH agonist (GnRHa), e.g. Lupron® and (2) GnRH-antagonist, e.g. Ganirelix®. GnRHa must be offered to women who have a low risk of OHSS. The two classes of medications are described below:

   i. *Use of GnRH agonists*: With the introduction of new technologies, besides the human menopausal gonado-tropins (hMGs) (Menopur®), pure FSH gonadotropins and recombinant FSH and LH gonadotropins are also currently available. The gonadotropins are administered in the dosage varying from 150 IU/day to 450 IU/day, depending on the patient's age and history of previous ovulatory response.[11,12] The response to GnRHa is mainly monitored using daily serum oestradiol (E_2) determination and later using pelvic ultrasonography. Once most of the follicles reach 17–18 mm in diameter, the gonadotropins are discontinued. Trigger injection with administration of hCG (urinary or recombinant) in the dosage of 10,000 IU is given that evening and oocyte retrieval is performed 35 hours later.

   ii. *Use of GnRH antagonists*: The GnRH antagonists can be used for ovulation induction in two protocols known as the flare-up protocol and the luteal-phase protocol. In the flare-up protocol, high doses of GnRH antagonists are administered during the early follicular phase of the cycle. The flare-up protocol has the advantage of causing transitory elevation of FSH, which occurs during the first 4 days of the follicular phase. This elevation helps in the follicular recruitment process.

   In the luteal-phase protocol, GnRH antagonist is started on the 17th or 21st day of the menstrual cycle. The GnRH antagonists are the latest generation of drugs that block LH secretion without a flare-up effect. Use of GnRH antagonists has the advantage of blocking the LH surge at the periovulatory period; therefore, premature luteinisation or spontaneous LH surge does not occur. As a result, the pituitary gland is not downregulated at the beginning of the menstrual cycle, due to which smaller amounts of gonadotropins are required to stimulate ovulation. Another advantage with this protocol is the prevention of OHSS.

2. *Stimulating the development of multiple follicles*: FSH products can be exogenously administered for stimulating the development of multiple eggs. Selective oestrogen receptor modulators, such as clomiphene or tamoxifen, can also help in achieving development of multiple follicles. These drug protocols are described as follows:

   • *Clomiphene citrate protocol*: In the clomiphene citrate only protocol, clomiphene citrate is administered in the doses of 50–150 mg for 5–7 days, starting from the 2nd day of the menstrual cycle. The ovarian response is monitored using pelvic ultrasonography and serial determinations of serum E_2 and LH levels. Oocyte retrieval must be performed within 24–26 hours after the LH surge. The advantages of the clomiphene citrate protocol include low cost and a very low risk of development of OHSS. The major disadvantages associated with this protocol include low oocyte yield (1–2 per cycle), high cancellation rate (25–50%) and low pregnancy rate.

   • *Use of clomiphene citrate with hMG protocol*: The combination of clomiphene citrate and hMG protocol is also sometimes used. This has an advantage of increasing the number of recruited follicles. The dose of clomiphene citrate is similar to that described above, while that of hMG is 150 IU, administered for a period of 2–7 days after the clomiphene citrate. Frequent monitoring with pelvic ultrasonography and daily determinations of E_2 and LH levels are performed. When the follicle reaches a size of 17–18 mm, hCG (10,000 IU intramuscularly) must be administered in order to complete the oocyte maturation. Oocyte aspiration should be performed 35 hours after the hCG injection. The advantage of the combined protocol is an increase in the number of recruited follicles. The disadvantages of the protocol are premature luteinisation, spontaneous LH surge (20–50%) and high cancellation rate (15–50%).

- *Use of hMG only*: The protocol comprising hMGs only involves the administration of hMG for ovarian stimulation.

3. *Initiation of ovulation*: Human chorionic gonadotropin is used for initiating the final maturation of the eggs and for starting the ovulatory cascade. It is administered when the follicles are likely to be mature (i.e. two or more follicles with a mean diameter of 18 mm or more and a serum oestradiol level of 200 pg/mL per codominant follicle). Both urinary and recombinant hCG preparations and GnRHa can be used to trigger ovulation.[13]

Various Protocols

Depending on the time duration for which various ovulation-inducing agents are administered, the stimulation protocols could be either long protocol or short protocol (Fig. 76.1).

Long Protocols

Long protocols involve commencing medications in the menstrual cycle before the IVF cycle. This usually involves the administration of either a GnRHa or GnRH antagonist or OCPs. GnRHa are usually preferred over GnRH antagonists for the long protocol because of their low cost.

❖ *Long protocol using GnRH agonist*: In this, the GnRHa is administered daily for about 2 weeks or until downregulation is complete. Administration of GnRHa helps in inhibiting the production of pituitary gonadotropins, thereby maximising control of the cycle. Pituitary suppression of LH secretion helps in preventing the surge of endogenous LH prior to full maturation of the cohort of ovarian follicles. The most commonly used GnRHa in the United States is leuprolide acetate in the daily dosage of 0.5–1 mg subcutaneously. Measurement of oestradiol levels (<30 pg/mL) helps in verifying the occurrence of downregulation. When

stimulation begins, hMG (or FSH), or both are administered in the dosage of 225–300 IU/day subcutaneously to stimulate follicular growth, with the GnRHa being continued at a lower dose to prevent a premature surge in LH secretion. The hMG dose is subsequently adjusted according to follicular growth as determined by TVS. Serum oestradiol concentrations are also determined because they are indicative of granulosa cell proliferation. In a 'step-down' protocol, the starting dose of gonadotropin is high and this is followed by gradual reductions in dose during the cycle depending on the response. In a 'step-up' protocol, the starting dose of gonadotropin is low and is then gradually increased during the cycle depending on the response.

❖ *Gonadotropin-releasing hormone agonist flare protocol*: This protocol is usually used in patients who are poor responders to stimulation. This protocol involves the administration of GnRHa in combination with ovarian stimulation, so that the initial agonistic response of the GnRHa can be used for ovarian stimulation.

Short Protocols

'Short protocols' refer to a regimen in which medications are started at the time of the natural menstrual cycle. Stimulation is achieved with hMG or FSH and spontaneous ovulation is blocked with either a GnRHa or with a GnRH antagonist. GnRH antagonists are preferred over GnRHa for the short protocol.

❖ *Short protocol using GnRH antagonist*: Administration of GnRH antagonists results in more rapid pituitary desensitisation in comparison to the GnRHa. In cases where GnRH antagonist is used, no pretreatment with an agonist is required. In cases of short protocol, the stimulation is begun at the time of menses, whereas in cases of long protocol, the stimulation is begun after a variable period of pretreatment with oral contraceptives. An antagonist is administered when the follicles are large (typically >14 mm in greatest diameter) and there is a risk of premature ovulation. Daily injections of the antagonist are then continued until hCG has been administered.

Poor Responders to Ovarian Stimulation

Increasing attention is now being focussed on women who are unable to produce an optimal number of follicles in response to ovulation induction. Such women are also termed as 'poor responders'. Though the definition of a poor responder has not been universally defined, it generally includes women who are unsuccessful in producing an optimal number of follicles (usually ≤3, having a diameter of ≥18 mm) in response to induction of ovulation. In a first practical attempt at standardising the definition of poor ovarian responders (POR), the ESHRE working group has proposed a standardised, simple and reproducible definition for POR, which has been published in the recent issue of the journal, Human Reproduction.[14] This criteria for defining POR is also known as the Bologna criteria. In accordance with the Bologna criteria, at least two of the following three features must be present:

1. Advanced maternal age or any other risk factor for POR

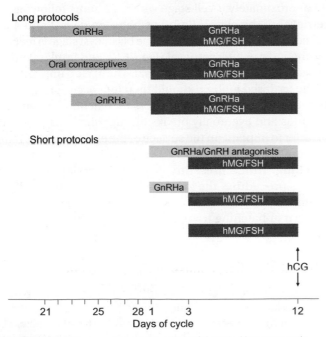

Fig. 76.1: Diagrammatic representation of short and long protocols

Abbreviations: hMG, human menopausal gonadotropin; GnRHa, gonadotropin-releasing hormone agonist

2. A previous POR
3. An abnormal ovarian reserve test (ORT).

Apart from the above three criteria, in the absence of advanced maternal age or abnormal ORT, the patient can be defined as a poor responder if she has two episodes of poor ovarian response even after maximal stimulation. Although one stimulated cycle is necessary for diagnosing POR, patients with advanced age or abnormal ORT may be considered as poor responders, because both the factors suggest the possibility of decreased ovarian reserve. They, therefore, serve as markers of poor stimulation cycle outcomes. Such patients should be classified as 'expected poor responders'.

The group reached the conclusion that such a comprehensive criteria is likely to assist the researchers in selecting a homogenised population for future studies, having a lower bias due to spurious POR definitions. This would facilitate the comparison of results for reaching precise decisions.

Presently, there is inadequate evidence supporting the routine use of any particular intervention in form of pituitary downregulation with either GnRHa or anatagonists, ovarian stimulation, or adjuvant therapy for the management of poor responders to controlled ovarian stimulation in IVF.[15,16] Better evidence from good-quality randomised, double-blinded multicentric trials would be required in future to arrive at a definite conclusion.

Follicular Aspiration

Oocytes are aspirated from the ovary 34–36 hours following administration of hCG. Initially, all aspirations were performed under laparoscopic guidance. However now, follicular aspirations are commonly performed under ultrasonographic guidance, both transabdominal as well as transvaginal. The transvaginal route for follicular aspiration has presently become the preferred procedure in most IVF programmes. The procedure of follicular aspiration comprises of the following steps:

❖ The oocyte aspiration is usually performed under heavy sedation, while the patient has been placed in the dorsal lithotomy position. Some type of analgesia or anaesthesia (most commonly, IV propofol) is commonly used.
❖ The vaginal wall is washed with saline, following which a 5–9 MHz ultrasonographic probe with a sterile cover and attached needle guide is inserted inside the vagina. This helps in localising the ovaries and the follicles.
❖ A 17-gauge needle is subsequently passed via the needle guide through the vaginal fornix into the ovaries in order to aspirate the follicular fluid.
❖ Once the fluid has been aspirated out, it is sent to the IVF laboratory as soon as possible.

Oocyte Classification

Following their aspiration, the oocytes are graded according to the appearance of the corona-cumulus complex. The presence of a polar body (metaphase II stage) and/or germinal vesicle (prophase stage) is a determining factor for the short preincubation time prior to the insemination. The degenerated oocytes are those which are atretic or have a fractured zona. The last category must constitute fewer than 15% of the total oocytes obtained.

Sperm Preparation and Oocyte Insemination

A semen sample is obtained after a 3–5 days period of sexual abstinence immediately prior to the oocyte retrieval. The procedure of sperm preparation involves removal of certain components of the ejaculate (i.e. seminal fluid, excess cellular debris, leucocytes, morphologically abnormal sperms, etc.) along with the retention of the motile fraction of sperms. For most specimens, the motile portion of the sperms is separated via the process of centrifugation through a discontinuous density gradient system. The sperms are incubated for 60 minutes in an atmosphere of 5% carbon dioxide in air. Finally, the supernatant containing motile fraction of sperms is removed. Sperm concentration and motility are determined. A final number of 200,000 motile sperms in a small volume of culture media with a layer of mineral oil on top are added to the oocytes in order to achieve fertilisation in vitro. The optimum number of hours for which the sperm and oocytes must be incubated has yet not been determined.

Embryo Culture

The inseminated oocytes are incubated in an atmosphere of 5% carbon dioxide in air with 98% humidity. Fertilisation of the oocyte is confirmed when two pronuclei and extrusion of the second polar body can be observed within the zygote nearly 18 hours after insemination. The fertilised embryos are transferred into growth media and placed in the incubator. No further evaluation is performed over the next 24 hours. A 4–8 cell stage, pre-embryo is observed approximately 36–48 hours after insemination. Since the individual cells of each embryo or 'blastomeres' divide every 12–14 hours, the embryo reaches an approximately 8-cell stage within 72 hours following the retrieval of the eggs.[17] Embryos between days 2 and 4 are called 'cleavage stage embryos'. The blastocyst stage is reached by about day 5 after retrieval (Fig. 76.2), and implantation is expected by day 7 after egg retrieval. The in vitro implantation of the fertilised embryo should therefore occur prior to this. In the naturally occurring process of 'hatching', an embryo expands and eventually breaks through the zona pellucida in order to implant on the surface of the endometrium. If this process is artificially simulated in vitro, it is known as 'assisted hatching', which presently is a controversial procedure. In this procedure, the zona pellucida is mechanically or chemically opened at about day-3 embryo stage to help the embryo in hatching from the zona and get implanted over the endometrium.

Embryo Transfer

The procedure of embryo transfer is performed within 72 hours after oocyte insemination at the cleavage stage, when the embryo has become approximately 8–16 cells in size. The next most common time for transfer is the day 5 transfer at the blastocyst stage. The embryo quality must be assessed at both the stages. Major advantages of blastocyst stage transfer

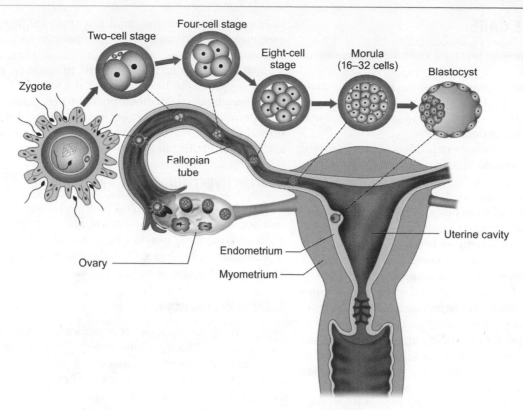

Fig. 76.2: Formation of the blastocyst stage of the embryo

are the ability to perform preimplantation genetic diagnosis and the reduction in the rate of multiple pregnancies with single blastocyst transfer. The embryo transfer is usually performed transcervically under the guidance of TAS. The embryos should be loaded with 15–20 µL of culture media at the time of transfer. The endometrial thickness at the time of embryo transfer should be preferably more than 5 mm. The catheter is advanced up to the fundus of the endometrial cavity and then withdrawn slightly. The embryos are ejected into the miduterine cavity, approximately 1–2 cm away from the fundus. Touching the catheter to the top uterine cavity is thought to induce uterine cramping, thereby reducing the success rate of the procedure. Subsequent to the embryo transfer, the patient must be on bed rest for about 20 minutes. Having bed rest for more than 20 minutes duration following embryo transfer is not likely to improve the outcome of IVF treatment. The usual number of embryos transferred depends on a number of factors including maternal age, the number of oocytes retrieved and availability of embryos for cryopreservation.[18,19] While transferring more than one embryo increases the chance for a pregnancy, it also increases the chance of multiple pregnancy. In order to reduce the chances of multifoetal gestation, number of embryos transferred has been limited to two at most of the IVF centres.[20] The present trend is towards transferring a single high-quality embryo.

Cryopreservation

Cryostorage of supernumerary embryos can be offered if there are more than two embryos. Embryos in excess of those which would be safely transferred can be cryopreserved for future use.[21] Both slow freezing and vitrification (ultrarapid freezing) have been found to be safe and effective methods of cryopreservation.

Management of the Luteal Phase

Once the embryo has reached the endometrial cavity, endometrial receptivity plays a major role in determining the success or failure of embryo implantation after IVF. Following 36–72 hours after oocyte retrieval, the endometrium must be supplemented with progesterone in order to maintain the luteal phase.[22-27] Supplementation with exogenous progesterone is especially required because superovulation and follicular aspiration at the time of oocyte retrieval is likely to have induced an abnormal endocrine milieu. Several progesterone preparations are available for use, e.g. natural progesterone in oil base for intramuscular injection, vaginal progesterone suppositories, and gels and capsules of micronised progesterone to be used vaginally or sublingually. The route of administration of progesterone does not appear to be significant.[28] The optimum duration of progesterone supplementation has yet not been established. Normally, progesterone supplementation is continued for approximately 2 weeks. In case the pregnancy test result is positive, progesterone must be continued until the 12th week of gestation. hCG should not be routinely administered for luteal phase support following IVF treatment because of the increased likelihood of OHSS.

CHAPTER 76

POSTPROCEDURE CARE

The following steps need to be taken after the completion of the procedure of IVF:

* Postprocedure, the patient can resume her regular daily activities. Neither physical activity nor diet has been shown to have any influence upon the success of embryo implantation or conception.
* In most of the cases, the patient is advised some form of rest or reduced physical activity following the embryo transfer.
* The patient must be counselled that there may be passage of a small amount of clear or bloody fluid from the vagina shortly after the procedure. She must be assured that this is normal and not a sign that the embryos are being expelled.
* She may also experience minor symptoms such as breast tenderness and engorgement, bloating, constipation, etc. These may occur due to the elevated levels of hormones associated with ovarian stimulation, and due to the supplemental hormones used for luteal phase support.
* Mild cramping and abdominal bloating can commonly occur. However, the woman must be counselled to immediately consult her clinician in cases of moderate or severe pain because this may be related to infection, ovarian torsion, other causes of abdominal pain (such as appendicitis, OHSS, etc.). Doppler ultrasound may be required to establish the diagnosis in these cases. Pelvic pain occurring weeks after IVF should be evaluated as in any woman with acute pain.
* *Monitoring for pregnancy*: Pregnancy is diagnosed by identifying rising serum hCG levels after the embryo transfer. If pregnancy occurs, hCG levels start rising approximately 1–2 days following implantation, which normally occurs within 7–8 days following oocyte retrieval. Serial hCG measurements are performed to monitor whether the rise is normal and consistent with a normal developing intrauterine pregnancy.
* Negative hCG level, even 14 days after oocyte retrieval, is a strong indication of a failed IVF cycle. In these cases, the luteal phase supplementation is stopped. Menstruation commonly occurs after 1–3 days.
* If the hCG test is found to be positive, ultrasound evaluation of pregnancy is usually begun at 6 weeks of gestational age. This is the time when the foetal heartbeat may first be detected. The patient is usually referred for obstetric care at any time after that.

 COMPLICATIONS

Some disadvantages associated with the procedure include:

* High cost of the procedure[29]
* Administration of certain medications to the woman and performance of certain procedures on her.
* Increased rates of multiple pregnancy and other complications related to the procedure.

Maternal morbidity and mortality rate directly related to IVF per se are low. Complications are primarily related to hormonal stimulation and egg retrieval, and include complications such as OHSS, thromboembolism, infection, abdominal bleeding, adnexal torsion, allergic reaction, anaesthetic complications, ectopic pregnancy, etc. If the IVF cycle proves to be successful, the woman is at risk of usual pregnancy-related complications (e.g. pre-eclampsia or eclampsia, haemorrhage, amniotic fluid embolism, thromboembolism, sepsis, etc.). Some of the complications associated with ART or IVF are described next.[30,31]

Ovarian Hyperstimulation Syndrome

Ovarian hyperstimulation syndrome is an iatrogenic condition that occurs in patients undergoing ovulation induction with hMG or controlled ovarian hyperstimulation for assisted reproductive technologies. OHSS has been discussed in details in Chapter 74 (Polycystic Ovarian Disease).

Ectopic Pregnancy

Ectopic pregnancy is another complication which can occur as a result of ART with an incidence of 1–3% of pregnancies being ectopic following assisted reproduction. It has been described in details in Chapter 35 (Ectopic Pregnancy). It can be diagnosed when there is lack of visualisation of a gestational sac in the uterine cavity above the discriminatory threshold of hCG, and should also be suspected when β-hCG titres are not rising normally. Generally, the mean doubling time for the β-hCG titre in a normal pregnancy is 48 hours. An abnormal rise, plateau or decline in the β-hCG levels may be associated with ectopic pregnancy.[32] Ectopic pregnancy can be managed with non-surgical management using methotrexate in selective patients and traditional laparoscopic salpingectomy or salpingostomy in symptomatic patients.

Iatrogenic Multiple Pregnancy

Widespread use of ART over the past few decades has been associated with an increase in the iatrogenic multifoetal gestations. Since multifoetal gestations are associated with their own risks and complications, their occurrence in association with infertility treatment has to be regarded as an adverse outcome. Some foetal complications associated with multifoetal gestations include a higher incidence of miscarriage, preterm deliveries, congenital malformations, discordancy and IUGR, all of which increase the perinatal morbidity. Multifoetal gestations may also be associated with a higher incidence of maternal complications such as pre-eclampsia, anaemia, labour difficulties, postpartum haemorrhage, failed lactation, psychological disturbances in a woman, etc.

Strategies to Reduce the Risk of Multiple Pregnancies

Some of the strategies which have been adopted to reduce the risk of multiple pregnancies during ARTs are as follows:

* *Elective single embryo transfer*: Recently, transfer of one embryo has been found to be associated with a high

PART III

chance of live birth. As a result, elective single embryo transfer has been recommended as the standard of care in the ART cycles.[33-39]

❖ *Excess oocyte aspiration and vitrification*: Results of a recent meta-analysis have shown that the cycles with three or four follicles do not result in any substantial gain in pregnancy rate, but are associated with an increased rate of multiple pregnancies. A less aggressive ovarian stimulation serves as an effective method for preventing excessive multifollicular growth and therefore reducing the risk of multiple pregnancies in ovarian stimulation. The application of excess oocyte retrieval and vitrification (oocyte cryopreservation) may further improve the cost-effectiveness of stimulated IUI by effectively reducing the rate of multiple pregnancies, at the same time offering additional chances of pregnancy.

❖ *Multifoetal pregnancy reduction*: Multifoetal pregnancy reduction (MFPR) techniques have been promoted to reduce high-order pregnancies to twin gestation, with the aim of improving perinatal outcomes. The technique of MFPR appears to work as an effective treatment option by reducing the rate of pregnancy loss, antenatal complications, preterm birth, caesarean delivery, low birthweight babies and neonatal death.

❖ *Other strategies*: Other strategies for prevention of multiple pregnancies as a result of ovulation stimulation include cycle cancellation, coasting, aspiration of follicles before the administration of hCG and switching to IVF in an IUI cycle. Coasting is a method involving withdrawal of exogenous gonadotropins until there is a decline in serum oestradiol levels.

Oncogenic Risk Related to Assisted Reproductive Technology

Recently, there have been reports showing increased prevalence of perinatal problems associated with ART. Evidence obtained from animal experiments raises concerns that infertility and its treatment with ART (processes such as ovarian stimulation, culture of gametes and embryos) may be associated with an increased oncogenic risk (ovarian cancer, breast cancer, etc.) in both women and their offsprings.[40,41] Although there appears to be a possible risk of ART treatment causing oncogenesis, this has not been proven. The oncogenic risks are minimal, especially with the use of short stimulation protocols nowadays. Nevertheless, long-term studies and follow-up are required to reach any definitive conclusion.

CLINICAL PEARLS

❖ According to the recommendations by the NICE and the HFEA (UK),[1,3] a policy of single embryo transfer must be adopted to reduce the chances of multifoetal gestation with IVF. In all cases of IVF where a top-quality blastocyst is available, single embryo transfer should be preferably used. If no top-quality embryos are available, two embryos can be transferred. In women aged more than 40 years, if a top-quality embryo is not available, no more than two embryos should be transferred during any one cycle of IVF treatment. When considering double embryo transfer, the couple must be counselled regarding the risks of multiple pregnancy associated with this strategy.

❖ The main causes for failure to achieve pregnancy with IVF are poor embryos, poor receptivity of the endometrium and poor efficiency of embryo transfer.

❖ In the UK, women are not offered natural cycle IVF treatment.

❖ Ultrasound monitoring of ovarian response must be offered as an integral part of the IVF treatment cycle.

EVIDENCE-BASED MEDICINE

❖ Presently, there is insufficient evidence to recommend the use of alternative ART such as GIFT and ZIFT in preference to IVF in couples with unexplained fertility problems or male factor fertility problems.[3]

❖ Women undergoing IVF treatment must be informed that the available evidence does not support the continuation of any form of treatment for luteal phase support beyond 8 weeks of gestation.[3]

❖ *Outcome*: The cause of infertility affects IVF outcome. Rate of live birth is the highest in women having ovulatory dysfunction and lowest amongst those with diminished ovarian reserve. Success rate of IVF appears to vary depending upon the patient's race and ethnicity. IVF amongst the Black, Asian and Hispanic women has been found to be associated with lower live birth rate in comparison to the white women. In 2011 in the United States, amongst all fresh non-donor ART cycles, 29% resulted in a live birth.[42] This is higher than the fecundability of natural conception cycles in the general population, where the live birth rate per natural cycle is about 27.7 %.

REFERENCES

1. Human Fertilisation and Embryology Authority (HFEA). (2011). Fertility treatment in 2011: trends and figures. [online] Available from www.hfea.gov.uk/docs/HFEA_Fertility_Trends_and_Figures_2011_-_Annual_Register_Report.pdf. [Accessed September, 2016].
2. Steptoe PC, Edwards RG. Birth after the reimplantation of a human embryo. Lancet. 1978;2(8085):366.
3. National Institute of Clinical Excellence (NICE). (2013). NICE Clinical Guidelines. Fertility problems: assessment and treatment. [online] Available from www.nice.org.uk/guidance/cg156. [Accessed October, 2016]
4. De Vos A, Polyzos NP, Verheyen G, Tournaye H. Intracytoplasmic morphologically selected sperm injection (IMSI): a critical and evidence-based review. Basic Clin Androl. 2013;23:10.
5. Jurema MW, Nogueira D. In vitro maturation of human oocytes for assisted reproduction. Fertil Steril. 2006;86(5):1277-91.
6. Johnson N, van Voorst S, Sowter MC, Strandell A, Mol BW. Surgical treatment for tubal disease in women due to undergo fertilisation. Cochrane Database Syst Rev. 2010;(1):CD002125.

CHAPTER 76

7. van Rooij IA, Bancsi LF, Broekmans FJ, Looman CW, Habbema JD, te Velde ER. Women older than 40 years of age and those with elevated follicle stimulating hormone levels differ in poor response rate and embryo quality in in vitro fertilization. Fertil Steril. 2003;79(3):482-8.

8. Younglai EV, Holloway AC, Foster WG. Environmental and occupational factors affecting fertility and IVF success. Hum Reprod Update. 2005;11(1):43-57.

9. Martin JS, Nisker JA, Tummon IS, Daniel SA, Auckland JL, Feyles V. Future in vitro fertilization pregnancy potential of women with variably elevated day 3 follicle-stimulating hormone levels. Fertil Steril. 1996;65(6):1238-40.

10. Paulson RJ, Marrs RP. Ovulation stimulation and monitoring for in vitro fertilization. Curr Probl Obstet Gynecol Infert. 1986;10:497.

11. Albuquerque LE, Tso LO, Saconato H, Albuquerque MC, Macedo CR. Depot versus daily administration of gonadotrophin-releasing hormone agonist protocols for pituitary down regulation in assisted reproduction cycles. Cochrane Database Syst Rev. 2013;1:CD002808.

12. Al-Inany HG, Youssef MA, Aboulghar M, Broekmans F, Sterrenburg M, Smit J, et al. Gonadotrophin releasing hormone antagonists for assisted reproductive technology. Cochrane Database Syst Rev. 2011;(5):CD001750.

13. Al-Inany HG, Aboulghar M, Mansour R, Proctor M. Recombinant versus urinary human chorionic gonadotrophin for ovulation induction in assisted conception. Cochrane Database Syst Rev. 2005;(2):CD003719.

14. Ferraretti AP, La Marca A, Fauser BC, Tarlatzis B, Nargund G, Gianaroli L, et al. ESHRE consensus on the definition of 'poor response' to ovarian stimulation for in vitro fertilization: the Bologna criteria. Hum Reprod. 2011;26(7):1616-24.

15. Shanbhag S, Aucott L, Bhattacharya S, Hamilton MA, McTavish AR. Interventions for 'poor responders' to controlled ovarian hyperstimulation (COH) in in-vitro fertilisation (IVF). Cochrane Database Syst Rev. 2007;(1):CD004379.

16. Belaisch-Allart J, Testart J, Frydman R. Utilization of GnRH agonists for poor responders in an IVF programme. Hum Reprod. 1989;4(1):33-4.

17. Mahadevan MM. Optimization of culture conditions for human in vitro fertilization and embryo transfer. Semin Reprod Endocrinol. 1998;16(3):197-208.

18. Mains L, Van Voorhis BJ. Optimizing the technique of embryo transfer. Fertil Steril. 2010;94(3):785-90.

19. Abou-Setta AM, D'Angelo A, Sallam HN, Hart RJ, Al-Inany HG. Post-embryo transfer interventions for in vitro fertilization and intracytoplasmic sperm injection patients. Cochrane Database Syst Rev. 2009;(4):CD006567.

20. Practice Committee of Society for Assisted Reproductive Technology, Practice Committee of American Society for Reproductive Medicine. Guidelines on number of embryos transferred. Fertil Steril. 2008;90(5 Suppl):S163-4.

21. Ethics Committee of the American Society for Reproductive Medicine. Disposition of abandoned embryos: a committee opinion. Fertil Steril. 2013;99(7):1848-9.

22. Practice Committee of the American Society for Reproductive Medicine. Progesterone supplementation during the luteal phase and in early pregnancy in the treatment of infertility: an educational bulletin. Fertil Steril. 2008;89(4):789-92.

23. Glujovsky D, Pesce R, Fiszbajn G, Sueldo C, Hart RJ, Ciapponi A. Endometrial preparation for women undergoing embryo transfer with frozen embryos or embryos derived from donor oocytes. Cochrane Database Syst Rev. 2010;(1):CD006359.

24. Hubayter ZR, Muasher SJ. Luteal supplementation in in vitro fertilization: more questions than answers. Fertil Steril. 2008;89(4):749-58.

25. Kyrou D, Fatemi HM, Zepiridis L, Riva A, Papanikolaou EG, Tarlatzis BC, et al. Does cessation of progesterone supplementation during early pregnancy in patients treated with recFSH/GnRH antagonist affect ongoing pregnancy rates? A randomized controlled trial. Hum Reprod. 2011;26(5):1020-4.

26. Daya S, Gunby J. Luteal phase support in assisted reproduction cycles. Cochrane Database Syst Rev. 2004;(3):CD004830.

27. van der Linden M, Buckingham K, Farquhar C, Kremer JA, Metwally M. Luteal phase support for assisted reproduction cycles. Cochrane Database Syst Rev. 2011;(10):CD009154.

28. Zarutskie PW, Phillips JA. A meta-analysis of the route of administration of luteal phase support in assisted reproductive technology: vaginal versus intramuscular progesterone. Fertil Steril. 2009;92(1):163-9.

29. Hull MG. Effectiveness of infertility treatments: choice and comparative analysis. Int J Gynaecol Obstet. 1994;47(2):99-108.

30. Serour GI, Aboulghar M, Mansour R, Sattar MA, Amin Y, Aboulghar H. Complications of medically assisted conception in 3,500 cycles. Fertil Steril. 1998;70(4):638-42.

31. Schenker JG, Ezra Y. Complications of assisted reproductive techniques. Fertil Steril. 1994;61(3):411-22.

32. Ankum WM, Mol BW, Van der Veen F, Bossuyt PM. Risk factors for ectopic pregnancy: a meta-analysis. Fertil Steril. 1996;65(6):1093-9.

33. Prevention of twin pregnancies after IVF/ICSI by single embryo transfer. ESHRE Campus Course Report. Hum Reprod. 2001;16(4):790-800.

34. Pinborg A. IVF/ICSI twin pregnancies: risks and prevention. Hum Reprod Update. 2005;11(6):575-93.

35. Nakhuda GS, Sauer MV. Addressing the growing problem of multiple gestations created by assisted reproductive therapies. Semin Perinatol. 2005;29(5):355-62.

36. Söderström-Anttila V, Vilska S. Five years of single embryo transfer with anonymous and nonanonymous oocyte donation. Reprod Biomed Online. 2007;15(4):428-33.

37. Gerris J, De Neubourg D, Mangelschots K, Van Royen E, Vercruyssen M, Barudy-Vasquez J, et al. Elective single day 3 embryo transfer halves the twinning rate without decrease in the ongoing pregnancy rate of an IVF/ICSI programme. Hum Reprod. 2002;17(10):2626-31.

38. van Rumste MM, Custer IM, van der Veen F, van Wely M, Evers JL, Mol BW. The influence of the number of follicles on pregnancy rates in intrauterine insemination with ovarian stimulation: a metaanalysis. Hum Reprod Update. 2008;14(6):563-70.

39. Ombelet W, Camus M, de Catte L. Relative contribution of ovarian stimulation versus in vitro fertilization and intracytoplasmic sperm injection to multifetal pregnancies requiring reduction to twins. Fertil Steril. 2007;88(4):997-9.

40. Stewart LM, Holman CD, Hart R, Bulsara MK, Preen DB, Finn JC. In vitro fertilization and breast cancer: is there cause for concern? Fertil Steril. 2012;98(2):334-40.

41. Källén B, Finnström O, Lindam A, Nilsson E, Nygren KG, Olausson PO. Malignancies among women who gave birth after in vitro fertilization. Hum Reprod. 2011;26(1):253-8.

42. Society for assisted reproductive technology (SART). (2011). In vitro fertilization rates. [online] Available from www.sartcorsonline.com/rptCSR_PublicMultYear.aspx? ClinicPKID=0. [Accessed October, 2016].

Primary Ovarian Insufficiency

INTRODUCTION

Primary ovarian insufficiency (POI) also known as premature ovarian failure, premature menopause, or early menopause occurring in nearly 1% of women is an important cause of hypergonadotropic hypogonadism.[1] The human ovary functions as both a reproductive organ and an endocrine organ, wherein both these functions are tightly coupled.

Each month, highly coordinated hormonal and ovarian morphological changes develop and release a mature oocyte that is ready for fertilisation. In case fertilisation does not occur, menstruation occurs, a hallmark of healthy ovarian function during the reproductive years. A disruption of this process may result in anovulation and ovarian steroid hormone deficiency. Ageing is associated with a decline in the number of ovarian follicles, menstrual irregularities, ovarian hormonal deficiency, anovulation and decreased fertility. This eventually results in a complete and irreversible cessation of menses known as menopause, which usually occurs at the mean age of 51 years. Normally, in women aged 40 years or older, there is a physiological decline in ovarian function with ageing. This transition phase is known as the perimenopause or the menopausal transition.

Ovarian insufficiency can be defined as failure of the ovary to function adequately in a woman younger than 40 years, in its role either as an endocrine organ or as a reproductive organ.[2] As described by the WHO, ovarian insufficiency can be defined as either primary or secondary. Primary ovarian insufficiency is caused by a primary disorder in the ovary due to which it fails to function normally. Secondary ovarian insufficiency, on the other hand, is due to secondary causes, most commonly due to the failure of hypothalamus and pituitary to provide appropriate gonadotropin stimulation.

AETIOLOGY

In majority of cases, the underlying cause is not identified. The known causes are described next.[3]

❖ *Genetic causes*: Genetic aberrations, which could involve the X chromosome or autosomes. Though a large number of genes have been screened as candidates for causing POI; only few clear causal mutations have been identified. Some of these genes include fragile site mental retardation 1 gene (FMR1), FSH receptor (FSHR) gene, etc.

❖ *Autoimmune causes*: POI commonly occurs in association with other autoimmune disorders of endocrine system (e.g. thyroid, hypoparathyroid, diabetes mellitus, Addison's disease, etc.) as well as non-endocrine system (e.g. idiopathic thrombocytopenic purpura, vitiligo, alopecia, autoimmune haemolytic anaemia, pernicious anaemia, systemic lupus erythematosus, rheumatoid arthritis, Crohn's disease, Sjögren syndrome, primary biliary cirrhosis, etc.). Presence of antiovarian antibodies has been observed in several cases of POI. However, their specificity and pathogenic role presently remains uncertain.

❖ *Iatrogenic causes*: POI may sometimes develop following surgical, radiotherapeutic or chemotherapeutic interventions (cytotoxic chemotherapy), e.g. that required in cases of malignancies.

❖ *Environmental factors*: Environmental factors involved in the pathogenesis of POI may include viral infections, toxins, etc. However, their mechanism of action presently remains uncertain.

DIAGNOSIS

Clinical Presentation

Primary ovarian insufficiency is a condition characterised by primary or secondary amenorrhoea, hypo-oestrogenism, and elevated serum gonadotropin levels in women younger than 40 years. The woman must be enquired about the date of her last spontaneous menstrual cycle. Prior history of infection, surgery, radiotherapy, chemotherapy, history suggestive of any autoimmune disorders, thyroid or adrenal disorders, etc., which may serve as the likely aetiology of POI also needs to be enquired. Family history of POI needs to be asked because women whose mothers give a history of premature ovarian failure are likely to be at an increased risk.

General Physical Examination

❖ *Signs of hypo-oestrogenism*: There may be signs suggestive of hypo-oestrogenism such as dryness of skin and vaginal atrophy. For details related to the symptoms of premature menopause, kindly refer to Chapter 60 (Menopause and Hormone Replacement Therapy)

❖ *Signs suggestive of hypothyroidism*

❖ *Signs suggestive of autoimmune diseases*: There may be signs suggestive of autoimmune diseases such as Addison's disease, thyroid disorders, etc.

Investigations

The following investigations can be done in cases of POI.[4]

❖ *Serum FSH levels*: The diagnosis of POI is based on finding of amenorrhoea before the age of 40 years associated with FSH levels in the menopausal range. Since the FSH levels are likely to significantly fluctuate in a patient, measurement of serial levels is usually advised. Two or three measurements of FSH levels at 6 weeks intervals are likely to be sufficient. High serum FSH levels along with low serum oestradiol levels help in confirming the diagnosis of POI.

❖ *Screening for autoimmune disorders*: Screening for associated autoimmune disorders is important because these disorders may be commonly linked with POI. Autoantibody screen including thyroid and adrenal antibodies must be performed.

❖ *Karyotyping*: Karyotypic analysis is particularly important in early onset disease and helps in excluding any genetic cause for POI. Genetic screen for fragile X syndrome (FRAXA) premutation must also be performed.

❖ *Thyroid function tests*: These are useful because thyroid involvement is a common association.

❖ *Tests for adrenal function*: Tests for adrenal function, such as the synacthen test, renal function test and CT scan, may also be required.

❖ *Bone mineral density scan*: Bone mineral density scan [dual-energy X-ray absorptiometry (DEXA)] is a very useful investigation even if the patient has only recently attained menopause.

❖ *Testing for ovarian reserve*: Tests used for assessing ovarian reserves commonly include tests such as antral follicle count and levels of anti-müllerian hormone (AMH). However, none of these tests are able to predict the likelihood of a woman developing premature ovarian insufficiency.

❖ *Pelvic ultrasound*: Pelvic ultrasound may help in delineating small ovaries with little or no follicular activity.

❖ *Ovarian biopsy*: Use of ovarian biopsy is unlikely to change the management plan, therefore it is rarely required.

MANAGEMENT

The principle of management in cases of POI basically involves the use of HRT and infertility treatment.[5] In addition, the associated pathology needs to be assessed and managed. Long-term follow-up may be required for monitoring the patients taking HRT. Management also involves taking steps for preventing the development of POI in patients predicted to be at a high risk.

Preventing the Development of POI in Young Women Exposed to Gonadotoxic Chemotherapy

In some cases, it is possible to predict the development of premature menopause, e.g., patients undergoing anticancer treatment with chemotherapy. Various treatment options for preventing premature ovarian failure in these have been reviewed by Blumenfeld (2003).[6] Cryopreservation of embryo, ovarian tissue and oocytes appears to be a promising strategy for cases where ovarian failure is predictable in future, e.g. women undergoing treatment for cancer.[6,7] Oocyte cryopreservation and subsequent intracytoplasmic sperm injection has resulted in pregnancies and live births in patients with POI.[8,9] Use of cryopreserved embryos is likely to be associated with a high pregnancy rate of 30% per transfer.[10]

Cotreatment with gonadotropin-releasing hormone agonists (GnRHa) to suppress the pituitary-gonadal axis is likely to protect the germinal epithelium against the cytotoxic effects of chemotherapy, thereby preventing the development of POI during cytotoxic chemotherapy.[11,12] Use of apoptotic inhibitors, such as sphingosine-1-phosphate, is also likely to have radioprotective and chemoprotective effect against germ cell death. These agents probably act by inhibiting the signalling events involved in apoptotic process, thereby protecting the patient from POI.[13-15]

Treatment for Infertility

There is a 5–10% chance of spontaneous ovarian activity in women with POI having normal karyotype. The possibility of spontaneous ovarian activity and subsequent pregnancy must be explained to the patient. Symptomatic women with POI requiring HRT, who are still hoping for natural conception, may be prescribed sequential HRT because this does not have any contraceptive effect. On the other hand, effective contraceptive advice must be provided to women with POI who wish to avoid conception.

There is no proven effective treatment for infertility in cases of POI. In cases where natural conception is not possible, the only proven means for conception is assisted conception with donated oocytes.[16-19] Adoption and oocyte donation are amongst the available options, but require appropriate guidance and counselling.

Use of Barrier Contraception in Women Who Wish to Avoid Pregnancy

Natural oestrogens used in HRT are unlikely to prevent any spontaneous ovulatory activity. Moreover, ovulation and pregnancy may occur in women with POI using the combined oral contraceptives. Barrier contraceptives are therefore recommended for women with POI who wish to avoid pregnancy.

Hormonal Replacement Therapy

Hormonal replacement therapy can be administered via oral, transdermal, subcutaneous, or vaginal routes. A particular HRT regimen should be based on the individual patient's preferences. Combined OCPs can also be used as the oestrogen replacement. Long-term HRT is required for alleviation of menopausal symptoms (e.g. vasomotor instability, sexual dysfunction, mood, fatigue, etc.). HRT also helps in preventing long-term health sequel of oestrogen deficiency, such as osteoporosis.[20] Oestrogen replacements are usually continued up to 50 years of age, following which the risk and benefit of continuing the treatment are reviewed. [21]

At the time of administration of oestrogen replacement therapy, if the uterus is still present, addition of progestogens in the form of sequential (10–14 days each month) or continuous combined preparations can be done to provide endometrial protection. Progestins can be administered via oral or transdermal routes. An alternative to this involves the use of Mirena® intrauterine system, which is licensed for 4 years of use in the UK. Continuous progestin regimen helps in preventing menstrual blood flow, whereas sequential regimens ensure monthly menstrual bleed, which may provide psychological benefit to some young women. Use of the type of progestins may vary from the more potent ones such as norethisterone to comparatively less potent ones such as dydrogesterone.

In cases where there is persistent fatigue and loss of libido persists despite optimised oestrogen replacement therapy, androgen replacement may prove to be a useful therapy.[22,23] For details related to HRT, kindly refer to Chapter 60 (Menopause and Hormone Replacement Therapy).

Prevention of Bone Loss

❖ Oestrogen therapy helps in reducing the risk of osteoporosis and fractures. Adequate bone protection can be achieved with low-dose HRT.
❖ The general measures advised for prevention of bone loss include performance of weight-bearing exercises regularly, consumption of adequate diet rich in calcium and vitamin D, and avoidance of activities such as smoking and alcohol abuse, which may promote bone loss. Calcium and vitamin D supplementation may be offered in women who appear to be deficient in these minerals.
❖ Women with osteoporosis or osteopenia, who cannot tolerate or those who refuse HRT can be prescribed non-hormonal treatment including biphosphonates,

strontium, raloxifene, etc. However, these preparations must not be used in those with normal bone density.
❖ Bone mineral density should be preferably monitored with DEXA scans to help identify the women with osteoporosis who may require specific additional intervention.

Psychological Support

Women also require personal and emotional support to deal with impact of diagnosis on their health and relationships.

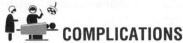

COMPLICATIONS

Earlier than expected oestrogen deficiency is likely to result in several serious health consequences contributing to increased mortality and morbidity at an earlier age. Women with premature menopause are likely to be associated with nearly 50% increased risk of mortality in comparison to women having menopause at an average age of 50 years. Some of these complications associated with premature menopause are as follows:

❖ *Cardiovascular disease*: Hypo-oestrogenism due to POI is probably related to an increased risk of ischaemic heart disease in women attaining menopause prior to the age of 40 years in comparison to the women undergoing menopause between the age of 52 to 55 years. Hypo-oestrogenism is likely to increase the risk of ischaemic heart disease due to the following causes:
  • Endothelial dysfunction resulting in progression of atherosclerosis
  • Dyslipidaemia resulting in altered lipid profile
  • Reduced insulin sensitivity and metabolic syndrome.

Initiation of oestrogen replacement therapy immediately after commencement of menopause at the young age is likely to significantly reduce the risk of mortality, heart failure, or myocardial infarction.[24] Oestrogen replacement can be administered in the form of HRT or synthetic ethinyl oestradiol in the form of combined OCPs.

❖ *Osteoporosis*: There is an acceleration of bone loss following menopause. Therefore, earlier the occurrence of menopause in life, lower would be the bone density later in life. Methods for prevention of osteoporosis have been described previously in the text.
❖ *Cognitive impairment*: This may include complications such as dementia and Parkinsonism. Patients with early menopause are likely to be associated with a high risk of impaired cognitive function.
❖ *Psychological sequel*: Diagnosis of POI may be associated with distressing long-lasting psychological effects such as anxiety, depression, psychological distress and overall reduced feeling of well-being. The patients must be made aware of the POI support groups such as the Daisy network and the POI Support Group to help her regain a sense of control and confidence.
❖ *Impaired sexual functioning*: Women with premature ovarian function may be associated with several psychosexual problems such as decreased level of sexual

CHAPTER 77

fulfilment, reduced arousal, lower frequency of sexual encounters, dyspareunia, etc. Besides the oestrogen replacement therapy, psychosexual counselling may also be required in these cases.

❖ *Subfertility*: There may be occasional resumption of ovarian activity in some women, resulting in continuation of irregular periods. As previously mentioned, spontaneous pregnancies are likely to occur in 5–10% of karyotypically normal women with idiopathic POI.

❖ *Association with autoimmune conditions*: Premature ovarian insufficiency may be often associated with other autoimmune conditions such as hypothyroidism, Addison's disease, diabetes mellitus, vitiligo, pernicious anaemia, systemic lupus erythematosus, rheumatoid arthritis, myasthenia gravis, etc. In some cases there may be a presence of antiovarian and antiadrenal antibodies. Patients should be treated for the specific autoimmune disease, which may be present.

CLINICAL PEARLS

❖ There is no role of ovarian biopsy or ultrasound in making the diagnosis of POI.

❖ Intermittent ovarian function can sometimes occur in women with POI and pregnancies may occasionally occur. It is not possible to predict the likelihood of recovery of ovulation in cases of POI.

❖ Besides the several complications related with premature ovarian failure, it also offers protective effect on the development of breast malignancy.

EVIDENCE-BASED MEDICINE

❖ Presently, assisted conception with donated oocytes is the only means for fertility treatment in POI that carries high success rate.[16-19]

❖ The available evidence has failed to demonstrate any significant improvement in ovulation and pregnancy rates using various therapeutic options (e.g. gonadotropins suppression using GnRHa, oestradiol, oral contraceptives, etc.) in patients with POI. [25-30]

REFERENCES

1. Goswami D, Conway GS. Premature ovarian failure. Hum Reprod Update. 2005;11(4):391-410.
2. Shelling AN. Premature ovarian failure. Reproduction. 2010; 140(5):633-41.
3. Welt CK. Pathogenesis and causes of spontaneous primary ovarian insufficiency (premature ovarian failure). [online] Available from www.uptodate.com/contents/pathogenesis-and-causes-of-spontaneous-primary-ovarian-insufficiency-premature-ovarian-failure. [Accessed October, 2016].
4. Lentz G, Lobo RA, Gershenson D, Katz VL. Comprehensive Gynecology, 6th edition. Philadelphia, PA: Mosby Elsevier; 2012.
5. Rafique S, Sterling EW, Nelson LM. A new approach to primary ovarian insufficiency. Obstet Gynecol Clin North Am. 2012;39(4):567-86.
6. Blumenfeld Z. Gynaecologic concerns for young women exposed to gonadotoxic chemotherapy. Curr Opin Obstet Gynecol. 2003;15(5):359-70.
7. Poirot C, Vacher-Lavenu MC, Helardot P, Guibert J, Brugieres L, Jouannet P. Human ovarian tissue cryopreservation: indications and feasibility. Hum Reprod. 2002;17(6):1447-52.
8. Chen C. Pregnancy after human oocyte cryopreservation. Lancet. 1986;1(8486):884-6.
9. Borini A, Bonu MA, Coticchio G, Bianchi V, Cattoli M, Flamigni C. Pregnancies and births after oocyte cryopreservation. Fertil Steril. 2004;82(3):601-5.
10. Abdalla HI, Baber RJ, Kirkland A, Leonard T, Studd JW. Pregnancy in women with premature ovarian failure using tubal and intrauterine transfer of cryopreserved zygotes. Br J Obstet Gynaecol. 1989;96(9):1071-5.
11. Blumenfeld Z, Avivi I, Linn S, Epelbaum R, Ben-Shahar M, Haim N. Prevention of irreversible chemotherapy-induced ovarian damage in young women with lymphoma by a gonadotrophin-releasing hormone agonist in parallel to chemotherapy. Hum Reprod. 1996;11(8):1620-6.
12. Blumenfeld Z, Dann E, Avivi I, Epelbaum R, Rowe JM. Fertility after treatment for Hodgkin's disease. Ann Oncol. 2002;13 (Suppl 1):138-147.
13. Morita Y, Perez GI, Paris F, Miranda SR, Ehleiter D, Haimovitz-Friedman A, et al. Oocyte apoptosis is suppressed by disruption of the acid sphingomyelinase gene or by sphingosine-1-phosphate therapy. Nat Med. 2000;6(10):1109-14.
14. Spiegel S, Kolesnick R. Sphingosine 1-phosphate as a therapeutic agent. Leukemia. 2002;16(9):1596-602.
15. Tilly JL, Kolesnick RN. Sphingolipids, apoptosis, cancer treatments and the ovary: investigating a crime against female fertility. Biochim Biophys Acta. 2002;1585(2-3):135-8.
16. Asch R, Balmaceda J, Ord T, Borrero C, Cefalu E, Gastaldi C. Oocyte donation and gamete intrafallopian transfer as treatment for premature ovarian failure. Lancet. 1987;1(8534): 687.
17. Oskarsson T, Edgar DH, Whalley KM, Mills JA. Clinical and biochemical pregnancy in two respective recipients without ovarian function following gamete intrafallopian transfers using oocytes from a single donor. Scott Med J. 1990;35(4):114-5.
18. Rotsztejn DA, Remohi J, Weckstein LN, Ord T, Moyer DL, Balmaceda JP, et al. Results of tubal embryo transfer in premature ovarian failure. Fertil Steril. 1990;54(2):348-50.
19. van Kasteren Y. Treatment concepts for premature ovarian failure. J Soc Gynecol Investig. 2001;8(1 Suppl Proceedings): S58-9.
20. Davis SR. Premature ovarian failure. Maturitas. 1996;23(1):1-8.
21. Armitage M, Nooney J, Evans S. Recent concerns surrounding HRT. Clin Endocrinol (Oxf). 2003;59(2):145-55.
22. Mazer NA. Testosterone deficiency in women: etiologies, diagnosis, and emerging treatments. Int J Fertil Womens Med. 2002;47(2):77-86.
23. Arlt W. Management of the androgen-deficient woman. Growth Horm IGF Res. 2003;13 (Suppl A):S85-9.
24. Schierbeck LL, Rejnmark L, Tofteng CL, Stilgren L, Eiken P, Mosekilde L, et al. Effect of hormone replacement therapy on cardiovascular events in recently postmenopausal women: randomised trial. BMJ. 2012;345:e6409.

25. van Kasteren YM, Schoemaker J. Premature ovarian failure: a systematic review on therapeutic interventions to restore ovarian function and achieve pregnancy. Hum Reprod Update. 1999;5(5):483-92.

26. Taylor AE, Adams JM, Mulder JE, Martin KA, Sluss PM, Crowley WF. A randomized, controlled trial of estradiol replacement therapy in women with hypergonadotropic amenorrhea. J Clin Endocrinol Metab. 1996;81(10):3615-21.

27. Kreiner D, Droesch K, Navot D, Scott R, Rosenwaks Z. Spontaneous and pharmacologically induced remissions in patients with premature ovarian failure. Obstet Gynecol. 1988;72(6):926-8.

28. Rebar RW, Connolly HV. Clinical features of young women with hypergonadotropic amenorrhea. Fertil Steril. 1990;53(5): 804-10.

29. Blumenfeld Z, Halachmi S, Peretz BA, Shmuel Z, Golan D, Makler A, et al. Premature ovarian failure—the prognostic application of autoimmunity on conception after ovulation induction. Fertil Steril. 1993;59(4):750-5.

30. Chatterjee R, Mills W, Katz M, McGarrigle HH, Goldstone AH. Induction of ovarian function by using short-term human menopausal gonadotrophin in patients with ovarian failure following cytotoxic chemotherapy for haematological malignancy. Leuk Lymphoma. 1993;10(4-5):383-6.

CHAPTER 77

Fertility Preservation

INTRODUCTION

With the increasing incidence of malignancy in the Western population, there has been a rise in the number of both men and women undergoing treatment for malignancy. Due to early detection and improved cancer treatment protocols, more than 75% of young cancer patients nowadays are able to survive for long term.[1] The most common cancer of the female reproductive system is breast cancer. Other cancers commonly encountered in the women include leukaemia, melanomas, lymphomas, cervical and ovarian cancer. In men belonging to the reproductive age group, the most common type of cancers encountered include testicular germ cell tumours followed by leukaemia and Hodgkin's lymphoma.

Treatment of malignancy may be associated with gonadal dysfunction and fertility problems (e.g. premature ovarian failure).[1] In male gonads, germ cells are much more sensitive to irradiation and chemotherapy in comparison to the Leydig cells. Radiation doses as low as 0.1–1.2 Gy can impair spermatogenesis. Thus, infertility is a more common adverse effect of cancer treatment than hypogonadism.

Some malignancies are particularly susceptible towards causing fertility-related problems. For example, persistent azoospermia may commonly occur following treatment for Hodgkin's lymphoma. Nevertheless, many of the patients who are diagnosed with cancer during their childhood or adult life may be desirous of future fertility.

There are many methods for fertility preservation, which can be employed in such patients to ensure the prospects of their future fertility. Patients at risk for hypogonadism and infertility should be identified prior to treatment, and become candidates for one of the available methods for gonadal preservation. During follow-up of the cancer patients, the oncologists should routinely discuss these issues with the patient. Fertility issues in such patients should be managed by a multidisciplinary team comprising of an oncologist, gynaecologist, infertility specialist, etc.

Fertility preservation is the process, which involves protecting the eggs, sperms, or reproductive tissue of an individual so that they can be utilised for having biological children in the future. It is an attempt to help patients (e.g. cancer patients), who have been predicted to lose their fertility in foreseeable future, to retain their ability to procreate.[2] This option assumes special significance due to an increase in the survival rate of cancer patients.

INDICATIONS

Indications for preservation of fertility are described next.

Loss of Fertility due to Cancer Treatment

Fertility preservation procedures are indicated when the loss of fertility usually due to cancer treatment in near future is predicted. Certain types of chemotherapy and radiation treatment to the pelvic area for cancer treatment are likely to affect the reproductive health. Chemotherapeutic drugs which are likely to be associated with moderate-to-high risk of damage to the ovaries include procarbazine and alkylating drugs such as cyclophosphamide, ifosfamide, busulfan, melphalan, chlorambucil and chlormethine, doxorubicin and platinum analogues such as cisplatin and carboplatin. On the other hand, chemotherapeutic drugs with low risk of gonadotoxicity include drugs such as vincristine and vinblastine (plant derivatives), bleomycin and dactinomycin (antibiotics), and methotrexate, mercaptopurine, cytarabine and 5-fluorouracil (antimetabolites). Chemotherapy is likely to damage the primordial follicles. Following chemotherapy, the ovaries atrophy due to the replacement of cortical stromal cells with collagen.

Radiotherapy, particularly, which is directed to the pelvis can also adversely affect the ovarian reserve. Radiotherapy to the pelvis can also cause disruption of the uterine vasculature, reduced muscular elasticity, impaired uterine blood flow and endometrial damage. This may be associated with adverse obstetric consequences such as increased risk of miscarriage, low birth weight, premature delivery, etc.

Decline in Fertility due to Ageing

Advanced maternal age (>35 years) may be associated with a decline in fertility. Options for fertility preservation, such as cryopreservation of oocytes or ovarian tissue may also be used to prevent infertility, as well as birth defects, associated with advancing age of the mother.

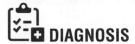 **DIAGNOSIS**

Clinical Presentation

For many cancer patients, the decline in reproductive function is temporary. On the other hand, many men and women, may not regain fertility following cancer treatment. In fact, some of the patients undergoing serious radiation, chemotherapy, or surgery may experience symptoms resembling menopause (in women) or andropause (in men), which indicate reproductive damage. In women, reduced oestrogen levels as a result of ovarian deficiency lead to reduced bone density, altered thermoregulatory mechanism, mood changes, reduced libido, etc. Men with testicular insufficiency also experience similar symptoms such as reduced libido, changes in temperature control, etc.

While considering the various options for fertility preservation, a detailed history must be taken from the patient regarding her age, menstrual history, previous pregnancies, desire for future fertility, whether or not she has a partner or spouse, the cancer location, its staging, prognosis, potential for metastasis to the reproductive organs, proposed treatment options, predicable side effects in the future, time available for fertility preservation, probability for delaying the initiation of cancer therapy, patient's general condition, baseline ovarian reserve, etc.

Investigations

Since the type of fertility option to be used in the patient depends on the patient's baseline ovarian reserves, tests for measuring ovarian reserves need to be performed. If the woman is found to have a reduced ovarian reserve, or the natural fertility appears to be unlikely, the fertility specialist should resort to the option of assisted reproductive technology (ART). Options of adoption and surrogacy can also be considered in these cases. Various options for testing ovarian reserve are as follows:

❖ *Baseline FSH levels*: The most commonly used tests for measuring ovarian reserves include baseline FSH levels between day 2 and day 5 of the menstrual cycle. Since the levels of FSH can commonly fluctuate, two or three measurements of FSH levels at 6 weeks intervals are usually advisable. However, nowadays other tests for ovarian reserve such as levels of anti-müllerian hormone (AMH) and antral follicle count are commonly being used.

❖ *Levels of anti-Müllerian hormone*: In women with cancer, measurement of the levels of AMH, which is an indicator of ovarian reserve, is useful for predicting the long-term loss of ovarian function following chemotherapy or radiotherapy.[3,4] This in turn helps in planning the future fertility preservation strategies. AMH levels can be measured at any stage of the menstrual cycle.

❖ *Sonography*: Ultrasound evaluation of ovaries helps in providing an estimate of total antral follicle count and measurement of ovarian volume.

❖ *Response to ovarian stimulation*: Poor ovarian response to stimulation by gonadotropins is an indicator of low ovarian reserve.

 MANAGEMENT

❖ Management should preferably be by a multidisciplinary team comprising of an oncologist, fertility specialist, gynaecologist, clinical psychologist, etc. All decisions must be taken following a close discussion with the family and the partner. Management plan should be devised in such a way, which helps in prolonging the patients' life, but also helps improve their quality of life, as well as their social and psychological well-being.

❖ Clinical psychologist is likely to play a vital role in counselling the patients and their families.

❖ Patients desirous of future fertility must be provided an explanation about the various fertility preserving options. Patients should be referred to the fertility specialist who can counsel them appropriately prior to the initiation of treatment.

Fertility Preserving Options

The type of fertility option which would be helpful for the patient depends upon various factors such as pubertal stage of the patient, baseline ovarian reserve, time available for preservation of fertility, whether the patient is in a stable relationship with a partner who is willing to offer his sperms, or if the patient is willing to accept donor sperms, etc. A number of fertility-preserving options are available for men, women, and children, which have been described next.

Fertility-preserving Options for Men

Presently, there are no options for preservation of fertility in prepubertal boys. Cryopreservation of testicular tissue from prepubertal males is presently under experimental stages. Sperm banking or cryopreservation of sperms can be used as an option in postpubertal boys.[5] Sperms can be obtained through masturbation, electroejaculation or surgical retrieval. Men or boys with testicular cancer have an excellent chance of survival and may be interested in future fertility. If cisplatinum-based chemotherapy is used, nearly all patients are likely to become azoospermic.[6] However, in majority of the patients, recovery of spermatogenesis occurs within 4 years. Also, the semen quality returns to baseline in most patients within 2 years of undergoing prophylactic radiation therapy for seminoma. In all these cases, cryopreservation of sperms serves as a suitable option for fertility preservation.

On the other hand, in men with persistent poor semen quality, ARTs [IVF and intracytoplasmic sperm injection (ICSI)] may be useful for achieving fertility. ARTs have also greatly improved the chance of pregnancy with cryopreserved sperm.

Sperm cryopreservation or sperm banking: This involves storage of frozen semen samples for future use. For postpubescent boys and men, sperms can be obtained through masturbation. On the other hand, for prepubescent boys, sperms can be sometimes obtained through epididymal sperm aspiration, testicular sperm extraction or electroejaculation and then stored for future use.[7] The option of semen cryopreservation should be used even if the specimen is extremely poor, but at least one viable sperm is present. The cryopreserved sperms can be stored for an initial period of 10 years. However, cryostorage of sperms beyond 10 years can be offered for men who remain at the significant risk of malignancy.

Gonadal shielding: Radiation treatment for cancer, especially the one which is directed to the pelvic region, can cause damage to the gonads. Protecting the gonads (testicles) with a lead shield may be helpful in some cases.

Fertility-preserving Options for Women

Cryopreservation of embryos: The eggs from the woman are fertilised with the sperms from her partner or a donor in a laboratory through the process of IVF. The resulting embryos are frozen and stored for future use. In future when the woman is ready to initiate pregnancy, the embryo is thawed and implanted into the uterus for maturation and birth. Donor sperm can be used in cases where the woman does not have a partner.

Cryopreservation of embryos following IVF is the method of choice associated with high success rates. While this option is the most common fertility preservation method in postpubescent women, it is not available to prepubescent girls, who do not have mature eggs that can be fertilised. Moreover, this procedure requires hormonal stimulation for a period of 2 weeks to augment maturation of eggs. Therefore, this method cannot be used for female patients who have hormone-sensitive cancers (e.g. breast cancer, ovarian cancer, etc.).[8] Alternative methods of hormonal stimulation (e.g. letrozole or tamoxifen) may be used for women with hormone-sensitive cancers. Also, this method can only be used if the woman has a male partner or the donor sperms are acceptable to the woman.

A cycle of controlled ovarian hyperstimulation (COH) can be used before retrieving the occytes from the patient's ovaries. hCG is routinely used for triggering final oocyte maturation in the normal IVF cycles. However, use of hCG for COH in the context of cryopreserved oocytes may be associated with an increased risk of ovarian hyperstimulation syndrome (OHSS). Use of GnRH agonists (GnRHa) rather than hCG in COH treatment regimens in combination with oocyte or embryo cryopreservation where the cycle has been downregulated with a GnRH antagonist is a better strategy. This is likely to be associated with a reduced risk of complications and similar birth rates in comparison to those cycles where hCG is used for induction ovulation.[9]

Controlled ovarian stimulation and cryopreservation of oocytes: This is the most established method for female fertility preservation. The process of cryopreservation of oocytes is similar to the cryopreservation of embryos, except that in these cases, a cycle of COH is performed following which the woman's unfertilised eggs are retrieved, frozen and then stored. COH is usually required for a period of 2 weeks before oocyte retrieval can be performed. Preservation of the oocytes may be technically challenging due to the size and structural complexities of the oocyte. Effectiveness of oocyte preservation depends on the number of oocytes obtained because each oocyte is associated with 3–5% chances of successful pregnancy.

Cryopreservation of the ovarian tissue followed by transplantation: Strips of cortical ovarian tissue can also be cryopreserved. Generally no more than 50% of one ovary should be removed for the purpose of cryopreservation. Following the completion of treatment, this tissue is later reimplanted into the body so as to enable the encapsulated immature follicles to complete their maturation. This option can be particularly useful in prepubertal girls or in women who require treatment for cancer within a minimum of 2 weeks and cannot wait for controlled ovarian stimulation. Cryopreservation and transplantation of the ovarian tissues should be preferably carried out at specialised centres due to the risk of ischaemic damage to the tissues at the time of implantation and revascularisation. Moreover, there is a theoretical risk reintroduction of malignant tumour cells at the time of transplantation.

Third-party reproduction: Alternatives for bearing biological children, such as IVF using donor eggs or donor sperms, can be performed in patients with impaired infertility (e.g. those undergoing treatment for malignancy). The resulting embryo can be implanted into the woman's uterus after stimulating the uterine endometrium with hormones to prepare for the development of the embryo.

Gonadal shielding: This process is similar to gonadal shielding for men. The only difference being that in these cases ovaries rather than testicles are protected with a lead screen.

Ovarian transposition: Ovarian transposition is a procedure used for preserving fertility in girls with cancer. It is indicated for patients with tumours requiring pelvic radiation at doses of 42.0–58.4 Gy, a dosage much higher than that can bring about the loss of ovarian function (4–20 Gy), for example, in the cases of cervical cancer, ovaries can be transposed to reduce the radiation exposure to the ovaries.[10,11] Ovarian transposition is usually performed with the help of minimally invasive surgery or open surgery in cases where concomitant resection of the abdominal tumour is performed. Based on the type of tumour and the direction of the radiation field, the ovaries are moved and placed in the paracolic gutters (when the radiation field reaches the midline) or contralateral to the tumour or in line with the iliac crests. Nevertheless, the procedure may fail to protect the ovaries in 10–14% of cases.

Gonadotropin-releasing hormone agonists for ovarian protection: Role of GnRHa for protecting the ovaries at the time of chemotherapy currently remains obscure.[12-15] Presently, there are no high-level, evidence-based recommendations for preservation of fertility or of ovarian function using GnRHa. There are ongoing trials to assess the role of ovarian protection by using GnRHa. However, their results are still awaited. Nevertheless, the premenopausal women undergoing chemotherapy should be counselled regarding the various options for ovarian preservation, including the use of GnRHa therapy and OCPs.

COMPLICATIONS

Increased risk of arterial thrombotic events: Individuals with cancer are likely to be associated with an increased risk of arterial thrombotic events such as stroke, myocardial infraction, peripheral arterial embolisation, etc. in comparison to the general population. This risk is further increased in women undergoing COH for fertility preservation. Furthermore, such women are also at an increased risk of developing OHSS. As previously mentioned in the text, use of GnRHa rather than hCG for triggering final oocyte maturation at the time of attempting COH (where the cycle has been downregulated with a GnRH antagonist) in conjunction with oocyte or embryo cryopreservation is likely to be associated with a reduced risk of OHSS.

Prophylaxis with anticoagulants can also be administered to the selected subgroups of women, especially those having risk factors for hypercoagulability or those who do develop OHSS in the early stages.[16]

CLINICAL PEARLS

❖ The two main aspects of fertility preservation include minimisation of the effect of cancer treatment on the individual's fertility and provision of effective options for storing gametes, embryos or germinal tissues.

❖ Alkylating agents, such as cyclophosphamide and procarbazine, are most damaging to the germ cells. Radiation therapy, especially whole-body irradiation, is also associated with the risk of permanent sterility.

❖ Some of the options for fertility preservation, e.g. sperm, oocyte and embryo cryopreservation, are available only to adult individuals who have gone through puberty and have mature sperm and eggs. However, options such as gonadal shielding and ovarian transposition can also be used for children who have not gone through puberty.

❖ Cryopreservation of semen before the commencement of cancer treatment is currently one of the most important methods for preserving future male fertility.

EVIDENCE-BASED MEDICINE

❖ The present evidence has indicated that the treatment results with cryopreserved semen in fathers who had been treated for cancer in the past are generally good and comparable with that of IVF and ICSI in the normal population.[5,7] So far, there is no evidence to indicate an increased risk of congenital abnormalities or malignancies in children born from fathers who had cancer treatment is the past. Nevertheless, close follow-up is necessary in such pregnancies, especially in children born after IVF or ICSI.

❖ The present evidence indicates that use of GnRHa rather than hCG for final maturation induction at the time of attempting COH (where the cycle has been downregulated with a GnRH antagonist) in conjunction with oocyte or embryo cryopreservation is unlikely to be associated with any difference in the rate of live birth in comparison to those cycles where hCG is used for final maturation induction of the oocytes. Furthermore, this strategy is likely to be associated with a reduced incidence of OHSS. This is in contrast to fresh cycles where usage of GnRHa rather than hCG is associated with a lower live birth rate in COH treatment regimens where the cycle has been downregulated using a GnRH antagonist.[9]

❖ Presently, there is controversial evidence to indicate that suppression of folliculogenesis using GnRH analogues during chemotherapy is likely to preserve the ovaries.[12-15] Meta-analysis by Ben-Aharon et al. has shown that treatment with GnRHa is effective in reducing amenorrhea rates in patients undergoing chemotherapy (RR = 0.26, 95% CI = 0.14–0.49).[12] Use of GnRHa is also likely to be associated with a higher pregnancy rate. However, the advantage of GnRHa was demonstrated only by the observational studies and not by the RCTs. Several randomised trials are ongoing to outline the role and mechanism of GnRHa in preserving the ovarian function at the time of chemotherapy.[13] Moreover, the use of GnRHa and OCPs is not associated with any serious side effects. In fact, GnRHa can even reduce the incidence of chemotherapy-induced complications, such as severe menometrorrhagia, etc.[14] There is a requirement for large RCT with adequate follow-up in future to prove the efficacy of GnRHa as fertility preserving agents.

REFERENCES

1. Brydøy M, Fosså SD, Dahl O, Bjøro T. Gonadal dysfunction and fertility problems in cancer survivors. Acta Oncol. 2007;46(4):480-9.

2. Klock SC, Zhang JX, Kazer RR. Fertility preservation for female cancer patients: early clinical experience. Fertil Steril. 2010;94(1):149-55.

3. Broer SL, Broekmans FJ, Laven JS, Fauser BC. Anti-Müllerian hormone: ovarian reserve testing and its potential clinical implications. Hum Reprod Update. 2014;20(5):688-701.

4. Grynnerup AG, Lindhard A, Sørensen S. Recent progress in the utility of anti-Müllerian hormone in female infertility. Curr Opin Obstet Gynecol. 2014;26(3):162-7.

5. Ohl DA, Sonksen J. What are the chances of infertility and should sperm be banked? Semin Urol Oncol. 1996;14(1):36-44.

6. Dohle GR. Male infertility in cancer patients: Review of the literature. Int J Urol. 2010;17(4):327-31.

7. Fosså SD, Aass N, Molne K. Is routine pre-treatment cryo-preservation of semen worthwhile in the management of patients with testicular cancer? Br J Urol. 1989;64(5):524-9.

8. Cruz MR, Prestes JC, Gimenes DL, Fanelli MF. Fertility preservation in women with breast cancer undergoing adjuvant chemotherapy: a systematic review. Fertil Steril. 2010;94(1):138-43.

9. Youssef MA, Van der Veen F, Al-Inany HG, Mochtar MH, Griesinger G, Nagi Mohesen M, et al. Gonadotropin-releasing hormone agonist versus HCG for oocyte triggering in antagonist-assisted reproductive technology. Cochrane Database Syst Rev. 2014;(10):CD008046.

10. Irtan S, Orbach D, Helfre S, Sarnacki S. Ovarian transposition in prepubescent and adolescent girls with cancer. Lancet Oncol. 2013;14(13):e601-8.

11. Howard FM. Laparoscopic lateral ovarian transposition before radiation treatment of Hodgkin disease. J Am Assoc Gynecol Laparosc. 1997;4(5):601-4.

12. Ben-Aharon I, Gafter-Gvili A, Leibovici L, Stemmer SM. Pharmacological interventions for fertility preservation during chemotherapy: a systematic review and meta-analysis. Breast Cancer Res Treat. 2010;122(3):803-11.

13. Clowse ME, Behera MA, Anders CK, Copland S, Coffman CJ, Leppert PC, et al. Ovarian preservation by GnRH agonists during chemotherapy: a metaanalysis. J Womens Health (Larchmt). 2009;18(3):311-9.

14. Blumenfeld Z, von Wolff M. GnRH-analogues and oral contraceptives for fertility preservation in women during chemotherapy. Hum Reprod Update. 2008;14(6):543-52.

15. Beck-Fruchter R, Weiss A, Shalev E. GnRH agonist therapy as ovarian protectants in female patients undergoing chemotherapy: a review of the clinical data. Hum Reprod Update. 2008;14(6):553-61.

16. Somigliana E, Peccatori FA, Filippi F, Martinelli F, Raspagliesi F, Martinelli I. Risk of thrombosis in women with malignancies undergoing ovarian stimulation for fertility preservation. Hum Reprod Update. 2014;20(6):944-51.

Unexplained Infertility

INTRODUCTION

Unexplained infertility or idiopathic infertility can be defined as cases in which no cause for infertility has been found upon the standard infertility testing, and the couple fails to achieve pregnancy after 12 months of attempting conception (6 months in women 35 years and older). According to the Practice Committee of the American Society for Reproductive Medicine (ASRM) guidelines for standard infertility evaluation, standard infertility testing includes tests for confirmation of ovulation, tests for confirmation of tubal patency, and tests for uterine factor and semen analysis.[1] In some cases, if required, tests for ovarian reserve and laparoscopic examination may also be performed. These tests, however, are no longer done as part of the routine fertility workup. Introduction of additional tests for identifying potential causes of infertility is not cost-effective and is unlikely to change the management plan. The current rate of unexplained infertility varies from 15% to 30% for couples with a female partner under the age of 35 years. This rate can increase to about 50% with the age of female partner increasing to 40 years or above.[2]

AETIOLOGY

As per the definition of unexplained infertility, its cause remains unknown. The abnormalities are likely to be present, but remain undetected using the standard tests. Slight functional changes in follicle development, ovulation and the luteal phase may be responsible for unexplained infertility. Some likely risk factors for unexplained infertility are as follows:[3]

❖ *Failure of ovulation*: Ovum could not be released at the optimum time for fertilisation or ovum may not be able enter the fallopian tube
❖ *Poor quality of the egg*: It is progressively being acknow-ledged that egg quality of the ovum is of prime importance for successful conception. Poor egg quality may be associated with poor quality embryos.
❖ *Failure of fertilisation*: Failure of fertilisation may occur because sperm may not be able to reach the egg
❖ *Failure of implantation*: Transport of the zygote till the uterine endometrium may be disturbed, or there may be failure of implantation
❖ *Increased age of the female partner*: The possibility of unexplained infertility is considerably increased in women above the age of 35 years. This is probably related to a decline in the oocyte count and poor egg quality with the woman's increasing age. Women of advanced maternal age are likely to have poor-quality eggs having reduced capability for normal and successful fertilisation.
❖ *Mild endometriosis*: Some experts believe that the infer-tility associated with mild endometriosis belongs to the 'unexplained' category because a cause and effect relationship between mild endometriosis and fertility problems has not been definitely established.

It is also possible that no defect is actually present in cases of unexplained infertility and it just represents the lower extreme of the normal distribution of fertility. This is so because the likelihood of pregnancy without treatment amongst couples with unexplained infertility is less than that of fertile couples but is greater than zero.

The exact mechanism behind unexplained infertility is yet not clear. Polymorphisms in the genes related to folate pathways could be one reason for fertility complications in some women with unexplained infertility.[4] Aberrations in the sperm DNA methylation patterns may be responsible for infertility amongst normozoospermic men.[5] Epigenetic modifications in sperm may be partially responsible for infertility. Altered epigenetic profiles (e.g. histone-to-protamine exchange, aberrant epigenetic reprogramming postfertilisation, etc.) have been identified in sperms from men with oligozoospermia and oligoasthenoteratozoospermia.[6] Genetic and environmental factors are also likely to have negative effects on epigenetic processes controlling implan-tation, placentation and foetal growth.

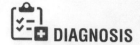

DIAGNOSIS

Clinical Presentation

General Physical Examination

Body mass index: Measurement of BMI is important in these cases because women having BMI in the range of 19–30 kg/m² before commencing assisted reproduction are likely to have higher success rates in comparison to the women having BMI outside this range.

Investigations

As per the definition of unexplained infertility, the following investigations should be done before making the diagnosis of unexplained infertility:[7]

- ❖ Tests for the evaluation of ovulation (urinary LH ovulation predictor kits and mid-luteal serum progesterone testing)
- ❖ Tests for the evaluation of tubal patency (hysterosalpingo-graphy)
- ❖ Tests for the evaluation of uterine factor (pelvic ultrasound)
- ❖ Semen analysis.

In some selected cases, tests for ovarian reserve and laparoscopic examination may be required.

- ❖ *Tests for ovarian reserve*: Women with advanced age (≥35 years) or history of prior ovarian surgery are at an increased risk for diminished ovarian function or reserve. Ovarian function can be assessed with the help of tests such as day 3 serum FSH and oestradiol levels, clomiphene citrate challenge test, and/or an ultrasonographic ovarian antral follicle count.[1]
- ❖ *Role of laparoscopy in infertility evaluation:* While in the past, laparoscopy used to be the part of basic infertility workup, nowadays, laparoscopic examination of pelvis is reserved only for selected cases. According to ASRM guidelines, laparoscopy should be performed in women with unexplained infertility having signs and symptoms of endometriosis or in suspected cases of reversible adhesive tubal disease.[1]

MANAGEMENT

The treatment for unexplained infertility is therefore, by definition, pragmatic because there is no underlying specific defect or functional impairment. The management strategies most commonly used in the cases of unexplained infertility include, expectant observation with timed intercourse and lifestyle changes, clomiphene citrate, intrauterine insemination (IUI), and controlled ovarian hyperstimulation (COH) with IUI and IVF. The optimal treatment strategy needs to be based on individual patient characteristics such as age of the female partner, side-effect profile, cost considerations, etc. Each of these treatment strategies have been described next in detail.

Expectant Management

Expectant management comprises no medical treatment and forms the first line of management in cases of unexplained infertility. It involves the use of timed intercourse and lifestyle changes for helping the couples achieve natural conception. Expectant management is likely to be useful in younger couples with short duration of infertility. The female partner should be counselled to achieve a normal BMI (between 19 kg/m² and 30 kg/m²), reduce caffeine intake to no more than two cups of coffee daily (250 mg daily), and reduce alcohol intake to no more than four standardised drinks per week.[8] Although expectant management is associated with the lowest cost, it results in the lowest fecundity or fertility rates per cycle. Therefore, this method can be considered inferior to the commonly available reproductive techniques described next. A retrospective analysis of 45 published studies by Guzick et al. has shown that the combined pregnancy rates per initiated cycle vary between 1.3% to 4.1% in the untreated groups. This rate is likely to be the lowest in comparison to other treatment interventions.[9] In a study from Netherlands, cumulative chances of pregnancy over a 12-month period in the couples with unexplained infertility while waiting for an IVF or ICSI, varied between 10% to 15%.[10] Expectant management may serve as a useful option for couples with unexplained infertility in which the female partner is young and has a good ovarian reserve.

Intrauterine Insemination

Intrauterine insemination of the sperms in the uterus at around the time of ovulation is the most commonly used treatment option in case of unexplained infertility. IUI is likely to be associated with higher chances of natural conception in cases of unexplained infertility in comparison to the other causes of infertility.[11] It can be performed in combination with natural ovulation timed with LH kit and ovulation stimulation using clomiphene citrate or injectable gonadotropins. Though IUI in combination with ovarian stimulation is likely to be more effective than the use of IUI alone, it is likely to be associated with a higher risk of complications, e.g. multiple pregnancies.[12]

Intrauterine insemination can also be used in cases where the male partner is diagnosed with ejaculatory dysfunction or mild male factor infertility or where the female partner is diagnosed with mild endometriosis. Moreover, IUI with donor sperms can be used as a treatment option in cases of single women, lesbians or in heterosexual couples where the male partner is diagnosed with aspermia.[13] IUI can also be used as an option in couples who are unable to or would find it very difficult to have vaginal intercourse because of a clinically diagnosed physical disability or those with psychosexual problems who are using partner or donor sperm.

Women with unexplained infertility who fail to conceive even after six cycles of donor or partner insemination must be offered a further six cycles of unstimulated IUI before being considered for IVF.

To further increase the efficacy of IUI in couples with unexplained infertility, many techniques have been tried. One such technique is pertubation which is likely to improve the efficacy of IUI through mechanical as well as anti-inflammatory effect on the spermatozoa. In a prospective, randomised, open study, it was shown that preovulatory pertubation treatment with low-dose local anaesthetic agent during clomiphene citrate and insemination cycles for couples with unexplained infertility is likely to significantly enhance the clinical pregnancy rate. Moreover, this procedure was well-tolerated and no complications were noted.[14] The combined treatment of clomiphene citrate, pertubation and insemination can be used as a cost-effective, first-line treatment for couples with unexplained infertility.

Controlled Ovarian Hyperstimulation

Both clomiphene citrate and gonadotropins have been used for COH, in combination with IUI or alone.

Clomiphene Citrate

Use of clomiphene citrate for ovarian stimulation in women with unexplained infertility who are already ovulating is unlikely to be effective. Moreover, the treatment with clomiphene citrate is costly and has been neither shown to shorten the time to pregnancy nor increase the rate of live birth.[15] Treatment with clomiphene citrate tablets along with IUI has been shown to be useful in improving the fertility rates, but not the pregnancy rates in couples with unexplained infertility or surgically corrected endometriosis.[16]

The association between infertility and minimal to mild endometriosis is controversial and poorly understood. A retrospective, controlled cohort study has shown that COH and IUI shortly after laparoscopic excision of endometriosis is as effective as COH and IUI in patients with unexplained subfertility.[17]

Nevertheless, clomiphene citrate has been commonly used for the treatment of unexplained infertility in the UK. Though the previous evidence based on a number of small randomised trials supports the use of clomiphene in the cases of unexplained subfertility and the NICE fertility guidelines (UK) approve the use of clomiphene citrate for cases of unexplained infertility, the present evidence indicates that the use of clomiphene citrate is not likely to be more effective in comparison to the expectant management.[15] Therefore, administration of clomiphene (without insemination) is usually not recommended for treatment of women over the age of 35 years with unexplained infertility. Moreover, before commencing treatment with clomiphene citrate, its high cost and potential side effects (e.g. risk of multiple pregnancy, threefold increased risk of ovarian cancer if used for >12 cycles) should be discussed with the patient.[18]

Gonadotropin Injections

Use of gonadotropins may be associated with an increased risk of multiple pregnancy. IVF rather than IUI with gonadotropins is preferred for women in whom clomiphene citrate with IUI has failed. An RCT (FASTT trial) has shown that the addition of gonadotropins to IUI cycle is not likely to be associated with any additional benefit.[19]

Assisted Reproductive Technologies and In Vitro Fertilisation

The most successful, but at the same time, most expensive treatment of unexplained infertility consists of the spectrum of assisted reproductive technology including IVF, with or without ICSI. IVF serves as the treatment of choice for unexplained infertility when the less costly, but also less effective treatment modalities described previously have failed.[20] IVF is likely to be associated with high success rates in young women with unexplained infertility having normal ovarian reserves. IVF remains the treatment of choice in longstanding unexplained infertility and, when coupled with the use of elective single embryo transfer, can help minimise the risk of multiple pregnancies. Data from randomised trials confirming the superiority of IVF over expectant management is limited.[21]

If the woman (below the age of 40 years) with unexplained infertility does not conceive even after three cycles of IUI, IVF can be considered. IVF can also be offered if expectant management fails to be successful after a period of 2 years. In these cases, IVF appears to be more cost-effective. In addition to offering the highest success rate, IVF also helps in explaining the cause of infertility in some of these couples. In some IVF programmes, ICSI is performed in all couples with unexplained infertility. On the other hand, other IVF programmes may perform ICSI in 50% of the retrieved oocytes. ICSI helps in dealing with an undetected fertilisation problem.

Last Options

In the women in whom none of the above options appear to be successful, one of the following strategies can be adopted as the last resort for achieving pregnancy: ovulation induction with the aromatase inhibitor (e.g. letrozole), pregnancy with donor egg, gestational surrogacy, adoption, etc.

COMPLICATIONS

- ❖ *Complications associated with ovarian stimulation:* Ovarian stimulation may be associated with complications such as ovarian hyperstimulation syndrome, multiple pregnancy, increased cost, etc.
- ❖ Pregnancies following IUI are likely to be associated with higher risk of obstetric complications such as pre-eclampsia, abruptio placentae, preterm labour, multifoetal gestation, emergency caesarean section and induction of labour.[22]

CLINICAL PEARLS

- ❖ The prognosis for spontaneous pregnancy in couples with unexplained infertility is better than in those with diagnosed causes of infertility.

CHAPTER 79

❖ Women with an advanced age or history of prior ovarian surgery are at risk for diminished ovarian function or reserve.

❖ The longer the duration of infertility, the less likely is it for the couple to conceive on their own. After 5 years of infertility, a couple with unexplained infertility has less than a 10% chance for success on their own.

EVIDENCE-BASED MEDICINE

❖ Though IVF is commonly used for the treatment of unexplained infertility, presently there is little evidence to support the efficacy of IVF in comparison to other management strategies such as expectant management, IUI alone and IUI along with ovarian stimulation. IVF is likely to be more effective than the use of expectant management, IUI alone as well as the combination of IUI with ovarian stimulation in women who have had previous unsuccessful treatment. However, the results have to be interpreted with caution. Before considering IVF for management of unexplained infertility, clinicians and couples need to balance the invasive nature of IVF and its costs against chances of success with other treatment modalities.[20,21] Also, presently there is limited evidence regarding the adverse effects related with the use of these various interventions in cases of unexplained infertility.

❖ The available evidence does not indicate any significant difference in the rates of live birth in couples with unexplained infertility treated with IUI (both with and without ovarian hyperstimulation) in comparison to those couples treated with timed intercourse.[12,15]

REFERENCES

1. The Practice Committee of the American Society for Reproductive Medicine. Optimal evaluation of the infertile female. Fertil Steril. 2006;86(5 Suppl):S264-7.
2. The Practice Committee of the American Society for Reproductive Medicine. Effectiveness and treatment for unexplained infertility. Fertil Steril. 2006;86(5 Suppl):S111-4.
3. Kamath MS, Bhattacharya S. Demographics of infertility and management of unexplained infertility. Best Pract Res Clin Obstet Gynaecol. 2012;26(6):729-38.
4. Altmäe S, Stavreus-Evers A, Ruiz JR, Laanpere M, Syvänen T, Yngve A, et al. Variations in folate pathway genes are associated with unexplained female infertility. Fertil Steril. 2010;94(1):130-7.
5. Aston KI, Uren PJ, Jenkins TG, Horsager A, Cairns BR, Smith AD, et al. Aberrant sperm DNA methylation predicts male fertility status and embryo quality. Fertil Steril. 2015;104(6):1388-97.e1-5.
6. Dada R, Kumar M, Jesudasan R, Fernández JL, Gosálvez J, Agarwal A. Epigenetics and its role in male infertility. J Assist Reprod Genet. 2012;29(3):213-23.
7. Quaas A, Dokras A. Diagnosis and treatment of unexplained infertility. Rev Obstet Gynecol. 2008 Spring;1(2):69-76.
8. Barbieri RL. The initial fertility consultation: recommendations concerning cigarette smoking, body mass index, and alcohol and caffeine consumption. Am J Obstet Gynecol. 2001;185(5):1168-73.
9. Guzick DS, Sullivan MW, Adamson GD, Cedars MI, Falk RJ, Peterson EP, et al. Efficacy of treatment for unexplained infertility. Fertil Steril. 1998;70(2):207-13.
10. Eijkemans MJ, Lintsen AM, Hunault CC, Bouwmans CA, Hakkaart L, Braat DD, et al. Pregnancy chances on an IVF/ICSI waiting list: a national prospective cohort study. Hum Reprod. 2008;23(7):1627-32.
11. Veltman-Verhulst SM, Hughes E, Ayeleke RO, Cohlen BJ. Intrauterine insemination for unexplained subfertility. Cochrane Database Syst Rev. 2016;(2):CD001838.
12. Bhattacharya S, Harrild K, Mollison J, Wordsworth S, Tay C, Harrold A, et al. Clomifene citrate or unstimulated intrauterine insemination compared with expectant management for unexplained infertility: pragmatic randomized control trial. BMJ. 2008;337:a716.
13. National Institute of Clinical Excellence (NICE). (2013). Fertility problems: assessment and treatment. Clinical guideline [CG156]. [online] Available from www.nice.org.uk/guidance/cg156 [Accessed October, 2016].
14. Hughes E, Brown J, Collins JJ, Vanderkerchove P. Clomiphene citrate for unexplained subfertility in women. Cochrane Database Syst Rev. 2010;(1):CD000057.
15. Deaton JL, Gibson M, Blackmer KM, Nakajima ST, Badger GJ, Brumsted JR. A randomized, controlled trial of clomiphene citrate and intrauterine insemination in couples with unexplained infertility or surgically corrected endometriosis. Fertil Steril. 1990;54(6):1083-8.
16. Werbrouck E, Spiessens C, Meuleman C, D'Hooghe T. No difference in cycle pregnancy rate and in cumulative live-birth rate between women with surgically treated minimal to mild endometriosis and women with unexplained infertility after controlled ovarian hyperstimulation and intrauterine insemination. Fertil Steril. 2006;86(3):566-71.
17. Wordsworth S, Buchanan J, Mollison J, Harrild K, Robertson L, Tay C, et al. Clomifene citrate and intrauterine insemination as first-line treatments for unexplained infertility: are they cost-effective? Hum Reprod. 2011;26(2):369-75.
18. Edelstam G, Sjösten A, Bjuresten K, Ek I, Wånggren K, Spira J. A new rapid and effective method for treatment of unexplained infertility. Hum Reprod. 2008;23(4):852-6.
19. Reindollar RH, Regan MM, Neumann PJ, Levine BS, Thornton KL, Alper MM. A randomized clinical trial to evaluate optimal treatment for unexplained infertility: the fast track and standard treatment (FASTT) trial. Fertil Steril. 2010;94(3):888-99.
20. Pandian Z, Gibreel A, Bhattacharya S. In vitro fertilisation for unexplained subfertility. Cochrane Database Syst Rev. 2015;(11):CD003357.
21. Sitti-Amina AA, Mares P. Recent data on the treatment of unexplained infertility with clomiphene citrate, intrauterine insemination, and in vitro fertilization. Contracep Fertil Sex. 1997;25(2):95-100.
22. Pandian Z, Bhattacharya S, Templeton A. Review of unexplained infertility and obstetric outcome: a 10 year review. Hum Reprod. 2001;16(12):2593-7.

Urogynaecological and Pelvic Floor Abnormalities

GYNAECOLOGY

Urogenital Prolapse

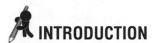 **INTRODUCTION**

Uterine prolapse can be described as a descent or herniation of the uterus into or beyond the vagina. Uterine prolapse is best considered under the broader heading of 'pelvic organ prolapse,' which also includes abnormalities, such as cystocele, urethrocele, enterocele and rectocele. Anatomically, the vaginal vault has three compartments: (1) an anterior compartment (consisting of the anterior vaginal wall), (2) a middle compartment (cervix) and (3) a posterior compartment (posterior vaginal wall). Weakness of the anterior compartment results in cystocele and urethrocele, whereas that of the middle compartment, in the descent of uterine vault or uterine prolapse and enterocele. The weakness of the posterior compartment results in rectocele.[1] There is no medical cure for prolapse, except that in some cases, pessaries can be used to provide temporary relief against symptoms of prolapse. The only definitive cure for prolapse is surgery. Surgery helps in providing relief against symptoms of prolapse by restoring pelvic anatomy, sexual functioning and human physiologic functions (micturition and defecation).[2] Since uterine prolapse is not a life-threatening condition, surgery is indicated only if the patient feels that her condition is severe enough that it warrants correction. Mild prolapse, which is rarely symptomatic, does not require surgical correction. Surgery is usually advised in women over 40 years, unless it is contraindicated or hazardous on account of some medical disorders. Various surgical options which can be used in cases of prolapse are tabulated in Box 80.1. Although the choice of procedure largely depends on the surgeon's preference and experience, the gynaecologist needs to consider numerous factors, such as the patient's general health status, degree and type of uterine prolapse, requirement for preservation or restoration of coital function, concomitant intrapelvic disease and the patient's desire for preservation of menstrual and reproductive functions. The choice of surgery depends on numerous factors summarised here:

❖ Degree of prolapse
❖ Areas specific for prolapse
❖ Desire for future pregnancies
❖ Desire to maintain future sexual function
❖ Presence of concomitant medical conditions
❖ Preservation of vaginal function
❖ Woman's age and general health status
❖ Patient's choice (i.e. desire for surgery or no surgery)
❖ Severity of symptoms
❖ Patient's suitability for surgery
❖ Presence of other pelvic conditions requiring simultaneous treatment, including urinary or faecal incontinence
❖ Presence or absence of urethral hypermobility
❖ History of previous pelvic surgery.

Aim of surgery is to restore the pelvic anatomy and human physiologic functions, such as micturition, defecation and sexual functioning. A careful preoperative evaluation should be carried out in order to identify all concomitant defects associated with uterine prolapse, which should be repaired in order to avoid recurrence of prolapse in future. In patients with advanced degree of prolapse, additional procedures like transvaginal sacrospinous ligament fixation, transabdominal sacral colpopexy or colpectomy with colpocleisis may be required to provide adequate support to the vaginal vault.

Box 80.1: Surgical options which can be used in cases of prolapse

❑ Vaginal hysterectomy, posterior culdoplasty, colporrhaphy
❑ Vaginal hysterectomy, closure of enterocele sac, total colpectomy, colporrhaphy, colpocleisis
❑ Combined vaginal colporrhaphy and abdominal hysterectomy
❑ Moschcowitz culdoplasty, sacral colpopexy and suprapubic urethrocolpopexy
❑ Manchester operation
❑ Vaginal repair and uterine suspension
❑ Abdominal sling surgery

Table 80.1: Baden-Walker Halfway system for evaluation of pelvic organ prolapse

Stage	Definition
0	Normal position for each respective site
I	Descent of the cervix to any point in the vagina above the introitus
II	Descent of the cervix up to the introitus
III	Descent of the cervix halfway past the hymen
IV	Total eversion or procidentia

Evaluation of the Degree of Prolapse

Baden-Walker Halfway System

Uterine prolapse can be classified into four stages based on Baden-Walker halfway system as described in Table 80.1. This is the system which is commonly used for evaluation of pelvic organ prolapse. Another important system, which is often used for evaluation of pelvic organ prolapse, is the pelvic organ prolapse quantification (POP-Q) system for quantification of pelvic prolapse and is described next.

POP-Q System for Quantification of Pelvic Prolapse

In 1966, the International Continence Society defined the POP-Q system for quantification of pelvic prolapse. This system is based on a series of site-specific measurements of the woman's pelvic organ support system in relation to the hymen in each of the segments. This system is based on the measurement of six points, which are located with reference to the plane of the hymen: two on the anterior vaginal wall (Aa and Ba), two in the apical vagina (C and D) and two on the posterior vaginal wall (Ap and Bp). All these six points are measured with the patient engaged in maximum protrusion and have been illustrated in Figure 80.1.[1]

While assessing the degree of prolapse using the POP-Q system, the hymenal plane is defined as zero (Table 80.2). The anatomical position of these points from the hymen is measured in centimetres. Points above the hymen are described with a negative number, whereas the points below the hymen are described using a positive number. It is important to remember that these various measurements can change in accordance with the position of the patient, e.g. whether the patient was standing or in lithotomy position or whether she was asked to strain. Thus, it is important to mention the patient's position at the time of taking measurements. If the POP-Q examination is performed, firstly the genital hiatus and the perineal body are measured during the Valsalva manoeuvre. The total vaginal length (TVL) is the only measurement made while the patient is not engaged in Valsalva manoeuver. It is measured by placing the marked ring forceps at the vaginal apex and noting the distance to the hymen. The apical points C and D are then measured during maximal Valsalva effort. The anterior and posterior vaginal walls are next visualised and lastly the points Aa, Ba, Ap and Bp are, respectively, measured. The urethra is also evaluated during anterior vaginal wall assessment. If the posterior vaginal wall descends, attempts must be made to determine whether rectocele or enterocele is present. The POP-Q staging system is shown in Table 80.2.

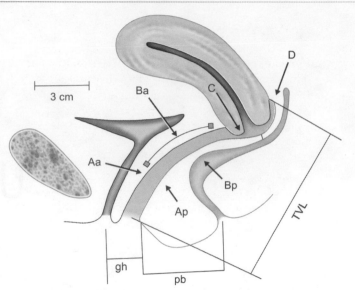

Fig. 80.1: POP-Q system for quantification of pelvic prolapse[1]

Abbreviation: POP-Q, pelvic organ prolapse quantification

Point Aa: This is the point on the anterior vaginal wall in the midline and lies 3 cm above the external urethral meatus, corresponding to the proximal location of the urethrovesical crease; Point Ap: This point is located 3 cm proximal to the hymen on the posterior vaginal wall; Point Ba: This point represents the most distal edge of cervix or vaginal cuff; Point Bp: This point represents the most distal position of the upper portion of the posterior vaginal wall from the vaginal cuff; Point C: This point either represents the most distal edge of the cervix or the leading edge of the vaginal cuff after total hysterectomy; Point D: This represents the location of posterior fornix in a woman who still has a cervix; Total vaginal length (TVL): This is the greatest depth of vagina (in centimetres) when points C and D are reduced to their fullest position; The genital hiatus (gh) is measured from the middle of the external urethral meatus to the midline of the posterior hymenal ring. The perineal body (pb) is measured from the posterior margin of the genital hiatus to the mid-anal opening.

Table 80.2: POP-Q staging system for pelvic organ prolapse

Stage of prolapse	Definition
Stage 0	No prolapse is demonstrated. Points Aa, Ap, Ba and Bp are all 3 cm above the hymenal ring (value = −3) and either points C or D is at a position above the hymen that is equal to or within 2 cm of total vaginal length (TVL). Thus, the quantitation value for point C or D is ≤ −(TVL − 2 cm)
Stage I	The criteria for stage 0 are not met, but all the points are >1 cm above the level of the hymen (i.e. its quantitation value is ≤ −1 cm)
Stage II	The most distal portion of the prolapse protrudes to a point to or above 1 cm above the hymen but no more than 1 cm beyond the hymen (i.e. its quantitation value ≥1 cm but ≤ +1 cm)
Stage III	The most distal portion of the prolapse protrudes at least 1 cm below the plane of hymen but protrudes no further than 2 cm less than the TVL (in cm), i.e. its quantitation value is > +1 cm but < +(TVL − 2 cm)
Stage IV	Complete eversion of the total length of the lower genital tract is demonstrated. The distal portion of the prolapse protrudes to within 2 cm of the TVL, i.e. its quantitation value is ≥ +(TVL− 2) cm

Abbreviation: POP-Q, pelvic organ prolapse quantification

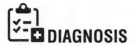 AETIOLOGY

Uterine prolapse usually occurs in postmenopausal and multiparous women, in whom the pelvic floor muscles and the ligaments that support the female genital tract have become slack and atonic. Injury to the pelvic floor muscles during repeated childbirths, causing excessive stretching of the pelvic floor muscles and ligaments acts as a major risk factor for causing reduced tone of the pelvic floor muscles.[3] Reduced oestrogen levels following menopause is another important cause for atonicity and reduced elasticity of the muscles of pelvic floor. Prolapse can also occur in nulliparous women due to conditions such as spina occulta and split pelvis.

Indications of various surgeries performed for prolapse are listed in Box 80.2.[4,5]

DIAGNOSIS

Clinical Presentation

❖ Minor prolapse can be asymptomatic.
❖ The main complaint in cases of uterovaginal prolapse is a feeling of something coming down the vagina, sensation of lump in the vagina, a feeling of pelvic insecurity and low backache. The symptoms are relieved by lying flat.
❖ Bloodstained vaginal discharge may be present in the cases of procidentia and decubitus ulcerations.

Box 80.2: Indications for various surgeries performed for uterine prolapse[4,5]

Hysterectomy
❑ Removal of a non-functioning organ in postmenopausal women
❑ Concomitant uterine or cervical pathology (e.g. large fibroid uterus, endometrial carcinoma, etc.)
❑ Patient desires removal of the uterus

Anterior colporrhaphy
❑ Presence of cystocele, urethrocele or a cystourethrocele
❑ Repair of anterior defects

Posterior colpoperineorrhaphy
❑ Presence of a rectocele
❑ Repair of posterior defects

Manchester operation
❑ Childbearing function is not required
❑ Malignancy of the endometrium has been ruled out
❑ Absence of urinary tract infection
❑ Presence of a small cystocele with only a first- or second-degree prolapse
❑ Absence of an enterocele
❑ Symptoms of prolapse are largely due to cervical elongation
❑ Patient requires preservation of menstrual function

Le Fort colpocleisis
❑ No sexual activity at present or no plans for sexual activity in future
❑ Patient is medically fragile

❖ Urinary symptoms, such as difficulty in passing urine and recurrent UTIs, may be associated with cystocele and cystourethrocele.
❖ Presence of rectocele may be associated with symptoms such as difficulty with defecation or incomplete defecation.

Investigations

The diagnosis of pelvic prolapse is established on the basis of history and clinical examination. Routine investigations, which must be ordered prior to surgery, include CBC with haematocrit, urine routine and microscopy, kidney function tests, chest X-ray and ultrasound examination.

 SURGICAL MANAGEMENT

Principles of Surgery for Pelvic Organ Prolapse

The following principles must be taken into consideration, while undertaking surgery for pelvic organ prolapse:[6,7]

❖ At the time of clinical examination, when the patient is made to bear down, the site of primary damage appears first, followed by the sites of secondary damage. The gynaecologist must take special note of this site of primary damage. The primary site of damage should be identified first and over-repaired in order to reduce the chances of recurrence.
❖ The gynaecologist must repair all relaxations of the supporting tissues, even if they are minor in order to prevent recurrence in the future.
❖ The strength of the various support structures should be evaluated. Even the relatively weak structures can be used, but they must not be used to provide dependable support at the time of reconstruction surgery.
❖ As far as possible, the surgeon must try to create a normal anatomy. Normal vaginal length should be maintained because a shortened vagina is likely to prolapse again.
❖ The vagina should be suspended in its normal posterior direction over the levator plate and rectum, pointing into the hollow of the sacrum, towards S3 and S4. The surgeon should avoid suspending the vaginal vault anteriorly to the abdominal wall.
❖ The cul-de-sac should be closed and rectocele repaired in all cases. A posterior colpoperineorrhaphy should be preferably performed in all cases, where possible. Repair of the lower posterior vaginal wall provides some support to the anterior vaginal wall and also lengthens the vagina. When performed in properly selected patients, anterior colporrhaphy serves as an effective procedure for treating stress incontinence, which may be commonly associated with anterior cystocele. A vaginal hysterectomy may not always be indicated in a patient, in whom the primary aim is to repair a cystocele. In fact, a vaginal hysterectomy with anterior colporrhaphy may produce a variety of disorders of the bladder function, including stress urinary incontinence, detrusor instability and other voiding difficulties.

Removal of uterus helps in facilitating the repair of an enterocele. The choice of surgery for repair of enterocele and massive eversion of vagina includes perineorrhaphy. A hysterectomy with colporrhaphy and colpopexy works well for the patient with prolapse, who wishes to preserve coital interest. Colpocleisis can be considered for patients in whom preservation of the sexual functioning is not important. When the uterosacral ligaments are long and strong, the addition of McCall or New Orleans type of culdoplasty will help to re-establish the vaginal length. The McCall's culdoplasty involves attaching the uterosacral cardinal ligament complex to the peritoneal surface. The sutures are attached in such a way so that when they are tied, the uterosacral cardinal ligaments are drawn towards the midline. This helps in closing off the cul-de-sac. Additionally, when the sutures are tied, the posterior vaginal apex is drawn up to a higher position, thereby supporting the vaginal vault.

❖ Various abdominal surgeries for prolapse include sling operations, closure or repair of enterocele, sacrocolpopexy (suspension of the vaginal apex to the sacral promontory), anterior colpopexy (stitching of vagina to the ileopectineal ligament), colposuspension (fixation of the vaginal vault to the abdominal wall via a fascial strip or mersilene tape) and paravaginal repairs.

Preoperative Preparation

❖ Medical treatment for chronic cough or constipation must be administered.
❖ If decubitus ulceration is present over the prolapsed tissue, it first needs to be treated by the application of glycerine acriflavine pack or ring pessaries.
❖ Surgery must be undertaken only when the associated infections (UTI, PID, etc.) have been aggressively treated.
❖ Preoperative oestrogen therapy must be given, especially to the elderly postmenopausal patients, in whom vaginal epithelium is thin and inflamed.
❖ Full dose of antibiotics (80 mg of gentamycin, 1 g of ampicillin and 500 mg of metronidazole) must be administered 2 hours before surgery to prevent postoperative pelvic infections.
❖ Recent advances in pelvic imaging such as MRI prior to surgery helps in making various measurements such as the urethrovesical angle, descent of the bladder base, quality of the levator muscles and the relationship between the vagina and its lateral connective tissue attachments.
❖ A urinalysis should be performed prior to surgery for evaluation of UTI, especially if the patient reports any dysfunction of the lower urinary tract.
❖ In the presence of symptoms of incontinence or voiding dysfunction, urodynamic assessment of filling and voiding function is generally indicated.
❖ Preoperative assessment in case of Le Fort colpocleisis comprises undertaking a vaginal smear and endometrial curettage for ruling out any pathology, particularly malignancy. In long-standing cases, an intravenous pyelogram may be required because of the tendency towards associated hydroureter and hydronephrosis due to kinking of the ureter. Cystoscopy and renal function tests are also essential in long-standing cases to rule out concomitant renal pathology.

Steps of Surgery

Anterior Colporrhaphy

Anterior colporrhaphy operation is one of the most commonly performed surgeries to repair a cystocele and cystourethrocele.[8,9] This surgery is usually performed under general or regional anaesthesia.

Principles of anterior colporrhaphy: Anterior colporrhaphy comprises of the following steps:
❖ Excision of a portion of relaxed anterior vaginal wall
❖ Mobilisation of bladder
❖ Pushing the bladder upwards after cutting the vesico-cervical ligament
❖ Permanently supporting the bladder by tightening the pubocervical fascia.

Steps of surgery: Steps for anterior colporrhaphy comprise of the following:
❖ A speculum is inserted into the vagina to expose it during the procedure. Traction is applied on the cervix using Allis forceps, in order to expose the anterior vaginal wall.
❖ An inverted T-shaped incision is made in the anterior vaginal wall, starting with a transverse incision on the bladder sulcus.
❖ Through the midpoint of this transverse incision, a vertical incision is given, which extends up to the urethral opening.
❖ The vaginal walls are reflected to either side, to expose the bladder and vesicovaginal fascia. Bladder is pushed upwards, and the vaginal skin is separated from the underlying fascia.
❖ The overlying vesicovaginal and pubocervical fascia is plicated with interrupted 0 catgut sutures to correct the vaginal wall laxity and to close the hiatus through which the bladder herniates.
❖ Redundant portion of the vaginal mucosa is cut on either side.
❖ Cut margins of vagina are apposed together.
❖ In women suffering from stress incontinence, a Kelly's suture to plicate the bladder neck, helps to correct stress incontinence.[10] Figures 80.2A to F illustrate the sequence of events in the repair of a midline defect cystocele.

Posterior Colporrhaphy and Colpoperineorrhaphy

While repairing the rectocele, most surgeons also perform a posterior colporrhaphy. This process involves non-specific midline plication of the rectovaginal fascia after reducing the rectocele. The lax vaginal tissue over the rectocele is excised. The medial fibres of the levator ani are then pulled together, approximated and sutured over the top of rectum.

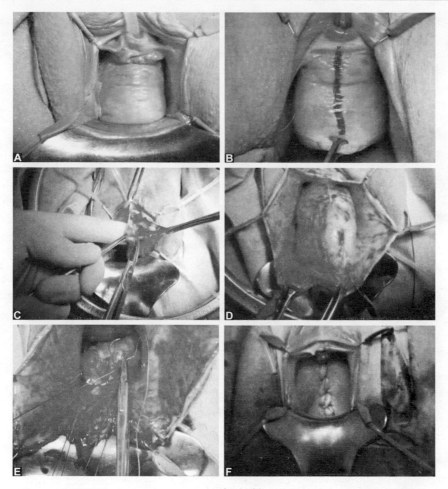

Figs 80.2A to F: (A) Appearance of cystocele just before giving the incision; (B) Skin incision is given over the skin overlying the cystocele; (C) Dissection of the underlying fascia; (D) Dissection of the underlying fascia is continued until the midline defect in pubocervical fascia is visualised; (E) The tissue under the bladder is plicated and pulled together in the midline, thus reducing the bulge. Following the reduction, excess vaginal skin is then cut off, which can create a shortened or constricted vagina; (F) Closure of the vaginal epithelium *(For colour version, see Plate 6)*

This helps in restoring the calibre of the hiatus urogenitalis and strengthening the perineal body. An adequate amount of perineum is also created, which helps in separating the hiatus urogenitalis from the anal canal. Though this surgery is quite effective in the treatment of the rectocele, these patients often suffer from dyspareunia following surgery. The surgical procedure for rectocele repair is illustrated in Figures 80.3A to F.

Manchester Repair

Manchester repair is performed in those cases where removal of the uterus is not required.[11]

Procedure: The procedure for Manchester repair (also called Fothergill operation) is shown in Figures 80.4A to E, and it comprises of the steps, described next in details.

❖ Anterior colporrhaphy is firstly performed
❖ The bladder is dissected from the cervix. A circular incision is given over the cervix
❖ The attachment of Mackenrodt ligaments to the cervix on each side are exposed, clamped and cut
❖ The vaginal incision is then extended posteriorly round the cervix

❖ The cervix is amputated and posterior lip of cervix is covered with a flap of mucosa
❖ The base of cardinal ligament is sutured over the anterior surface of cervix
❖ The raw area of the amputated cervix is then covered
❖ Colpoperineorrhaphy is ultimately performed to correct the posterior and perineal defects.

Abdominal Sling Surgery

Sling operations are especially useful in women, desirous of retaining their childbearing function, who are suffering from second-degree or third-degree prolapse. These surgeries aim at buttressing the weakened ligaments (e.g. Mackenrodt and uterosacral ligaments) with help of synthetic tapes such as nylon and Dacron that are used for forming slings to support the uterus.[12]

Principle of sling surgery: With a fascial strip or prosthetic material (mersilene tape or Dacron), the cervix is fixed to the abdominal wall, sacrum or pelvis.

Commonly performed abdominal sling surgery: The most commonly performed abdominal sling surgery is abdominal cervicopexy.[13]

CHAPTER 80

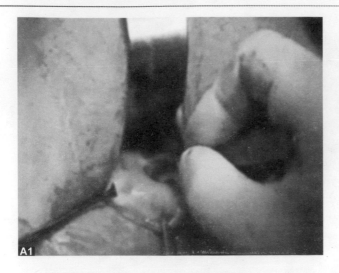

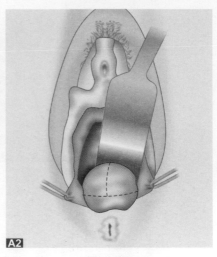

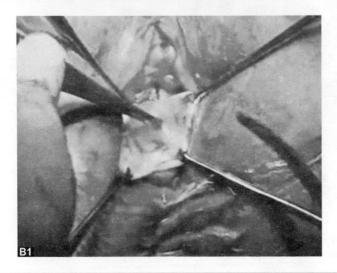

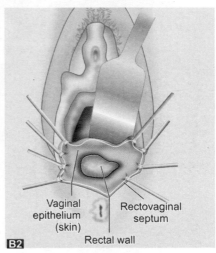

Vaginal
epithelium
(skin)

Rectovaginal
septum

Rectal wall

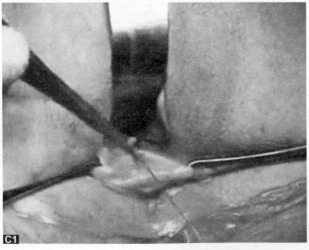

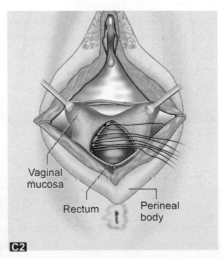

Vaginal
mucosa

Rectum

Perineal
body

Figs 80.3A to C (For colour version, see Plate 7)

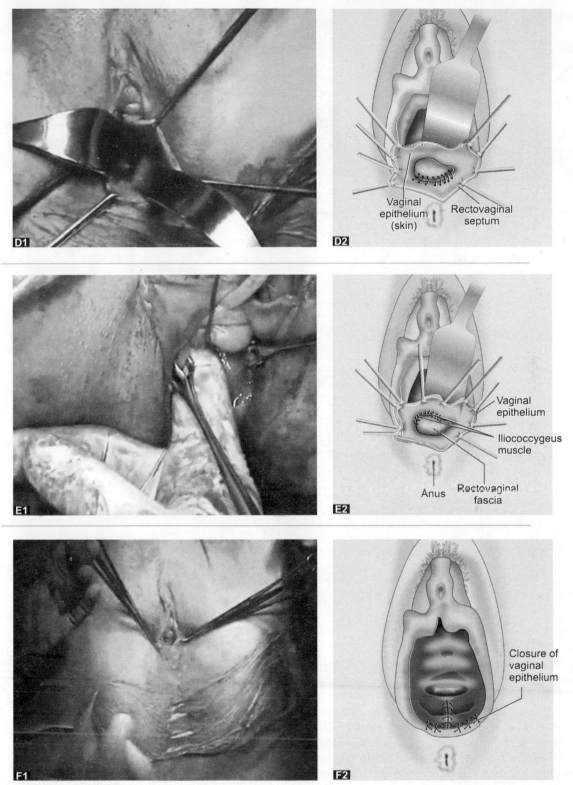

Figs 80.3A to F: Procedure of posterior colporrhaphy and colpoperineorrhaphy: (A1 and A2) Rectocele identified and skin incised: a bulge is apparent on the bottom (posterior) floor of the vagina. The dotted line represents the skin incision, about to be performed in this posterior repair procedure; (B1 and B2) Identification of the fascia break: the rectocele exists because of a break in the supportive layer known as the rectovaginal fascia. The defect is readily identified and the rectal wall is found protruding through this break in the rectovaginal fascia; (C1 and C2) The rectovaginal fascia is reattached to the perineal body, where the distal defect was located; (D1 and D2) The rectovaginal fascial defect has been repaired; (E1 and E2) The rectovaginal fascia is reattached to the iliococcygeal muscles bilaterally with permanent sutures; (F1 and F2) Closure of the vaginal epithelium (skin) completes the operation *(For colour version, see Plate 7)*

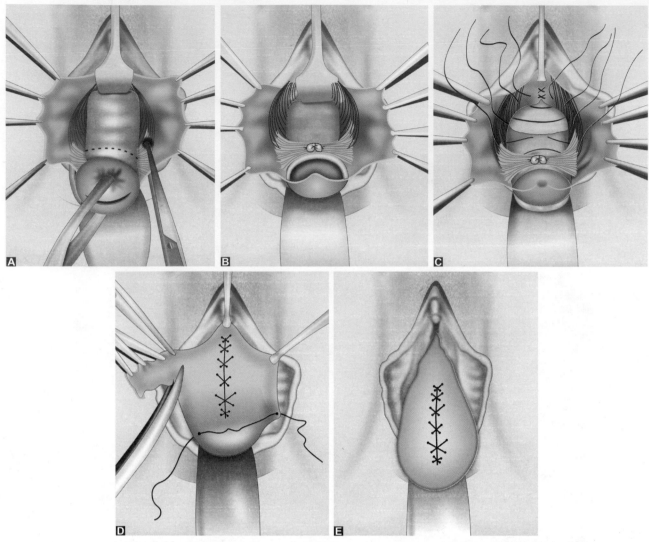

Figs 80.4A to E: Steps of Manchester repair; (A) The bladder is dissected from the cervix. A circular incision is given over the cervix. The base of cardinal ligament is exposed, clamped and cut; (B) The cervix is amputated and posterior lip of cervix is covered with a flap of mucosa. The base of cardinal ligament is sutured over the anterior surface of cervix; (C) Approximation of pubovesicocervical fascia in the midline; (D) The fascial approximation has been completed and excessive vaginal mucosa has been excised; (E) Vaginal mucosa has been closed

Abdominal Cervicopexy

Two musculofascial slings are obtained from the rectus sheath after giving transverse incisions and elevating the fascia from the midline outwards and laterally up to the lateral border of rectus abdominis muscle on either side. The uterus is brought into view after opening the peritoneum in the midline. The uterovesical fold of peritoneum is incised and bladder mobilised from the front of uterine isthmus. The medial ends of the sling are directed retroperitoneally between the two layers of broad ligament up to the space created in front of the uterine isthmus. The slings are pulled and anchored here with the help of non-absorbable sutures after ensuring adequate correction of the uterine position. Nowadays, surgeons are commonly using 12 inches long mersilene or nylon tapes instead of the tapes fashioned from the rectus sheath. Purandare and Mhatre's modification of this surgery involved attaching the tape posteriorly to the cervix, close to the attachments of the uterosacral ligaments.

Uterine Suspension

Vault prolapse is a delayed complication of both abdominal and vaginal hysterectomy when the supporting structures, i.e. paravaginal fascia and levator ani muscles become weak and deficient. It may also result from failure to identify and repair an enterocele during hysterectomy. Uterine suspension procedures involve putting the uterus back into its normal position. Various types of uterine suspensions can be performed either via the abdominal or vaginal route. This may be done by reattaching the pelvic ligaments to the lower part of the uterus to hold it in place (e.g. sacrospinous colpopexy).[14] Another technique uses special materials which act like sling in order to support the uterus in its proper position (abdominal sacral colpopexy). Recent advances include performing these procedures laparoscopically, thereby considerably reducing postoperative pain and facilitating speedy recovery.

Abdominal sacral colpopexy: This procedure comprises suspending the vault to the sacral promontory extraperitoneally using various grafts such as harvested fascia lata, abdominal fascia, dura mater, Marlex, Prolene, Gore-tex, Mersilene or cadaveric fascia lata (Figs 80.5A and B). Injury to the ureter, bladder, sigmoid colon and middle sacral artery should be avoided. Bleeding is the most serious complication of sacral colpopexy due to injury to the presacral venous plexus or the middle sacral artery while operating in the presacral space. The aim of surgery is to restore the normal pelvic anatomy as far as possible. At the end of the surgery, normal vaginal length should be maintained with its axis directed towards S3-S4 vertebra. Abdominal sacral colpopexy has the highest cure rate for vault prolapse, probably because of the use of graft tissue with high strength and not relying on the patient's own tissue that may not be strong enough to hold up the vaginal vault. As a result, sacral colposcopy can also be considered in patients who have had previous failed operations, older patients with poor tissue or patients with large defects or severe prolapse.

Transvaginal sacrospinous ligament fixation: In this method, the vaginal apex is attached, using permanent sutures, to the sacrospinous ligament. The posterior vaginal wall is opened vertically, following which a window space is created between the vagina and the rectum towards the right sacrospinous ligament. Using Deschamps ligature carrier, a synthetic ligature is used for fixing the vaginal vault to the sacrospinous ligament, 3–5 cm away from the ischial spine (Figs 80.6A and B). The suture must be placed through the ligament, rather than around it. The two most serious complications from sacrospinous ligament fixation are haemorrhage and nerve injury as a result of damage to the pudendal neurovascular bundle. Thus, the surgeon must try to avoid injuring the pudendal bundle and the inferior gluteal vessels as far as possible.

Postoperative Care

In the postoperative period, the following instructions must be given to the patient:

* ❖ The patient must be instructed in the postoperative period that she may experience slight vaginal spotting and difficulty in passing urine or stools.
* ❖ Appropriate antibiotics, analgesics and IV fluids must be administered.
* ❖ In order to prevent the problem of bladder distension once the catheter is removed, the patient must be advised to void 'by the clock,' after every 2–3 hours for about 15–20 days following surgery. If the residual urine volume after the removal of catheter is more than 50 mL, the catheter must be passed again.

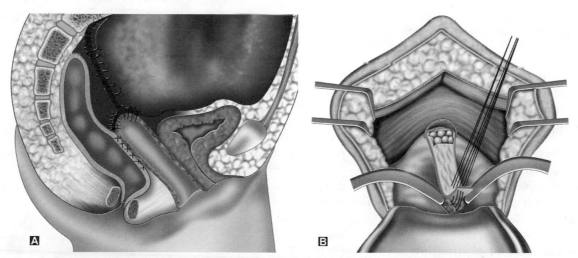

Figs 80.5A and B: Abdominal sacral colpopexy. (A) Lateral view; (B) Surgery as visualised from the abdominal incision (superior view)

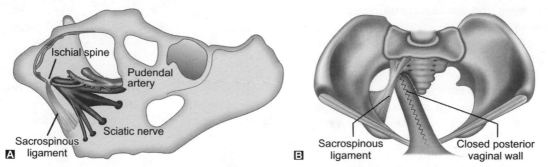

Figs 80.6A and B: (A) The sacrospinous ligament must be penetrated 3–5 cm medial to the ischial spine at the point marked by 'X'; (B) Transvaginal sacrospinous ligament fixation

CHAPTER 80

❖ In order to avoid straining of pelvic floor muscles, the patient must be advised to take precautions to help prevent constipation. Consuming a high-fibre diet is the best way of avoiding constipation. If constipation still develops, she can be prescribed stool softeners.

❖ The patient may experience vaginal and pelvic discomfort in the first week following surgery. This can be largely avoided by sitting in sitz baths (hot salt-water baths) once or twice daily.

❖ The patient should be asked to avoid sexual intercourse and lifting heavy weights for the first 6 weeks following surgery.

❖ The patient is instructed to come for a follow-up visit at 15 days and then again after 6 weeks to assess if the surgical wound has properly healed and whether the patient can resume her normal day-to-day activities.

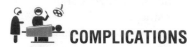

COMPLICATIONS

Complications due to Uterine Prolapse

Uterine prolapse, if not corrected, can interfere with bowel, bladder and sexual functions and result in the development of the following complications:

❖ Ulceration
❖ Infection or sepsis (including due to pessary use)
❖ Urinary incontinence
❖ Constipation
❖ Fistula formation
❖ Postrenal failure
❖ Decubitus ulceration.

Intraoperative Complications of Anterior Colporrhaphy

Intraoperative complications associated with the procedure of anterior colporrhaphy are as follows:[15]

❖ Excessive bleeding, requiring blood transfusion may occur. There can be development of a haematoma in the anterior vagina (especially after vaginal or paravaginal repair)
❖ Injury to the bladder or urethra in the course of dissection
❖ Ureteral damage or obstruction occurs rarely (0–2% incidence) usually with very large cystoceles or with apical prolapse
❖ Other rare complications include intravesical or urethral suture placement and fistula formation (either urethro-vaginal or vesicovaginal)
❖ Development of erosions, draining sinuses or chronic areas of vaginal granulation tissue, especially if permanent sutures or mesh material is used for the repair
❖ Urinary tract infections can commonly occur
❖ Voiding difficulty can occur after anterior vaginal wall prolapse repair. Treatment comprises of bladder drainage or intermittent self-catheterisation until spontaneous voiding resumes, usually within 6 weeks
❖ Sexual function may be positively or negatively affected by vaginal operations for anterior vaginal wall prolapse.

CLINICAL PEARLS

❖ The most important risk factor for the development of prolapse is the loss of strength of the pelvic support structures. Muscles [levator ani, coccygeus, obturator internus, piriformis, superficial transverse perineal muscles and deep transverse perineal muscles (Figs 80.7 and 80.8)] and ligaments of the pelvic floor [transverse cervical ligaments, uterosacral ligament, pubocervical ligament, pubourethral ligament and pelvic fascia (Fig. 80.9)] are the main source of support to the pelvic structures. Minor support is provided by the broad ligament and round ligaments.

❖ The supports for different parts of vagina have been summarised in Table 80.3.

❖ The perineal body, a pyramid-shaped fibromuscular structure lying at the midpoint between the vagina and the anus, assumes importance in providing support to the pelvic organs as it provides attachment to the following eight muscles of the pelvic floor: superficial and deep transverse perineal muscles; levator ani muscles of both the sides; bulbocavernosus anteriorly and the external anal sphincter posteriorly (Fig. 80.10).

❖ Expectant management, including the pelvic floor exercises (Kegel exercises) and vaginal pessaries are currently the mainstay of non-surgical management amongst patients with mild-degree uterine prolapse, with no or minimal symptoms.

EVIDENCE-BASED MEDICINE

Innovations in Surgery for Uterine Prolapse

Use of prosthetic material for prolapse surgery: Synthetic and biological prosthetic material is nowadays commonly being

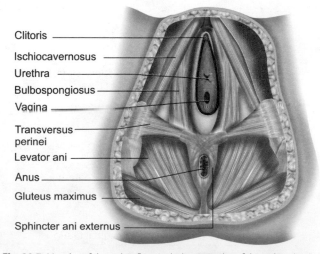

Clitoris
Ischiocavernosus
Urethra
Bulbospongiosus
Vagina
Transversus perinei
Levator ani
Anus
Gluteus maximus
Sphincter ani externus

Fig. 80.7: Muscles of the pelvic floor including muscles of the pelvic diaphragm (levator ani muscle); muscles of the urogenital diaphragm (deep transverse perineal muscle); superficial muscles of the pelvic floor (superficial transverse perineal muscle, external anal sphincter and bulbospongiosus)

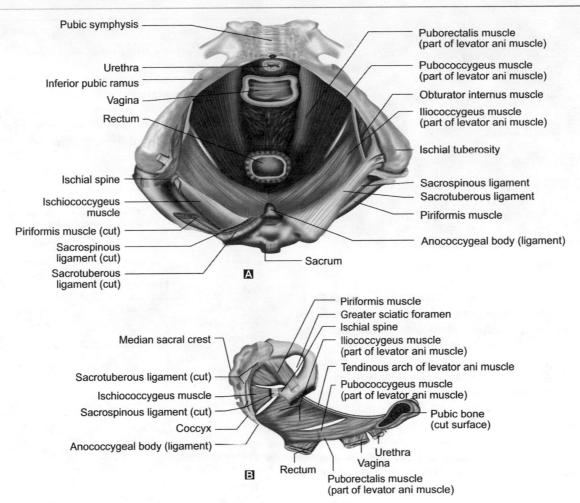

Figs 80.8A and B: Levator ani muscle: (A) Inferior view; (B) Lateral view

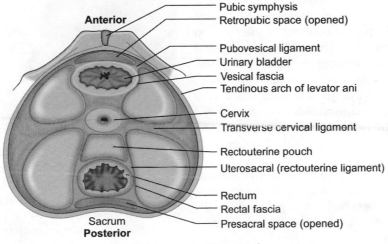

Fig. 80.9: Ligaments of the pelvic floor

Table 80.3: Different levels of support for vaginal tissue

Different levels of support of vagina	Support elements
Level I (for proximal one-third of vagina)	Cardinal and the uterosacral ligaments
Level II (for middle one-third of vagina)	Paravaginal fascia
Level III (for distal one-third of vagina and the introitus)	Levator ani and perineal muscles

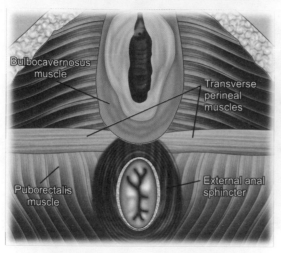

Fig. 80.10: Attachments of perineal body

PART III

used in cases of pelvic reconstructive surgery, especially in cases where women experience recurrence or in cases of repeat surgery. Anterior colporrhaphy with graft augmentation either involves use of a prosthetic material to help support the anterior vaginal wall or placement of a piece of polyglactin 910 mesh into the fold of imbricated bladder wall below the trigone and apical portion of the vaginal vault.[16]

Vaginal or paravaginal repair can also be carried out with graft augmentation. The various types of prosthetic material which is being used for prolapse surgery has been listed in Box 80.3. The objective of paravaginal defect repair for anterior vaginal wall prolapse is to reattach the detached lateral vaginal wall to its normal place of attachment at the level of the white line or 'arcus tendineus fasciae pelvis' which is done using a vaginal or retropubic approach.

Transobturator tension-free vaginal mesh techniques can also be used for management of anterior vaginal wall prolapse. These techniques facilitate a tension-free placement of an allograft, xenograft or polypropylene mesh implant without trimming of the vagina or suturing of the mesh to the vagina. The involved 'systems' allow selective application of anterior, posterior or total vaginal implants. Therefore, the requirement for hysterectomy is potentially eliminated. The mesh implants have arms that are delivered with trocars or special devices through anatomical landmarks via the obturator membrane or the ischiorectal fossa. Some of the currently available commercial kits have been listed in Table 80.4. Figure 80.11 shows perigee system for transobturator cystocele repair. The graft is depicted in the centre and has the dimensions of 5 × 10 cm. The graft has four arms that come out laterally and are attached to the pelvic sidewalls with the help of needles. The pink needles are the superior needles, which are used for attaching the bladder neck arms. The grey needles are the inferior needles, which are used for attaching the apical arms of the graft to the arcus tendineus. Figures 80.12A and B show that the graft has been placed in position under the bladder. It provides an entire new floor of support for the bladder from side-to-side. The skin of vagina is closed over the graft. The tissue in growth occurs rapidly causing the graft to get incorporated and soon become a part of patient's anatomy. High rate of anatomical cure due to the

Box 80.3: Various types of prosthetic material being used for prolapse surgery

Synthetic material
- ❑ Non-absorbable (Marlex, Prolene)
- ❑ Absorbable polyglactin (Vicryl)

Biological materials
- ❑ Autologous material (rectus fascia, fascia lata)
- ❑ Xenografts (porcine dermis or porcine small intestine submucosa)

New systems
- ❑ Polypropylene tapes
- ❑ Apogee and perigee

Table 80.4: Commercial transvaginal mesh kits available

Company	Device	Implant material
American Medical Systems Inc., Minnetonka, MN	Apogee/Perigee	Intepro polypropylene InteXen porcine dermis
Gynecare/Ethicon, Johnson & Johnson, Somerville, NJ	Anterior Prolift	Gynemesh-PS polypropylene
CR Bard Inc., Murray Hill, NJ	Avaulta-Plus	Polypropylene + porcine collagen

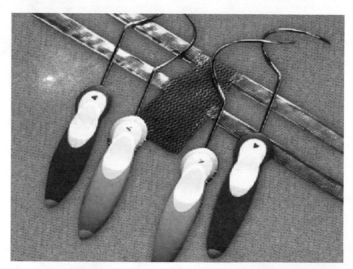

Fig. 80.11: Perigee system for transobturator cystocele repair
(For colour version, see Plate 7)

use of tension-free vaginal tape (TVT) has been demonstrated in the uncontrolled short-term case studies. These techniques are still awaiting safety and efficacy studies. Nevertheless, they are still increasingly being used in clinical practice.[17] Before undertaking the procedure, the patients must be counselled regarding the serious adverse results of transvaginal mesh repair including pain, dyspareunia, etc.

Laparoscopic surgery for prolapse: Nowadays, laparoscopic procedures are commonly being performed for the cases of prolapse. Some of these are described next.

❖ Cervicopexy or sling operations with or without laparoscopic paravaginal repair or vaginal repair

❖ Vaginal hysterectomy/laparoscopic vaginal hysterectomy/laparoscopic hysterectomy/total laparoscopic hysterectomy along with colposuspension

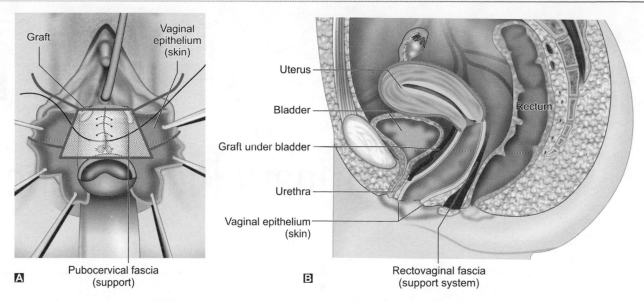

Figs 80.12A and B: Graft has been placed in position under the bladder. (A) Front view; (B) Side view

* Vaginal hysterectomy/laparoscopic vaginal hysterectomy/laparoscopic hysterectomy/total laparoscopic hysterectomy along with laparoscopic pelvic reconstruction
* Rectocele repair and levatorplasty
* Enterocele repair with suturing of uterosacral ligaments
* Anterior or posterior colpopexy.

All types of sling operations can be performed by laparoscopy. Associated vaginal or paravaginal defects can also be repaired via laparoscopic route. Vaginal anterior and posterior colporrhaphy can be done either before or after laparoscopy. Laparoscopic vault suspension culdoscopy can be performed along with vaginal hysterectomy, laparoscopic-assisted vaginal hysterectomy, laparoscopic hysterectomy and total laparoscopic hysterectomy. This helps in correcting mild laxity and prevents vault prolapse. Advantages of laparoscopic surgery for prolapse include small incision, better view, minimal packing, minimal bowel and tissue handling, short recovery period, less pain and insignificant scar tissue formation.

REFERENCES

1. Bump RC, Mattiasson A, Bø K, Brubaker LP, DeLancey JO, Klarskov P, et al. The standardization of terminology of female pelvic organ prolapse and pelvic floor function. Am J Obstet Gynecol. 1996;175(1):10-7.
2. Brown JS, Waetjen LE, Subak LL, Thom DH, Van den Eeden S, Vittinghoff E. Pelvic organ prolapse surgery in the United States, 1997. Am J Obstet Gynecol. 2002;186(4):712-6.
3. Elancey JO. Anatomy and biomechanics of genital prolapse. Clin Obstet Gynecol. 1993;36(4):897-909.
4. Jones HW, Rock JA (Eds). Surgery for correction of defects in pelvic support and pelvic fistulas. Te Linde's Operative Gynecology, 10th edition. Philadelphia: JB Lippincott; 2008. pp. 720-3.
5. Kaser O, Ikg FA, Hirsch HA. Atlas of Gynecologic Surgery, 2nd edition. New York: Thieme-Stratton; 1985. pp. 6.1-6.9.
6. Lentz GM. Anatomic defects of the abdominal wall and pelvic floor: abdominal and inguinal hernias, cystocele, urethrocele, enterocele, rectocele, uterine and vaginal prolapse and rectal incontinence: Diagnosis and Management. In: Katz VL, LentzGM, Lobo RA, Gershenson DM (Eds). Comprehensive Gynecology, 5th edition. Philadelphia: Mosby Elsevier; 2007.
7. Loret de Mola JR, Carpenter SE. Management of genital prolapse in neonates and young women. Obstet Gynecol Surv. 1996;51(4):253-60.
8. Morley GW. Treatment of uterine and vaginal prolapse. Clin Obstet Gynecol. 1996;39(4):959-69.
9. Nichols DH, Milley PS, Randall CL. Significance of restoration of normal vaginal depth and axis. Obstet Gynecol. 1970;36(2):251-6.
10. Rush CB, Entman SS. Pelvic organ prolapse and stress urinary incontinence. Med Clin North Am. 1995;79(6):1473-9.
11. Ranny B. Enterocele, vaginal prolapse, pelvic hernia: recognition and treatment. Am J Obstet Gynecol. 1981;140(1): 53-61.
12. Barrington JW, Edwards G. Posthysterectomy vault prolapse. Int Urogynecol J Pelvic Floor Dysfunct. 2000;11(4):241-5.
13. Ryan KJ, Berkowitz RS, Barbieri RL, Dunaif A (Eds). Kistner's Gynecology and Women's Health, 7th edition. St. Louis, MO: Mosby; 1999.
14. Campbell MF, Walsh PC, Retik AB. Campbell's Urology, 8th edition. Philadelphia: Elsevier Science; 2002.
15. Weber AM, Walters MD, Piedmonte MR. Sexual function and vaginal anatomy in women before and after surgery for pelvic organ prolapse and urinary incontinence. Am J Obstet Gynecol. 2000;182(6):1610-5.
16. Walter JE; Urogynaecology Committee, Lovatsis D, Walter JE, Easton W, Epp A, et al. Transvaginal mesh procedures for pelvic organ prolapse. J Obstet Gynaecol Can. 2011;33(2):168-74.
17. Altman D, Väyrynen T, Engh ME, Axelsen S, Falconer C; Nordic Transvaginal Mesh Group. Nordic transvaginal mesh group short-term outcome after transvaginal mesh repair of pelvic organ prolapse. Int Urogynecol J Pelvic Floor Dysfunct. 2008;19:787-93.

CHAPTER 80

Urinary Incontinence

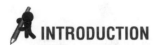 INTRODUCTION

Urinary incontinence (UI) can be defined as an involuntary loss of urine, which is a social or hygienic problem and can be demonstrated with objective means. It can occur as a result of an abnormality in the function of the lower urinary tract or due to other illnesses, which may cause leakage in different situations. There are two main types of UI: (1) stress incontinence and (2) urge incontinence.

Stress Incontinence

Stress urinary incontinence (SUI) can be defined as involuntary leakage of urine occurring during conditions resulting in an increase in intra-abdominal pressure (exertion, sneezing, coughing or exercise), which causes the intravesical pressure to rise higher than what the urethral closure mechanisms can withstand (in the absence of detrusor contractions).

Urge Incontinence

Urge urinary incontinence can be defined as involuntary leakage of urine accompanied by or immediately preceded by urgency. The corresponding urodynamic term is detrusor overactivity, which is evident in form of involuntary detrusor contractions at the time of filling cystometry. Urge incontinence is caused by uninhibited contractions of the detrusor muscle.

Stress urinary incontinence is the most common form of UI.[1] Urodynamic diagnosis of stress incontinence is termed as genuine stress incontinence. When UI markedly disrupts the woman's life and the symptoms of stress incontinence do not respond to conservative management and/or pharmacological therapy, surgical treatment may be the only option. Various surgical procedures for stress incontinence share the common goal of stabilising the bladder neck and proximal urethra. This support can be commonly achieved with the help of a sling, a piece of human or animal tissue or a synthetic tape, which the surgeon places in order to support the bladder neck and urethra. Nowadays, mid-urethral sling surgeries, those using the retropubic or the transobturator approaches are commonly used. Both these approaches are designed to reduce or eliminate stress incontinence in women.

Surgery for urge incontinence should be considered only in severe and refractory cases and includes bladder augmentation procedures, denervation procedures, urinary diversion, sacral neuromodulation, etc.

AETIOLOGY

Urinary incontinence usually has a multifactorial aetiology and includes the following:[2-10]

❖ Structural and functional disorders involving the bladder, urethra, ureters and surrounding connective tissues
❖ Disorders of the spinal cord or CNS (stroke, multiple sclerosis and Parkinson's disease)
❖ Some cases of UI may be pharmacologically induced (e.g. sedatives, anticholinergic drugs, antispasmodics, α-adrenergic agonists, α-blockers, calcium channel blockers, etc.).
❖ Stress incontinence can occur due to two separate aetiologies: (1) anatomic hypermobility of the urethra and (2) intrinsic sphincter deficiency (ISD) or weakness.
❖ Damage to the nerves, muscle and connective tissue of the pelvic floor is important in the genesis of stress incontinence. Weakening of pelvic connective tissues due to repeated childbirths (especially vaginal deliveries with episiotomy) appears to be an important mechanism.
❖ Genitourinary atrophy due to hypo-oestrogenism (especially in relation to menopause)
❖ Urge incontinence is usually caused due to uninhibited contractions of the detrusor muscle.

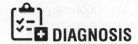 **DIAGNOSIS**

Clinical Presentation

The patient with UI can present as follows:
- ❖ Involuntary loss of urine (either triggered by stress or associated with urgency). This may present as a social and/or hygienic problem. The complaints may be minor and situational or severe, constant and debilitating.
- ❖ There may be associated symptoms of faecal incontinence and/or pelvic organ prolapse.
- ❖ During the initial clinical assessment, the woman's UI should be classified as SUI, urge UI or overactive bladder (OAB), or mixed UI so that the treatment can be instituted based on the type of incontinence.

General Physical Examination

The examination is tailored based on each specific case history. The following parameters must be recorded for each patient: height, weight, BP and pulse. The grading system for UI as devised by Stamey (1970) is described in Table 81.1.

Pelvic Examination

Pelvic floor muscles must be assessed to confirm their contractility. Assessment for pelvic prolapse must also be done.

Investigations

- ❖ *Urine dipstick test*: This must be done to detect the presence of blood, glucose, protein, leucocytes, nitrites, etc. in the urine.
- ❖ *Urine culture and sensitivity*: Midstream urine sample for culture and sensitivity may be required in the suspected cases of UTI.
- ❖ *Assessment of residual urine*: Postvoid residual volume can be measured by bladder scan or catheterisation in women with symptoms suggestive of voiding dysfunction or recurrent UTI.
- ❖ *Assessment of quality of life*: Various incontinence-specific quality-of-life scales, which can be used for evaluating the quality of life, include International Consultation on Incontinence Questionnaire (ICIQ), Bristol Female Lower Urinary Tract Symptoms (BFLUTS) questionnaire, Incontinence Quality of Life (I-QOL) questionnaire, Stress and Urge Incontinence and Quality of Life Questionnaire (SUIQQ), Urinary Incontinence Severity Score (UISS), Stress-related leak, Emptying ability, Anatomy, Protection, Inhibition, Quality of life, Mobility and Mental status incontinence classification System (SEAPI-QMM), Kings Health Questionnaire (KHQ), etc.
- ❖ *Maintenance of bladder diary*: The patients should be asked to maintain bladder diaries noting down the pattern of urination and incontinence every day.
- ❖ *Urodynamic testing*: Multichannel filling and voiding cystometry may be performed before surgery in women with a clinical suspicion of detrusor overactivity, symptoms suggestive of voiding dysfunction or anterior compartment prolapse or those who had surgery for stress incontinence in the past. If the diagnosis remains unclear after conventional urodynamic studies, ambulatory urodynamics or videourodynamics may be considered.

 MANAGEMENT

General Management

- ❖ *Multidisciplinary team approach*: Urinary incontinence should be preferably managed by a multidisciplinary team comprising a urogynaecologist, a urologist with a subspecialist interest in female urology, specialist nurse, a specialist physiotherapist, occupational therapist, etc.
- ❖ *Lifestyle changes*: This includes simple lifestyle modifications such as reduction in the intake of caffeine, modification of high or low fluid intake, weight reduction (in women with BMI >30 kg/m²).
- ❖ *Physical therapies*: This includes exercises for training the muscles of pelvic floor (in form of at least eight contractions three times a day for a period of 3 months) in cases of stress or mixed incontinence. Electrical stimulation and/or biofeedback therapy can be considered in women who are unable to actively contract the muscles of pelvic floor. Electrical stimulation, however, should not be used in combination with the training of pelvic floor muscles or in the treatment of women with OAB.
- ❖ *Behavioural therapy*: Behavioural therapy in the form of bladder training for a period of minimum 6 weeks serves as the first-line treatment in case of women with urge or mixed UI. If bladder training does not appear to work on its own, multicomponent behavioural therapy including OAB drugs along with bladder training can be considered.
- ❖ *Nerve stimulation*: Presently, there is insufficient evidence to recommend the use of transcutaneous posterior tibial nerve or transcutaneous sacral nerve stimulation for the routine treatment of cases of OAB. Percutaneous posterior tibial nerve stimulation can be sometimes used in cases of OAB (e.g. failure of conservative management including treatment with OAB drugs, or the woman does not desire therapy with botulinum toxin A).

Table 81.1: Grading system for urinary incontinence

Grade	Definition
0	Continent
1	Loss of urine with sudden increase in abdominal pressure, but not in bed at night
2	Incontinence worsens with lesser degree of physical stress
3	Incontinence with walking, standing erect from sitting position or sitting up in bed
4	Total incontinence occurs and urine is lost without relation to physical activity or position

❖ *Alternative conservative management options*: This involves the use of absorbent products, urinals, toileting aids, catheters, etc., as an adjunct to ongoing therapy or for the long-term management of UI only after other treatment options have been explored. Bladder catheterisation (intermittent or indwelling urethral or suprapubic catheterisation) should be considered for women in whom incontinence is due to persistent urinary retention or there is presence of symptomatic infection or renal dysfunction, and in whom other treatment modalities have failed.

PHARMACOLOGICAL THERAPY

Stress Incontinence

Drugs used for the treatment of stress incontinence may include α-adrenoceptor agonists (e.g. phenylpropanolamine, norephedrine, ephedrine, midodrine, methoxamine, etc.), β-adrenoreceptor agonists (clenbuterol), duloxetine, etc.

❖ *Alpha-adrenoreceptor agonists*: These include drugs which act on α-adrenergic receptors that are present on the bladder neck and proximal urethra.[11] Alpha-adrenergic agonists help in increasing the bladder outlet resistance by contracting the bladder neck. Therefore, these agents are beneficial for the treatment of women with mild to moderately severe stress incontinence. Since these agents cause the contraction of bladder neck smooth muscles, they are also likely to be useful in cases of urge incontinence. However, these drugs may sometimes be associated with potentially severe and life-threatening side effects such as haemorrhagic stroke, hypertension, anxiety, insomnia, headache, tremor, weakness, palpitations, cardiac arrhythmias, etc.[11]

❖ *Duloxetine/venlafaxine*: Both duloxetine and venlafaxine are combined inhibitors of serotonin or norepinephrine reuptake, which may help in strengthening the effects of serotonin and norepinephrine on the storage mechanisms of the lower urinary tract. Duloxetine may be considered as a second-line treatment option for women with SUI preferring pharmacological therapy over surgical treatment or those who are not suitable for surgical treatment. However, it should not be considered as a first-line treatment option for women with predominant SUI. If duloxetine is prescribed, the women must be counselled about its adverse effects such as agitation, hallucinations, loss of co-ordination, neck rigidity, easy bruising, unusual bleeding, difficulty in micturition, difficulty in concentration, severe allergic reaction, etc.

Urge Incontinence

Pharmacological therapy forms the first line of management in cases of urge incontinence and includes the following drugs:

❖ *Anticholinergic agents*: These help in controlling urge incontinence by causing relaxation of the overactive detrusor muscles in the bladder wall. These may include drugs such as tolterodine, tropsium, solifenacin, propantheline bromide, atropine, hyoscyamine, etc. Anticholinergic drugs may be associated with adverse effects such as dry mouth and constipation.

❖ *Tricyclic antidepressants*: They possess both central and peripheral anticholinergic effect as well as α-adrenergic agonist effect and central sedative effect, which can help decrease bladder contractility and increase urethral resistance.[12] The resultant clinical effect is bladder muscle relaxation and increased urethral sphincter tone. The most commonly used drug in cases of OAB is imipramine and doxepin. Tricyclic antidepressants can produce side effects such as rashes, hepatic dysfunction, jaundice, agranulocytosis, weakness, fatigue, tremors, postural hypotension, arrhythmias, etc.

❖ *Drugs with mixed actions*: These may include drugs such as oxybutynin, propiverine, dicyclomine, flavoxate, etc. Of these various drugs, oxybutynin is commonly used in the dosage of 5 mg, 2–4 times per day.

❖ *Alpha-adrenoreceptor antagonists*: These include drugs such as alfuzosin, doxazosin, prazosin, terazosin, tamsulosin, etc.

❖ *Beta-adrenoreceptor agonists*: These include drugs such as salbutamol, terbutaline, etc. Theoretically, use of β-adrenergic blocking agents should unmask or potentiate an α-adrenergic effect, resulting in an increased urethral resistance.[13] Few initial studies showed the successful effect of β-adrenergic blocking agents, such as propranolol in the treatment of incontinence.[13,14] However, subsequent studies could not demonstrate the efficacy of propranolol in the treatment of incontinence. Additionally, propranolol can result in some major potential side effects such as heart failure and increased airway resistance.

❖ *Other drugs*: Other drugs used in cases of OAB include baclofen, capsaicin, resiniferatoxin, botulinum toxin, oestrogen, desmopressin, etc.

- *Vasopressin analogues/desmopressin*: Desmopressin is an artificial version of the antidiuretic hormone, which can be used for suppressing the nocturnal urine production in women with UI or OAB. It can be administered in the form of an oral formulation or a nasal spray. Its use can result in side effects such as headache, abdominal pain, nausea, and nasal congestion, and nosebleeds (with the nasal spray). It should be used with caution in women with cystic fibrosis and preferably be avoided in those over 65 years of age with cardiovascular disease or hypertension.

- *Oestrogens*: Systemic HRT must not be offered for the treatment of UI. Use of intravaginal oestrogens can be considered for the treatment of OAB symptoms in postmenopausal women with vaginal atrophy. Although oestrogens may not influence the pharmacological mechanism of urethral continence directly, they can indirectly affect pharmacologic interactions in the lower urinary tract, such as receptor sensitivity, density and neurotransmitter metabolism.[15-17] They may also alter the vascular and connective tissue elements of the urethral wall, which play an important role in the maintenance of urethral continence.

- *Botulinum toxin A*: Injection of the bladder wall with botulinum toxin A can be offered to women with OAB caused by proven detrusor overactivity, which has not responded to conservative management (including pharmacotherapy) following a discussion with the multidisciplinary team. The risks and benefits of treatment with botulinum toxin, such as the likelihood of being symptom free or experiencing a reduction in symptoms, the potential requirement for clean intermittent catheterisation for a variable period of time after the effect of the injections has worned off, etc., need to be explained to the women before taking their informed consent for administration of botulinum toxin A. Usually 200 units of botulinum toxin A are initially offered. However, 100 units of botulinum toxin A can be considered for women who would prefer a dose with a lower chance of catheterisation, but simultaneously with a reduced chance of success. If the treatment proves to be effective, the patient should be called for a follow-up at 6 months.

SURGICAL MANAGEMENT

Stress Incontinence

Surgery forms the mainstay of treatment for cases of stress incontinence. Before offering a particular surgical procedure to the woman, the risks and benefits of the different treatment options should be explained to the patient with the help of information leaflets. If conservative medical management for SUI has failed, the surgical options which can be considered for the patient include the following:[18-23]

- ❖ Suburethral slings (bladder neck slings and mid-urethral sling)
- ❖ Retropubic bladder neck colposuspension (especially Burch colposuspension)
- ❖ Injection of urethral bulking agents.

The advent of synthetic tapes especially that of the tension-free vaginal tapes (TVTs) has further revolutionised the surgery for stress incontinence.[24-28] Several newer modifications of these tapes are available nowadays, such as the transobturator tapes (TOTs) and crossover tapes. The advantage, which the sling surgery has over the previously used surgeries (especially Burch procedure), is the potential of sling surgery to treat ISD in addition to the urethral hypermobility. Since some element of ISD seems to be mandatory for a leak, it is nearly always present in cases of stress incontinence and is commonly the cause for long-term recurrence. As a result, nowadays, most surgeons favour sling surgery over Burch colposuspension.

Indications for Surgery

Indications for sling surgery are as follows:
- ❖ Various forms of stress incontinence, especially those with ISD
- ❖ Stress incontinence with concomitant pelvic organ prolapse

- ❖ Failed procedures such as needle suspension or Burch colposuspension
- ❖ Women with a urethral diverticulectomy or urethral loss such as after a urethra-vaginal fistula repair (an autologous sling is preferred over synthetic sling in these cases).

Preoperative Preparation

Preoperative evaluation involves taking the complete history from the patient and performing a complete general physical examination, focussing on the following parameters:
- ❖ *Type of incontinence*: Whether the symptoms are suggestive of stress incontinence, urge incontinence or mixed (both the types).
- ❖ *Performance of tests for confirmation of stress incontinence*:
  - *Cough stress test or urinary stress test*: In this test, the patient with stress incontinence is asked to perform a Valsalva manoeuvre (the effort to breathe out forcibly while the mouth and nose are firmly closed or the vocal cords are pressed together) or cough. Instantaneous leakage of urine with cough or Valsalva manoeuvre is suggestive of SUI. Delayed leakage of urine is usually suggestive of incontinence due to detrusor overactivity.
  - *Measurement of the postvoidal residual volume*: In this test, the patient with a full bladder is asked to void as she normally would, without requirement of an additional effort to fully empty the bladder. Following voiding, the residual urine in the bladder is measured by either catheterisation or bladder sonography. Generally, a postvoidal residual volume of greater than 200 cc may be suggestive of voiding dysfunction or detrusor weakness.
- ❖ The patient must be asked to maintain a complete voiding diary.
- ❖ The surgeon also needs to determine if there is any associated voiding dysfunction suggestive of ISD. This might have an impact on the surgical management plan to be followed as well as the future prognosis because the patients with ISD do not have as good a long-term outcome with any procedure in comparison to those patients having predominant hypermobility. A patient with an underactive detrusor may be associated with the likelihood of voiding difficulty following surgical treatment of incontinence.
- ❖ The clinician must assess the pelvic anatomy including strength of the muscles of pelvic floor. The surgeon must also determine if there is any associated pelvic floor dysfunction such as cystocele, enterocele, rectocele, anal sphincter incompetence or vault prolapse. In case any such dysfunction is present, it must be taken care of at the time of surgery.
- ❖ Performance of urodynamic studies may provide important diagnostic and prognostic information and must be performed prior to any invasive therapy. Urodynamic evaluation is not necessary for many women with uncomplicated SUI. Urodynamic testing may prove to be useful in cases where the symptoms are not consistent with physical examination findings or in women having mixed or complicated incontinence situations.

❖ Oestrogen replacement therapy prior to surgery may enhance urethral, bladder and vaginal tissue integrity.

❖ Treatment of various underlying medical disorders such as asthma, chronic obstructive pulmonary disease (COPD), diabetes, chronic constipation, etc. must be undertaken prior to surgery.

❖ Good nutrition helps to maximise tissue integrity and support good healing.

❖ *Patient counselling*: This must comprise of thorough discussion of risks, benefits, anticipated success rates and potential common complications related to the procedure.

❖ Patient is placed in the lithotomy position under general or spinal anaesthesia for surgery.

Intraoperative Details

The various types of surgeries, which can be performed for stress incontinence, are described next in details.

Suburethral Sling

A suburethral sling is a sling that is inserted through a small vaginal incision and placed either at the bladder neck, mid-urethra or proximal urethra for the purpose of supporting the urethra in women with SUI. There are two types of suburethral slings: (1) bladder neck slings and (2) mid-urethral slings.

Bladder Neck Sling

Also known as a proximal urethral sling, this sling is placed at the level of the proximal urethra and bladder neck. This procedure is usually performed using both a vaginal and abdominal incision. These slings can be made of either biological materials (including the patient's own tissue) or synthetic mesh. The bladder neck slings are also referred to as pubovaginal slings when the arms of the sling material are affixed to the anterior rectus fascia rather than the pubic bone or Cooper's ligament. Pubovaginal slings involve the use of autologous fascia, which can be harvested from the patient's rectus sheath or alternatively from the patient's thigh (fascia lata).

Mid-urethral Sling

This is a suburethral sling that is inserted via a small vaginal incision and placed at the level of the mid-urethra in a tension-free manner. This surgery involves the interplay of three structures: (1) pubourethral ligaments; (2) suburethral vaginal tissues; and (3) the pubococcygeus muscle. Though there can be several variations of these procedures, all involve placement of a synthetic mesh. Based on the route of placement, i.e. whether a retropubic or a transobturator approach is used, these procedures can be classified as follows:

❖ Retropubic method: Tension-free vaginal tape

❖ Transobturator approach: Transobturator tape.

When offering a synthetic mid-urethral tape procedure to the patient, surgeons should consider using those procedures and devices for which there is availability of high-quality evidence regarding the efficacy and safety of the particular method. Surgeons should preferably use a device for which they have received appropriate training.

Retropubic approach: There are several commercially available kits and one commonly used technique is the TVT. In this technique, one trocar is placed through a vaginal suburethral incision lateral to the urethra and brought out suprapubically through a skin incision (Figs 81.1A to E). The TVT devices are associated with a 71% cure rate at 11.5 years.[29]

Transobturator approach: This approach was introduced to reduce the risks related to injury to the lower urinary tract and vascular structures, which can be associated with traversing the retropubic space. Various kits for this approach are available, each containing a needle and a mesh design sling material made up of polypropylene. In this surgery, the sling material is directed bilaterally through the obturator foramen underneath the mid-urethra (Figs 81.2A to D). The point of entry overlies the proximal tendon of adductor longus muscle.

Based on the method of needle placement, the trans-obturator procedures can be of two types:

1. An 'in-to-out' approach: Needle placement begins inside the vagina and is directed outwards.
2. An 'out-to-in' approach: Needle placement begins outside the vagina and is directed inwards.

Initially, when the transobturator sling procedure was introduced, an 'out-to-in' approach was used. However, this approach was associated with several complications such as injury to the bladder, urethra, etc. The 'in-to-out' approach was then introduced with the aim of reducing injury to the lower urinary tract.

However, in this approach, the needle travels to the obturator neurovascular bundle. Though each method has theoretical advantages, the possibility of injury cannot be completely excluded. Nevertheless, the transobturator approach serves as an effective day-surgery technique with potentially lower rate of bladder injury. However, some retrospective studies have shown that it may show limited effectiveness in patients having urodynamic criteria for ISD.[23,24]

Pubovaginal Sling Surgery

This surgery comprises of following steps (Figs 81.3A to G):

❖ *Harvesting the strip of rectus fascia*: In this surgery, firstly, a strip of rectus fascia is harvested by making a 3-inch long transverse incision just above the pubis below the pubic hairline down to the surface of the rectus fascia. The rectus fascia is dissected free of subcutaneous tissue from the above and freed from the muscles below to fashion out a rectus fascia sling, which is about 12–16 cm long and 2 cm in width. Once the entire dissection is complete, the fascial strip is excised and placed in a basin of saline. A helical stitch is placed using a 0 gauge delayed-absorbable polypropylene sutures at each end of the fascial strip. The abdominal wound is packed temporarily and the vaginal surgery is begun.

❖ *Identification of bladder neck*: A Foley catheter is inserted into the bladder. The bladder neck can be identified by inserting a Foley catheter inside the urethra. Applying gentle traction on the Foley catheter and palpation of the balloon would help in delineation of bladder neck.

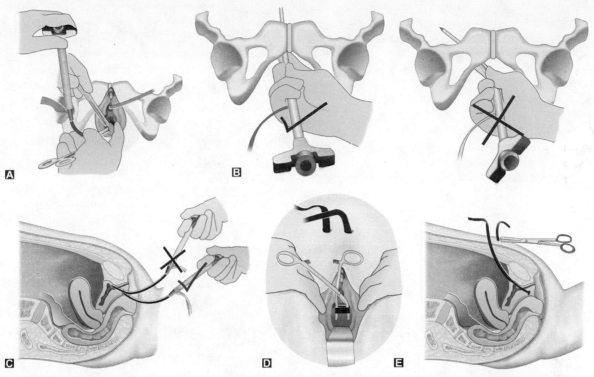

Figs 81.1A to E: Tension-free vaginal tape surgery. (A) Placing the needle through the submucosal tunnel; (B) Correct and incorrect positioning of the transducer; (C) Correct and incorrect positioning of hand and the transducer; (D) Setting mesh tension; (E) Bringing the tape out through the suprapubic abdominal incision and trimming the tape

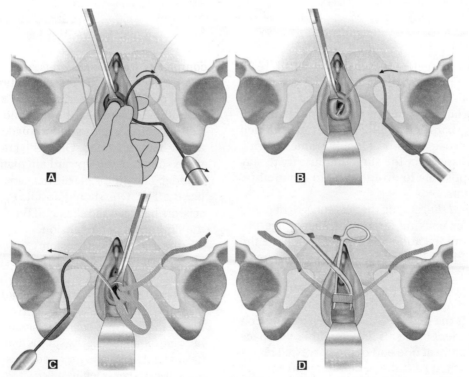

Figs 81.2A to D: Tension-free obturator tape. (A) Introduction of the needle; (B) Passage of the needle; (C) Placing the tape; (D) Setting mesh tension

❖ *Vaginal dissection to reach the pubic bone*: A vertical incision or a gently curved horizontal incision (~5–6 cm long) is made about 2 cm below the urethral meatus on the anterior vaginal wall superficial to the pubocervical fascia (Fig. 81.3B). The edges of the incision are held using Allis forceps, and a combination of sharp and blunt dissection is used to lift the vaginal epithelium off the underlying fibromuscular layer. The plane corresponding to the undersurface of the anterior vaginal wall is identified by noting the characteristic shiny white

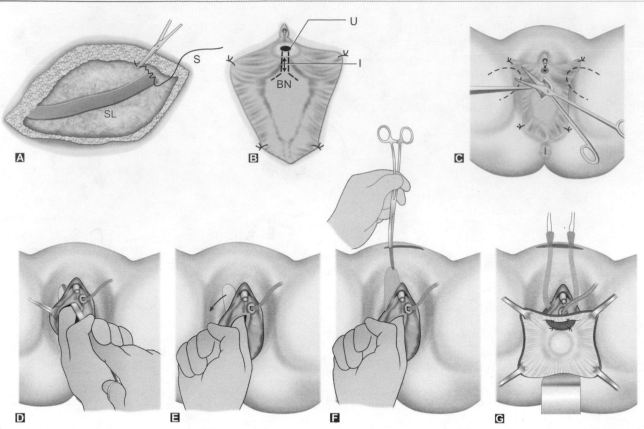

Figs 81.3A to G: Pubovaginal sling surgery. (A) Harvesting the strip of rectus fascia: Prolene no. 1 mattress suture (S) should be placed at each end of the sling (SL); (B) A short vertical incision (I) is made below the urethra (U) over the bladder neck (BN); (C) A combination of sharp and blunt dissection is performed until the finger can palpate the ischiopubic ramus; (D) Entry into the space of Retzius; (E) Palpation of the pubic bone; (F) Placement of the strip of fascia; (G) Suturing the fascial sling in place

appearance. Blunt dissection is then performed to create a space up to the pubic bone by entering the space of Retzius. The dissection is carried out using the dissecting scissors, pointing laterally until the pubic bone is reached. A combination of sharp and blunt dissection is performed until the finger can palpate the ischiopubic ramus. During this part of the dissection, the surgeon must try to stay as far lateral as possible to avoid injury to the urethra, bladder and ureters.

❖ *Placing the urethral sling*: Using the surgeon's right hand, a long dressing or packing forceps or needle ligature carrier is used from the abdominal side to perforate the rectus sheath caudal to the prior harvest incision. Simultaneously, the surgeon's left index finger is placed in the vagina to bluntly retract the bladder neck medially. The forceps is placed against the back of pubic bone and advanced towards the vagina. Concurrently, the surgeon guides the instrument using his fingers within the space of Retzius. The suture at one end of the harvested rectus fascial strip is grasped with the penetrating forceps and threaded up through the abdominal incision on the side of urethra. A similar procedure is repeated on the other side with the other end of the sling. As a result, the fascial sling lies positioned beneath the bladder neck. The sling is fixed beneath the bladder neck using 3–4 delayed absorbable sutures. Two small stab wounds are made in the rectus fascia just above the pubis and the sling is brought through them on either side.

❖ *Placing the sling in a tension-free manner*: Sutures attached to the sling are then tied together above the rectus sheath. While tying the knot, a space of two- or three-finger breadth is left between the knot and the fascia to prevent future complications such as bladder neck obstruction and urinary retention. Once the knot has been secured, there should be no upward angulation of the urethra or bladder. The sling is placed in a tension-free manner, just like the TVT. One should be able to place a heavy pair of scissors between the sling and the urethra to ensure that the sling is not under tension.

❖ *Closure of the vaginal incision*: Cystoscopy is performed to ensure that the urinary tract is safe and there has been no bladder perforation or obstruction of urethra. The vagina is then closed using 2-0 chromic catgut sutures in a running fashion. Some surgeons may prefer to close the vagina before the sling has been tied since adequate access may become difficult once the sling is tied and the bladder neck has moved up to a higher and a less accessible location. A Foley catheter is left in place.

❖ *Closure of the abdominal incision*: At the end of surgery, the abdominal incision is closed using interrupted silk sutures.

Minimally Invasive Slings

Modification of TVT and TOT procedures is observed with minimally invasive slings, sometimes also known as the microslings or minislings. In this technique, a small incision is made in the vagina, through which an 8-cm long strip of polypropylene synthetic mesh is placed across and beneath the mid-urethra. Since the mesh is not threaded through the retropubic space, it helps in avoiding potential vascular injury.

Retropubic Bladder Neck Colposuspension

All these procedures are performed through lower abdominal incision and involve the attachment of periurethral and perivesical endopelvic fascia (vaginal wall adjacent to mid-urethra and bladder neck) to some other supporting structure in the anterior pelvis (Table 81.2 and Fig. 81.4). These procedures are also referred to as retropubic urethropexy. Nowadays, some of these procedures are performed through laparoscopic and robotic surgery. These procedures had been long considered as the gold standard for the surgical treatment of stress incontinence, with 1-year continence rates varying between 85% and 90%.[30] Some complications commonly associated with retropubic urethropexy include detrusor overactivity, urinary retention and in case of Marshall-Marchetti-Krantz procedure, osteitis pubis.

Injection of Urethral Bulking Agents

Periurethral injections are performed under local anaesthesia and involve administration of various types of materials around the periurethral tissues to facilitate their coaptation under conditions of increased intra-abdominal pressure. Various

Table 81.2: Various supporting structures in different types of retropubic bladder neck colposuspension procedures

Name of surgical procedure	Supporting structure in the anterior pelvis
Paravaginal procedure	Arcus tendineus
Modified Marshall-Marchetti-Krantz procedure	Back of pubic symphysis
Burch colposuspension	Iliopectineal ligament (Cooper's ligament)
Turner-Warwick vaginal obturator shelf procedure	Fascia over obturator internus

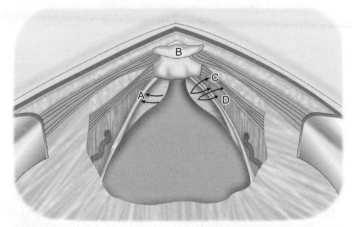

Fig. 81.4: Point of attachment of endopelvic fascia during bladder neck suspension procedures. (A) Arcus tendineus; (B) Periosteum of the pubic symphysis; (C) Iliopectineal ligaments (Cooper's ligaments); (D) Obturator internus fascia

bulking agents have been used including collagen, carbon-coated zirconium, ethylene vinyl alcohol, polydimethylsiloxane, polytetrafluoroethylene and glutaraldehyde cross-linked bovine collagen (Contigen®). Indications for periurethral injection of bulking agents include the following:

❖ Patients who would be unable to tolerate surgery
❖ Patients who do not desire surgery
❖ Patients with recurrent or refractory incontinence with previous history of sling surgery for stress incontinence.

Use of Artificial Urinary Sphincter

Use of an artificial urinary sphincter should be considered for the management of SUI in women in case of the failure of surgery. This helps in preventing long-term morbidity.

Postoperative Care

❖ Voiding trials are begun as soon as the patient is comfortable, usually on the first or second postoperative day.
❖ Bladder drainage is an essential aspect of postoperative care. Most patients are able to void spontaneously in 3–7 days.
❖ Measures must be taken to control chronic cough and to avoid or treat constipation.
❖ The patient should avoid lifting anything heavier than 10 pounds for 12 weeks.
❖ The patient must be instructed to avoid smoking and other activities that may repetitively stress the pelvic floor, resulting in long-term failure of the procedure.
❖ Patients who have undergone surgery for urinary continence should be called for a follow-up visit within 6 months. Vaginal examination should be performed during this visit to exclude erosion.

COMPLICATIONS

❖ *Haemorrhage:* Bleeding is usually from the perivesical venous plexus. Haemorrhage can occur in nearly 2% cases undergoing retropubic procedures.
❖ *Urinary tract and visceral injury:* Bladder injuries can commonly occur with the laparoscopic approach. Injury to the ureter can occur due to kinking or angulation during the retropubic procedures. Injury to the bowel can also sometimes occur. Various complications, which may especially occur with the use of mid-urethral sling surgeries, include mesh erosion, urinary retention, de novo UI, and vascular, bowel and lower urinary tract injury. Of the various injuries to the urinary tract, bladder perforation is the most common.[31]
❖ *Urinary tract infection:* These are especially associated with postoperative voiding difficulties resulting in prolonged catheterisation.
❖ *Wound infection:* Prophylactic antibiotics in the form of a single dose of a broad-spectrum agent are usually effective.
❖ *Osteitis pubis:* This is a self-limited inflammation of the pubic bone related to placement of foreign body material such as sutures, etc. Osteomyelitis can rarely occur.

❖ *Urogenital fistula*: This is also a rare complication.

❖ *Nerve injuries*: Injuries to various nerves such as common peroneal, sciatic, obturator, femoral, saphenous and ilioinguinal nerves have been reported.

❖ *Voiding dysfunction*: This may manifest in the form of slow or poor urinary stream or in the inability to void.

❖ *Detrusor overactivity*: De novo detrusor overactivity may at times develop postoperatively.

❖ *Pelvic organ prolapse*: Rate of enterocele formation may be as high as 8% following surgery. Rate of rectocele formation also may be increased.

❖ *Other complications*: These may include complications such as dyspareunia, chronic suprapubic pain, sinus tract formation, etc.

CLINICAL PEARLS

❖ Urinary incontinence is a condition which may seriously influence the physical, psychological and social well-being of affected individuals.

❖ Stress urinary incontinence is the most common form of UI. Urodynamic diagnosis of stress incontinence is termed as genuine stress incontinence.

❖ Some researchers have used microwave energy to heat the connective tissue lateral to the bladder neck and proximal urethra, resulting in the shrinkage of the tissue, which provides better support to the bladder neck, thereby helping in the correction of stress incontinence.

❖ Urodynamic studies for evaluation of detrusor overactivity include uroflowmetry, filling cystometry, pressure-flow voiding studies, urethral pressure profilometry and determination of leak-point pressure.

❖ Intravesical pharmacotherapy with naturally occurring pungent substances such as capsaicin, resiniferatoxin, etc. may be helpful in cases of urge incontinence.

EVIDENCE-BASED MEDICINE

❖ Nowadays, mid-urethral sling procedures are commonly used. Mid-urethral slings are as effective as other surgical treatments for SUI, but with a shorter operative duration and a lower risk of certain postoperative complications.[26,32] Mid-urethral slings are associated with considerably reduced morbidity and voiding dysfunction in comparison to the bladder neck slings. Therefore, bladder neck slings (also known as pubovaginal slings) are used only in those women where the mid-urethral slings are contraindicated or are unsuccessful. Moreover, mid-urethral slings are associated with several advantages such as high short-term cure rate and better quality of life.[33-39]

❖ Of the two approaches (retropubic and transobturator approach) commonly used in cases of mid-urethal sling surgeries, both the approaches appear to offer comparable results.[40-45] Despite these favourable comparisons, abundant long-term data regarding the efficacy of trans-obturator approach are lacking.

❖ Pubovaginal rectus fascia slings have excellent long-term results with more than 80% of the patients remaining continent beyond 5 years of surgery.[46]

❖ Some surgical procedure which were commonly used previously, but are rarely used nowadays for treatment of incontinence include anterior colporrhaphy with Kelly's plication[47] transabdominal paravaginal repair, transvaginal needle suspension procedures,[48] etc.

REFERENCES

1. Haylen BT, de Ridder D, Freeman RM, Swift SE, Berghmans B, Lee J, et al. An International Urogynecological Association (IUGA)/International Continence Society (ICS) joint report on the terminology for female pelvic floor dysfunction. Neurourol Urodyn. 2010;29(1):4-20.

2. Luber KM. The definition, prevalence, and risk factors for stress UI. Rev Urol. 2004;6(Suppl 3):S3-9.

3. Norton PA. Etiology of genuine stress incontinence. In: Brubaker LT, Saclarides TJ (Eds). The Female Pelvic Floor: Disorders of Function and Support. Philadelphia: Davis; 1996. pp. 153-7.

4. Peschers U, Schaer G, Anthuber C, Delancey JO, Schuessler B. Changes in vesical neck mobility following vaginal delivery. Obstet Gynecol. 1996;88(6):1001-6.

5. Thom DH, van den Eeden SK, Brown JS. Evaluation of parturition and other reproductive variables as risk factors for urinary incontinence in later life. Obstet Gynecol. 1997;90(6):983-9.

6. Meyer S, Schreyer A, DeGrandi P, Hohlfeld P. The effects of birth on urinary continence mechanisms and other pelvic-floor characteristics. Obstet Gynecol. 1998;92(4 Pt 1):613-8.

7. Snooks SJ, Badenock DF, Tiptaft RC, Swash M. Perineal nerve damage in genuine stress incontinence: an electrophysiology study. Br J Urol. 1985;57(4):422-6.

8. Smith ARB, Hosker GL, Warrell DW. The role of pudendal nerve damage in the aetiology of genuine stress incontinence in women. Br J Obstet Gynecol. 1989;96(1):29-32.

9. Allen RE, Hosker GL, Smith ARB, Warrell DW. Pelvic floor damage and childbirth: a neurophysiological study. Br J Obstet Gynaecol. 1990;97(9):770-9.

10. Handa VL, Harris TA, Ostergard DR. Protecting the pelvic floor: obstetric management to prevent incontinence and pelvic organ prolapse. Obstet Gynecol. 1996;88(3):470-8.

11. Rovner ES, Wein AJ. Drug treatment of voiding dysfunction. In: Cardozo L, Staskin D (Eds). Textbook of Female Urology and Urogynecology, 1st edition. London: Isis Medical Media; 2001. pp. 357-407.

12. Barlett DM, Wein AJ. Voiding dysfunction: diagnosis, classification and management. In: Gillenwater JY, Grayhack JT, Howards ST, Duckett JW (Eds). Adult and Pediatric Urology, 2nd edition. St. Louis: Mosby Year Book; 1991. pp. 1001-99.

13. Gleason D, Reilly R, Bottaccinin M, Pierce MJ. The urethral continence zone and its relation to stress incontinence. J Urol. 1974;112(1):81-8.

14. Kaisary AU. Beta adrenoceptor blockade in the treatment of female stress urinary incontinence. J Urol. 1984;90(5):351-3.

15. Hodgson BJ, Dumas S, Bolling DR, Heesch CM. Effect of estrogen on sensitivity of rabbit bladder and urethra to phenylephrine. Invest Urol. 1978;16(1):67-9.

16. Levin RM, Shofer FS, Wein AJ. Estrogen-induced alterations in the autonomic responses of the rabbit urinary bladder. J Pharmacol Exp Ther. 1980;215(3):614-8.

17. Larsson B, Andersson K, Batra S, Mattiasson A, Sjogren C. Effects of estradiol on norepinephrine-induced contraction, alpha adrenoreceptor number and norepinephrine content in the female rabbit urethra. J Pharmacol Exp Ther. 1984;229(2):557-63.

18. Kane AR, Nager CW. Midurethral slings for stress UI. Clin Obstet Gynecol. 2008;51(1):124-35.

19. Dmochowski RR, Blaivas JM, Gormley EA, Juma S, Karram MM, Lightner DJ, et al. Update of AUA guideline on the surgical management of female stress UI. J Urol. 2010;183(5):1906-14.

20. Jonsson Funk M, Levin PJ, Wu JM. Trends in the surgical management of stress UI. Obstet Gynecol. 2012;119(4):845-51.

21. Walters MD, Karram MM. Sling procedures for stress UI. In: Walters MD, Karram MM (Eds). Urogynecology and Reconstructive Pelvic Surgery, 3rd edition. Philadelphia: Mosby Elsevier; 2007. p. 197.

22. Smith T, Chang D, Dmochowski R, Hilton P, Nilsson CG, Reid FM, et al. Surgery for urinary incontinence in women. In: Abrams P, Cardozo L, Khoury S, Wein A (Eds). Incontinence. Plymouth, UK: Health Publication Ltd; 2009.

23. Leach GE, Dmochowski RR, Appell RA, Blaivas JG, Hadley HR, Luber KM, et al. Female Stress UI Clinical Guidelines Panel summary report on surgical management of female stress UI. The American Urological Association. J Urol. 1997;158(3):875-80.

24. Anger JT, Weinberg AE, Albo ME, Smith AL, Kim JH, Rodríguez LV, et al. Trends in surgical management of stress UI among female Medicare beneficiaries. Urology. 2009;74(2):283-7.

25. Trabuco EC, Klingele CJ, Weaver AL, McGree ME, Lightner DJ, Gebhart JB. Preoperative and postoperative predictors of satisfaction after surgical treatment of stress UI. Am J Obstet Gynecol. 2011;204(5):444.e1-6.

26. Schimpf MO, Rahn DD, Wheeler TL, Patel M, White AB, Orejuela FJ, et al. Sling surgery for stress UI in women: a systematic review and metaanalysis. Am J Obstet Gynecol. 2014;211(1):71.e1-71.e27.

27. Ward KL, Hilton P, UK, Ireland TVT Trial Group. Tension-free vaginal tape versus colposuspension for primary urodynamic stress incontinence: 5-year follow up. BJOG. 2008;115(2):226-33.

28. Cody J, Wyness L, Wallace S, Glazener C, Kilonzo M, Stearns S, et al. Systematic review of the clinical effectiveness and cost-effectiveness of tension-free vaginal tape for treatment of urinary stress incontinence. Health Technol Assess. 2003;7(21):iii, 1-189.

29. Nilsson CG, Palva K, Rezapour M, Falconer C. 11 years prospective follow-ups of tension free vaginal tape procedure for the treatment of stress of UI. Int Urogynecol J Pelvic Floor Dysfunct. 2008;19(8):1043-7.

30. Lapitan MC, Cody JD, Grant A. Open retropubic colposuspension for UI in women. Cochrane Database Syst Rev. 2009;(2):CD002912.

31. Morton HC, Hilton P. Urethral injury associated with minimally invasive mid-urethral sling procedures for the treatment of stress UI: a case series and systematic literature search. BJOG. 2009;116(8):1120-6.

32. Ogah J, Cody JD, Rogerson L. Minimally invasive synthetic suburethral sling operations for stress UI in women. Cochrane Database Syst Rev. 2009;(4):CD006375.

33. Paick JS, Ku JH, Shin JW, Son H, Oh SJ, Kim SW. Tension-free vaginal tape procedure for UI with low Valsalva leak point pressure. J Urol. 2004;172(4):1370-3.

34. Meschia M, Pifarotti P, Buonaguidi A, Gattei U, Spennacchio M. Tensionfree vaginal tape (TVT) for treatment of stress UI in women with low-pressure urethra. Eur J Obstet Gynecol Reprod Biol. 2005;122(1):118-21.

35. Goktolga U, Atay V, Tahmaz L, Yenen MC, Gungor S, Ceyhan T, et al. Tension-free vaginal tape for surgical relief of intrinsic sphincter deficiency: results of 5-year follow-up. J Minim Invasive Gynecol. 2008;15(1):78-81.

36. Sinha D, Blackwell A, Moran PA. Outcome measures after TVT for mixed UI. Int Urogynecol J Pelvic Floor Dysfunct. 2008;19(7):927-31.

37. Rezapour M, Ulmsten U. Tension-free vaginal tape (TVT) in women with mixed UI—a long-term follow-up. Int Urogynecol J Pelvic Floor Dysfunct. 2001;12(Suppl 2):S15-8.

38. Paick JS, Ku JH, Kim SW, Oh SJ, Son H, Shin JW. Tension-free vaginal tape procedure for the treatment of mixed UI: significance of maximal urethral closure pressure. J Urol. 2004;172(3):1001-5.

39. Lim HS, Kim JM, Song PH, Kim HT, Jung HC. Impact of the midurethral sling procedure on quality of life in women with UI. Korean J Urol. 2010;51(2):122-7.

40. deTayrac R, Deffieux X, Droupy S, Chauveaud-Lambling A, Calvanèse-Benamour L, Fernandez H. A prospective randomized trial comparing tension-free vaginal tape and transobturator suburethral tape for surgical treatment of stress UI. Am J Obstet Gynecol. 2004;190(3):602-8.

41. Miller JJ, Botros SM, Akl MN, Aschkenazi SO, Beaumont JL, Goldberg RP, et al. Is transobturator tape as effective as tension-free vaginal tape in patients with borderline maximum urethral closure pressure? Am J Obstet Gynecol. 2006;195(6):1799-804.

42. Laurikainen E, Valpas A, Kivelä A, Kalliola T, Rinne K, Takala T, et al. Retropubic compared with transobturator tape placement in treatment of UI: a randomized controlled trial. Obstet Gynecol. 2007;109(1):4-11.

43. O'Connor RC, Nanigian DK, Lyon MB, Ellison LM, Bales GT, Stone AR. Early outcomes of mid-urethral slings for female stress UI stratified by Valsalva leak point pressure. Neurourol Urodyn. 2006;25(7):685-8.

44. Richter HE, Albo ME, Zyczynski HM, Kenton K, Norton PA, Sirls LT, et al. Retropubic versus transobturator midurethral slings for stress incontinence. N Eng J Med. 2010;362(22):2066-76.

45. Morey AF, Medendorp AR, Noller MW, Mora RV, Shandera KC, Foley JP, et al. Transobturator versus transabdominal midurethral slings: a multi-institutional comparison of obstructive voiding complications. J Urol. 2006;175(3 Pt 1):1014-7.

46. Benson JT, Lucente V, McClellan E. Vaginal versus abdominal reconstructive surgery for the treatment of pelvic support defects: a prospective randomized study with long-term outcome evaluation. Am J Obstet Gynecol. 1996;175(6):1418-21.

47. Thaweekul Y, Bunyavejchevin S, Wisawasukmongchol W, Santingamkun A. Long term results of anterior colporrhaphy with Kelly plication for the treatment of stress UI. J Med Assoc Thai. 2004;87(4):357-60.

48. Glazener CM, Cooper K. Bladder neck needle suspension for UI in women. Cochrane Database Syst Rev. 2004;(2):CD003636.

CHAPTER 81

Urinary Tract Infection

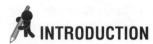

INTRODUCTION

Urinary tract infections (UTIs) involve a spectrum of infections ranging from asymptomatic bacteriuria to severe pyelonephritis. UTI can be classified as complicated or uncomplicated. Uncomplicated UTI can be defined as UTI in which infection occurs without any underlying structural or functional abnormality of the urinary tract (kidneys, ureter, bladder and urethra). Complicated UTI, on the other hand, occurs in the presence of an underlying anatomical or functional abnormality of the urinary tract.[1] As a result, the outcome of a complicated UTI is more serious than expected in comparison to its occurrence in individuals not having any identified risk factors (i.e. uncomplicated UTI).

The classification system for UTI by the European Association of Urology, also known as ORENUC, is based on the clinical presentation of the UTI and its associated host risk factors.[2] The various categories are as follows:

❖ **O**: No known or associated risk factor, e.g. healthy premenopausal women
❖ **R**: Recurrent risk factor for UTI, but there is no risk of severe outcome, e.g. promiscuous sexual behaviour, use of contraceptive devices, controlled diabetes mellitus, etc.
❖ **E**: Extra-urogenital risk factor, with risk of more severe outcome, e.g. pregnancy, poorly controlled diabetes mellitus, etc.
❖ **N**: Nephropathic disease, with risk of more severe outcome, e.g. relevant renal insufficiency, polycystic nephropathy, etc.
❖ **U**: Urological risk factor, with risk of more severe outcome, which can be resolved with therapy, e.g. ureteral obstruction due to stone, stricture, etc., temporary short-term urinary tract catheter, etc.
❖ **C**: Permanent urinary catheterisation and non-resolvable urological risk factor, with risk of more severe outcome, e.g. non-resolvable urinary obstruction and poorly controlled neurogenic bladder.

In adults, uncomplicated UTIs fall under categories O, R and partially E, while complicated UTIs mainly fall in categories N, U and C.

Other entities commonly related with UTIs in clinical practice include recurrent UTI and asymptomatic bacteriuria. Recurrent UTI can be defined as presence of three or more episodes of UTI during a period of 1 year or 2 episodes of infection within a 6 months period. If the recurrent episodes of UTI are caused by the same organism following adequate therapy, this is known as relapse.

Asymptomatic bacteriuria, on the other hand, refers to the presence of bacteria in the urine of asymptomatic women. Bacteria must be present in the quantities of at least 100,000 CFU/mL of urine in at least two consecutive voided specimens. Asymptomatic bacteriuria does not usually cause renal disease or damage. Treatment for asymptomatic bacteriuria is likely to increase the risk of subsequent symptomatic UTIs, hence, it is not usually recommended.

AETIOLOGY

Urinary tract infections occur when the urinary tract becomes infected by bacteria. In most cases, bacteria enter the urinary tract via the urethra. The majority of uncomplicated UTIs are caused by *Escherichia coli* (causing 70–95% cases), with organisms such as *Proteus mirabilis, Klebsiella spp., Staphylococcus saprophyticus, Pseudomonas, Serratia* and *Enterococci* accounting for rest of the cases.[3] Possible risk factors for the development of recurrent UTI are tabulated in Table 82.1.

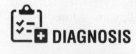

DIAGNOSIS

Clinical Presentation

Clinical signs and symptoms consistent with uncomplicated UTI are described next.

Table 82.1: Possible risk factors for recurrent urinary tract infections (UTIs) in women

Young and premenopausal women	Postmenopausal and elderly women
• Sexual intercourse • Use of spermicide with condoms or contraceptive diaphragms • A new sexual partner • Maternal history of UTI • History of UTI during childhood • Medical conditions such as diabetes, obstruction of the urinary tract as a result of calculi, etc.	• History of UTI before menopause • Urinary incontinence • Atrophic vaginitis due to oestrogen deficiency • Cystocele • Increased postvoid residual urine volume • Blood group antigen, urine secretory status • Weakened immune system • Urine catheterisation and functional status deterioration in elderly women

- ❖ Dysuria
- ❖ Increased frequency or urgency of micturition
- ❖ Back pain or costovertebral angle tenderness
- ❖ Cloudy or foul-smelling urine
- ❖ Presence of RBCs in the urine
- ❖ General malaise, lower abdominal pain and tiredness
- ❖ Usually, there is no accompanying vaginal discharge or irritation in cases of uncomplicated UTI. In presence of vaginal discharge, alternative diagnoses such as STDs and vulvovaginitis, usually due to *Candida*, must be considered.

The symptoms which may occur in the presence of upper UTIs include the following:

- ❖ High temperature of 38°C (100.4°F) or above
- ❖ Pain on the sides or back
- ❖ Shivering and chills
- ❖ General malaise, nausea and tiredness
- ❖ Confusion
- ❖ Agitation or restlessness.

There is usually no requirement for investigations in uncomplicated UTI. Empirical treatment with an antibiotic must be commenced, in otherwise, healthy women aged less than 65 years presenting with severe or greater than or equal to three symptoms of UTI.[4]

Investigations

- ❖ *Urine routine or microscopy*: Parameters which can be assessed at the time of urine routine or microscopic examination include its colour, appearance and smell, presence of ions and trace elements, proteins, enzymes, blood cells, WBCs, small molecules (glucose, ketone bodies, bilirubin, etc.).
- ❖ *Urine culture and sensitivity*: Urine culture helps in isolating the causative organism and providing antibiotic sensitivity for guiding antimicrobial treatment. Conventional laboratory practice in the UK determines aerobic bacteria in the urine at a value of greater than or equal to 10^4 CFU/mL.[5] Urine cultures are recommended in patients having risk factors for complicated UTIs and in the following situations:[3]
  - • Suspected acute pyelonephritis

- • Symptoms not resolving within 2–4 weeks after completion of antibiotic treatment
- • Women presenting with atypical symptoms
- • Pregnant women
- • Male patients with suspected UTI.
- ❖ *Dipstick test*: Urine dipstick test for detecting the presence of nitrites and leucocytes can be used for diagnosing UTI. The probability of having UTI is particularly high if the dipstick test is positive for both. Urine dipstick analysis serves as a reasonable alternative to urine culture for diagnosing the cases of acute uncomplicated cystitis. Urine dipstick tests can be used for guiding treatment in otherwise healthy women under 65 years of age presenting with mild or less than or equal to two symptoms of UTI.

MANAGEMENT

PREVENTION

In order to prevent the development of UTI, the patient should be asked to observe the following precautions:

- ❖ Avoiding the use of perfumed bubble bath, soap or talcum powder, especially around the genitals.
- ❖ Emptying her bladder as soon as possible after having sexual intercourse or as soon as she has an urge to micturate and taking care to always empty her bladder fully.
- ❖ *Staying adequately hydrated*: Drinking plenty of fluids is likely to help the patient feel better.
- ❖ Using another method of contraception rather than using a contraceptive diaphragm or condoms with spermicidal lubricant.
- ❖ Wearing underwear made from cotton, rather than synthetic material such as nylon, and avoiding tight-fitting jeans and trousers.
- ❖ Use of methenamine hippurate must be considered in women without any known abnormalities of the upper renal tract to prevent the development of symptomatic UTI.[6]

TREATMENT

Complicated Urinary Tract Infections

The treatment strategy for complicated UTIs depends upon the severity of the illness. Hospitalisation is often necessary in these cases. Numerous IV and oral antimicrobial treatment options are available. Majority of patients with serious UTIs require initial IV therapy due to the likelihood of bacteraemia or sepsis or impaired gastrointestinal absorption. While there are no contemporary guidelines for treatment of these infections, targeted therapy should be initiated once susceptibility data for the causative organisms are known.[7] Agents commonly prescribed include aminoglycosides, β-lactam or β-lactamase inhibitor combinations, imipenem, advanced-generation cephalosporins and fluoroquinolones.

Fluoroquinolones are often recommended when conventional agents have failed or are not appropriate due to concerns related to toxicity or hypersensitivity, or in cases of high resistance. Many experts agree that empirical therapy for the institutionalised or hospitalised patient with a serious UTI should include an IV antipseudomonal agent due to an increased risk of urosepsis.

Uncomplicated Urinary Tract Infections

❖ *Pain killers*: Over-the-counter painkillers such as paracetamol or ibuprofen can help to reduce the pain. However, there is no evidence demonstrating the efficacy of over-the-counter pain killers in such women.

❖ *Antibiotics*: Uncomplicated UTIs are normally treated with a short course of antibiotics. An appropriate antibiotic should be selected either empirically or based on the results of culture and sensitivity. The drug should also be able to reach an appropriate concentration within the urinary tract.[8,9] The recommended treatment of first choice in cases of uncomplicated UTI is nitrofurantoin in the dosage of 50 mg every 6-hourly or 100 mg 12-hourly for 5 days. Scottish Intercollegiate Guidelines Network (SIGN) and Health Protection Agency (HPA) recommend the use of nitrofurantoin or 3-day course of trimethoprim sulfamethoxazole [160/800 mg (1 double-strength tablet) twice-daily for 3 days] (first-line therapy) for empirical treatment of uncomplicated UTI amongst non-pregnant women of any age group.[5,10] In case of the failure of first-line therapy, the second-line treatment comprises of performing urine culture and prescribing against the urine culture results. Particular care should be taken when prescribing nitrofurantoin to elderly patients, who may be at an increased risk of toxicity. Non-pregnant women with symptoms or signs of acute uncomplicated UTI can be treated with a course of ciprofloxacin for 7 days or co-amoxiclav for 14 days (second-line therapy). Use of broad spectrum antibiotics (e.g. co-amoxiclav, quinolones and cephalosporins) should be preferably avoided due to an increased risk of development of antibiotic resistance, *Clostridium difficile* infection, methicillin-resistant *Staphylococcus aureus* (MRSA), resistant UTIs, etc. Women with lower UTI, who are prescribed nitrofurantoin, must not be simultaneously advised to take alkalinising agents (such as potassium citrate) because minimum inhibitory concentration (MIC) of this drug rises with an increase in pH. There is no need to treat non-pregnant women (of any age) having asymptomatic bacteriuria with an antibiotic.

In a few regions, the uropathogen resistance rates to the fluoroquinolones have exceeded 10–25%.[11] This has made empirical therapy with fluoroquinolones difficult. β-lactams are not recommended because of suboptimal clinical and bacteriological results compared with those of non-β-lactams. If a β-lactam is chosen, it should be administered for at least 7 days.

Treatment of Urinary Tract Infections in Pregnancy

In case of a pregnant woman presenting with the symptoms of UTI, a standard quantitative urine culture should be routinely performed during the first antenatal visit. Presence of bacteriuria in urine must be confirmed with a second urine culture. Testing with dipstick should not be used for screening for bacterial UTI during the first or subsequent antenatal visits during pregnancy. Pregnant women with symptomatic UTI should be treated with an antibiotic. Choice of antibiotic therapy must be based on the results of culture and sensitivity and the local guidelines. A 7-day course of treatment is usually adequate. A urine culture should be preferably performed after 7 days, following the completion of antibiotic therapy to confirm bacteriological cure.

Asymptomatic bacteriuria detected during pregnancy must also be treated with a 3–7 day course of antibiotic because such treatment is likely to reduce the risk of complications such as preterm deliveries, low-birthweight babies, etc.[12] Antibiotics such as penicillin or cephalosporins or nitrofurantoin are unlikely to have any toxic effects or an increased risk of congenital malformations in pregnant women during the first or second trimester. However, nitrofurantoin may be associated with a very low risk of haemolysis in women with glucose-6-phosphate dehydrogenase deficiency. Therefore, its use must be avoided in the third trimester. Sulphonamides should also be avoided during the third trimester due to the risk of hyperbilirubinaemia and kernicterus.

Moreover, trimethoprim must not be prescribed to pregnant women during the first trimester or in the women with established folate deficiency, low dietary folate intake, or women taking other folate antagonists because trimethoprim may cause adverse effects in presence of folate deficiency. Similarly, use of flouroquinolones should also be avoided during early pregnancy due to its adverse effect on the foetal cartilage.

Treatment of Recurrent Urinary Tract Infection

Various strategies for the prevention of recurrent UTI infection have been previously described in the text. Use of cranberry juice or probiotics is often advised for the prevention of recurrent UTI. However, there is currently little evidence to suggest that drinking cranberry juice or using probiotics is likely to significantly reduce the woman's chances of developing UTI.[13,14] A Cochrane review by Albert et al. (2004) has shown that continuous antibiotic prophylaxis for 6–12 months is likely to reduce the rate of UTI during prophylaxis in comparison to placebo.[15] However, no difference in the incidence of UTI is observed following the discontinuation of the antibiotic therapy. Moreover, the women who received antibiotic therapy were associated with a high risk of adverse events. The available evidence also shows that long-term use of antibiotics in individuals with recurrent UTI is associated with little benefit. On the other hand, its use may be associated with an increased risk of microbial resistance. Therefore, this strategy is best avoided.[16] The available evidence also shows that the use of vaginal oestrogen preparations (vaginal cream, tablets or ring) can be considered in the postmenopausal women with urogenital atrophy suffering from recurrent UTI.[17]

COMPLICATIONS

❖ *Renal scarring*: Though the outcome of UTI is usually benign, infection in the early childhood may sometimes result in renal scarring, which may lead to several complications in adulthood including hypertension, proteinuria, renal damage and sometimes even chronic renal failure, requiring treatment with dialysis.

❖ *Spread of infection*: Lower UTIs are usually not a cause for major concern. Upper UTIs, on the other hand, can be serious if left untreated, as they could damage the kidneys or spread to the bloodstream, respectively, resulting in the development of pyelonephritis and septicaemia.

❖ *Adverse effect of UTI on pregnancy*: Urinary tract infection in pregnancy can result in adverse outcomes such as preterm births, low-birthweight infants, foetal growth restriction, increased perinatal mortality, etc. UTI in pregnancy can also be associated with maternal adverse outcomes such as chorioamnionitis and endometritis.

CLINICAL PEARLS

❖ Uncomplicated lower UTI remains one of the most commonly treated infections amongst women in the primary care. UTIs are most commonly seen in sexually active young women.

❖ Treatment of patients with serious complicated UTIs presently remains challenging.

❖ Women may be more likely to acquire UTIs because they have a shorter urethra, which is closer to anus, in comparison to men.

❖ It is important to rule out the diagnosis of urogenital tuberculosis and/or malignancy in the patients presenting with persistent, non-resolving symptoms of UTI.

❖ *Escherichia coli* remains the chief uropathogen in acute cases of community-acquired uncomplicated UTIs.

❖ Use of antimicrobial therapy must be based on the results of culture and sensitivity.

EVIDENCE-BASED MEDICINE

❖ There is currently little evidence to suggest that drinking cranberry juice or using probiotics is likely to significantly reduce the woman's chances of developing UTI. A recent Cochrane review has indicated that the use of cranberry juice is less effective in the treatment of UTI as was indicated by previous studies.[13] Women should be advised that intake of cranberry capsules may be more convenient than juice and high-strength capsules are likely to be most effective.

❖ Despite the lack of adequate evidence showing reduction in UTI using probiotics, the use of probiotics is likely to be useful for prevention of recurrent UTI in women.[14] Larger well-designed randomised trials are required in future to demonstrate the beneficial effect of probiotics in comparison to antibiotics in cases of UTI.

❖ The available evidence shows that the clinical outcomes for UTIs treated with antibiotics are better in comparison to those treated with a placebo.[8]

❖ The available evidence supports the use of fluoroquinolones for serious UTIs.[18] Presently, the most commonly used fluoroquinolone is ciprofloxacin. Recently, its once-daily extended-release tablet formulation has been introduced.

❖ The available evidence indicates that 3 days of treatment with antibiotics is as effective as 5–10 days of antibiotic therapy for attaining symptomatic cure in cases of uncomplicated UTI treatment.[19] However, longer duration of therapy is more effective in obtaining bacteriological cure. Longer duration of antibiotic therapy is also associated with an increased risk of adverse effects.

REFERENCES

1. Salvatore S, Salvatore S, Cattoni E, Siesto G, Serati M, Sorice P, et al. Urinary tract infections in women. Eur J Obstet Gynecol Reprod Biol. 2011;156(2):131-6.
2. Grabe M, Bartoletti R, Bjerklund Johansen TE, Cai T, Çek M, Köves B, et al. (2015). Guidelines on Urological Infections. [online] Available from uroweb.org/wp-content/uploads/19-Urological-infections_LR2.pdf. [Accessed January, 2017].
3. Foxman B. Epidemiology of urinary tract infections: incidence, morbidity, and economic costs. Am J Med. 2002;113(Suppl 1A):5S-13S.
4. Flores-Mireles AL, Walker JN, Caparon M, Hultgren SJ. Urinary tract infections: epidemiology, mechanisms of infection and treatment options. Nat Rev Microbiol. 2015;13(5):269-84.
5. Health Protection Agency, British Infection Association. Management of Infection Guidance for Primary Care for Consultation and Local Adaptation. London: Health Protection Agency; 2010.
6. Lee BS, Simpson JM, Craig JC, Bhuta T. Methenamine hippurate for preventing urinary tract infections (Cochrane Review). Cochrane Database Syst Rev. 2012;(10):CD003265.
7. Wagenlehner FM, Naber KG. Current challenges in the treatment of complicated urinary tract infections and prostatitis. Clin Microbiol Infect. 2006;12(Suppl 3):67-80.
8. Gupta K, Hooton TM, Naber KG, Wullt B, Colgan R, Miller LG, et al. International clinical practice guidelines for the treatment of acute uncomplicated cystitis and pyelonephritis in women: A 2010 update by the Infectious diseases Society of America and the European Society for microbiology and infectious diseases. Clin Infect Dis. 2011;52(5):e103-20.
9. Guay DR. Contemporary management of uncomplicated urinary tract infections. Drugs. 2008;68(9):1169-205.
10. Scottish Intercollegiate Guidelines Network (SIGN). Management of suspected bacterial urinary tract infection in adults. Edinburgh: SIGN; 2012.
11. Miller LG, Tang AW. Treatment of uncomplicated urinary tract infections in an era of increasing antimicrobial resistance. Mayo Clin Proc. 2004;79(8):1048-53.

12. Smaill FM, Vazquez JC. Antibiotics for asymptomatic bacteriuria in pregnancy. Cochrane Database Syst Rev. 2007;(2):CD000490.

13. Jepson RG, Williams G, Craig JC. Cranberries for preventing urinary tract infections. Cochrane Database Syst Rev. 2012;(10):CD001321.

14. Schwenger EM, Tejani AM, Loewen PS. Probiotics for preventing urinary tract infections in adults and children. Cochrane Database Syst Rev. 2015;(12):CD008772.

15. Albert X, Huertas I, Pereiró II, Sanfélix J, Gosalbes V, Perrota C. Antibiotics for preventing recurrent urinary tract infection in non-pregnant women. Cochrane Database Syst Rev. 2004;(3):CD001209.

16. Williams G, Craig JC. Long-term antibiotics for preventing recurrent urinary tract infection in children. Cochrane Database Syst Rev. 2011;(3):CD001534.

17. Perrotta C, Aznar M, Mejia R, Albert X, Ng CW. Oestrogens for preventing recurrent urinary tract infection in postmenopausal women. Cochrane Database Syst Rev. 2008;(2):CD005131.

18. Carson C, Naber KG. Role of fluoroquinolones in the treatment of serious bacterial urinary tract infections. Drugs. 2004;64(12):1359-73.

19. Milo G, Katchman EA, Paul M, Christiaens T, Baerheim A, Leibovici L. Duration of antibacterial treatment for uncomplicated urinary tract infection in women. Cochrane Database Syst Rev. 2005;(2):CD004682.

SECTION 15

Gynaecological Oncology

GYNAECOLOGY

Endometrial Cancer

INTRODUCTION

Endometrial cancer develops from the lining of the uterus, this lining is known as the endometrium. It is the most common gynaecologic cancer and the fourth most common cancer amongst women. Approximately, 1 in every 50 women is likely to get affected with the endometrial cancer. The most common symptom associated with endometrial cancer is abnormal uterine bleeding (AUB).[1] Endometrial cancer usually affects women after menopause, commonly in the age group of 50–65 years.

Most cases of endometrial cancer are histologically of adenomatous type. The endometrioid type of adenocarcinoma accounts for about 80% of endometrial cancers. The endometrial cancers can be of different grades (G1, G2 and G3) based on the degree of cellular differentiation, anaplasia and glandular architecture, with higher grade of tumour associated with a worse prognosis. There appear to be two distinct pathogenetic types of endometrial cancer: type I and type II tumours. The first tumour type is typically seen in younger perimenopausal women and comprises approximately 80% of the cases. This cancer occurs in the background of oestrogen stimulation and endometrial hyperplasia. Classification of endometrial hyperplasia based on the latest classification system published by WHO in 2014 is described in Table 83.1.[2] Type I tumours are well-differentiated and are associated with a better prognosis in comparison to the other type.

On the other hand, the other pathogenetic variety occurs in postmenopausal women with atrophic endometrium. These cancers are often poorly differentiated and associated with a worse prognosis. These tumours comprise nearly 20% cases

Table 83.1: Classification of endometrial hyperplasia proposed by WHO (2014)[2]

New term	Synonyms	Genetic changes	Coexistent invasive endometrial carcinoma	Progression to invasive carcinoma
Hyperplasia without atypia	Benign endometrial hyperplasia; simple non atypical endometrial hyperplasia; complex non-atypical endometrial hyperplasia; simple endometrial hyperplasia without atypia; complex endometrial hyperplasia without atypia	Low level of somatic mutations in scattered glands with morphology on histopathological examination (HPE) staining showing no changes	<1%	RR = 1.01–1.03
Atypical hyperplasia/ endometrioid intraepithelial neoplasia	Complex atypical endometrial hyperplasia; simple atypical endometrial hyperplasia; endometrial intraepithelial neoplasia (EIN)	Many of the genetic changes typical for endometrioid endometrial cancer are present, including: micro satellite instability; PAX2 inactivation; mutation of PTEN, KRAS and CTNNB1 (β-catenin)	25–33%	RR = 14–45

and may also include tumours of non-endometrioid histology such as serous, clear cell, mucinous, squamous, transitional cell, mesonephric and undifferentiated tumours.

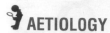

AETIOLOGY

The most important risk factor for endometrial cancer is hyper-oestrogenism or exposure to unopposed oestrogen, both endogenous and exogenous. Other risk factors for endometrial cancer include:

❖ Woman of low parity or nulliparous women
❖ Early menarche and late menopause (associated with prolonged exposure to oestrogen)
❖ Unopposed and unsupervised administration of HRT
❖ Chronic anovulation associated with dysfunctional uterine bleeding (DUB), infertility and PCOS
❖ Use of tamoxifen (for breast cancer) is associated with an increased risk of endometrial hyperplasia
❖ Triad of diabetes, obesity and hypertension increases the risk of cancer.

Role of Tamoxifen in the Pathogenesis of Breast Cancer

Tamoxifen is a non-steroidal antioestrogen, which has been successfully used for the treatment of breast cancer in selected patients. Tamoxifen was originally introduced as an adjuvant treatment of the postmenopausal women with advanced breast cancer disease. However, now the drug is also available for the palliative treatment of premenopausal women with oestrogen receptor (ER) positive disease.[3] Due to its high proven efficacy and the low incidence of side effects, tamoxifen appears to be an ideal agent as an adjuvant therapy for women with node-positive breast cancer.[4] Tamoxifen has been shown to decrease the overall progression of the disease and prevent its spread into the contralateral breast. However, the extended use of tamoxifen has raised questions related to its long-term safety, especially its impact on the ovarian function and its oestrogenic effect over the endometrium, bone and cardiovascular system in premenopausal women, and the potential risks to the foetus if pregnancy occurs. Presently, there are no reports about teratogenicity of tamoxifen in the pregnant women. Nevertheless, tamoxifen should not be used if the patient is pregnant. Also, the physicians must counsel women, taking tamoxifen, about the probable risk to pregnancy in case she conceives. Concerns regarding the occurrence of increased bone density and decreased risk of coronary heart disease due to a decline in the circulating cholesterol levels with the long-term administration of tamoxifen appear to be superfluous. Due to its oestrogenic activities, tamoxifen appears to serve a valuable role as a HRT for all postmenopausal women following a diagnosis of breast cancer. However, due to its oestrogenic action on the uterine endometrium, tamoxifen may be associated with an increased risk of developing endometrial carcinoma.[5]

First results from the International Breast Cancer Intervention Study (IBIS-I), a randomised prevention trial, have shown that use of prophylactic tamoxifen is likely to reduce the risk of breast cancer by nearly one-third.[6] However, use of tamoxifen may be associated with an increased risk of thromboembolic disease. As a result of deaths due to non-breast cancer-related causes, such as thromboembolism, the risk:benefit ratio of tamoxifen is yet not clear. Continued follow-up of the currently on-going trials and initiation of new well-designed trials is essential in future.

Long-term use of tamoxifen due to its oestrogenic effects on the endometrium is likely to result in endometrial proliferation, as well as a spectrum of benign and malignant changes in the endometrium, including endometrial hyperplasia (both simple and atypical), polyps and endometrial cancer. Therefore, the women receiving tamoxifen should be closely monitored by TVS and hysteroscopy to detect development of any endometrial pathologies.[7] However, office hysteroscopy, where biopsy cannot be taken, is not useful for diagnosis of endometrial abnormalities in women taking tamoxifen.

While there have been only a few reports till date of endometrial carcinoma following adjuvant therapy with tamoxifen, any instance of AUB or spotting in women on tamoxifen therapy should be followed up with an endometrial biopsy. A pipelle biopsy is appropriate as the first line of investigation. However, negative results on pipelle biopsy are equivocal. Use of TVS for assessment of endometrial thickness can be considered in these cases after taking into account the fact that tamoxifen is likely to have a sonolucent effect on both the uterine endometrium and myometrium, thereby resulting in false-positive reports. Therefore, in these cases hysteroscopy serves as the investigation of choice because it allows direct inspection of the endometrium, thereby allowing the clinician to take full thickness endometrial biopsies.[8] On the other hand, presently there is no clinical or cost-effective method for endometrial screening of asymptomatic women. Also, there is no evidence to indicate that asymptomatic women taking tamoxifen should be screened for endometrial changes.

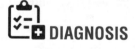

DIAGNOSIS

Clinical Presentation

❖ *Bleeding abnormalities*: The most common bleeding abnormalities include menorrhagia or irregular bleeding in perimenopausal women and postmenopausal bleeding (PMB).
❖ *Risk factors*: Risk factors related to the development of endometrial cancer, which can be elicited at the time of taking history are tabulated in Box 83.1.
❖ *Features indicative of presence of endometrial malignancy*: The pointers in the history of bleeding, indicative of underlying malignancy in case of AUB include the following:
  • Sudden change in the bleeding pattern
  • Irregular bleeding
  • Intermenstrual bleeding
  • Postcoital bleeding
  • Dyspareunia, pelvic pain
  • Lower extremity oedema, which could be secondary to metastasis.

Box 83.1: Risk factors related to the development of endometrial cancer

- ❑ Patients older than 35 years of age
- ❑ Overweight or obesity
- ❑ Unopposed exposure of endometrial cavity to oestrogens (both endogenous and exogenous)
- ❑ More than 35 days between two consecutive periods
- ❑ History of diabetes or hypertension
- ❑ History of intake of medications such as tamoxifen
- ❑ Nulliparous women or those with low parity
- ❑ Early menarche or late menopause
- ❑ Non-ovulatory cycles as seen in cases of anovulatory DUB or PCOS
- ❑ Lynch II syndrome

Abbreviations: DUB, dysfunctional uterine bleeding; PCOS, polycystic ovarian syndrome

General Physical Examination

Body mass index: Obese women (with increased BMI) are more likely to be suffering from endometrial malignancies. Obesity increases the levels of free oestrogen in the body by decreasing the levels of serum hormone-binding proteins. Moreover, aromatisation of the androgen, epiandrostenedione to oestrone occurs in peripheral fat.

Blood pressure: Increased blood pressure could be related with an increased risk for endometrial cancer.

Per Speculum Examination

Sometimes metastatic vaginal growth may be visible.

Pelvic Examination

- ❖ Uterus may appear to be bulky due to associated fibroid or pyometra
- ❖ In advanced stages, the growth may be observed to be protruding through the os.

Investigations

- ❖ *Cytological examination*: This includes investigations such as endometrial biopsy, endometrial aspiration, fractional curettage, etc.
- ❖ *Transvaginal ultrasound*: It is especially indicated in the women at high risk for endometrial cancer. If TVS is not available then an endometrial sample should be taken. Measurement of the endometrial thickness is not a replacement for biopsy. Measurement of endometrial thickness on TVS has become a routine investigation in patients with AUB, especially those belonging to the postmenopausal age groups. If the endometrial thickness on TVS is greater than 5 mm (Fig. 83.1), an endometrial sample should be taken to exclude endometrial hyperplasia. Increased endometrial thickness on TVS examination is an indication for further follow-up by saline infusion sonography (SIS) or hysteroscopic-guided endometrial biopsy. Histopathological examination is especially important in these cases to rule out endometrial hyperplasia, atypia and carcinoma. Endometrial sampling is not usually required in case the endometrial thickness is

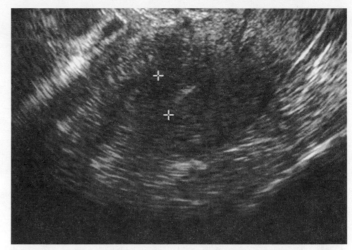

Fig. 83.1: Abnormal endometrial thickness (7 mm) on transvaginal sonography in a 65-year-old patient with abnormal uterine bleeding

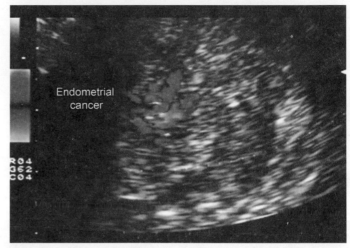

Fig. 83.2: Thick heterogeneous endometrium with proliferation of blood vessels on colour Doppler. This was found to be advanced stage of endometrial cancer *(For colour version, see Plate 8)*

less than 4 mm. In premenopausal women with suspected endometrial neoplasia, sonographic measurement of endometrial thickness is not used as an alternative to endometrial sampling. Doppler ultrasound in case of malignancy may reveal a low-resistance index (Fig. 83.2).

- ❖ *Endometrial studies*: In case the endometrial thickness is more than 5 mm on TVS examination, endometrial studies should be done in order to exclude endometrial hyperplasia.[9] Endometrial sampling is usually performed with an office endometrial biopsy, which can be performed in an outpatient setting, most commonly using a pipelle device, without any requirement for anaesthesia and is a non-invasive approach.[10] Indications for endometrial biopsy are enlisted in Box 83.2.
- ❖ *Hysteroscopy*: Hysteroscopy with biopsy can be regarded as the 'gold standard' investigation for the diagnosis of AUB. Hysteroscopy with biopsy provides the most comprehensive evaluation of the endometrium and is recommended for use in any woman with equivocal or suspicious findings on biopsy or ultrasonography. Hysteroscopy allows for direct visualisation of the endometrial cavity along with the facility for directed biopsy.

Box 83.2: Indications for endometrial biopsy

❑ Endometrial thickness on TVS is ≥4 mm (in postmenopausal women)
❑ Persistent intermenstrual bleeding
❑ Abnormal uterine bleeding in a woman >35 years of age
❑ Abnormal uterine bleeding in postmenopausal women
❑ Treatment failure or ineffective treatment
❑ Patients having high-risk factors for the development of endometrial cancer
❑ There is a pelvic mass and the uterus is >10 weeks' gestation in size
❑ There is a pelvic mass and no facility for urgent ultrasound scan is available

❖ *Investigations for evaluating the spread of cancer*: In case the diagnosis of endometrial cancer has been confirmed, the following investigations are performed to evaluate the spread of cancer:[11]

- Blood tests (haematocrit)
- Kidney and liver function tests
- Chest X-ray
- Computed tomography
- Magnetic resonance imaging (Fig. 83.3).

DIFFERENTIAL DIAGNOSIS

❖ Senile endometritis, tubercular endometritis
❖ Atypical hyperplasia, endometrial polyps
❖ Lesions such as cervical cancer may also cause PMB.

MANAGEMENT

Cancer Staging

The detailed FIGO staging of endometrial cancer and stage-wise treatment is described in Table 83.2.[12]

For patients with stage I and II cancer, the treatment of choice is an extrafascial total abdominal hysterectomy (TAH) and bilateral salpingo-oophorectomy (BSO), with lymph node sampling. Removal of a vaginal cuff is usually not required in these cases. The removed tumour specimen is examined for tumour size, depth of myometrial invasion and extension into the cervix. Endocervical glandular involvement should be considered as stage I and no longer as stage II. In cases of cervical stromal involvement, the treatment options include laparoscopic radical hysterectomy with pelvic lymphadenectomy or TAH with BSO with or without lymphadenectomy followed by postoperative radiotherapy.

Pelvic lymphadenectomy may be done in selective cases. This procedure is often used for establishing the presence of extra-uterine disease and as a therapeutic procedure. The results of the ASTEC (A Study in the Treatment of Endometrial Cancer) surgical trial has indicated that pelvic lymphadenectomy cannot be recommended as routine

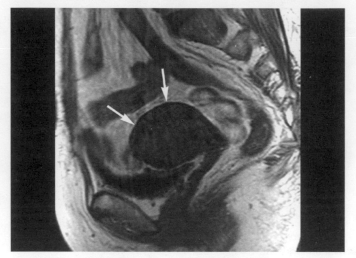

Fig. 83.3: MRI scan showing endometrial adenocarcinoma

procedure in addition to TAH and BSO for therapeutic purposes in cases of endometrial carcinoma.[13] Pelvic lymphadenectomy is not likely to cause an improvement in the overall or recurrence-free survival in women with early endometrial cancer. Indications for pelvic lymph node sampling are enlisted in Box 83.3. In these conditions, lymph node sampling must be done even if the lymph nodes are clinically negative. Laparoscopically assisted vaginal hysterectomy with BSO and laparoscopic retroperitoneal lymph node sampling is being tried at certain centres in place of the conventional abdominal surgery.

Presently, there is no clear agreement regarding the advantages of laparoscopically assisted surgery (LAS) versus open surgery (OS) for early stage endometrial cancer. Several studies have shown that a laparoscopic procedure is likely to be clinically and economically effective alternative to open surgery.[14-18] A meta-analysis of RCTs has shown that LAS is likely to be associated with certain advantages such as fewer postoperative complications (e.g. thromboembolism, postoperative infections, etc.), reduced requirement for blood transfusion, lower amount of blood loss and shorter duration of hospital stay. However, it is likely to be associated with a longer operative period especially if the surgeon is not sufficiently experienced. Also, no significant difference was found in terms of recurrence and survival in comparison to the open surgery. Therefore, if performed by suitably specialised surgeons in selected patients, LAS can be considered as an effective and safe procedure for patients with early stage endometrial cancer.

The results of the LAP-2 trial (conducted in the timeframe between 1996 and 2005), the largest American RCT by the Gynecologic Oncology Group (GOG) comparing laparoscopic with open hysterectomy has shown that laparoscopic-assisted hysterectomy serves as an acceptable alternative to laparotomy for the treatment of early stage uterine cancer.[19] Despite the established short-term advantages of the laparoscopic surgery, there was no consensus regarding the survival benefits of laparoscopic-assisted surgical procedures for endometrial cancer. However, recently, initial survival data from LAP2, which was reported at the 41st annual meeting of

Table 83.2: FIGO staging of endometrial cancer and stage-wise treatment[12]

Stage	Characteristics	Treatment
Stage 0	Cases of endometrial hyperplasia	Total abdominal hysterectomy (TAH) with salpingo-oophorectomy
Stage I (Grade 1, 2, or 3)	Cancer confined to the corpus uteri IA: Tumour limited to endometrium or invades less than one-half of the myometrium IB: Tumour invades one-half or more of the myometrium	Extrafascial TAH and bilateral salpingo-oophorectomy with lymph node sampling. Removal of a vaginal cuff is usually not required in these cases. In the cases where lymph nodes are involved, postoperative radiotherapy may be required
Stage II (Grade 1, 2, or 3)	Tumour involves the stromal connective tissue of cervix, but does not extend beyond the uterus*	Radiation therapy (brachytherapy) is followed by surgery. External radiotherapy may be applied based on the histopathological findings. Alternatively, the surgeon may perform radical hysterectomy with bilateral salpingo-oophorectomy and pelvic lymphadenectomy
Stage III (Grade 1, 2, or 3)	_Local and/or regional spread:_ IIIA: Invasion of serosa and/or adnexa and/or positive peritoneal cytology IIIB: Vaginal metastases IIIC: Metastases to pelvic and/or para-aortic lymph nodes 　IIIC1: Regional lymph node metastasis to pelvic lymph nodes 　IIIC2: Regional lymph node metastasis to para-aortic lymph nodes, with or without positive pelvic lymph nodes	For stage III tumours, the treatment involves TAH and salpingo-oophorectomy with selective lymphadenectomy, biopsies of suspicious areas, omental biopsy and debulking of tumour followed by radiotherapy. Chemotherapy with doxorubicin in the dosage of 60 mg/m² and other drugs including cisplatin and paclitaxel is also being tried
Stage IV (Grade 1, 2, or 3)	_Tumour becomes widespread:_ IVA: Invasion of bladder and/or bowel mucosa (bullous oedema is not sufficient to classify a tumour as T4) IVB: Distant metastases, including intra-abdominal metastases and/or inguinal lymph nodes. It excludes metastasis to para-aortic lymph nodes, vagina, pelvic serosa or odnera	Treatment has to be individualised in those with stage IV tumours because cancer in this stage is usually non-operable. Usually, palliative therapy comprising of a combination of surgery, radiotherapy, hormone therapy or chemotherapy is required

*Endocervical glandular involvement should be considered as stage I and no longer as stage II.

Box 83.3: Indications for pelvic lymph node sampling

❏ The tumour histology is known to be clear cell type, serous, squamous or poorly differentiated grade III endometrioid type
❏ Cut section shows that the myometrium has been invaded to more than half of its thickness
❏ The tumour has extended to the cervix or isthmus
❏ Size of the tumour is >2 cm
❏ There is an evidence of extrauterine disease

the Society of Gynecologic Oncologists (SGO), has indicated identical 3-year overall survival rates amongst the patients undergoing laparotomy and laparoscopy.[20]

Surgery alone may serve as an appropriate treatment option for patients with stage IA (G1 and G2) tumours, in whom there is no evidence of invasion of the lymphovascular space, cervix or isthmus; peritoneal cytology is negative, and there is no evidence of metastasis. In all the other patients, some form of adjuvant radiotherapy is indicated. This method helps in bringing about a significant reduction in the incidence of vaginal vault recurrence. Postoperative radiotherapy for early stage endometrial carcinoma is likely to reduce the locoregional cancer recurrence but is unlikely to affect the overall survival.[21] Radiotherapy, however, is likely to increase treatment-related morbidity. Postoperative radiotherapy is, therefore, not indicated in patients with stage-1 endometrial carcinoma below 60 years and patients with grade-2 tumours having superficial invasion.[22]

Radical hysterectomy has no place in the management of early stage endometrial cancer. For stage II tumours, radical hysterectomy with BSO and pelvic lymphadenectomy is the most commonly used treatment modality. However, some gynaecologists prefer to use the same standard surgical approach, as described for stage I disease, followed by appropriate pelvic or extended field external and intravaginal irradiation. Following surgery for stage I or IIA endometrial carcinoma, recurrence of cancer can frequently occur particularly in the vagina. Postoperative radiotherapy is frequently used to prevent this recurrence. Results from the ASTEC and EN.5 trials have shown that use of external beam radiotherapy (EBRT) in preventing isolated local recurrence is associated with only a small absolute benefit.[23] Moreover, there may be toxic systemic side effects. EBRT cannot be therefore recommended as part of routine treatment for women with intermediate-risk or high-risk early-stage endometrial cancer.

The study by PORTEC (Post Operative Radiation Therapy in Endometrial Carcinoma) study group has shown that vaginal brachytherapy (VBT) is as effective as EBRT in prevention of vaginal recurrence.[24] Moreover, it is associated with fewer adverse effects (e.g. gastrointestinal toxic effects) and improved quality of life in comparison to ERBT. VBT can be considered for the adjuvant treatment of choice for patients with endometrial carcinoma of high-intermediate risk.

Patients with stage IBG3 and stage IIA (G1 and G2) tumours are given either pelvic irradiation or vaginal cuff irradiation.

Box 83.4: Indications of radiotherapy

- ❑ *Postoperative vaginal irradiation*
  - Stage IA G3 tumours
  - Stage IB G1 and G2 tumours
  - Stage IB G3 and stage IIA (G1 and G2) tumours
- ❑ *External pelvic irradiation*
  - Tumours in stage IC (all grades), stage IIA (G3) and stage IIB (all grades), stage IIIA (all grades) or those with lymphovascular space invasion
  - All patients with positive lymph nodes
  - Patients with documented para-aortic and common iliac lymph node involvement
  - Selected IVA patients

For those with tumours in stage IC (all grades), stage IIA (G3) and stage IIB (all grades), stage IIIA (all grades) or those with lymphovascular space invasion, external pelvic irradiation of 50 Gy is recommended in addition to vaginal irradiation. This may also be suitable for selected IVA patients. Various indications for radiotherapy are listed in Box 83.4. Patients with documented para-aortic and common iliac lymph node involvement are additionally given extended field irradiation in the dosage of 45 Gy. Patients with stage IV disease with intraperitoneal spread may require whole abdominal irradiation along with systemic chemotherapy.

For stage III growths, the goal of surgery is TAH and BSO with selective lymphadenectomy, biopsies of suspicious areas, omental biopsy and debulking of tumour followed by radiotherapy.

Stage IV cancers are usually non-operatable. Treatment has to be individualised in those with stage IV tumours. Usually, a combination of surgery, radiotherapy, hormone therapy or chemotherapy is required. Chemotherapy with doxorubicin in the dosage of 60 mg/m^2 and other drugs including cisplatin and paclitaxel is also being tried. Medroxyprogesterone acetate administered in the dosage of 1 g weekly, acts as an adjuvant to chemotherapy.

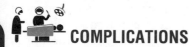

COMPLICATIONS

Complications Associated with Endometrial Cancer

Complications associated with endometrial cancer per se include the following:

- ❖ Pyometra
- ❖ Uterine enlargement
- ❖ Menorrhagia, PMB, intermenstrual bleeding, etc.
- ❖ Anaemia due to blood loss and cancer cachexia
- ❖ Uterine perforation.

Complications Associated with Therapy

Therapeutic modalities like surgery, radiotherapy and chemotherapy can result in numerous complications. Some of these complications are described here.[1]

Complications due to Radiotherapy

During the acute phase of pelvic radiation, the surrounding normal tissues, such as the intestines, the bladder and the perineum skin are often affected. As a result, radiotherapy to the pelvic area can cause side effects, such as tiredness, diarrhoea, dysuria, etc. These side effects can vary in severity depending on the strength of the radiotherapy dose and the length of treatment. Some of these complications are described next.

Cystourethritis: Inflammation of bladder and urethra can result in complications, like dysuria, increased urinary frequency and nocturia. Antispasmodics medicines are often helpful in providing symptomatic relief. Urine should be examined for possible infection. If UTI is diagnosed, therapy should be instituted without delay.

Gastrointestinal effects: Gastrointestinal side effects due to radiotherapy include diarrhoea, abdominal cramping, rectal discomfort, bleeding, etc. Diarrhoea can be either controlled by loperamide (Imodium®) or diphenoxylate (Lomotil®). Small steroid containing enemas are prescribed to alleviate symptoms resulting from proctitis.

Soreness of skin: Radiotherapy can result in erythema and desquamation of skin.

Tiredness: Radiotherapy can result in extreme tiredness. Therefore, the patient must be advised to take as much rest as possible.

Bowel complaints: In a small number of cases, the bowel may be permanently affected by the radiotherapy, resulting in continued diarrhoea. The blood vessels in the bowel can become more fragile after radiotherapy treatment, resulting in haematochezia.

Vaginal stenosis: Radiotherapy to the pelvis can cause narrowing and shortening of the vaginal orifice, thereby making the sexual intercourse difficult or uncomfortable. This problem can be overcome by prescribing oestrogen creams to the patient. Using vaginal dilators or having regular penetrative sexual intercourse often helps in maintaining the suppleness of the vaginal orifice.

Lymphoedema: Lymphoedema resulting in the swelling of one or both the legs can commonly occur as a complication of radiotherapy or due to the cancer per se in advanced stages.

Side Effects due to Chemotherapy

Chemotherapy can cause side effects which may be slightly worse if it is given alongside radiotherapy. Chemotherapy can temporarily reduce the number of normal blood cells, resulting in development of symptoms including increased susceptibility to infection, easy fatigability, anaemia, etc. Other side effects, which the chemotherapy drugs can cause, may include oral ulcerations (stomatitis), nausea, vomiting and alopecia. Nausea and vomiting can be well controlled with effective antiemetic drugs. Regular use of mouthwashes is important in treating the mouth ulcerations.

Complications due to Surgery

Some complications related to surgery (hysterectomy) include the following:

❖ *Premature menopause*: Removal of ovaries in young patients can result in symptoms related to premature menopause.

❖ *Urinary dysfunction*: The most frequent complication of radical hysterectomy is urinary dysfunction, as a result of partial denervation of the detrusor muscle.

❖ *Other complications*: Other complications resulting from surgery may include shortened vagina, ureterovaginal and rectovaginal fistulas, haemorrhage, infection, bowel obstruction, stricture and fibrosis of the intestine or rectosigmoid colon and bladder, formation of seromas in the femoral triangle, DVT, pulmonary embolism, myocardial infarction, etc.

Complications Related to Radical Vulvectomy and Bilateral Inguinal Lymphadenectomy

Some specific complications related to such surgery are as follows:

❖ *Wound infection*: In case of groin dissection, the most important cause of immediate postoperative morbidity is wound infection, necrosis and breakdown. This can be considerably reduced by adopting a separate incision approach.

❖ *Wound breakdown*: This occurs due to the skin loss at the margins of the groin incision. This complication can be reduced by removing lesser amounts of skin and reducing the undermining of the skin flaps. Suction drainage also helps in reducing the morbidity.

❖ *Lymphoedema of the lower extremities*: This may occur in patients who have undergone dissection of inguinal and deep pelvic group of lymph nodes.

❖ *Late complications*: Late complications can occur in the form of chronic leg oedema, recurrent lymphangitis or cellulitis of the leg. Introital stenosis in the long run can result in dyspareunia.

CLINICAL PEARLS

❖ Patients who are at an increased risk of development of endometrial malignancy include patients with triad of hypertension, diabetes and obesity and those with chronic anovulation (e.g. PCOS), atypical glandular cells of undetermined significance (AGUS) on Pap smear, new-onset menorrhagia, etc.

❖ Dedicated PMB clinics in the UK are used for providing rapid-access outpatient services (e.g. transvaginal scanning) to the women with PMB. Women with abnormal TVS results at the time of their first assessment should be offered endometrial biopsy and/or outpatient hysteroscopy.

❖ The overall beneficial effects of tamoxifen in patients with breast cancer are greater than its risk, especially that related to endometrial proliferation and the likely potential of causing endometrial carcinoma.

❖ Complete investigations must be performed in patients on tamoxifen who experience AUB.

❖ Radiotherapy is mainly used as an adjuvant therapy following surgery in cases of endometrial cancer. This therapy is likely to reduce the risk of vaginal recurrence.

❖ Both the therapies such as lymphadenectomy and radiotherapy may result in the development of lymphoedema, an important treatment related complication.

EVIDENCE-BASED MEDICINE

❖ The available evidence indicates that the use of tamoxifen is likely to substantially improve the 10-year survival rate in women with ER-positive breast cancer. At the same time, it is likely to cause a non-significant increase in the risk of endometrial cancer by a factor of 4 after nearly 5 years of treatment with tamoxifen.[3-6]

❖ While women having tamoxifen who have AUB or spotting should be followed up with an endometrial biopsy and/or hysteroscopy, presently there is no evidence to indicate that asymptomatic women taking tamoxifen should be screened for endometrial changes. Presently, there is no clinical or cost-effective method for endometrial screening of asymptomatic women.[3-6]

❖ The available evidence indicates that ultrasound measurement of endometrial thickness alone cannot be used for accurately ruling out the presence of endometrial cancer. However, measurement of both the endometrial layers thickness of less than or equal to 5 mm on TVS helps in ruling out the presence of endometrial pathology with a good certainty.[9]

❖ The present evidence indicates that pelvic lymphadenectomy cannot be recommended as routine procedure in addition to TAH and BSO for treatment in all cases of early endometrial carcinoma because the procedure is unlikely to cause an improvement in the overall or recurrence-free survival in such women.[13]

REFERENCES

1. Souhami R, Tobias J. Cancer and its Management, 5th edition. Oxford, UK: Blackwell Publishing Ltd; 2005.

2. Zaino R, Carinelli SG, Ellenson LH, et al. Tumours of the uterine corpus: epithelial tumours and precursors. In: Kurman RJ, Carcanglu ML, Herrington CS, Young RH (Eds). WHO Classification of Tumours of Female Reproductive Organs, 4th edition. Lyon: WHO Press; 2014. pp. 125-26.

3. Jordan VC. The role of tamoxifen in the treatment and prevention of breast cancer. Curr Probl Cancer. 1992;16(3):129-76.

4. Early Breast Cancer Trialists' Collaborative Group. Tamoxifen for early breast cancer: an overview of the randomised trials. Lancet. 1998;351(9114):1451-67.

5. Ceci O, Bettocchi S, Marello F, Nappi L, Chiechi LM, Laricchia L, et al. Sonographic, hysteroscopic, and histologic evaluation of the endometrium in postmenopausal women with breast cancer receiving tamoxifen. J Am Assoc Gynecol Laparosc. 2000;7(1):77-81.

CHAPTER 83

6. Cuzick J, Forbes J, Edwards R, Baum M, Cawthorn S, Coates A, et al. First results from the International Breast Cancer Intervention Study (IBIS-I): a randomized prevention trial. Lancet. 2002;360(9336):817-24.

7. Ceci O, Bettocchi S, Marello F, Di Venere R, Pellegrino AR, Laricchia L, et al. Hysteroscopic evaluation of the endometrium in postmenopausal women taking tamoxifen. J Am Assoc Gynecol Laparosc. 2000;7(2):185-9.

8. Timmerman D, Deprest J, Bourne T, Van den Berghe I, Collins WP, Vergote I. A randomized trial on the use of ultrasonography or office hysteroscopy for endometrial assessment in postmenopausal patients with breast cancer who were treated with tamoxifen. Am J Obstet Gynecol. 1998; 179(1):62-70.

9. Gupta JK, Chien PF, Voit D, Clark TJ, Khan KS. Ultrasonographic endometrial thickness for diagnosing endometrial pathology in women with postmenopausal bleeding: a metaanalysis. Acta Obstet Gynecol Scand. 2002;81(9):799-816.

10. Reagan MA, Isaacs JH. Office diagnosis of endometrial carcinoma. Prim Care Cancer. 1992;12:49-52.

11. Mettlin C, Jones G, Averette H, Gusberg S.B, Murphy Gerald P. Defining and updating the American Cancer Society guidelines for the cancer-related checkup: prostate and endometrial cancers. CA Cancer J Clin. 1993;43(1):42-6.

12. Pecorelli S. Revised FIGO staging for carcinoma of the vulva, cervix, and endometrium. Int J Gynaecol Obstet. 2009;105(2):103-4.

13. ASTEC study group, Kitchener H, Swart AM, Qian Q, Amos C, Parmar MK. Efficacy of systematic pelvic lymphadenectomy in endometrial cancer (MRC ASTEC trial): a randomized controlled trial. Lancet. 2009;373(9658):125-36.

14. Childers JM, Surwit EA. Combined laparoscopic and vaginal surgery for the management of two cases of stage I endometrial cancer. Gynecol Oncol. 1992;45(1):46-51.

15. Eltabbakh GH, Shamonki MI, Moody JM, Garafano LL. Laparoscopy as the primary modality for the treatment of women with endometrial carcinoma. Cancer. 2001;91(2): 378-87.

16. Kim DY, Kim MK, Kim JH, Suh DS, Kim YM, Kim YT, et al. Laparoscopic-assisted vaginal hysterectomy versus abdominal hysterectomy in patients with stage I and II endometrial cancer. Int J Gynecol Cancer. 2005;15(5):932-7.

17. Ghezzi F, Cromi A, Bergamini V, Uccella S, Beretta P, Franchi M, et al. Laparoscopic management of endometrial cancer in nonobese and obese women: a consecutive series. J Minim Invasive Gynecol. 2006;13(4):269-75.

18. Yu CK, Cutner A, Mould T, Olaitan A. Total laparoscopic hysterectomy as a primary surgical treatment for endometrial cancer in morbidly obese women. BJOG. 2005;112(1):115-7.

19. Walker JL, Piedmonte MR, Spirtos NM, Eisenkop SM, Schlaerth JB, Mannel RS, et al. Laparoscopy compared with laparotomy for comprehensive surgical staging of uterine cancer: Gynecologic Oncology Group Study LAP2. J Clin Oncol. 2009;27(32):5331-6.

20. Walker JL, Piedmonte MR, Spirtos NM, Eisenkop SM, Schlaerth JB, Mannel RS, et al. Recurrence and survival after randomization to laparoscopy versus laparotomy for comprehensive surgical staging of uterine cancer: Gynecologic Oncology Group LAP2 Study. J Clin Oncol. 2012;30(7):695-700.

21. Creutzberg CL, van Putten WL, Koper PC, Lybeert ML, Jobsen JJ, Wárlám-Rodenhuis CC, et al. Surgery and postoperative radiotherapy versus surgery alone for patients with stage-1 endometrial carcinoma: multicentre randomised trial. PORTEC Study Group. Post Operative Radiation Therapy in Endometrial Carcinoma. Lancet. 2000;355(9213):1404-11.

22. Johnson N, Cornes P. Survival and recurrent disease after postoperative radiotherapy for early endometrial cancer: systematic review and meta-analysis. BJOG. 2007;114(11):1313-20.

23. The ASTEC/EN.5 writing committee on behalf of the ASTEC/EN.5 Study Group Adjuvant external beam radiotherapy in the treatment of endometrial cancer (MRC ASTEC and NCIC CTG EN.5 randomised trials): pooled trial results, systematic review, and meta-analysis. Lancet. 2009;373(9658):137-46.

24. Nout RA, Smit VT, Putter H, Jürgenliemk-Schulz IM, Jobsen JJ, Lutgens LC, et al. Vaginal brachytherapy versus pelvic external beam radiotherapy for patients with endometrial cancer of high-intermediate risk (PORTEC-2):an open-label, non-inferiority, randomised trial. Lancet. 2010;375(9717):816-23.

Ovarian Neoplasia (Benign and Malignant)

BENIGN OVARIAN MASSES

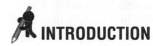

INTRODUCTION

Ovarian neoplasms (tumours) can be neoplastic or physiological. Neoplastic lesions of the ovary can be either benign or malignant in nature. Most ovarian tumours (80–85%) are benign and occur in the women between 20 years to 44 years.[1] Non-neoplastic cysts of ovary are also extremely common and can occur at any age (early reproductive age until perimenopause). These cysts are also known as functional cysts and include follicular cysts, corpus luteum cysts and theca lutein cysts.

The most common neoplastic growths of the ovary include the epithelial tumours, which can be of the following histopathological types:

❖ Serous tumours, which are similar to the epithelium of fallopian tube (most common subtype)

❖ Mucinous tumours, which are similar to the endocervical mucosa

❖ Endometrial tumours, which are similar to the endometrium

❖ Clear cell (mesonephroid) tumours

❖ Brenner tumours, which contain cells similar to the transitional epithelium of the bladder.

The WHO classification of different types of the epithelial tumours has been detailed in Box 84.1.[2] Most malignant ovarian cancers are derived from the surface epithelium of the ovary. Serous and mucinous cystadenocarcinomas are the most common types of invasive epithelial ovarian cancers (EOCs) accounting for nearly 65–70% of cases. Non-epithelial ovarian cancer (e.g. germ cell tumours such as ovarian teratomas and sarcomas) are much less common. Germ cell tumours usually affect younger women and tend to behave very differently from other types of ovarian cancer. While germ cell tumours may account for 15–20% cases of malignant ovarian tumours, sex cord stromal tumours account for 5–10%

cases. Metastatic ovarian cancer arising from non-ovarian primary cancer may account for further 5% of the cases.

Serous Tumours

Serous cystadenomas and cystadenocarcinomas are amongst the most common cystic ovarian neoplasms accounting for nearly 50% of all the ovarian neoplasms. Out of these, 60–70% are benign, whereas 20–25% are malignant. These tumours are characterised by the presence of papillary excrescences both on the surface and within the loculi. In case of carcinoma, the papillary excrescences are coarse and friable and may spread to the peritoneal surface. The benign tumours may contain straw-coloured fluid, while this fluid may be bloodstained in case of malignant tumours.

Mucinous Tumours

Mucinous tumours are multiloculated which commonly contain loculi filled with mucinous contents. If the tumour ruptures, it may result in the formation of pseudomyxoma peritonei.

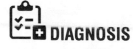

DIAGNOSIS

Clinical Presentation

❖ An adnexal mass may be detected at the time of routine pelvic examination or may present with symptoms that could be related to the presence of the mass per se or due to cyst accidents such as torsion, haemorrhage, rupture, etc. For example, torsion of the cyst may be associated with severe pain along with gastrointestinal symptoms.

❖ A pelvic mass may often result in pelvic pain, which may radiate down to the inner aspect of legs.

❖ Acute abdominal tenderness along with guarding, rigidity and other signs of peritonitis may be associated with rupture or haemorrhage of large cystic masses. In extreme cases, there may be signs of shock.

Box 84.1: WHO histological classification of neoplastic ovarian growths (major groups only)[2]

I. Common epithelial tumours
  A. Serous tumours
    1. Benign
    2. Of borderline malignancy (carcinomas of low malignant potential)
    3. Malignant
  B. Mucinous tumours
    1. Benign
    2. Of borderline malignancy (carcinomas of low malignant potential)
    3. Malignant
  C. Endometrioid tumours
    1. Benign
    2. Of borderline malignancy (carcinomas of low malignant potential)
    3. Malignant
  D. Clear cell (mesonephroid) tumours
    1. Benign
    2. Of borderline malignancy (carcinomas of low malignant potential)
    3. Malignant: Carcinoma and adenocarcinoma
  E. Brenner tumours
    1. Benign
    2. Of borderline malignancy (proliferating)
    3. Malignant
  F. Mixed epithelial tumours
    1. Benign
    2. Of borderline malignancy
    3. Malignant
  G. Undifferentiated carcinoma
  H. Unclassified epithelial tumours
II. Sex cord stromal tumours
  A. Granulosa-stromal cell tumours
  B. Androblastomas, Sertoli-Leydig cell tumours
    1. Well differentiated
    2. Of intermediate differentiation
    3. Poorly differentiated (sarcomatoid)
    4. With heterologous elements
  C. Gynandroblastoma
  D. Unclassified
III. Germ cell tumours
  A. Dysgerminoma
  B. Endodermal sinus tumour
  C. Embryonal carcinoma
  D. Polyembryoma
  E. Choriocarcinoma
  F. Teratomas
  G. Mixed forms
IV. Lipid (lipoid) cell tumours
V. Gonadoblastoma
  A. Pure
  B. Mixed with dysgerminoma or other form of germ cell tumour
VI. Soft tissue tumours not specific to ovary
VII. Unclassified tumours
VIII. Secondary (metastatic) tumours
IX. Tumour-like conditions

❖ Diagnosis of the condition is established on the basis of findings of history and clinical examination. Information regarding the duration and rate of growth of the adnexal mass helps in establishing if the mass is benign or malignant. Family history is also important because of genetic association with malignancy. Duration of use of OCPs is important because women taking the contraceptive pill are at a reduced risk of developing ovarian cancer.

❖ A complete general physical, abdominal, pelvic and rectal examination must be performed in these cases.

Investigations

❖ Routine blood investigations such as CBC, blood group and cross-match, serum electrolytes, blood urea, amylase levels, LFTs, etc.

❖ Urine tests including urine pregnancy test (to exclude pregnancy) and urine for culture and sensitivity

❖ *Tumour markers:* High levels of tumour markers such as cancer antigen (CA)-125 levels could be associated with malignancy. CA-125 is a surface glycoprotein found on the surface of ovarian cancer cells and on some normal tissues. However, measurement of CA-125 should not be used as a stand alone test to diagnose ovarian cancer because estimation of CA-125 levels is associated with low specificity. It can also be raised in presence of benign conditions like endometriosis, tuberculosis, leiomyomas, liver or kidney disease, pelvic inflammatory disease, etc.

❖ *Imaging tests:* Imaging investigations, which need to be done in cases of an ovarian mass, include ultrasound or MRI examination. A pelvic ultrasound, particularly TVS helps in delineating the morphology and dimensions of the adnexal mass. Features on ultrasound, which point towards the benign or malignant nature of the mass, have been discussed later in the chapter.

MANAGEMENT

❖ *Immediate surgical intervention:* This may be specifically required in cases when an ovarian cyst presents with acute symptoms probably due to some complication such as rupture, haemorrhage, torsion, etc. Patients with peritonitis or hypovolemic shock need to be urgently resuscitated.

❖ *Classifying the adnexal mass as benign or malignant:* The most important step of management in these cases comprises of classifying the adnexal mass as benign or malignant. An algorithm illustrating the use of imaging for the evaluation of ovarian masses is shown in Flow chart 84.1. An ovarian mass observed on ultrasound examination does not require further imaging characterisation if it is obviously malignant, e.g. presence of concurrent omental implants, other evidence of peritoneal disseminated disease, lymphadenopathy, pleural effusion, hydronephrosis, etc. Also, simple unilocular cysts less than 5–6 cm in size, with no solid components in a premenopausal woman, are likely to be benign and do not require further imaging. Simple cysts that are larger may warrant additional imaging during the

Flow chart 84.1: Evaluation of adnexal lesion observed on ultrasound imaging studies

future follow-up visit to document whether these cysts have undergone resolution. This is particularly important because such cysts can undergo torsion and may need to be removed surgically if they persist. On the other hand, lesions found in postmenopausal women and those that have solid components on ultrasound examination require further evaluation, usually within 6 weeks.

Management Based on Risk of Malignancy Index-I

An estimation of the risk of malignancy is essential for the assessment of an ovarian mass. At present, the most widely used index, Risk of Malignancy Index-I (RMI-I) for evaluation of malignancy is based on parameters such as CA-125 levels, menopausal status and ultrasound scores. This has been described in details in Chapter 17 (Malignancy during Pregnancy). The use of RMI is endorsed by both RCOG and NICE guidelines in the UK.[3-5] Based on the RMI index, these patients can be categorised as high risk, intermediate risk or low risk and are discussed next in details.[6,7] If the RMI is high (>250), the women must be referred to a gynaecological oncologist for management in the cancer centre. Here, the woman must be preferably managed by a multidisciplinary team. In case the RMI is low (<25), the woman must be managed by a general gynaecologist, while a woman with moderate RMI (25–250) should be preferably managed in a cancer unit.

Low-risk Patients

Simple cysts less than 5 cm in diameter and serum CA-125 levels of less than 25 IU/mL should be conservatively managed. In these cases, the risk of malignancy is less than 3%. Conservative management involves measurement of serum 125 levels and ultrasound scans every 4 months for 1 year. Low-risk patients are usually managed by a general gynaecologist. If the woman requests surgery in these cases, laparoscopic oophorectomy serves as a useful option.

Intermediate-risk Patients

These cases are associated with approximately 20% risk of malignancy and should be managed in a cancer unit. Laparoscopic oophorectomy is useful in selected cases. Patients with intermediate risk of malignancy should be considered for laparoscopic management only if the operator is skilled enough and there are facilities for prompt frozen section.[8] In case the malignancy is revealed, a complete surgical staging procedure must be undertaken in a cancer centre.

High-risk Patients

According to the RCOG guidelines, if the serum CA-125 levels are more than 200 units/mL in premenopausal women, there are high chances of malignancy, with the risk of malignancy being as high as nearly 75%.[3] In such women, discussion with a gynaecological oncologist is recommended.[9] These patients should be managed in a cancer centre and require a full staging laparotomy. Role of laparoscopy for management of ovarian cancer is yet not proven and is not a routine procedure in the UK.

❖ *IOTA Group Model*: A specific model comprising the ultrasound parameters, derived from the International Ovarian Tumour Analysis (IOTA) Group, which is likely to be associated with increased sensitivity and specificity in detection of malignancy, is also commonly used. For further details, kindly refer to Chapter 17 (Malignancy during Pregnancy).

❖ *Management in premenopausal women*: In case of premenopausal women, if the adnexal mass does not show any feature of malignancy (i.e. the mass is freely mobile, cystic in consistency and of regular contour) a period of observation of no more than 2 months can be allowed during which hormonal suppression with OCPs can be used. A benign mass would regress, while a malignant mass would be persistent and would mandate surgical removal.

❖ *Management in postmenopausal women*: Ovarian masses in postmenopausal women should be assessed with the help of CA-125 levels, transvaginal and grey scale sonography. Conservative management should be adopted in case of cysts less than 5 cm in diameter and CA-125 levels of less than 30 IU/mL. These women can be followed up for 1 year with the help of regular TVS and CA-125 levels.

❖ *Conservative laparoscopic surgery*: Laparoscopic surgery should be considered in cases where there is a low risk of malignancy on preoperative evaluation. Laparoscopic management should be undertaken by a suitably qualified laparoscopic surgeon. Laparoscopic aspiration of the cyst either for therapeutic or diagnostic purposes must not be done. In postmenopausal women, laparoscopic management of low-risk ovarian cysts should preferably involve bilateral oophorectomy rather than cystectomy. The ovaries should be removed intact in a bag without the cyst rupturing into the peritoneal cavity.

COMPLICATIONS

Common complications associated with ovarian cysts include intracystic haemorrhage, rupture and torsion. On the other hand, complications such as infection, necrosis, fistula and hernia are rare.

CLINICAL PEARLS

❖ Ultrasound examination, particularly TVS is the single important investigation for predicting whether the mass is benign or malignant.

❖ The RMI is used for stratifying the patients with an adnexal mass on the basis of the likely risk of malignancy, thereby identifying patients who need to be referred to a gynaecological oncologist.

❖ Laparotomy and a complete surgical staging carried out by a trained gynaecological oncologist appear to offer the best prognosis to the patient with a malignant ovarian mass.

EVIDENCE-BASED MEDICINE

❖ Presently, there is no evidence to indicate the routine role for investigation modalities such as 3D or Doppler ultrasound, MRI, CT scan or PET in the management of ovarian masses.[10]

❖ The available evidence has demonstrated the safety and efficacy of laparoscopic surgery for the management of benign ovarian masses.[3,4]

OVARIAN CANCER

INTRODUCTION

Ovarian cancer is the fourth most common cause of cancer-related deaths in women and is the seventh most common cancer diagnosed. An estimated 200,000 cases and 125,000 deaths due to ovarian cancer occur worldwide annually. Its incidence is highest amongst the high-resource countries, with the incidence being 9.3 per 100,000 women.[11] There were 7,284 new cases of ovarian cancer in the UK in the year 2013 and nearly 4,200 deaths due to ovarian cancer in the year 2014.[12] This type of cancer develops most often in women aged 50–70 years. Nearly 80% of the cancers are epithelial cell cancers which originate from the surface epithelium of the ovaries. Other types of ovarian cancers include germ cell tumours, sex cord stromal cell tumours and metastatic cancers. Primary peritoneal cancer and primary fallopian tube cancer are rare malignancies but share many similarities with ovarian cancer. Also, clinical management of these three types of cancers is similar. Therefore, they follow a common staging system. Fallopian tube cancer has also been discussed in details in Chapter 87 (Rare Cancers of the Female Genital Organs).

AETIOLOGY

Some of the risk factors for ovarian cancer are as follows:
❖ Old age, nulliparity, having the first child late in life
❖ Early menarche, late menopause
❖ Family history of cancer of the uterus, breast or large intestine. Mutations of the gene BRCA-1 (chromosome-17) and BRCA-2 (chromosome 13) are commonly implicated in its pathogenesis.
❖ Risk increases with age (up to 70 years)
❖ Multiple ovulation in the IVF programme.

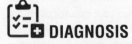

DIAGNOSIS

Clinical Presentation

Many women with ovarian cancer may not have any symptoms, until the cancer is in an advanced stage. Clinical presentation in case of EOC is described in Table 84.1.[13] Moreover, if the symptoms do appear they may be vague such as lower abdomen pain or discomfort, indigestion, bloating, loss of appetite, backache, cachexia, anaemia, etc.

Table 84.1: Clinical presentation in case of epithelial ovarian cancer

Acute presentation	Subacute presentation
• Pleural effusion: Shortness of breath • Bowel obstruction: Severe nausea and vomiting • Venous thromboembolism	• Adnexal mass: Discovered on a routine pelvic examination or an imaging study performed for another indication • Pelvic and abdominal symptoms: Bloating, urinary urgency or frequency, difficulty in eating or early satiety, pelvic or abdominal pain

On general physical examination, either of the following groups of lymph nodes may be enlarged: supraclavicular group, axillary group or inguinal group of lymph nodes.

Abdominal Examination

A lump may be palpated on the abdominal examination. The malignant ovarian tumours are often bilateral, solid, irregular, fixed and may present with ascites. An upper abdominal mass (omental cake) may also be present. Assessment of the hepatic enlargement must also be done.

Pelvic Examination

An adnexal mass, separate from the uterus, may be felt on pelvic examination. Fixed nodules may be palpated in the Pouch of Douglas (POD) on the vaginal examination. A per rectal examination must also be performed.

Breast and Chest Examination

Both the breasts should be examined for the presence of any lump or nodule. This is especially important due to the familial association of breast cancer with ovarian cancer. A chest examination should be carried out to particularly rule out pleural effusion.

Investigations

Tests for Assessing the Likelihood of Malignancy and Planning the Extent of Surgery

❖ *Ultrasonography:* Presence of solid tumours with a thick capsule and papillary projections is suggestive of malignancy. Table 84.2 categorises ovarian masses based on the features as observed on ultrasound examination. Ultrasound examination should not only include the assessment of pelvis, but also of the kidneys and liver. The possibility of a non-ovarian primary cancer is increased in the presence of liver parenchymal metastasis. Significant hydronephrosis in the kidneys can also be identified on ultrasound examination.

❖ *Chest imaging:* This may help in the identification of pleural effusion and the possibility of metastatic disease because occult metastasis to the diaphragm may be recognised in nearly 8% cases.

❖ *CT, MRI scan (of both the abdomen and pelvis):* CT scan helps in outlining the extent of upper abdominal disease, thereby helping in guiding the further course of management: primary surgery or chemotherapy. MRI of the pelvis also helps in surgical planning by determining the involvement of large bowel and/or pelvic sidewalls in the malignant disease process.

❖ Biopsy of the tumour tissue.

❖ Examination of the ascitic fluid.

❖ *Levels of CA-125:* The levels of this antigen have been found to be raised in nearly 80% cases of epithelial cancers.

❖ *Levels of carcinoembryonic antigen (CEA):* Presence of raised levels of CEA is indicative of gastrointestinal malignancy.

❖ *Levels of alpha-foetoprotein (AFP) and β-hCG:* Measurement of the levels of these two markers is particularly important in young women less than the age of 40 years, due to an increased prevalence of germ cell malignancy in the first 2 decades of life.

Tests for Assessing the Anaesthetic Fitness

These may include the following tests:
❖ Full blood count
❖ Kidney function tests: Blood urea and serum creatinine
❖ Serum electrolytes
❖ Liver function tests (including total protein and albumin levels).

MANAGEMENT

Management for ovarian cancer initially includes taking history, conducting physical examination and evaluation

Table 84.2: Categorisation of ovarian masses

Risk category	Ultrasound features	Management options
High risk	Features of malignancy, i.e. presence of solid components, nodular, thick septations (>2–3 mm); size >10 cm	Surgical exploration
Intermediate risk	Not completely anechoic and/or unilocular, but there are no definite features of malignancy (e.g. a mass with thin septations or low level echoes or size of the mass between 5 cm to 10 cm)	Management must be based upon coexisting tumour marker levels, risk factors and symptoms. Many women may be managed with surveillance, but surgical exploration should be performed if clinically significant risk factors or symptoms are observed. Surgical exploration may be performed in women with a 5–10 cm mass who also have symptoms suggestive of ovarian cancer
Low risk	Anechoic unilocular fluid-filled cysts with thin walls	Surveillance rather than surgery is recommended in these cases because the risk of malignancy is less than the risk of complications associated with surgical exploration

PART III

Box 84.2: Aims of performing a surgical procedure

❑ Obtaining the tissue for biopsy to help confirm the diagnosis
❑ Assessing the extent of disease (i.e. surgical staging)
❑ Attempting optimal cytoreduction (which may be essential for successful treatment especially in advanced cases)

Box 84.3: Women who are poor candidates for aggressive initial surgical cytoreduction

❑ Patients with a complex ovarian cyst in whom an extraovarian primary tumour has not been excluded
❑ Imaging findings suggestive of an extensive disease (liver or pulmonary metastases, disease in the porta hepatis, massive ascites, etc.)
❑ Women with a poor performance status (e.g. elderly patients or those having medical comorbidities)

of serum CA-125 levels in combination with imaging (ultrasound, MRI and CT). Neither imaging results nor CA-125 levels alone are sufficiently accurate in diagnosing ovarian cancer. The diagnosis and management of ovarian carcinoma requires surgical exploration. The staging of ovarian cancer is done at the time of exploratory laparotomy. Surgical staging is particularly important because subsequent treatment and prognosis is determined by the disease stage. Patients with advanced stage disease must go through debulking or cytoreductive surgery to remove as much of the tumour and its metastasis as possible, provided the patient is medically fit for a major surgery. Surgery is almost always performed in all women with suspected ovarian cancer, even when advanced. Aims of performing a surgical procedure are listed in Box 84.2. Primary surgical cytoreduction (usually without any chemotherapy) forms the preferred management plan for patients with stage I and II ovarian cancer. Primary surgical cytoreduction followed by systemic chemotherapy is the preferred initial management for women with stage III or IV EOC. However, there are some exceptions to the diagnosis via initial aggressive cytoreduction, which are listed in Box 84.3. Such patients must be treated with neoadjuvant chemotherapy. The FIGO system (2014), used for cancer staging, is summarised in Table 84.3.[14]

Prevention

Screening for Ovarian Cancer

Presently research studies are being carried out to assess whether ovarian cancers can be detected at an early stage so that they can be treated more effectively. Some of the tests, which are being considered in various research trials, include estimation of CA-125 levels or performing a TVS. The aim of these research trials is to evaluate if either of these tests might help in the diagnosis of women with an early stage ovarian cancer. It is important to identify an appropriate screening test because survival rates from ovarian cancer are related to the stage at diagnosis. 5-year survival rates of over 90% have been reported for the minority of women with stage I disease. Since presently, it is not known whether these screening tests could help in detection of ovarian cancers at an earlier stage; currently, there exists no National Screening Programme for ovarian cancer.

Definitive Therapy

The treatment of a patient with ovarian cancer must be planned by a multidisciplinary team comprising a gynaecological oncologist, a clinical or medical oncologist, radiologist, pathologist, a gynaecological oncology nurse specialist, dietician, physiotherapist, occupational therapist

and clinical psychologist or counsellor. The issues, which need to be discussed with the patient before undertaking therapy, include the type and extent of treatment the patient would receive; the advantages and disadvantages of the treatment; any other treatment options that may be available and any significant risks or side effects of the treatment.

Stage IA (Grade I Disease)

Primary treatment for stage I EOC is surgical, i.e. a total abdominal hysterectomy and a bilateral salpingo-oophorectomy and surgical staging. The uterus and contralateral ovary can be preserved in woman with stage IA, grade I disease who desire to preserve their fertility. However, such women must be periodically monitored with routine pelvic examinations and determination of serum CA-125 levels.

Stage IA and IB (Grade II and III) and Stage IC

Treatment options in this case include additional chemotherapy or radiotherapy besides surgery as described earlier. Chemotherapy is the more commonly used option and comprises either single agent or multiagent chemotherapy. The most commonly used single agent chemotherapy in the past was melphalan which was administered orally on a 'pulse' basis for 5 consecutive days, every 28 days. Radiotherapy could be administered either in the form of intraperitoneal (IP) radiocolloids (P32) or whole abdominal radiation. According to the current treatment recommendations, the treatment must be in form of either cisplatin or carboplatin or combination therapy of either of these drugs with paclitaxel for three to four cycles.

Fertility preservation (unilateral salpingo-oophorectomy) can be considered as an option for women with stage IA EOC. Even if conservative surgery is being planned, full surgical staging should be performed.

The staging should include collection of peritoneal washings, omentectomy, appendectomy and lymph node biopsies. A thorough abdominal exploration and biopsy of any abnormal areas must be performed. Endometrial biopsy should also be performed to exclude endometrial cancer. At the time of surgery, the contralateral ovary is not usually biopsied, if it appears to be normal. Young women with a well-differentiated lesion of one ovary, who have undergone conservative surgery, must go through hysterectomy and removal of the remaining ovary upon completion of their families, or by the age of 35 years.

Table 84.3: Staging of carcinoma ovaries, fallopian tube and peritoneum based on TNM and FIGO staging systems[14]

Primary tumour		
TNM categories	**FIGO stage**	**Stages**
TX		Primary tumour cannot be assessed
T0		No evidence of primary tumour
T1	I	Tumour limited to ovaries (one or both) or fallopian tube(s)
T1a	IA	Tumour limited to one ovary or fallopian tube; capsule intact, no tumour on ovarian surface. No malignant cells in ascites or peritoneal washings
T1b	IB	Tumour limited to both ovaries or fallopian tubes; capsules intact, no tumour on ovarian surface. No malignant cells In ascites or peritoneal washings
T1c	IC	Tumour limited to one or both ovaries or fallopian tube with any of the following: Capsule ruptured, tumour on ovarian surface, malignant cells in ascites or peritoneal washings
T1c1	IC1	Surgical spill
T1c2	IC2	Capsule ruptured before surgery or presence of the tumour cells on ovarian or fallopian tube surface
T1c3	IC3	Malignant cells in the ascites or peritoneal washings
T2	II	Tumour involves one or both ovaries or fallopian tube with pelvic extension (below pelvic brim) or primary peritoneal cancer
T2a	IIA	Extension and/or implants on uterus and/or tube(s) and/or ovaries
T2b	IIB	Extension to and/or implants on other pelvic tissues
T3	III	Tumour involves one or both ovaries or fallopian tubes, or primary peritoneal cancer, with cytologically or histologically confirmed spread to the peritoneum outside the pelvis and/or metastasis to the retroperitoneal lymph nodes
	IIIA1	Positive retroperitoneal lymph nodes only (cytologically or histologically proven)
	IIIA1(i)	Metastasis up to 10 mm in greatest dimension
	IIIA1(ii)	Metastasis more than 10 mm in greatest dimension
T3a	IIIA2	Microscopic extrapelvic (above the pelvic brim) peritoneal involvement with or without positive retroperitoneal lymph nodes
T3b	IIIB	Macroscopic peritoneal metastasis beyond the pelvis up to 2 cm in greatest dimension, with or without metastasis to the retroperitoneal lymph nodes
T3c	IIIC	Macroscopic peritoneal metastasis beyond the pelvis more than 2 cm in greatest dimension, with or without metastasis to the retroperitoneal lymph nodes (includes extension of tumour to capsule of liver and spleen without parenchymal involvement of either organ)
T4	IV	Growth involving one or both the ovaries with distant metastasis. If pleural effusion is present, there must be a positive cytological test result to allot a case to stage IV; parenchymal liver metastasis also equals stage IV
Regional lymph nodes (N)		
TNM categories	**FIGO stages**	**Stages**
NX		Regional lymph node metastasis
N0		No regional lymph node metastasis
N1	IIIC	Regional lymph node metastasis
Distant metastasis (M)		
TNM categories	**FIGO stages**	**Stages**
M0		No distant metastasis
M1	IV	Distant metastasis (excludes peritoneal metastasis

Abbreviations: TNM, tumour, node and metastasis; FIGO, International Federation of Gynecology and Obstetrics

Stage II, III and IV

Debulking surgery or cytoreductive surgery is performed in these cases. This involves an initial exploratory procedure with the removal of as much disease as possible (both tumour and the associated metastatic disease).

Cytoreductive Surgery

Cytoreductive surgery (Box 84.4) includes abdominal hysterectomy and bilateral salpingo-oophorectomy, complete omentectomy and resection of metastatic lesions from the peritoneal surface.[15] The gynaecologist must take the biopsies or remove some of the lymph nodes in the abdomen and pelvis. They may also have to remove the omentum, appendix and part of the peritoneum. Resection of rectosigmoid colon should be attempted in women with bulky abdominal disease in case maximal cytoreduction appears to be a likely option. Bowel surgery is of little value in case of grossly unresectable disease, except for relieving gastrointestinal obstruction. Gastrointestinal surgery can add significant morbidity to

Box 84.4: The procedure of cytoreductive surgery

Preoperative preparation
❑ Nutritional assessment
❑ Assessment of intercurrent medical diseases, which should be under optimum control (e.g. good glycaemic control in women with diabetes)
❑ Preoperative laboratory tests
  – A complete blood count
  – Liver and renal function tests
  – Serum electrolytes, glucose
  – Coagulation tests
  – Baseline CA-125 levels
  – Chest radiograph
  – Electrocardiogram
  – Computed tomography of the abdomen
  – Liver imaging helps to determine whether metastatic disease, if present, is confined to surface implants or whether a partial hepatic resection of parenchymal disease may be required

Surgery
❑ Abdominal hysterectomy and bilateral salpingo-oophorectomy
❑ Complete omentectomy
❑ Collection of ascitic fluid (if present) or collection of peritoneal washings (after instillation of normal saline in the paracolic gutters)
❑ Resection of metastatic lesions from the peritoneal surface
❑ Biopsy of the lymph nodes in the abdomen and pelvis
❑ Random biopsies are taken from peritoneal surfaces, including the pouch of Douglas, bladder peritoneum, paracolic gutters, and bowel mesentery
❑ Diaphragm should be biopsied or scraped for cytology
❑ Any adhesions or peritoneal surface irregularities must be biopsied
❑ Pelvic and para-aortic node sampling
❑ Appendectomy

Postoperative preparation
❑ Maintenance of fluid electrolyte balance

Box 84.5: Potential benefits of cytoreduction in women with epithelial ovarian cancer

❑ Removal of bulky disease helps in rapidly improving the disease-related symptoms (e.g. abdominal pain, increased abdominal girth, dyspnoea, early satiety, etc.) and the quality of life.
❑ Removal of tumour bulk may help improve host immune competence by reducing the production of immunosuppressive cytokines (e.g. interleukin-10, vascular endothelial growth factor), which are normally produced by the tumour tissue.
❑ Reduction of tumour bulk helps in reducing the tumour burden (which now becomes well perfused and therefore mitotically active), thereby maximising the effect of chemotherapeutic agents.

surgical treatment. In case the patient has ascites, ascitic fluid must be collected and sent for cytological examination. In case of absence of ascites, peritoneal washings must be collected after instillation of normal saline in the paracolic gutters. At the time of surgery, exploratory laparotomy is carried out in a systematic manner in which the status of various organs such as pelvic organs, small and large intestine, mesentery, appendix, stomach, liver, gallbladder, spleen, omentum, diaphragm, the entire peritoneum, retroperitoneal structures such as the kidneys, pancreas and lymph nodes, are assessed. The affected adnexa should be removed intact and a frozen section must be obtained to confirm the diagnosis. Biopsies must be taken from all suspicious areas. If suspicious areas cannot be obviously seen, multiple random biopsies are taken from peritoneal surfaces, including the POD, bladder peritoneum, paracolic gutters and bowel mesentery, to help detect micrometastases. The diaphragm should be biopsied or scraped for cytology. Any adhesions or peritoneal surface irregularities should also be sampled.

The omentum is resected rather than biopsied. Resection of the omental cake must be performed even when optimal cytoreduction is not possible in order to reduce the tumour bulk and postoperative ascites formation. Pelvic and para-aortic node sampling is performed to exclude the possibility of microscopic stage III disease. Suspicious nodes are removed. Lymph nodes are randomly sampled in case there are no suspicious nodes. Para-aortic nodes, especially those above the inferior mesenteric artery, are involved more commonly than pelvic nodes. Appendectomy is performed as part of the routine staging procedure. Cytoreduction can be a complicated surgery and should ideally be done by a specialist gynaecological oncologist. The goal of cytoreductive surgery is resection of the primary tumour and all the metastatic disease. If this is not possible, the goal must be to reduce the tumour burden by resection of the tumour to an 'optimal status'. Potential benefits of aggressive primary surgical management (cytoreduction) in women with EOC are listed in Box 84.5.

Optimal Cytoreduction

The Gynecologic Oncology Group (GOG) (2004) has defined optimal cytoreduction as leaving residual disease having less than 1 cm maximum tumour diameter. The volume of residual disease remaining after cytoreductive surgery shows an inverse correlation with the survival rates. Therefore, in cases where it is technically feasible, all visible tumour tissue must be resected at the time of initial surgery. Cytoreduction must preferably be performed by gynaecologic oncologists experienced in this surgery so as to achieve optimal cytoreduction. If the initial surgical attempt at cytoreduction was not an optimal one then chemotherapy followed by secondary surgical cytoreduction may be beneficial, but survival is not as high as that achieved with optimal cytoreduction at the time of primary surgery. A second attempt at cytoreduction after chemotherapy for suboptimally debulked disease is usually not as successful as an aggressive initial surgical debulking. However, if the initial surgical attempt at cytoreduction was not a maximal surgical effort then chemotherapy followed by secondary surgical cytoreduction might be beneficial. The two modalities used in the postoperative treatment of newly diagnosed advanced stage EOC are IV chemotherapy alone or a combination of IV and IP chemotherapy. A choice between these options is dependent on the amount of disease remaining after surgery. Combination IV/IP treatment is reserved for women with optimally cytoreduced EOC. On the other hand, patients with suboptimal cytoreduction (having greater than 1 cm of residual disease following surgery) are treated with IV chemotherapy instead of IP because the IP administered chemotherapy drugs have limited penetration into larger tumours. For patients with no clinical evidence of disease and negative tumour markers at the completion of chemotherapy, a reassessment laparotomy or 'second-look' surgery may be performed.

Second-look laparoscopy: Many patients who undergo cyto-reductive surgery and chemotherapy may have no evidence of disease at the completion of the treatment. In order to detect the presence of subclinical disease, a second-look surgery is often performed. This is usually in form of laparotomy, though laparoscopy is sometimes performed. The technique of second-look laparotomy is essentially identical to that for the staging laparotomy. Multiple cytological specimens and biopsies of the peritoneal surface must be performed, particularly in any areas of previously documented tumour. Additionally, any adhesions or surface irregularities must also be sampled. Biopsy specimen must be taken from the pelvic sidewalls, cul-de-sac, bladder, paracolic gutters, residual omentum and the diaphragm. A pelvic and para-aortic lymph node dissection should be performed for those patients whose nodal tissues have not been previously removed. Second-look laparotomies have not been shown to influence patient's survival. Therefore, these should be performed only in research settings where second-line or salvage therapies are undergoing clinical trials. Various second-line therapies include secondary cytoreduction, whole abdominal irradiation, secondary chemotherapy and IP instillation of radiocolloids.

Radiation Therapy

Radiation therapy is not commonly used for the treatment of ovarian cancer. Whole abdominal radiation therapy appears to be a useful option for patients with metastatic disease that is microscopic or completely resected. The current evidence suggests that the whole abdominal radiation is inappropriate for the patients with macroscopic residual disease. Radiotherapy may be rarely used to treat an area of cancer that has come back after surgery and chemotherapy, when other treatment options are no longer appropriate. It can also be used as palliative therapy in order to reduce bleeding or symptoms of pain and discomfort. It has been successfully used in the treatment of recurrent germ cell tumours that are very radiosensitive. Radioactive isotopes of gold (Au 198) or phosphorus (P 32) have been used intraperitoneally in combination with external radiotherapy.

Primary Surgery versus Interval Debulking Surgery following Neoadjuvant Chemotherapy in Advanced Stage Disease

Two multicentric randomised trials, European Organisation for Research and Treatment of Cancer (EORTC) and chemotherapy or upfront surgery (CHORUS) have investigated whether the strategy of performing primary surgery followed by chemotherapy or that of performing interval debulking surgery after neoadjuvant chemotherapy (3–4 cycles of chemotherapy administered prior to surgery) is likely to result in better survival rates and a more complete cytoreductive surgery.[16,17] The results of these trials have shown that the patients undergoing primary cytoreductive surgery followed by chemotherapy are likely to have similar outcomes in terms of survival to the patients, with advanced ovarian cancer, or those with poor performance status or those with large tumour burden, undergoing interval debulking surgery following neoadjuvant chemotherapy. Interval debulking is associated with reduced morbidity and lesser number of major resections. Patients with no residual disease following cytoreductive surgery and those who respond to platinum-based chemotherapy (platinum-sensitive) are likely to have a better survival rate. Results from the EORTC trial have also shown that the patients with stage IIIC and less extensive metastatic tumours are likely to have higher survival rates with primary surgery, in comparison to those with stage IV disease and large metastatic tumours.

Chemotherapy

Various indications for chemotherapy are enumerated in Box 84.6. Chemotherapy is often recommended after surgery for women with moderate- or high-grade ovarian cancer or those with stage IB or IC cancer. Generally, six sessions of chemotherapy are given, over 5–6 months. In advanced-stage ovarian cancer, chemotherapy is sometimes given before surgery (neoadjuvant chemotherapy), to shrink any residual tumour. Women who are given neoadjuvant chemotherapy are given three cycles of chemotherapy before the surgery, followed by three further cycles after the surgery. In case of stage IV cancer with distant metastasis, chemotherapy is the main treatment modality, which is used. In women with early stage ovarian cancer, chemotherapy is given after surgery to reduce the chance of the cancer recurrence. Though chemotherapy cannot guarantee that the cancer will not come back, it does help in reducing the risk of disease recurrence.

International Collaboration on Ovarian Neoplasms (ICON) study, a multicentre, open randomised trial has helped in determining that platinum-based adjuvant chemotherapy helps in improving overall survival and delaying recurrence in women with early-stage EOC having poor prognostic factors or in patients receiving adjuvant chemotherapy if they had not been completely staged at the time of surgery.[18] EORTC Adjuvant ChemoTherapy in Ovarian Neoplasm (ACTION) collaborators from a randomised phase III trial have also shown similar findings. The benefit of adjuvant chemotherapy appeared to be limited to patients with non-optimal staging, i.e. patients with more risk of unappreciated residual disease.[19]

> **Box 84.6:** Indications for chemotherapy
>
> ❏ Early stage ovarian (stage IB or IC) cancer (after surgery in order to reduce the chance of the cancer recurrence): Adjuvant chemotherapy
> ❏ Moderate or high-grade ovarian cancer (after surgery)
> ❏ Neoadjuvant chemotherapy before surgery in advanced stage ovarian cancer
> ❏ Stage IV cancer with distant metastasis

CHAPTER 84

A systematic review and meta-analysis by Winter Roach has demonstrated that chemotherapy is likely to confer significant benefit both in terms of overall and disease-free survival.[20] Platinum-based chemotherapy should be offered to reduce risk of recurrence except in women where adequate surgical staging has revealed a well-differentiated disease confined to one or both ovaries with intact capsule. Presently, for patients with high-risk early-stage disease and for advanced-stage ovarian cancer, the recommended treatment is chemotherapy comprising of platinum-taxane combination for six cycles. Platinum-based therapy is likely to be more effective than the non-platinum-based chemotherapy. Moreover, the use of combination therapy is likely to improve the survival rates in comparison to the use of platinum alone.

Types of Chemotherapy

Intraperitoneal chemotherapy: Chemotherapy can be instilled directly into the abdomen and pelvis through a thin tube. The drugs destroy the cancer cells in the abdomen and pelvis. Use of IP chemotherapy is likely to extend the overall survival by 12–17 months in women with advanced ovarian cancer who have been completely cytoreduced. Presently, the role of IP chemotherapy remains unclear and it is not widely used probably due to its high rate of toxicity. According to the results of a new study, OV21/PETROC trial, a randomised phase II trial, presented at the 2016 American Society of Clinical Oncology (ASCO) Annual Meeting, a combination of IP (carboplatin based) and intravenous chemotherapy is likely to be more effective than IV chemotherapy alone in women with optimally resected advanced ovarian cancer following neoadjuvant chemotherapy.[21] This therapy is not only well tolerated, it also helps in reducing the progressive disease rate by nearly 19% at 9 months.

Systemic chemotherapy: Systemic chemotherapy may be either taken in orally or injected intravenously. The drugs enter the bloodstream and destroy or control cancer throughout the body. IV chemotherapy is given as a session of treatment, usually over several hours. This is followed by a rest period of a few weeks, which allows the patient's body to recover from any side effects of the treatment. Together, the treatment and the rest periods are known as a cycle of chemotherapy. Most women are given six cycles of chemotherapy.

Intravenous chemotherapy: Presently, platinum- and taxane-based combination therapy has been recommended as the first-line treatment for EOC.[22,23] For patients with advanced EOC, IV carboplatin [dosed by AUC (area under the curve) = 6 (range 5–7.5)] is administered with IV paclitaxel (175 mg/m² over 3 hours) repeated every 3 weeks for six cycles. Phase III studies have demonstrated that carboplatin produces response rates and survival outcomes similar to cisplatin. Moreover, the use of carboplatin is associated with reduced toxicity in comparison with cisplatin. The recent trend is, therefore, to replace cisplatin with carboplatin. Since the renal and gastrointestinal toxicities of carboplatin are modest compared to those with cisplatin, the patients being treated with carboplatin do not require prehydration as that required by cisplatin.

- ❖ Docetaxel (75 mg/m²) and carboplatin (AUC = 5) IV every 3 weeks for six cycles. Due to the potential risk of neutropenia, the use of prophylactic growth factors during therapy is also recommended.
- ❖ Cisplatin (75 mg/m²) plus paclitaxel (135 mg/m² over 24 hours) every 3 weeks for six cycles. Dose-dense treatment comprises of carboplatin (AUC = 6 on day 1) and weekly paclitaxel (80 mg/m² days 1, 8 and 15) every 3 weeks for six cycles.

There is currently no role for the addition of a third chemotherapeutic agent in addition to carboplatin and paclitaxel. A randomised, phase 3 trial conducted by the GOG (2006) has shown that the combination of intravenous paclitaxel with IP cisplatin and paclitaxel in comparison with intravenous paclitaxel plus cisplatin alone is likely to improve survival in patients with optimally debulked stage III ovarian cancer.[24]

Alternative regimens include the following:

- ❖ *Incorporation of angiogenesis inhibitors (bevacizumab)*: Presently, there has been increased interest towards the incorporation of angiogenesis inhibitors (bevacizumab) and other vascular endothelial growth factor (VEGF) targeting agents into the first-line treatment for patients with EOCs. Bevacizumab is humanised monoclonal antibody which binds with VEGF, thereby preventing it from binding to its receptor. This blocks growth and maintenance of blood vessels feeding the cancer cells. The Gynecologic Cancer Inter Group (GCIG) ICON7 (International Collaborative Ovarian Neoplasm) trial, a multicentric RCT and the complementary GOG-0218 (ClinicalTrials.gov number, NCT00262847) have indicated that incorporation of bevacizumab to platinum and taxane-based chemotherapy improves progression-free survival but not the overall survival rates or the quality of life in patients with stage IV disease and those with residual disease following surgery.[25] Therefore, the use of angiogenesis inhibitors along with chemotherapy in the first-line setting for treatment of EOC is presently not recommended by most clinicians. Women with EOCs who are treated with bevacizumab may be associated with complications such as new or worsening hypertension, proteinuria, thrombotic events, bleeding, altered wound healing, gastrointestinal perforation, etc.[26] Early detection of these complications, especially gastrointestinal perforation might help in reducing the morbidity and mortality associated with the use of bevacizumab.
- ❖ *Novel angiogenesis-inhibiting agents*: There have been several ongoing clinical trials evaluating other anti angiogenic agents for treatment of women with EOC. Some of these agents are enumerated in Table 84.4.

Treatment of Recurrent Disease

The management in case of relapsed or recurrent ovarian cancer is decided based upon the platinum-free interval (PFI). This can be defined as the extent of time that has passed between the completion of platinum-based treatment and the recognition of the disease relapse. Based on the amount of PFI, patients can be classified as follows:

- ❖ *Patients with a PFI of 6 months or longer*: Such patients are considered to have 'platinum-sensitive' disease. A

Table 84.4: Novel angiogenesis-inhibiting agents

Angiogenesis-inhibiting agents	Description
Aflibercept (VEGF-Trap)	A fusion protein which binds to both VEGF receptors, VEGFR1 and VEGFR2
Trebananib/AMG386	An angiopoietin antagonist (peptide-Fc fusion protein) which prevents angiopoietin-1 and angiopoietin-2 from binding to their tyrosine kinase receptors
Nintedanib (BIBF 1120)	An oral angiokinase inhibitor which aims at VEGFR-1, -2, and -3, PDGFR-α/β, FGFR-1, -2, and -3, members of the sarcoma viral oncogene homologue (Src) family, and fms-like tyrosine kinase 3
Pazopanib	A novel antiangiogenic agent which specifically targets VEGFR-1, -2, and -3, PDGFR-α/β, FGFR-1 and -3, and c-kit
Cediranib (AZD 2171)	A novel antiangiogenic agent which specifically targets VEGFR-1, -2, and -3, PDGFR-α/β, FGFR-1 and c-kit.

Abbreviations: VEGFR, vascular endothelial growth factor receptors; PDGFR, platelet-derived growth factor receptors; FGFR, fibroblast growth factor receptors

combination of cisplatin and taxol is the drug of choice in these cases.

❖ *Patients with a PFI of less than 6 months*: Such patients are considered to have 'platinum-resistant' disease. For the patients who experience disease recurrence, chemotherapy is the mainstay of treatment. Surgery is reserved only for selective cases. Patients with 'platinum-sensitive' disease have a high probability of responding again to platinum-based treatment at the time of relapse. For women with recurrent 'platinum-resistant' disease, second-line chemotherapy comprising of combinations different to carboplatin, with or without the addition of taxol, are usually indicated. Sequential single agent chemotherapy with pegylated liposomal doxorubicin, which is not associated with significant side effects (e.g. hair loss, myelosuppression, etc.), is usually used in 4-weekly cycles. Single agent regimens are usually adopted due to their ease of administration and low toxicity. Other chemotherapeutic agents without cross-resistance, which can be used in these cases, include gemcitabine, anthracyclines, topoisomerase inhibitors (etoposide, topotecan) and others (e.g. tamoxifen). Second-line chemotherapy regimens are associated with a much lower response rate in comparison to the first-line chemotherapeutic regimens.

Follow-Up after Treatment for Ovarian Cancer

Follow-up is usually in the form of regular tests to check the level of CA-125 in the patient's blood. Often, the CA-125 level will begin to rise before any clinical symptoms suggestive of cancer recurrence develop. In the MRC OV05/EORTC 55955 collaborative trial, it was shown that institution of early treatment on the basis of increased CA-125 concentrations is not likely to be associated with a survival benefit in

Table 84.5: Different types of tumour markers being tried to detect cancer recurrence

Epithelial tumours	Germ cell tumours	Stromal tumours
• CA-125 antigen • BRCA-1 and BRCA-2 • Carcinoembryonic antigen • Galactosyltransferase • Tissue polypeptide antigen	• Alpha-foetoprotein • Human chorionic gonadotropin	• Inhibin

comparison with delayed treatment on the basis of clinical recurrence.[27] Therefore, the value of routine measurement of CA-125 in the follow-up of patients with ovarian cancer who attain a complete response after first-line treatment presently remains unclear.

Therefore, presently, the measurement of CA-125 levels has limited role in deciding the management of cancer recurrence. As a result, presently the treatment for cancer recurrence is delayed until she starts showing symptoms, or the results of an examination or scan make it clear that the cancer has come back. Different types of tumour markers (Table 84.5), based on the histological pattern of the tumour, are being tried under research settings. If the cancer comes back, treatment is usually given with chemotherapy. Many different types of chemotherapy can be used for women in this situation. The same chemotherapy drugs that were given initially can be used or different ones may be tried. Occasionally, it may be possible to remove tumours using surgery. Radiotherapy may be used to treat particular areas or to relieve symptoms.

COMPLICATIONS

❖ *Poor prognosis*: Cancer of the ovaries has the worst prognosis in comparison to any other type of gynaecologic cancer. As a result, it is the fifth most common cause of cancer deaths in women.
❖ *Metastasis*: The ovarian cancer is one of the most aggressive types of cancers, which can spread directly to the surrounding tissues, through the lymphatic system to other parts of the pelvis and abdomen and through the bloodstream to the distant body organs, mainly the liver and lungs.
❖ Ascites and/or pleural effusion and/or peritonitis
❖ *Side effects related to chemotherapy*: These include anorexia, bone marrow damage, constipation, diarrhoea, hair loss, increased risk of infection, etc.

CLINICAL PEARLS

❖ Protective factors for ovarian cancer include multiparity, breastfeeding, use of OCPs and anovulation.
❖ The gold standard treatment of ovarian cancer comprises of laparotomy followed by maximal reduction of the tumour mass. The surgical staging is followed by definite

surgery or debulking, which is usually followed by chemotherapy or radiotherapy.

❖ Patients with early-stage disease associated with high-risk factors (e.g. poor degree of differentiation, capsular penetrance, presence of surface excrescences, malignant ascites, cyst rupture, etc.) usually require additional therapy, especially adjuvant chemotherapy. On the other hand, patients with low-grade stage IA and IB disease usually do not require any adjuvant chemotherapy.

❖ Adequate surgical staging in apparent early-stage ovarian cancer is one of the most important components of management in cases of ovarian cancer.

❖ Ovarian cancer rarely causes vaginal bleeding. Therefore, in presence of abnormal vaginal bleeding, full assessment of the cervix and uterus including an outpatient endometrial biopsy must be carried out because the ovarian mass in these cases may be the site of secondary spread from a primary cervical or endometrial carcinoma.

❖ Primary surgery in cases of ovarian cancer not only helps in establishing the cancer diagnosis and staging, but also helps in achieving optimal cytoreduction with an effort to remove the bulk of tumour. The amount of residual tumour remaining following cytoreduction acts as one of the most important prognostic factors for survival of women with EOC.

❖ Gynecologic Oncology Group currently defines 'optimal status' as having residual tumour nodules each measuring 1 cm or less in maximum diameter, with complete cytoreduction (microscopic disease) being the desirable ideal surgical outcome.

EVIDENCE-BASED MEDICINE

❖ High-quality evidence indicates that platinum-based adjuvant chemotherapy is effective in prolonging survival in women with early-stage (FIGO stage I/IIa) EOC. Presently, it remains unclear whether adjuvant chemotherapy is likely to be similarly beneficial in women with low- and intermediate-risk early-stage disease as women with high-risk disease. Treatment of women with low- and intermediate-risk early-stage disease should be individualised to taking into account the various individual factors.[28]

❖ *Treatment of borderline ovarian tumours*: Borderline ovarian tumours are usually associated with a low mortality rate and chances of recurrence. Bilateral cystectomy may be offered to women with bilateral borderline ovarian tumours diagnosed intraoperatively who are wishing to conceive in the future. Presently, there is insufficient evidence to support the use of any specific adjuvant therapy for the treatment of borderline ovarian tumours. Future RCTs evaluating the role of adjuvant therapy with optimally dosed newer chemotherapy drugs are required, particularly for advanced borderline ovarian tumours.[29]

❖ *Ultra-radical or extensive surgery for ovarian cancer*: Presently, there is low-quality evidence, which suggests that ultra-radical surgery may result in better survival rates in cases of ovarian cancer. However, it remains unclear whether ultra-radical surgery causes significant changes in progression-free survival, quality of life and morbidity in comparison to the standard surgery in patients with ovarian cancer. Sufficiently powered or well-designed RCTs comparing ultra-radical surgery with standard surgery in the future are required.[30]

REFERENCES

1. Scully RE. Tumors of the ovary and maldeveloped gonads. Atlas of Tumor Pathology, Second Series, Fascicle 16. Washington, DC: Armed Forces Institute of Pathology; 1979.
2. IARC. WHO classification of tumours of female reproductive organs. 2014.
3. Royal College of Obstetricians and Gynaecologists. Management of suspected ovarian masses in premenopausal women. Green-top Guideline No. 62. London: RCOG Press; 2011.
4. Royal College of Obstetricians and Gynaecologists. Ovarian cysts in postmenopausal women. Guideline No. 34. London: RCOG Press; 2010.
5. National Institute of Clinical Excellence. Ovarian cancer: recognition and initial management. Clinical Guideline cg 122. London: NICE; 2011.
6. Vaughan S, Coward JI, Bast RC, Berchuck A, Berek JS, Brenton JD, et al. Rethinking ovarian cancer: recommendations for improving outcomes. Nat Rev Cancer. 2011;11(10):719-25.
7. Department of Health: NHS executive. (1999). Guidance on Commissioning Cancer Services Improving Outcomes in Gynaecological Cancers: the good practice manual. [Online] Available from stratog.rcog.org.uk/files/rcog-corp/elearn/38695/49861/doh_improvingoutcomes.pdf. [Accessed October, 2016].
8. Ratnavelu ND, Brown AP, Mallett S, Scholten RJ, Patel A, Founta C, et al. Intraoperative frozen section analysis for the diagnosis of early stage ovarian cancer in suspicious pelvic masses. Cochrane Database Syst Rev. 2016;(3):CD010360.
9. Vernooij F, Heintz P, Witteveen E, van der Graaf Y. The outcomes of ovarian cancer treatment are better when provided by gynaecologic oncologists and in specialized hospitals: a systematic review. Gynecol Oncol. 2007;105(3):801-12.
10. Sohaib SA, Mills TD, Sahdev A, Webb JA, Vantrappen PO, Jacobs IJ, et al. The role of magnetic resonance imaging and ultrasound in patients with adnexal masses. Clin Radiol. 2005;60(3):340-8.
11. Ferlay J, Shin HR, Bray F, Forman D, Mathers C, Parkin DM. Estimates of worldwide burden of cancer in 2008: GLOBOCAN 2008. Int J Cancer. 2010;127(12):2893-917.
12. Cancer Research UK. (2014). Ovarian cancer statistics. [online] Available from www.cancerresearchuk.org/health-professional/cancer-statistics/statistics-by-cancer-type/ovarian-cancer#F43xzSjr9Bzx3Ibe.99. [Accessed October, 2016].
13. Souhami R, Tobias J (Eds). Cancer and Its Management, 5th edition. Oxford, UK: Wiley-Blackwell; 2005.
14. Prat J, FIGO Committee on Gynecologic Oncology. Staging classification for the cancer of ovary, fallopian tube and peritoneum. Int J Gynecol Obstet. 2014;124(1):1-5.
15. Elattar A, Bryant A, Winter-Roach BA, Hatem M, Naik R. Optimal primary surgical treatment for advanced epithelial ovarian cancer. Cochrane Database Syst Rev. 2011;(8):CD007565.

16. van Meurs HS, Tajik P, Hof MH, Vergote I, Kenter GG, Mol BW, et al. Which patients benefit most from primary surgery or neoadjuvant chemotherapy in stage IIIC or IV ovarian cancer? An exploratory analysis of the European Organisation for Research and Treatment of Cancer (EORTC) 55971 randomised trial. Eur J Cancer. 2013;49(15):3191-201.

17. Kehoe S, Hook J, Matthew N, Jayson GC, Kitchener H, Lopes T, et al. Primary chemotherapy versus primary surgery for newly diagnosed advanced ovarian cancer (CHORUS): an open-label, randomised, controlled, non-inferiority trial. Lancet. 2015;386(9990):249-57.

18. International ovarian neoplasm (ICON) collaborators. International Collaborative ovarian neoplasm trial I: a randomized trial of adjuvant chemotherapy in women with early stage ovarian cancer. J Natl Cancer Inst. 2003;95(2):125-32.

19. Trimbos JB, Vergote I, Bolis G, Vermorken JB, Mangioni C, Madronal C, et al. Impact of adjuvant chemotherapy and surgical staging in early stage ovarian carcinoma: European Organisation for research and treatment of cancers –adjuvant chemotherapy in ovarian neoplasm trial. J Natl Cancer Inst. 2003;95(2):113-25.

20. Winter-Roach B, Hooper L, Kitchener H. Systematic review of adjuvant therapy for early stage (epithelial) ovarian cancer. Int J Gynecol Cancer. 2003;13(4):395-404.

21. OV21/PETROC: a randomized Gynecologic Cancer Intergroup (GCIG) phase II study of intraperitoneal (IP) versus intravenous (IV) chemotherapy following neoadjuvant chemotherapy and optimal debulking surgery in epithelial ovarian cancer (EOC). J Clin Oncol. 2016;34(Suppl; abstr LBA5503).

22. McGuire WP, Hoskins WJ, Brady MF, Kucera PR, Partridge EE, Look KY, et al. Cyclophosphamide and cisplatin compared with paclitaxel and cisplatin in patients with stage III and IV ovarian cancer. N Engl J Med. 1996;334(1):1-6.

23. Armstrong DK, Bundy B, Wenzel L, Huang HQ, Baergen R, Lele S, et al. Intraperitoneal cisplatin and paclitaxel in ovarian cancer. N Engl J Med. 2006;354(1):34-43.

24. Markman M, Bundy BN, Alberts DS, Fowler JM, Clark-Pearson DL, Carson LF, et al. Phase III trial of standard-dose intravenous cisplatin plus paclitaxel versus moderately high-dose carboplatin followed by intravenous paclitaxel and intraperitoneal cisplatin in small-volume stage III ovarian carcinoma: an intergroup study of the Gynecologic Oncology Group, Southwestern Oncology Group, and Eastern Cooperative Oncology Group. J Clin Oncol. 2001;19:1001-7.

25. Perren TJ, Swart AM, Pfisterer J, Ledermann JA, Pujade-Lauraine E, Kristensen G, et al. A Phase 3 Trial of Bevacizumab in Ovarian Cancer. N Engl J Med. 2011;365:2484-96.

26. Burger RA, Brady MF, Bookman MA, Fleming GF, Monk BJ, Huang H, et al. Incorporation of bevacizumab in the primary treatment of ovarian cancer. N Engl J Med. 2011;365(26):2473-83.

27. Rustin GJ, van der Burg ME, Griffin CL, Guthrie D, Lamont A, Jayson GC, et al. Early versus delayed treatment of relapsed ovarian cancer (MRC OV05/EORTC 55955): a randomised trial. Lancet. 2010;376(9747):1155-63.

28. Lawrie TA, Winter-Roach BA, Heus P, Kitchener HC. Adjuvant (post-surgery) chemotherapy for early stage epithelial ovarian cancer. Cochrane Database Syst Rev. 2015;(12):CD004706.

29. Faluyi O, Mackean M, Gourley C, Bryant A, Dickinson HO. Interventions for the treatment of borderline ovarian tumours. Cochrane Database Syst Rev. 2010;(9):CD007696.

30. Ang C, Chan KK, Bryant A, Naik R, Dickinson HO. Ultra-radical (extensive) surgery versus standard surgery for the primary cytoreduction of advanced epithelial ovarian cancer. Cochrane Database Syst Rev. 2011;(4):CD007697.

CHAPTER 84

Cervical Intraepithelial Neoplasia

INTRODUCTION

Cervical intraepithelial neoplasia (CIN) can be described as the preinvasive stage of cancer cervix. It denotes a continuum of disorders ranging from mild through moderate to severe dysplasia and carcinoma in situ (CIS). Cancer of cervix usually is the end stage of the spectrum of these disorders. CIN can be considered as a precancerous lesion in which a part or the full thickness of the stratified squamous cervical epithelium is replaced by cells showing varying degrees of dysplasia. This is different from the invasive cancer, as in this case the basement membrane remains intact whereas in case of invasive cancer, the basement membrane is penetrated. CIN is a premalignant condition of the uterine cervix that arises from the area of metaplasia in the transformation zone at the squamocolumnar junction (Fig. 85.1).

Since cervix is an easily accessible organ, and there is existence of simple screening tests for preinvasive cervical conditions, the incidence of cervical cancer has greatly reduced in the developed countries, where there is availability of effective cervical cancer screening programmes. Diagnosis of cervical dysplasia or CIN is mainly based on cytological screening, Papanicolaou test (Pap) smear or liquid-based cytology (LBC) of the population. The implementation of NHS Cancer Screening Programme (NHSCSP) in 1988 has prevented nearly 4,500–5,000 deaths due to cervical cancer per annum in the UK.[1-3]

According to the WHO, cervical dysplasia has been categorised into mild, moderate, or severe dysplasia and a separate category called CIS. The term 'cervical intraepithelial neoplasia' was introduced by Richart (1968). CIN1 represents mild-to-moderate dysplasia; CIN2 is an intermediate grade and CIN3, severe dysplasia or carcinoma in situ. CIN therefore represents a continuum of changes from CIN1 to CIN3 and invasive cancer. However, according to the most recent classification that is the Bethesda system, all cervical epithelial precursor lesions have been divided into two groups: low

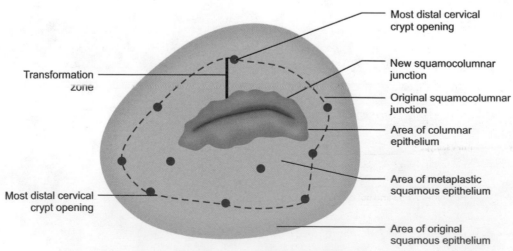

Most distal cervical crypt opening

New squamocolumnar junction

Original squamocolumnar junction

Area of columnar epithelium

Transformation zone

Area of metaplastic squamous epithelium

Most distal cervical crypt opening

Area of original squamous epithelium

Fig. 85.1: Identification of the squamocolumnar junction

grade squamous intraepithelial lesion (LSIL) and high-grade squamous intraepithelial lesion (HSIL).[4] LSIL corresponds to CIN1 and HSIL includes CIN2 and CIN3.

Amongst the European community, the second highest incidence of CIN has been recorded in the UK. Since the year 2002, there has been an increase in the incidence rates of CIN by 60% amongst the women aged 25–34 years. This increase could be attributed to causes such as an increase in HPV infection, increase in the proportion of women initiating sexual activity before the age of 16 years, increase in the incidence of smoking amongst women, increase in the immigrant population from countries with no cervical screening programme. Approximately 3.1 million women were screened in England in between the years 2014–2015. [5]

AETIOLOGY

Infection with HPV is an important causative factor for cervical cancer.[6] HPVs are a group of viruses which contain more than 100 viruses. Infection with HPV has been considered as one of the most important causes for the development of preinvasive and invasive lesions of the cervix.[7] HPVs infect the stratified squamous epithelium of skin and mucous membranes, where they cause benign lesions, some of which have the potential to progress to invasive cancer. While some of these viruses belong to low-risk group and produce wart like, benign growths or papillomas, some types of high-risk HPV have been found to be associated with certain types of cancers, particularly cervical cancer. The presence of the virus may cause morphological abnormalities in the epithelium, including papillomatosis, parakeratosis and koilocytosis.

Human papillomaviruses are usually transmitted sexually and nearly 40 types of HPV can be sexually transmitted and infect the genital area, including the cervix, vagina, vulva, anus and penis. Different HPV types and their association with cancer are shown in Table 85.1.[8] HPV infections are usually asymptomatic and therefore majority of infections remain unnoticed. Most genital warts are caused by HPV types 6 and 11. Certain HPV types account for nearly 90% of high-grade intraepithelial lesions and cancer. The high-risk types (e.g. HPV 16, 18, 31, 33, 35, 39, 45, 51, 52, 56, 58, 59, 68, etc.) may cause flat, abnormal growths in the genital area and on the cervix.[9-11] While infection with low-risk HPV viruses is benign, subclinical, self-limited and usually regresses spontaneously,

persistent cervical infection (infection that lasts for an interval of 6 months or longer) with a high-risk HPV types, especially HPV16 and HPV18, is the most important risk factor for progression to high-grade dysplasia. The HPV types 16 and 18 are most commonly found in association with invasive cancer, CIN2 and CIN3 and nearly 47% of women with cancer in all stages. The interval between the acquisition of HPV infection and malignant progression usually takes at least 10 years and is frequently longer. Cervical cancer is, therefore, very uncommon in women under 25 years; the incidence rises progressively for women over 25 years and is highest for women over 40 years.

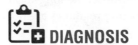 DIAGNOSIS

Clinical Presentation

Presence of dysplasia may be associated with minimal findings on clinical examination.

Per Speculum Examination

On inspection, the cervix often appears normal, or there may be cervicitis or erosion, which bleeds on touch.

Investigations

The various methods for screening of cervical cancer are summarised in Flow chart 85.1 and are described next in details.

Cytologic Screening Test

The most important investigation, which helps in detection of cervical cancer in its preinvasive stage, is the Pap smear. Pap smear involves cytological analysis of the cells from the squamocolumnar junction, which is an area of rapid cell turnover, squamous metaplasia and the site of oncogenic transformation. In young women of childbearing age, the squamocolumnar junction is usually readily visible on the ectocervix. With age as the cervical epithelium matures, the squamocolumnar junction may recede within the endocervical canal. As a result, the squamocolumnar junction may be difficult to visualise and to be adequately sampled.

Table 85.1: Human papillomavirus (HPV) types and their association with cancer[8]

Association with cancer	HPV subtype
High-risk HPV subtypes	HPV types 16, 18, 31, 33, 39, 45, 51, 52, 56, 58, 59, 68, 69, 73 and 82
Probable high risk	HPV types 26, 53 and 66
Intermediate risk	HPV types 30, 31, 33, 35, 39, 51, 52, 58, 66
Low-risk HPV subtypes	HPV types 6 and 11 (mainly cause genital warts), 40, 42, 43, 44, 54, 61, 70, 72, 81 and CP6108

Flow chart 85.1: Screening tools for cervical cancer

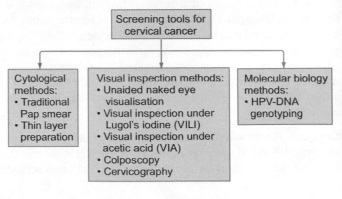

The risks of cervical cancer screening using the conventional Pap smear include the occurrence of false-negative as well as false-positive test results. False-negative test results imply that screening test results may appear to be normal even though cervical cancer is present. This may delay the patient from seeking medical care even if she has symptoms suggestive of cancer. False-positive test results occur when screening test results appear to be abnormal even though no cancer is present. This can cause unnecessary patient's anxiety. Also, a false-positive test may be followed by more invasive tests and procedures such as colposcopy, cryotherapy or loop electrosurgical excision procedure (LEEP), which are associated with their own risks. Furthermore, the long-term effects of these procedures on fertility and pregnancy are not known.

Until recently, the Pap smear had remained the principal technology for preventing cervical cancer. However, following a review of the presently published literature, LBC has now been incorporated within the UK national screening programme to further improve the efficacy of cytological screening test. Two systems are presently available, the ThinPrep® and SurePath®. There is some evidence that liquid-based cytological methods offer following advantages over traditional smear techniques:[12-14]

❖ A reduction in the proportion of inadequate specimens
❖ An improvement in sensitivity rates: During clinical trials, use of ThinPrep® was associated with a reduction in the number of ambiguous interpretations and an increased detection rate of dysplasias by nearly 13%. The use of LBC has mainly helped in reducing the number of inadequate smears from around 9% to around 1%. It also helps in increasing the detection of true dyskaryosis. This has reduced the need to recall women for a repeat smear.
❖ A possible reduction in interpretation time of specimens
❖ Reduction in the number of false-negative test results by optimising the collection and preparation of cervical cells
❖ With LBC, it is possible to perform reflex testing such as HPV DNA or p16 immunocytochemistry without taking a repeat sample.

Liquid-based cytology has now become the standard test in the NHSCSP.[15-17] While the conventional 'Pap smear' involves direct preparation of the slide from the cervical scrape obtained, the procedure of 'ThinPrep®' involves making a suspension of cells from the sample, which is then used to produce a thin layer of cells on a slide. In this technique, the sample is taken using a plastic spatula, which could be either an endocervical brush or a cervical broom, also known as the cervex. Using this technique, the cells collected from the cervix are placed in a preservative fluid, which is then sent to the laboratory rather than being directly spread onto a slide. At the laboratory, the sample is treated to remove unwanted material (blood, mucus and inflammatory material) and then a thin layer of the cell suspension is placed on the slide for inspection.

Cervical smear abnormalities: A new classification for abnormal cervical cytology adopted by the NHSCSP and the British Association for Cytopathology since 2013 is described

Table 85.2: Summary of changes in terminology[18]

Previous terminology (BSC 1986)	New terminology
Borderline change	Borderline change in squamous cells Borderline change in endocervical cells
Mild dyskaryosis Borderline change with koilocytosis	Low-grade dyskaryosis
Moderate dyskaryosis	High-grade dyskaryosis (moderate)
Severe dyskaryosis	High-grade dyskaryosis (severe)
Severe dyskaryosis/?Invasive	High-grade dyskaryosis/?invasive squamous carcinoma
?Glandular neoplasia	?Glandular neoplasia of endocervical type ?Glandular neoplasia (non-cervical)

in Table 85.2.[18] Previously in the UK, the British Society for Clinical Cytology (1986) classification was being used for reporting cervical cytology. Elsewhere, throughout the world other classification systems are used, particularly the Bethesda Classification, which was introduced in the US in 1991. The new classification system adopted by the NHSCSP helps in reducing the gap between these two systems, thereby enabling international comparisons.

The new classification for abnormal cervical cytology incorporates the following changes:
❖ Division of the 'borderline change' into 'squamous' and 'endocervical' categories
❖ Division of dyskaryosis into 'low-grade' and 'high-grade' categories
❖ Division of glandular neoplasia into 'endocervical' and 'non-cervical' categories.

National Health Service Cancer Screening Programme

National Health Service cancer screening programme (Flow chart 85.2) helps in identifying individuals who appear healthy, but may be at an increased risk of developing cervical cancer in future. No screening test is perfect and each test may be associated with a number of false positives and false negatives. NHSCSP is available to all the women in England who are aged 25–64 years. All eligible women who are registered with a GP automatically receive an invitation for cervical screening by mail. Woman's first invitation for routine screening must be sent out 6 months before her 25th birthday, i.e. at the age of 24 and half years. This ensures that the woman would be screened by her 25th birthday. All subsequent invitations for screening must be sent approximately 6 weeks before the woman's test due date. Women, who are between the ages of 25–49 years, receive an invitation after every 3 years. On the other hand, women who are aged between 50 to 64 years receive an invitation after every 5 years. Though slightly more costly, 3-yearly cervical screening programme is likely to significantly prevent more cancers than 5-yearly screening programme in younger women.[19,20] After 65 years of age, invitation can be sent to women who have had recent abnormal tests. Screening can be performed on request for women who have not had an adequate screening test since the age of 50 years.[18]

Flow chart 85.2: Screening protocol algorithm and colposcopy management recommendations cytology with HPV triage and test of cure (TOC)

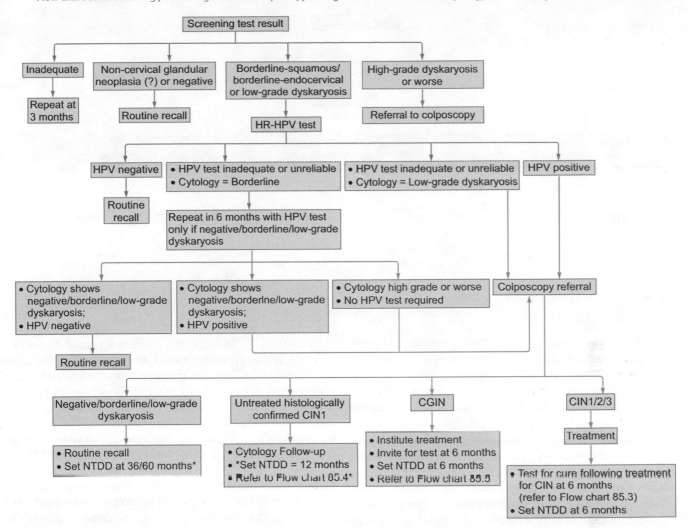

Abbreviations: NTDD, next test due date; CIN, cervical intraepithelial neoplasia; CGIN, cervical glandular intraepithelial neoplasia; HR-HPV, high-risk human papillomavirus

*Women more than 60 years who are cytology negative, HPV positive and have a satisfactory and negative colposcopy can be removed from the programme. Women more than 60 years who show borderline/low-grade dyskaryosis, HPV positive and have a satisfactory and negative colposcopy should consider large loop excision of the transformation zone (LLETZ) if decline recall at 60 months.

The Advisory Committee on Cervical Screening (ACCS), advised the Department of Health (DH) to increase the age for cervical screening from 20 years to 25 years taking into account the newly available evidence illustrating the unbeneficial effect of screening below the age of 25 years.[21] Amongst the women under the age of 25 years, the prevalence of HPV infection is high. As a result, HPV-associated cellular changes are quite common amongst the sexually active women in this age group.[22] However, majority of low-grade abnormalities related to HPV infection detected in cytology samples taken from women under the age of 25 years are likely to regress spontaneously with time.[23] As a result, the incidence of cervical cancer in this age group is very low.[20, 24,25] Screening of women under the age of 25 years, therefore, may result in a large number of referrals to colposcopy for further investigation. This may be the cause of increased levels of anxiety for these women. Additionally, unnecessary treatment may be administered by the colposcopist for abnormalities that are anyway likely to resolve on their own without any

further intervention. Treatment-related complication may result in obstetric complications with future pregnancy, e.g. large loop excision of the transformation zone (LLETZ) may result in preterm labour.[26-31] Recently available conflicting evidence has shown that the risk of preterm delivery in women treated by colposcopy within the NHS in England is significantly lower than that reported in studies from other countries.[32,33] Therefore, screening of teenagers cannot be justified.

Human Papilloma Virus Triage and Test of Cure

Test of cure (TOC) protocol following treatment for CIN1 is illustrated in Flow chart 85.3. Under the high-risk HPV (HR-HPV) triage protocol, women whose cervical samples are reported to be showing borderline changes (of squamous or endocervical type) or low-grade dyskaryosis are subjected to a reflex HR-HPV test. The available evidence shows that HR-HPV testing using Hybrid Capture® 2 assay [Qiagen

Flow chart 85.3: Test of cure following treatment for CIN

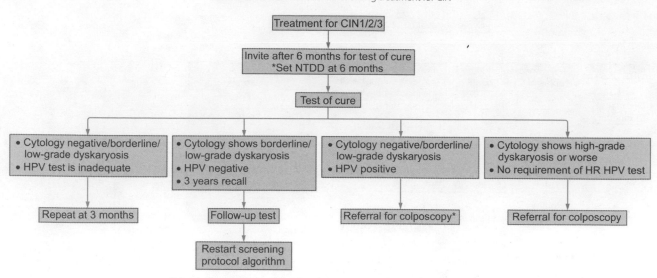

Abbreviations: NTDD, next test due date; CIN, cervical intraepithelial neoplasia

* Women who are HR-HPV positive and have borderline/low-grade dyskaryosis or negative cytology are referred back to colposcopy . If colposcopy report is satisfactory or negative, she can be recalled after 3 years.

Gaithersburg, Incorporation, MD, USA (previously Digene Corporation)] technique is a more sensitive screening test than either cytological or colposcopic examination.[34-36]

Following this test, women who are HPV positive are referred to colposcopy. On the other hand, those who are HR-HPV negative are returned to routine recall. Women whose cervical sample is reported as high-grade dyskaryosis or worse are referred directly for colposcopic examination without being subjected to a HR-HPV test. National rollout of HR-HPV triage for women with borderline or low-grade cytology results and HR-HPV test of cure was completed in 2013. Incorporation of HPV triage into the NHSCSP appears to be a practical option, which is acceptable to women. HPV triage helps in reducing the requirement for repeat cytology and enables effective use of colposcopy services.[37] This, however, results in an increased pressure on the workforce due to an overall increase in the referral to colposcopic services. Introduction of the HPV triage tool has resulted in introducing homogeneity in the referral system of the screening programme. This has also helped in reducing the time period of treatment and surveillance from an average of 12 years to 9 months.[38]

Under the HR-HPV 'test of cure' protocol, women with all grades of CIN following treatment are invited for screening after 6 months of treatment. During this screening test, women with the findings of negative, borderline change (of squamous or endocervical type), or low-grade dyskaryosis on cytological analysis are subjected to an HR-HPV test. If the HR-HPV test is negative, the woman is recalled for a screening test in 3 years (irrespective of age). She can then be returned to routine recall if the subsequent test result is cytologically negative. Women who are HR-HPV positive are referred back to colposcopy. Women whose cytological analysis reveals high-grade dyskaryosis or worse are referred directly for colposcopic examination without an HR-HPV test.

High-risk HPV as the primary screening test in the cervical cancer screening programme is associated with an increased sensitivity and efficacy in comparison with the use of LBC alone. Also, it helps in increasing the intervals between screening rounds so that the woman may be required to attend the screening tests less frequently. The ARTISTIC trial investigated 24,510 women aged 25–64 years over two screening rounds, approximately 3 years apart (2001–03 and 2004–07) within the NHSCSP in the region of Greater Manchester.[39] The results of this study showed that the primary screening with HR-HPV is likely to detect more than 90% cases of CIN2, CIN3 and invasive cancer. The combination of LBC and additional HR-HPV testing over two screening rounds is likely to be 25% more sensitive than cytology alone for the detection of CIN3+ or CIN2+. It is also 25% more sensitive than LBC in detecting borderline changes. However, in these cases, it is less specific than LBC. The results of the study also showed that the use of HPV testing in a population-based screening programme as a primary screening method in combination with the cytology triage served as the most cost-effective method. Primary HR-HPV screening with cytology triage serves as an effective way to classify women greater than 25 years of age on the basis of their risk for CIN3+. This is based on the results of the VUSA-screen study (Vrije Universiteit medical centre SAltro laboratory population-based cervical screening), which has shown that HR-HPV positive women with normal cytology are at a lower risk of CIN3+ in comparison to the HR-HPV positive women with abnormal cytology. On the other hand, negative HR-HPV test offers 50% better protection against the presence of CIN3 lesions in comparison to negative cytology.[40] HR-HPV, therefore, seems as a feasible alternative to cytological screening. Repeat cytological examination is, however, required after 1 year for HPV-positive women with normal cytology before they can be returned for routine screening. However, routine screening for HPV infection is yet not recommended.

Results of the US Athena study has shown that HPV testing along with separate HPV16 and HPV18 genotype detection serves as an alternative, more sensitive, and efficient strategy for detection of CIN3+ in comparison to the other screening methods based solely on the cytology.[41] It has also been shown that the reduced specificity of HR-HPV DNA testing can be improved by the addition of HR-HPV genotyping. The POBASCAM (Population Based Screening Study Amsterdam) study has revealed the genotype-specific differences in clearance rates at 6 and 18 months. The lowest clearance rates in women with normal cytology were observed for the genotypes, HPV16, HPV18, HPV31 and HPV33. Amongst women who did not clear their HPV infection, persistence of HPV16 infection is likely to be associated with increased detection rates of CIN3 or greater.[42] Genotyping, therefore, should be associated with an increase in surveillance following referral of women positive for HR-HPV types 16/18. On the other hand, a more conservative approach can be adopted for the follow-up of women positive for the remaining HR-HPV types.

Colposcopy

Colposcopy may be used as a primary investigation in countries, which do not have a well-organised screening system. In the UK, colposcopy is used as a secondary investigation because of the presence of a well-organised screening system. In the UK, following women must be referred for the colposcopic examination:

❖ Woman found to be positive for HR-HPV along with the presence of borderline or low-grade dyskaryosis on cytological testing
❖ Women whose cytological analysis reveals high-grade dyskaryosis or worse.

While the cytological analysis detects abnormal cells, colposcopy helps in locating the abnormal lesions. A colposcope is like a small microscope with a light and enables the gynaecologist to perform a thorough examination of the cervix.[43] The adjunctive colposcopic imaging technologies, which are newly available in the NHS, include dynamic spectral imaging system (DySIS) and near infrared imaging system (NIRIS).[44] DySIS is a digital video colposcope which uses dynamic spectral imaging to evaluate the blanching effect of acetowhitening, following the application of acetic acid to the epithelium. NIRIS, on the other hand, uses near-infrared light to scan the epithelial tissues. As per the recommendations by the NICE guidelines, DySIS can be used within the NHSCSP because it is cost-effective.[44] On the other hand, NICE does not recommend the use of NIRIS because it is not cost-effective.

Colposcopy is an office-based procedure during which the cervix is examined under illumination and magnification before and after application of dilute acetic acid and Lugol's iodine. The characteristic features of malignancy and premalignancy on colposcopic examination include changes such as acetowhite areas, abnormal vascular patterns, mosaic pattern, punctuation and failure to uptake iodine

stain. Endocervical sampling may accompany colposcopy, particularly in non-pregnant women where the cytology shows atypical glandular cells or adenocarcinoma in situ. Satisfactory colposcopy requires visualisation of the entire squamocolumnar junction and transformation zone for the presence of any visible lesions. Both a regular white light and a green light are used during colposcopy. The green filter enhances visualisation of blood vessels by making them appear darker in contrast to the surrounding epithelium. The colposcopic examination helps in the following:

❖ When abnormal cells have been detected on cytology, location and extent of abnormal lesions on the cervix can be assessed with the help of colposcopy.
❖ Biopsy can be taken from the areas of abnormality.
❖ Conservative surgery (e.g. conisation) can be performed under colposcopic guidance.
❖ Colposcopic examination can also be performed during follow-up examination of cases that have undergone conservative therapy.

Procedure

❖ The patient is placed in the lithotomy position.
❖ Under all aseptic precautions, a speculum is inserted inside the vagina.
❖ The colposcope is brought into the position. The perineum, vulva, vagina and cervix must be examined for presence of lesions using the colposcope's white light and then green light.
❖ The entire cervix must be viewed both under the low- and high-power magnification. Higher-power magnification helps in visualisation of small details and features.
❖ Cervix is visualised after the application of both dilute 5% acetic acid and Lugol's iodine in order to enhance any abnormal epithelial findings. Both acetic acid and Lugol's iodine are applied onto the cervix with the help of a cotton swab and allowed to remain there for at least 30 seconds.
❖ Under white light, the cervix is visualised for acetowhite changes. The location of the squamocolumnar junction, transformation zone, abnormal and atypical vessels and areas of acetowhite changes are recorded. On application of Lugol's iodine, the areas of abnormalities such as those with squamous metaplasia, leucoplakia as well as neoplastic tissue do not take up iodine stain and become yellowish in appearance, whereas the normal glycogen containing cervical cells turn deep brown. A scoring system such as 'the Reid's Colposcopic Index' may be used to help the colposcopist in classifying the colposcopic appearance.
❖ The cervix is re-examined under the green light, which helps in accentuating the margins of the acetowhite areas and in identifying the abnormal blood vessels.

DIFFERENTIAL DIAGNOSIS

❖ Cervicitis
❖ Infection of the cervix (HPV, HSV, *Treponema pallidum*, etc.)

- ❖ Tubercular lesions of cervix
- ❖ Hyperkeratosis and parakeratosis
- ❖ Endocervical polyps
- ❖ Squamous papillomas
- ❖ Cervical endometriosis.

MANAGEMENT

STRATEGIES FOR PREVENTION

Prevention of Human Papillomavirus Infection

Most important way to prevent the occurrence of cervical cancer is to eliminate risk for genital HPV infection by refraining from any genital contact with another infected individual. For those who want to remain sexually active, a long-term, mutually monogamous relationship with an uninfected partner is the strategy, which is most likely to prevent genital HPV infection. Presently, it is not known whether condoms can provide any protection against HPV infection, because areas not covered by a condom can be infected by HPV.

Use of Condoms

Though the use of condoms is unlikely to reduce the rates of HPV infection, its use has been found to be useful in preventing potentially precancerous changes in the cervix. Exposure to semen has been found to be associated with an increased risk of precancerous changes, especially CIN3. Therefore, use of condoms does help in providing some protection.[45]

Nutritional Advice

Consumption of high amounts of fruits and vegetables (at least five portions) has been found to be associated with a reduced risk of persistent HPV infection. Consumption of high levels of antioxidants, particularly vitamin A, E and C has also been found to exert a protective role. Higher circulating levels of carotenoids have been found to be associated with a significant decrease in the clearance time of type-specific HPV infection, particularly during the early stages of infection (≤120 days). Another foodstuff, which has been observed to exert a protective role in the development of cancer cervix, is folic acid. High levels of folic acid have been found to be inversely related with the risk of developing HPV infection. Some studies have shown that lower levels of antioxidants coexisting with low levels of folic acid increases the risk of CIN development. Improving folate status in subjects at risk of getting infected or already infected with high-risk HPV may have a beneficial impact in the prevention of cancer. However, presently, the role of various antioxidants and other foodstuffs in cancer prevention is not yet clear.

HUMAN PAPILLOMAVIRUS VACCINATION PROGRAMME

Identification of a viral agent such as HPV as a cause of disease(s) implies that successful prophylactic or therapeutic intervention against the viral agent would be able to prevent the disease(s) it causes. The aim of vaccination could be either to prevent the disease (prophylactic use) or treat it (therapeutic use). Prophylactic vaccination aims to prevent the infection either by targeting the viral capsid protein or prevent the early spread of infection through production of neutralising antibodies. Therapeutic vaccination, on the other hand, helps in enhancing the host's cell-mediated immunity in order to attack the established infection.

Presently, there are two vaccines available for preventing HPV infection. Both bivalent and quadrivalent HPV vaccines are available, which are highly efficient in preventing CIN2, CIN3, or adenocarcinoma in situ caused by HPV16 and 18 in women between 15 years and 26 years of age. Of these two vaccines, the first is a quadrivalent vaccine, called Gardasil®, developed by Merck and Company, New Jersey, USA, which is effective against four strains of HPV (6, 11, 16 and 18). This vaccine has gained approval from the FDA and has been made available in the market since June 2006. Gardasil® has also been approved in the European Union. The vaccine is indicated for women aged 9–26 years and provides protection against genital warts and gynaecologic cancer.[46] Gardasil® is also indicated in boys and men between the age of 9–26 years for prevention of anal cancer and genital warts. However, there is no evidence to suggest that vaccination of the boys is likely to alter the rates of CIN or HPV infection.

Gardasil® is administered through a series of three intra-muscular injections over a period of 6 months. No major adverse effects have been found to be associated with this vaccine, though the first day syncope and skin infections (after 2 weeks) have been observed in some patients.

The second vaccine called Cervarix® is a bivalent vaccine (effective against the HPV strains, 16 and 18) that has been developed by GlaxoSmithKline, Middlesex, UK, and gained FDA approval in 2009. This vaccine is also given in three doses over a 6-month period. For both the vaccines, three separate doses are needed. The second and third doses are given at 2 months and 6 months after the first dose. The high cost of both these vaccine has been a cause for concern.

Though both these vaccines provide protection against the subsequent HPV infection, they do not provide protection against an active infection and cannot be used for treating CIN. HPV infection peaks in early 20s and the cervical cancer occurs in the 40s. Since both the vaccines only work if they are administered before HPV infection actually occurs, this vaccine is specifically targeted at girls and women between the ages of 9–26 years, before they become sexually active. However, neither of these HPV vaccines has been proven to provide complete protection against persistent infection with other HPV types, some of which may cause cervical cancer. Despite this fact, widespread vaccination has the potential to reduce cervical cancer deaths around the world by nearly 70% if all women were to be given this vaccine. There are no major side effects associated with HPV vaccination except for redness, pain and swelling at the injection site and raised temperature. Despite of receiving HPV vaccination, women who are over the age of 25 years are advised to have a cervical smear test before they are immunised with the vaccine. They would still require attending their routine cervical smear test, because there are other types of HPV linked with cervical cancer, which the vaccines are not active against.

Several RCTs are now available which suggest that these vaccines are likely to have prophylactic efficacy against CIN lesions associated with HPV16 or HPV18 infection and thus could be used for prevention against preinvasive and invasive cervical disease.[47-49] Thus, vaccination is likely to result in reduced rates of HPV-related cancers. However, the duration of protection provided by these vaccines presently remains unknown. It is likely to vary anywhere between 5 years to 20 years. Therefore, presently there are no clear guidelines regarding the requirement for booster vaccines.

The HPV vaccination programme in the NHS started in 2008 and was organised through schools. Initially, only the bivalent vaccine, Cervarix® was available through the NHS and the quadrivalent vaccine, Gradasil® was available only on a private basis. However, since September 2012, Gradasil® has been adopted by the NHS, as per the recommendations by the Department of Health.

TREATMENT OF DYSPLASTIC CHANGES

Though the high-grade lesions (CIN2/3) must be treated, presently it remains unclear whether or not CIN1 lesions should be treated because nearly 60% of the CIN1 lesions are likely to resolve spontaneously on their own. Treatment of CIN lesions can involve either ablative techniques (involving destruction of the area of abnormality) or excisional techniques (involving removal of the area of abnormality). Flow chart 85.4 illustrates the protocol for management of histologically confirmed CIN1. Though most of the ablative and excisional methods are associated with success rates

varying between 90% to 98% (except for cryotherapy), the available evidence does not indicate the superiority of one treatment method over the other.[50]

The various treatment options, which are available, are as follows:

❖ *Ablative methods*: Local destructive methods such as cryosurgery, fulguration or electrocoagulation and laser ablation. Ablative methods which destroy the abnormal tissue, do not provide the surgeon with a specimen of abnormal tissue, which can be examined on histopathology.

❖ *Excisional methods*: Excision of the abnormal tissue with cold knife conisation, laser conisation, LLETZ, LEEP and needle excision of transformation zone (NETZ). Removal of the transformation zone is likely to provide a large tissue sample for histopathological examination.

❖ *Surgical options*: Surgical options such as therapeutic conisation, hysterectomy or hysterectomy with removal of vaginal cuff can be used if CIS extends to the vaginal vault.

Locally Destructive Methods

Locally destructive or ablative methods are used in the following circumstances:

❖ There is no evidence of microinvasion or invasive cancer on cytology, colposcopy, endocervical curettage or biopsy.

❖ The lesion can be visualised completely and is located on the ectocervix, and there is no involvement of the endocervix.

❖ The results of colposcopy and endocervical curettage indicate the presence of high-grade cervical dysplasia.

Cryosurgery

Cryosurgery is a locally destructive OPD procedure in which the dysplastic cells are destroyed using freezing agents [CO_2

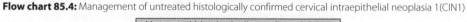

Flow chart 85.4: Management of untreated histologically confirmed cervical intraepithelial neoplasia 1(CIN1)

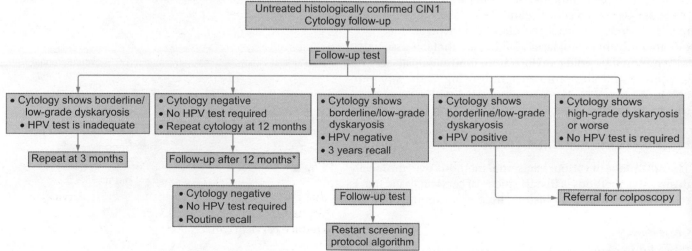

Abbreviation: CIN, cervical intraepithelial neoplasia

*The management of women with abnormal cytology during this follow-up test is similar to that at the first 12 month repeat test.

(–60°C) and nitrous oxide (–80°C)]. The optimal temperature required for effective tissue destruction must be in the range from –20°C to –30°C. A cryoprobe is used, usually without any anaesthesia or analgesia and causes destruction of the cells by crystallization of intercellular fluid.[51] It uses the 'freeze-thaw-freeze' technique in which an ice ball is achieved 5 mm beyond the edge of the probe. The cryoprobe is applied over the area of abnormality for over 9 minutes and destroys the tissue up to the depth of about 4–5 mm. The time required for the procedure is related to the pressure of gas. The higher the pressure of gas, faster is the rate of ice ball formation. Overall, cryosurgery is a relatively safe procedure with fewer complications.

Success rates of cryotherapy for treating CIN3 disease varies between 77% to 93%. Therefore, it appears to be a reasonable option for the treatment of low-grade and not high-grade disease. Its use is, therefore, suitable in the low-resource settings.

Electrocoagulation

Electrocoagulation is a locally destructive procedure in which the dysplastic cells are destroyed using temperature over 700°C. The procedure is quite painful and is therefore usually performed under general anaesthesia. The abnormal tissues are destroyed up to the depth of about 8–10 mm.[52] This procedure can be associated with numerous complications including recurrence of the lesions, bleeding, sepsis, cervical stenosis and indrawing of the squamocolumnar junction within the cervical canal.

Laser Ablation

Laser ablation is a locally destructive OPD procedure, usually done under local anaesthesia, which uses laser energy to destroy the dysplastic cells by boiling, steaming and exploding the cells. The extensive heat energy liberated causes incineration of the protein and mineral content of the tissues, resulting in a charred appearance at the base of exposed area. The main advantage of this method is that the tissue can be ablated up to the depth of about 7 mm, which is the location of the deepest endocervical gland. Thus, laser ablation can be used in lesions with extensive glandular involvement.

Other advantages of laser ablation are that it is associated with minimal bleeding, no infection, minimal postlaser scar formation and does not cause indrawing of the squamo-columnar junction. It is also associated with a rapid post-treatment healing phase.

Excision of the Abnormal Tissue

The advantage of various excisional methods over the locally destructive methods is that the piece of cervical tissue that is removed can be sent for histopathological examination.

Cone Biopsy

Cone biopsy serves as both a diagnostic and therapeutic procedure. The procedure involves the removal of the entire area of abnormality. It is capable of providing tissue for histopathological examination. The cone biopsy may be performed under general or local anaesthesia. This method involves obtaining a wide cone of excision including the entire outer margin of the lesion and the entire endocervical lining. Indications for cone biopsy are as follows:

❖ The area of the abnormality is large, or its inner margin has receded into the cervical canal.
❖ The limits of the lesion cannot be visualised by colposcopy.
❖ The squamocolumnar junction is not completely observable on colposcopy.
❖ There is discrepancy between the findings of cytology and colposcopy.
❖ There is a suspicion of microinvasion based on the results of biopsy, colposcopy or cytology.
❖ The findings of endocervical curettage are positive for CIN2 or CIN3.
❖ Colposcopist is unable to rule out invasive cancer.

Cold-knife Conisation

This procedure is performed with help of a scalpel under anaesthesia (either regional or general) and comprises of the following steps:

❖ The patient is placed in dorsal lithotomy position.
❖ A colposcopic examination may be performed prior to the procedure, and the area of transformation zone may be demarcated using Lugol's iodine or 3–5% acetic acid.
❖ Under all aseptic precautions, the anterior lip of the cervix may be grasped with help of a single tooth tenaculum.
❖ A vasoconstrictor solution [vasopressin (0.5 U/mL) or 1:200,000 epinephrine solution] may be injected into the cervix at this time in order to reduce intraoperative blood loss, thereby improving the exposure at the time of surgery.
❖ A circumferential incision is made just lateral to the outer limit of the transformation zone, usually starting from the posterior side, using a long-handled scalpel with a No. 11 blade (Fig. 85.2). The desired circular incision is made in the region surrounding the endocervical canal using

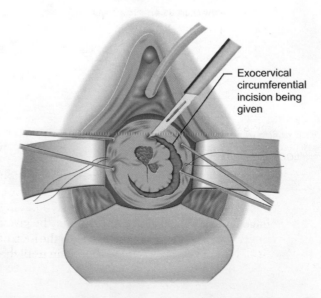

Exocervical circumferential incision being given

Fig. 85.2: Making a circular incision over the exocervix at the time of cone biopsy

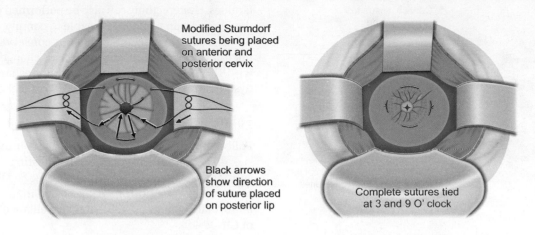

Fig. 85.3: Application of Sturmdorf sutures following cold-knife conisation

a slight sawing motion, preferably including the entire transformation zone and/or the area of abnormality by inserting the scalpel blade to the desired depth, in the direction slightly towards the endocervical canal. Mayo's scissors can be used to complete and deepen the incision.

❖ Following excision, the cone bed can be sutured using the modified Sturmdorf type sutures (Fig. 85.3). A rolled gauze pack soaked in ferric subsulphate solution can be placed inside the cervical canal to reduce the amount of bleeding. This pack must be removed by the patient within 12–24 hours.

Laser Excision

This method employs the use of laser energy for obtaining the cone biopsy. In this method, with the help of a colposcope, the margin around the outer limit of the transformation zone may be marked by making a series of dots using carbon dioxide laser (Fig. 85.4). The incision is deepened circumferentially by passing the laser beam progressively across the tissues. The planned outer margin of the cone is circumferentially deepened to the extent depending on the amount of exposure. This is done with a smaller spot size (0.5–1 mm) and a high power density (1,000–1,500 watts/cm²).

As an alternative technique, the surgeon may plan ablation after marking the outer and inner margins of the planned area of ablation and dividing it into quadrants (Fig. 85.5). Starting from the posterior side, each quadrant is vapourised to a depth of 5–7 mm using a power density of 500–1,000 watts/cm².

Large Loop Excision of the Transformation Zone

The LLETZ stands for 'large loop excision of the transformation zone'. In the USA, this procedure is called LEEP—loop electrosurgical excision procedure. This method basically uses low voltage diathermy (30–40 watts) and may be given at the same time as colposcopy. In this procedure, the loop of wire is advanced into the cervix lateral to the lesion until the required depth is reached.[53] The loop is then taken across to the opposite side and a cone of tissue is removed. The area of abnormal cells is removed completely using a loop of wire

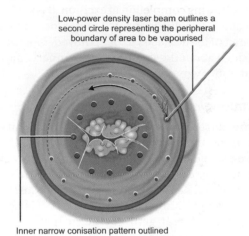

Fig. 85.4: Marking surgical boundaries for laser cervical conisation with the help of circle of dots

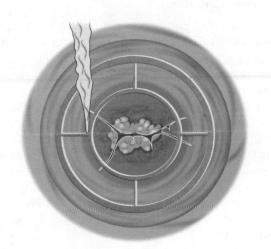

Fig. 85.5: Laser vapourisation of the cervix in which the areas planned for vapourisation-conisation are marked according to quadrants. Each quadrant is vapourised at a time

CHAPTER 85

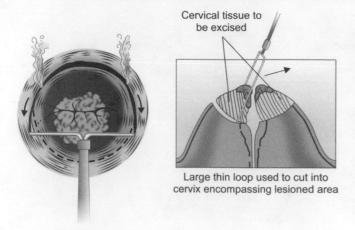

Cervical tissue to be excised

Large thin loop used to cut into cervix encompassing lesioned area

Fig. 85.6: Large loop excision of the transformation zone

and electrosurgery (Fig. 85.6). An endocervical curettage is performed following completion of excision. It is an outpatient treatment and is usually performed under local anaesthesia. If a large area of tissue needs to be removed, or if the patient is very anxious about the treatment, the surgery may also be performed under general anaesthesia.

Loop Electrosurgical Excision Procedure

In this procedure, a thin wire loop that carries an electric current is used to remove abnormal areas of the cervix. The excised area of the cervix removed is sent to the laboratory for histopathological examination. This electric energy is also used to coagulate the blood vessels on the surface of the cervix. LEEP is even simpler than LLETZ and is applicable anywhere in the lower genital tract, whereas LLETZ is applicable only to the cervix.

Surgical Options

These include therapeutic conisation, hysterectomy or hysterectomy with removal of vaginal cuff.

Therapeutic Conisation

The procedure of conisation not only provides tissue for histopathological study, but can also serve as a therapeutic procedure. Conisation includes the entire outer margin of the cervix and endocervical lining, short of internal os. A smaller cone may be desirable in young women as it helps in avoiding complications such as abortion or preterm labour. Complications associated with the procedure include bleeding, sepsis, cervical stenosis, abortion and preterm labour. Conisation may also be done in cases of endocervical dysplasia, when transformation zone cannot be completely visualised or when there is discrepancy in findings between the findings of cytology, colposcopy and biopsy.

Hysterectomy

Hysterectomy is considered as the treatment of last resort in cases of recurrent high-grade CIN. It may serve as an appropriate option in older and parous women who have attained menopause or those who have completed their

families. Hysterectomy can also be performed when it appears that the woman would not be able to comply with the follow-up or recurrence occurs following conservative therapy, if microinvasion exists or if the dysplastic changes are associated with the presence of other pathologies such as fibroids, dysfunctional uterine bleeding (DUB) or uterine prolapse.

Follow-up after Therapy

Follow-up in cases of treatment for either high-risk or low-risk disease comprises of HR-HPV testing. There occurs a substantial evidence base supporting the fact that HPV testing is advantageous both in triage of women with equivocal abnormal cytology as well as for surveillance after treatment of CIN lesions. [18]

Cervical Glandular Intraepithelial Neoplasia

Glandular preinvasive disease or adenocarcinoma in situ or high-grade cervical glandular intraepithelial neoplasia (CGIN) of cervix is a rare condition, which may be diagnosed by chance. Neither colposcopy nor cytology is a reliable method for diagnosis of this condition. The disease may co-exist with squamous preinvasive disease in nearly 30% cases. Although the condition can involve the entire endocervical canal, lesions most commonly occur with 1 cm of the squamocolumnar junction. [54] Treatment usually comprises of conisation with disease-free margins. Management protocol for the women adequately treated for CGIN is described in Flow chart 85.5.

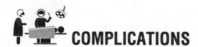

COMPLICATIONS

Progression to Invasive Cancer

The main complication of dysplastic cervical changes is progression to cervical cancer if the condition is left untreated.

Procedural Complications

Complications resulting from cone biopsy are as follows:

❖ *Intraoperative and postoperative bleeding*: Major intra-operative complications rarely occur during cone biopsy. Bleeding may be sometimes heavy and conservative measures (e.g. application of sutures, use of cautery and application of ferric subsulphate paste) are usually helpful in these cases for controlling haemorrhage. The surgeon may be seldom required to resort to more invasive procedures such as application of a cerclage type stitch, internal iliac artery embolisation or ligation, or hysterectomy in case the bleeding becomes very severe.

❖ *Uterine perforation*: Uterine perforation is a rare complication, which is more likely to occur in cases when the uterus is acutely anteflexed or atrophied (postmenopausal women). Extension of the perforation in lateral direction may result in laceration of the uterine artery. In uncommon circumstances, injuries such as broad ligament haematoma or laceration of the bladder and rectum may occur. In these

PART III

Flow chart 85.5: Management of women adequately treated for cervical glandular intraepithelial neoplasia (CGIN)

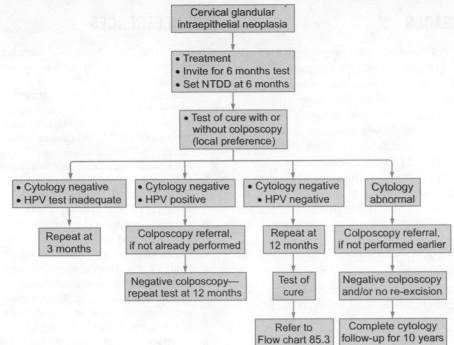

cases, laparoscopy or even laparotomy may be required for management.

❖ *Postoperative bleeding*: Bleeding shortly after surgery may be due to inadequate intraoperative haemostasis or a result of vasodilation due to the wearing off of the effect of the vasoconstrictor solution. Delayed haemorrhage may occur 1–2 weeks after surgery and may be due to dissolution of sutures or erosion of a blood vessel during the healing process. This bleeding can be controlled with the help of conservative measures (previously described) or uterine packing. Occasionally, surgical haemostasis under anaesthesia may be required.

❖ *Infection*: Infection occurs rarely if the procedure is performed observing aseptic surgical precautions. Prophylactic antibiotics are usually not required prior to the procedure. However, antibiotics may be prescribed following the procedure if the clinician suspects a risk of infection or in high-risk cases (e.g. history of gonorrhoea, PID, etc.). The infection may manifest in many ways, including local cervical inflammation, endometritis, parametritis, salpingitis, pelvic abscess, etc.

❖ *Reproductive effects of treatment*: Cervical surgery involves removal or destruction of tissue, which may cause many adverse results (Box 85.1), thereby affecting the reproductive outcomes. Some of the adverse reproductive outcomes, which may occur following the surgical procedures, are as follows:
  • *Infertility*: Refer to Box 85.1 for the likely causes of infertility and adverse reproductive outcomes in these cases.
  • *Second trimester pregnancy loss*: Previous history of cervical conisation is associated with an increased risk of second trimester pregnancy loss.

Box 85.1: Causes of adverse reproductive outcomes in cases of cervical surgery

❑ *Alteration of cervical mucus*: Removal of cervical glands may undesirably affect fertility by changing the cervical mucus, which is required for normal sperm migration and sustainability.

❑ *Premature dilatation of cervix*: Removal or destruction of a large portion of the collagen matrix that forms the cervical stroma may decrease the tensile strength, thereby causing the cervix to dilate prematurely during pregnancy.

❑ *Increased risk of ascending infection*: Removal of tissue and loss of cervical glands and cervical mucus may theoretically increase the risk of ascending infection.

❑ *Loss of cervical plasticity*: This may make the membranes more vulnerable to rupture, thereby resulting in preterm PROMs.

❑ *Cervical stenosis*: Scarring from cervical surgery may result in cervical stenosis. This may cause difficulty in cervical dilatation during labour, which may partially or completely obstruct the uterine cavity, interfering with the menstrual flow. In severe cases, haematometra or pyometra can occur. In pregnant women with cervical stenosis, the cervix may fail to dilate normally during labour.

  • *Preterm premature rupture of membranes*: The risk of preterm PROMs may be increased in some women undergoing CIN treatment procedures.
  • *Preterm delivery and perinatal mortality*: Preterm PROMs associated with various treatment procedures for CIN may result in increased risk for preterm delivery and increased perinatal mortality.

❖ *Late complications*: Late complications of conisation may include complications such as cervical insufficiency and cervical stenosis.

CHAPTER 85

CLINICAL PEARLS

❖ The severe varieties of dysplasia may progress to invasive cancer in about 10–30% of cases in 5–10 years time. Therefore, the peak incidence of occurrence of dysplasias appears to be 10 years earlier than that of frank invasive cancer.

❖ Human papillomavirus infection is commonly prevalent amongst women less than 25 years of age. However, it rarely causes cancer. Nevertheless, almost all cases of cervical cancer are caused by HPV infection.

❖ The principle of management of the new NHS cervical screening programme is to keep the low-risk woman in the community and to refer the high-risk woman for colposcopic examination.

❖ Satisfactory colposcopy requires visualisation of the entire squamocolumnar junction and transformation zone for presence of any visible lesions.

❖ High-grade squamous intraepithelial lesion changes have the greatest risk of turning cancerous in the future, thus these need to be definitively treated. Other types of changes also may require further testing, but may not need treatment.

❖ Though the various ablative and excisional procedures can be used as a treatment option for CIN2 and CIN3, the preferred treatment option for CIN2 and CIN3 is LEEP. Most of the ablative and excisional procedures described previously can be performed on an OPD basis.

❖ Neither colposcopy nor cervical cytology serves as a reliable method for detection of cervical glandular disease.

EVIDENCE-BASED MEDICINE

❖ Presently, there is no evidence to indicate that cervical cancer screening programmes would be able to reduce the mortality related to cervical cancer.[18] The benefit of screening is illustrated by the extrapolation of data showing a reduction in incidence and mortality related to cervical cancer in the areas of Northern Europe (e.g. Iceland, Denmark, Finland, etc.) having a well-organised screening programme. On the other hand, countries with no organised screening programme (e.g. Norway) continue to show an increase in the incidence of both these parameters.

❖ The available evidence indicates that the 3-yearly cervical screening programme is likely to substantially prevent more cancers in comparison to 5-yearly screening programme amongst younger women (belonging to the age-group between 25 and 49 years), with slightly increased healthcare costs.[17,18]

❖ The available evidence does not indicate the superiority of one treatment methodology (except cryotherapy) over the other for management of cases of CIN. The success rates of most treatment modalities vary between 90% to 98%, except for cryotherapy whose success rate varies between 77% to 93%.[50]

REFERENCES

1. Peto J, Gilham C, Fletcher O, Matthews FE. The cervical cancer epidemic that screening has prevented in the UK. Lancet. 2004;364(9430):249-56.

2. Sasieni PD, Cuzick J, Lynch-Farmery E. Estimating the efficacy of screening by auditing smear histories of women with and without cervical cancer. The national coordinating network for cervical screening. Br J Cancer. 1996;73(8):1001-5.

3. Herbert A. Cervical screening in England and Wales: its effect has been underestimated. Cytopathology. 2000;11(6):471-9.

4. Solomon D, Davey D, Kurman R, Moriarty A, O'Connor D, Prey M, et al. The 2001 Bethesda System: terminology for reporting results of cervical cytology. JAMA. 2002;287:2114-9.

5. Cervical Screening Programme, England: Statistics for 2014-15. The Health and Social Care Information Centre, November 2015.

6. Walboomers JM, Jacobs MV, Manos MM, Bosch FX, Kummer JA, Shah KV, et al. Human papilloma virus is a necessary cause of invasive cervical cancer worldwide. J Pathol. 1999;189(1):12-9.

7. Bosch FX, Lorincz A, Muñoz N, Meijer CJ, Shah KV. The causal relation between human papillomavirus and cervical cancer. J Clin Pathol. 2002;55(4):244-65.

8. de Villiers EM, Fauquet C, Broker TR, Bernard HU, zur Hausen H. Classification of papillomaviruses. Virology. 2004;324(1):17-27.

9. Diaz ML. Human Papilloma Virus––Prevention and Treatment. Obstet Gynecol Clin North Am. 2008;35(2):199-217.

10. Lombard I, Vincent-Salomon A, Validire P, Zafrani B, de la Rochefordière A, Clough K, et al. Human papillomavirus genotype as a major determinant of the course of cervical cancer. J Clin Oncol. 1998;16(8):2613-9.

11. Schiffman MH, Bauer HM, Hoover RN, Glass AG, Cadell DM, Rush BB. Epidemiologic evidence showing that human papillomavirus infection causes most cervical intraepithelial neoplasia. J Natl Cancer Inst. 1993;85(12):958-64.

12. Zhu J, Norman I, Elfgren K, Gaberi V, Hagmar B, Hjerpe A, et al. A comparison of liquid-based cytology and Pap smear as a screening method for cervical cancer. Oncol Rep. 2007;18(1):157-60.

13. de Bekker-Grob EW, de Kok IM, Bulten J, van Rosmalen J, Vedder JE, Arbyn M, et al. Liquid-based cervical cytology using ThinPrep technology: weighing the pros and cons in a cost-effectiveness analysis. Cancer Causes Control. 2012;23(8):1323-31.

14. Cox JT. Liquid-based cytology: evaluation of effectiveness, cost-effectiveness, and application to present practice. J Natl Compr Canc Netw. 2004;2(6):597-611.

15. Mayor S. NHS cervical screening programme to introduce liquid based cytology. BMJ. 2003;327(7421):948.

16. Whitley MW. Cervical cancer screening: liquid based cytology is successful. BMJ. 2003;327(7407):161-2.

17. The Health and Social Care Information Centre. (2014). Announcement of methodological changes to Cervical Screening Programme, England, Statistics for 2013-14. [online] Available from www.content.digital.nhs.uk/media/15458/Cervical-Screening-Programme-Methodological-Change-Notice/pdf/MethChange201404_CervicalScreening2013-14.pdf. [Accessed October, 2016].

18. Public Health England. NHS Cervical Screening Programme Colposcopy and Programme Management NHSCSP Publication number 20, 3rd edition. Sheffield: NHSCP; 2016.

19. Herbert A, Stein K, Bryant TN, Breen C, Old P. Relation between the incidence of invasive cervical cancer and the screening interval: is a five-year interval too long? J Med Screen. 1996;3(3):140-5.

20. Sasieni P, Adams J. Effect of screening on cervical cancer mortality in Wales and England: analysis of trends with an age cohort model. BMJ. 1999;318(7193):1244-5.

21. Minutes of an extraordinary meeting of the ACCS to re-examine current policy on cervical screening for women aged 20 to 24 years taking account of any new evidence and to make recommendations to the National Cancer Director and Ministers, 19 May 2009. [online] Available from www.cancerscreening.nhs.uk/cervical/cervical-review-minutes-20090519.pdf [Accessed December, 2016].

22. Collins S, Mazloomzadeh S, Winter H, Blomfield P, Bailey A, Young LS, et al. High incidence of cervical human papillomavirus infection in women during their first sexual relationship. BJOG. 2002;109:96-8.

23. Sasieni P, Castanon A, Cuzick J. Impact of cervical screening on young women: a critical review of the literature (NHSCSP Publication No 31). Sheffield: NHS Cancer Screening Programmes; 2010.

24. Sasieni P, Adams J, Cuzick J. Benefit of cervical screening at different ages: evidence from the UK audit of screening histories. Br J Cancer. 2003;89(1):88-93.

25. Sasieni P, Castanon A, Cuzick J. Effectiveness of cervical screening with age: Population based case-control study of prospectively recorded data. BMJ. 2009;339:b2968.

26. Kyrgiou M, Koliopoulos G, Martin-Hirsch P, Arbyn M, Prendiville W, Paraskevaidis E. Obstetric outcomes after conservative treatment for intraepithelial or early invasive cervical lesions: systematic review and meta-analysis. Lancet. 2006;367(9509):489-98.

27. Bruinsma F, Lumley J, Tan J, Quinn M. Precancerous changes in the cervix and risk of subsequent preterm birth. BJOG. 2007;114:70-80.

28. Arbyn M, Kyrgiou M, Simoens C, Raifu AO, Koliopoulos G, Martin-Hirsch P, et al. Perinatal mortality and other severe adverse pregnancy outcomes associated with treatment of cervical intraepithelial neoplasia: meta-analysis. BMJ. 2008;337:a1284.

29. Jakobsson M, Gissler M, Sainio S, Paavonen J, Tapper AM. Preterm delivery after surgical treatment for cervical intraepithelial neoplasia. Obstet Gynecol. 2007;109(2 Pt 1):309-13.

30. Jakobsson M, Gissler M, Paavonen J, Tapper AM. Loop electrosurgical excision procedure and the risk for preterm birth. Obstet Gynecol. 2009;114(3):504-10.

31. Noehr B, Jensen A, Frederiksen K, Tabor A, Kjaer SK. Loop electrosurgical excision of the cervix and subsequent risk for spontaneous preterm delivery: a population-based study of singleton deliveries during a 9-year period. Am J Obstet Gynecol. 2009;201(1):33.e1-6.

32. Cruickshank M, Flannelly G, Campbell DM. Fertility and pregnancy outcome following large loop excision of the cervical transformation zone. Br J Obstet Gynaecol. 1995;102(6):467-70.

33. Castanon A, Brocklehurst P, Evans H, Peebles D, Singh N, Walker P, et al. Risk of preterm birth after treatment for cervical intraepithelial neoplasia among women attending colposcopy in England: retrospective-prospective cohort study. BMJ. 2012;345:e5174.

34. Kelly RS, Patnick J, Kitchener HC, Moss SM. HPV testing as a triage for borderline or mild dyskaryosis on cervical cytology: results from the Sentinel Sites study. Br J Cancer. 2011;105(7):983-8.

35. Paraskevaidis E, Arbyn M, Sotiriadis A, Diakomanolis E, Martin-Hirsch P, Koliopoulos G, et al. The role of HPV DNA testing in the follow-up period after treatment for CIN: a systematic review of the literature. Cancer Treat Rev. 2004;30(2):205-11.

36. Cuzick J, Arbyn M, Sankaranarayanan R, Tsu V, Ronco G, Mayrandf M, et al. Overview of Human Papillomavirus-Based and Other Novel Options for Cervical Cancer Screening in Developed and Developing Countries. Vaccine. 2008;26(10):K29-41.

37. Arbyn M, Martin-Hirsch P, Buntinx F, Van Ranst M, Paraskevaidis E, Dillner J. Triage of women with equivocal or low-grade cervical cytology results: a meta-analysis of the HPV test positivity rate. J Cell Mol Med. 2009;13(4):648-59.

38. NHSCSP. HPV triage and test of cure implantation. NHSCSP good practice guide No. 3, 2011.

39. Kitchener HC, Almonte M, Thomson C, Wheeler P, Sargent A, Stoykova B, et al. HPV testing in combination with liquid-based cytology in primary cervical screening (ARTISTIC): a randomised controlled trial. Lancet Oncol. 2009;10(7):672-82.

40. Rijkaart DC, Berkhof J, van Kemenade FJ, Coupe VM, Rozendaal L, Heideman DA, et al. HPV DNA testing in population-based cervical screening (VUSA-Screen study): results and implications. Br J Cancer. 2012;106:975-81.

41. Castle PE, Stoler MH, Wright TC Jr, Sharma A, Wright TL, Behrens CM. Performance of carcinogenic human papillomavirus (HPV) testing and HPV16 or HPV18 genotyping for cervical cancer screening of women aged 25 years and older: a subanalysis of the ATHENA study. Lancet Oncol. 2011;12(9):880-90.

42. Bulkmans NW, Berkhof J, Bulk S, Bleeker MC, van Kemenade FJ, Rozendaal L, et al. High-risk HPV type-specific clearance rates in cervical screening. Br J Cancer. 2007;96(9):1419-24.

43. Apgar BS, Rubin MM, Brotzman GL. Principles and techniques of the colposcopic examination. In: Apgar BS, Brotzman GL, Spitzer M (Eds). Colposcopy Principles and Practice: An Integrated Textbook and Atlas. Philadelphia: WB Saunders; 2002. pp. 115-32.

44. Adjunctive colposcopy technologies for examination of the uterine cervix--DySIS and Niris Imaging System. London: NICE; 2012.

45. Hogewoning CJ, Bleeker MC, van den Brule AJ, Voorhorst FJ, Snijders PJ, Berkhof J, et al. Condom use promotes regression of cervical intraepithelial neoplasia and clearance of human papilloma virus: A randomized clinical trial. Int J Cancer. 2003;107:811-6.

46. Klein NP, Hansen J, Chao C, Velicer C, Emery M, Slezak J, et al. Safety of quadrivalent human papillomavirus vaccine administered routinely to females. Arch Pediatr Adolesc Med. 2012;1:1-9.

47. Paavonen J, Jenkins D, Bosch FX, Naud P, Salmerón J, Wheeler CM, et al. Efficacy of a prophylactic adjuvanted bivalent L1 virus-like-particle vaccine against infection with human papillomavirus types 16 and 18 in young women: an interim analysis of a phase III double-blind, randomized controlled trials. Lancet. 2007;369(9580):2161-70.

48. Koutsky LA, Ault KA, Wheeler CM, Brown DR, Barr E, Alvarez FB, et al. A controlled trial of a human papillomavirus type 16 vaccine. N Engl J Med. 2002;347(21):1645-51.

49. Joura EA, Leodolter S, Hernandez-Avila M, Wheeler CM, Perez G, Koutsky LA, et al. Efficacy of a quadrivalent prophylactic

human papillomavirus (types 6, 11, 16 and 18) L1 virus-like particle vaccine against high-grade vulval and vaginal lesions: a combined analysis of three randomized clinical trials. Lancet. 2007;369(9574):1693-702.

50. Martin-Hirsch PP, Paraskevaidis E, Bryant A, Dickinson HO, Keep SL. Surgery for cervical intraepithelial neoplasia. Cochrane Database Syst Rev. 2010;(6):CD001318.

51. Sammarco MJ, Hartenbach EM, Hunter VJ. Local anesthesia for cryosurgery of the cervix. J Reprod Med. 1993;38:170-2.

52. Herzog TJ, Williams S, Adler LM, Rader JS, Kubiniec RT, Camel HM, et al. Potential of cervical electrosurgical excision procedure for diagnosis and treatment of cervical intraepithelial neoplasia. Gynecol Oncol. 1995;57:286-93.

53. Prendiville W, Cullimore J, Norman S. Large loop excision of the transformation zone (LLETZ). A new method of management for women with cervical intraepithelial neoplasia. Br J Obstet Gynecol. 1989;96:1054-60.

54. Wright TC, Massad LS, Dunton CJ, Spitzer M, Wilkinson EJ, Solomon D. 2006 consensus guidelines for the management of women with cervical intraepithelial neoplasia or adenocarcinoma in situ. J Low Genit Tract Dis. 2007;11: 223-39.

Invasive Cervical Cancer

INTRODUCTION

Cervical cancer is the fourth most common type of cancer amongst women, with an estimated 528,000 new cases and 266,000 deaths occurring from cervical cancer worldwide in 2012.[1] Cervical cancer accounted for nearly 7.5% of all female cancer deaths. These statistics reflect the global estimates for cervical cancer in the developed countries. In the developing countries, where women do not have access to cervical cancer screening and prevention programmes, cervical cancer remains the second most common type of cancer. In UK, cervical screening has been carried out since 1960s. As a result, the incidence of cervical cancer in the UK has fallen by nearly 45% since 1975 and the mortality rate due to cervical cancer fell to 2.4 per 100,000 deaths in 2011.[2]

On the other hand, nearly 90% of deaths due to cervical cancer occur in the less developed region. It has become the most commonly diagnosed cancer amongst the women in Southern Africa and Central America. Mortality due to cervical cancer generally increases with the woman's age, with the highest number of deaths occurring in women in their late 70s.

Cervical cancer usually affects women aged 35–55 years, but it can also affect women as young as 20. Though there is a decline in the incidence of cervical cancer in the older age groups (60–70 years), the incidence of cervical cancer again peaks in the 80-years age group.[3] Cancer of the cervix involves the squamous epithelium of cervix, and typically begins at the transformation zone between the ectocervix and endocervix. Women who are infected with high-risk HPV genital subtypes (especially HPV 16 and HPV 18) are associated with an increased risk of malignant transformation. Widespread use of the Papanicolaou (Pap) smear has dramatically reduced the incidence of cervical cancer in developed countries. As a result, cervical cancer has become relatively uncommon in developed countries having intensive cytologic screening programmes.

AETIOLOGY

Some risk factors for cervical cancer are as follows:[4,5]
* History of having STDs such as Herpes simplex
* Infection with human papilloma virus (16, 18, 31, 33) or condylomata
* Young age at the time of first sexual intercourse (coitus before the age of 18 years)
* Delivery of the first child before the age of 20 years
* Having multiple sexual partners
* Multiparity with poor birth spacing between pregnancies
* Poor personal hygiene and low socioeconomic status
* History of smoking cigarettes or drug abuse
* History of disorders of immune system (e.g. AIDS)
* History of having preinvasive lesions.

DIAGNOSIS

Clinical Presentation

There may be no symptoms in the early stages of cancer and the woman may be completely asymptomatic. The cervical lesion may be detected at the time of routine Pap smear. The most common symptoms indicative of cervical cancer, which need to be elicited, include the following:[6]
* History of abnormal bleeding, spotting, or watery discharge in between periods or after intercourse. A history of postcoital bleeding must specifically raise the suspicion of cervical cancer.
* Often there is also a foul smelling vaginal discharge and discomfort during intercourse
* The presentation could be in the form of postmenopausal bleeding
* In advanced stages of cancer there may be symptoms like pelvic pain, loss of appetite, weight loss, fatigue, back pain, leg pain, leg swelling, bleeding from the vagina, leaking of urine or faeces from the vagina and bone fractures.

General Physical Examination

No specific finding may be detected on the general physical examination. Chronic bleeding may be associated with anaemia. Advanced stages of cancer may be associated with cancer cachexia, lymphadenopathy or pedal oedema. Evaluation of supraclavicular, axillary and inguinofemoral nodes is important to exclude the metastatic disease.

Per Speculum Examination

On per speculum examination, cervix must be carefully inspected for presence of any suspicious lesions. Vaginal fornices must also be closely inspected. Squamous cell cancers of the ectocervix may appear as proliferative or cauliflower-like, vascular, friable growth, which bleeds on touch; ulcerative lesions; or as flat indurated areas. The growth may undergo ulceration and necrosis, which may result in an offensive foul smelling vaginal discharge. In case of an invasive cancer, the cervix may appear firm and expanded on per speculum examination. This finding, however, needs to be confirmed on digital examination.

A per speculum examination may be helpful in detection of abnormal lesions over the cervix. It also enables the gynaecologist to simultaneously take the punch biopsy of the suspected lesion. On vaginal examination, both fungating and ulcerative cervical lesions may be identified. Uterus may appear bulky due to occurrence of pyometra in advanced stage when the cervix gets blocked by growth.

Rectal Examination

A rectovaginal examination is also essential in cases of suspected cervical malignancy. This examination may help the examiner to identify nodules or masses, which indicate the possibility of locally invasive disease. The rectal examination may reveal thickening and induration of uterosacral ligaments and evaluation of parametrial extension of the disease (identified in form of parametrial nodularity). It is also useful for assessing cervical consistency and size, particularly in patients with endocervical disease.

Investigations

❖ *Pap smear*: Pap smear is able to accurately detect cervical cancers in up to 90% of the cases in the early stages, even before the symptoms have developed.
❖ *Colposcopic examination and biopsy*: In case an abnormality is detected on pap smear, a colposcopic examination and biopsy may be performed to further confirm the diagnosis.
❖ *Tissue biopsy*: Histopathological examination helps in establishing the accurate diagnosis. Different types of biopsies, which can be performed are punch biopsy, endo-cervical curettage, cone biopsy, etc.[7]
❖ *Imaging studies*: These include ultrasound (trans-abdominal, transvaginal and colour Doppler) and CT examination (Figs 86.1 to 86.5).
❖ *Investigations for staging*: Various investigations which help in the staging include cystoscopy, chest X-ray, sigmoidoscopy, CT, MRI, barium enema, bone and liver scans and PET.

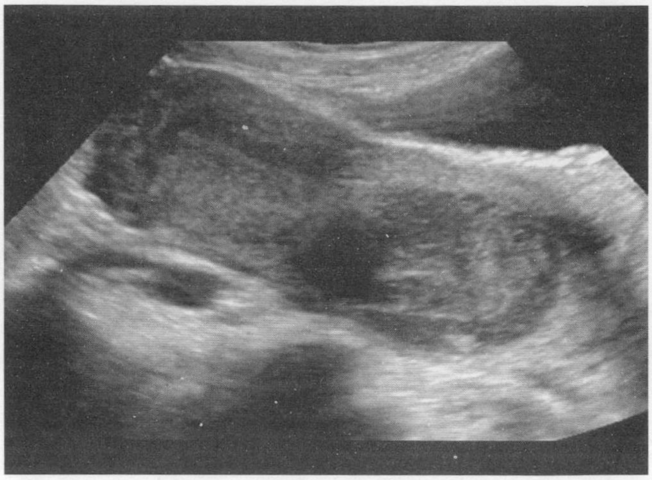

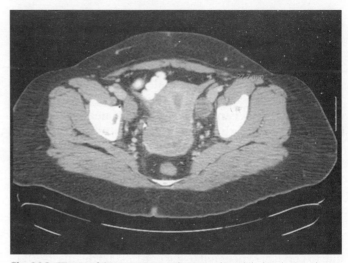

Fig. 86.1: Transabdominal sonography showing solid heterogeneous cervical mass

Fig. 86.2: CT scan of the same patient showing a large lobulated cervical mass with central hypoattenuation

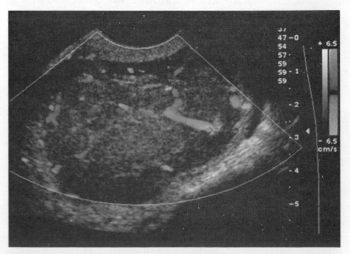

Fig. 86.3: Colour Doppler of the same patient showing randomly distributed irregular vessels in the mass arising from the posterior aspect of the cervix (For colour version, see Plate 8)

PART III

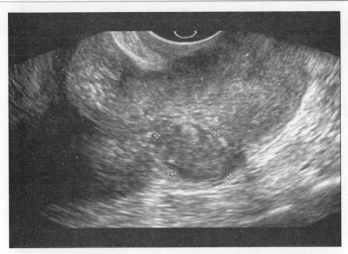

Fig. 86.4: TVS of cervix of a 47-year-old patient with severe suprapubic pain. TVS shows presence of a solid cervical mass measuring 3 × 2 × 2.5 cm

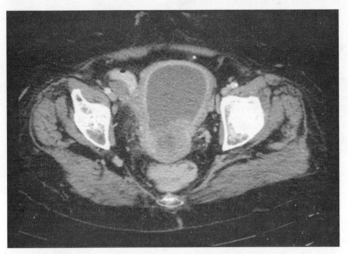

Fig. 86.5: CT scan of the same patient showing spread of the cancer

DIFFERENTIAL DIAGNOSIS

❖ Ulcerative growths such as tubercular and syphilitic ulcers
❖ Fibroid polypus
❖ Sarcoma of the cervix (rarely).

Biopsy of the cervical lesion helps in establishing the diagnosis in most of the cases.

MANAGEMENT

Staging system for cervical cancer as devised by FIGO and TNM staging systems is described in Table 86.1.[8-10]

The treatment of cervical cancer varies with the stage of the disease (Table 86.2). For early invasive cancer, surgery is the treatment of choice.[11] In more advanced cases, radiation combined with chemotherapy is the current standard of care.[12] In patients with disseminated disease, chemotherapy or radiation provides symptom palliation.

Definitive Treatment for Invasive Cancer

The treatment of cervical cancer varies with the stage of the disease. While radiotherapy can be used for all stages of cervical cancer, for early invasive cancer (stage I and IIA disease), surgery is the treatment of choice.[11] In more advanced cases, radiation combined with chemotherapy is the current standard of care.[12] In patients with disseminated disease, chemotherapy or radiation provides symptom palliation. Palliative radiotherapy is often useful for controlling bleeding, pelvic pain and urinary or partial large bowel obstructions resulting from pelvic disease. The 5-year survival rate of cancer cervix treated with either radiation therapy or radical hysterectomy is 85%. Recent improvements in the treatment of cervical cancer include use of adjuvant chemoradiation in patients discovered to have high-risk cervical cancer after radical hysterectomy and in patients with locally advanced cervical cancer.

Depending on the staging and grading of the cervical cancer, various treatment options are summarised in Table 86.2 and are described here in details.

Stage IA Tumours

As described before, stage IA tumours are mainly diagnosed by microscopic examination. The risk of nodal metastasis in the early invasive tumours (stage IA1) is quite low, only about 0.5%; therefore, the prognosis in these cases is quite good. 5-year survival rate exceeds 95% with appropriate treatment.[13] The recommended therapy for stage IA1 tumours without lymphovascular space invasion who are not desirous of future fertility is type I hysterectomy (extrafascial hysterectomy). If lymphovascular space invasion (LVSI) is found, a modified radical hysterectomy (type II hysterectomy) with pelvic lymphadenopathy is an appropriate and effective treatment option. For early stage cervical cancer (stage IA), a modified radical hysterectomy with pelvic lymphadenectomy is recommended rather than primary chemoradiation. Conisation with clear margins may be considered adequate in young patients with stage IA disease who want to conserve their uterus. For effective treatment, there must not be any evidence of LVSI and both endocervical margins and curettage findings must be negative for cancer or dysplasia. If endocervical margins or curettage is positive for dysplasia or malignancy, further treatment is necessary because these findings are predictive of residual disease. Also, the patients undergoing conisation require close follow-up, including cytology, colposcopy and endocervical curettage. Radical trachelectomy or radical type II hysterectomy with pelvic lymphadenectomy may be recommended in cases with stage IA2 disease. The risk of lymph node involvement with stage IA2 disease is as high as 8%, indicating the need for lymphadenectomy, which may be performed via any one of the following routes: vaginal, abdominal, laparoscopic, or robotic. In young women desirous of childbearing, conservative treatment comprising of laparoscopic lymphadenectomy followed by vaginal trachelectomy can be done. Radical

Table 86.1: TNM and FIGO staging systems for cervical cancer staging[8-10]

TNM stage	FIGO stage	Stage description
Tx	–	Primary tumour cannot be assessed
T0	–	No evidence of primary tumour
Tis	0	Carcinoma in situ
T1	I	Cervical carcinoma confined to uterus (extension to corpus should be disregarded)
T1a	IA	Invasive carcinoma diagnosed only by microscopy
		All macroscopically visible lesions—even with superficial invasion—are T1b/IB. Stromal invasion with a maximal depth of 5.0 mm measured from the base of the epithelium and a horizontal spread of 7.0 mm or less. Vascular space involvement, venous or lymphatic, does not affect classification
T1a1	IA1	Measured stromal invasion 3 mm or less in depth and 7 mm or less in lateral spread
T1a2	IA2	Measured stromal invasion more than 3 mm but not more than 5 mm with a horizontal spread 7 mm or less
T1b	IB	Clinically visible lesion confined to the cervix or microscopic lesion greater than IA2
T1b1	IB1	Clinically visible lesion 4 cm or less in greatest dimension
	IB2	Clinically visible lesion more than 4 cm
T2	II	Cervical carcinoma invades beyond uterus but not to pelvic wall or to the lower third of vagina
T2a	IIA	Tumour without parametrial invasion
T2b	IIB	Tumour with parametrial invasion
T3	III	Tumour extends to the pelvic wall and/or involves the lower third of the vagina and/or causes hydronephrosis or non-functioning kidney
T3a	IIIA	Tumour involves lower third of vagina; no extension to pelvic wall
T3b	IIIB	Tumour extends to pelvic wall and/or causes hydronephrosis or non-functioning kidney
–	IV	Cervical carcinoma has extended beyond the true pelvis or has involved (biopsy proven) bladder mucosa or rectal mucosa. Bullous oedema does not qualify as a criterion for stage IV disease
T4	IVA	Spread to adjacent organs (bladder, rectum, or both)
M1	IVB	Distant metastasis
*Lymph nodes**		
NX	–	Regional lymph nodes cannot be assessed
N0	–	No regional lymph nodes metastasis
N1	–	Regional lymph nodes metastasis

*Regional lymph nodes (N) include paracervical, parametrial, hypogastric (obturator), common, internal and external iliac, presacral and sacral group of lymph nodes.

Table 86.2: Summary of treatment of invasive cervical carcinoma

Cervical cancer stage	Therapeutic option
Stage 0	Loop electrosurgical excision procedure (LEEP), laser therapy, conisation and cryotherapy
Stage IA1	Conisation or type I hysterectomy
Stage IA2	Radical trachelectomy or radical type II hysterectomy with pelvic lymphadenectomy
Stage IB1 (invasion >5 mm, <2 cm)	Radical trachelectomy or radical type III hysterectomy with pelvic lymphadenectomy
Stage IB2	Radical type III hysterectomy with pelvic and para-aortic lymphadenectomy or primary chemoradiation
Stage IIA1 and IIA2	Radical type III hysterectomy with pelvic and para-aortic lymphadenectomy or primary chemoradiation
Stage IIB, IIIA and IIIB	Primary chemoradiation
Stage IVA	Primary chemoradiation or primary exenteration
Stage IVB	Primary chemotherapy with or without radiotherapy

trachelectomy is rapidly emerging as a surgical management option in women with stage IA2 and IB1 disease who desire preservation of uterus and fertility.[14,15] The procedure of trachelectomy involves the removal of whole or at least 80% of the cervix, upper vagina and lymph nodes in the pelvis and cutting the Mackenrodt's ligament on either side. A radical trachelectomy can be performed abdominally, vaginally, or using laparoscopic or robotic surgery. Patients who are ideal candidates for this procedure have tumours less than 2 cm in diameter. This procedure may be accompanied by pelvic lymphadenectomy and cervical cerclage placement. Although, complications associated with the procedure are uncommon, women who are able to conceive after surgery are likely to develop preterm labour or late miscarriages. Presently, the experience with this technique is limited. Although, early results with this technique look promising, it is uncertain whether the long-term outcome would be similar to that of traditional therapy.

Stage IB and IIA Tumours

The treatment option for early stage cervical cancer (stage IB1) is primarily surgical treatment rather than primary chemoradiation. Treatment options for stage IB2 and stage IIA are surgical treatment or primary chemoradiation. Surgery in these cases comprises of radical type III hysterectomy with pelvic and para-aortic lymphadenectomy. Radiotherapy can be either in the form of external beam and intracavitary radiotherapy. Though presently there is not enough evidence, nevertheless, primary radiotherapy does not appear to be an adequate treatment for cervical cancer in comparison to primary surgery. Radiotherapy must be used as the primary treatment for only those women who are poor candidates for surgery due to the presence of medical comorbidities or poor functional status. Adjuvant radiotherapy may be, however, required for the cases with intermediate risk, defined by the Sedlis' criteria (Box 86.1).

Adjuvant chemoradiation rather than adjuvant radiotherapy alone is recommended for women with high-risk factors (Peters' criteria), which include the following:[16]

❖ Pathologically involved lymph nodes
❖ Microscopic parametrial invasion
❖ Positive surgical margins.

In these cases, single agent cisplatin, rather than a combination of cisplatin with 5-fluorouracil must be administered in conjunction with radiotherapy.[17,18]

Women with cervical cancer belonging to reproductive age group who wish to preserve their fertility and have a lesion size less than or equal to 2 cm and no lymph node metastases, uterus-preserving surgery is a reasonable treatment option.

Stage IIB, III and IV Tumours

In stage IIB, III and IV cancer as the tumour invades local organs; radiation therapy has become the mainstay of treatment. However, in some cases combination of chemotherapy and radiotherapy is employed. Patients with distant metastases (stage IVB) also require chemotherapy with or without radiotherapy to control systemic disease. Recently, the combination of cisplatin and topotecan is being preferred rather than use of single-agent cisplatin. Adult dose of cisplatin is 50–100 mg/m² IV quarterly 3 weeks. Cisplatin can result in side effects such as hypersensitivity, renal failure, peripheral neuropathy and bone marrow suppression. Adult dose of topotecan is 1.5 mg/m²/day IV for 5 days quarterly 4 weeks. In advanced cases of cervical cancer, the most extreme surgery, called pelvic exenteration in which all of the organs of the pelvis, including the bladder and rectum are removed, may be employed.

Various Available Treatment Options

Surgery

Various types of surgical options which can be used in cases of cervical cancer are described in Table 86.3 and Figure 86.6.[19] Previously, surgery commonly included a radical hysterectomy (Wertheims hysterectomy or Schauta vaginal hysterectomy). The hysterectomy originally described by Wertheims is less extensive than type II radical hysterectomy, commonly performed nowadays. Wertheims hysterectomy involves removal of the entire uterus, both adnexa, medial one-third of parametrium, uterosacral ligaments, upper 2–3 cm cuff of the vagina, dissection of pelvic lymph nodes and selective removal of enlarged lymph nodes. This is in contrast to type II radical hysterectomy, which also includes pelvic lymphadenectomy. Para-aortic lymphadenectomy is performed if the para-aortic nodes are found to be suspicious for metastatic disease at the time of pelvic lymphadenectomy. Oophorectomy is usually not necessary in premenopausal women with squamous cell carcinoma of cervix because

Box 86.1: Sedlis' criteria for defining women at intermediate risk of cancer recurrence following surgery

❑ Presence of lymphovascular space invasion (LVSI) plus deep one-third cervical stromal invasion and tumour of any size
❑ Presence of LVSI plus middle one-third stromal invasion and tumour size ≥2 cm
❑ Presence of LVSI plus superficial one-third stromal invasion and tumour size ≥5 cm
❑ No LVSI but deep or middle one-third stromal invasion and tumour size ≥4 cm

Table 86.3: Classification of radical hysterectomy[19]

Classification	Description
Type I radical hysterectomy (simple/extrafascial hysterectomy)	Removal of the uterus and cervix, but not the parametria or more than the upper vaginal margin
Modified radical or type II radical hysterectomy	Removal of the entire uterus, both adnexa, medial half of cardinal and uterosacral ligaments, upper 2–3 cm cuff of the vagina and pelvic lymphadenectomy
Type III radical hysterectomy (originally described by Meigs in 1944)	Removal of the entire uterus, both adnexa, most of the cardinal and uterosacral ligaments, upper one-third of the vagina and pelvic lymphadenectomy
Type IV radical hysterectomy (extended radical hysterectomy)	Periureteral tissues, superior vesicle artery and as much as three-fourths of the vagina and paravaginal tissue are excised (in addition to structures removed in type III radical hysterectomy)
Type V radical hysterectomy (partial exenteration)	In addition to the structures removed in type IV hysterectomy, portion of distal ureter and bladder are also removed

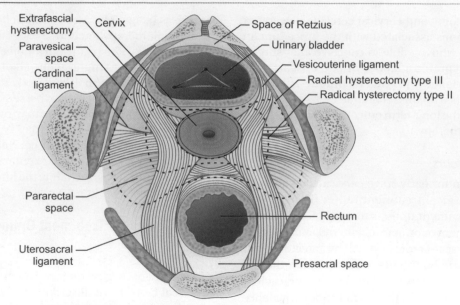

Fig. 86.6: Different types of hysterectomies which can be used in cases of cancer cervix

ovarian metastases are quite uncommon with squamous cell cancer. However, ovarian metastasis may commonly occur in adenocarcinoma. Therefore, consideration must be given towards the removal of ovaries in these cases.

Recently, it has been shown that patients with parametrial involvement, positive pelvic nodes, or positive surgical margins may benefit from a postoperative combination of cisplatin containing chemotherapy and pelvic radiation. Presence of close vaginal margins, defined as tumour less than or equal to 0.5 cm from the vaginal margins of resection in the radical hysterectomy specimen performed for stage IA2, IB, or IIA cervical cancer serves as an important prognostic for deciding whether or not the patient requires adjuvant therapy. Adjuvant therapy following surgery is especially important in high-risk patients with stage 1B and IIA cervical cancer undergoing surgery.[20-25]

Schautas operation is an extended vaginal hysterectomy consisting of removal of the entire uterus, adnexa, most of the vagina and medial portion of the parametrium. This may be preceded by laparoscopic pelvic lymphadenectomy or followed later by extraperitoneal (Taussigs) lymphadenectomy. Alternately, postoperative pelvic radiotherapy may also be given. The type II radical hysterectomy differs from type III radical hysterectomy in the following ways:

❖ The uterine artery is transected at the level of ureter, thereby, preserving the ureteral branch to the ureter
❖ The cardinal ligament is not divided near the sidewall, but instead is divided close to its midportion near the ureteral dissection
❖ The anterior vesicouterine ligament is divided, but the posterior vesicouterine ligament is conserved
❖ A smaller margin of vagina is removed.

A prospective randomised trial has shown that both class II and class III radical hysterectomies are equally effective in surgical treatment of cervical carcinoma.[26] However, class II radical hysterectomy is likely to be associated with a lower risk of late complications.

Surgery versus Radiotherapy

There are advantages to the use of surgery instead of radio-therapy, particularly in younger women in whom conversation of ovaries is important. Fibrosis and reduced vascularity resulting from radiation therapy can result in chronic bladder and bowel problems, which may be difficult to treat. Moreover, sexual dysfunction can commonly occur following radiation because of vaginal shortening, fibrosis and atrophy of the epithelium. Radical hysterectomy is reserved for women who are in good physical condition. Lesions larger than 4 cm should not preferably be operated because these patients would require postoperative radiotherapy.

Chemoradiation

Chemoradiation helps in covering the benefits of systemic chemotherapy along with the benefits of regional radiation therapy. Use of chemotherapy helps in sensitising the cells to radiation therapy. Use of chemoradiation has been found to be associated with a significant improvement in progression free survival as well as the overall survival at 43 months. Cisplatin-based chemotherapy forms the treatment of choice in patients with advanced stage cervical cancer. Chemoradiation has been found to be superior to radiation alone.

Radiation Therapy

Radiation may be used to treat cancer that has spread beyond the pelvis, or cancer that has returned. Patients who receive radiotherapy must be closely monitored to assess response to treatment. Tumour may be expected to regress for up to 3 months following radiotherapy. Radiation therapy can be either external or internal.

Internal radiation therapy: Internal radiation therapy also known as brachytherapy involves placing the selectron tubes inside the patient's vagina. This method helps in delivering radiation directly to the cervix and the surrounding areas.

The radioactive balls in the selectron tube can be withdrawn into the machine when other people come into the patient's room. This helps in keeping the dose of radioactivity to visitors and nurses as low as possible. Based on the current evidence, NICE (2006) supports the use of high-dose rate (HDR) brachytherapy for carcinoma of the cervix, provided that the patient has given consent and the arrangements for monitoring the patient are in place.[27] Prior to the procedure, the patients must receive appropriate counselling and pain management. HDR brachytherapy helps in reducing the radiation hazard to staff, and also helps in reducing the length of inpatient treatment. For delivering HDR brachytherapy to the cervix, applicators are placed in the cervix and connected to an afterloading machine which delivers high-dose radiation, usually for a few minutes. The treatment is often repeated several times, a few days apart, on an outpatient basis. While this procedure delivers a high dose of radiation to the cervix and the adjacent areas, tissues and organs more than a few centimetres away receive a low dose of radiation. Virtually all HDR brachytherapy is given in combination with external-beam radiation therapy.

External radiation therapy: External radiation therapy involves administration of radiation beams from a large machine onto the body where the cancer is located. CT scan is often used for ensuring the accurate targeting of the external radiation beam. External radiotherapy is normally administered on an outpatient basis. The treatments are usually given from Monday to Friday, with a rest at the weekend.

Chemotherapy

The most commonly employed chemotherapy regimens use cisplatin, 5-fluorouracil, carboplatin, ifosfamide, paclitaxel, cyclophosphamide, etc. and is usually used as a palliative therapy.[28] Chemotherapy is sometimes used in the form of neoadjuvant chemotherapy. This method involves use of chemotherapy before surgery or radiotherapy, to shrink the cancer and to make these treatments more effective.

Pelvic Exenteration

If the cancer recurs in the pelvis after radiation therapy, the gynaecologist may need to resort to surgery for removing all pelvic organs. This procedure cures up to 50% of women. This is a major operation that involves removing all of the structures in the pelvic area, including the uterus, cervix, vagina, ovaries, bladder and the rectum. This operation may involve creating two stomas: (1) a colostomy and (2) a urostomy. The operation also involves reconstructing a new vagina.

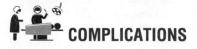

COMPLICATIONS

Complications due to cervical cancer per se and its treatment are as follows:[29]
- Infertility

Table 86.4: Complications due to radical hysterectomy

Acute complications	Chronic complications
• Blood loss • Fistula formation (ureterovaginal/vesicovaginal fistulas) • Pulmonary embolus • Small bowel obstruction • Febrile morbidity (due to pelvic infection, urinary tract infection, wound infection, pelvic abscess, phlebitis, etc.	• Bladder dysfunction (particularly difficulty in voiding) • Lymphocyst formation • Lymphoedema • Premature menopause

- Therapy-related complications: Complications related to treatment modalities such as surgery, chemotherapy and radiotherapy
- Cancer recurrence and metastatic spread
- High rate of mortality and morbidity.

Complications due to Surgery

Complications which may occur due to radical hysterectomy are tabulated in Table 86.4. Other complications which can occur as a result of surgery are as follows:
- *Premature menopause*: Removal of ovaries in young patients can result in symptoms related to premature menopause.
- *Urinary dysfunction*: The most frequent complication of radical hysterectomy is urinary dysfunction as a result of partial denervation of the detrusor muscle.
- *Other complications*: Other complications resulting from surgery may include shortened vagina, ureterovaginal and rectovaginal fistulas, haemorrhage, infection, bowel obstruction, stricture and fibrosis of the intestine or rectosigmoid colon and bladder.

Complications due to Radiotherapy and Chemotherapy

Complications as a result of radiotherapy and chemotherapy, which are commonly used for cancer treatment, have been discussed in details in Chapter 85 (Cervical Intraepithelial Neoplasia).

CLINICAL PEARLS

- Regular testing with Pap smears and HPV vaccination can help prevent cervical cancer. Advent of prophylactic vaccines against types HPV types 16/18 is likely to reduce the risk of cervical cancer by as much as 40%.
- Cone biopsy or excisional treatment alone can be used for the treatment of early micro-invasive disease.
- Both surgery and radiotherapy are associated with similar overall 5-year and disease-free survival rates, in cases of stage IB and IIA disease.

- Use of both surgery and adjuvant radiotherapy is associated with higher morbidity rates in comparison to the use of either surgery or radiotherapy alone.
- Though use of chemoradiation helps in improving survival in comparison to radiotherapy alone in cases with advanced disease, it is associated with greater amount of side-effects.

EVIDENCE-BASED MEDICINE

- *Adjuvant therapy following radical hysterectomy for patients with stage IB and IIA cervical cancer*: Due to the high incidence of distant metastases in high-risk patients undergoing radical hysterectomy, the surgeon must consider the administration of adjuvant systemic chemotherapy in addition to radiation therapy following surgery. This is especially important in high-risk patients with presence of poor prognostic factors such as lymph node metastasis, large lesions (>4 cm in diameter), histologic grade, race (non-Caucasian), and age (>40 years). The incidence of severe gastrointestinal or genitourinary tract complications is not likely to be increased in patients undergoing combination adjuvant therapy in comparison to those undergoing surgery alone. However, the incidence of lymphoedema is increased in patient's undergoing adjuvant radiation therapy. Although adjuvant radiation therapy is unlikely to result in any serious complications, the extent to which this therapy improves local control rates and survival in high-risk patients presently remains unclear. [20-24]
- *Role of neoadjuvant chemotherapy*: Long-term follow-up of the first randomised trial using neoadjuvant chemotherapy [comprising three courses consisting of 50 mg/m^2 cis-platinum, 1 mg/m^2 vincristine, and 25 mg/m^2 bleomycin (days 1–3) at 10-day intervals] for stage Ib squamous carcinoma of the cervix has shown increased survival rates as a result of improved operability with free survival margins. [25]
- *Vaginal radical trachelectomy, a fertility-preserving surgery for the treatment of early-stage cervical cancer*: The available evidence has shown that vaginal radical trachelectomy (VRT) serves as an effective fertility-sparing option for selective group of women with early-stage cervical cancer. [14,15] VRT is likely to be associated with a low incidence of recurrence and acceptable rates of conception. However, the procedure is likely to be associated with a high rate of obstetric complications such as premature labour and miscarriages.

REFERENCES

1. International Agency for Research on Cancer. (2012). GLOBOCAN: All Cancers (excluding non-melanoma skin cancer) Estimated Incidence, Mortality and Prevalence Worldwide in 2012. [online] Available from www.globocan.iarc.fr/Pages/fact_sheets_cancer.aspx. [Accessed September, 2016].

2. Cannistra SA, Niloff JM. Cancer of the uterine cervix. N Engl J Med. 1996;334(16):1030-8.

3. Adami, HO, D Hunter, D Trichopoulos (Eds). Textbook of Cancer Epidemiology, 2nd edition. New York: Oxford University Press; 2002.

4. DiSaia PJ, Creasman WT. Clinical Gynecologic Oncology, 5th edition. St. Louis: Mosby; 1997.

5. Parazzini F, Chatenoud L, La Vecchia C, Negri E, Franceschi S, Bolis G. Determinants of risk of invasive cervical cancer in young women. Br J Cancer. 1998;77(5):838-41.

6. Elkas J, Farias-Eisner R. Cancer of the uterine cervix. Curr Opin Obstet Gynecol. 1998;10(1):47-50.

7. Irvin W, Taylor P. Biopsy of lesions of the female genital tract in the ambulatory setting. J Long Term Eff Med Implants. 2004;14(3):185-99.

8. Pecorelli S, Zigliani L, Odicino F. Revised FIGO staging for carcinoma of the cervix. Int J Gynaecol Obstet. 2009;105(2):107-8.

9. Pecorelli S. Revised FIGO staging for carcinoma of the vulva, cervix, and endometrium. Int J Gynaecol Obstet. 2009;105(2):103-4.

10. National Comprehensive Cancer Network NCCN. (2013). Clinical Practice Guidelines in Oncology: Cervical Cancer V3. [online]. Available from www.nccn.org/professionals/physician_gls/pdf/cervical.pdf. [Accessed October, 2016].

11. Bansal N, Herzog TJ, Shaw RE, Burke WM, Deutsch I, Wright JD. Primary therapy for early-stage cervical cancer: radical hysterectomy vs radiation. Am J Obstet Gynecol. 2009;201(5):485.e1-9.

12. Monk BJ, Wang J, Im S, Stock RJ, Peters WA, Liu PY, et al. Rethinking the use of radiation and chemotherapy after radical hysterectomy: a clinical-pathologic analysis of a Gynecologic Oncology Group/Southwest Oncology Group/Radiation Therapy Oncology Group trial. Gynecol Oncol. 2005;96(3):721-8.

13. Nuovo J, Melnikow J, Willan AR, Chan BK.Treatment outcomes for squamous intraepithelial lesions. Int J Gynaecol Obstet. 2000;68(1):25-33.

14. Plante M, Renaud MC, Hoskins IA, Roy M. Vaginal radical trachelectomy: a valuable fertility-preserving option in the management of early-stage cervical cancer. A series of 50 pregnancies and review of the literature. Gynecol Oncol. 2005;98(1):3-10.

15. Shepherd JH, Spencer C, Herod J, Ind TE. Radical vaginal trachelectomy as a fertility-sparing procedure in women with early-stage cervical cancer-cumulative pregnancy rate in a series of 123 women. BJOG. 2006;113(6):719-24.

16. Peters WA, Liu PY, Barrett RJ, Stock RJ, Monk BJ, Berek JS, et al. Concurrent chemotherapy and pelvic radiation therapy compared with pelvic radiation therapy alone as adjuvant therapy after radical surgery in high-risk early-stage cancer of the cervix. J Clin Oncol. 2000;18(8):1606-13.

17. Omura GA, Blessing JA, Vaccarello L, Berman ML, Clarke-Pearson DL, Mutch DG. Randomized trial of cisplatin versus cisplatin plus mitolactol versus cisplatin plus ifosfamide in advanced squamous carcinoma of the cervix: A Gynecologic Oncology Group study. J Clin Oncol. 1997;15(1):165-71.

18. Rose PG, Bundy BN, Watkins EB, Thigpen JT, Deppe G, Maiman MA, et al. Concurrent cisplatin-based radiotherapy and chemotherapy for locally advanced cervical cancer. N Engl J Med. 1999;340(15):1144-53.

19. Mota F, Vergote I, Trimbos JB, Amant F, Siddiqui N, Del Rio A, et al. Classification of radical hysterectomy adopted by the Gynecological Cancer Group of the European Organization

for Research and Treatment of Cancer. Int J Gynecol Cancer. 2008;18(5):1136-8.

20. Estape RE, Angioli R, Madrigal M, Janicek M, Gomez C, Penalver M. Close vaginal margins as a prognostic factor after radical hysterectomy. Gynecol Oncol. 1998;68(3):229-32.

21. Wertheim MS, Hakes TB, Daghestani AN, Nori D, Smith DH, Lewis JL. A pilot study of adjuvant therapy in patients with cervical cancer at high risk of recurrence after radical hysterectomy and pelvic lymphadenectomy. J Clin Oncol. 1985;3(7):912-6.

22. Soisson AP, Soper JT, Clarke-Pearson DL, Berchuck A, Montana G, Creasman WT. Adjuvant radiotherapy following radical hysterectomy for patients with stage IB and IIA cervical cancer. Gynecol Oncol. 1990;37(3):390-5.

23. Kinney WK, Alvarez RD, Reid GC, Schray MF, Soong SJ, Morley GW, et al. Value of adjuvant whole pelvis radiation after Wertheim's hysterectomy for early stage squamous carcinoma of the cervix with pelvic nodal metastasis: a matched-control study. Gynecologic Oncol. 1989;34(3):258-62.

24. Rotman M, Sedlis A, Piedmonte MR, Bundy B, Lentz SS, Muderspach LI, et al. A phase III randomized trial of postoperative pelvic irradiation in Stage IB cervical carcinoma with poor prognostic features: follow-up of a gynecologic oncology group study. Int J Radiat Oncol Biol Phys. 2006;65(1):169-76.

25. Sardi JE, Giaroli A, Sananes C, Ferreira M, Soderini A, Bermudez A, et al. Long-term follow-up of the first randomized trial using neoadjuvant chemotherapy in stage Ib squamous carcinoma of the cervix: the final results. Gynecol Oncol. 1997;67(1):61-9.

26. Landoni F, Maneo A, Cormio G, Perego P, Milani R, Caruso O, et al. Class II versus class III radical hysterectomy in stage IB-IIA cervical cancer: a prospective randomized study. Gynecol Oncol. 2001;80(1):3-12.

27. National Institute for Health and Clinical Excellence (NICE). (2006). High dose rate brachytherapy for carcinoma of the cervix. Interventional Procedure Guidance 160. [online] Available from www.nice.org.uk/guidance/ipg160. [Accessed October, 2016].

28. Thigpen JT, Vance R, Puneky L, Khansur T. Chemotherapy as a palliative treatment in carcinoma of the uterine cervix. Semin Oncol. 1995;22(2 Suppl 3):16-24.

29. Rubin P, Williams JP (Eds). Clinical Oncology: A Multi-disciplinary Approach for Physicians and Students, 8th edition. Philadelphia, PA, USA: WB Saunders; 2001.

Rare Cancers of the Female Genital Organs

VAGINAL CANCER

 INTRODUCTION

Vaginal cancer is a disease in which malignant cells mainly involve the vagina. It is a rare gynaecologic malignancy and accounts for less than 1% of all cancer deaths amongst women in the UK (2014).[1] When found in early stages, it can often be cured. There are two main types of vaginal cancer: squamous cell carcinoma (80–90%) and adenocarcinoma (4–10%). Vaginal cancer is found most often in women aged 60 years or older, typically following the cessation of sexual activity. Its incidence peaks between the ages of 70 to 80 years. Only 10–15% of patients are below 50 years. Prognosis of the disease depends on several factors, such as the patient's age, tumour histologic type, ethnicity and tumour stage. Ethnic groups such as Black, Asian or Pacific Islander, and Hispanic women are more likely to be diagnosed with late-stage disease. Also these groups of women are likely to have lower 5-year relative survival rates in comparison to the White, non-Hispanic, women.[2]

AETIOLOGY

Risk factors for vaginal cancer are as follows:
❖ The leading risk factor for vaginal intraepithelial neoplasia (VAIN).
❖ Exposure to diethylstilbestrol in utero (clear cell adeno-carcinoma)
❖ Aged 60 years or more
❖ Trophic ulcers in women with procidentia
❖ Prolonged and neglected use of ring pessary in cases of prolapse
❖ Infection with HPV (especially HPV type 16 virus)
❖ History of cervical dysplasia or cervical cancer
❖ Exposure to radiation for the treatment of cervical cancer.

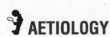 **DIAGNOSIS**

Clinical Presentation

The patient may present with the following clinical symptoms:
❖ Abnormal vaginal bleeding or discharge, which is not related to the menstrual periods
❖ Pain during sexual intercourse
❖ Pain in the pelvic area
❖ A lump in the vagina
❖ Bladder or bowel symptoms (in case of involvement of these structures).

Per Speculum Examination

Areas of involvement may be visible as diffuse, velvety, raised lesions or whitish ulcerative patches. They may bleed on touch. Invasive cancers are more likely to be located in the upper one-third of the vagina in comparison to the less invasive ones.[3] Cervix must be carefully examined to exclude cervical involvement.

Pelvic Examination

Pelvic examination along with the rectal examination helps in determining the extent of spread.

Investigations

❖ *Pap smear*: Cytological examination for identification of intraepithelial lesions
❖ Staining with Schiller's iodine
❖ Colposcopic examination
❖ *Biopsy*: If a Pap smear shows abnormal cells, a biopsy may be performed during colposcopy. An adequate biopsy should be taken in such a way so that it includes the entire thickness of the vaginal epithelium. This is especially

important because depth of invasion of the tumour into the vaginal mucosa and muscle is significant for staging the disease

❖ *Other investigations*: Investigations such as a chest X-ray, cystoscopy, proctoscopy, barium enema, CT scan, MRI, etc. may be done to evaluate the spread of cancer.

DIFFERENTIAL DIAGNOSIS

❖ Vaginal condyloma or vaginal endometriosis
❖ Vaginitis or vaginal inflammation
❖ Metastatic lesions in vagina as a result of primary growth in cervix, endometrium, etc.

MANAGEMENT

Staging and treatment of vaginal cancer is described in Table 87.1.

Early-stage Cancer

If staged early, radical surgery as well as radiation therapy can be curative. Surgery in these cases includes wide local excision or total vaginectomy with vaginal reconstruction.[4] Radiotherapy in the form of both external beam and brachytherapy plays a crucial role in management of most patients with disease beyond VAIN. Such patients should receive a substantial component of external irradiation prior to intracavitary brachytherapy in the dosage of 60–70 cGy. In case the lesion is present in the lower third of vagina, pelvic and inguinal lymphadenectomy may be required.

A retrospective review, comprising of 301 patients with vaginal carcinoma, by Chyle et al. (1996) has shown that vaginal carcinoma poses a therapeutic challenge.[5] In most centres in the UK, standard treatment for vaginal cancer is radiotherapy. Radiotherapy is likely to cause preservation of vaginal anatomy, which also imparts certain psychological benefits to the patient. However, preservation of the vaginal function after treatment of invasive vaginal cancer rarely occurs.[6] Many studies have shown that radiation therapy serves as an effective treatment for patients with vaginal carcinoma, particularly Stage I.[5-9]

Advanced Cases

More advanced stages are treated with a combination of radiation therapy with surgery, similar to the cases of cervical cancer. However, vaginal cancer is associated with poorer survival rates in comparison to cervical cancer. Radical surgery in more advanced cases comprises of radical vaginectomy, lymph node dissection and/or possibly pelvic exenteration. Radiotherapy in these cases comprises of intracavitary brachytherapy along with external beam radiation, especially if there is involvement of pelvic or inguinal group of lymph nodes.

Table 87.1: Staging and treatment of vaginal cancer

Cancer stage	Description	Treatment
Stage 0 (carcinoma in situ) [vaginal intraepithelial neoplasia (VAIN)]	Squamous cell cancer is found in tissue lining the interior of vagina	• Wide local excision, with or without a skin graft • Partial or total vaginectomy, with or without a skin graft • Topical chemotherapy (fluorouracil cream) • CO_2 laser surgery • Internal radiation therapy
Stage I	Cancer limited to the vaginal walls	• Internal radiation therapy, with or without external radiation therapy to lymph nodes or large tumours • Wide local excision or vaginectomy with vaginal reconstruction. Radiation therapy may be given after surgery • Vaginectomy and lymphadenectomy, with or without vaginal reconstruction. Radiation therapy may be given after the surgery
Stage II	Cancer has spread from the vaginal walls to the tissues around the vagina but not up to pelvic side walls	• Both internal and external radiation therapy to the vagina, with or without external radiation therapy to the lymph nodes • Vaginectomy or pelvic exenteration, with or without radiation therapy
Stage III	Cancer has spread from the vagina to the lymph nodes in the pelvis or groin, or to the pelvic walls, or both	Both internal and external radiation therapy, with or without surgery
Stage IVA	Extension beyond the true pelvis, with or without the involvement of the pelvic lymph nodes, bladder and/or the rectum	Both internal and external radiation therapy, with or without surgery
Stage IVB	Distant metastasis such as the lungs. Cancer may also have spread to the distant lymph nodes	Radiation therapy as palliative therapy to relieve symptoms and improve the quality of life. Chemotherapy may also be given

Follow-up

Follow-up is required following treatment in cases of vaginal cancer after every 3 months for a period of first 2 years. This is likely to help in the detection of recurrence, as well as of management of treatment-related morbidity in case of their occurrence. Following this, the patient must be examined at every 6-monthly intervals for another 3 years.

CHAPTER 87

COMPLICATIONS

Complications associated with vaginal carcinoma are as follows:[9]

❖ *Metastasis*: Metastasis of vaginal cancer can occur to distant organs, such as lung, liver, etc.
❖ *Therapy-related complications*: Complications related to treatment modalities such as radiation, surgery and chemotherapy.

 CLINICAL PEARLS

❖ Vaginal intraepithelial neoplasia is a recognised pre-cancerous condition affecting the vagina. The majority of women with high-grade VAIN 3 have a history of premalignant or malignant disease of the cervix.
❖ Diagnosis of vaginal cancer can be established with certainty, only in presence of a normal cervix.
❖ The prognosis in these cases depends upon the cancer stage, grade and the tumour size.
❖ New types of treatment are being tested in clinical trials. These include radiosensitisers which make tumour cells more sensitive to radiation therapy.
❖ Treatment of recurrent vaginal cancer may include pelvic exenteration and radiation therapy.

 EVIDENCE-BASED MEDICINE

❖ *Radiation therapy for early-stage vaginal cancer*: Due to the rarity of vaginal cancer, there is limited published evidence in the form of RCTs. Limited evidence is available in the form of case-controlled series and retrospective reviews. Case series support the use of surgery in selected cases. Management of Stage I and II squamous vaginal cancer patients with surgery followed by selective radiotherapy is likely to be associated with good 5-year survival rates and local tumour control.[4] On the other hand, many retrospective studies have shown that excellent outcomes can be achieved with definitive radiation therapy for invasive squamous cell carcinoma of the vagina.[5,0]
❖ *Vaginal intraepithelial neoplasia*: It is a rare asymptomatic disorder involving the upper third of the vagina, with the high-grade lesion (VAIN 3) being potentially premalignant. There is limited clinical evidence regarding the optimal management of VAIN.[10-12] Ablative treatment with laser or 5-fluorouracil cream is usually unsatisfactory. Treatment of VAIN 3 with high-dose-rate brachytherapy in a dosage of 34–45 Gy is associated with a low rate of recurrence and complications.

CANCER OF THE FALLOPIAN TUBES

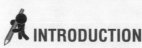 **INTRODUCTION**

Fallopian tube cancer, also known as tubal cancer, develops in the fallopian tubes that connect the ovaries and the uterus. This cancer was once thought to be rare, but it is believed that most cancers previously labelled 'ovarian cancer' were actually fallopian tube cancers, which originated from the fimbrial end of the fallopian tube. It is associated with an extremely poor prognosis with a few long-term survivors. It is frequently associated with the malignancy of upper genital tract.

Primary adenocarcinoma is the most common histological type of primary fallopian tube cancer.[13] The management of fallopian tube cancer is similar to that of the epithelial ovarian cancer. However, unlike ovarian cancer, fallopian tube cancer is not routinely suspected and its treatment may be delayed. Therefore, it often appears to have a worse prognosis in comparison to the ovarian cancer.

The most common type of tumour is an adenocarcinoma and typically affects women between the ages of 50 to 60 years. It is bilateral in nearly one-third cases.

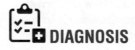 **AETIOLOGY**

❖ Due to the rareness of this cancer, little is known regarding the definitive aetiology, diagnosis and treatment of fallopian tube cancer.
❖ Women who have inherited the *BRCA1* gene (linked with the development of ovarian and breast cancer) are also at an increased risk of developing fallopian tube cancer.[14]
❖ It is more common in nulliparous menopausal women.

DIAGNOSIS

Clinical Presentation

❖ Fallopian tube cancer usually presents as a virulent ovarian cancer or as a benign pelvic mass. Almost all cases are diagnosed at the time of surgery or autopsy.
❖ There may be abnormal vaginal bleeding or amber coloured discharge, especially after menopause.
❖ There may be abdominal pain or a feeling of pressure in the abdomen.

Pelvic Examination

A pelvic mass at the time of diagnosis may be present in up to two-thirds of patients.

Investigations

Since the cancer of fallopian tubes is extremely rare, the diagnosis is mainly reached on the basis of suspicion.

Various investigations which must be done in these cases include the following:[15]

* *Pap smear*: Unreliable test for the diagnosis of fallopian tube cancer
* *Uterine biopsy*: Negative findings on the biopsy of the uterine curettings and a negative hysteroscopic examination in a patient with postmenopausal bleeding should raise the suspicion of fallopian tube cancer
* *Imaging*: Transvaginal ultrasound may show presence of an adnexal mass. Doppler flow velocimetry may show low resistance blood flow in the mass
* *CA-125 test*: An estimated 85% of women with gynaecological disease have increased levels of CA-125.

DIFFERENTIAL DIAGNOSIS

* Pyosalpinx
* Tubercular lesion of the tube
* Other malignancies of genital tract such as endometrial, cervical, vaginal, etc.

MANAGEMENT

Some authorities believe that fallopian tube cancer could be an extension of the high-grade serous cancer of the ovaries, which originates in the fimbria of the fallopian tubes and spreads to the surface of the ovaries. Similarly, some peritoneal cancers may begin in the fallopian tubes. Therefore, these three cancers appear to be linked and follow a common staging system, which is discussed in details in Chapter 84 [Ovarian Neoplasia (Benign and Malignant)].

Primary treatment for fallopian tube cancer usually involves surgery and comprises of total abdominal hysterectomy with bilateral salpingo-oophorectomy, pelvic lymph node sampling and omentectomy.[16] Postoperative adjuvant therapy with radiotherapy, chemotherapy and hormonal therapy with progestogens may be required depending upon the spread of cancer.

Aggressive cytoreductive surgery must be followed by chemotherapy and second-look laparotomy. However, the clinical value of second-look laparotomy presently remains controversial because of eventual relapse in a significant proportion of patients and poor survival following negative second-look laparotomy.[17-19]

In advanced stages of fallopian cancer, survival can be prolonged by using platinum-based chemotherapy. The use of platinum-based chemotherapy (cisplatin/carboplatin, etc.) presently appears as an effective adjuvant therapy for both early stages and advanced stages.[20-22] Use of a paclitaxel-based chemotherapy regimen is also likely to significantly improve survival in patients with fallopian tube cancer who have undergone cytoreductive surgery.[23-25]

COMPLICATIONS

* *Metastasis*: This is a highly malignant tumour which spreads rapidly to the surrounding as well as distant tissues.
* *High mortality rate*: Prognosis is poor with the 5-year cure rate of approximately 25%.

CLINICAL PEARLS

* Surgical staging is an important aspect of treatment in these cases
* Since fallopian tube cancer is so rare, and its symptoms are non-specific and can resemble ovarian or peritoneal cancer, it can be difficult to diagnose
* The prognosis in cases of fallopian cancer is generally regarded as very poor and is usually similar to that of ovarian carcinoma
* It is more common for fallopian tube cancer to arise as a result of metastasis from cancer in other parts of the body, such as the ovaries or peritoneum, rather than for cancer to actually originate in the fallopian tubes as a primary growth.

EVIDENCE-BASED MEDICINE

* *Platinum-based chemotherapy*: Optimal primary treatment of fallopian tube cancer is still not well-defined, and there is little evidence regarding the efficacy of cisplatin-based combination chemotherapy. The CAP regimen comprising of cyclophosphamide (500 mg/m²), adriamycin (50 mg/m²) and cisplatin (50 mg/m²) appears to be active in the treatment of primary fallopian tube carcinoma and yields response rates comparable to those reported for epithelial ovarian cancer [20-25]
* *Second-look laparotomy*: Many retrospective reviews have shown that second-look laparotomy or laparoscopy following cytoreductive surgery and platinum-based combination chemotherapy in patients with fallopian tube cancer provides useful prognostic information in patients with tubal cancer. Nearly 80% of patients who have a negative second-look following platinum-based chemotherapy are likely to remain disease-free.[17,18] Study by Littell et al. (2006) has shown that high rate of recurrent disease following negative second-look laparotomy, and the lack of effective second-line treatment in patients with persistent disease, represent major condemnations of this procedure.[19] On the other hand, Rose et al. (1990) have shown that second-look laparoscopy or laparotomy may be useful if found to be positive.[15] Due to the conflicting results of the studies delineating the role of second-look laparotomy in cases of fallopian tube cancer, there is a requirement of well-designed randomised trials in future. This, however appears to be difficult due to the rarity of this cancer.

REFERENCES

1. Cancer research UK. (2014). Statistics of vaginal cancer. [online] Available from www.cancerresearchuk.org/health-professional/cancer-statistics/statistics-by-cancer-type/vaginal-cancer. [Accessed October, 2016].
2. Wu X, Matanoski G, Chen VW, Saraiya M, Coughlin SS, King JB, et al. Descriptive epidemiology of vaginal cancer incidence and survival by race, ethnicity, and age in the United States. Cancer. 2008;113(10 Suppl):2873-82.
3. Creasman WT. Vaginal cancers. Curr Opin Obstet Gynecol. 2005;17(1):71-6.
4. Tjalma WA, Monaghan JM, de Barros Lopes A, Naik R, Nordin AJ, Weyler JJ. The role of surgery in invasive squamous carcinoma of the vagina. Gynecol Oncol. 2001;81(3):360-5.
5. Chyle V, Zagars GK, Wheeler JA, Wharton JT, Delclos L. Definitive radiotherapy for carcinoma of the vagina: outcome and prognostic factors. Int J Radiat Oncol Biol Phys. 1996;35(5):891-905.
6. Lilic V, Lilic G, Filipovic S, Visnjic M, Zivadinovic R. Primary carcinoma of the vagina. J BUON. 2010;15(2):241-7.
7. Perez CA, Grigsby PW, Garipagaoglu M, Mutch DG, Lockett MA. Factors affecting long-term outcome of irradiation in carcinoma of the vagina. Int J Radiat Oncol Biol Phys. 1999;44(1):37-45.
8. Frank SJ, Jhingran A, Levenback C, Eifel PJ. Definitive radiation therapy for squamous cell carcinoma of the vagina. Int J Radiat Oncol Biol Phys. 2005;62(1):138-47.
9. Johnston GA, Klotz J, Boutselis JG. Primary invasive carcinoma of the vagina. Surg Gynecol Obstet. 1983;156(1):34-40.
10. MacLeod C, Fowler A, Dalrymple C, Atkinson K, Elliott P, Carter J. High-dose-rate brachytherapy in the management of high-grade intraepithelial neoplasia of the vagina. Gynecol Oncol. 1997;65(1):74-7.
11. Diakomanolis E, Stefanidis K, Rodolakis A, Haidopoulos D, Sindos M, Chatzipappas I, et al. Vaginal intraepithelial neoplasia: report of 102 cases. Eur J Gynaecol Oncol. 2002;23(5):457-9.
12. Audet-Lapointe P, Body G, Vauclair R, Drouin P, Ayoub J. Vaginal intraepithelial neoplasia. Gynecol Oncol. 1990;36(2):232-9.
13. Singhal P, Odunsi K, Rodabaugh K, Driscoll D, Lele S. Primary fallopian tube carcinoma: a retrospective clinicopathologic study. Eur J Gynaecol Oncol. 2006;27(1):16-8.
14. Liapis A, Michailidis E, Deligeoroglou E, Kondi-Pafiti A, Konidaris S, Creatsas G. Primary fallopian tube cancer--a ten year review. Clinicopathological study of 12 cases. Eur J Gynaecol Oncol. 2004;25(4):522-4.
15. Rose PG, Piver MS, Tsukada Y. Fallopian tube cancer. The Roswell Park experience. Cancer. 1990;66(12):2661-7.
16. Friedrich M, Villena-Heinsen C, Schweizer J, Holländer M, Stieber M, Schmidt W. Primary tubal carcinoma: a retrospective analysis of four cases with a literature review. Eur J Gynaecol Oncol. 1998;19(2):138-43.
17. Barakat RR, Rubin SC, Saigo PE, Lewis JL, Jones WB, Curtin JP. Second-look laparotomy in carcinoma of the fallopian tube. Obstet Gynecol. 1993;82(5):748-51.
18. Cormio G, Gabriele A, Maneo A, Marzola M, Lissoni A, Mangioni C. Second-look laparotomy in the management of fallopian tube carcinoma. Acta Obstet Gynecol Scand. 1997;76(4):369-72.
19. Littell RD, Hallonquist H, Matulonis U, Seiden MV, Berkowitz RS, Duska LR. Negative laparoscopy is highly predictive of negative second-look laparotomy following chemotherapy for ovarian, tubal, and primary peritoneal carcinoma. Gynecol Oncol. 2006;103(2):570-4.
20. Takeshima N, Hasumi K. Treatment of fallopian tube cancer. Review of the literature. Arch Gynecol Obstet. 2000;264(1):13-9.
21. Morris M, Gershenson DM, Burke TW, Kavanagh JJ, Silva EG, Wharton JT. Treatment of fallopian tube carcinoma with cisplatin, doxorubicin, and cyclophosphamide. Obstet Gynecol. 1990;76(6):1020-4.
22. Cormio G, Maneo A, Gabriele A, Zanetta G, Losa G, Lissoni A. Treatment of fallopian tube carcinoma with cyclophosphamide, adriamycin, and cisplatin. Am J Clin Oncol. 1997;20(2):143-5.
23. Pectasides D, Barbounis V, Sintila A, Varthalitis I, Dimitriadis M, Athanassiou A. Treatment of primary fallopian tube carcinoma with cisplatin-containing chemotherapy. Am J Clin Oncol. 1994;17(1):68-71.
24. Gemignani ML, Hensley ML, Cohen R, Venkatraman E, Saigo PE, Barakat RR. Paclitaxel-based chemotherapy in carcinoma of the fallopian tube. Gynecol Oncol. 2001;80(1):16-20.
25. Pectasides D, Pectasides E, Papaxoinis G, Andreadis C, Papatsibas G, Fountzilas G, et al. Primary fallopian tube carcinoma: results of a retrospective analysis of 64 patients. Gynecol Oncol. 2009;115(1):97-101.

Vulvar Cancer and Vulval Pain Syndromes

VULVAR CANCER

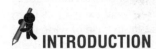

INTRODUCTION

Vulvar cancer, which affects the vulva (region of female external genitalia including various anatomical structures such as labia majora, mons pubis, labia minora, clitoris, vestibule and the vaginal introitus), is the fourth most common gynaecologic cancer, accounting for 3–4% of these cancers in the United States. In the United Kingdom, nearly 800 cases of vulvar cancer are diagnosed every year.[1] Vulvar cancer usually occurs after menopause. The average age at diagnosis is 70 years. Vulvar cancer can, however, also occur in a proportion of younger women (under 50 years of age). Therefore, the clinician must always keep the diagnosis of vulvar cancer in mind even when a younger patient presents with a vulvar lesion. The most common histological subtype of vulvar cancer is squamous cell cancer.[2] Melanoma of vaginal cancer is the second most common type of malignancy arising from the vulva.

Microinvasive carcinoma of vulva can be described as lesions less than or equal to 2 cm with less than 1 mm of stromal invasion.[3] When the degree of stromal invasion is greater than 1 mm, there is a high probability of lymph node metastasis. In 50% of cases, presentation is in the form of a lump or a mass along with a long-standing history of pruritus, which may be related to vulvar dystrophy. In 60% of the cases, the lesion is in labia majora; 20% of the cases in labia minora; 12% cases in the clitoris; and 6% cases in the perineum. The vulvar cancer can spread by direct extension to the adjacent structures, such as vagina, urethra and anus, by lymphatic route to adjacent lymph nodes and via haematogenous route to distant organs such as lungs, liver and bone. Lymphatic metastasis occurs early in the disease and most commonly occurs to the inguinal group of lymph nodes. From here, the spread can occur to the femoral group

of lymph nodes. Depending on the extent and type of the cancer, vulvectomy is performed. Lymphadenectomy may be also done depending upon the involvement of lymph nodes. For early stage cancers, such treatment is usually all that is required. However, for more advanced cancers, radiation therapy, along with cisplatin is usually required. After the removal of the cancerous tissues, surgical reconstruction of the vulva and vagina may be performed.

AETIOLOGY

Vulvar cancer can be of two types based on the predisposing factors. The first type may develop from vulvar intraepithelial neoplasia (VIN) caused by HPV infection. Observational studies have reported a wide variation in the rate of malignant potential of VIN.[4,5] This type of vulvar cancer has been increasing in prevalence amongst young women.

The second type, which more often occurs in older women, is not related to HPV infection. This type may develop from vulvar non-neoplastic epithelial disorders as a result of chronic inflammation (e.g. lichen sclerosus). Aetiopathology of vulvar cancer can be attributed to the following factors:

* *Precancerous dysplastic changes*: The risk factors for developing vulvar cancer include presence of precancerous or dysplastic changes, e.g. lichen sclerosus, VIN, etc. in the vulvar tissues. VIN3 is a potentially preinvasive condition. However, the risk of progression to malignancy remains unknown. Lichen sclerosus, also known as lichen sclerosus et atrophicus, is a vulval inflammatory dermatosis associated with an increased risk of progression to malignancy. Though the exact risk of malignant transformation remains unknown, it is estimated that approximately 4 out of every 100 women with lichen sclerosus may develop this malignancy.
* *Infection with human papilloma virus*: An association of vulvar cancer with HPV infection has been found in approximately 30% cases of vulvar malignancy.

❖ *Molecular biology event*: Variations in the cell cycle regulatory protein, p53 has been thought to be the cause of malignancy in approximately 30% cases.

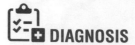

DIAGNOSIS

Diagnosis of vulvar cancer is established on the basis of the findings described next in details.[6]

Clinical Presentation

❖ *Symptoms*: In 50% of cases, presentation is in the form of a lump or a mass along with a long-standing history of pruritus and vulvar soreness, which may be related to vulvar dystrophy. Sometimes, there may be presence of a friable mass which may be painful and bleeds on touch.
❖ *General physical examination*: A complete general physical examination must be performed including the palpation of inguinal lymph nodes for the presence of lymphadenopathy.
❖ *Per speculum examination*: There may be a lesion in labia majora, labia minora, clitoris, perineum, vagina, urethra, anus, etc.
❖ *Pelvic examination*: This may help to detect abnormalities in the cervix, uterus and adnexa.

Investigations

❖ *Biopsy of the abnormal area over the vulva*: A full thickness biopsy should be preferably taken from the area of abnormality, including the interface between the area of abnormality and the apparently normal surrounding skin.
❖ Pap smear to be obtained from the cervix because a cervical carcinoma may coexist with a vulvar malignancy.
❖ Colposcopic examination of the cervix and vagina.
❖ Wedge biopsy of the lesions is commonly performed. In case the lesion is less than 1 cm in diameter, an excisional biopsy may be performed.
❖ *CT or MRI scan*: CT scan and/or MRI examination helps in ruling out the presence of any obvious pelvic lymphadenopathy.

DIFFERENTIAL DIAGNOSIS

❖ Paget's disease of the vulva
❖ Vulvar intraepithelial neoplasia
❖ Non-neoplastic vulvar lesions such as lichen sclerosis, squamous cell hyperplasia and vulvar vestibulitis
❖ Infectious lesions (e.g. herpes simplex virus, HPV, syphilis, etc.).

MANAGEMENT

Treatment in cases of vulvar carcinoma needs to be individualised on the basis of extent of tumour spread and lymph node involvement. Such cases should preferably be managed by a specialised gynaecological oncologist. All the cases of vulvar cancer must be discussed at the local specialist gynaecological oncology multidisciplinary meeting.

Staging of Vulvar Cancer

The International Federation of Gynecology and Obstetrics (FIGO) staging of vulvar cancers is described in Table 88.1. Staging involves resection of the primary tumour(s) and inguinofemoral lymphadenectomy.

SURGICAL TREATMENT OF VULVAR CANCER

Surgical procedures for the treatment of vulvar cancer include wide local excision, simple partial vulvectomy, radical partial vulvectomy, en block radical vulvectomy and radical complete vulvectomy (Figs 88.1A to C).[8-14] Of the various surgical procedures used, the en block dissection, which was commonly used previously, has now largely been abandoned. In current practice, radical local excision is preferred over radical vulvectomy. This approach conserves vulvar anatomy and encourages wound healing. Wide local excision is used for microinvasive tumours of the vulva. In case of wide local excision, 1–2 cm surgical margins are obtained around the lesion. This ensures the attainment of pathological disease free margin of approximately 8 mm due to the shrinkage of tissues as a result of pathological fixation. This is associated with a zero rate of local recurrence.

With radical partial vulvectomy, tumour containing portions of vulva are completely removed. Skin margins of

Table 88.1: Staging of vulvar cancer[7]

Stage	Description
I	Tumour confined to the vulva
IA	Tumour ≤2 cm in size, confined to the vulva or perineum and with stromal invasion ≤1.0 mm and no nodal metastasis
IB	Lesions >2 cm in size with stromal invasion >1.0 mm confined to the vulva or perineum with negative nodes
II	Tumour of any size with extension to the adjacent perineal structures (one-third lower urethra, one-third lower vagina, anus) with negative nodes
III	Tumour of any size with extension to the adjacent perineal structures (one-third lower urethra, one-third lower vagina, anus) with positive inguinofemoral lymph nodes
IIIA	Either with 1 lymph node metastasis ≥5 mm or 1–2 lymph node metastasis(es) (<5 mm)
IIIB	With 2 or more lymph node metastasis (≥5 mm) or 3 or more lymph node metastasis (<5 mm)
IIIC	Having positive nodes with extracapsular spread
IV	Tumour invades other regional (two-thirds upper urethra, two-thirds upper vagina) or distant structures
IVA	Tumour invades any of the following: Upper urethral and/or vaginal mucosa, bladder mucosa, rectal mucosa or the tumour is fixed to the pelvic bone or there are fixed or ulcerated inguinofemoral lymph nodes
IVB	Any distant metastasis including pelvic lymphadenopathy

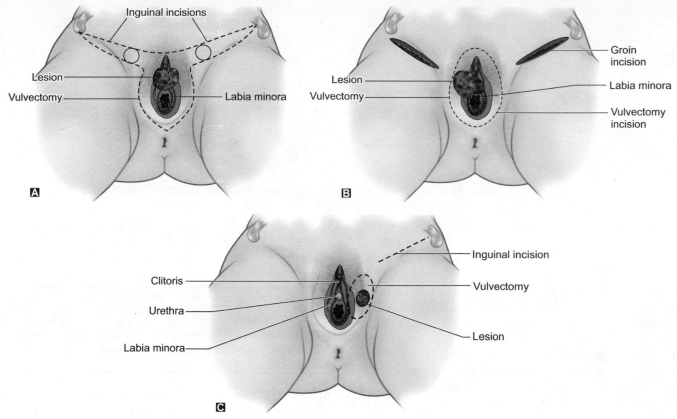

Figs 88.1A to C: Different types of surgical approaches: (A) Single butterfly incision for en bloc radical vulvectomy and groin dissection; (B) Three separate skin incisions for radical complete vulvectomy and groin dissection; (C) Two separate skin incisions for radical partial vulvectomy with ipsilateral inguinofemoral lymphadenectomy

1–2 cm are usually obtained and the excision extends deep till the perineal membrane. In radical complete vulvectomy, 1–2 cm margins are obtained around a large vulvar tumour and the dissection is completed down till the perineal membrane. Vulvar defects created as a result of surgery can be closed with the help of skin grafts, advancement flaps or rotational flaps. The procedure of radical partial or radical complete vulvectomy is often accompanied by lymphadenectomy. This dissection usually involves the excision of both superficial inguinal and deep femoral nodes in order to maximise the detection of metastatic disease. Previously, all patients diagnosed with vulvar cancer were staged and treated with an en bloc radical vulvectomy and bilateral inguinofemoral lymphadenectomy through a butterfly incision. This procedure has nowadays, largely, become obsolete because it is associated with high rates of morbidity, such as poor wound healing, lymphoedema, adverse effects on body image and sexual dysfunction. Both the techniques of radical partial vulvectomy and radical complete vulvectomy, which are commonly used nowadays, employ two or three separate incisions. The first incision is made to perform a radical local excision (a radical partial vulvectomy, radical hemivulvectomy, or modified radical vulvectomy) and involves resection of the primary tumour with 1 cm clinical margins laterally and a dissection down to the perineal membrane (deep fascia of the urogenital diaphragm). The excision can be unilateral in most cases. The other (and separate) incisions are for the inguinofemoral

lymphadenectomy, which may be unilateral or bilateral depending on the primary vulvar tumour. This approach helps in keeping the intervening skin bridge intact, which aids in conserving vulvar anatomy and speeding up wound healing. This is also likely to reduce the morbidity rates without compromising survival.[10]

Microinvasive or Superficially Invasive Vulvar Cancer

In these cases, the depth of tumour invasion is up to 1 mm and the risk of nodal involvement is virtually zero. These tumours are treated with wide local excision.

Stage IA

In these cases, the risk of inguinal metastasis is negligible. Lymphadenectomy is not indicated for these patients with a low risk for lymph node metastasis. Depth of tumour invasion is the best predictor for the risk of nodal involvement. Cases where the depth of tumour invasion is more than 1 mm are associated with a high risk of lymph nodal involvement.

Stage IB to Stage II

These patients require radical resection of the primary tumour and assessment of the inguinofemoral lymph nodes. A more conservative approach at the time of surgery is favoured. Stage IB lesions can be managed with radical partial vulvectomy. An inguinofemoral lymphadenectomy

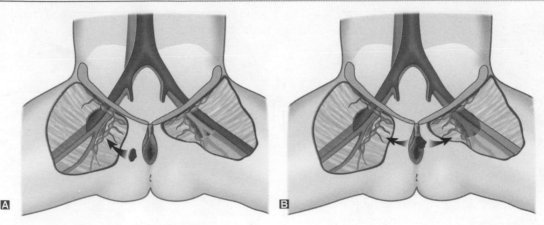

Figs 88.2A and B: Lymphatic spread of the vulvar lesions: (A) Lateral vulvar lesions spread to the ipsilateral group of lymph nodes; (B) Midline vulvar lesions can spread to the lymph nodes of both the groins

(which may be either unilateral or bilateral depending on the location of the valvular lesions) may be required. Most ipsilateral vulvar lesions defined as lesions located 1–2 cm of the midline can be managed with an ipsilateral inguino-femoral lymphadenectomy. Midline lesions located within 1–2 cm of the midline require bilateral inguinofemoral lymphadenectomy.[15] Lesions greater than 2 cm or those having extension to the lower perineal structures are best managed with a radical partial excision. This includes anterior hemivulvectomy with distal urethrectomy and bilateral inguinofemoral lymphadenectomy.

Lateral Vulval Tumours

Lateral vulval tumours can be defined as those in which the medial border lays at least 2 cm lateral to the midline (a line between clitoris and anus). Lateral vulvar lesions spread initially to the ipsilateral superficial inguinal lymph nodes, whereas midline lesions can spread to both groins (Figs 88.2A and B). Therefore, in the lateral tumours, initially only an ipsilateral lymph node dissection is done. If ipsilateral lymph nodes are negative, involvement of contralateral lymph nodes is rare. However, in case the ipsilateral lymph nodes are involved, dissection of contralateral lymph nodes must be undertaken.

Inguinofemoral Lymphadenectomy

Inguinofemoral lymphadenectomy is the standard approach for evaluation of the lymph nodes in women with vulvar cancer. Metastasis to the lymph nodes can be considered as an important prognostic factor in case of vulvar cancers because inguinofemoral lymphadenectomy is associated with high morbidity rates. Therefore, assessment for lymph node is especially essential for staging. Superficial inguinal lymph nodes are assessed by dissecting below the inguinal ligament along the fascia lata to reach the fossa ovalis. Superficial inguinal lymph node dissection, which removes lymph nodes only above the cribriform fascia, is likely to be associated with a higher rate of recurrence in comparison with inguinofemoral dissection which also removes tissues below

Box 88.1: Criteria for unilateral lymphadenectomy
❑ Primary lesion <2 cm
❑ Lesion is lateral in location (>2 cm from the vulvar midline)
❑ There are no palpable groin nodes on examination
❑ Squamous histology

the cribriform fascia. An inguinofemoral lymphadenectomy should, therefore, consist of removal of both the inguinal (superficial) and femoral (deep) lymph nodes.

Wherever possible, unilateral rather than bilateral lympha-denectomy must be performed, because it is associated with reduced postoperative morbidity. Unilateral lymphadenectomy can be performed for women with disease that meets the criteria enlisted in Box 88.1.

When unilateral lymphadenectomy is performed, the nodes should be sent for intraoperative frozen pathology evaluation. In case the lymph nodes are found to be positive for cancer, contralateral lymphadenectomy should be performed. Adjuvant radiotherapy can be performed in cases where further surgery may not appear as a feasible option.

As previously mentioned, inguinofemoral lymph node dissection for vulvar cancer is associated with a high rate of morbidity. Primary radiotherapy to the groin, on the other hand, is likely to result in lower morbidity. However, the available evidence related to the efficacy of primary radiotherapy to the groin has shown conflicting results in terms of groin recurrences and survival. In a study by Gynecologic Oncology Group (GOG), 58 patients with squamous carcinoma of the vulva and non-suspicious (N0-1) inguinal nodes were randomised to receive either groin dissection or groin radiation, each in combination with radical vulvectomy. The study was closed prematurely when the results of short-term monitoring revealed an excessive number of groin relapses in the group of patients receiving groin radiation regimen. Groin radiation was found to be significantly inferior to groin dissection in patients with squamous carcinoma of the vulva having negative nodes.[16] A Cochrane review by Van der Velden has shown that primary radiotherapy to the groin results in lower morbidity but may be associated with a higher risk of groin recurrence and reduced survival in comparison to surgery.[17] However, the studies included in this review comprised of a small number of patients and there were criticisms regarding the depth of radiotherapy applied. Therefore, these findings need to be validated by larger RCTs in future using a standardised method of radiotherapy. However, until better evidence is available, surgery should be considered as the treatment of choice for the groin nodes in women with vulvar cancer. Individual patients, who are not physically able to withstand surgery, may be treated with primary radiotherapy.

An important development in the treatment of vulvar cancer is that the selective dissection of a solitary node or nodes (termed as sentinel node biopsy) can help in reducing surgical morbidity and at the same time accurately assessing the nodal involvement. The basic principle of this approach is that the first lymph node to receive lymphatic drainage from the tumour site is sentinel lymph node.[18] Therefore, this is likely to be the first site of malignant lymphatic spread. If a sentinel lymph node is devoid of malignancy, it implies the absence of lymph node metastasis. Radionuclide scanning is usually done to identify the sentinel lymph node. This involves injection of a marking dye or radioactive substance, injected by a tumoural or peritumoural injection, through the afferent lymphatic vessels draining the primary tumour to the sentinel lymph node. This technique has led to a shift in practice towards unilateral lymphadenectomy, whenever possible. The GROningen INternational Study on Sentinel nodes in Vulvar cancer (GROINSS-V) is a recently published prospective non-blinded observational study by Van der Zee et al. to investigate the safety and clinical utility of the sentinel node procedure in early-stage vulvar cancer patients. The results of this study have shown that negative sentinel node in early-stage vulvar cancer patients is associated with a low rate of recurrence, excellent survival rates and minimal treatment-related morbidity. It is recommended that sentinel node dissection, performed by a quality-controlled multidisciplinary team, should be included as part of the standard treatment in selected patients with early-stage vulvar cancer.[19] Sentinel lymph node biopsy is presently an active area of investigation and is nowadays being increasingly utilised. Currently, the GOG 270 study has joined the GROINSS VII study, addressing the management of women with positive sentinel nodes, i.e. whether they should be managed by a full groin dissection or radiation therapy.[20]

Stage III Vulvar Cancer

Such patients include those with node positive cancer. Patients with resectable primary vulvar cancer, which is metastatic to the lymph nodes benefits from postoperative pelvic and groin irradiation. Radiotherapy is typically begun 3–4 weeks after the surgery to allow adequate wound healing. Some clinicians prefer adding platinum-based chemotherapy to radiation therapy. However, if nodes are fixed to the femoral vessels or other vital structures, resection of the primary tumour and inguinofemoral lymphadenectomy may not be possible. Furthermore, surgery may not be possible in presence of other comorbidities or medical ill-health. In these situations,

primary radiation therapy is preferred. In case the patients are candidates for chemotherapy, chemoradiation is preferred over primary radiation therapy.

Stage IVA Vulvar Cancer

These locally advanced vulvar cancers may involve the upper urethra, bladder, or rectal mucosa or pubic bone and may or may not have associated positive inguinal lymph node or fixed ulcerated lymph nodes. Occasionally, such patients can be treated with radical primary surgery. However, more often due to size and location of the tumour, some form of exenterative surgical procedure may be required to remove the entire lesion with adequate margins. Such unresectable, locally advanced vulvar cancers can be treated with chemoradiation.[21] Preoperative cisplatin-based chemoradiation may be required in the following cases:

❖ Extensive primary lesion that may require pelvic exenteration

❖ *Inoperable primary tumours*: In cases where the patient does not have fixed groin nodes, pretreatment inguino-femoral lymphadenectomy may help determine the requirement for groin irradiation. The surgical approach chosen depends upon the size and extent of the lesion and has been summarised in Table 88.2.

Treatment of Positive or Narrow Margins

For patients with tumour at or close to the surgical margins (≤8 mm) identified at final pathologic analysis, re-excision must be performed. For those patients who do not want to undergo repeat surgery, radiation therapy may serve as a reasonable alternative.

Table 88.2: Summary of treatment for vulvar cancer

Tumour stage	Extent of spread	Treatment
T1 lesions	No extension to adjacent perineal structures, i.e. lower/distal one-third urethra, lower/distal one-third vagina, anus	Radical local excision
T2 lesions	Extension to adjacent perineal structures	Modified radical vulvectomy (e.g. modified radical hemivulvectomy, modified radical anterior vulvectomy, modified radical posterior vulvectomy)
T3 lesions	Extension to any of the following: Upper/proximal two-thirds of urethra, upper/proximal two-thirds vagina, bladder mucosa, rectal mucosa, or tumour is fixed to pelvic bone	Most of these patients are treated with chemo-radiation followed by a selective procedure that is individualised to the patient on the basis of size and location of the residual tumour. In selected patients where chemoradiation is unsuccessful, exenteration with colostomy or urethral diversion appears to be a feasible option

Involved Groin Nodes on Examination

Patients presenting with suspicious or bulky groin nodes, who are candidates for surgery can be considered for nodal debulking followed by chemoradiation.

Radiation Therapy

Patients who are not candidates for any form of surgical excision (e.g. due to medical frailty or comorbidities) should receive primary radiation therapy (total dose of radiation should be between 60 Gy and 70 Gy).

Adjuvant Radiation Therapy

Adjuvant radiation therapy is performed in the following high-risk cases:

❖ Tumour size more than 4 cm
❖ Evidence of lymphovascular invasion
❖ Close or positive surgical margins
❖ Pathologic involvement of lymph nodes.

Primary Chemoradiation

For patients who are candidates for chemotherapy, some experts prefer to administer chemoradiation in patients with vulvar cancer who have tumours that might not be technically resectable without being at significant risk for postoperative morbidity. Surgical excision of the primary site is not necessary in patients with complete response. The bilateral inguinofemoral lymph nodes may be included within the treatment target volume for these patients.

Patients who are not candidates for surgery and are deemed not to be candidates for chemotherapy should receive primary radiation therapy or chemoradiation. Appropriate candidates for chemoradiation include patients with the following:

❖ Anorectal, urethral or bladder involvement (in an effort to avoid colostomy and urostomy)
❖ Disease that is fixed to the bone
❖ Gross inguinal or femoral node involvement (regardless of whether a debulking lymphadenectomy was previously performed).

Use of chemoradiation is associated with higher survival benefits in comparison to the use of radiotherapy alone. Use of single-agent cisplatin with radiotherapy is usually preferred. Concurrent use of fluorouracil (5-FU) alone or in combination with cisplatin or mitomycin-C is also being considered.

Post-treatment Surveillance

The optimal surveillance strategy has not been established. However, some commonly used recommendations are as follows:

❖ Serial review of symptoms and physical examination of the vulva, skin bridge and inguinal nodes.
❖ For early stage disease, this should be done every 6 months for the first 2 years and then annually.
❖ For advanced stage disease, this should be done every 3 months for the first 2 years, then every 6 months for years 3 through 5, and then annually.

❖ Cervical cytology (or vaginal cytology, if the cervix has been removed) annually.

For patients with locally advanced vulvar cancer who undergo surgery and have evidence of high-risk features (i.e. two or more microscopically positive groin lymph nodes, one or more macroscopically involved lymph nodes, or any evidence of extracapsular spread) on follow-up, some experts recommend the use of adjuvant radiation therapy. However, other experts prefer to treat these patients with chemoradiation.

 COMPLICATIONS

❖ Metastasis to distant organs such as lungs, liver, pelvic bones, etc.
❖ Complications related to surgery such as wound infection, sexual dysfunction, venous thromboembolism, etc.
❖ *Complications related to radical vulvectomy and bilateral inguinal lymphadenectomy*: Some specific complications related to such surgery are as follows:
  • *Immediate postoperative morbidity*: In case of groin dissection, the most important cause of immediate postoperative morbidity is wound infection, necrosis and breakdown. This can be considerably reduced by adopting a separate incision approach.
  • *Wound breakdown*: This occurs due to the skin loss at the margins of the groin incision. This complication can be reduced by removing lesser amounts of skin and reducing the undermining of the skin flaps. Suction drainage also helps in reducing the morbidity.
  • *Lymphoedema of the lower extremities*: This may occur in patients who have undergone dissection of inguinal and deep pelvic group of lymph nodes.
  • *Late complications*: Late complications can occur in the form of chronic leg oedema, recurrent lymphangitis or cellulitis of the leg. Introital stenosis in the long run can result in dyspareunia.

 CLINICAL PEARLS

❖ In cases of vulvar cancer, the most common site of involvement is the labia majora.
❖ Investigation of cases with post-menopausal bleeding should also include examination of vulva because sometimes vulvar cancer can present as friable masses which bleed upon touch.
❖ Presently, the treatment of choice in cases of invasive vulvar cancer is radical wide excision and selective inguinal lymphadenectomy based on its stage and location, which has now replaced the previously performed surgery, en bloc radical vulvectomy with bilateral inguinofemoral lymphadenectomy. Cases of vulvar cancer should be preferably managed in a cancer centre.
❖ Lymphadenectomy is usually required in all the cases except in superficially invasive squamous cancers. Inguinal-femoral lymphadenectomy remains the procedure of

choice. On the other hand, pelvic lymphadenectomy is not required for cases of vulvar cancer.

❖ At the time of inguinofemoral lymphadenectomy, in cases of vulvar cancer, sparing the long saphenous vein helps in reducing the morbidity related to lymphoedema.

EVIDENCE-BASED MEDICINE

❖ Since vulvar cancer is a relatively uncommon malignancy, good quality evidence in the form of randomised trials is unavailable. Most of the evidence available at present is in the form of observational studies and case series. Variations in the observational studies have reported that the malignant potential of VIN to vary between 5% to 80%.[4,5]

❖ The present evidence indicates that surgical dissection of inguinal lymph nodes rather than radiotherapy is essential in cases of early stage vulvar cancer where the depth of tumour invasion is greater than 1 mm.[16,17]

VULVAR PAIN SYNDROME

INTRODUCTION

Vulvodynia or vulvar pain syndrome has been defined by the International Society for the Study of Vulvovaginal Diseases (ISSVD) as 'vulvar discomfort, most often described as burning pain, occurring in the absence of relevant visible findings or a specific, clinically identifiable, neurologic disorder'.[22] Before making the diagnosis of vulvodynia, other causes of vulval pain such as infections, vulval dermatoses, etc. must be excluded.

Depending on the anatomical site of pain, ISSVD has categorised vulvodynia as generalised or localised (e.g. generalised vulvodynia, hemivulvodynia, clitorodynia, etc.), and on the basis of triggering factor as provoked, unprovoked or a combination of the two. ISSVD classification of vulval pain is described in Table 88.3.[23,24]

Table 88.3: International Society for the Study of Vulvovaginal Diseases classification of vulval pain[23,24]

Pain related to a specific cause	Pain not related to a specific cause (vulvodynia)

• Infections (e.g. candidiasis, herpes, etc.)
 • Inflammation (e.g. lichen planus, lichen sclerosus, immunobullous disorders, etc.)
 • Neoplastic disorders (e.g. Paget's disease, squamous cell carcinoma, etc.)
 • Neurological disorders (e.g. herpes neuralgia, spinal nerve compression, etc.)
	• Generalised
	   – Provoked (sexual/non-sexual)
	   – Unprovoked
	   – Mixed
	 • Localised
	   – Provoked (vestibulodynia)
	   – Unprovoked
	   – Mixed

Flow chart 88.1: Aetiology of vulvodynia

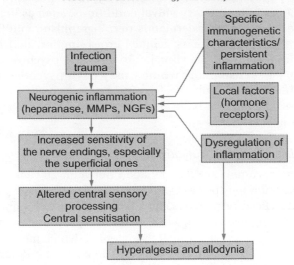

Abbreviations: MMP, matrix metalloproteinases; NGF, nerve growth factor

AETIOLOGY

Clinical pain in vulvodynia can be either inflammatory or neuropathic in origin (Flow chart 88.1). Inflammatory pain is associated with tissue damage and injury, whereas neuropathic pain is caused by damage to either the central or peripheral nervous system. Inflammatory pain is clinically characterised by sensory hypersensitivity which may be associated with hyperalgesia (exaggerated response to noxious substances and allodynia (altered pain sensation). Neuropathic pain, on the other hand, may or may not be associated with hyperalgesia and allodynia.

Localised Provoked Vulvodynia

Localised provoked vulvodynia, also known as vestibulodynia, was formerly known as vulvar vestibulitis syndrome. Aetiology of localised provoked vulvodynia is likely to be multifactorial. A recurrent history of vulvovaginal candidiasis is the most commonly reported feature.[25]

Unprovoked Vulvodynia

Unprovoked vulvodynia is also known as dysesthetic vulvodynia; the aetiology of unprovoked vulvodynia remains unknown and the condition is best managed as a chronic pain syndrome.

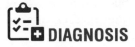

DIAGNOSIS

Clinical diagnosis of vulvodynia is made on history and examination.

Clinical Presentation

An accurate history needs to be elicited and clinical examination needs to be performed in order to differentiate between various subtypes of vulvodynia and for excluding other vaginal conditions which may be responsible for pain (e.g. inflammatory vulval conditions, such as lichen sclerosis, seborrhoeic dermatitis, dermographism, aphthous ulceration, lichen planus, genital herpes simplex, etc.). It is also important for the clinician to elicit the psychosexual history because many women may have psychosexual dysfunction and require referral to psychosexual services. In case the diagnosis is not clear, the patient must be referred to a vulval service or clinic.

Localised Provoked Vulvodynia

Affected women are usually aged between 20 years and 40 years and may present with the history of provoked pain, e.g. superficial dyspareunia, intolerance to the use of tampons, pain during gynaecological examination, etc. Sometimes, there may be severe introital dyspareunia, which may make sexual intercourse impossible for the couple. A delay of 6 months following the onset of symptoms is considered prior to making the diagnosis of vestibulodynia.

Symptoms: Vestibulodynia is characterised by vestibular tenderness upon light touch. This hyperaesthesia can be generalised throughout the vestibule or can sometimes be more localised. The patient may experience itching or the sensation of dryness. There may be elevated tone of the muscles of pelvic floor or vaginismus.

Signs: Focal tenderness may be elicited by gentle applying a cotton wool tip bud or a Q-tip applicator at the introitus or around the clitoris. There are usually no signs of an acute inflammatory process. Mild erythema may sometimes be present.

Unprovoked Vulvodynia

Symptoms: There may be long-standing pain, the cause of which remains unexplained. The pain may be associated with urinary symptoms such as interstitial cystitis.[26] The pain may also be associated with rectal, perineal and/or urethral discomfort because there may be an overlap with other perineal pain syndromes. Superficial dyspareunia is not frequently reported in these cases because many women may be sexually inactive.

Signs: The vulva usually appears normal at the time of examination.

Investigations

Clinical diagnosis of vulvodynia is established on the basis of history and examination following various investigations to exclude the other treatable causes of vulval pain.

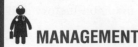

MANAGEMENT

❖ *Multidisciplinary approach*: A multidisciplinary approach to patient care, comprising a gynaecologist, dermatologist, physiotherapist, sexual therapist or counsellor, and a gynaecologic surgeon in cases of vulvodynia is recommended by the British Society for the Study of Vulval Disease (BSSVD).[27,28]

❖ *Pain management*: One of the main aims of management in these cases is to reduce vulval or vestibular tenderness. Patient may be referred to a pain clinic in cases of treatment-resistant unprovoked vulvodynia.

❖ *Psychosexual counselling*: Referral to psychosexual clinic may be required if the patient needs psychosexual counselling.

❖ *General measures*: The patient must be reassured and adequately counselled regarding the condition. Written information in form of leaflets should be preferably provided to the patient. The patient should be counselled to maintain strict vulval hygiene.

Localised Provoked Vulvodynia

❖ *Topical agents*: The patient should be counselled to avoid contact with all kinds of irritating factors in order to reduce chances of contact sensitivity. The patient should be advised to use emollient soap substitute. Topical local anaesthetics, e.g. 5% lidocaine ointment or 2% lidocaine gel should be cautiously used because they can cause irritation. This gel should be applied 15–20 minutes prior to penetrative sex and it must be washed off just prior to sex. Alternatively, a condom can be used by the partner to reduce the risk of transfer of lidocaine gel, resulting in penile numbness. In absence of the availability of good quality evidence regarding the efficacy of a particular treatment modality for vulvodynia, lidocaine gel along with the use of vaginal dilators act as the first-line treatment modality in cases of vulvodynia.[29] Other topical agents which are commonly used include steroid and antifungal creams. However, their use has been found to be associated with variable results.

❖ *Physical therapies*: This includes therapies such as pelvic floor muscle biofeedback, vaginal transcutaneous electrical nerve stimulation (TENS), vaginal trainers, etc.[30-32]

❖ *Psychological counselling*: This can involve the use of cognitive behaviour therapy. Counselling sessions by a clinical psychologist can help the patient cope up with pain.[33]

❖ *Pain modifiers*: Benefit of drugs such as tricyclic anti-depressants, gabapentin and pregabalin in cases of vulvodynia presently remains unclear. Their use may be beneficial in some women.

❖ *Surgery*: Modified vestibulectomy may be considered as a last resort in cases where other treatment measures have proved to be unsuccessful.[34,35] This surgery involves excision of a horseshoe-shaped area of vestibule and inner fold of labia followed by the dissection of posterior vaginal wall (Fig. 88.3). Women who respond to the application of lidocaine gel prior to sexual activity are likely to have a more successful outcome with this surgery. Postoperative psychosexual counselling is likely to further improve the outcomes of this surgery.

❖ *Biofeedback therapy*: Biofeedback therapy using surface electromyographic signals from the pelvic floor is likely to help women with vestibulodynia, probably by overcoming

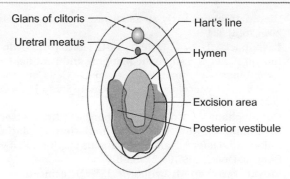

Fig. 88.3: Modified posterior vestibulectomy

Labels: Glans of clitoris — Uretral meatus — Hart's line — Hymen — Excision area — Posterior vestibule

the dysfunction of the muscles of pelvic floor. Use of both computerised electromyographic as well as portable electromyographic biofeedback therapy is likely to cause a significant improvement in pelvic floor dysfunction as well as contractility of the muscles of pelvic floor.[36] However, the machine for delivering this biofeedback therapy is not routinely available in the UK and therefore an adequate experience regarding its use is lacking. An RCT by Bergeron et al. (2001) comprising of 78 subjects compared three different treatment modalities: (1) 12 weeks trial of group cognitive-behavioural therapy, (2) 12 weeks trial of surface electromyographic biofeedback and (3) vestibulectomy for the treatment of vulvar vestibulitis.[37] All the three treatment modalities showed statistically significant reductions in the pain scores, measures of psychological adjustment and sexual function, post-treatment and at the time of 6-month follow-up visit. Also the group undergoing vestibulectomy was found to be significantly more successful in terms of reduction in pain scores in comparison to the two other groups. However, the deceptive superiority of vestibulectomy needs to be carefully inferred with because seven women who had been assigned to vestibulectomy did not go ahead with the surgery. Findings suggest that women with dyspareunia can benefit from both surgical and behavioural interventions. However, patients are likely to prefer a behavioural approach rather than a surgical one.

Unprovoked Vulvodynia

❖ *Topical agents*: Various topical agents such as emollient soap substitute, topical local anaesthetic agents, etc. have been tried in cases of unprovoked vulvodynia without much evidence of benefit.

❖ *Pain modifiers*: Tricyclic antidepressants have proved to be useful in the management of chronic pain related to unprovoked vulvodynia. Amitriptyline is frequently considered as the first-line treatment. Dosage should be increased by small increments starting at 10 mg up to 100 mg daily, based on the patient's response.[38] However, the beneficial effect of amitriptyline has not been demonstrated by a recent randomised study.[39] If the patient appears to be unresponsive to amitriptyline or is unable to tolerate its side effects, gabapentin or pregabalin may be used.[40-43]

❖ Cognitive behavioural therapy and psychotherapy[44]

❖ Acupuncture[45]

❖ *Surgery*: Surgery is usually contraindicated in the cases of unprovoked vulvodynia.

Follow-up

Patients with vulvodynia must be followed up on the basis of their clinical requirements. Long-term follow-up and psychological support may be required in the future.

COMPLICATIONS

Vulvodynia can be associated with the following complications:

❖ *Sexual dysfunction*: There may be sexual dysfunction problems such as reduced sexual arousal, negative sexual feelings, reduced spontaneous interest in sex, etc.

❖ *Psychosexual dysfunction*: There may be psychosexual problems such as vaginismus, anorgasmia, etc.

❖ *Psychological morbidity*: Since vulvodynia is a chronic disease, such patients are likely to experience increased psychological problems, e.g. anxiety, depression, etc.

❖ *Reduced quality of life*: There may be reduced quality of life as a result of psychological disability, severe preoccupation with the pain and limitation of daily activities.

CLINICAL PEARLS

❖ Non-tenderness of the labial skin is a defining feature of vestibulodynia

❖ The diagnosis of vulvodynia is one of exclusion

❖ Long-term use of topical agents such as steroids and antifungal creams in cases of vulvodynia should be avoided because of the risk of development of irritant dermatitis

❖ If the patient does not respond to the various management options, she must be referred to the local vulval services

❖ Of the various therapies that have been recommended for use in cases of vestibulodynia, none has proven successful

❖ Amitriptyline and gabapentin are treatment of choice in cases of unprovoked vulvodynia. On the other hand, surgery is usually contraindicated in these cases. Surgery may, however, be suitable in well-selected cases of vestibulodynia.

EVIDENCE-BASED MEDICINE

❖ Presently, good quality evidence regarding the effective mode of treatment in cases of vulvodynia is missing. Most of the presently available studies are methodologically flawed or are of low quality. Though many agents are commonly used, evidence supporting a specific application is lacking.[29]

❖ Recent evidence has indicated that the novel anticonvulsant agent gabapentin may prove to be useful in the treatment of cases of unprovoked generalised vulvodynia probably due to the fact that it represents an unexplained neuropathic process.[40-43] It is also associated with a low side effects profile.

REFERENCES

1. Judson PL, Habermann EB, Baxter NN, Durham SB, Virnig BA. Trends in the incidence of invasive and in situ vulvar carcinoma. Obstet Gynecol. 2006;107(5):1018-22.

2. Carter JS, Downs LS. Vulvar and vaginal cancer. Obstet Gynecol Clin North Am. 2012;39(2):213-31.

3. Ghurani GB, Penalver MA. An update on vulvar cancer. Am J Obstet Gynecol. 2001;185(2):294-9.

4. Jones RW, Rowan DM, Stewart AW. Vulvar intraepithelial neoplasia: aspects of the natural history and outcome in 405 women. Obstet Gynecol. 2005;106(6):1319-26.

5. van Seters M, van Beurden M, de Craen AJ. Is the assumed natural history of vulvar intraepithelial neoplasia III based on enough evidence? A systematic review of 3322 published patients. Gynecol Oncol. 2005;97(2):645-51.

6. Alkatout I, Schubert M, Garbrecht N, Weigel MT, Jonat W, Mundhenke C, et al . Vulvar cancer: epidemiology, clinical presentation, and management options. Int J Womens Health. 2015;7:305-13.

7. Pecorelli S. Revised FIGO staging for carcinoma of the vulva, cervix, and endometrium. Int J Gynaecol Obstet. 2009;105(2):103-4.

8. DiSaia PJ, Creasman WT, Rich WM. An alternate approach to early cancer of the vulva. Am J Obstet Gynecol. 1979;133(7): 825-32.

9. Stehman FB, Look KY. Carcinoma of the vulva. Obstet Gynecol. 2006;107(3):719-33.

10. Rouzier R, Haddad B, Atallah D, Dubois P, Paniel BJ. Surgery for vulvar cancer. Clin Obstet Gynecol. 2005;48(4):869-78.

11. De Hullu JA, Hollema H, Lolkema S, Boezen M, Boonstra H, Burger MP, et al . Vulvar carcinoma. The price of less radical surgery. Cancer. 2002;95(11):2331-8.

12. Ansink A, van der Velden J. Surgical interventions for early squamous cell carcinoma of the vulva. Cochrane Database Syst Rev. 2000;(2):CD002036.

13. Fuh KC, Berek JS. Current management of vulvar cancer. Hematol Oncol Clin North Am. 2012;26(1):45-62.

14. Morgan MA, Mikuta JJ. Surgical management of vulvar cancer. Semin Surg Oncol. 1999;17(3):168-72.

15. Gonzalez Bosquet J, Magrina JF, Magtibay PM, Gaffey TA, Cha SS, Jones MB. Patterns of inguinal groin metastases in squamous cell carcinoma of the vulva. Gynecol Oncol. 2007;105(3):742-6.

16. Stehman FB, Bundy BN, Thomas G, Varia M, Okagaki T, Roberts J, et al. Groin dissection versus groin radiation in carcinoma of the vulva: a Gynecologic Oncology Group study. Int J Radiat Oncol Biol Phys. 1992;24(2):389-96.

17. van der Velden J, Fons G, Lawrie TA. Primary groin irradiation versus primary groin surgery for early vulvar cancer. Cochrane Database Syst Rev. 2011;(5):CD002224.

18. Ayhan A, Celik H, Dursun P. Lymphatic mapping and sentinel node biopsy in gynaecological cancers: a critical review of literature. World J Surg Oncol. 2008;6:53.

19. Van der Zee AG, Oonk MH, De Hullu JA, Ansink AC, Vergote I, Verheijen RH, et al. Sentinel node dissection is safe in the treatment of early-stage vulvar cancer. J Clin Oncol. 2008;26(6):884-9.

20. Levenback CF, Ali S, Coleman RL, Gold MA, Fowler JM, Judson PL, et al. Lymphatic Mapping and Sentinel Lymph Node Biopsy in Women With Squamous Cell Carcinoma of the Vulva: A Gynecologic Oncology Group Study. J Clin Oncol. 2012;30(31):3786-91.

21. Cunningham MJ, Goyer RP, Gibbons SK, Kredentser DC, Malfetano JH, Keys H. Primary radiation, cisplatin and 5-flourouracil for advanced squamous carcinoma of vulva. Gynecol Oncol. 1997;66(2):258-61.

22. Moyal-Barracco M, Lynch PJ. ISSVD terminology and classification of vulvodynia: a historical perspective. J Reprod Med. 2004;49(10):772-7.

23. Haefner HK. Report of the international society for the study of vulvovaginal terminology and classification of vulvodynia. J Low Genit Tract Dis. 2007;11(1):48-9.

24. McKay M. Subsets of vulvodynia. J Reprod Med. 1988;33(8): 695-8.

25. Farmer MA, Talor AM, Bailey AL, Tuttle AH, MacIntyre LC, Milagrosa ZE, et al. Repeated vulvovaginal fungal infections cause persistent pain in a mouse model of vulvodynia. Sci Transl Med. 2011;3(101):101ra91.

26. Peters K, Girdler B, Carrico D, Ibrahim I, Diokno A. Painful bladder syndrome/interstitial cystitis and vulvodynia: a clinical correlation. Int Urogynecol J Pelvic Floor Dysfunct. 2008;19(5):665-9.

27. Nunns D, Mandal D, Byrne M, McLelland J, Rani R, Cullimore J, et al. Guidelines for the management of vulvodynia. Br J Dermatol. 2010;162(8):1180-5.

28. Spoelstra SK, Dijkstra JR, van Driel MF, Weijmar Schultz WC. Long-term results of an individualized, multifaceted, and multidisciplinary therapeutic approach to provoked vestibulodynia. J Sex Med. 2011;8(2):489-96.

29. Friedrich EG. Therapeutic studies on vulval vestibulitis. J Reprod Med. 1988;33(6):514-8.

30. Gentilcore-Saulnier E, McLean L, Goldfinger C, Pukall CF, Chamberlain S. Pelvic floor muscle assessment outcomes in women with and without provoked vestibulodynia and the impact of a physical therapy program. J Sex Med. 2010;7(2 Pt 2):1003-22.

31. Murina F, Bianco V, Radici G, Felice R, Di Martino M, Nicolini U. Transcutaneous electrical nerve stimulation to treat vestibulodynia: a randomised controlled trial. BJOG. 2008;115(9):1165-70.

32. Murina F, Bernorio R, Palmiotto R. The use of amielle vaginal trainers as adjuvant in the treatment of vestibulodynia: an observational multicentric study. Medscape J Med. 2008;10(1):23.

33. Desrochers G, Bergeron S, Khalife S, Dupuis MJ, Jodoin M. Provoked vestibulodynia: psychological predictors of topical and cognitive-behavioral treatment outcome. Behav Res Ther. 2010;48(2):106-15.

34. Tommola P, Unkila-Kallio L, Paavonen J. Long-term follow up of posterior vestibulectomy for treating vulvar vestibulitis. Acta Obstet Gynecol Scand. 2011;90(11):1225-31.

35. Eva LJ, Narain S, Orakwue CO, Luesley DM. Long-term follow-up of posterior vestibulectomy for treating vulvar vestibulitis. J Reprod Med. 2008;53(6):435-40.

36. Glazer HI, Rodke G, Swencionis C, Hertz R, Young AW. Treatment of vulval vestibulitis syndrome with electro-myographic biofeedback of pelvic floor musculature. J Reprod Med. 1995;40(4):283-90.

37. Bergeron S, Binik YM, Khalifé S, Pagidas K, Glazer HI, Meana M, et al. A randomized comparison of group cognitive—behavioral therapy, surface electromyographic biofeedback, and vestibulectomy in the treatment of dyspareunia resulting from vulvar vestibulitis. Pain. 2001;91(3):297-306.

38. Reed BD, Caron AM, Gorenflo DW, Haefner HK. Treatment of vulvodynia with tricyclic antidepressants: efficacy and associated factors. J Low Genit Tract Dis. 2006;10(4):245-51.

39. Brown CS, Wan J, Bachmann G, Rosen R. Self-management, amitriptyline, and amitriptyline plus triamcinolone in the management of vulvodynia. J Womens Health (Larchmt). 2009;18(2):163-9.

40. Harris G, Horowitz B, Borgida A. Evaluation of gabapentin in the treatment of generalized vulvodynia, unprovoked. J Reprod Med. 2007;52(2):103-6.

41. Jerome L. Pregabalin-induced remission in a 62-year-old woman with a 20-year history of vulvodynia. Pain Res Manag. 2007;12(3):212-4.

42. Boardman LA, Cooper AS, Blais LR, Raker CA. Topical gabapentin in the treatment of localized and generalized vulvodynia. Obstet Gynecol. 2008;112(3):579-85.

43. Ben-David B, Friedman M. Gabapentin therapy for vulvodynia. Anesth Analg. 1999;89(6):1459-60.

44. Masheb RM, Kerns RD, Lozano C, Minkin MJ, Richman S. A randomized clinical trial for women with vulvodynia: Cognitive-behavioral therapy vs. supportive psychotherapy. Pain. 2009;141(1-2):31-40.

45. Powell J, Wojnarowska F. Acupuncture for vulvodynia. J R Soc Med. 1999;92(11):579-81.

CHAPTER 88

SECTION 16

Gynaecological Infections

GYNAECOLOGY

Sexually Transmitted Infections

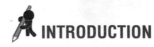

INTRODUCTION

Sexually transmitted infections (STIs) are an important cause for women presenting with a history of vaginal discharge. Other causes of vaginal discharge have been discussed in Chapter 90 (Vaginal Discharge). In the cases of STIs, it is especially important for the clinician to elicit sexual history from the patient in a sensitive and non-judgemental manner. While taking the sexual history from the patient, it is particularly important for the clinician to ask the patient about the kind of relationship she has with her partners, homosexual or heterosexual. History of different sexual practices, e.g. oral or anal sex also needs to be taken. Specialist services for the management of STI in the UK are available at the genitourinary medicine (GUM) clinic which is located in most of the major towns and cities. Strong links must be developed with this department to improve the overall management of STIs within each gynaecology unit. Some basic principles and practices of GUM are as follows:

* *Maintenance of confidentiality*: Maintenance of patient's confidentiality is of utmost importance and the patient's details must not be disclosed to other patients or even other healthcare professionals without the patient's informed consent. All NHS employees are required to abide by the Caldicott's principles of confidentiality, commissioned in 1997 by the Chief Medical Officer of England.[1] The patient's medical records are not to be made available to other healthcare professionals outside the department, including the patient's GP, except by the patient's explicit consent.
* *Provision of information*: The patients should be provided with clear and accurate written information pertaining to their conditions as well as the long-term implications of the condition for themselves as well as their partner. The patients with STIs should be advised not to have sexual intercourse until their treatment as well as the treatment and follow-up of their partner has been completed.

* *Screening for other STIs*: Patient with one STI may be at risk of other STIs also. Therefore, the patient should be screened for other STIs as well. Before performing these tests, informed consent must be taken from the patient after explaining her about nature of the procedure and the follow-up procedure in case the test comes out as positive.
* *Partner notification*: Partner notification or contact tracing is an essential component for the management of STIs. This is a process through which the sexual contacts of a patient with an STI are informed that they may be at risk, following which they are then offered screening, and treatment if indicated. Partner notification or contact tracing is a method of targeted case-finding which aims at diagnosing and treating undiagnosed, often asymptomatic infection, thereby reducing reinfection of the index patient, and preventing the transmission of STIs in the community. It also provides an opportunity to discuss the practice of safer sex with the patient and her partner. The term 'partner notification' reflects the basic approach in which the patients inform their partners themselves about the risk of STI. This term has now replaced the term, 'contact tracing'.[2] During the process of partner notification, patients pass on the medical slips, containing a nationally agreed code for each STI to their partners, which they have been given at the time of treatment. The partners can then present these slips at any GUM clinic in the UK and they would be appropriately managed.
* *Contact tracing*: This is a process through which the health workers directly contact the sexual contacts on the index patient with STI and then manage them appropriately.

CHLAMYDIAL INFECTION

INTRODUCTION

Chlamydia trachomatis is a gram-negative, aerobic, intracellular pathogen which is typically coccoid or rod-shaped.

However, it is different from other bacteria because it requires growing cells in order to remain viable. Chlamydia cannot be grown on an artificial medium because it cannot synthesise its own adenosine triphosphate (ATP) molecules. *C. trachomatis* can be considered as one of the most common causes for STI, worldwide, in association with blindness and infertility. In the UK, *C. trachomatis* is the most common bacterial STI, affecting both sexually active men and women equally. There exists the National Chlamydia Screening programme (NCSP) in the UK, specifically targeting sexually active young individuals under the age of 25 years.

AETIOLOGY

Chlamydia has a very unique life cycle (Fig. 89.1) which alternates between a non-replicating, infectious, elementary body (EB) and a replicating, non-infectious and reticulate body (RB). The EB, which is metabolically inactive, can be considered equivalent to the spore and helps in transmitting the disease. The infectious EB attaches to the host cells. Following the entry into the cell, it gets differentiated into a RB. Once inside a cell, the EB germinates as the result of interaction with glycogen and gets converted into its reticulate form. The reticulate form divides by binary fission every 2–3 hours and has an incubation period of about 7–21 days in its host.[3] Within 40–48 hours, the RBs transform back into infective EBs, which are subsequently released from the infected cell through the process of exocytosis and infect the neighbouring cells.

DIAGNOSIS

Clinical Presentation

❖ The majority of women with chlamydial infection remain asymptomatic. However, some women may develop vaginal discharge, dysuria, abdominal pain, increased urinary frequency, urgency, urethritis and cervicitis.[4]

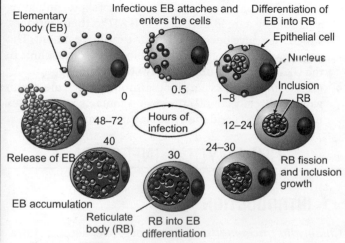

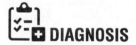

Fig. 89.1: Life cycle of *Chlamydia trachomatis*

❖ Infection of the urethra is often associated with chlamydial infection of the cervix.
❖ Chlamydia is very destructive to the fallopian tubes. If left untreated, nearly 30% of women with chlamydia may develop PID.[5] Pelvic infection often results in symptoms such as fever, pelvic cramping, abdominal pain or dyspareunia. Pelvic infection can often lead to infertility or even absolute sterility. Tubal destruction due to chlamydial infection may also result in an increased incidence of tubal pregnancy.
❖ Pelvic inflammatory disease due to *C. trachomatis* is associated with higher rates of consequent tubal infertility, ectopic pregnancy, and chronic pelvic pain in comparison with PID caused by other infections such as gonorrhoea. Occasionally, patients with chlamydial infection may develop an inflammation of the liver capsule and adjacent peritoneal surfaces resulting in perihepatitis. This is also known as Fitz-Hugh-Curtis syndrome. *Neisseria gonorrhoeae* not only causes similar clinical syndromes as *C. trachomatis* but also coexists in a significant percentage of patients with chlamydial infection. Therefore, women undergoing testing for *C. trachomatis* should also be simultaneously tested for *N. gonorrhoeae*.
❖ Amongst men, infection with *C. trachomatis* can result in urethritis and epididymitis.
❖ It can also cause arthritis or Reiter's syndrome in both the sexes.

Investigations

❖ *Nucleic acid amplification testing*: Nucleic acid amplification testing (NAAT) using either PCR or transcription-mediated amplification (TMA) of vulvovaginal swabs in women can be considered as the test of choice for establishing the diagnosis of chlamydial infection.[6] This is a highly sensitive test (90–95% sensitivity), which can be useful in various situations, including the medicolegal cases. First-catch urine samples and endocervical swabs (if available) can also be used. If amplification techniques are unavailable, tests such as antigen detection and genetic probe methods can be applied to endocervical or urethral swabs for diagnosing chlamydial infection.
❖ *Polymerase and ligase chain reactions*: Newer tests such as polymerase and ligase chain reactions, DNA probe and DNA amplification are also being used.
❖ *Immunoassay*: Rapid tests for chlamydia may be used for establishing the diagnosis in low-resource settings. ELISA are no longer recommended in the UK.

MANAGEMENT

Prevention

The National Chlamydia Screening Programme in the UK aims at preventing and controlling chlamydial infection through early diagnosis and treatment of asymptomatic infection. It aims at reducing the onward transmission to sexual partners and preventing the consequences of untreated infection. Under this programme, all sexually active individuals under the age of 25 years are educated about chlamydia, and provided access to sexual health services to help reduce the risk of infection or transmission. It is recommended that sexually active young individuals under the age of 25 years be annually screened for chlamydial infection or whenever they change partner. If an individual test is positive for chlamydia, resting should be done again at 3 months following treatment. Screening for chlamydia should be offered as an integrated component of the existing sexual and reproductive health services including primary care-based services, community contraceptive services, abortion services, etc. There is also a provision for internet-based testing and pharmacy-based testing to ensure that young people have universal access to testing.

Under this programme, home-based methods of screening involving the self-collected first-void urine specimen and vulvovaginal swabs have been found to be acceptable. These are likely to improve the universal screening rates. RCTs have demonstrated a reduction in the risk of PID amongst the women screened for *C. trachomatis*.[7,8]

Medical Treatment

❖ Treatment of chlamydia involves the use of broad-spectrum antibiotics, with the most commonly used antibiotic being azithromycin in a single dosage of 1 g per orally. Alternatively, doxycycline can be used orally in the dosage of 100 mg BID for 7 days.
❖ The combination of cofoxitin and ceftriaxone with doxycycline or tetracycline also proves to be useful.
❖ Erythromycin or amoxicillin in TID or QID dosage may also be given during pregnancy.
❖ Use of protective barrier such as condoms often helps to prevent the spread of the infection.
❖ Chlamydial infection, similar to gonorrhoea, can infect the infant during passage through the infected birth canal, leading to serious eye damage or pneumonia. Due to this, all newborns born to women infected with *C. trachomatis* must be treated with eye drops containing a broad-spectrum antibiotic (e.g. tetracycline), which kills chlamydia.
❖ *Follow-up*: The patient should be called for a follow-up, 6 weeks following the completion of treatment to check for partner notification, reinforcing health education, assessing the efficacy of treatment and exclusion of reinfection. Test for cure is usually not required unless the patient is pregnant, non-compliant or re-exposure is suspected.
❖ *Chlamydial infection during pregnancy*: Use of antibiotics such as quinolones and tetracyclines is usually not advised during pregnancy. Amoxicillin in the dosage of 500 mg three times a day for 7 days appears to be a reasonable alternative. Use of clindamycin and azithromycin can also be considered during pregnancy. As per the recommendations of BNF, use of azithromycin during pregnancy must be restricted to only those situations where no other alternative is available.

COMPLICATIONS

❖ Pelvic infection can often lead to infertility or even absolute sterility.
❖ Tubal destruction due to chlamydial infection may also result in an increased incidence of tubal pregnancy.
❖ Chlamydial infection during pregnancy may be associated with an increased incidence of premature births.[9]
❖ At the time of delivery, chlamydial infection may be transmitted to the foetus resulting in an increased risk of serious eye damage (neonatal conjunctivitis or ophthalmia neonatorum) or pneumonia in the infant. Also, there may be an increased risk of uterine infection in the mother.

CLINICAL PEARLS

❖ Gonorrhoea and chlamydia are bacterial STDs, which are frequently found together
❖ Uncomplicated chlamydial infection is not an indication for the removal of an intrauterine device (IUD) or intra-uterine system (IUS)
❖ Following the exposure to *C. trachomatis*, there exists a 2-week window period, following which the NAAT test comes out positive in the infected individuals. Therefore, the infected patients are usually advised to return for a repeat NAAT test 2 weeks following the last exposure.

GENITAL HERPES

INTRODUCTION

Genital herpes is a viral infection caused by the HSV (most commonly HSV II) which is transmitted through sexual contact. Two types of viruses are commonly associated with Herpes lesions: HSV I and HSV II.[10] HSV I is commonly responsible for causing herpes blisters in the perioral region (orolabial herpes), while HSV II is more commonly associated with lesions in the genital or the perianal area.

AETIOLOGY

Infection due to herpes could be either primary or recurrent (due to reactivation of the latent primary infection). Primary genital herpes infection spreads only by direct person-to-person contact. The virus enters through the mucous membrane of the genital tract via microscopic tears. From there, the virus travels to the nerve roots near the spinal cord and settles down permanently. Here, the virus becomes latent and get periodically reactivated at intervals resulting in either symptomatic or asymptomatic infection. This, however, may be associated with infectious viral shedding.

DIAGNOSIS

Clinical Presentation

Diagnosis is usually based on clinical examination. Genital herpes is suspected when multiple painful blisters and vesicles are present on the external genitalia including the vulva, vagina, cervix, perianal area or inner thigh, which ultimately develop into shallow and painful ulcers within a period of 2–6 weeks. They are frequently accompanied by itching and mucoid vaginal discharge. There may be associated vulval pain. In case of primary infection, these symptoms can be very severe, resulting in swelling, ulceration and infection of the vulva. Ulceration may also occur in the cervix. Primary infection may also be occasionally associated with tender inguinal lymphadenopathy, which is commonly due to secondary infection.

Following the exposure to the virus, there is an incubation period, which generally lasts from 3 days to 7 days before development of lesions begin. Prior to this, there are no symptoms and the virus cannot be transmitted to others. The primary infection may be associated with constitutional symptoms like fever, malaise, vulval paresthesia, itching or tingling sensation on the vulva and vagina followed by redness of the skin. Finally, the formation of blisters and vesicles begins, which eventually develop into shallow and painful ulcers within a period of 2–6 weeks. When the blisters break, they are usually very painful to touch. These lesions peak in 7 days and last for approximately 2 weeks. The outbreak is self-limited and usually heals without scarring. From the beginning of itching, until the time of complete healing of the ulcer, the infection is definitely contagious.

Recurrent infection, on the other hand, is less severe and self-limiting, and occasionally may be even asymptomatic.

Investigations

❖ *Cytological tests*: The blister fluid may be sent directly to the laboratory in the viral culture medium. However, this test is not very sensitive and may be associated with a high false negative rate of nearly 50%.
❖ *Immunological tests*: Immunological blood tests for detecting antibodies are not commonly used for making a diagnosis.
❖ *Other diagnostic tests*: Other diagnostic tests such as PCR and HSV NAAT screening tests are being used to identify HSV in some laboratories and are associated with higher sensitivity in comparison to the viral culture.
❖ *Biopsy*: The Tzanck smear is a rapid, fairly sensitive and inexpensive method for diagnosing HSV infection. Smears are preferably prepared from the base of the lesions and stained with 1% aqueous solution of toluidine blue 'O' for 15 seconds. Positive smear is indicated by the presence of multinucleated giant cells with faceted nuclei and homogeneously stained 'ground glass' chromatin (Tzanck cells).

MANAGEMENT

Treatment of genital herpes helps in shortening the duration of attack, preventing the occurrence of complications and reducing the risk of transmission. Various steps for management in these cases include the following:

❖ *General measures*: This involves drinking large quantity of water to dilute the urine, thereby reducing pain on micturition. Other general measures which help in reducing pain include use of saline bath analgesic drugs such as NSAIDs, etc. and use of topical anaesthetic gel.
❖ *Oral antiviral medications*: Oral antiviral medications, such as aciclovir (200 mg five times a day), famciclovir (250 mg three times a day) or valaciclovir (500 mg twice daily), which prevent the multiplication of the virus, are commonly used.[11] All these drugs help in reducing the severity and duration of episodes. However, they do not alter the natural history of the disease. Local application of aciclovir provides local relief and accelerates the process of healing. In severe cases, aciclovir can be administered intravenously in the dosage of 5 mg/kg body weight every 8 hourly for 5 days.
❖ The couple is advised to abstain from intercourse starting right from time of experiencing prodromal symptoms until total re-epithelisation of the lesions occurs.
❖ Supervision of a GUM specialist may be required for administration of suppressive antiviral therapy in case the patient suffers more than six attacks each year.
❖ Although topical agents do exist, they are generally less effective than oral formulations and therefore are not routinely used. However, it is important for the clinician to remember that there is still no curative medicine available for genital herpes and the above-mentioned antiviral drugs only help in reducing the severity of symptoms and duration of outbreaks.
❖ Since the initial infection with HSV tends to be the most severe episode, an antiviral medication is usually recommended. Though the use of these medications can significantly help in reducing pain and decreasing the length of time until the sores heal, treatment of the first infection does not appear to provide protection against the future episodes. In contrast to a new outbreak of genital herpes, recurrent herpes episodes tend to be milder in intensity. In these cases, the benefit of antiviral medication is derived only if therapy is started immediately prior to the outbreak or within the first 24 hours of the outbreak. Thus, the antiviral drug must be provided to the patient well in advance and the patient is instructed to begin treatment as soon as she experiences the preoutbreak 'tingling' sensation or as soon as the blisters appear.
❖ Herpes can be spread from one part of the body to another during an outbreak. Therefore, it is important to instruct the patient not to touch her eyes or mouth after touching the blisters or ulcers. She must be asked to scrupulously

wash her hand. Clothing that comes in contact with ulcers should not be shared with others.

❖ Couples who want to minimise the risk of transmission should always use condoms if a partner is infected. Such couples must be instructed to avoid all kinds of sexual activity, including kissing, during an outbreak of herpes.

Management of Genital Herpes during Pregnancy

❖ Women with suspected herpes during pregnancy should be preferably referred to a GUM specialist. For details regarding the management of pregnant women with herpes infection, kindly refer to Chapter 20 (Infection during Pregnancy).

❖ Maternal herpes infection acquired during the first or second trimester is not associated with an increased risk to the foetus. However, maternal infection during the first trimester may be associated with an increased risk of miscarriage. Aciclovir via oral or IV route may be administered in these cases. However, aciclovir is not licensed for use during pregnancy.[12]

❖ The risk of the neonate to acquire HSV infection at the time of delivery from maternal viral shedding is most likely to occur with new maternal herpes infection acquired during the third trimester.

❖ Pregnant women with active herpetic lesion after 34 weeks of pregnancy must be preferably delivered by caesarean section. This is so because the risk of viral shedding during labour is very high in these cases, thereby resulting in vertical transmission to the foetus which may lead to the development of neonatal herpes. Continuous administration of aciclovir (400 mg TDS) in the last month of pregnancy helps in reducing the risk of clinical recurrence at term and thereby requirement for caesarean delivery.[13]

❖ Women who have herpes and are pregnant can have a vaginal delivery as long as they are not experiencing symptoms or actually having an active outbreak while in labour. Pregnant women with active herpetic lesion must be preferably delivered by caesarean section.[13]

COMPLICATIONS

❖ *Urinary retention*: This may occur due to autonomic neuropathy or due to local reaction around the vulva and urethra because of severe vulval pain. Suprapubic catheterisation may be required in these cases.

❖ *Postherpetic neuralgia*: This may be the cause of chronic vulval pain.

CLINICAL PEARLS

❖ Cases of severe primary genital herpes infection should be considered as a genitourinary emergency. Such patients should also be referred to GUM clinic for ongoing treatment and partner notification.

❖ There is still no curative medicine available for genital herpes and the antiviral drugs only help in reducing the severity of symptoms and duration of outbreaks.

❖ Herpes can be spread from one part of the body to another through tissue fluids. Thorough hand washing is a must during outbreaks in order to prevent the spread of infection.

EVIDENCE-BASED MEDICINE

❖ Though aciclovir is not licensed for use during pregnancy, the available evidence supports the safety of this drug during pregnancy.[12]

❖ There is conflicting evidence to show that the continuous administration of aciclovir (400 mg TDS) in the last month of pregnancy helps in reducing the risk of clinical recurrence at term and the risk of neonatal herpes, thereby requirement for caesarean delivery.[13]

❖ There is no good quality evidence to indicate that caesarean section in case of the symptoms of herpes after 34 weeks of gestation helps in preventing the risk of neonatal herpes infection. If the membranes have ruptured for more than 4 hours, caesarean section may not prevent the vertical transmission of herpes infection. Nevertheless, British Association for Sexual Health and HIV (BASHH), recommends that caesarean delivery should be performed even though the evidence regarding its effectiveness is lacking.[13]

GONORRHOEA

INTRODUCTION

Gonorrhoea is an STD, which is derived from the Greek words gonos (seed) and rhoia (flow) implying 'flow of seeds' and is caused by the bacterium *N. gonorrhoeae*. Gonorrhoea is spread through contact with the penis, vagina, mouth or anus. It can also be spread from mother to baby at the time of delivery.

AETIOLOGY

The disease is characterised by adhesion of the gonococci to the surface of urethra or other mucosal surfaces. The gonococci penetrate through the intercellular spaces between the columnar epithelial cells and reach the subepithelial connective tissue by the 3rd day of infection. Gonococci usually penetrate the columnar epithelial cells because the stratified squamous epithelium is relatively resistant to infection. Thus, infection usually does not occur in young prepubertal girls; however, severe vulvovaginitis can still sometimes occur in prepubertal girls. The incubation period is 2–8 days.

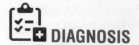

DIAGNOSIS

Clinical Presentation

❖ The most common clinical presentation of the disease in men is acute urethritis resulting in dysuria and a purulent penile discharge. Lesions due to gonorrhoea are summarised in Figure 89.2. The infection may extend along the urethra to the prostate, seminal vesicles and epididymis, resulting in complications such as epididymitis, prostatitis, periurethral abscesses and chronic urethritis. The infection may spread to the periurethral tissues, resulting in formation of abscesses and multiple discharging sinuses (watering-can perineum).

❖ In women, the primary site of infection is the endocervix and the infection commonly extends to the urethra and vagina, giving rise to mucopurulent discharge. Symptomatic patients commonly experience vaginal discharge, dysuria and abdominal pain. Gonorrhoea can rarely cause intermenstrual bleeding or menorrhagia as a result of endometritis.

❖ The infection may extend to Bartholin's glands, endometrium and fallopian tubes. The gonococci can typically ascend to the fallopian tubes at the time of menstruation or after instrumentation [for medical termination of pregnancy (MTP)] giving rise to acute salpingitis.[14] Acute salpingitis may be followed by PID. This may be associated with a high probability of sterility if not treated adequately. Peritoneal spread occasionally occurs and may produce a perihepatic inflammation, resulting in Fitz-Hugh-Curtis syndrome.

❖ Usually no abnormal findings are present on clinical examination. Men may rarely show epididymal tenderness or balanitis.[15]

Investigations

❖ *Nucleic acid amplification tests*: These tests show higher sensitivity than culture in both symptomatic and asymptomatic cases of gonorrhoea.

❖ *Culture and sensitivity*: Culture using an endocervical and urethral swab specimen provides maximum sensitivity. Patients in whom NAAT is positive must be confirmed for gonorrhoea by culture on selective medium (which has been impregnated with antibiotics).[16]

MANAGEMENT

Uncomplicated Anogenital Infection in Adults

Treatment comprises using the following antibiotics: Ceftriaxone 500 mg IM or cefixime 400 mg (oral if IM dose is contraindicated or refused) or spectinomycin 2 g IM as a single dose. Doxycycline 100 mg BID for 7 days or azithromycin 1 g PO (single dose) is usually added with a third-generation cephalosporin.[17] This addition is recommended even if chlamydial infection is negative because its use may help delay the onset of resistance to cephalosporins. Due to emerging antibiotic resistance against *N. gonorrhoeae,* an antibiotic should be chosen in such a way that it is able to eliminate infection in at least 95% of cases in the local community.

Pregnant or Breastfeeding Mothers

Treatment comprises using the following antibiotics: Ceftriaxone 500 mg IM single dose with azithromycin 1 g PO or spectinomycin 2 g IM as a single dose with azithromycin 1 g PO.

Use of quinolone or tetracycline antibiotics is usually not advisable during pregnancy. Use of azithromycin is advisable only under circumstances where adequate alternatives are not available.

Follow-up

At least one follow-up visit is recommended to ensure resolution of infection and partner notification. Test of cure using NAAT test is usually recommended after 2 weeks of completion of treatment due to concerns regarding the emerging antibiotic resistance.

COMPLICATIONS

❖ The infection may extend along the urethra to the prostate, seminal vesicles and epididymis, resulting in complications such as epididymitis, prostatitis, periurethral abscesses and chronic urethritis.

❖ The infection may spread to the periurethral tissues, resulting in formation of abscesses and multiple discharging sinuses (watercan perineum).

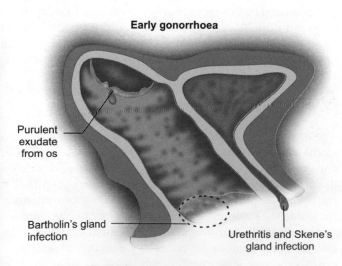

Early gonorrhoea

Purulent exudate from os

Bartholin's gland infection

Urethritis and Skene's gland infection

Fig. 89.2: Lesions due to gonorrhoea

- Acute salpingitis may be followed by PID. This may be associated with a high probability of sterility, if not treated adequately.
- Peritoneal spread occasionally occurs and may produce a perihepatic inflammation, resulting in Fitz-Hugh-Curtis syndrome.
- As a result of vertical transmission to the foetus, gonorrhoea can cause severe conjunctivitis, also known as ophthalmia neonatorum. This is a notifiable disease in the UK.
- Disseminated haematogenous gonococcal infection, which rarely occurs, can result in complications such as arthralgia, arthritis, tenosynovitis, skin lesions, etc.

CLINICAL PEARLS

- Nucleic acid amplification testing serves as a test of choice for asymptomatic individuals with gonorrhoea.
- In the UK, significant levels of resistance have developed for *N. gonorrhoeae* to the antibiotics such as penicillin, tetracyclines and ciprofloxacin.
- Since coinfection with *C. trachomatis* can occur in nearly 40% cases, women should be simultaneously screened for *C. trachomatis*.

SYPHILIS

INTRODUCTION

Syphilis is an STD caused by the spirochete *Treponema pallidum*. Syphilis infection could be acquired or congenital. Though the route of transmission of acquired syphilis is almost always through sexual contact, sometimes congenital syphilis can occur via transmission from mother to child in utero. The incubation period of the disease varies between 9 to 90 days.

DIAGNOSIS

Clinical Presentation

- The acquired disease comprises of an early stage and a late stage of infection. Early infection is typically characterised by three phases: (1) primary, (2) secondary and (3) early latent phase (<2 years of infection). Late stage of infection includes late latent phase (>2 years of infection) and the tertiary phase.
- *Primary phase*: Primary lesions appear approximately 10–90 days after the initial exposure. Primary lesion, also known as a chancre, often appears at the point of contact, usually the external genitalia. The chancre of syphilis is a firm, painless, relatively avascular, circumscribed, indurated and superficially ulcerated lesion. The chancre of syphilis is often termed as 'hard chancre' in order to

distinguish it from the 'soft sore' caused by *Haemophilus ducreyi*. The 'hard chancre' of syphilis usually persists for about 4–6 weeks and heals spontaneously.
- In most patients, a painless regional lymphadenopathy develops within 1–2 weeks after the appearance of the chancre. As a result, the regional lymph nodes often become swollen, discrete, rubbery and non-tender.
- *Secondary phase*: Secondary syphilis occurs approximately 1–6 months after the primary infection. This stage is typically characterised by a 'flu-like' syndrome, lymphadenopathy and the appearance of symmetrical reddish-pink non-itchy rashes on the trunk and extremities. The rash can involve the palms of the hands and the soles of the feet. In moist areas of the body, such as the anus and vagina, the rash often develops into flat, broad, whitish lesions known as condylomata lata. Mucous patches may also appear on the genitals or in the mouth. All of the lesions of secondary stage are infectious and harbour active treponema organisms and therefore patients in this stage are most contagious. Other common symptoms of this stage include fever, malaise, sore throat, weight loss, headache, meningismus, enlarged lymph nodes, etc.
- *Latent syphilis*: Following the secondary stage, there often occurs a period of quiescence known as 'latent syphilis'. No clinical manifestations are evident during this phase and all the lesions of secondary stage have disappeared. The diagnosis during this period is possible only by serological tests. In many cases, this phase is followed by natural cure.
- *Tertiary syphilis*: In some cases, manifestations of tertiary syphilis may appear after several years. Tertiary syphilis usually occurs 1–10 years after the initial infection and is characterised by the formation of gummas, which are soft, tumour-like balls of granulomatous inflammation. Other characteristic features of untreated tertiary syphilis include neuropathic joint disease (characterised by degeneration of joint surfaces resulting in loss of proprioception), neurosyphilis and cardiovascular syphilis.
- *Congenital syphilis*: For details related to congenital syphilis, kindly refer to Chapter 39 (Foetal Infection).

Investigations

- Dark-field microscopy
- *Non-treponemal tests*: Kahn's test, rapid plasma regain (RPR) and VDRL
- *Treponemal tests*: Microhaemagglutination assay for *T. pallidum* antibodies (MHA-TP), and fluorescent treponemal antibody absorption (FTA-ABS).

MANAGEMENT

- Women with syphilis should be preferably managed in GUM clinic
- All women must be offered screening for other STIs including HIV
- Primary, secondary and early latent stages of syphilis can generally be treated with a single-dose IM injection of 2.4 million units benzathine penicillin-G, which is

unlicensed in the UK. Alternatively, a single dose of azithromycin can be administered in a single dosage as the second-line therapy. On the other hand, cases of neurosyphilis can be treated with procaine penicillin-G along with concomitant oral probenecid as the first-line therapy[18]

❖ *Management in pregnant women*: In the third trimester of pregnancy, second dose of benzathine penicillin-G must be administered 1 week after the first dose.

COMPLICATIONS

Transplacental passage of treponemal infection at any stage of pregnancy may lead to complications such as polyhydramnios, stillbirths, miscarriage, preterm labour, hydrops, congenital syphilis, etc.

CLINICAL PEARLS

❖ The chancre of syphilis is often termed as 'hard chancre' in order to distinguish it from the 'soft sore' caused by *H. ducreyi*.

❖ All of the lesions of secondary stage are infectious and harbour active treponema organisms and therefore patients in this stage are most contagious.

❖ The rash of secondary syphilis can involve the palms of the hands and the soles of feet.

❖ Jarisch-Herxheimer reaction may occur in nearly 40% patients with syphilis treated with penicillin. In pregnant patients, this reaction can cause symptoms such as fever, uterine contractions, foetal heart decelerations, etc.

REFERENCES

1. The Caldicott Committee. (1997). The Caldicott Report. [online] Available from www.dh.gov.uk/en/Publicationsandstatistics/Publications/PublicationsPolicyAndGuidance/DH_4068403. [Accessed October, 2016].
2. Ward H, Bell G. Partner notification. Medicine (Abingdon). 2014;42(6):314-7.
3. Stamm WE, Jones RB, Batteiger BE. Chlamydia trachomatis (trachoma, perinatal infections, lymphogranuloma venereum, and other genital infections). In: Mandell GL, Bennett JE, Dolin R (Eds). Principles and Practice of Infectious Disease, 6th edition. Philadelphia, PA: Elsevier; 2005. pp. 2239-55.
4. Gaydos CA, Howell MR, Pare B, Clarke KL, Ellis DA, Hendrix RM, et al. Chlamydia trachomatis infections in female military recruits. N Engl J Med. 1998;339(11):739-44.
5. Geisler WM. Duration of untreated, uncomplicated Chlamydia trachomatis genital infection and factors associated with chlamydia resolution: a review of human studies. J Infect Dis. 2010;201(Suppl 2):S104-13.
6. Handsfield HH, Jasman LL, Roberts PL, Hanson VW, Kothenbeutel RL, Stamm WE. Criteria for selective screening for Chlamydia trachomatis infection in women attending family planning clinics. JAMA. 1986;255(13):1730-4.
7. Scholes D, Stergachis A, Heidrich FE, Andrilla H, Holmes KK, Stamm WE. Prevention of pelvic inflammatory disease by screening for cervical chlamydial infection. N Engl J Med. 1996;334(21):1362-6.
8. Ostergaard L, Andersen B, Møller JK, Olesen F. Home sampling versus conventional swab sampling for screening of Chlamydia trachomatis in women: a cluster-randomized 1-year follow-up study. Clin Infect Dis. 2000;31(4):951-7.
9. Rours GI, Duijts L, Moll HA, Arends LR, de Groot R, Jaddoe VW, et al. Chlamydia trachomatis infection during pregnancy associated with preterm delivery: a population-based prospective cohort study. Eur J Epidemiol. 2011;26(6):493-502.
10. Langenberg AG, Corey L, Ashley RL, Leong WP, Straus SE. A prospective study of new infections with herpes simplex virus type 1 and type 2. Chiron HSV Vaccine Study Group. N Engl J Med. 1999;341(19):1432-8.
11. Corey L, Benedetti J, Critchlow C, Mertz G, Douglas J, Fife K, et al. Treatment of primary first-episode genital herpes simplex virus infections with acyclovir: results of topical, intravenous and oral therapy. J Antimicrob Chemother. 1983;12(Suppl B):79-88.
12. Girard M. Safety of acyclovir in general practice: a review of the literature. Pharmacoepidemiol Drug Saf. 1996;5(5):325-32.
13. Royal College of Obstetricians and Gynaecologists (RCOG) or British Association for Sexual health and HIV (BASHH) Guidelines. Management of genital herpes in pregnancy. London: RCOG Press; 2014.
14. World Health Organization. Tubal infertility: serologic relationship to past chlamydial and gonococcal infection. World Health Organization Task Force on the prevention and Management of Infertility. Sex Transm Dis. 1995;22(2):71-7.
15. Cecil JA, Howell MR, Tawes JJ, Gaydos JC, McKee KT, Quinn TC, et al. Features of Chlamydia trachomatis and Neisseria gonorrhoeae infection in male Army recruits. J Infect Dis. 2001;184(9):1216-9.
16. Ressel GW. CDC releases 2002 guidelines for treating STDs: Part I. Diseases characterized by vaginal discharge and PID. Am Fam Physician. 2002;66(9):1777-8.
17. Centers for Disease Control and Prevention (CDC). (2011). Sexually Transmitted Disease Surveillance 2010. [online] Available from www.cdc.gov/std/stats10/surv2010.pdf. [Accessed November, 2016].
18. Workowski KA, Berman S, Centers for Disease Control and Prevention (CDC). Sexually transmitted diseases treatment guidelines, 2010. MMWR Recomm Rep. 2010;59(RR-12):1-110.

Vaginal Discharge

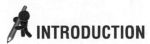

INTRODUCTION

Vaginal discharge is one of the most common presenting complaints faced by the gynaecologists in clinical practice, which can be caused by physiological or pathological causes (Table 90.1). The most important challenge for the gynaecologist is to differentiate between the pathological and physiological causes of discharge. If a pathological cause of discharge is suspected, the gynaecologist needs to diagnose the exact cause for vaginal discharge.

AETIOLOGY

Various causes of pathological vaginal discharge are enlisted in Table 90.2. Vulvovaginitis can be considered as one of the most common causes for pathological vaginal discharge, irritation and itching in women. Nearly 90% of cases of vaginitis are secondary to bacterial vaginosis, vulvovaginal candidiasis (VVC) and trichomoniasis. Bacterial vaginosis, which is not an STD, is the most common cause of vaginal discharge amongst women.[1] The second most common cause of vaginal discharge is candidiasis, which is also not sexually transmitted. It is often misdiagnosed by both the women and their healthcare professionals.

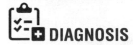

DIAGNOSIS

Clinical Presentation

Diagnostic features of the most common causes of vaginitis have been described in Table 90.3.[2,3]

Investigations

Laboratory investigations for documentation of the aetiology of vaginitis are required before initiation of therapy. In a patient presenting with vaginal discharge, the following investigations need to be carried out.[3]

Pregnancy Test

Pregnancy test must be done to rule out pregnancy because certain treatment medicines might be contraindicated during pregnancy.

Microscopic Examination

If the findings of the history and/or physical examination suggest that the patient has vaginitis, a sample of the vaginal discharge should be obtained for gross and microscopic examinations. Microscopic examination of normal vaginal discharge mainly shows squamous epithelial cells, polymorphonuclear leucocytes and microorganisms related to the *Lactobacillus* species. Pathological vaginal discharge could be associated with the presence of candidal buds or hyphae in case of candidal infection or presence of motile trichomonads in case of infection with *Trichomonas vaginalis*. Clue cells (epithelial cells studded with adherent coccobacilli) may be observed in cases of bacterial vaginosis. Presence of a large number of polymorphonuclear cells without any evidence of candidal species, trichomonads, or clue cells is highly suggestive of cervicitis.

Wet mount preparation: Preparation of wet mount is an easy, reliable method for the screening of infection. In this method, the sample of the discharge is placed on the slide with a drop of saline. The slide is covered with a cover slip and then examined microscopically using low power (for WBCs, RBCs and epithelial cells) and then under high power to look for trichomonads, clue cells, pseudohyphae, *Lactobacillus* and WBCs . The saline should be at room temperature, and microscopy should be performed within 10–20 minutes to reduce the possibility of loss of any trichomonads. Viewing the specimen should not be delayed, since drying could change the result. For example, trichomonads may lose their motility, if the wet smear dries. Following the wet mount preparation, the slide must be examined using 10% potassium hydroxide (KOH) solution.

Table 90.1: Differentiation between physiological and pathological causes of vaginal discharge

Characteristic	Physiological vaginal discharge	Pathological vaginal discharge
Discomfort to the patient	Does not usually cause any discomfort to the patient (except for hygiene problems)	Usually causes significant distress and irritation to the patient
Colour of the discharge	Translucent to whitish in colour	May vary in colour from dirty white to yellowish green
Association of itching	Is not associated with itching	May be associated with itching
Variations in the amount of discharge during the different phases of menstrual cycle	Amount of discharge may vary in different phases of menstrual cycle	Amount of discharge does not vary in different phases of menstrual cycle
Smell of the discharge	Not foul smelling	May be foul smelling

Table 90.2: Causes of pathological vaginal discharge

Infective discharge	Other causes for discharge
• Vulvovaginal candidiasis • Vaginitis caused by *Trichomonas vaginalis, Chlamydia trachomatis* • Sexually transmitted disease (*Neisseria gonorrhoeae*) • Bacterial vaginosis • Acute PID • Postoperative pelvic infection • Postabortal/postpartum sepsis *Less common causes* • Human papilloma virus • Primary syphilis • *Mycoplasma genitalium* • *Ureaplasma urealyticum* • *Escherichia coli*	• Retained tampon or condom • Chemical irritation • Allergic responses • Ectropion • Endocervical polyp • Intrauterine device *Less common causes* • Atrophic changes • Physical trauma • Vault granulation tissue • Vesicovaginal fistula • Rectovaginal fistula • Neoplasia (cervical, vulvar, vaginal or endometrial)

Table 90.3: Features of the most common causes of vaginitis[2,3]

Characteristic features	Bacterial vaginosis	Vulvovaginal candidiasis	Trichomoniasis
Causative organism	Alteration of normal vaginal pH resulting in the proliferation of organisms which are normally suppressed such as *Haemophilus vaginalis, Gardnerella mobiluncus, Mycoplasma hominis, Gardnerella vaginalis, Peptostreptococcus spp.*, etc.[4]	In most of the cases (80–92%), infecting agent is the yeast *Candida albicans*	It is caused by the protozoa *Trichomonas vaginalis*
Signs and symptoms	Thin, greyish to off-white coloured discharge; unpleasant 'fishy' odour, with odour especially increasing after sexual intercourse. The discharge is usually homogeneous and adheres to vaginal walls	Thick, white (curd-like) discharge with no odour[5]	Copious, malodorous, yellow-green (or discoloured) discharge, pruritus and vaginal irritation, dysuria, no symptoms in 20–50% of affected women[6]
Physical examination	Normal appearance of vaginal tissues; greyish-white coloured discharge may be adherent to the vaginal walls	• Vulvar and vaginal erythema, oedema and fissures • Thick, white discharge that adheres to vaginal walls	• Vulvar and vaginal oedema and erythema, 'strawberry' cervix in up to 25% of affected women • Frothy, purulent discharge
Vaginal pH (normal ≤4.5)	Elevated (>4.5)	Normal	Elevated (>4.5)
Microscopic examination of wet-mount and potassium hydroxide (KOH) preparations of vaginal discharge	'Clue cells' (vaginal epithelial cells coated with coccobacilli): few lactobacilli, occasional motile, curved rods, belonging to *Mobiluncus* species	Pseudohyphae, mycelial tangles or budding yeast cells	Motile trichomonads Many polymorphonuclear cells
'Whiff' test (Normal = no odour)	Positive	Negative	Can be positive
Additional tests	Amsel's criteria (Box 90.1) is positive in nearly 90% of affected women with bacterial vaginosis	KOH microscopy, Gram stain, culture	Deoxyribonucleic acid (DNA) probe tests: sensitivity of 90% and specificity of 99.8% Culture: sensitivity of 98% and specificity of 100%

Box 90.1: Amsel's diagnostic criteria for bacterial vaginosis

❏ Thin, homogeneous discharge
❏ Positive 'Whiff' test
❏ Presence of 'clue cells' on microscopic examination
❏ Vaginal pH >4.5

KOH preparation: The slide is prepared by placing a drop of vaginal secretion on a slide with a drop of 10–20% KOH and using a coverslip to protect the microscope lens. A coverslip is placed on the slide, and air or flame dried before examination is carried out under the microscope. KOH, by dissolving the non-fungal elements, is useful for detection of candidal hyphae, mycelial tangles and spores. The test is positive in 50–70% of women with candidal infection. This is particularly useful in diagnosis of candidal vaginitis. Following the examination of the slide, the KOH Whiff test is performed.

KOH Whiff Test

Smelling (whiffing) the slide immediately after applying KOH is useful for detecting the fishy (amine) odour of bacterial vaginosis. The odour results from the liberation of amines and organic acids produced from the alkalisation of anaerobic bacteria. A positive Whiff test or amine test is suggestive of bacterial vaginosis.[7]

Nitrazine pH Paper

Nitrazine pH paper is used to evaluate the pH of vaginal discharge sample which is collected at the time of per speculum examination. The normal vaginal pH ranges between 3.8 and 4.2. The gynaecologist must remember that both blood and cervical mucus are alkaline in nature and their presence may alter the pH of a vaginal sample. The pH level is also high in cases with atrophic vaginitis. A pH greater than 4.5 is found in 80–90% of patients with bacterial vaginosis and frequently in patients with trichomoniasis. VVC is normally associated with a pH of less than 4.5.

Alternative Options to Microscopic Examination

In case the microscopic examination is not available, commercial diagnostic testing methods [e.g. rapid antigen and nucleic acid amplification test (NAAT)] may be used for confirming the clinical diagnosis of bacterial vaginosis or trichomonas vaginitis.[8] However, none of these methods are sufficiently sensitive for detecting candidal organisms. For confirming the diagnosis of candidal species, vaginal culture must be obtained.

Vaginal Culture

Vaginal culture may help to diagnose the exact aetiology in case of a bacterial or fungal infection. If the microscopic examination for candidal species is negative, vaginal culture for *Candida* species must be done because microscopic examination is not sufficiently sensitive to exclude the diagnosis of candida organisms in symptomatic patients.

In case of clinical suspicion of trichomonal infection, diagnostic test card using NAAT, if available, may serve as a reasonable alternative to culture.

Cervical Culture

In a woman with purulent vaginal discharge, culture of cervical secretions is important for establishing the diagnosis of cervicitis, typically due to *Neisseria gonorrhoeae* or *Chlamydia trachomatis*.

MANAGEMENT

Management plan for a patient presenting with vaginal discharge is described in Flow chart 90.1 and the treatment of various causes of vaginal discharge is summarised in Table 90.4.[9]

Bacterial Vaginosis

Treatment for bacterial vaginosis consists of prescription of antibiotics. All pregnant women with symptomatic bacterial vaginosis must undergo treatment to obtain relief from bothersome symptoms. Commonly used treatment options for both pregnant and non-pregnant women are tabulated in the Table 90.6.[7,10,11] While previously, some clinicians avoided the use of metronidazole in the first trimester because of its potential to cross the placenta, the Centers for Disease Control and Prevention (CDC) no longer discourages the use of metronidazole in the first trimester. Moreover, routine screening and treatment of all pregnant women with asymptomatic bacterial infection to prevent preterm birth and its consequences is not presently recommended by the ACOG, United States Preventive Services Task Force (USPSTF) and CDC.

A few of the routinely used antibiotics include the following:

❖ *Metronidazole*: The WHO has recommended metronidazole as the first-line therapy for the treatment of bacterial vaginosis. A 7-day course of metronidazole (500 mg BD) is effective in nearly 85% cases. Vaginal therapy with 0.75% metronidazole gel (5 g once daily for 5 days) has been found to be as effective as oral metronidazole.[12] The choice of whether to use oral or vaginal therapy should be based upon patient preference. The oral metronidazole can cause some minor, but unpleasant side effects, such as anorexia, nausea, metallic taste, abdominal cramps, headache, glossitis, dryness of mouth, dizziness, rashes, transient neutropenia, etc. Despite of these side effects, it is believed to be the most effective treatment. Tinidazole is an antibiotic that appears to have fewer side effects than metronidazole and is also effective in treating bacterial vaginosis. Ornidazole, 500 mg vaginal tablet daily for 7 days is another effective option. Use of vaginal tablets helps in avoiding first pass metabolism. Treatment of male sexual partners of affected women is not required.

Flow chart 90.1: Management plan for a patient presenting with vaginal discharge

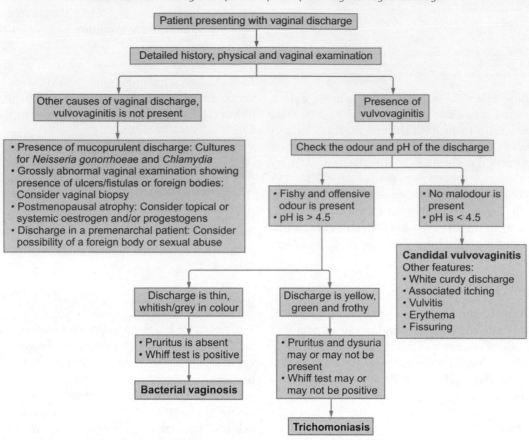

Table 90.4: Treatment summary of various causes of vaginal discharge

Treatment regimens	Bacterial vaginosis	Vulvovaginal candidiasis	Trichomoniasis
Acute regimens	• Metronidazole (Flagyl), 500 mg orally twice daily for 7 days, forms the first-line treatment or • *Clindamycin phosphate vaginal cream (2%)*: Application of one full applicator (5 g) intravaginally each night for 7 days or • *Metronidazole gel 0.75% (Metrogel-vaginal)*: Application of one full applicator (5 g) intravaginally twice daily for 5 days	Topical antifungal agents (Table 90.5) or Fluconazole 150 mg orally, single dose	Metronidazole, 2 g orally in a single dose
Alternative regimens	Metronidazole, 2 g orally in a single dose or Clindamycin (Cleocin), 300 mg orally twice daily for 7 days or metronidazole 375 mg TID, orally for 7 days	Boric acid powder in size-0 gelatin capsules intravaginally once or twice daily for 2 weeks	Metronidazole, 200 mg orally thrice daily for 7 days
Pregnancy	Metronidazole, 250 mg orally three times daily for 7 days (recommended regimen)	Only topical azole agents such as clotrimazole, miconazole, terconazole, and tioconazole intravaginally for 7–10 days	Metronidazole, 2 g orally in a single dose (usually not recommended in first trimester)
Recurrence	Retreat with an alternative regimen	*For four or more episodes of symptomatic vulvovaginal candidiasis annually*: Initial acute intravaginal regimen for 10–14 days followed immediately by maintenance regimen for at least 6 months (e.g. ketoconazole, 100 mg orally once daily)	Metronidazole, 2 g orally once daily for 3–5 days (Note that treatment of sexual partners increases cure rate)

Table 90.5: Topical antifungal therapy for candida vulvovaginitis

Antifungal drugs	Intravaginal cream preparation
Butoconazole	2% cream: Application of 5 g/day intravaginally for 3 days
Clotrimazole	1% cream: Application of 5 g/day intravaginally for 7–14 days
Miconazole	2% cream: Application of 5 g/day intravaginally for 7 days
Tioconazole	5% ointment: Application of 5 g intravaginally in a single application
Terconazole	0.4% cream: Application of 5 g/day intravaginally for 7 days 0.8% cream: Application of 5 g/day intravaginally for 3 days
Antifungal drugs	**Intravaginal suppository**
Clotrimazole	• 100 mg vaginal tablet, one tablet per day intravaginally for 7 days • 500 mg vaginal tablet, one tablet administered intravaginally in a single dose application • Clotrimazole 100 mg vaginal tablet, two tablets per day intravaginally for 3 days
Miconazole	200 mg vaginal suppository per day for 3 days or 100 mg vaginal suppository per day for 7 days
Nystatin	1,00,000 unit vaginal tablet (Mycostatin), one tablet per day intravaginally for 14 days
Terconazole	80 mg vaginal suppository, one suppository per day for 3 days

Table 90.6: Treatment options for women with bacterial vaginosis

Pregnant women	Non-pregnant women
• Metronidazole 500 mg orally twice daily for 7 days • Metronidazole 250 mg orally three times daily for 7 days • Clindamycin 300 mg orally twice daily for 7 days • Intravaginal preparations of metronidazole and clindamycin are avoided by some experts during pregnancy	• Metronidazole 500 mg twice daily orally for 7 days • Metronidazole gel 0.75% (5 g) once daily vaginally for 5 days • Clindamycin 2% vaginal cream once daily at bed time for 7 days • Clindamycin 300 mg twice per day orally for 7 days • Clindamycin 100 mg vaginal suppositories at bed time for 3 days • Clindamycin bioadhesive cream (Clindesse®) 2% as a single vaginal dose of 5 g of cream containing 100 mg of clindamycin phosphate

❖ *Lincosamides*: Vaginal clindamycin cream, 2% (cleocin), or oral clindamycin, 300 mg twice daily for 7 days is effective.

❖ *Ampicillin*: Ampicillin 500 mg TDS or cephalosporins 500 mg BID for 7 days is also effective.

❖ *Tetracyclines*: Tetracycline 500 mg, four times a day or doxycycline 100 mg twice daily for 7 days is effective.

Candidal Infection

Antifungals: Imidazoles and triazoles are presently the most extensively used antifungal drugs for treatment of VVC. Imidazole antifungal agents, which can be used in form of creams and pessaries for treatment of VVC, include butoconazole, clotrimazole and miconazole. Some of these agents are freely available over the counter. Trizole agents include systemically acting agents such as fluconazole.

A single dose of triazole antifungals (e.g. 150 mg of fluconazole) has also been shown to be effective in most cases. Alternatively, topical azole antifungal agents can be applied daily for 7–14 days. Oral fluconazole in the dosage of 150 mg every 72 hours for three doses serves as an effective therapy for severe or complicated vulvovaginitis. This should be then followed by weekly doses for a few weeks. The underlying predisposing factors must be corrected to provide long-term relief. In cases of recurrent VVC, initial therapy should be with 150 mg of oral fluconazole every 72 hours for three doses, followed by maintenance dosage of fluconazole 150 mg once every week for 6 months. If oral fluconazole does not appear as a feasible option, a topical azole or an alternative oral azole (e.g. itraconazole) followed by maintenance therapy with topical antifungal agents must be instituted for 6 months.[13] Most clinicians prefer not to use fluconazole during pregnancy due to an increased risk of major congenital malformations. Administration of oral azoles during the first trimester is not recommended due to the risk of development of various birth defects such as abnormalities of cranium, face, bones, and heart after first trimester exposure to high-dose therapy (400–800 mg/day). Most clinicians, however, prefer to use topical formulations of imidazole (clotrimazole and miconazole) and triazole antifungals during pregnancy. Systemic absorption of these topical medications is minimal, posing little risk of transfer to the unborn baby. Topical nystatin is another safe alternative to azole antifungals that can be used during the first trimester of pregnancy. Since nystatin has negligible systemic absorption, there are unlikely to be any major malformations associated with the use of this drug. The recommended dose of nystatin during pregnancy is 1,00,000 units intravaginally once daily for 2 weeks. For symptomatic relief of redness or itching, short-term use of a low-potency topical corticosteroid is also considered as a safe option during pregnancy.

Corticosteroids: Topical corticosteroids are commonly prescribed to alleviate symptoms such as itchiness and redness, which may commonly occur in cases of VVC.

Treatment of sexual partners: Although sexual transmission of *Candida* species can occur, the present available evidence does not support treatment of sexual partners in cases of VVC. However, in woman with recurrent vulvovaginitis, this issue presently remains controversial.

Box 90.2: Criteria of complicated candidal infection

❑ Severe signs or symptoms of vulvovaginitis
❑ Identification of *Candida* species other than *C. albicans*, particularly *C. glabrata*
❑ Pregnancy, poorly controlled diabetes, immunosuppression, debilitation
❑ History of recurrent (≥4 per year) culture-verified vulvovaginal candidiasis

Breastfeeding women: The American Academy of Pediatrics (AAP) considers the use of fluconazole to be safe in breast-feeding infants. Also, nystatin can be used in nursing mothers because it does not enter the breast milk.

Complicated VVC: Complicated VVC includes recurrent or severe disease, or when there is the presence of adverse factors in the host (e.g. immunocompromised host). This also includes persistent infection with species other than *Candida albicans* (e.g. *C. glabrata, C. tropicalis,* etc.) due to the increasing use of over-the-counter antifungal medications.[14] Criteria for complicated candida infection are described in Box 90.2. By the time complicated VVC is diagnosed, the patient has already received conventional therapy with azoles and nystatin. Culture and sensitivity is usually advised in order to isolate the involved organism. However, in case of emergency situation, if infection with *C. glabrata* is suspected, while awaiting the culture results, it is a reasonable choice to administer the patient either nystatin or, if not available, miconazole nitrate 1,200 mg on alternate days. This can be used with oral itraconazole 200 mg daily for 2 weeks. Otherwise, treatment involves use of various salvage therapies. The aim of these 'salvage' therapies is to eradicate the organism from the vagina. Due to this, prolonged treatment for at least 2 weeks is necessary in most of the cases. There are, however, no randomised studies available and the optimum length of treatment presently remain unclear.

Salvage treatment: The optimal salvage therapy to be used in these patients is presently not known. One approach may be to use oral systemic fungicidal therapy in combination with topical therapy to penetrate into vaginal epithelia. The various salvage treatment options, which can be employed, are as follows:[15]

❖ *First-line salvage therapy*: The first-line salvage therapy can be considered as the use of intravaginal flucytosine (5FC) for 2–3 weeks in combination with amphotericin or nystatin (both being polyene antibiotics)

❖ *Second-line salvage therapy*: Following the failure of 5FC or nystatin, the next step is the administration of intravaginal boric acid. The typical dose of boric acid in case of VVC caused by *C. glabrata* is 600 mg intravaginally per night for 14 consecutive nights.[16] One should remember that boric acid capsules if swallowed orally can prove to be fatal. Presently, there is little evidence regarding the safety of boric acid in women at the time of pregnancy. Unless the vaginal epithelium is severely excoriated, only a limited amount of boric acid is systemically absorbed. Therefore, in most of the cases, the amount absorbed through the vaginal mucosa is minimal and risk to the unborn foetus is negligible.

❖ *Third-line salvage therapy*: The next treatment step presently remains unclear. Most clinicians consider a prolonged course, i.e. 4 weeks of either 5FC or nystatin or boric acid, but there is currently no strong evidence to support this.

❖ *Fourth-line salvage therapy*: If the patient still has persistent infection, the next step may depend on the susceptibility profile of the isolate *C. glabrata* which will usually remain susceptible to 5FC and moderately susceptible to azoles. In case there is resistance to 5FC, it would be a wise decision to use either boric acid or vaginal pessaries containing topical imidazoles, e.g. clotrimazole 500 mg or miconazole nitrate 1,200 mg on alternate days alongside intensive oral treatment. Systemic therapy with triazoles, such as voriconazole, posaconazole or high-dose fluconazole can also be considered. The length of course is unclear, but this may be dictated by the patient's ability to tolerate the drug.

❖ *Fifth-line salvage therapy*: If the patient still remains infected, then they may be effectively incurable. Suppressive vaginal boric acid may be a useful option here.

❖ For treatment of vaginitis caused by *C. krusei*, treatment comprises of intravaginal clotrimazole, miconazole, or terconazole for 7–14 days. For treatment of vaginitis caused by all other species of *Candida*, conventional dosage of fluconazole is preferred.

Vaginal Trichomoniasis

Metronidazole in the dose of 200 mg TDS or 375 mg BID must be prescribed to both the partners for a period of 7 days. The CDC, however, recommends a single dose of 2 g of metronidazole. This single dose regimen has been found to be associated with a greater cure rate varying from 90% to 95% in comparison to the week-long treatment with either 250 mg TID or 375 mg BID of metronidazole.[17] Additionally, the single-dose regimen is more convenient to take in comparison to 7-day regimen and is associated with better patient compliance. Since trichomoniasis is largely believed to be an STD, both the partners should be advised to avoid intercourse or use a condom during the course of therapy.[18] An alternative to metronidazole could be to prescribe tinidazole in the dose of 300 mg BD for 7 days or secnidazole in a single dose of 1,000 mg daily for 2 days.[19] The husband should be treated simultaneously, especially if the woman develops recurrent infection. Use of metronidazole is contraindicated during pregnancy and lactation.

During early pregnancy, the following may be used: vinegar douches to lower the vaginal pH, trichofuran suppositories and betadine gel.

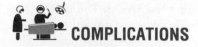

COMPLICATIONS

General Complications

These may include the following:
❖ Pelvic inflammatory disease
❖ Intrauterine infections

- ❖ Chorioamnionitis
- ❖ Postpartum endometritis
- ❖ Vaginitis emphysematous
- ❖ Preterm labour
- ❖ Premature rupture of membranes
- ❖ Newborn infections
- ❖ Low-birthweight babies.

Complications Specific to Bacterial Vaginosis

Some complications related to bacterial vaginosis are as follows:

- ❖ *Pelvic inflammatory disease*: Infection with bacterial vaginosis can cause PID, which can result in complications such as an increased frequency of endometritis, abnormal Papanicolaou (Pap) smears, abdominal pain, uterine bleeding, and uterine and adnexal tenderness. Performance of an invasive gynaecological procedure or surgery in a patient with bacterial vaginosis may result in the development of vaginal cuff cellulitis, PID and endometritis.
- ❖ *Pregnancy-related complications*: Bacterial vaginosis during pregnancy can result in complications like premature labour, preterm birth, low-birthweight babies, chorioamnionitis, postpartum endometritis, ectopic pregnancy and postcaesarean section wound infections.[20]
- ❖ Bacterial vaginitis in postpartum women can be associated with complications such as endometrial bacterial colonisation, plasma-cell endometritis, postpartum fever, postabortal infection, etc.
- ❖ Bacterial vaginosis can also be associated with post-hysterectomy vaginal cuff cellulitis.
- ❖ Bacterial vaginosis may act as a risk factor for acquisition and transmission of various STDs such as HIV, HSV type 2, gonorrhoea, and chlamydial infection.
- ❖ Bacterial vaginosis may also serve as a risk factor in development of precancerous cervical lesions.

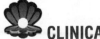

CLINICAL PEARLS

- ❖ The physiological vaginal discharge is formed by sloughing epithelial cells, normal bacteria and vaginal transudate. The quality and quantity of this physiological vaginal discharge may vary even in the same woman over different phases of menstrual cycle.
- ❖ In case of VVC and trichomoniasis, ideally, both the partners should be treated and be advised to avoid intercourse or use a condom during the course of therapy.
- ❖ For treatment of vaginal trichomoniasis, use of metronidazole is contraindicated during pregnancy and lactation. During early pregnancy, vinegar douches to lower the vaginal pH, trichofuran suppositories and Betadine® gel can be used.

EVIDENCE-BASED MEDICINE

- ❖ *Oral versus intravaginal administration of antifungal agents*: Present evidence does not indicate any significant difference in clinical cure rates of antifungals administered by the oral or intravaginal routes for the treatment of uncomplicated vaginal candidiasis.[13] Also, there is no evidence regarding the relative safety of oral or intravaginal antifungals for the treatment of uncomplicated vaginal candidiasis. The decision for prescription or recommendation for the purchase of a particular oral or intravaginal antifungal preparation should be based on the factors such as safety, cost, treatment preference and previous history of adverse reaction to one route of administration.[15]
- ❖ *Treatment of recurrent vulvovaginal candidiasis*: A systemic review and meta-analysis has shown that fluconazole in the dosage of 150 mg weekly, administered orally for 6 months served as an effective prophylaxis against recurrent vulvovaginal candidiasis.[21]

REFERENCES

1. Anderson MR, Klink K, Cohrssen A. Evaluation of vaginal complaints. JAMA. 2004;291(11):1368-79.
2. Carr PL, Felsenstein D, Friedman RH. Evaluation and management of vaginitis. J Gen Intern Med. 1998;13(5):335-46.
3. Sobel JD. Vaginitis. N Engl J Med. 1997;337(26):1896-903.
4. Chiaffarino F, Parazzini F, DeBesi P, Lavezzari M. Risk factors for bacterial vaginosis. Eur J Obstet Gynecol Reprod Biol. 2004;117(2):222-6.
5. Eckert LO, Hawes SE, Stevens CE, Koutsky LA, Eschenbach DA, Holmes KK. Vulvovaginal candidiasis: Clinical manifestations, risk factors, management algorithm. Obstet Gynecol. 1998;92(5):757-65.
6. Hammill HA. Trichomonas vaginalis. Obstet Gynecol Clin North Am. 1989;16(3):531-40.
7. Krohn MA, Hillier SL, Eschenbach DA. Comparison of methods for diagnosing bacterial vaginosis among pregnant women. J Clin Microbiol. 1989;27(6):1266-71.
8. Eschenbach DA, Hillier SL. Advances in diagnostic testing for vaginitis and cervicitis. J Reprod Med. 1989;34(8 Suppl):555-64.
9. Haefner HK. Current evaluation and management of vulvovaginitis. Clin Obstet Gynecol. 1999;42(2):184-95
10. Joesoef M, Schmid G. Bacterial vaginosis. In: Joesoef M, Schmid G (Eds). Clinical Evidence. London: BMJ Publishing Group; 2001. p. 887.
11. Morris M, Nicoll A, Simms I, Wilson J, Catchpole M. Bacterial vaginosis: a public health review. BJOG. 2001;108(5):439-50.
12. Hager WD, Brown ST, Kraus SJ, Kleris GS, Perkins GJ, Henderson M. Metronidazole for vaginal trichomoniasis. Seven-day vs singledose regimens. JAMA. 1980;244(11):1219-20.
13. Watson MC, Grimshaw JM, Bond CM, Mollison J, Ludbrook A. Oral versus intravaginal imidazole and triazole antifungal treatment of uncomplicated vulvovaginal candidiasis. Cochrane Database Syst Rev. 2001;(1):CD002845.
14. Horowitz BJ, Giaquinta D, Ito S. Evolving pathogens in vulvovaginal candidiasis: Implications for patient care. J Clin Pharmacol. 1992;32(3):248-55.

CHAPTER 90

15. Davies S, Johnson E, White D. How to treat persistent vaginal yeast infection due to species other than Candida albicans. Sex Transm Infect. 2013;89(2):165-6.

16. Guaschino S, De Seta F, Sartore A, Ricci G, De Santo D, Piccoli M. Efficacy of maintenance therapy with topical boric acid in comparison with oral itraconazole in the treatment of recurrent vulvovaginal candidiasis. Am J Obstet Gynecol. 2001;184(4):598-602.

17. Hanson JM, McGregor JA, Hillier SL, Eschenbach DA, Kreutner AK, Galask RP, et al. Metronidazole for bacterial vaginosis. A comparison of vaginal gel vs. oral therapy. J Reprod Med. 2000;45(11):889-96.

18. Lossick JG, Kent HL. Trichomoniasis: Trends in diagnosis and management. Am J Obstet Gynecol. 1991;165(4 Pt 2):1217-22.

19. Forna F, Gulmezoglu AM. Interventions for treating trichomoniasis in women. Cochrane Database Syst Rev. 2003; (2):CD000218.

20. Hillier SL, Nugent RP, Eschenbach DA, Krohn MA, Gibbs RS, Martin DH, et al. Association between bacterial vaginosis and preterm delivery of a low-birth-weight infant. The Vaginal Infections and Prematurity Study Group. N Engl J Med. 1995;333(26):1737-42.

21. Rosa MI, Silva BR, Pires PS, Silva FR, Silva NC, Silva FR, et al. Weekly fluconazole therapy for recurrent vulvovaginal candidiasis: a systematic review and meta-analysis. Eur J Obstet Gynecol Reprod Biol. 2013;167(2):132-6.

Pelvic Inflammatory Disease

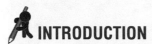 INTRODUCTION

Pelvic inflammatory disease (PID) represents a spectrum of infections and inflammatory disorders of the uterus, fallopian tubes and adjacent pelvic structures. This spectrum includes infections such as endometritis, salpingitis, tubo-ovarian abscess (TOA) and oophoritis. Five stages of PID as described by Gainesville are shown in the Table 91.1.[1]

Salpingitis is the inflammation of the fallopian tube, which is most commonly caused by an infection. The tubes become swollen, hyperaemic and oedematous. Some discharge of seropurulent fluid may occur from the fimbrial end of the tube. Initially, as the fimbrial end of the tube is open, pus discharge pours out into the pelvic cavity resulting in the formation of pelvic abscess.[2] Eventually, with the sealing of fimbrial end by fibrinous exudates, there is accumulation of pus in the tubal lumen, resulting in the formation of pyosalpinx. Involvement of ovaries, along with the tubes and presence of adhesions results in the development of TOA.

AETIOLOGY

Pelvic inflammatory disease occurs as a result of spread of microorganisms from the cervix upwards to the superior portion of genital tract such as fallopian tubes, ovaries and other adjacent structures resulting in the development of endometritis, salpingitis, parametritis, oophoritis, TOA and/or pelvic peritonitis, which form the spectrum of PID. *Chlamydia trachomatis* is responsible for approximately 25–50% cases of PID, whereas *Neisseria gonorrhoeae* is responsible for about 10–20% cases.[3,4] Mixed infection with both aerobic and anaerobic micro-organisms (*Gardnerella vaginalis, Bacteroides, Peptostreptococcus, Peptococcus, Prevotella, Atopobium, Leptotrichia,* etc.) may also be responsible for a substantial number of cases. Risk factors for occurrence of PID include sexual activity with multiple sexual partners, young age, procedures requiring cervical and uterine instrumentation such as intrauterine device insertion, endometrial biopsy, and dilation and curettage (D&C).

Pelvic inflammatory disease is typically associated with gonorrhoeal and chlamydial infection. Formation of peritoneal adhesions secondary to PID can compromise the motility of the fallopian tubes. Furthermore, obstruction of the distal end of the fallopian tubes results in accumulation of the normally secreted tubal fluid, creating distension of the tube. This subsequently causes damage to the epithelial cilia and may result in development of hydrosalpinx.

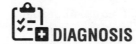 DIAGNOSIS

The features which are suggestive of a diagnosis of PID include the following described next.[3-6]

Clinical Presentation

Patients with PID may present with the following symptoms:
* Lower abdominal pain or tenderness (typically bilateral)
* Fever, nausea, vomiting and malaise
* Back pain
* Abnormal uterine bleeding (including postcoital and intermenstrual bleeding, menorrhagia, etc.)

Table 91.1: Stages of pelvic inflammatory disease[1]

Disease stage	Description
I	Acute salpingitis without peritonitis
II	Acute salpingitis with peritonitis
III	Acute salpingitis with superimposed tubal occlusion or TOA or ESR >50 mL/h
IV	Ruptured TOA or generalised peritonitis or septicaemia
V*	Adult respiratory distress syndrome

Abbreviations: TOA, tubo-ovarian abscess; ESR, erythrocyte sedimentation rate
*Suggested addition to the original classification

❖ Unusual or foul smelling, purulent vaginal or cervical discharge
❖ Dysuria and dyspareunia (typically deep).

Physical Examination

❖ *Pulse rate*: This may be increased due to fever
❖ *Temperature*: The body temperature may be elevated to more than 101°F (>38.3°C).

Abdominal Examination

There may be bilateral lower abdominal tenderness.

Pelvic Examination

❖ There may be cervical, uterine or adnexal tenderness on pelvic examination
❖ Uterus may be retroverted and immobile
❖ The appendages may be thickened and tender to touch.

Investigations

❖ *Blood investigations*: This must include a CBC along with differential leucocyte count and haematocrit. Blood culture may be required in cases of bacteraemia. Blood urea, serum electrolytes and levels of CRP may also be done. Diagnosis of PID is suggested by an elevated ESR or raised levels of CRP. However, these tests are non-specific.[7]
❖ Culdocentesis may be required to rule out ectopic pregnancy or to establish the diagnosis of ectopic pregnancy.
❖ *Laparoscopic examination*: This is not routinely required in cases of PID.
❖ *Urine investigations*: This must include urine pregnancy test in order to rule out pregnancy amongst the women of child-bearing age group. A routine urine analysis is also required to rule out infection.
❖ *Cervical culture*: This is required to rule out gonorrhoea and chlamydial infection. The absence of infection at this site, however, does not exclude PID because it is associated with a poor positive predictive value.[8]
❖ *Imaging studies such as ultrasound, CT and MRI*: A pelvic ultrasound may help in diagnosing complications such as ovarian cysts, TOAs, hydrosalpinx, pyosalpinx, ovarian torsion, ectopic pregnancy, etc. (Figs 91.1 to 91.3). TOA appears as a complex cystic adnexal mass with thick irregular walls and septations.
❖ *Screening for sexually-transmitted diseases*: All sexually active patients should be offered screening for sexually transmitted infections including HIV.[9]

DIFFERENTIAL DIAGNOSIS

❖ Appendicitis
❖ Ectopic pregnancy
❖ Haemorrhagic ovarian cysts, ovarian torsion
❖ Endometriosis, urinary tract infection
❖ Irritable bowel disease, cholecystitis, nephrolithiasis.

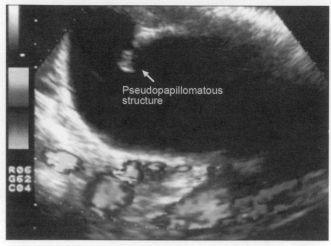

Fig. 91.1: Chronic hydrosalpinx: Dilated fallopian tube with thin-walled incomplete septations (*For colour version, see Plate 8*)

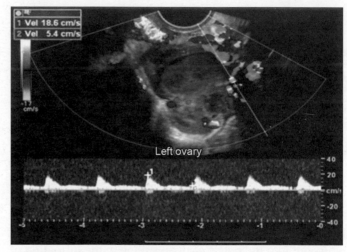

Fig. 91.2: Tubo-ovarian mass: Complex cystic solid structure showing prominent vascular perfusion with low-moderate vascular impedence on colour flow Doppler (*For colour version, see Plate 8*)

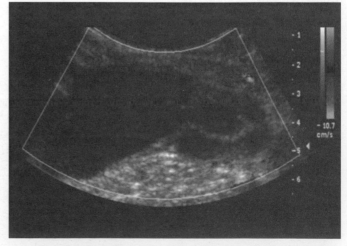

Fig. 91.3: Retort-shaped tubal mass suggestive of hydrosalpinx (*For colour version, see Plate 8*)

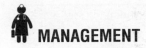

MANAGEMENT

General Management

❖ Patients, especially those with severe disease must be advised to take rest
❖ Suitable analgesia should be provided
❖ Patients should be advised to avoid unprotected intercourse until they, and their partner(s), have completed treatment and follow-up
❖ Accurate written information in the form of leaflets must be provided to the patient with particular emphasis on the long-term implications on their own health as well as their partner(s) due to PID, such as the future risk of infertility, chronic pelvic pain or ectopic pregnancy. They should be provided an explanation regarding the type of treatment being administered and its possible adverse effects. They should be counselled that clinically more severe disease is likely to be associated with a greater risk of future complications. Also, repeat episodes of PID are associated with an exponential increase in the risk of infertility. Administration of early treatment is likely to lower the risk of future fertility problems. The importance of screening her sexual contacts for STIs and treating them needs to be emphasised. She must be advised to use barrier contraception in future to reduce the risk of PID.

Medical Management

Medical therapy mainly comprises of broad-spectrum antibiotic therapy, covering organisms such as *N. gonorrhoeae*, *C. trachomatis* as well as a variety of aerobic and anaerobic bacteria commonly isolated from the upper genital tract in women with PID.[3,4]

The available evidence does not indicate superiority of one treatment regimen over the other.[10,11] A multicentric RCT, the PEACH (Pelvic Inflammatory Disease Evaluation and Clinical Health) randomised trial evaluating the effectiveness of inpatient and outpatient treatment strategies amongst women with mild-to-moderate PID has shown no significant difference in reproductive outcomes between women randomised to receive inpatient treatment and those randomised to outpatient treatment. Thus, outpatient therapy is likely to be as effective as inpatient treatment for patients with clinically mild-to-moderate PID. The choice of an appropriate treatment regimen may be influenced by factors enlisted in Box 91.1. Medical treatment mainly comprises of using antibiotics, pain-killers

---

Box 91.1: Indicators for appropriate treatment regimen in cases of pelvic inflammatory disease

❑ Local antimicrobial sensitivity patterns
❑ Local epidemiology of specific infections in the patient's residential setting
❑ Cost involved
❑ Patient's preference and compliance
❑ Patterns of disease severity

---

and IV fluids. In case of requirement for parenteral antibiotic therapy, hospital admission is necessary. The evidence-based antibiotic regimens (both inpatient and outpatient) for treatment of PID are shown in Box 91.2.[12-26]

Intravenous therapy is recommended for patients with severe PID (e.g. pyrexia >38°C, clinical signs of TOA, signs of pelvic peritonitis, etc.). IV therapy should be continued until 24 hours after clinical improvement and then switched to oral. Metronidazole is included in some regimens to improve coverage for anaerobic bacteria. Anaerobes are relatively more prevalent in cases of severe PID. Therefore, patients with mild or moderate PID are unlikely to be infected with anaerobic bacteria. In these cases, metronidazole may be discontinued, especially if the patient is unable to tolerate it.

Quinolones such as ofloxacin and moxifloxacin should be avoided in patients who are at an increased risk of gonococcal PID (e.g. when the patient's partner has gonorrhoea) due to an increase in quinolone resistance against gonococcal infection in the UK. Quinolones should also be avoided as first-line empirical treatment for PID in areas where more than 5% cases of PID are caused by quinolone resistant *N. gonorrhoeae*.

Levofloxacin is the isomer of ofloxacin and has the advantage of once daily dosing (500 mg OD for 14 days). It may be used as a more convenient alternative to ofloxacin.[20]

Replacing intramuscular ceftriaxone with an oral cephalosporin (e.g. cefixime) is not recommended because there is no clinical trial evidence to support its use. Also, oral administration may be associated with lower efficacy due to low tissue levels of this drug. Due to the reports of reduced susceptibility of *N. gonorrhoeae* to cephalosporins, the use of parenteral-based regimens is recommended in cases of gonococcal PID in order to maximise tissue levels and overcome low-level antibiotic resistance.

Surgical Management

Indications for surgery in cases of PID are enumerated in Box 91.3.[27] Drainage of a TOA can be done through minimal invasive surgery. Laparoscopy may also help in the early disease resolution through the division of adhesions.[28] However, ultrasound-guided aspiration of pelvic fluid collections is likely to be less invasive and may be equally effective.[29,30]

Pelvic Inflammatory Disease in Pregnant or Breastfeeding Patients

Pelvic inflammatory disease in pregnancy is associated with an increase in both maternal and foetal morbidity. Therefore, parenteral therapy is advised in pregnancy. However, none of the suggested evidence-based regimens have proved to be safe in this situation. Administration of the recommended antibiotic therapy during very early pregnancy is associated with a low risk because any significant drug toxicity during this period is likely to result in a failed implantation.

Treatment of Sexual Partners

Current male partners of women with PID should be contacted and offered health advice, screening and treatment

Box 91.2: Recommended antibiotic regimens for pelvic inflammatory disease[12-26]

Recommended outpatient regimen
Ceftriaxone 500 mg* IM in a single dose
Plus
Doxycycline 100 mg orally twice a day for 14 days
With or without
Metronidazole 400 mg orally twice a day for 14 days
Or
Cefoxitin† 2 g IM in a single dose and probenecid, 1 g orally administered concurrently in a single dose
Plus
Doxycycline 100 mg orally twice a day for 14 days
With or without
Metronidazole 500 mg orally twice a day for 14 days
Or
Other parenteral third-generation cephalosporin (e.g. ceftizoxime or cefotaxime)
Plus
Doxycycline 100 mg orally twice a day for 14 days
With or without
Metronidazole 500 mg orally twice a day for 14 days
Alternative outpatient regimens (in case of allergy, intolerance, etc.)
Intramuscular ceftriaxone 500 mg immediately, followed by azithromycin 1 g/week for 2 weeks
Or
Oral moxifloxacin 400 mg once daily for 14 days
Recommended inpatient regimens
Parenteral regimen A
Ceftriaxone 2 g IV every 12 h
Or
Cefoxitin 2 g IV every 6 h
Plus
Doxycycline 100 mg orally or IV every 12 h*
Plus
Oral metronidazole 400 mg twice daily for a total of 14 days

Parenteral regimen B
Clindamycin 900 mg IV every 8 h
Plus
Gentamicin§ loading dose IV or IM (2 mg/kg of body weight), followed by a maintenance dose (1.5 mg/kg) every 8 h. This can be substituted with a single daily dosing (7 mg/kg) followed by either oral clindamycin 450 mg 4 times daily or oral doxycycline 100 mg twice daily plus oral metronidazole 400 mg twice daily to complete 14 days

Cefoxitin must be discontinued 24 h after improvement in the patient's symptoms and doxycycline must be continued in the dosage of 100 mg PO BID for a total of 14 days. If tubo-ovarian abscess is present, clindamycin or metronidazole can be added for better anaerobic coverage.
Alternative inpatient regimens (in case of allergy, intolerance, etc.)
IV ofloxacin 400 mg BD
Plus
IV metronidazole 500 mg TID for 14 days
Or
IV ciprofloxacin 200 mg BD
Plus
IV (or oral) doxycycline 100 mg BD
Plus
IV metronidazole 500 mg TID for 14 days

---

*Clinical trial data support the use of cefoxitin for the treatment of PID but this agent is not easily available in the UK so ceftriaxone, which has a similar spectrum of activity, is recommended.
†The dose of ceftriaxone has been increased to 500 mg stat to reflect the reduced sensitivity of *Neisseria gonorrhoeae* to cephalosporins and the current UK treatment guidelines for uncomplicated gonorrhoea.
§Gentamicin levels along with the renal function tests need to be monitored if this regimen is used.

PART III

Box 91.3: Indications for surgical intervention in cases of pelvic inflammatory disease[27]

- Lack of response or intolerance to oral therapy
- Clinically severe disease
- Acute spreading peritonitis resistant to medical treatment
- Presence of a pyoperitoneum
- Intestinal obstruction
- Drainage of a pelvic abscess
- Ruptured tubo-ovarian abscess
- Suspected intestinal injury
- Removal of septic products of conception from the uterine cavity
- Concomitant pregnancy

for gonorrhoea and chlamydia preferably in a genitourinary medicine clinic. Other recent sexual partners (within 6 months period of onset of symptoms) may also be traced and offered screening. If gonorrhoea or chlamydia is diagnosed in the male partner, it should be treated suitably alongside with the index patient. Since many cases of PID are not associated with gonorrhoea or chlamydia infection, broad-spectrum empirical therapy should also be offered to male partners, e.g. azithromycin 1 g single dose. If screening for gonorrhoea is not available, additional specific antibiotics effective against *N. gonorrhoeae* should be offered, e.g. ceftriaxone 500 mg single dose IM. Partners should be advised to avoid intercourse until they and the index patient have completed the course of treatment.

Women with Concomitant Human Immunodeficiency Virus Infection

Women with HIV may have more severe symptoms associated with PID but respond well to standard antibiotic therapy. Therefore, no change in treatment recommendations is required in HIV-infected patients in comparison to those not infected with HIV.[30-32] Hospital admission and parenteral therapy may be required in those with a clinically severe disease. Before prescription of specific antibiotics, their interactions with antiretroviral drugs need to be considered.

Pelvic Inflammatory Disease with Intrauterine Device In Situ

If an IUCD is in situ in cases of PID, its removal can be considered if this is likely to improve short-term clinical outcomes or there is no improvement in the symptoms even after 3 days of antibiotic administration.[33] The decision to remove the IUCD needs to be balanced between the risk of pregnancy in those who have had otherwise unprotected intercourse in the preceding 7 days and the improvement in clinical outcomes with its removal. Hormonal emergency contraception may be considered for some women in this situation.[33,34]

Follow-up

Cases with moderate or severe PID should be particularly reviewed at 72 hours. They should ideally be showing a substantial improvement in clinical symptoms and signs at this time, if they have been receiving appropriate medical care. In case they fail to show significant improvement, they require further investigations, parenteral therapy and/or surgical intervention.

Further, review 2–4 weeks after therapy may be useful to ensure that there is adequate clinical response to treatment, the patient is compliant with oral antibiotics and to repeat pregnancy test, if clinically indicated. This is also the period when the patient's sexual contacts should be screened and treated. The patient and her partner or sexual contacts should be made aware of the significance of PID and its sequelae.

COMPLICATIONS

- ❖ Ectopic pregnancy
- ❖ Infertility
- ❖ Chronic pelvic pain
- ❖ Tubo-ovarian abscess
- ❖ Pelvic adhesions
- ❖ Distension of ampullary portion more than that of the isthmic portion results in the development of a fluid-filled or pus-filled retort-shaped mass, respectively, known as the hydrosalpinx and pyosalpinx.
- ❖ Rarely, there may be an upwards spread of infection, resulting in the development of peritonitis, paralytic ileus, subdiaphragmatic and perinephric abscess, Fitz-Hugh-Curtis syndrome, etc. The Fitz-Hugh-Curtis syndrome (Fig. 91.4) comprises of right upper quadrant pain associated with perihepatitis and may occur in some women with PID. Although laparoscopic division of hepatic adhesions has been attempted in some cases, presently there is insufficient evidence to justify its routine use in cases beyond uncomplicated PID.

CLINICAL PEARLS

- ❖ Pelvic inflammatory disease almost exclusively occurs in sexually active women and amongst adolescents.
- ❖ Symptoms related to PID are usually worse at the end of a menstrual period and for a few days afterwards.
- ❖ A diagnosis of PID and empirical antibiotic treatment should be considered in sexually active young (under 25) non-pregnant woman who experience recent onset of bilateral lower abdominal pain associated with local tenderness on bimanual vaginal examination.
- ❖ Tubo-ovarian abscess can be defined as the collection of pus involving the tubes and the ovary.
- ❖ The major clinical significance of a hydrosalpinx is its adverse effect on fertility, thereby resulting in a reduced pregnancy rate.

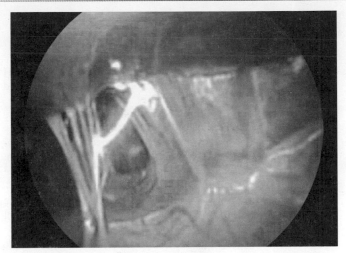

Fig. 91.4: Fitz-Hugh-Curtis syndrome *(For colour version, see Plate 8)*

- ❖ A hydrosalpinx, although sterile, can be reinfected at a later date leading to the development of a pyosalpinx.

EVIDENCE-BASED MEDICINE

- ❖ Patients with PID may present with symptoms or may be asymptomatic. Even when present, clinical symptoms and signs lack adequate sensitivity and specificity in establishing the diagnosis of PID. The positive predictive value of a clinical diagnosis is 65–90% in comparison to the laparoscopic diagnosis.[4-6]
- ❖ Presently, there is no or minimal evidence to indicate that laparoscopic adhesiolysis in cases of Fitz-Hugh-Curtis syndrome is superior to the use of antibiotic therapy alone.[3]
- ❖ Presently, there is insufficient evidence to recommend a specific regimen or empirical therapy in cases of PID in pregnant women. The antibiotic regimen used should preferably comprise of agents effective against gonorrhoea, chlamydia and anaerobic infections after taking into account local antibiotic sensitivity patterns. All the recommended regimens are of similar efficacy. There is no evidence indicating the superiority of one antibiotic regimen over the other.[10,11]
- ❖ Though the available good-quality evidence supports the use of moxifloxacin in cases of PID due to its high efficacy, it is not commonly used due to the high risk of complications such as hepatic reactions and other serious risks (such as QT interval prolongation).[20,22,23] Oral moxifloxacin should, therefore, be used only when it is considered inappropriate to use the other commonly used antibacterial agents for PID or when these treatment options have failed.
- ❖ There is no clear evidence of the superiority of any one of the suggested regimens over the others for patients with PID. Therefore, patients known to be allergic to one of the suggested regimens should be treated with an alternative.[10,11]

REFERENCES

1. Paruk F. Pelvic inflammatory disease. In: Kurger TF, Botha MH (Eds). Clinical Gynaecology, 3rd edition. Cape Town: Juta and Co. Ltd.; 2007. pp. 166-76.

2. Brunham RC, Gottlieb SL, Paavonen J. Pelvic inflammatory disease. N Engl J Med. 2015;372(21):2039-48.

3. Templeton A. The Prevention of Pelvic Infection: Recommendations Arising from the 31st RCOG Study Group. London: RCOG Press; 1996. pp. 267-70.

4. Bevan CD, Johal BJ, Mumtaz G, Ridgway GL, Siddle NC. Clinical, laparoscopic and microbiological findings in acute salpingitis: report on a United Kingdom cohort. Br J Obstet Gynaecol. 1995;102(5):407-14.

5. Morcos R, Frost N, Hnat M, Petrunak A, Caldito G. Laparoscopic versus clinical diagnosis of acute pelvic inflammatory disease. J Reprod Med. 1993;38(1):53-6.

6. Centers for Disease Control. (2006). Sexually Transmitted Diseases Treatment Guidelines 2006. Morbidity and Mortality Weekly Report. [online] Available from www.cdc.gov/mmwr/preview/mmwrhtml/rr5511a1.htm. [Accessed October, 2016].

7. Miettinen AK, Heinonen PK, Laippala P, Paavonen J. Test performance of erythrocyte sedimentation rate and C- reactive protein in assessing the severity of acute pelvic inflammatory disease. Am J Obstet Gynecol. 1993;169(5):1143-9.

8. Yudin MH, Hillier SL, Wiesenfeld HC, Krohn MA, Amortegui AA, Sweet RL. Vaginal polymorphonuclear leukocytes and bacterial vaginosis as markers for histologic endometritis among women without symptoms of pelvic inflammatory disease. Am J Obstet Gynecol. 2003;188(2):318-23.

9. Ross JD, Ison CA. UK National Screening and Testing Guidelines for STIs. Sex Transm Infect. 2006;82(Suppl IV): iv1-iv5.

10. Ness RB, Soper DE, Holley RL, Peipert J, Randall H, Sweet RL, et al. Effectiveness of inpatient and outpatient treatment strategies for women with pelvic inflammatory disease: results from the Pelvic Inflammatory Disease Evaluation and Clinical Health (PEACH) Randomized Trial. Am J Obstet Gynecol. 2002;186(5):929-37.

11. Ness RB, Trautmann G, Richter HE, Randall H, Peipert JF, Nelson DB, et al. Effectiveness of treatment strategies of some women with pelvic inflammatory disease: a randomized trial. Obstet Gynecol. 2005;106(3):573-80.

12. Arredondo JL, Diaz V, Gaitan H, Maradiegue E, Oyarzún E, Paz R, et al. Oral clindamycin and ciprofloxacin versus intramuscular ceftriaxone and oral doxycycline in the treatment of mild-to- moderate pelvic inflammatory disease in outpatients. Clin Infect Dis. 1997;24(2):170-8.

13. Hemsell DL, Little BB, Faro S, Sweet RL, Ledger WJ, Berkeley AS, et al. Comparison of three regimens recommended by the Centers for Disease Control and Prevention for the treatment of women hospitalized with acute pelvic inflammatory disease. Clin Infect Dis. 1994;19(4):720-7.

14. Martens MG, Gordon S, Yarborough DR, Faro S, Binder D, Berkeley A. Multicenter randomized trial of ofloxacin versus cefoxitin and doxycycline in outpatient treatment of pelvic inflammatory disease. Ambulatory PID Research Group. South Med J. 1993;86(6):604-10.

15. Walker CK, Kahn JG, Washington AE, Peterson HB, Sweet RL. Pelvic inflammatory disease: meta-analysis of antimicrobial regimen efficacy. J Infect Dis. 1993;168(4):969-78.

16. Wendel GD, Cox SM, Bawdon RE, Theriot SK, Heard MC, Nobles BJ. A randomized trial of ofloxacin versus cefoxitin and doxycycline in the outpatient treatment of acute salpingitis. Am J Obstet Gynecol. 1991;164(5 Pt 2):1390-6.

17. Soper DE, Brockwell NJ, Dalton HP. Microbial etiology of urban emergency department acute salpingitis: treatment with ofloxacin. Am J Obstet Gynecol. 1992;167(3):653-60.

18. Peipert JF, Sweet RL, Walker CK, Kahn J, Rielly-Gauvin K. Evaluation of ofloxacin in the treatment of laparoscopically documented acute pelvic inflammatory disease (salpingitis). Infect Dis Obstet Gynecol. 1999;7(3):138-44.

19. Isaacson DM, Fernadez JA, Frosco M, Foleno BD, Goldschmidt RM, Amaratunga D, et al. Levofloxacin: A review of its antibacterial activity. Recent Res Devel in Antimicrob Agents Chemotherapy. 1996;1:391-439.

20. Judlin P, Liao Q, Liu Z, Reimnitz P, Hampel B, Arvis P. Efficacy and safety of moxifloxacin in uncomplicated pelvic inflammatory disease: the MONALISA study. BJOG. 2010;117(12):1475-84.

21. Savaris RF, Teixeira LM, Torres TG, Edelweiss MI, Moncada J, Schachter J. Comparing ceftriaxone plus azithromycin or doxycycline for pelvic inflammatory disease: a randomized controlled trial. Obstet Gynecol. 2007;110(1):53-60.

22. Bevan CD, Ridgway GL, Rothermel CD. Efficacy and safety of azithromycin as monotherapy or combined with metronidazole compared with two standard multidrug regimens for the treatment of acute pelvic inflammatory disease. J Int Med Res. 2003;31(1):45-54.

23. Heystek M, Ross JD, PID Study Group. A randomised double-blind comparison of moxifloxacin and doxycycline/metronidazole/ciprofloxacin in the treatment of acute, uncomplicated pelvic inflammatory disease. Int J STD AIDS. 2009;20(10):690-5.

24. Ross JD, Cronje HS, Paszkowski T, Rakoczi I, Vildaite D, Kureishi A, et al. Moxifloxacin versus ofloxacin plus metronidazole in uncomplicated pelvic inflammatory disease: results of a multicentre, double blind, randomised trial. Sex Transm Infect. 2006;82(6):446-51.

25. Witte EH, Peters AA, Smit IB, van der Linden MC, Mouton RP, van der Meer JW, et al. A comparison of pefloxacin/metronidazole and doxycycline/metronidazole in the treatment of laparoscopically confirmed acute pelvic inflammatory disease. Eur J Obstet Gynecol Reprod Biol. 1993;50(2):153-8.

26. Heinonen PK, Teisala K, Miettinen A, Aine R, Punnonen R, Grönroos P. A comparison of ciprofloxacin with doxycycline plus metronidazole in the treatment of acute pelvic inflammatory disease. Scand J Infect Dis Suppl. 1989;60:66-73.

27. Reich H, McGlynn F. Laparoscopic treatment of tuboovarian and pelvic abscess. J Reprod Med. 1987;32(10):747-52.

28. Aboulghar MA, Mansour RT, Serour GI. Ultrasonographically guided transvaginal aspiration of tuboovarian abscesses and pyosalpinges: an optional treatment for acute pelvic inflammatory disease. Am J Obstet Gynecol. 1995;172(5): 1501-3.

29. Corsi PJ, Johnson SC, Gonik B, Hendrix SL, McNeeley SG, Diamond MP. Transvaginal ultrasound-guided aspiration of pelvic abscesses. Infect Dis Obstet Gynecol. 1999;7(5):216-21.

30. Cohen CR, Sinei S, Reilly M, Bukusi E, Eschenbach D, Holmes KK, et al. Effect of human immunodeficiency virus type 1 infection upon acute salpingitis: a laparoscopic study. J Infect Dis. 1998;178(5):1352-8.

31. Bukusi EA, Cohen CR, Stevens CE, Sinei S, Reilly M, Grieco V, et al. Effects of human immunodeficiency virus 1 infection on microbial origins of pelvic inflammatory disease and on efficacy of ambulatory oral therapy. Am J Obstet Gynecol. 1999;181(6):1374-81.

32. Irwin KL, Moorman AC, O'Sullivan MJ, Sperling R, Koestler ME, Soto I, et al. Influence of human immunodeficiency virus infection on pelvic inflammatory disease. Obstet Gynecol. 2000;95(4):525-34.

33. Altunyurt S, Demir N, Posaci C. A randomized controlled trial of coil removal prior to treatment of pelvic inflammatory disease. Eur J Obstet Gynecol Reprod Biol. 2003; 107(1):81-4.

34. Soderberg G, Lindgren S. Influence of an intrauterine device on the course of an acute salpingitis. Contraception. 1981; 24(2):137-43.

CHAPTER 91

SECTION 17

Pregnancy Prevention

GYNAECOLOGY

Contraception (Temporary and Permanent)

INTRODUCTION

The goal of family planning is to enable couples and individuals to freely choose how many children to have and when to have them. This can best be done if the healthcare attendant provides them with a full range of safe and effective contraceptive methods and gives them sufficient information to ensure that they are able to make informed choices. Various contraceptive methods are based on three general strategies: (1) prevention of ovulation; (2) prevention of fertilisation or (3) prevention of implantation. Various methods for contraception are described in Box 92.1. Efficacy of different contraceptive agents is described in Figure 92.1. Amongst these, are various methods, which provide long-term contraception and need to be administered less than once per month or cycle. As a result, they are more cost-effective than the combined hormonal methods of contraceptions. Some such long-acting reversible contraceptives (LARC) include the following:

❖ Non-hormonal methods [intrauterine devices (IUDs) or IUCDs]
❖ Hormonal systems [intrauterine systems (IUS)]
❖ Progestogen-only injectable contraception
❖ Progestogen-only implants.

These various methods would be subsequently dealt with in the text.

INDICATIONS

Contraception may be required for the following conditions:
❖ Postponement of first pregnancy
❖ Birth spacing and control
❖ Prevention of pregnancy.

MANAGEMENT

The detailed use of each contraceptive has been described individually. The United Kingdom Medical Eligibility Criteria

---

Box 92.1: Various methods of contraception

Temporary methods
❑ Natural regulation of fertility
❑ Barrier methods
❑ Hormonal contraception
  – Combined hormonal contraception (CHC)
    ◊ Combined oral contraceptive pills (COCPs):
      - Monophasic pills (each tablet containing a fixed amount of oestrogen and progestogen)
      - Biphasic pills (each tablet containing a fixed amount of oestrogen, while the amount of progestogen increases in the luteal phase of the cycle)
      - Triphasic pills (the amount of oestrogen may be fixed or variable, while the amount of progestogen increases over three equally divided phases of the cycle)
    ◊ Evra® patch
    ◊ NuvaRing®
  – Progestogen-only contraception
    ◊ Progestin-only pill (POP)
    ◊ Injections (Depo-Provera®)
    ◊ Implants (Norplant® I and II)
    ◊ Patches
    ◊ Vaginal rings
❑ Intrauterine contraceptive devices
❑ Emergency (postcoital) contraception
Permanent methods
❑ Sterilisation
❑ Female sterilisation
❑ Vasectomy

(UKMEC) for the use of various contraceptive methods, adapted from the WHO medical eligibility criteria (WHOMEC), has been described in Table 92.1.[1,2] This classification system (Categories 1–4) is applicable for all hormonal methods, intrauterine devices (copper IUD and levonorgestrel IUD), emergency contraception and barrier methods. Classification systems for the fertility awareness-based methods, and male and female sterilisation are different and are described in Tables 92.2 and 92.3, respectively. UKMEC for the use of

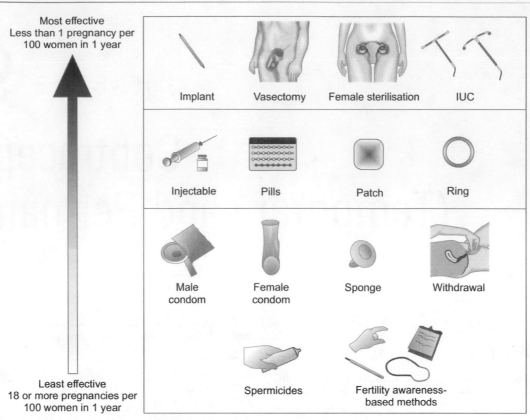

Fig. 92.1: Efficacy of different contraceptive agents

Abbreviation: IUC, intrauterine contraception

Table 92.1: UK medical eligibility criteria (UKMEC) for contraceptive use[1]

Category	Description
UKMEC 1	A condition where there is no restriction for the use of the contraceptive method
UKMEC 2	A condition where the advantages of using the method generally outweigh the theoretical or proven risks
UKMEC 3	A condition where the theoretical or proven risks usually outweigh the advantages of using the method
UKMEC 4	A condition that represents an unacceptable health risk if the contraceptive method is used

Table 92.2: Definitions of UK categories for fertility awareness-based methods[1]

UK category		Fertility awareness-based methods
A	Accept	There is no medical reason to deny the particular fertility awareness method to a woman in this circumstance
C	Caution	The method is normally provided in a routine setting, but with extra preparation and precautions. For the various fertility awareness-based methods, special counselling of the couple may be required to ensure correct use of the method
D	Delay	Use of the method should be delayed until the condition is evaluated or changes. Alternative temporary methods of contraception should be offered

Table 92.3: Definitions of UK categories for sterilisation[1]

UK category		Sterilisation
A	Accept	There is no medical reason to deny sterilisation to a man or woman in this circumstance
C	Caution	The procedure is normally provided in a routine setting, but with extra preparation and precautions
D	Delay	Use of the method should be delayed until the condition is evaluated or changes. Alternative temporary methods of contraception should be offered
S	Special	The procedure should be undertaken in a setting with an experienced surgeon and staff, equipment needed to provide general anaesthesia, and other back-up medical support. For these conditions, the capacity to decide on the most appropriate procedure and the method of anaesthesia is also required. Alternative temporary methods of contraception should be provided, if referral is required or there is otherwise any delay

different contraceptive methods in presence of various medical disorders can be obtained from the website of the faculty of sexual and reproductive health (www.FSRH.org).[1]

PART III

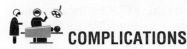

COMPLICATIONS

The specific complications associated with different types of contraceptives have been individually described.

CLINICAL PEARLS

❖ The prescription of a contraceptive device must be individualised

❖ The type of contraception, which must be prescribed to a particular patient, is the one that provides effective contraception, acceptable cycle control and is associated with least side effects.

COMBINED HORMONAL CONTRACEPTION

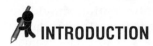

INTRODUCTION

Oral Contraceptive Pills

There are two main types of hormonal contraception, first being the combined hormonal contraception (CHC) (containing both oestrogen and progestogen), commonly available as combined oral contraceptive pills (COCPs), patch and an intravaginal ring, and the second being the formulations containing progestogen only. Three types of COCPs formulations are available: (1) monophasic pills; (2) biphasic pills and (3) triphasic pills. The dosage of oestrogen and progestogen is changed during the various phases of cycle in biphasic and triphasic pills, thereby imitating the body's cyclical variation in the hormonal levels. Most traditional COCPs are contained in a compact package of 21 active pills and 7 inactive pills (or no pills) and are taken as 21/7 regimens. The most commonly used such formulation in the UK is Yasmin®, which comprises of 3 mg drospirenone (DRSP) and 0.03 mg ethinyl oestradiol. Some COCPs formulations which are not consumed as 21/7 regimens have been introduced in the UK. Some such newly available contraceptive pills include, Zoely® and Qlaira®.

Zoely®: Zoely® is a type of hormonal contraception containing two active ingredients, 1.5 mg ethinyl oestradiol and 2.5 mg nomegestrol acetate (NOMAC). It has been marketed in the UK since May 2013. Ethinyl oestradiol present in Zoely® is identical to the endogenous human 17 β-oestradiol, while nomegestrol acetate is a progestogenic agent with strong antigonadotropic and mild anti-androgenic properties. It is taken as a 24/4 regimen, having 24 active tablets followed by 4 inactive pills. There is no pill-free interval. Randomised trials have shown that OCP containing combination of NOMAC and ethinyl oestradiol (e.g. Zoely®) is likely to provide high contraceptive efficacy with acceptable

Table 92.4: Dosage of various hormones in Qlaira®

No. of pills	Colour	Dosage of oestradiol valerate	Dosage of dienogest
First two pills	Dark yellow	3 mg oestradiol	–
3rd to 7th pill	Medium red	2 mg oestradiol	2 mg dienogest
8th to 24th pill	Light yellow	2 mg oestradiol	3 mg dienogest
25th and 26th pill	Dark red	1 mg oestradiol	–
27th and 28th pill	White (placebo pills)	–	–

cycle control similar to that of COCPs containing a combination of DRSP and ethinyl oestradiol.[3] The overall adverse event profile of these two types of OCP formulations was also found to be similar. Some women taking Zoely® may experience side effects such as weight gain and acne. Withdrawal bleeding associated with Zoely® is shorter and lighter in comparison to other hormonal agents. Withdrawal bleeding may be sometimes completely absent with Zoely®.

Qlaira®: Qlaira® is a COCP containing oestradiol valerate (E2V) and dienogest (DNG) in the dosage as described in Table 92.4. This pill delivers 17-β oestradiol which is similar to that released in the body. It is taken as 26/2 regimen, further reducing the pill free interval to 2 days. Reduction in the pill-free interval is likely to result in a decline in the oestrogen withdrawal symptoms such as mood changes, headache, menstrual loss, pelvic pain, etc.

Qlaira® (E2V and DNG) has proven to be safe, effective and well-tolerated in three large-scale clinical trials conducted across Europe and North America.[4-7] Qlaira® is associated with a failure rate of 0.4 per 100 women year (WY) which is similar to that reported with the conventional COCP. Majority of women using Qlaira® are satisfied with its use. Use of Qlaira® is likely to result in a bleeding profile similar to that of an ethinyl oestradiol-based combined oral contraceptive (COC).[8] Qlaira® is well tolerated and associated with a low incidence of adverse events and serious adverse events similar to other low-dose oral contraceptices.[7]

Women treated with Qlaira® are likely to experience a shorter, lighter episode of withdrawal bleeding. Withdrawal bleeding may be frequently absent.[4] Some women may be concerned about the absence of withdrawal bleeding, so they need to be counselled regarding the fact that the presence or absence of withdrawal bleeding with Qlaira® treatment may not always be an indicator of contraceptive efficacy. Qlaira® has proven to be useful for the treatment of heavy menstrual bleeding (HMB).[7] Clinical trials have shown that use of Qlaira® serves as an oral, non-invasive, reversible and fertility-conserving treatment, which helps in causing a significant, rapid and sustained reduction in the menstrual blood loss by approximately 90% after 6 months of treatment in comparison with baseline data.[9,10]

Evra® Patch

This is the first transdermal patch contraceptive releasing 20 µg of oestradiol and 150 µg of norelgestromin every

CHAPTER 92

24 hours. It is applied weekly for 3 weeks followed by a patch free interval. Its efficacy, cycle control and side-effects profile is similar to that of other COCPs.[11,12] An RCT has shown that extended use of the Evra® transdermal patches (weekly application for 12 consecutive weeks, 1 patch-free week and 3 more consecutive weekly applications) is likely to delay menses and result in fewer bleeding days in comparison to the cyclical use (four consecutive cycles of 3 weekly applications and 1 patch-free week) of these patches. This regimen may represent a useful alternative for women who prefer fewer episodes of withdrawal bleeding.[13] Therefore, extended use of Evra® patches may represent a useful alternative for women preferring fewer episodes of withdrawal bleeding.

NuvaRing®

NuvaRing® is a combined hormonal contraceptive vaginal ring made up of flexible plastic material (ethylene-vinyl acetate copolymer) manufactured by Merck and is available on prescription. It releases 120 µg of etonogestrel and 15 µg of ethinyl oestradiol daily. It is 54 mm in diameter and 4 mm in thickness. Contraceptive efficacy, cycle control and compliance of NuvaRing® has been found to be higher in comparison to COCPs.[14] The incidence of side effects such as breast tenderness, headache and nausea is comparable to the conventional COCPs containing 30 µg of ethinyl oestradiol. However, women using NuvaRing® are likely to experience a higher rate of local complications such as vaginitis, leucorrhoea, foreign body sensation, expulsion, etc.

AETIOLOGY

Combined hormonal contraceptive methods act through following mechanisms:

❖ Prevention of ovulation
❖ Thickening of mucus at the cervix so that sperms cannot pass through
❖ Changing the environment of the uterus and fallopian tubes to prevent fertilisation and/or implantation.

MANAGEMENT

❖ Patient assessment prior to prescription of combined hormonal contraception (CHC): Before prescription a thorough history should be taken, including potential contraindications, smoking history and medications. The physical examination should include a blood pressure measurement.
❖ A pelvic examination is not mandatory before prescription
❖ Adequate counselling prior to initiation of CHCs may help to improve compliance and adherence.

Prescription

Yasmin®

❖ Conventionally, the COCPs must be started during the first day of the menstrual cycle.

❖ Once a woman has started taking a COCPs, it is important for her to be consistent and take the pill regularly at the same time each day.
❖ Women who use a 21-day preparation need to take the pills for 21 days followed by a 7-day pill-free interval. She should be cautioned not to exceed the 7-day pill-free interval between packs.

• If the woman forgets to take one or two tablets of 21-day preparation, e.g. Yasmin®, she should take the most recent pill as soon as she remembers and then continue to take the remaining pills as usual. This may mean taking two pills on the same day (one at the time of remembering and other at the regular time) or even both at the same time.
• If the woman forgets to take three or more tablets, she should take the most recent pill as soon as she remembers and then continue to take the remaining pills as usual. She should be advised to use condoms or abstain from sexual activities until she takes the pills for 7 days continuously.
• Additionally, if the woman misses taking a pill in week 1 (first 7 days), the pill-free interval has been extended. Emergency contraception should be considered if she had unprotected sexual activity during the pill-free interval in the week 1. Also, if the woman misses taking the pills in week 3, it is important to avoid extending the pill-free interval. In these cases, she should be counselled to finish all the remaining active pills in the pack, omit the pill-free interval and start the new pack from the next day.
• Backup method of contraception (e.g. condoms, foam) may be required in case the woman exceeds the pill-free interval of 7 days; experiences a serious adverse effect or requires protection from STDs.

Zoely®

❖ If the woman has not been using any hormonal contraceptive method in the past month, she should start taking Zoely® on first day of her menstrual bleeding. When doing so, no additional contraceptive measures are necessary. She needs to take one pill every day for a period of 28 days (24 active pills + 4 placebo pills). The successive pack must be started immediately after finishing the previous pack without having a break in the daily tablet intake and irrespective of presence or absence of withdrawal bleeding.
❖ If the woman has been using any of the hormonal contraceptive method (ring, patch or COCP) in the past month, she should start with Zoely® preferably on the day after the last active tablet (of her previous COC). At the latest, Zoely® must be started on the day following the usual tablet-free or placebo tablet interval of her previous COC. In case a vaginal ring or transdermal patch has been used, the woman should start using Zoely® preferably on the day of removal, but at the latest when the next application would have been due.
❖ The missed pill guidelines for Zoely® are as follows:
• *Pill missed on days 1–7*: The missed pill must be taken as soon as possible and extra precautions must be observed for next 1 week.

- *Pill missed on days 8–17*: The last missed pill must be consumed as soon as possible. Rest of the pack must be finished in a similar manner.
- *Pill missed on days 18–24*: In these cases, the four inactive pills must be omitted and the next packet must be started straight away.

Qlaira®

If the woman has not been previously taking hormonal contraceptive agents in the past month, she should start taking Qlaira® from the first day of her menstrual bleeding. If she had been previously taking some form of combined hormonal contraceptive (COCP, vaginal ring, or transdermal patch), she should start with Qlaira® on the day after the last active tablet of her previous COC. In case a vaginal ring or transdermal patch has been used, the woman should start using Qlaira® on the day of removal. In case the woman forgets to take a pill for more than 12 hours, the missed pill regimen is as follows:

- ❖ *Pill missed on days 1–17*: The missed pill must be taken immediately as soon as the woman remembers it. The subsequent pill must be taken at the usual time even if it means taking two pills at the same time. Rest of the packet must be consumed in a similar manner. Use of additional contraceptive method or abstinence must be practiced for 9 days rather than 7 days as in case of conventional 21/7 regimen COCPs.
- ❖ *Pill missed on days 18–24*: Rest of packet must be discarded. The woman must start taking the first pill from a new packet and this packet must be consumed in a usual manner. Use of additional contraceptive method or abstinence must be practiced for 9 days.
- ❖ *Pill missed on days 25 and 26*: The missed tablet must be taken immediately. The next tablet must be taken at the usual time even if it means taking two tablets on the same day. Additional contraceptive protection is not required in these cases.
- ❖ *Pill missed on days 27 and 28*: The forgotten tablets must be discarded and rest of the tablets continued in a normal way. No additional contraception is required.

Evra® Patch

As previously described, an Evra® patch must be applied weekly for 3 weeks followed by a patch free interval. In case the woman forgets to apply a patch for more than 12 hours, the missed patch regimen is as follows:

- ❖ If the woman applies the patch late during week 1, she should apply a new patch as soon as she remembers. If she is more than 48 hours late in the application of the new patch, new patch must be applied as soon as she remembers. However, a backup method for contraception must be used for a week following the application of the new patch. If during this period, the patient has a sexual intercourse without using a backup method, she should use emergency contraception.
- ❖ *If the woman applies the patch late during week 2 or 3*:
  - If she is less than 48 hours late in changing her patch, she should be advised to change it as soon as she remembers. She should change to her next patch as she would have normally done.
  - If she is more than 48 hours days late in changing her patch, she should change it as soon as she remembers it and then wear it for 1 week. She should then continue to change to the next patch on the same day of the next week.
  - A backup method for contraception must be used for a week following the application of the new patch. If during this period, the patient has a sexual intercourse without using a backup method, she should use emergency contraception.
- ❖ If the woman forgets to apply the patch on time during the 4th week, she should be advised to remove the patch when she remembers. A new patch must be applied on her regular patch change day.

NuvaRing®

The ring is placed inside the vagina for every 3 weeks followed by a ring-free interval of 1 week. Subsequently, a new ring must be inserted.

Follow-up

Follow-up visit in cases of CHC is required after 6 weeks to check patient compliance and well-being.

Extended and Continuous Regimens of Combined Oral Contraceptive Pills

The efficacy of COCPs may be reduced if the pills are missed at the beginning of the pack, in this manner extending the days without the active pills. This increases the risk of ovulation, thereby increasing the failure rate of the pills. Continuous or extended use of OCPs is likely to reduce this risk of ovulation by reducing the number of active pills which are missed when the pack is delayed. Continuous or extended use of COCPs, respectively, involves continuous intake of active contraceptive pills without any period of inactive pills or greatly increasing the interval at which inactive pills are taken. Some OCP products, which have been approved for extended or continuous contraception include, Seasonale®, Seasonique® and Lybrel®. Seasonale® contains 84 days of active pills and 7 days of inactive pills. Seasonique® contains 84 days of active pills and 7 days of low-dose oestrogen pills. Lybrel® contains a full year of active pills with no inactive pills. A Cochrane review has shown that bleeding pattern with extended or continuous regimens is similar to that of cyclic regimens. Nevertheless, the women with extended or continuous regimens may at times experience bothersome uterine bleeding. Extended or continuous use regimens are also likely to reduce menstrual symptoms, including dysmenorrhoea and premenstrual symptoms.[15]

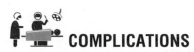

COMPLICATIONS

Minor side effects: These include clinical features such as irregular bleeding, breast tenderness, nausea, weight gain and mood changes. One of the major problems associated with combined hormonal preparations is poor compliance and discontinuation.

Major risks: These include side effects such as venous thromboembolism, myocardial infarction, stroke, gallbladder disease, breast cancer, cervical cancer, etc.

The patient should be counselled to report any adverse effects related to the use of COCPs, which can be remembered with the mnemonic *ACHES*:

A—Abdominal pain (severe)

C—Chest pain (severe), cough, shortness of breath or sharp pain upon breathing

H—Headache (severe), dizziness, weakness or numbness (especially one-sided)

E—Eye problems (complete loss of or blurring of vision)

S—Severe leg pain (calf or thigh).

 ## CLINICAL PEARLS

❖ The use of COCPs provides a protective effect against the development of ovarian and endometrial cancer and probably even colorectal cancer.

❖ Use of COCPs is a highly effective method of reversible contraception, with the failure rate being approximately 0.1 per 100 WYs of use.

❖ Combined oral contraceptive pills do not provide any protection against STDs or HIV infection.

❖ Normal menstrual cycles are likely to occur in 99% of the women within 6 months of stopping the pills. However, return of fertility may be slightly late due to delayed return of ovulation.

❖ Combined hormonal contraceptive agents such as Zoely® and Qlaira® are non-enzyme inducing agents. Therefore, antibiotics can be easily used in patients using these hormonal contraceptive agents.

❖ Women may or may not experience withdrawal bleeding while using hormonal methods of contraception.

 ## EVIDENCE-BASED MEDICINE

❖ There is no evidence that the COCPs cause teratogenic effects if taken inadvertently during pregnancy.[16-19]

❖ The available evidence demonstrates that extended and continuous cycle OCPs are likely to have efficacy similar to that of classic 21 + 7 cyclic OCPs.[20-22]

PROGESTOGEN-ONLY PILL

 ## INTRODUCTION

Progestogen-only containing contraceptive methods are available in various formulations:

❖ Progestogen-only pill (POP) or minipill

❖ Subdermal contraceptive implants (Norplant® I, II and implanon)

❖ Progestogen-only injectables (POI), e.g. depot medroxyprogesterone acetate (DMPA)

❖ Intrauterine system (Mirena® and progestasert).

Progestogen-only pills shall be discussed here. Other types of progestogen-only contraceptive methods have been subsequently discussed in the chapter. There are two different types of POP:

1. *Three-hour progestogen-only pill*: These are traditional POPs, which must be taken within 3 hours of the same time each day. The POPs may contain 350 µg of norethisterone or 75 µg of norgestrel or 30 µg of levonorgestrel. Some examples of POPs include Femulen®, MicroNor®, Norgeston® and Noriday®.

2. *Twelve-hour progestogen-only pill*: These include desogestrel pill, such as Cerazette®, which must be taken within 12 hours of the same time each day.

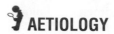 ## AETIOLOGY

Progestogen-only pills act through the following mechanisms: Thickening of cervical mucus, thereby reducing sperm viability and penetration

❖ Making the endometrium unfavourable to implantation

❖ *Inhibition of follicular development and ovulation*: This effect of POP is variable and may only occur in about 60% cases. However, in case of Cerazette®, desogestrel-only pill, the main mode of action is inhibition of ovulation.

 ## MANAGEMENT

Prescription

Progestogen-only pills must be started on the first day of menstrual cycles. Unlike the COCPs, these pills must be taken on a continuous basis without any breaks between packets. These must be consumed in accordance with a strict time schedule everyday (within 3 hours for traditional POPs vs 12 hours for Cerazette®). If a woman is more than 3 hours late taking a dose, she should take another pill as soon as she remembers. The next pill must be taken at the usual time. If the woman missed taking more than one pill, she just needs to take one pill as soon as she remembers. The next pill must be taken at the usual time. A backup method should be used for 2 days if a woman is more than 3 hours late taking a dose. Backup contraception should be considered during the first month when the woman first starts taking minipills and then at midcycle every month thereafter (the time when ovulation is likely to occur).

 ## COMPLICATIONS

❖ *Changes in the bleeding pattern*: Irregular bleeding, spotting, break through bleeding, amenorrhoea, etc.

❖ Depression, headache, migraine

❖ Weight gain and ectopic pregnancy

- ❖ Mastalgia (breast tenderness)
- ❖ Mood swings
- ❖ Abdominal cramps.

CLINICAL PEARLS

- ❖ Unlike the COCPs, minipills are not associated with an increased risk of complications such as venous thrombo-embolism, myocardial infraction, stroke, heart disease or breast cancer.
- ❖ Minipills are recommended over COCPs in women who are breastfeeding because they do not affect milk production. These pills can also be safely used in women of any age-group with a history of migraine (with or without aura).
- ❖ Effectiveness of POPs may vary between 0.3 per 100 WY and 8.0 per 100 WY. The efficacy of POPs is likely to be lower in older women (>40 years) in comparison to the younger women.
- ❖ Cerazette® is an oestrogen-free, progestogen-only oral contraceptive pill containing 75 μg of desogestrel.

EVIDENCE-BASED MEDICINE

- ❖ The available evidence suggests that the failure rates of the traditional POP and the desogestrel pill are similar. Amongst the breastfeeding women, the difference in efficacy between the traditional POPs and desogestrel is likely to be insignificant. Desogestrel, however, may be more effective than levonorgestrel in women, who are not breastfeeding. The potential for better efficacy of desogestrel is counterbalanced by its higher incidence of adverse events (e.g. irregular bleeding patterns) in comparison to levonorgestrel.
- ❖ The available evidence does not suggest that the efficacy of any POP is reduced in obese women weighing more than 70 kg.

INJECTABLE CONTRACEPTIVES (PROGESTOGENS)

INTRODUCTION

Injectable contraceptives comprise of delivering certain hormonal drugs in form of deep intramuscular injections into the muscles of arms or buttocks. Three types of injectable progestogen-only contraceptive formulations are available in the UK: (1) DMPA, intramuscular and subcutaneous formulations; and (2) norethisterone enanthate (NETEN) (Table 92.5).[23] Combined formulations of injectable contraceptives (e.g. Mesigyna®, Cyclofem®, etc.), containing both progestogen and oestrogen, are available in some countries of Asia, Africa and Latin America.

Table 92.5: Different types of injectable contraceptives

Name	Active ingredients	Dosage
Progestogen-only injectables (POIs)		
Depot-medroxyprogesterone acetate (DMPA) (progestogen-only); available as a Provera (most commonly used in the UK)	150 mg medroxyprogesterone acetate in an aqueous microcrystalline suspension	150 mg administered by deep IM injection after every 90 days/12 weeks
DMPA (progestogen-only) subcutaneous; available in the UK since June 2013	104 mg/0.65 mL, Sayana® Press formulation	This progestogen-only formulation is administered subcutaneously via a new delivery system, which is available in a prefilled injector, every 13 weeks (±7 days)
NETEN (progestogen-only); available as Noristerat and is licensed for short-term use in the UK	200 mg norethisterone enanthate in an oily preparation	It is administered via deep IM injection every 8 weeks/60 days

These preparations overcome the inconvenience of daily compliance required with POPs or COCP. This is a suitable method for women in whom oestrogens present health risks. Besides contraceptive benefit, injectable contraceptives also help in improving the symptoms of dysmenorrhoea and endometriosis.

AETIOLOGY

The mechanism of action of injectable progestogens is similar to that of POPs as described previously in the text.

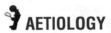

MANAGEMENT

Prescription

The intramuscular DMPA formulation must be injected into the thigh, buttocks or deltoid muscle four times a year (every 11–13 weeks) and provides pregnancy protection starting a week after the first injection. The subcutaneous DMPA injection can be administered over the anterior part of thigh, upper arm or abdomen. The ideal time for initiating DMPA injection is within 7 days of the onset of menses.

The injection site should not be massaged afterwards, since this may accelerate absorption of the drug. Since DMPA is an aqueous suspension, a DMPA vial must be shaken vigorously, before it is loaded into the syringe, to resuspend any active ingredient in the bottom of the vial. The syringe should then be checked to ensure that it contains the correct dosage. Any leakage from the syringe should be checked and kept under control.

COMPLICATIONS

* *Menstrual irregularities*: Disruptions of the menstrual cycle including amenorrhoea, prolonged menses, spotting between periods, and heavy or prolonged bleeding.
* *Other side effects*: These include adverse effects such as weight gain, headache, dizziness and low bone mass.

CLINICAL PEARLS

* Injectable contraceptive provide women with safe, highly effective and reversible contraceptive protection, with the failure rate being 0.1–0.4 per 100 WY g use.
* Contraceptive efficacy of these injectable formulations is not reduced by the simultaneous use of enzyme-inducing drugs (e.g. rifampicin, carbamazepine, phenytoin, etc.). Therefore, injection intervals need not be reduced in women taking these drugs.
* Progestogen-only injectables can be used by breastfeeding women at 6 weeks postpartum without adverse effects on nursing infants.
* Fertility is not impaired after discontinuation of DMPA or NETEN, although its return may be delayed.
* They do not provide protection against HIV and STDs.

EVIDENCE-BASED MEDICINE

* The available evidence shows subcutaneous preparation of DMPA-SC to be an effective and well-tolerated contraceptive option, having similar contraceptive efficacy and side-effects such as rates of bone loss, amenorrhoea, weight gain and return of fertility as the intramuscular preparation of DMPA-IM.[24] Use of DMPA-SC is especially beneficial for women on anticoagulant therapy because use of DMPA-IM in these women may result in development of haematoma. DMPA-SC may also be more useful amongst obese women.
* Concerns have been raised regarding the potential harmful effects of DMPA on the bone mineral density (BMD), especially amongst the women less than 18 years of age (who have yet not attained their peak bone mass) or amongst elderly women approaching menopause (when some bone loss is likely to occur). Although the use of DMPA is associated with loss of BMD, current evidence suggests that recovery of BMD occurs after discontinuation of DMPA. Moreover, there is no high-quality evidence to indicate the effect of DMPA on the potential risk of fractures in adolescents or adults later in life. The effect of DMPA on BMD and potential fracture risk should not prevent practitioners from prescribing DMPA or continuing use beyond 2 years. According to the guidelines by Medicines and Healthcare products Regulatory Agency (MHRA, UK) which are endorsed by the Faculty of Sexual and Reproductive Health (FSRH), the healthcare practitioner needs to balance the potential health risks associated with the adverse effects of DMPA on BMD against a woman's likelihood of pregnancy using other methods or no method, and the known negative health and social consequences associated with unintended pregnancy, particularly among adolescents.[25] DMPA can be used as the first-line contraception in women under the age of 18 years if all other options for contraception are considered to be unsuitable or unacceptable. Other methods of contraception should be preferably considered in women, having significant lifestyle and/or medical risk factors for osteoporosis.

SUBDERMAL PROGESTOGEN IMPLANTS

INTRODUCTION

Contraceptive implant is a method of birth control, where the device is inserted under the skin. Available subdermal implants are as follows:

* *Nexplanon®*: The only subdermal contraceptive implant in the UK
* Norplant® I and Jadelle® (Norplant® II) (not available in the UK).

These implants ensure slow, sustained release of progestogens. It is long-acting form of contraception, which is associated with minimal side effects.

Nexplanon®: Nexplanon® is a bioequivalent of implanon, which has largely replaced implanon and is the only subdermal implant available in the UK.[26] It comprises, a single radio-opaque small, soft rod, about 4 cm in length, containing 68 mg of etonogestrel in the membrane of ethylene vinyl acetate. It is licensed for 3 years of use.

Norplant® I: This contains six silastic capsules made up of siloxane of the size 34 mm × 2.4 mm, with each containing about 36 mg of levonorgestrel. Its effects last for approximately 5 years.

Norplant® II or Jadelle®: This comprises of two rods, each containing about 70 mg of levonorgestrel. The daily release of hormone is about 50 mg and it provides protection for 3–5 years. Though Norplant® I and II are not available in the UK, the healthcare professionals in the UK may encounter women from other countries using these implants.

AETIOLOGY

Mechanism of action of subdermal implants is as follows:
* Inhibition of ovulation
* Thickening of cervical mucus making it difficult for sperm to pass through
* Changes in the endometrium making the environment unfavourable for implantation.

MANAGEMENT

The implants are inserted on first day of the menstrual cycle. If the woman does not receive the implant on the first 5 days of her periods, a back-up method of contraception should be used for 1 week following insertion of the implant if the patient indulges in sexual intercourse. Following application of a local anaesthetic over the upper arm, a needle-like applicator is used to insert the Nexplanon® rod under the skin into the subdermal tissues on the upper side of the arm between biceps and triceps.[27] The average time required for insertion varies between half and one minute. A bandage must be kept on the site of insertion for about 24 hours afterwards.

This implant can be removed anytime the patient desires pregnancy. Since the capsules are non-biodegradable, they need removal at the end of use or earlier if the side effects are intolerable. Both insertion and removal of these implants require local anaesthesia and a small incision and must be performed by an experienced clinician. A small incision is made on the skin over the implant, which is then removed using forceps.

COMPLICATIONS

❖ *Bleeding abnormalities*: These may include problems such as menstrual irregularities, oligomenorrhoea, amenorrhoea, etc. Sexual history must be taken to establish the risk of STI amongst women who complain of problematic bleeding while using the subdermal implants. The patient must also be investigated for the presence of an underlying gynaecological pathology, especially if clinically indicated. In case the STIs and other gynaecological abnormalities have been ruled out, bleeding abnormalities can be treated using mefenamic acid or ethinyl oestradiol.
❖ *Weight gain*: This may occur between 5% and 15% of the women using subdermal implants.
❖ *Complications related to removal*: This could be related to implants which are deeply embedded, are non-palpable and have broken or migrated from their position. Since Nexplanon® is radiopaque, it can be identified with the help of 2D X-rays, CT scan, ultrasound and MRI.
❖ The main disadvantage associated with this form of contraception is that the woman cannot start or stop using this method on her own. Implants must be inserted in and removed by a specially trained practitioner.
❖ *Other changes*: This may include changes in the mood, loss of libido, acne, etc.
❖ Some amount of discomfort may be present for several hours following insertion.
❖ Removal is sometimes painful and often more difficult than insertion.
❖ Ectopic pregnancy can occur in approximately 1.3% patients.
❖ Pregnancy rate varies from 0.2 per 100 WY to 1.3 per 100 WY
❖ This is an expensive form of contraception.

CLINICAL PEARLS

❖ Return of fertility is almost immediate, following the removal of the implant.
❖ It does not harm the quality and quantity of the breast milk and can be used by nursing mothers starting 6 weeks after childbirth.
❖ Contraceptive efficacy of these implants is reduced by the simultaneous use of enzyme-inducing drugs (e.g. rifampicin, carbamazepine, phenytoin, etc.). Therefore, simultaneous use of condoms is recommended in these cases.
❖ Prophylactic antibiotics at the time of insertion or removal of implants are not required for prevention of endocarditis.

EVIDENCE-BASED MEDICINE

❖ There is little evidence to suggest that the use of subdermal implants have any clinically significant effect on the BMD.[28]
❖ The available evidence indicates that the risk of venous thrombosis is not significantly increased with use of subcutaneous implants.[29]

INTRAUTERINE CONTRACEPTIVE DEVICES

INTRODUCTION

Intrauterine contraceptive devices are flexible plastic devices, made up of polyethylene, which are inserted inside the uterine cavity for the purpose of contraception. Each device has a nylon thread which protrudes through the cervical canal into the vagina, where it can be felt by the patient or the doctor. Initially, biologically inert devices such as Lippes loop and saf-T-coil were introduced, which have now been withdrawn from the market. Newer devices are medicated and contain substances such as copper, progestogens, etc. Copper carrying devices include, copper T 200, copper 7, multiload, copper 250, copper T 380, copper T 220 and nova T. Their effective life varies from 3 years to 5 years. T-shaped IUCDs (Cu380 A or paraguard) which have copper on their arms, containing at least 380 mm² of copper can be considered as the IUCD of choice. They are likely to be most effective and have the longest duration of action (approximately 10–12 years). A state-of-the-art recent advance in intrauterine contraception has been the development of the SCu300A intrauterine ball (IUB).[30] This is a 3D, spherical copper IUCD, which is inserted and removed in the manner similar to the 2D T-shaped IUCDs. It is spherical in shape, which helps in reducing the likelihood of complications such as perforation, malposition and expulsion.

CHAPTER 92

Table 92.6: Comparison of size between Mirena® and Jaydess®

Type of IUS	Height (mm)	Breadth (mm)
Mirena®	32	32
Jaydess® (Skyla)®	30	28

Intrauterine contraceptive devices containing progestogen include progestasert, Levosert and Mirena®. These devices are known as IUS. Mirena®, the IUS available in the UK, is a type of progestogen-containing IUCD, having 52 mg of levonorgestrel, which is released at the rate of 20 µg/day. The effects of Mirena® last for about 5 years. It is sometimes also known as levonorgestrel-intrauterine system (LNG-IUS). Another levonorgestrel-containing IUS which has been recently introduced in the UK is Jaydess®, also known as Skyla® (Bayer). It is slightly smaller in size in comparison to Mirena® (Table 92.6). As a result, this device can be used in younger and even nulliparous women. Jaydess® contains 13.5 mg of levonorgestrel, which is released at the rate of 6–10 µg per day. It is licensed for use for a period of 3 years. It has a silver ring, which differentiates it from Mirena® on ultrasound and enables its visualisation by X-ray. Initial placement of Jaydess® is easier and less painful for women in comparison to Mirena®. However, bleeding profiles of both are similar.[31-33]

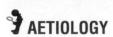

AETIOLOGY

The possible mechanisms of action of IUCD are as follows:
- ❖ Copper IUCD acts as a foreign body in the uterine cavity, which makes migration of spermatozoa difficult
- ❖ Increased release of prostaglandins provokes uterine contractility. This causes the fertilised egg to be rapidly propelled along the fallopian tube so that it reaches the uterine cavity before the development of chorionic villi and thus is unable to implant
- ❖ Leucocytic infiltration of the endometrium
- ❖ Presence of copper results in certain enzymatic and metabolic changes in the endometrial tissues, which may inhibit implantation of the fertilised ovum.

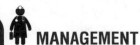

MANAGEMENT

Prior to Insertion

- ❖ *Informed consent*: Prior to insertion, informed consent should be obtained and the patient should be aware of the potential side effects, benefits and alternative methods of contraception. It should be emphasised to the patient that the IUCD does not provide protection against STIs or HIV.
- ❖ *Per speculum examination*: The cervix should be carefully inspected for any signs of infection prior to IUCD insertion. If there is any evidence of mucopurulent discharge or pelvic tenderness, cervical swabs should be sent for culture and sensitivity and IUCD insertion delayed until the infection (if present) has been treated
- ❖ *Pelvic examination*: A pelvic examination must be performed prior to the procedure to determine the position and the size of uterus.

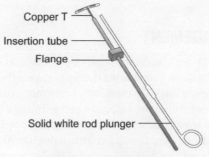

Fig. 92.2: Parts of a copper device

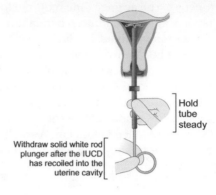

Fig. 92.3: Method of insertion of intrauterine contraceptive device

Insertion

- ❖ Various parts of a copper IUCD are shown in Figure 92.2, whereas the method for insertion is shown in Figure 92.3.
- ❖ Cervix is grasped with vulsellum or Allis forceps
- ❖ Length of the uterine cavity is determined with help of an uterine sound
- ❖ The copper device with an insertion tube is available in presterilised packs. The IUCD is mounted into the insertion tube and the flange on the insertion tube is adjusted according to the length of the uterine cavity
- ❖ The insertion tube is then passed into the uterine cavity through the cervix
- ❖ As the solid white rod plunger is put inside the insertion tube, the IUCD recoils within the uterine cavity
- ❖ After withdrawing the plunger, insertion tube is removed and the nylon thread is cut to the required length. The speculum and the forceps are then removed.

Postinsertion

- ❖ The patient is instructed to examine herself and feel for the thread every week
- ❖ A follow-up visit should be scheduled 6 weeks post-insertion for the exclusion of presence of infection, an assessment of any abnormal bleeding and evaluation of the patient and partner satisfaction
- ❖ An IUCD user should be instructed to contact her health-care provider if any of the following occur: IUCD's threads

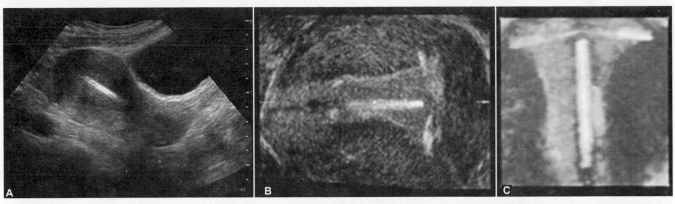

Figs 92.4A to C: (A) Two-dimensional ultrasound showing the presence of copper device in the uterine cavity; (B and C) Three-dimensional ultrasound showing the presence of an intrauterine copper device

cannot be felt; she or her partner can feel the lower end of the IUCD; she experiences persistent abdominal pain, fever, dyspareunia and/or unusual vaginal discharge, etc.

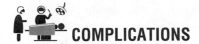

COMPLICATIONS

* *Difficulties at the time of insertion*: Immediate difficulties at the time of insertion include vasovagal attack, difficulty in insertion of the copper device and presence of uterine cramps. In case the patient experiences a vasovagal attack, the clinician must immediately abandon the procedure and remove the coil as well as the instruments; lower the patient's head end and elevate her legs; monitor the patient's pulse and blood pressure; administer oxygen to the patient and administer atropine IV in the dosage of 0.6 mg/mL (if the patient's heart rate is <40 beats/min or systolic BP is <90 mmHg).
* *Bleeding*: Irregular menstrual bleeding, spotting, menorrhagia, etc. are the most common side effects of copper containing IUCDs in the first month after insertion. Use of NSAIDs or tranexamic acid may be helpful. With the use of LNG-IUS, there may be irregular bleeding or spotting during the first 6–8 months following insertion. However, by 1 year, light bleeding or amenorrhoea usually ensues.
* *Pain or dysmenorrhoea*: Pain may be a physiological response to the presence of the copper-containing device, but the possibility of infection, malposition of the device (including perforation) and pregnancy should be excluded. The LNG-IUS has been associated with a reduction in menstrual pain.
* *Systemic hormonal side-effects*: These may be typically associated with the LNG-IUS and include side effects such as depression, acne, headache and breast tenderness
* *Functional ovarian cysts*: They may occur in up to 30% of LNG-IUS users and usually resolve spontaneously.
* *Uterine perforation*: Uterine perforation is a rare, but serious complication of IUCD insertion, occurring at a rate of 0.6–1.6 per 1,000 insertions. This may occur either at the time of insertion or at a later stage due to the embedment of the device into the myometrium and its subsequent

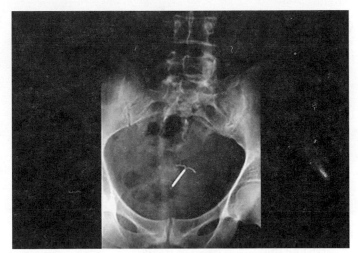

Fig. 92.5: An X-ray showing intrauterine device inside the abdominal cavity, confirming the diagnosis of uterine perforation

migration into the intra-abdominal cavity. If the IUCD strings are not seen in the cervical os, the device may have been expelled or may have perforated the uterine wall. If the IUCD strings cannot be found, ultrasound is the preferred method to identify the location of the IUCD (Figs 92.4A to C). If the device is not identified within the uterus or the pelvis, a plain X-ray of the abdomen should be performed to determine whether the device has perforated the uterine wall (Fig. 92.5)

* *Infection or pelvic inflammatory disease*: Infection at the time of insertion can result in the development of pelvic inflammatory disease (PID) in the long run. To prevent the occurrence of vaginal infection, IUCD users should continue to use condoms for protection against STDs. Overall risk for development of PID is low in women in whom IUCD has been inserted unless the women is at a high risk for STIs (e.g. history of multiple sexual partners in the last years). Such women must be offered testing for *Chlamydia trachomatis* at the minimum. If the results for STI testing are not available at the time of insertion, prophylactic antibiotics must be provided at least against Chlamydia.

CHAPTER 92

If the woman with IUCD in situ shows signs and symptoms suggestive of pelvic infection, appropriate antibiotics may be commenced, preferably after taking appropriate swabs. The device may require removal if the symptoms fail to improve even 72 hours after commencement of antibiotics.

Actinomycosis infection may also commonly occur and the presence of actinomyces-like organisms may be detected on the smear in these patients. If the woman shows no signs and symptoms of pelvic infection, there is no need to remove the IUCD or to commence antibiotics. Medical advice must be, however, sought if the symptoms of infection develop.

❖ *Expulsion*: Expulsion of the IUCD is most common in the first year of use (2–10% of users)
❖ *Ectopic pregnancy*: Ectopic pregnancy can sometimes occur with IUCD in situ.

CLINICAL PEARLS

❖ It is a highly effective method of contraception with the pregnancy rate being 2–6 per 100 WY.
❖ Though IUCD is commonly inserted in multiparous women, nulliparity is not a contraindication for IUCD use. It can be successfully used in carefully selected nulliparous women.
❖ If given a choice between levonorgestrel and copper IUCDs, the majority of women choose levonorgestrel-based IUCDs due to the lack of negative side-effects and the associated beneficial effects such as reduction in dysmenorrhoea and menstrual blood loss.
❖ Levonorgestrel-intrauterine system is often used as the first-line therapy in cases of HMB.
❖ Intrauterine contraceptive devices per se do not increase the risk of ectopic pregnancy. However, in women who conceive with an IUCD in place, the diagnosis of ectopic pregnancy should be excluded.
❖ The copper IUCD may decrease the risk of endometrial cancer.

EVIDENCE-BASED MEDICINE

❖ The available evidence indicates that amongst the various types of IUCDs, TCu380A or TCu380S appear to be more effective than other IUCDs.[34]
❖ There is no evidence to indicate that a particular type of IUCD is associated with a lower rate of complications such as expulsion rates, bleeding and pain in comparison to other IUCDs.[34]

NATURAL FAMILY PLANNING METHODS

INTRODUCTION

Also known as the fertility awareness methods, the natural family planning methods aim at controlling childbirth by instructing the couple to abstain from sexual intercourse during the fertile period of menstrual cycle. These methods are based on the fact that there are only few days during the menstrual cycle when conception can occur. Following ovulation, which occurs once in the menstrual cycle, the egg remains viable for 12–24 hours, whereas the sperm may remain viable for 2–5 days in the female genital tract. The fertile period must be, therefore, calculated by allowing for the survival time of the sperm and ovum.

Being natural, these methods are free of side effects associated with hormonal or intrauterine devices. These methods can also be used in cases of medical illnesses, which contraindicate the use of hormonal contraception. Some women may also choose natural methods on the basis of moral or religious grounds. Some of these methods are described next.

Calendar or rhythm method: In this method, the fertile period is calculated by subtracting 18 days from the shortest cycle and 10 days from the longest cycle after recording the cycle length for a minimum of six cycles. This would give the first and the last day of the fertile period, respectively. The couple must be instructed to abstain from sexual relations during this period. For example, if the shortest cycle is of 25 days and the longest cycle is of 36 days, then she should perceive the period of her maximum fertility to be starting from day 7 (25–18 = 7) through till day 26 (36–10 = 26). In order to avoid pregnancy, she should abstain from having sexual intercourse between day 7 and day 26.

Basal body temperature method: This method is based on the fact that basal body temperature (BBT) increases by 0.2–0.5°C following ovulation due to thermogenic effect of hormone progesterone (Fig. 92.6). The couple must be instructed that the safest way to use BBT for avoiding pregnancy is to avoid intercourse or use a barrier method during at least the first half of the menstrual cycle until 3 days after there has been a rise in BBT.

Ovulation method (cervical mucus or Billings method): This method is based on the fact that as the fertile time approaches, the cervical mucus increases in amount, becomes clearer in colour, wetter, stretchy and slippery (spinnbarkeit phenomenon). Following ovulation, the mucus usually becomes sticky, thicker and pasty in character and reduces in amount (Fig. 92.7). Sexual intercourse is considered safe during the days immediately following the menses until the cervical mucus attains the above-described characteristics. Thereafter, the couple must abstain from having sexual intercourse until the 4th day after the 'peak mucus day'.

Coitus interruptus (withdrawal): This is a method in which the man takes his penis out of the woman's vagina just before he ejaculates. Ejaculation may or may not take place afterwards. This technique, however, requires considerable control on the part of man.

Symptothermal method: This method includes the combination of calendar, BBT and cervical mucus methods.

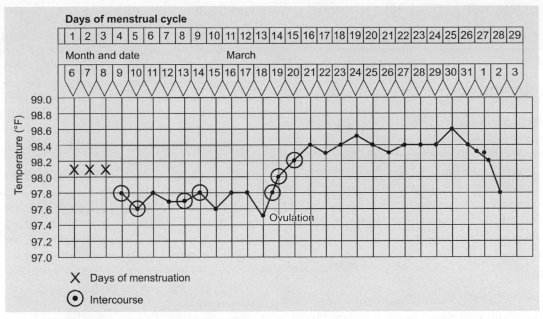

Days of menstrual cycle

Month and date   March

Fig. 92.6: Basal body temperature method

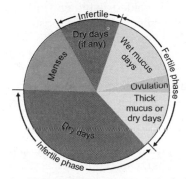

Fig. 92.7: Cervical mucus method

Lactational amenorrhoea method: There is only a 1–2% chance of becoming pregnant in lactating woman who fulfils the following three conditions:
1. She is breastfeeding her baby on demand, both day and night and not feeding him or her other foods or liquids regularly
2. Menses has not yet returned and
3. The baby is less than 6 months of age.

Women who fulfil these three conditions are naturally protected against pregnancy. Hence, this method is also considered as the natural family planning method.

Personal fertility monitors: Persona® monitor (Swiss Precision Diagnostics GmbH, Switzerland) is a *h*and-held device, which measures the woman's urine levels of oestrone-3-glucuronide and LH at home to determine the fertile period.[35] As a contraceptive device, Persona displays a green light during the infertile phase and a red light during the fertile phase. A symbol is also displayed in this device during the fertile phase which indicates the surge in LH and impending ovulation. Women may use these devices to prevent pregnancy by avoiding intercourse (or using back-up methods of contraception) during the phase when the red light is displayed.

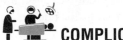

COMPLICATIONS

❖ These methods require a learning period, careful record keeping, periodic abstinence and partner's cooperation. These methods require long periods of sexual abstinence.
❖ They do not provide protection against HIV infection and other STDs.
❖ *High failure rate*: Perfect use is associated with a failure rate of 2%, whereas typical use is associated with a failure rate of 20%.

CLINICAL PEARLS

❖ Fertility awareness methods are natural and safe and there are no side effects.
❖ These methods are associated with high failure rates of approximately 20–25 pregnancies per 100 WY of use.
❖ The high failure rate associated with these methods commonly results due to irregular ovulation or irregular menstrual cycles.

EVIDENCE-BASED MEDICINE

The available evidence shows that the Persona® fertility monitor is likely to be effective in nearly 94% of women desiring to avoid pregnancy.[35] Additionally, an Italian study has shown that in nearly 95% cases, the fertile phase determined by the Persona® monitor is likely to correlate well with follicular growth and ovulation, as observed on ultrasound images and confirmed with serum levels of LH and progesterone.[36] However, further studies are required in future to show that use of personal fertility monitors may serve as a useful option for family planning.

CHAPTER 92

BARRIER METHOD OF CONTRACEPTION

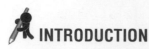 **INTRODUCTION**

Barrier method of contraception is moderately effective, but one of the commonly used methods of contraception. This methods aims at creating a type of barrier which prevents the sperm from meeting the ovum. Barrier contraceptives are associated with a failure rate of 9–30 per 100 WY of use.[37] Some of the commonly used contraception in the barrier method include, male condom, female condom, diaphragm, cervical cap, vaginal sponge and spermicides.

Male Condom

A male condom is a thin sheath made of latex or other materials. Men suffering from latex sensitivity can use condoms made of strong, soft, transparent polyurethane sheath (Fig. 92.8). The man puts the condom on his erected penis, while the condom holds the semen. After having sexual intercourse, the man must carefully take off the condom so that it does not leak. Each condom can be used only once.

Female Condom

This comprises of strong, soft, transparent polyurethane sheath, which is inserted in the vagina before sexual intercourse. It is approximately 15 cm in length and 7 cm in diameter. It has two flexible rings, the inner ring and an outer one (Fig. 92.9). The inner ring at the closed end of the condom eases insertion into the vagina, covering the cervix and holding the condom in place. The outer ring, which is larger than the inner one, stays outside the vagina and covers part of the perineum and labia during intercourse. Presently, there is only one brand of female condom available in the UK, known as Femidom®.

Diaphragm

A diaphragm is a shallow rubber dome made of latex or silicone with a firm flexible rim. It is available in different sizes ranging from 50 mm and 105 mm. Various types of cervical diaphragms include latex arcing spring, coil spring, flat spring and silicone wide seal rim. The latex arcing spring diaphragm has a firm rim, which makes its insertion in the posterior fornix easier. It is commonly used in cases of lax vagina. The rim of a coil spring diaphragm is soft and flexible, which does not form an arc when folded. This is usually used in women with tight vagina or those with moderate tone of vaginal muscles. The flat spring diaphragm is similar to coil spring, but has thinner and more delicate rim. It may be used in women with normal tone of vaginal muscles. Diaphragms are often used in combination with contraceptive jelly, spermicide, etc. It is immediately effective and reversible method of contraception, which can be inserted up to 6 hours before intercourse.

The application of a cervical diaphragm involves the following steps:

❖ The ring of the diaphragm is lubricated and then folded so that the two sides of ring are touching each other.
❖ The vulva is opened with one hand; the other hand is used to gently guide the folded diaphragm inside the vagina and to direct its placement toward the posterior fornix so that the dome of the diaphragm covers the cervical opening.
❖ The anterior rim of the diaphragm must be directly behind the pubic bone.

Patient education is an important parameter, which ensures patient compliance and the contraceptive effectiveness of the diaphragm. When the diaphragm is properly fitted, the patient should not be able to feel anything. The patient should be instructed to use spermicidal jelly inside the cup of diaphragm in order to improve its contraceptive efficacy. It should not have any holes or tear. After use, it must be removed, washed with soap and water, rinsed, dried and stored in an airtight container.

Cervical Cap

A cervical cap is a soft, deep rubber cup with a firm, round rim that fits snugly over the cervix. In Britain, one brand of

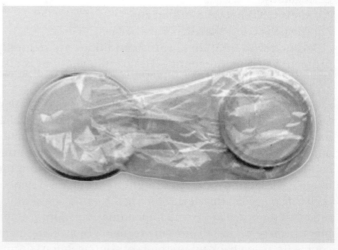

Fig. 92.8: An unrolled-up male condom made up of latex

Fig. 92.9: Female condom

cervical cap™ which is widely available in the NHS since 2014 is the silicone FemCap. The cap provides effective contraception for 48 hours and is manufactured in the sizes of 22 mm, 26 mm and 30 mm.

Spermicides

Two basic components of spermicides include active spermicidal agents such as surfactants (Nonoxynol-9, Octoxynol-9, Menfegol) and the base (carrier) agent such as foams, jellies, creams, foaming tablet, melting suppositories, aerosols, soluble films or vaginal suppositories. The woman must be instructed to insert the recommended dose of the spermicide deep into vagina to cover the cervix completely, just before sexual intercourse. A second dose of spermicide may be required if more than 1 hour passes before she has sexual intercourse.[38] An additional application of spermicides is needed for each additional act of intercourse.

Vaginal Contraceptive Sponge

Vaginal sponge is a safe, non-hormonal form of contraception, which provides protection for nearly 24 hours. Besides acting as a physical barrier, it also contains a spermicidal agent (nonoxynol-9). The sponges provide contraceptive action by two ways. One is by preventing the sperms from moving inside the cervix. Second is the presence of spermicide in the sponge, which causes immobilisation of the sperms.

The contraceptive sponge was marketed under the brand name of Today's® sponge in the United States, and the brand names of Protectaid® and Pharmatex® sponges in the UK. All these brands have been currently withdrawn from the US and UK markets, respectively.

COMPLICATIONS

Male condoms: Some of the complications include:
- ❖ Condoms can interrupt with sexual activity, thereby interfering with sexual pleasure
- ❖ Condoms may sometimes tear or leak and can cause an allergic reaction.

Female condoms: These may be expensive or limited in their availability and may be difficult to insert.

Diaphragm: It includes:
- ❖ The diaphragm is not an appropriate method if the man or woman has allergy to rubber, latex or spermicide, or if the woman has frequent urinary tract or bladder infections and/or anatomical abnormalities
- ❖ May be difficult to insert and remove
- ❖ May cause irritation in the vagina
- ❖ Urinary tract infection
- ❖ Localised pressure exerted by the diaphragm over the vaginal wall may result in the development of inflammatory reaction such as erosions, abrasions and sometimes even frank ulcers.

Cervical cap: It includes:
- ❖ Toxic shock syndrome

- ❖ Unpleasant odour
- ❖ Discomfort and awareness of the cap during coitus
- ❖ Accidental dislodgment.

Spermicides: These include:
- ❖ They may cause irritation in the vagina or on the penis, or an allergic reaction
- ❖ They cause interruption of sexual activity
- ❖ They do not provide protection against STDs.

CLINICAL PEARLS

- ❖ Latex condoms provide protection against STDs.
- ❖ Condoms also provide limited protection against HPV that can cause genital warts, thereby lowering the risk for development of cervical dysplasia and cancer.
- ❖ To increase the efficacy of condoms, the condoms can be lubricated with contraceptive cream or jelly prior to use.
- ❖ Condoms are not associated with any medical side effects, are inexpensive and easily accessible.
- ❖ The barrier methods are associated with a pregnancy rate of 10–14 per 100 WY of use.
- ❖ A diaphragm may reduce the risk of cervical cancer.
- ❖ Spermicides do not require a prescription; may be discontinued at any time and are safe.
- ❖ While using spermicides, douching should not be allowed for at least 6 hours after coitus.

EMERGENCY CONTRACEPTION

INTRODUCTION

Emergency contraception (EC) also known as 'postcoital contraception' or the 'morning-after pill' is a method of contraception which is used after intercourse and before the potential time of implantation. EC provides women with a safe means of preventing pregnancy following unprotected sexual intercourse (UPSI) or potential contraceptive failure. EC cannot be considered as an abortifacient. EC is a back-up method for occasional use, and should not be used as a regular method of birth control. The various methods used for EC are enumerated next. Of these, only the first three methods of EC are currently available in the UK:

1. *Progestogen-only emergency contraception*: This comprises the administration of a single dose of 1.5 mg levonorgestrel (levonelle 1500 or levonelle one-step or the morning after pill) as soon as possible after UPSI. It can be administered up to 96 hours outside the product license. The mode of action of levonorgestrel for the prevention of pregnancy is not fully understood. It probably acts through inhibition of ovulation and fertilisation and also through the alteration of the endometrial lining.

2. *Ulipristal acetate*: Ulipristal acetate (Ellaone®)is a selective progesterone receptor modulator. One tablet containing 30 mg of ulipristal acetate must be taken as soon as possible

CHAPTER 92

following UPSI or contraceptive failure, but no later than 120 hours. In case vomiting occurs within 3 hours, another tablet must be taken.

3. *Non-hormonal method*: This comprises of postcoital insertion of a copper containing IUCD.
4. *Use of COCPs, containing both oestrogen and progestin (Yuzpe's regimen)*: This method comprises of the oral administration of two doses of 100 µg ethinyl oestradiol and 500 µg levonorgestrel taken 12 hours apart. This can be considered as the least effective method for EC and was withdrawn from the UK market in October 2001.

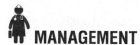

INDICATIONS

Indications for the use of EC are as follows:
❖ Unwanted pregnancy
❖ Failure to use a contraceptive method
❖ Condom breakage or leakage
❖ Dislodgement of a diaphragm or cervical cap
❖ Two or more missed birth control pills
❖ Injection of Depo-Provera® injection is late by 1 week or more
❖ Sexual assault when the woman had not been using reliable contraception.

MANAGEMENT

Prerequisites

❖ A pelvic examination is not a prerequisite to providing EC.
❖ There should be no history of recent PID and vaginal or cervical infection. According to the current recommendations by WHO, IUCDs must not be preferably inserted in women currently having PID, purulent cervicitis, active gonorrhoea or chlamydial infection.
❖ Prior to IUCD insertion for EC, women considered to be at the risk of STIs should be at least offered testing for *Chlamydia trachomatis* at the minimum. In case the results for STI testing are not immediately available at the time of IUCD insertion, prophylactic antibiotics (particularly against chlamydia) are recommended.

Method of Administration

Hormonal EC (levonorgestrel and uliprisal acetate) should be considered for any woman wishing to avoid pregnancy who presents within 5 days of unprotected or inadequately protected sexual intercourse. The dosages in which these hormonal preparations must be used have been previously described in the text. Although they have generally been used only up to 72 hours after intercourse, hormonal method of EC is effective when taken between 72 hours and 120 hours after unprotected intercourse.

A postcoital IUCD insertion can be considered up to 5 days after ovulation (in case the timing of ovulation can be determined). It is effective immediately after insertion.

IUCDs containing at least 380 mm² of copper have the lowest failure rates and should be the first-line choice, particularly if the woman intends to continue the IUCD as long-term contraception.

Drug Interaction and their Consequences on the Efficacy of Emergency Contraception

❖ Drugs inducing the liver enzymes (e.g. rifampin, griseofulvin, certain anticonvulsant drugs, Saint John's wort, certain antiretroviral drugs, etc.), which are likely to reduce the efficacy of OCPs, may also reduce the efficacy of emergency contraceptive pills (ECPs) such as levonorgestrel, ulipristal acetate, and combined ECPs. However, the efficacy of copper IUCDs remains unaffected by these drugs. Therefore, copper IUCDs can be offered to the women who are using these medications and also desire emergency contraception. If women using these medications still choose to use levonorgestrel EC (or if it is the only most easily available method), she should be advised to take the double dose of 3 mg. Use of ulipristal is not recommended in women using enzyme-inducing drugs.

❖ Ulipristal, being a progesterone receptor modulator, is likely to block the action of progestin, thereby reducing the efficacy of other hormonal contraceptives containing progestin. Study demonstrating this relationship is presently underway, but results have not yet been published. Presently, use of back-up method (abstinence or a barrier method) for 14 days following use of ulipristal is recommended amongst women continuing or starting progestin-only methods after use of ulipristal.[39]

❖ Use of ulipristal acetate with drugs which increase gastric pH (e.g. antacids, H_2 receptor, proton pump inhibitors, etc.) may reduce the absorption of ulipristal, thereby reducing its efficacy.

Repeated Use of Emergency Contraceptive Pills

Clinician should make sure that ECPs must not be repeatedly used as a routine method of contraception because of the availability of far more clinically effective and cost-effective methods for contraception. Women who present for EC and do not desire pregnancy in the near future must counselled to use a copper IUCD or another ongoing method of contraception of their choice.

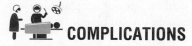

COMPLICATIONS

❖ Emergency contraceptive pills are associated with an excellent safety profile. No deaths or serious complications have been causally linked to any ECP regimen. Minor adverse effects have been commonly reported.
❖ The common side effects of hormonal EC are gastrointestinal and mainly include nausea, vomiting, dizziness and fatigue. Antiemetics such as meclizine can be used for controlling these side effects.

- Less common side effects of hormonal methods include headache, bloating, abdominal cramps, and spotting or bleeding.
- Ulipristal acetate can cause side effects such as abdominal pain and menstrual disorders (e.g. irregular vaginal bleeding, premenstrual syndrome, uterine cramps, etc.) .
- Possible complications of postcoital IUCD insertion include: pelvic pain, abnormal bleeding, pelvic infection, perforation and expulsion.

CLINICAL PEARLS

- Emergency contraception prevents pregnancy and does not interrupt previously established pregnancy.
- Emergency contraceptions are not a good option for providing long-term contraception .
- Emergency contraceptions do not protect against STDs.
- Emergency contraceptions do not increase the risk of ectopic pregnancy, nor do they affect future fertility.
- Presence of pregnancy (either confirmed or suspected) is a contraindication for the use of EC because it would not be effective in these cases.
- While levonorgestrel can be taken more than once in a cycle, use of ulipristal acetate for more than once in the cycle is not recommended.

EVIDENCE-BASED MEDICINE

- The available evidence indicates that ulipristal acetate is the most effective hormonal ECP. The available evidence has indicated the failure rate of ulipristal acetate to range between 0.9% and 2.1%, while that following the use of levonorgestrel to range from 0.6% to 3.1%.[40-43] The greater efficacy of ulipristal is probably due to the fact that it disrupts ovulation even after the beginning of the LH surge. On the other hand, levonorgestrel is ineffective after the beginning of the LH surge. Presently, there is no study comparing the efficacy of ulipristal acetate to IUCD (used for EC).
- While some research studies have shown that levonorgestrel ECPs may be effective up to 4 days after sexual intercourse, other studies have suggested that levonorgestrel ECPs are likely to be effective for up to 5 days after sexual activity. However, the efficacy may be reduced.[44]
- The available evidence points towards the use of copper IUCD as the most effective option for emergency contraception.[45] It is likely to be associated with a pregnancy rate of less than 0.1%, indicating that it helps in preventing almost all expected pregnancies. Furthermore, the copper IUCD is associated with an additional benefit of providing highly effective ongoing contraception if left in situ after placement for EC.

PERMANENT METHOD OF CONTRACEPTION

TUBAL STERILISATION

INTRODUCTION

Tubal sterilisation causes sterility by blocking a woman's fallopian tubes, thereby preventing the fertilisation of sperm with ovum. Dr J Blindell from London was the first to perform tubal ligation in 1823. This procedure can be either performed at the time of caesarean delivery or shortly after a normal vaginal delivery in the early postpartum period or as an interval procedure (6–12 weeks following delivery or thereafter). The most commonly used approach for performing interval tubal sterilisation in non-pregnant women is laparoscopic approach, using application of Falope rings. Periumbilical minilaparotomy, involving the ligation of tubes using Pomeroy's technique, has become the most widely practiced method in women undergoing tubal ligation in the immediate postpartum period.

SURGICAL MANAGEMENT

Preoperative Preparation

- *Complete preoperative workup*. This comprises of adequate history taking and general physical examination.
- *Investigations*: Urine analysis, urine pregnancy test and haematocrit with a CBC must be done. Other tests such as Papanicolaou test, gonorrhoea and chlamydia screening, ultrasonography, etc. may sometimes be required.
- *Preoperative counselling*: The procedure being practically irreversible, patients, especially those who are young, require preoperative patient counselling.
- *Written and informed consent*: After adequate counselling of the patient, written and informed consent from the patient is required in most countries.
- *Anaesthesia*: The procedure is usually performed under general anaesthesia, but can be sometimes also performed under local anaesthesia.

Steps of Surgery

- *Incision*: Although subumbilical minilaparotomy is the most common approach worldwide for postpartum procedures, laparoscopy is used most commonly for interval procedures in the US. In puerperal cases, where the uterus is felt per abdomen, the incision is made approximately 1 inch below the fundus. In interval ligations, the incision is made two finger breadths above the pubic symphysis. This incision could be midline, paramedian, or transverse.

❖ *Delivery of the tubes*: In case of laparotomy or minilaparotomy, the index finger is introduced through the incision and is passed across the posterior surface of the uterus and then to the posterior leaf of the broad ligament from where the tube is hooked out.

❖ *Tubal ligation*: Both the fallopian tubes can be obstructed (ligated or blocked) during laparotomy, minilaparotomy, hysteroscopy or laparoscopy. Tubal ligation is then performed by one of the following techniques:

  • *Pomeroy's technique*: Pomeroy's technique is the most commonly used technique for ligation. The technique has been illustrated in Figures 92.10A to D. The same procedure is then repeated on the other side and the tubal specimens obtained are submitted for histopathological examination. This technique is highly successful and the failure rate varies between 0.1% and 0.5%.

  • *Modified Pomeroy's technique*: If Pomeroy's technique is not used at the time of postpartum sterilisation, modified Pomeroy's technique is favourable to other techniques. Many modifications of the Pomeroy's technique have been described, of which the most commonly performed modification involves double ligation of each tube, thereby reducing the chances of failure.

  • *Laparoscopic obstruction of tubes*: Laparoscopic tubal ligation can be carried out using techniques such as mechanical blockage of tubes using Falope® rings or Filshie® clips. Electrodessication of tubes using electrosurgery can also be done.

❖ *Hysteroscopic sterilisation*: Procedure of tubal sterilization using hysteroscopic sterilisation is based on using a new device, 'Essure®', which helps in blocking the fallopian tubes (Figs 92.11A to C).[46-49] This device has been approved by the United States Food and Drug Administration (USFDA) and consists of using a small metallic implant, called the Essure® system. The device consists of polyethylene terephthalate fibres wrapped around a stainless steel core, surrounded by 24 coils of nickel-titanium alloy. Out of the 24 coils, 3–8 coils must be visible trailing in the uterine cavity, to confirm proper placement of the device.

  • *Adiana method*: This is another hysteroscopic method for female sterilisation. This method involves the use of radio frequency energy to cause thermal destruction of the inner lining of the fallopian tube. A non-absorbable silicone polymer micro insert is also introduced to cause blockage of the interstitial segment of the fallopian tube.

❖ *Closure of incision site*: After performing tubal ligation on both sides, the minilaparotomy incision is closed in layers. The patient is usually discharged within 24–48 hours of surgery.

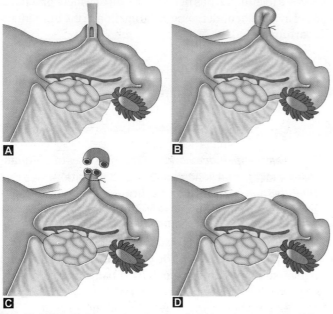

Figs 92.10A to D: Pomeroy's technique of tubal sterilisation: (A) The fallopian tube is grasped with Babcock clamp; (B) A loop is created, which is tied with No. 1 plain catgut sutures; (C) Excision of the loop; (D) Several months later, the ends of the tube get fibrosed, retracting from one another

Postoperative Care

❖ After undergoing tubal sterilisation, the patient must be instructed to come for a follow-up visit at 1–2 weeks postoperatively for examination of the surgical site and removal of non-absorbable sutures.

❖ The woman must also be instructed to notify her healthcare provider in case she has a missed period, developed fever (38°C or 100.4°F), an increasing or persistent abdominal pain or bleeding or purulent discharge from the incision site.

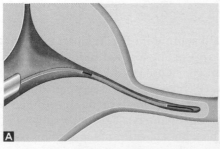 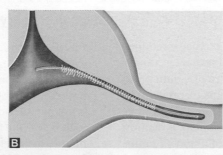 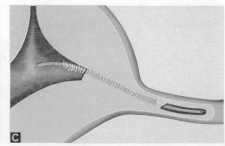

Figs 92.11A to C: Process of hysteroscopic sterilisation: (A) Hysteroscopic cannulation of tubal lumen; (B) Microinsert device inserted inside the tubal ostium; (C) Fibrosis develops over the 'Essure®' microinsert device over a period of time, resulting in tubal occlusion

PART III

COMPLICATIONS

❖ *Effects of anaesthesia*: In cases where general anaesthesia is used, the women are at risk of complications inherent to general anaesthesia.

❖ *Pain*: After undergoing laparoscopic sterilisation, the women may experience some degree of chest and shoulder pain due to pneumoperitoneum, which has been created prior to the insertion of trocar.

❖ *Bleeding and/or infection*: The laparoscopic procedure may be associated with complications such as infection, bleeding, wound infections, haematoma and severe infection, such as PIDs.

❖ *Injury to the body organs*: There is a risk of causing injury to the body organs such as gastrointestinal and genitourinary tract and major vessels, especially when the procedure is performed under laparoscopic guidance.

❖ *Failure of the procedure*: Although sterilisation is highly effective and considered the definitive form of pregnancy prevention, it has a failure rate of 0.1–0.8% during the first year usually due to incomplete closure of the tubes. At least one-third of these are ectopic pregnancies.

❖ *Mortality*: The risk of death from tubal sterilisation is 1–2 cases per 100,000 procedures; most of these are due to complications of general anaesthesia, especially hypoventilation.

❖ *Patient regret*: Sterilisation is intended to be permanent, but patient regret can commonly occur.

❖ *Post-tubal ligation syndrome*: This syndrome is a constellation of symptoms including pelvic discomfort, ovarian cystic changes and menorrhagia.

CLINICAL PEARLS

❖ The isthmic portion of the fallopian tube is the most commonly preferred site for all sterilisation procedures because of the relative ease of reanastomosis at this site, in case the reversal is required in future.

❖ Both laparoscopic sterilisation and minilaparotomy approach are associated with a very low risk of complications, when performed according to the accepted medical standards.

❖ Although the procedure of tubal sterilisation is practically irreversible in dire circumstances, the reversal can be attempted using microsurgical techniques.

❖ One of the major causes of failure of sterilisation is the inadvertent ligation of the round ligament, which is mistakenly identified as the fallopian tube.

VASECTOMY

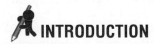

INTRODUCTION

Vasectomy is a procedure in which the vas deferens (tubes carrying sperms from the testicles and epididymis to the

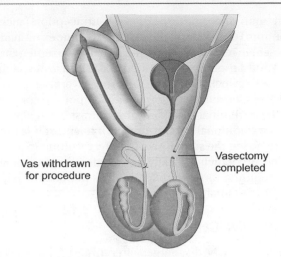

Fig. 92.12: The procedure of vasectomy

urinary tract and urethra) (Fig. 92.12) are surgically blocked to prevent the sperms from passing through and fertilising the egg at the time of sexual intercourse. For couples who do not want to have any more children, vasectomy is the safest and easiest form of permanent sterilisation.

SURGICAL MANAGEMENT

Preoperative Preparation

❖ The person must be instructed to wash meticulously and put on clean, snug underwear or a jock strap (support) before their appointment for surgery.

❖ The front portion of the scrotum may be shaved the night before surgery.

❖ Use of medication such as NSAIDs, aspirin, etc. can increase the risk of bleeding with vasectomy. Therefore, the patient must be advised not to use these medicines at least 10 days prior to surgery.

❖ *Informed consent*: The patient must be asked to sign a consent form prior to the procedure.

❖ *Counselling*: This is an essential component because vasectomy is practically a permanent method of contraception.

❖ In order to allow the possibility of reproduction in future via assisted reproductive technology after vasectomy, some men opt for cryopreservation of their sperms before sterilisation.

❖ The patient is asked to change into a sterile gown and lie on the examination table. The incision site is cleaned and draped taking all aseptic precautions.

❖ Local anaesthetic is injected over the scrotal region prior to the procedure.

❖ A scalpel is used to make two small incisions on each side of the scrotum at a location that allows the surgeon to bring out each vas deferens to the surface.

❖ The vasa deferentia are cut (sometimes a piece is removed), separated and then at least one side is sealed by suture ligation, cauterisation or clamping, before being dropped back into the scrotum.

CHAPTER 92

* The man must continue to use contraception (such as a condom) until laboratory and microscopic examination of his semen reveals azoospermia. Usually two semen analyses at 3 and 4 months are required to confirm azoospermia.
* The no-scalpel vasectomy is a less invasive, faster procedure and is associated with fewer complications in comparison to the traditional vasectomy. In contrast to a scalpel (used in the traditional surgery), a sharp haemostat is used for puncturing the scrotal sac, thereby resulting in a smaller 'incision' which typically limits infection, bleeding and haematoma formation. No stitches are usually required due to the small size of incision.

Postoperative Care

* The man can be discharged after surgery following 1 hour of observation period at the clinic. However, he should be instructed not to drive home by himself. He must be instructed to avoid lifting heavy weights or exercise for at least 1 week following the procedure.
* Pain relievers may be used in case of mild discomfort.
* In case of soreness over the incision site, the patient can be asked to apply an ice pack (wrapped in towel) to the scrotum for the first 24 hours after the procedure.
* The patient must be instructed to wear comfortable cotton briefs or an athletic supporter to help apply pressure and support to the incision site for 1–2 weeks after the procedure.

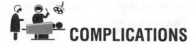

COMPLICATIONS

Vasectomy is associated with fewer complications in comparison to tubal sterilisation. Some of these include:
* Temporary bruising and haematoma formation
* *Postvasectomy pain syndrome*: This is characterised by chronic pain in the scrotal, pelvic and/or lower-abdominal regions and may develop immediately or several years after vasectomy
* Infection
* Sperm granuloma as a result of sperm leakage
* Epididymitis due to congestion of sperms at the epididymis.

CLINICAL PEARLS

* Vasectomy does not cause loss of masculinity.
* Vasectomy is highly effective, having a failure rate as low as 0.02–0.2%, which is less than that of tubal sterilisation. Except for complete abstinence, no method can be considered to be more effective than vasectomy in preventing pregnancy.

EVIDENCE-BASED MEDICINE

Faculty of Sexual and Reproductive Healthcare and RCOG (2014) recommend the use of no-scalpel vasectomy as this technique as well as its modifications can be considered as a type of minimally invasive vasectomy where the skin incision is less than or equal to10 mm.[50]

REFERENCES

1. Faculty of Sexual and Reproductive Health (FSRH). UK Medical Eligibility Criteria for Contraceptive Use. FSRH: London;2009.
2. World Health Organisation (WHO). Medical Eligibility Criteria for Contraception Use, 3rd edition. Geneva: WHO; 2008.
3. Mansour D, Verhoeven C, Sommer W, Weisberg E, Taneepanichskul S, Melis GB, et al. Efficacy and tolerability of a monophasic combined oral contraceptive containing nomegestrol acetate and 17β-oestradiol in a 24/4 regimen, in comparison to an oral contraceptive containing ethinylestradiol and drospirenone in a 21/7 regimen. Eur J Contracept Reprod Health Care. 2011;16(6):430-43.
4. Westhoff C, Kaunitz AM, Korver T, Sommer W, Bahamondes L, Darney P, et al. Efficacy, safety, and tolerability of a monophasic oral contraceptive containing nomegestrol acetate and 17β-estradiol: a randomized controlled trial. Obstet Gynecol. 2012;119(5):989-99.
5. Ahrendt HJ, Makalová D, Parke S, Mellinger U, Mansour D. Bleeding pattern and cycle control with an estradiol-based oral contraceptive: a seven-cycle, randomized comparative trial of estradiol valerate/dienogest and ethinyl estradiol/levonorgestrel. Contraception. 2009;80(5):436-44.
6. Fraser IS, Parke S, Mellinger U, Machlitt A, Serrani M, Jensen J. Effective treatment of heavy and/or prolonged menstrual bleeding without organic cause: pooled analysis of two multinational, randomised, double-blind, placebo-controlled trials of oestradiol valerate and dienogest. Eur J Contracept Reprod Health Care. 2011;16(4):258-69.
7. Nelson AL, Sampson-Landers C, Parke S, Jensen J. Efficacy of estradiol valerate/dienogest OC: results of 3 large studies in North America and Europe. Abstract plus poster presentation at 57th Annual Clinical Meeting of the American College of Obstetricians and Gynecologists. Chicago, IL: American College of Obstetricians and Gynecologists; 2009.
8. Palacios S, Wildt L, Parke S, Machlitt A, Römer R, Bitzer J. Efficacy and safety of a novel oral contraceptive based on oestradiol (oestradiol valerate/dienogest): A Phase III trial. Eur J Obstet Gynecol. 2010;149(1):57-62.
9. Parke S, Makalová D, Ahrendt H-J, Mansour D. Bleeding patterns and cycle control with a novel four-phasic combined oral contraceptive containing estradiol valerate and dienogest. Eur J Contracept Reprod Health Care. 2008;13(1):94-5.
10. Heads of Medicines Agencies. (2010). Qlaira® EU Summary of Product Characteristics. [online] Available from www.hma.eu/mri.html [Accessed November, 2016].
11. Jensen JT, Parke S, Mellinger U, Machlitt A, Fraser IS. Effective treatment of heavy menstrual bleeding with estradiol valerate and dienogest: a randomized controlled trial. Obstet Gynecol. 2011;117(4):777-87.
12. Goa KL, Warner GT, Easthope SE. Transdermal ethinylestradiol/norelgestromin: a review of its use in hormonal contraception. Treat Endocrinol. 2003;2(3):191-206.
13. Stewart FH, Kaunitz AM, Laguardia KD, Karvois DL, Fisher AC, Friedman AJ. Extended use of transdermal norelgestromin/ethinyl estradiol: a randomized trial. Obstet Gynecol. 2005; 105(6):1389-96.

14. Roumen FJ. Review of the combined contraceptive vaginal ring, NuvaRing®. Ther Clin Risk Manag. 2008;4(2):441-51.

15. Edelman A, Micks E, Gallo MF, Jensen JT, Grimes DA. Continuous or extended cycle vs. cyclic use of combined hormonal contraceptives for contraception. Cochrane Database Syst Rev. 2014;(7):CD004695.

16. Hook EB. Cardiovascular birth defects and prenatal exposure to female sex hormones: A re-evaluation of data from a large prospective study. Teratology. 1994;49(3):162-6.

17. Harlap S, Prywes R, Davies AM. Birth defects and oestrogens and progesterones in pregnancy. Lancet. 1975;1(7908):682-3.

18. Harlap S, Shiono PH, Ramcharan S. Congenital abnormalities in the offspring of women who used oral and other contraceptives around the time of conception. Int J Fertil. 1985;30(2):39-47.

19. Goujard J, Rumeau-Rouquette C. First trimester exposure to progestogen/estrogen and congenital malformations. Lancet. 1977;1(8009):482-3.

20. Anderson FD, Hait H. A multicenter, randomized study of an extended cycle oral contraceptive. Contraception. 2003;68(2):89-96.

21. Miller L, Hughes JP. Continuous combination oral contraceptive pills to eliminate withdrawal bleeding: a randomized trial. Obstet Gynecol. 2003;101(4):653-61.

22. Archer DF, Jensen JT, Johnson JV, Borisute H, Grubb GS, Constantine GD. Evaluation of a continuous regimen of levonorgestrel/ethinyl estradiol: phase 3 study results. Contraception. 2006;74(6):439-45.

23. Jain J, Jakimiuk AJ, Bode FR, Ross D, Kaunitz AM. Contraceptive efficacy and safety of DMPA-SC. Contraception. 2004;70(4):269-75.

24. Kaunitz AM, Darney PD, Ross D, Wolter KD, Speroff L. Subcutaneous DMPA vs. intramuscular DMPA: a 2-year randomized study of contraceptive efficacy and bone mineral density. Contraception. 2009;80(1):7-17.

25. Faculty of Sexual and Reproductive Health (FSRH). Progestogen-only Injectable Contraception Clinical Effectiveness Unit. FSRH: London; 2014.

26. Etonogestrel implant (Implanon) for contraception. Drug Ther Bull. 2001;39(8):57-9.

27. Adams K, Beal MW. Implanon: a review of the literature with recommendations for clinical management. J Midwifery Womens Health. 2009;54(2):142-9.

28. Pongsatha S, Ekmahachai M, Suntornlimsiri N, Morakote N, Chaovisitsaree S. Bone mineral density in women using the subdermal contraceptive implant Implanon for at least 2 years. Int J Gynaecol Obstet. 2010;109(3):223-5.

29. Lidegaard O, Hougaard NL, Skovlund CW, Løkkegaard E. Venous thrombosis in users of non-oral hormonal contraception: follow-up study, Denmark 2001-10. BMJ. 2012; 344: e2990.

30. Baram I, Weinstein A, Trussell J. The IUB, a newly invented IUD: a brief report. Contraception. 2014;89(2):139-41.

31. Nelson A, Apter D, Hauck B, Schmelter T, Rybowski S, Rosen K, et al. Two low-dose levonorgestrel intrauterine contraceptive systems: a randomized controlled trial. Obstet Gynecol. 2013;122(6):1205-13.

32. Apter D, Gemzell-Danielsson K, Hauck B, Rosen K, Zurth C. Pharmacokinetics of two low-dose levonorgestrel-releasing intrauterine systems and effects on ovulation rate and cervical function: pooled analyses of phase II and III studies. Fertil Steril. 2014;101:1656-62.

33. Gemzell-Danielsson K, Schellschmidt I, Apter D. A randomized, phase II study describing the efficacy, bleeding profile, and safety of two low-dose levonorgestrel-releasing intrauterine contraceptive systems and Mirena®. Fertil Steril. 2012;97(3):616-22.

34. Kulier R, O'Brien PA, Helmerhorst FM, Usher-Patel M, D'arcangues C. Copper containing, framed intra-uterine devices for contraception. Cochrane Database Syst Rev. 2007; (4):CD005347.

35. Guida M, Bramante S, Acunzo G, Pellicano M, Cirillo D, Nappi C. Diagnosis of fertility with a personal hormonal evaluation test. Minerva Ginecol. 2003;55(2):167-73.

36. Bonnar J, Flynn A, Freundl G, Kirkman R, Royston R, Snowden R. Personal hormone monitoring for contraception. Br J Fam Plann. 1999;24(4):128-34.

37. Mills A. Barrier contraception. Clin Obstet Gynaecol. 1984;11(3):641-60.

38. Hatcher RA, Warner DL. New condoms for men and women, diaphragms, cervical caps, and spermicides: overcoming barriers to barriers and spermicides. Curr Opin Obstet Gynecol. 1992;4(4):513-21.

39. Creinin MD, Schlaff W, Archer DF, Wan L, Frezieres R, Thomas M, et al. Progesterone receptor modulator for emergency contraception: A randomized controlled trial. Obstet Gynecol. 2006;108(5):1089-97.

40. Fine P, Mathe H, Ginde S, Cullins V, Morfesis J, Gainer E. Ulipristal acetate taken 48–120 hours after intercourse for emergency contraception. Obstet Gynecol. 2010;115(2 Pt 1):257-63.

41. Glasier AF, Cameron S, Fine P, Logan S, Casale W, Horn JV, et al. Ulipristal acetate versus levonorgestrel for emergency contraception: A randomised non-inferiority trial and meta-analysis. Lancet. 2010;375(9714):555-62.

42. Noé G, Croxatto HB, Salvatierra AM, Reyes V, Villarroel C, Muñoz C, et al. Contraceptive efficacy of emergency contraception with levonorgestrel given before or after ovulation. Contraception. 2011;84:486-92.

43. Novikova N, Weisberg E, Stanczyk FZ, Croxatto HB, Fraser IS. Effectiveness of levonorgestrel emergency contraception given before or after ovulation--a pilot study. Contraception. 2007;75(2):112-8.

44. Piaggio G, Kapp N, von Hertzen H. Effect on pregnancy rates of the delay in the administration of levonorgestrel for emergency contraception: a combined analysis of four WHO trials. Contraception. 2011;84:35-9.

45. Cleland K, Zhu H, Goldstuck N, Cheng L, Trussell J. The efficacy of intrauterine devices for emergency contraception: A systematic review of 35 years of experience. Hum Reprod. 2012;27(7):1994-2000.

46. Rosen DM. Learning curve for hysteroscopic sterilisation: lessons from the first 80 cases. Aust N Z J Obstet Gynaecol. 2004;44(1):62-4.

47. Levie MD, Chudnoff SG. Prospective analysis of office-based hysteroscopic sterilization. J Minim Invasive Gynecol. 2006;13(2):98-101.

48. Kerin JF, Cooper JM, Price T, Herendael BJ, Cayuela-Font E, Cher D, et al. Hysteroscopic sterilization using a micro-insert device: results of a multicentre Phase II study. Hum Reprod. 2003;18(6):1223-30.

49. Kerin JF, Munday DN, Ritossa MG, Pesce A, Rosen D. Essure hysteroscopic sterilization: results based on utilizing a new coil catheter delivery system. J Am Assoc Gynecol Laparosc. 2004;11(3):388-93.

50. RCOG and Faculty of Sexual and Reproductive Healthcare Clinical Guidance. Male and Female Sterilisation. London, UK; Faculty of Sexual and Reproductive Healthcare; 2014.

Medical Termination of Pregnancy

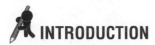

INTRODUCTION

Medical termination of pregnancy or induced abortion is often abbreviated as MTP. It is the medical method which enables a couple to get free from the unwanted pregnancy. In Great Britain, more than 2 lakh procedures are performed on an annual basis.[1,2] The law governing termination of pregnancy by medical practitioners in the UK is defined by four different Acts of Parliament:[3]

1. *The offences against the Person Act 1861*: Section 58 of this Act prohibits the unlawful medical or surgical induction of a miscarriage.
2. *The Infant Life (Preservation) Act 1929*: According to this act, it is an offence to 'destroy the life of a child capable of being born alive'. However, it also specifies that no person shall be found guilty of an offence under this section unless it is proved that the act which caused the death of the child was not done in good faith for the purpose only of preserving the life of the woman.
3. The Abortion Act 1967
4. The Human Fertilisation and Embryology Act 1990.

According to the Abortion Act 1967, an abortion must be performed within an NHS hospital or an approved clinic after informing the chief medical officer about the abortion. Pregnancy can only be terminated by a registered medical practitioner where two registered medical practitioners are of the opinion, formed in good faith (except in an emergency) that one of the stipulated grounds for abortion is being met. The Human Fertilisation and Embryology Act 1990 amended the 1967 Abortion Act. It introduced a time limit on most abortions of 24 weeks of gestation but permitted termination at any gestation on grounds of serious foetal anomaly.

Overview of Surgery

Surgical techniques in the first trimester practically comprise entirely of vacuum or suction techniques. The terms, 'vacuum curettage', 'uterine aspiration', or 'vacuum aspiration' are often used interchangeably. They all refer to evacuation of the uterus by suction, regardless of the source of the suction. Prior to the surgical evacuation, the cervix is often dilated.[4] Mechanical dilation using physical dilators is currently the most frequently used method of dilating the cervix. Other methods for dilatation include osmotic dilatation, using laminaria tents[5,6] or use of pharmacological dilatation using medications, such as misoprostol. Hegar's dilators, which are commonly used for cervical dilatation, are blunted instruments, having different sizes, of which different sizes vary by 1 mm. Misoprostol is a prostaglandin E_2 analogue, which has been approved by the United States Food and Drug Administration (USFDA) for prevention and treatment of gastric ulcers. This drug was contraindicated in pregnant women due to the risk of miscarriage. The side effect of this drug has been utilised and now it is extensively used for MTP, either alone or in combination with mifepristone or methotrexate. It can be administered by vaginal, oral or sublingual routes.

INDICATIONS

The five criteria for which an abortion can be carried out as defined by the Abortion Act 1967 (amended Human Fertilisation and Embryology Act 1990) include the following:

A. Continuation of pregnancy would involve risk to the life of the pregnant woman.
B. Termination of pregnancy is necessary to prevent grave permanent injury to the physical or mental health of the pregnant woman.
C. The pregnancy has not exceeded 24 weeks and that the continuation of pregnancy would involve risk greater than if the pregnancy was terminated or injury to the physical or mental health of the pregnant woman. Most of the abortions, which are carried out, fall under this category.
D. The pregnancy has not exceeded 24 weeks and that the continuation of pregnancy would involve risk greater than if the pregnancy was terminated or injury to the physical

or mental health of any existing child or children or the family of the pregnant woman.

E. There is a substantial risk that if the child was born, it would suffer from such mental or physical abnormalities to be seriously handicapped (Criteria E on the abortion notification form). Abortions done under this criteria are legal beyond 24 weeks. The most common causes for this are chromosomal abnormalities and congenital malformations, with the most important chromosomal abnormality for induced abortion in the UK being the Down's syndrome. Presently, there is no legal definition regarding what actually constitutes substantial risk or severe handicap.

MANAGEMENT

Preoperative Preparation

Patient counselling: Adequate counselling of the woman and her partner is essential, in order to enable her to make a free and fully informed decision. An informed consent from the woman or her guardian (in case of a minor patient) must be taken. Many women undergoing MTP may be apprehensive, frightened or guilty. Counselling may be especially required, in cases where pregnancies have resulted from abuse, coercion or assault. It is the duty of the surgeon, to ensure that the woman remains calm and relaxed during the procedure and should adopt a sympathetic attitude towards her. The woman should never be pressurised to proceed with the procedure, if she is not ready. Some women may require additional support, including access to the counselling services and social care.

❖ *Estimation of the gestational age*: The clinician can estimate the gestational age by calculating the period of amenorrhoea. The uterine size must be assessed by performing a bimanual examination. When the clinical estimate of gestational age disagrees with the period of amenorrhoea, the clinician must find out the reason for this discrepancy before proceeding. Uterine size may be larger than the period of gestation in cases, such as multiple pregnancy, hydramnios, uterine anomaly, uterine fibroids, a molar pregnancy or an ovarian tumour. In case the uterine size is considerably smaller than the duration of amenorrhoea, the likely explanations could be a false diagnosis of intrauterine pregnancy, where the patient may not be pregnant, may have a non-viable pregnancy or may have an ectopic pregnancy. An ultrasound examination can be performed to confirm the period of gestation. Many clinicians perform routine ultrasound examination before carrying out abortion. However, universal ultrasound examination has not been shown to be superior to selected ultrasound examination in the first trimester, in terms of complication rate. Therefore, routine use of preabortion ultrasound scanning is unnecessary.

❖ A complete medical history must be taken, in order to rule out the presence of the medical diseases, such as asthma, diabetes and the history of the drug allergy.

❖ Simple investigations, such as haemoglobin estimation, urine analysis and blood grouping (ABO, Rh) need to be done prior to the procedure.

❖ In case, where the procedure would be carried out under general anaesthesia (GA), investigations, such as blood sugar levels, kidney function tests, ECG and X-ray may be required.

❖ Cervical priming using 400 µg of vaginal or anal misoprostol, can be done prior to the procedure.[7-9]

❖ *Anaesthesia*: The procedure is usually carried out under local anaesthesia, using a paracervical block with 20 mL of 0.5% lignocaine.[10] Short GA may be used in the patients, who are very apprehensive. Many patients are likely to experience some discomfort during abortion, although the amount of pain usually varies from mild to moderate. In order to reduce the pain during and after the procedure NSAIDs, such as naproxen 550 mg, may be commonly prescribed before the procedure.[11,12] Vasoconstrictive agents, such as vasopressin (2 units) may be added to the local anaesthetic agent, which would help in reducing the amount of bleeding in second-trimester procedures. Atropine (0.5 mg) can also be mixed with the local anaesthetic agent to reduce vagal effects and prevent syncope and nausea. Vasovagal reaction is a complication, which can be produced in some women as a result of manipulation of the cervix.[13] This reaction may be associated with bradycardia, hypotension and possibly syncope. If the patient begins to show signs of vasovagal reaction, the surgeon should immediately stop the painful stimulus, give atropine 0.4–1.0 mg intravenously or subcutaneously, turn the patient to a more comfortable position and then monitor the vital signs, while the patient recovers. When the patient has fully recovered, the abortion procedure may be safely resumed. Solutions containing epinephrine must not be used because they have a risk of causing anxiety and cardiac arrhythmia.

❖ *Prophylactic antibiotics*: Prophylactic antibiotics must be preferably used during and after the procedure to reduce the risk of infective complications.[14] It has also been observed that the routine use of prophylactic antibiotics can help in preventing nearly 50% cases of postabortion endometritis.[15] Various antibiotic regimens, effective against *Chlamydia trachomatis* and anaerobes, which can be prescribed include the following:

• Metronidazole 1 g per rectally plus doxycycline 100 mg, orally, twice a day daily for a week commencing from the day of abortion.
 Or
• Metronidazole 1 g per rectally plus azithromycin 1 g orally on the day of abortion.
 Or
• Metronidazole 1 g rectally or 800 mg orally may be prescribed prior to or at the time of abortion for women who have tested negative for *C. trachomatis* infection.

❖ *Bladder catheterisation*: Bladder must be emptied prior to the procedure.

❖ *Cleaning and draping*: Shaving the perineum is not required, but the perineal hair must be trimmed. After taking all aseptic precautions, the area of perineum, mons and lower part of the abdomen must be cleaned and draped, using povidone-iodine or chlorhexidine solution. The surgeon must use the 'no-touch' technique, in which he or she must use sterile instruments and sterile gloves and take care never to touch that part of the instrument that would enter the uterus.

❖ *Advice related to contraception*: Advice related to future contraception is particularly important in order to prevent repeat terminations in future.

Actual Procedure

Surgery

Various options for performing MTP based on their period of gestation are given in Table 93.1 and Figure 93.1 and are discussed next in details.

Vacuum Aspiration

The procedure of vacuum aspiration comprises of the following described in Figures 93.2A to D.[16-18] Vacuum aspiration is an appropriate method for surgical abortion from 7 weeks to 15 weeks of gestation. Either electric or manual methods for vacuum aspiration may be used, as both the methods are equally effective and acceptable to both the women and their clinicians. Vacuum aspiration should preferably not be used if the period of gestation is less than

7 weeks due to high failure rates. Vacuum aspiration may also be performed from 14 weeks to 16 weeks of gestation, though dilatation and evacuation is more favourable during this period of gestation. In these cases, large-bore cannulae and suction tubing may be required to complete the procedure. For the period of gestation greater than 14 weeks, the procedure of surgical abortion should be preferably preceded by cervical preparation. During vacuum aspiration, the uterus should be emptied using the suction cannula and blunt forceps (if required).[19] The procedure should not be routinely completed by sharp curettage. It is usually recommended that access to ultrasound must be available at the time of the procedure. However, it is not routinely required in uncomplicated cases.

Cervical preparation prior to the procedure: Prior to 14 weeks of gestation, cervix should be preferably prepared by administering 400 µg of misoprostol vaginally, 3 hours prior to surgery or 2–3 hours sublingually prior to surgery.

Vaginal misoprostol can be administered either by the woman herself or by a clinician. After 14 weeks of gestation, osmotic dilators should be preferably used for cervical preparation.

Dilatation and Evacuation

When the period of gestation is greater than 14 weeks, surgical abortion by dilatation and evacuation (D&E), preceded by cervical preparation, appears to be the most appropriate procedure. In these cases, surgical abortion is performed using a combination of vacuum aspiration and specialised forceps for evacuation of uterine contents. RCOG recommends that D&E should be preferably performed under ultrasound guidance to reduce the risk of surgical complications.

Medical Abortion

For MTP using medicines, antiprogesterone (mifepristone) and prostaglandin analogues are usually used. Regimens using mifepristone and misoprostol in different dosage combinations are effective for inducing medical abortion at any period of gestation. While a single dose of misoprostol

Table 93.1: Various options for medical termination of pregnancy

First trimester	
Up to 9 weeks	Early medical abortion
10–11 weeks	Manual vacuum aspiration
7–15 weeks	Suction/vacuum aspiration under local or general anaesthesia
Second trimester	
15–20 weeks	Dilatation and evacuation
9+ to 24 weeks	Medical abortion

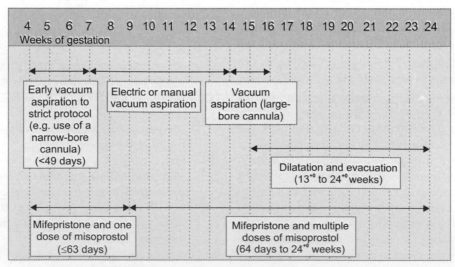

Fig. 93.1: Different methods for induced abortion in Great Britain

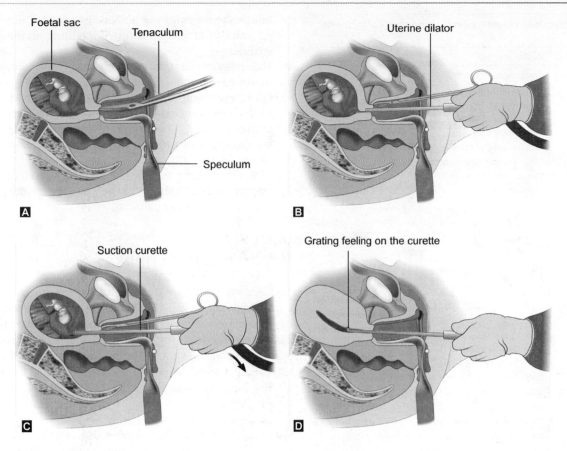

Figs 93.2A to D: Steps of the procedure of vacuum aspiration: (A) Retracting the posterior wall of the uterus with Sim's speculum and grasping the anterior lip with tenaculum; (B) Dilating the external cervical os with Hegar's dilator; (C) Insertion of Karman's cannula for producing suction; once the cannula has been inserted, the clinician must connect the cannula to a suction machine, which generates pressure equivalent to 60–70 mmHg. The cannula is rotated at an angle of 360° and moved back by 1–2 cm, back and forth, till the entire uterine cavity has been evacuated, and (D) The evacuation of the uterine contents is almost complete resulting in a grating feeling

may be sufficient in cases of early abortion, multiple doses of misoprostol may be required with an increasing period of gestation.

❖ *Medical abortion at less than or equal to 63 days of gestation (early medical abortion)*: The following regimen is recommended for early medical abortion: Administration of mifepristone 200 mg orally followed 24–48 hours later by misoprostol 800 µg by the vaginal, buccal or sublingual routes. If the period of gestation is less than or equal to 49 days, 200 mg oral mifepristone may be followed 24–48 hours later by 400 µg of oral misoprostol. For women in whom the period of gestation is between 50–63 days, if abortion does not occur 4 hours after the administration of misoprostol, a second dose of misoprostol 400 µg may be administered vaginally or orally (depending upon the patient's preference and amount of bleeding).

❖ *Medical abortion at 9–13 weeks of gestation*: The following regimen is recommended for medical abortion between 9 weeks to 13 weeks of gestation: Administration of mifepristone in the dosage of 200 mg orally followed 36–48 hours later by misoprostol 800 µg vaginally. A maximum of four further doses of misoprostol 400 µg may be administered at 3-hourly intervals, vaginally or orally.

❖ *Medical abortion at 13–24 weeks of gestation*: The following regimen is recommended for medical abortion between

13 weeks and 24 weeks of gestation: Administration of mifepristone 200 mg orally, followed 36–48 hours later by misoprostol 800 µg vaginally. This may be further followed by a maximum of four dosages of 400 µg of misoprostol orally or vaginally at 3-hourly intervals. If abortion still does not occur, mifepristone can be repeated 3 hours after the last dose of misoprostol. Misoprostol may be restarted 12 hours later.

One must, however, remember that all these regimens are presently unlicensed. Surgical evacuation of the uterus is not required routinely following medical abortion between 13 weeks to 24 weeks of gestation. It should be undertaken only if there is clinical evidence that the abortion is incomplete.

Comparison between medical and surgical abortion is summarised in Table 93.2. Medical abortion is defined as being successful if there is complete termination of pregnancy without the requirement of a surgical procedure. On the other hand, the procedure is considered unsuccessful in case there is requirement for a surgical process which may be the result of continuation of pregnancy, incomplete expulsion or heavy bleeding. If medical abortion fails, vacuum aspiration becomes essential. In summary, medical abortion may take several days, is not completely predictable, may be associated with heavy bleeding and severe cramping, which may last for a longer period and has a higher failure rate in comparison with the surgical method.

Table 93.2: Comparison between surgical and medical methods of abortion

Parameter	Medical abortion	Surgical abortion
The procedure itself	The process is more natural and may appear like a miscarriage. It may be associated with heavy bleeding and passage of clots for 3–4 days, following the administration of medicines	The procedure involves aspiration/evacuation of uterine contents and requires a single visit to the clinic which takes about 15–20 minutes
Follow-up visit	Many follow-up visits to the healthcare provider are required	A follow-up visit is essential and is usually fixed at 3–4 weeks' time
Duration of bleeding	The bleeding may last for 2 weeks or longer	Vacuum aspiration is associated with light to moderate bleeding, which may continue for a few days
Complications	Medical abortion has been found to be a safe and non-invasive process, associated with a lower rate of complications. It may be associated with minor complications such as bleeding and abdominal cramps	Though the complication rate is higher than that of medical abortion, serious complications usually do not occur in experienced hands
Time for completion	Takes longer time	Requires shorter time
Success rates	Medical abortion is successful in 97% cases	On the other hand, vacuum aspiration is more successful, the success rate being almost 99%
Required equipment	No requirement of any special equipment	Requirement of anaesthesia, vacuum aspiration machine and other instruments

Postoperative Care

❖ The patient must be observed in the recovery room for 2–3 hours before discharge.
❖ The patient's vital signs and blood loss must be regularly monitored.
❖ If the procedure is performed under GA, the patient can be discharged after a few hours, once she has stabilised.
❖ Non-immunised rhesus-negative women must be administered anti-D immunoglobulins preferably within 72 hours following the procedure. Prior to 20 weeks of gestation 250 IU must be administered and 500 IU thereafter.
❖ A woman who has undergone MTP must be counselled regarding the use of contraception in future, in order to prevent the reoccurrence of unwanted pregnancies. Immediate contraception in form of IUCD insertion or placement of a subdermal rod, intramuscular depot medroxyprogesterone acetate injections, etc. may be provided after the procedure depending on the patient's wishes.

❖ *Pain relief for abortion*: Women should routinely be offered medicines for pain relief (e.g. NSAIDs) during abortion. Oral paracetamol has not been shown to cause more pain relief in comparison to placebo. Therefore, its use during abortion is not recommended. Narcotic analgesia may be required in some women, particularly after 13 weeks of gestation.
❖ The patients are scheduled for a follow-up visit, 1–2 weeks after abortion, to check for the presence of any potential MTP-related complications.

COMPLICATIONS

Though small amount of cramping, pain and bleeding can commonly occur for 2–3 days after the procedure, severe degrees of persistent pain or amount of bleeding more than that associated with normal menstruation, especially in association with fever or fainting could be indicative of the underlying complications. Some of these are as follows:[20-33]
❖ Uterine perforation
❖ Infection
❖ Incomplete abortion
❖ Bleeding during and following the abortion
❖ Failure of procedure/continuing pregnancy
❖ Asherman's syndrome
❖ Cervical lacerations/cervical incompetence.

For further details, kindly refer to Chapter 36 (Spontaneous Miscarriage).

CLINICAL PEARLS

❖ Suction aspiration is the most commonly used method for termination of first trimester pregnancies.
❖ The most common reported chromosomal abnormality for induced abortions in the UK is Down's syndrome.
❖ Screening for chlamydial infection should be offered to all women undergoing induced abortion.
❖ Prophylactic antibiotics should be preferably offered during and after the procedure of surgical aspiration to prevent the development of infective complications.

EVIDENCE-BASED MEDICINE

❖ Sublingual administration of misoprostol has also been shown to be effective and the success rate have been found to be more or less similar to the vaginal administration of misoprostol for MTP using medicines.[34,35]
❖ Occasionally, the medical method may be associated with side effects such as nausea and vomiting, diarrhoea and abdominal cramps and rarely even fever. There are concerns related to excessive and prolonged bleeding,

undiagnosed ectopic pregnancy and teratogenic side effects. Moreover, these drugs can sometimes cross placenta, resulting in skull and limb deformities. [37]

❖ There is no evidence to suggest that there is an increased risk of psychological sequelae or future adverse reproductive outcome (ectopic pregnancy, infertility, pregnancy-related complication, etc.) with either method of induced abortion (medical or surgical).[36,37]

REFERENCES

1. Department of Health. Abortion Statistics, England and Wales: 2009. Statistical Bulletin 2010/1. London: Department of Health; 2010.
2. Information Services Division Scotland. Abortion Statistics, Year ending December 2009. Statistical Publication Note. Edinburgh: Information Services Division Scotland; 2010.
3. Royal College of Obstetricians and Gynaecologists (RCOG). . The Care of Women Requesting Induced Abortion. Evidence-based Clinical Guideline Number 7. London: RCOG; 2011.
4. Keder LM. Best practices in surgical abortion. Am J Obstet Gynecol. 2003;189(2):418-22.
5. Christin-Maitre S, Bouchard P, Spitz IM. Medical termination of pregnancy. N Engl J Med. 2000;342(13):946-56.
6. Parikh MN. Emergency Contraception, editorial. J Obs Gyn Ind. 2002;52:27-9.
7. Stubblefield PG. Surgical techniques of uterine evacuation in first- and second-trimester abortion. Clin Obstet Gynecol. 1986;13(1):53-70.
8. Blumenthal PD. Prospective comparison of Dilapan and laminaria for pretreatment of cervix in second trimester induction abortion. Obstet Gynecol. 1988;72(2):243-6.
9. Grimes DA, Ray IG, Middleton CJ. Lamicel versus laminaria for cervical dilation before early second trimester abortion a randomized clinical trial. Obstet Gynecol. 1987;69(6):887-90.
10. Carbonell JL, Velazco A, Rodriguez Y, Tanda R, Sánchez C, Barambio S, et al. Oral versus vaginal misoprostol for cervical priming in first trimester abortion: a randomized trial. Eur J Contracept Reprod Health Care. 2001;6(3):134-40.
11. Bugalho A, Bique C, Almeida L, Bergström S. Application of vaginal misoprostol before cervical dilation to facilitate first trimester pregnancy interruption. Obstet Gynecol. 1994;83(5 Pt 1):729-31.
12. EL-Refary H, Calder T, Wheatley DN, Templeton A. Cervical priming with prostaglandin E1 analogues, misoprostol and gemeprost. Lancet. 1994;343(8907):1207-9.
13. Mathai M, Sanghvi H, Guidotti RJ, et al. Paracervical Block in MCPC (P1). Geneva: WHO; 2000.
14. Stubblefield PG. Control of pain for women undergoing abortion. Suppl Int J Gynecol Obstet. 1989;3:131-40.
15. Suprato K, Reed S. Naproxen sodium for pain relief in first-trimester abortion. Am J Obstet Gynecol. 1984;150(8):1000-1.
16. Grimes DA. Management of Abortion in TeLinde's Operative Gynecology, 9th edition. Philadelphia: Lippincott Williams and Wilkins; 1997. p. 8.
17. Dajani AS, Taubert KA, Wilson W, Bolger AF, Bayer A, Ferrieri P, et al. Prevention of bacterial endocarditis: Recommendations by the American Heart Association. JAMA. 1997;277(22):1794-801.
18. Levallois P, Rioux JE. Prophylactic antibiotics for suction curettage abortion: results of a clinical controlled trial. Am J Obstet Gynecol. 1988;158(1):100-5.
19. Glick E. Surgical Abortion. Reno, Nevada: West End Women's Medical Group;1998. pp. 17-22.
20. Castadot RG. Pregnancy termination: Techniques, risks, and complications and their management. Fertil Steril. 1986;45(1):5-17.
21. Chen LH, Lai SF, Lee WH, Leong NK. Uterine perforation during elective first-trimester abortions: a 13-year review. Singapore Med J. 1995;36(1):63-7.
22. Grimes DA, Schulz KF, Cates WJ. Prevention of uterine perforation during curettage abortion. JAMA. 1984;251(16):2108-11.
23. Berek JS, Stubblefield PG. Anatomic and clinical correlates of uterine perforation. Am J Obstet Gynecol. 1979;135(2):181-4.
24. Lauerson NH, Birnbaum S. Laparoscopy as a diagnostic and therapeutic technique in uterine perforations during first-trimester abortions. Am J Obstet Gynecol. 1973;117(4):522-6.
25. Larrson PG, Platz-Christensen JJ, Theijls H, Forsum U, Påhlson C. Incidence of pelvic inflammatory disease after first-trimester legal abortion in women with bacterial vaginosis after treatment with metronidazole: a double-blind, randomized trial. Am J Obstet Gynecol. 1992;166(1 Pt 1):100-3.
26. Sands RX, Burnhill MS, Hakim-Elahi E. Postabortal uterine atony. Obstet Gynecol. 1974;43(4):595-8.
27. Fielding WL, Lee SY, Borten M, Friedman EA. Continued pregnancy after failed first-trimester abortion. Obstet Gynecol. 1984;63(3):421-4.
28. Pennes DR, Bowerman RA, Silver TM, Smith SJ. Failed first trimester pregnancy termination: Uterine anomaly as etiologic factor. J Clin Ultrasound. 1987;15(3):165-70.
29. Valle RF, Sabbagha RF. Management of first-trimester pregnancy termination failures. Obstet Gynecol. 1980;55(5):625-9.
30. World Health Organization. Maternal Health and Safe Motherhood Programme. Clinical Management of Abortion Complications: A Practical Guide. Geneva: WHO; 1994.
31. Lichtenberg ES, Grimes DA, Paul M. Abortion complications: Prevention and management. In: Paul M, Lichtenberg ES, Borgatta L, Stubblefield PG, Grimes DA (Eds). A Clinician's Guide to Medical and Surgical Abortion. New York: Churchill Livingstone; 1999. p. 197.
32. Grimes DA, Cates W. Complications from legally-induced abortion: a review. Obstet Gynecol Surv. 1979;34(3):177-91.
33. Molin A. Risk of damage to the cervix by dilation for first trimester induced abortion by suction aspiration. Gynecol Obstet Invest. 1993;35(3):152-4.
34. Hamoda H, Ashok PW, Flett GM, Templeton A. A randomised controlled trial of mifepristone in combination with misoprostol administered sublingually or vaginally for medical abortion up to 13 weeks of gestation. BJOG. 2005; 112(8):1102-8.
35. Dickinson JE, Jennings BG, Doherty DA. Mifepristone and oral, vaginal, or sublingual misoprostol for second-trimester abortion: a randomized controlled trial. Obstet Gynecol. 2014;123(6):1162-8.
36. Henshaw R, Naji S, Russell I, Templeton A. Psychological responses following medical abortion (using mifepristone and gemeprost) and surgical vacuum aspiration. A patient-centered, partially randomised prospective study. Acta Obstet Gynecol Scand. 1994;73(10):812-8.
37. Bygdeman M, Danielsson KG. Options for early therapeutic abortion: a comparative review. Drugs. 2002;62(17):2459-70.

CHAPTER 93

Index

Page numbers followed by *b* refer to box, *f* refer to figure, *fc* refer to flow chart, and *t* refer to table.

Tubo-ovarian abscess 831, 835
Tubo-ovarian mass
Tumour
  benign 759
  cells, malignant 712
  malignant 759
Tuohy's needle 428
Turner's syndrome 548, 549, 550, 651, 654, 657, 697
  stigmata of 673
Twin breech, management of 268
Twin gestation 223t, 310
  types of 217
Twin pregnancy 280
Twin presentation 435
Twin-to-twin transfusion syndrome 218, 321
Two-finger compression 523f
Typhoid 504

U

Ulceration 818
Ulipristal acetate 855-857
Ultrasonographic ovarian antral follicle count 716
Umbilical artery
  blood flow 380f
  Doppler 379, 481
  waveform analysis 381
Umbilical cord
  abnormalities 533
  haemangioma 393
Unfractionated heparin 35, 106
United Kingdom Medical Eligibility Criteria 841
United States Food and Drug Administration 858, 862
United States Preventive Services Task Force 825
Unprovoked vulvodynia 807, 808, 809
Unstable lie 279, 280
  aetiology 279
  complications 280
  diagnosis 280
  foetal causes 279
  management 280
  maternal causes 279
Untreated pyrexia 428
Ureaplasma 298
  urealyticum 227
Ureter 729
Urethra 730
  anatomic hypermobility of 734
  neck of 466
  vaginal fistula repair 737
Urethral bulking agents, injection of 737, 741
Urethral diverticulectomy 737
Urethral hypermobility 721
Urethral pressure profilometry 742
Urethral sling 740
  proximal 738
Urge incontinence 734, 736
Urinary catheter 437
Urinary catheterisation 744
Urinary dysfunction 757, 793
Urinary incontinence 730, 734, 735t, 742
  severity score 735
Urinary infection 34
Urinary obstruction 579
Urinary retention 34, 741
Urinary sphincter 741
  use of artificial 741
Urinary stress test 737
Urinary tract 444, 741
  complications 34, 579
  infection 31, 503, 579, 730, 741, 744-746

  recurrent 745t
  treatment of 746
  treatment of recurrent 746
  injury, lower 741
  lower 734, 736
  obstructive defects 402
Urine
  dipstick test 735
  pregnancy test 760
  test 45, 760
Urogenital atrophy
  mild 568
  moderate-to-severe 568
Urogenital diaphragm, muscles of 730
Urogenital fistula 742
Urogenital malformations 54
Urogenital sinus 540
Urogenital tract, infection of 502
Ursodeoxycholic acid 122
Uterine anomalies, classification of 668f
Uterine artery 792
  abnormal 379f
  blood flow
    patterns 379f
    normal 379f
  Doppler 378
  embolisation 603, 606-608, 610, 640
  ligation 494f
Uterine biopsy 799
Uterine bleeding
  abnormal 597, 751, 753f, 831
  causes of abnormal 597fc
  dysfunctional 598b, 752, 753, 782
Uterine cancer, history of 571
Uterine cavity 552, 851f
Uterine compression, bimanual 493f
Uterine contractions 411
Uterine endometrium 715
Uterine enlargement 756
Uterine evacuation, surgical 361
Uterine evaluation 601
Uterine factor 675, 715
  evaluation of 716
  infertility 667, 668
  treatment of 676
Uterine fibroids 302, 600
Uterine fundus, height of 410f
Uterine hyperactivity 616
Uterine incision 440, 441
  closure of 441
  location of 440
Uterine inversion 497
  degrees of 497f
Uterine leiomyomas 605
Uterine malformations 301, 360
Uterine massage, bimanual 491
Uterine myomas 605
Uterine natural killer cells 301
Uterine perforation 362, 756, 851, 851f
Uterine prolapse 721-723, 730
Uterine rupture 312, 424, 444
  types of 313
Uterine scar
  lower segment 440
  upper segment 440
Uterine septum 301
Uterine suspension 728
Uterine tamponade 363
Uterine trauma 638
Uterine tube, formation of 539f
Uterosacral ligament 730
  suturing of 733

Uterovaginal canal, mesoderm of 540f
Uterovaginal prolapse 723
Uterus 559, 716
  atonicity of 497
  lining of 751
  removal of 724
  rupture of 497
  tube, formation of 539f

V

Vaccination against cervical cancer 161
Vaccination programme 778
Vacuum aspiration 864
Vacuum delivery suction-cup devices, types of 448t
Vacuum devices, types of 448
Vagina 559, 566
  floor of 727
  formation of 540f
Vaginal assisted delivery 447
Vaginal atrophy 592
Vaginal birth 309, 311, 431
Vaginal bleeding, abnormal 796
Vaginal brachytherapy 755
Vaginal breech delivery 270
Vaginal canal 466
Vaginal cancer 796, 798
  staging of 797, 797t
  treatment of 797, 797t
Vaginal condyloma 797
Vaginal contraceptive sponge 855
Vaginal culture 825
Vaginal cytology 806
Vaginal delivery 465, 467
  instrumental 447
Vaginal discharge 47, 503, 815, 823, 824, 824t, 826fc
  causes of 824t, 826t
  pathological 823
Vaginal epithelial cells 592
Vaginal epithelium 592, 739
  closure of 725, 727
Vaginal examination 266, 278, 358, 366, 412, 503
  internal 316
Vaginal function, preservation of 721
Vaginal granulation tissue 730
Vaginal hysterectomy 723, 728, 732, 733
Vaginal incision, closure of 740
Vaginal injuries, repair of 494
Vaginal intraepithelial neoplasia 796, 798
Vaginal introitus, infibulation of 578f
Vaginal irradiation, postoperative 756
Vaginal mucosa 724, 728f
Vaginal oestrogen 560
Vaginal pessaries 730
Vaginal radical trachelectomy 794
Vaginal stenosis 756
Vaginal swab, high 490
Vaginal tears, repair of 468
Vaginal trichomoniasis 828
Vaginal vault 729
  apical portion of 732
Vaginal wall
  anterior 721, 722, 724, 730, 732, 739
  posterior 721, 722, 729
Vaginismus 589-591
Vaginitis
  causes of 824t
  emphysematous 829
Valproate 334
Valproic acid 333
Valsalva manoeuvre 722
Valvular heart disease 210

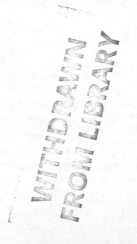
WITHDRAWN FROM LIBRARY

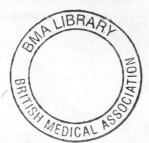
BMA LIBRARY
BRITISH MEDICAL ASSOCIATION